CONTEMPORARY

Oral and Maxillofacial Surgery

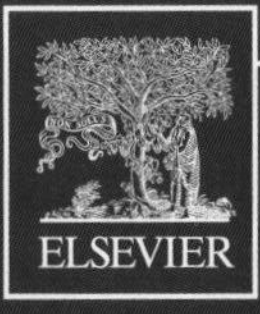

evolve

To access your Student Resources, visit:

http://evolve.elsevier.com/COMS

Evolve® Student Resources for ***Hupp, Ellis, Tucker: Comtemporary Oral and Maxillofacial Surgery,* Fifth Edition** offer the following features:

- **Video Clips of Basic Procedures**

http://evolve.elsevier.com/COMS

CONTEMPORARY
Oral and Maxillofacial Surgery

FIFTH EDITION

Editors

James R. Hupp, DMD, MD, JD, MBA, FACS, FACD, FICD

Dean, School of Dentistry
Professor, Oral and Maxillofacial Surgery
Professor of Surgery
Professor of Otolaryngology
School of Medicine
University of Mississippi Medical Center
Jackson, Mississippi

Edward Ellis III, DDS, MS

Professor, Division of Oral and Maxillofacial Surgery
University of Texas Southwestern Medical Center
Dallas, Texas

Myron R. Tucker, DDS

Private Practice, Oral and Maxillofacial Surgery
Charlotte, North Carolina
Adjunct Clinical Professor
Department of Oral and Maxillofacial Surgery
Louisiana State University,
New Orleans, Louisana

MOSBY

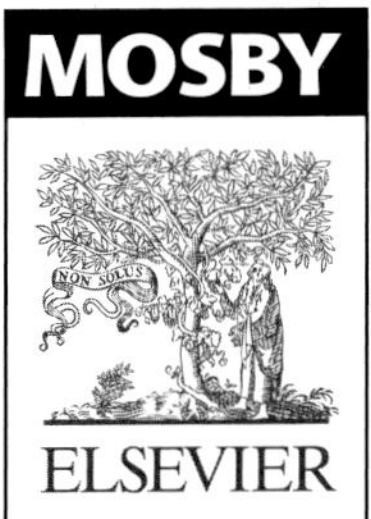

ELSEVIER

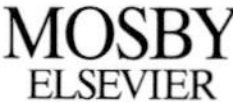

MOSBY
ELSEVIER

11830 Westline Industrial Drive
St. Louis, Missouri 63146

CONTEMPORARY ORAL AND MAXILLOFACIAL SURGERY,
FIFTH EDITION. ISBN: 978-0-323-04903-0

Notice

Knowledge and best practice in this field are constantly changing. As new research and experience broaden our knowledge, changes in practice, treatment and drug therapy may become necessary or appropriate. Readers are advised to check the most current information provided (i) on procedures featured or (ii) by the manufacturer of each product to be administered, to verify the recommended dose or formula, the method and duration of administration, and contraindications. It is the responsibility of the practitioner, relying on their own experience and knowledge of the patient, to make diagnoses, to determine dosages and the best treatment for each individual patient, and to take all appropriate safety precautions. To the fullest extent of the law, neither the Publisher nor the Editors assume any liability for any injury and/or damage to persons or property arising out of or related to any use of the material contained in this book.

The Publisher

Library of Congress Control Number: 2007937059

Vice President and Publisher: Linda Duncan
Senior Editor: John Dolan
Developmental Editor: Elizabeth Clark
Publishing Services Manager: Patricia Tannian
Project Manager: Claire Kramer
Text Designer: Paula Catalano
Cover Design Direction: Paula Catalano

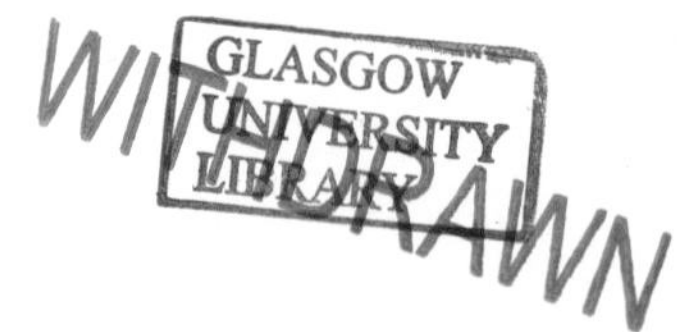

Printed in China
Last digit is the print number: 9 8 7 6 5 4 3 2 1

To all students of the specialty of oral and maxillofacial surgery.
Edward Ellis III

I dedicate my contributions to this book to Carmen, my wife and best friend; to our wonderfully talented and enjoyable children, Jamie, Justin, Joelle, and Jordan; and to my talented sister, Judy, and her supportive husband Bill Peer.
James R. Hupp

I dedicate my work on this textbook to my best friends: my wife, Jan, and Drs. Mark Ochs and Todd Mullikin.
I can't thank them enough for decades of guidance, constructive criticism, and enormous encouragement.
Myron R. Tucker

Contributors

Roger E. Alexander, DDS, FAAOMS, FACD, FICD
Professor
Department of Oral and Maxillofacial Surgery
Baylor College of Dentistry
Texas A&M Health Science Center
Dallas, Texas

Peter N. Demas, DMD, MD
Associate Professor
Oral and Maxillofacial Surgery
School of Dental Medicine
University of Pittsburgh
Pittsburgh, Pennsylvania

Bart C. Farrell, DDS, MD
Assistant Clinical Professor
Department of Oral and Maxillofacial Surgery
Louisiana State University Health Science Center
New Orleans, Louisiana
Private Practice
University Oral and Maxillofacial Surgery
Charlotte, North Carolina

Brian B. Farrell, DDS, MD
Assistant Clinical Professor
Department of Oral and Maxillofacial Surgery
Louisiana State University Health Science Center
New Orleans, Louisiana
Private Practice
University Oral and Maxillofacial Surgery
Charlotte, North Carolina

Thomas R. Flynn, DMD
Associate Professor
Oral and Maxillofacial Surgery
Harvard School of Dental Medicine
Assistant Visiting Surgeon
Oral and Maxillofacial Surgery
Massachusetts General Hospital
Boston, Massachusetts

Peter E. Larsen, DDS
Professor and Chair
Department of Oral and Maxillofacial Surgery
College of Dentistry
The Ohio State University
Chief of Pediatric Oral and Maxillofacial Surgery
Pediatric Dentistry
Children's Hospital of Columbus
Columbus, Ohio

Stuart E. Lieblich, DMD
Associate Clinical Professor
Oral and Maxillofacial Surgery
University of Connecticut School of Dental Medicine
Farmington, Connecticut
Senior Attending Staff
Oral and Maxillofacial Surgery
Hartford Hospital
Hartford, Connecticut

Edwin A. McGlumphy, DDS, MS
Associate Professor and Director of Implant Dentistry
Department of Restorative and Prosthetic Dentistry
College of Dentistry
The Ohio State University
Columbus, Ohio

Michael Miloro, DMD, MD
Professor of Surgery
Section Chief and Program Director
Leon F. Davis Distinguished Chair
Oral and Maxillofacial Surgery
University of Nebraska Medical Center
Omaha, Nebraska

Mark W. Ochs, DMD, MD
Professor and Chair
Department of Oral and Maxillofacial Surgery
School of Dental Medicine
University of Pittsburgh
Professor
Otolaryngology, Head and Neck Surgery
University of Pittsburgh Medical Center
Pittsburgh, Pennsylvania

Sterling R. Schow, DMD
Professor
Department of Oral and Maxillofacial Surgery
Baylor College of Dentistry
The Texas A&M University System Health Science Center
Dallas, Texas

Victoria J. Sterling, MA, JD
Senior Vice President
General Counsel
Oral and Maxillofacial Surgery National Insurance Company
Rosemont, Illinois

Preface

Oral and maxillofacial surgery is a continuously evolving area of health care. A multidisciplinary approach is necessary to meet the needs of most patients, making cooperation and coordination of care between the general dentist and medical and dental specialists essential to optimize care.

The primary purpose of *Contemporary Oral and Maxillofacial Surgery* is to present a comprehensive description of the basic oral surgery procedures that are performed in the office of the general practitioner. A secondary goal is to provide information on advanced and complex surgical management of patients typically referred to the specialist in oral and maxillofacial surgery. Primarily, this book is designed for use as an instructional text for the dental student, but the material is sufficiently comprehensive to serve as a reference book for general practitioners in private practice, general practice residents, and graduate students in other dental specialties. The resident, as well as the specialist in oral and maxillofacial surgery, will also find this book to be of value, especially the sections that relate to the medically compromised patients and to the concepts of team approach in the management of a variety of problems.

Contemporary Oral and Maxillofacial Surgery presents the fundamental principles of surgical and medical management of oral and maxillofacial surgery problems. The basic techniques of evaluation, diagnosis, and medical management are described in detail sufficient enough to allow immediate clinical application. The discussion of surgical techniques is extensively illustrated to help the reader readily understand these techniques. The large amount of detail is intended to enhance the reader's understanding of the biologic and the technical aspects of surgical procedures so that she or he can appropriately respond to surgical situations that are not "textbook cases."

This is the first edition produced without the direct involvement of former editor Larry J. Peterson, MS, DDS. However, Dr. Peterson's vision and concepts for this book remain evident. In the chapter he previously authored, many of his words are preserved. This work would not be the valued resource of information about oral and maxillofacial surgery without his past leadership.

The portions of the book that discuss complex oral and maxillofacial surgery procedures are written in an overview style, and no attempt has been made to describe these procedures in detail sufficient enough to allow the practitioner to actually learn the techniques.

For this fifth edition, the entire text was carefully reviewed and updated. Although certain chapters, such as the chapter on armamentarium, have few changes, other chapters, such as the endodontic surgery and infection chapters, were extensively revised. Also, the book is now in full color, which enhances the photographic images and techniques.

Part I has been updated to include the recent refinements in recommendations related to medical conditions as they relate to surgery.

In Part II, alterations have been made in the chapters on exodontia and postoperative management. A discussion of medicolegal issues related to health privacy laws appears.

In Part III, the chapter on dental implants has been completely updated in this rapidly advancing area.

Part IV, on infection, has been rewritten by a new author in light of current information on bacteria and antibiotics.

Parts V and VI, concerning pathology and trauma, have been updated to reflect current philosophies of treatment, including the newly recognized problem of jaw deterioration due to bisphosphonates.

Part VII, on dentofacial deformities, has undergone a rigorous revision to reflect the refinement and nuances of orthognathic surgery. A greater discussion on distraction osteogenesis is also provided.

Parts VIII and IX have been refined and updated.

The appendixes have also been updated to include current information.

Also new to this edition is an accompanying Evolve site (http://evolve.elsevier.com/COMS). This site will contain numerous instructional videos of basic surgical procedures. These videos will help reinforce procedures covered in the text. Students can watch the videos until they are comfortable with these procedures.

We hope readers and their patients will benefit from our contributions to this work, as well of those of our collaborating authors and the Elsevier production staff.

James R. Hupp
Edward Ellis III
Myron R. Tucker

ACKNOWLEDGMENTS

I acknowledge with gratitude all those who have helped shape my education and who continue to do so. These individuals are too numerous to list here, but they know who they are.

Edward Ellis III

My contributions to this book would not have been possible without the help of my terrific support staff at the University of Mississippi, Agnes Triplett and Helen Barnette, and Robert Gray, who did most of the photography for my contributions. I also appreciate all the help provided by the staff at Elsevier, including John Dolan, Elizabeth Clark, Julie Nebel, and Claire Kramer.

James R. Hupp

I would like to thank Ashley Tucker for the help she has given me on this publication (and many other things) and for her design of the book's cover.

Myron R. Tucker

Introduction

Oral and maxillofacial surgery is the specialty of dentistry that includes the diagnosis and surgical and adjunctive treatment of diseases, injuries, and defects, including both the functional and esthetic aspects of the hard and soft tissues of the oral and maxillofacial regions. This definition is intentionally broad and all-inclusive, primarily pertaining to the specialty of oral and maxillofacial surgery. The surgery performed in the office by general practitioners is usually much less extensive than that practiced by specialists in oral and maxillofacial surgery.

The scope of oral and maxillofacial surgery for the general practitioner is defined by several factors. The dentist's desire to perform surgical procedures is the first. Some dentists have little or no interest in doing surgical procedures, whereas other dentists enjoy it. The second factor is the dentist's training and experience in performing complex surgical procedures. A dentist may be interested in performing surgery for the removal of impacted teeth; however, without adequate surgical training and experience and the ability to deliver advanced forms of anesthesia, it would be unwise to do so. The third factor defining the scope of a dentist's surgical practice is the level of skill of the dentist. Even with a high interest level and with extensive training, a dentist who has little or no skill in the surgical arena or has let those skills go unused for a period of time should not perform complex surgical procedures. On the other hand, with a high level of interest, extensive training, and sufficient skill, the general practitioner can seriously consider performing more complex surgical procedures. The fourth and final factor is the availability of specialists in the dentist's vicinity. If specialists in oral and maxillofacial surgery are geographically separated from the general practitioner by a large distance, the general practitioner may wish to perform more surgical procedures and surgery of greater complexity than if there were a specialist relatively near.

It is important to note that the scope of oral and maxillofacial surgery practice for the general practitioner of dentistry is not usually defined by state law. Most state dental boards issue a single license for the practice of dentistry to both general practitioners and specialists. The general practitioner has the legal right to perform any oral and maxillofacial surgery procedure. Therefore each dentist must decide which surgical procedures to perform and which should be referred to a specialist, keeping in mind the best interests of the patient. The factors previously listed are those on which such decisions should be made.

The scope of oral and maxillofacial surgery for the general practitioner usually includes several surgical procedures. The extraction of erupted teeth and the removal of fractured roots are the procedures most often performed. On completion of dental school, every dentist should have adequate training, experience, and skill to provide these services. The dentist should be able to perform minor preprosthetic surgical procedures, which include most procedures that can be performed with local anesthesia in an office setting. The dentist should be able to manage minor infections of the teeth and soft tissues of the mouth. Because most odontogenic infections are minor, the reasonably experienced general dentist can manage them. The dentist should be able to evaluate the patient with an oral pathologic lesion and determine whether a biopsy is necessary. In many situations, the dentist should be the one who performs such a biopsy. Finally, the general dentist should have facility to manage traumatic injuries of the teeth and surrounding soft tissues. In many situations, definitive care must be provided by specialists, but initial care often can be provided by the general dentist.

The specialist in oral and maxillofacial surgery is a dentist who has had formal training in oral and maxillofacial surgery for 4 or more years after completing dental school. During this period, he or she has gained extensive experience in complex surgical and medical management and has received extensive training and experience in the diagnosis and surgical management of impacted teeth, as well as experience with the techniques of tooth extraction in patients with severe medical compromises. Important to the training of oral and maxillofacial surgeons is the acquisition of knowledge and skill in advanced and complex pain control methods, including intravenous sedation and ambulatory general anesthesia. In addition, the oral and maxillofacial surgeon receives extensive training and experience in the full evaluation and definitive care of the trauma patient, management of extensive odontogenic infections of the head and neck, management of oral and maxillofacial pathologic lesions (such as cysts and tumors of the jaws), diagnosis and management of dentofacial deformities (congenital, developmental, or acquired), complex maxillofacial preprosthetic surgery (including the use of dental implants), reconstruction with bone grafts of missing portions of the jaws, and management of facial pain and temporomandibular joint disorders.

Surgery does not require technical skill alone; it is a complex discipline that includes many factors. Surgical skill is the technical portion of the total surgical activity and accounts for less than one third of a surgeon's ability. Surgical judgment is the wisdom to make decisions about the need for surgery and the management of the patient undergoing a surgical procedure. Most important, the discipline of surgery includes the diagnosis of the surgical problem; the preparation of the patient, both psychologically and physiologically, for the procedure; the timing of the operation for the patient's maximal benefit; the adjustment and modification of standard surgical procedures to fit the individual needs of each patient; and, finally, the supportive postoperative care that is essential for an uneventful recovery from the surgical procedure.

To be excellent, a surgeon must be technically skilled but must also have strong components of humanism, kindness, humility, and compassion. It is important that he or she have a great deal of insight into the patient's concerns regarding the upcoming surgical procedure. The surgeon must take advantage of this insight and project an image of caring about these concerns, which all patients have. This humanistic approach will be the most important factor in the patient's judgment of the surgeon's overall skill. The excellent surgeon must have good surgical judgment, which is a measure of both maturity and surgical experience. Finally, the surgeon must have great respect for soft tissue, as well as hard tissue. Surgeons with little respect for tissue will cause patients to have a longer recuperation and a higher incidence of complications.

The excellent surgeon must reflect on these characteristics by knowing when to operate, where to perform the operation anatomically, and how to technically perform the procedure. Equally important, the surgeon, whether a generalist or a specialist, must know when not to operate. As the beginning surgeon enters training, he or she should observe teachers for examples of surgical maturity. He or she should look for teachers who emphasize surgical finesse over surgical force. He or she should observe how surgeons, whether they are other students or senior faculty, help anxious patients through a surgical procedure by expressing concern and interest in the patient as a person, as well as how they perform the technical portion of the surgery.

Contents

*The editors wish to acknowledge the past contributions of the late Larry Peterson, DDS, MS. It was his vision that shaped the creation of this publication, now in its fifth edition, and made it the leading textbook in the area of oral and maxillofacial surgery. Other authors have rewritten the chapters authored by Dr. Peterson in prior editions, but his influence is still strong in the organization and words used.

PART I

Principles of Surgery

Surgery is a discipline based on principles that have evolved from basic research and centuries of trial and error. These principles pervade every area of surgery, whether oral and maxillofacial, periodontal, or neurosurgery. Part I provides basic information about patient evaluation and surgical concepts, which together form the necessary foundation for the discussions of the specialized surgical techniques presented in succeeding chapters in this book.

Many patients have medical conditions that affect wound healing and their ability to tolerate oral and maxillofacial surgery. Chapter 1 discusses the process of evaluating the health status of patients. The chapter also describes methods of altering surgical treatment plans to accommodate patients with common medical problems.

Preventing medical emergencies in the patient undergoing oral and maxillofacial surgery or other forms of dentistry is typically easier than managing emergencies once they occur. Chapter 2 discusses the means of recognizing and managing medical emergencies in the dental office. Just as important, Chapter 2 also provides information about measures to lessen the likelihood of emergencies.

Contemporary surgery is guided by a set of principles, the majority of which apply no matter where in the human body they are put into practice. Chapter 3 covers the most important principles for those practitioners who perform surgery of the oral cavity, jaws, and face.

Surgery always leaves a wound, whether one was initially present or not. Although obvious, this fact is often forgotten by the inexperienced surgeon, who may act as if the surgical procedure is complete once the final suture has been tied and the patient leaves. The surgeon's responsibility to the patient continues until the wound created during surgery has healed; therefore an understanding of wound healing is important for anyone who intends to create wounds surgically or to treat accidental wounds. Chapter 4 presents basic wound-healing concepts, particularly as they relate to oral surgery.

The work of Semmelweiss and Lister in the 1800s made clinicians aware of the microbial origin of postoperative infections, thereby changing surgery from a last resort to a more predictably successful endeavor. The advent of antibiotics designed to be used for systemic effect further advanced surgical science, allowing completely elective surgery to be performed at low risk. However, pathogenic communicable organisms still exist that, when the epithelial barrier is breached during surgery, can cause wound infections or systemic infectious diseases. The most serious examples are the hepatitis B and the human immunodeficiency viruses. Chapter 5 describes the means of minimizing the risk of significant wound contamination and the spread of infectious organisms among individuals. This includes thorough decontamination of the surgical instruments, disinfection of the room in which surgery is performed, lowering of bacterial counts in the operative site, and adherence to infection control principles by the members of the surgical team—in other words, aseptic technique.

CHAPTER 1

Preoperative Health Status Evaluation

JAMES R. HUPP

CHAPTER OUTLINE

The extent of the medical history and the physical examination and laboratory evaluation of patients requiring ambulatory dentoalveolar surgery differs from that necessary for a patient requiring hospital admission for surgical procedures. A patient's primary care physician typically performs comprehensive histories and physical examinations of patients; it is impractical and of little value for the dentist to duplicate this process. However, the dental health care provider must discover the presence or history of medical problems that may affect the safe delivery of care, as well as any conditions specifically affecting the health of the oral and maxillofacial region.

Dentists are educated in the basic sciences and preclinical medical sciences, particularly as they relate to the maxillofacial region. This special expertise in medical topics as they relate to the oral region makes dentists valuable resources in a community health care delivery team. The responsibility that this designation carries is that dentists must be capable of recognizing and appropriately managing pathologic oral conditions. To maintain this expertise, a dentist must keep informed of new developments in medicine, be vigilant when treating patients, and be prepared to communicate a thorough but succinct evaluation of the oral health of patients to other health care providers.

MEDICAL HISTORY

An accurate medical history is the most useful information a clinician can have when deciding whether a patient can safely undergo planned dental therapy. The dentist must also be prepared to predict how a medical problem will alter a patient's response to planned anesthetic agents and surgery. If obtaining the history is done well, the physical examination and laboratory evaluation of a patient usually play minor roles in the presurgical evaluation. The standard format used for recording the results of medical histories and physical examinations is illustrated in Box 1-1.

The medical history interview and the physical examination should be tailored to each patient, considering the patient's medical problems, age, intelligence, and lifestyle; the complexity of the planned procedure; and the anticipated anesthetic methods.

BOX 1-1

Standard Format for Recording Results of History and Physical Examinations

1. Biographic data
2. Chief complaint and its history
3. Medical history
4. Social and family medical histories
5. Review of systems
6. Physical examination
7. Laboratory and radiographic/imaging examinations

Biographic Data

The most important information to obtain initially from a patient is biographic data. These data include the patient's full name, address, age, gender, and occupation, as well as the name of the patient's primary care physician. The clinician uses this information, along with an impression of the patient's intelligence and personality, to assess the patient's reliability. This is important because the validity of the medical history provided by the patient depends primarily on the reliability of the patient as a historian. If the identification data or patient interview gives the clinician reason to suspect that the medical history will be unreliable, alternative methods of obtaining the necessary information should be found. A reliability assessment should continue throughout the entire history interview and physical examination, with the interviewer looking for illogical, improbable, or inconsistent patient responses that might suggest the need for corroborating information.

Chief Complaint

Every patient should be asked to state the chief complaint. This can be accomplished on a form the patient completes, or the patient's answers should be transcribed (preferably verbatim) into the dental record during the initial interview by a staff member or dentist. This statement helps the clinician establish priorities during history taking and treatment planning. In addition, by having patients formulate a chief complaint, one encourages them to clarify for themselves and the clinician why they desire treatment. Occasionally a hidden agenda may exist for the patient, consciously or subconsciously. In such circumstances, subsequent information elicited from the patient interview may reveal the true reason the patient is seeking care.

History of Chief Complaint

The patient should be asked to describe the history of the present complaint or illness, particularly its first appearance, any changes since its first appearance, and its influence on or by other factors. Descriptions of pain should include onset, intensity, duration, location, and radiation, as well as factors that worsen and mitigate the pain. In addition, an inquiry should be made about constitutional symptoms such as fever, chills, lethargy, anorexia, malaise, and weakness associated with the chief complaint.

This portion of the health history may be straightforward, such as a 2-day history of pain and swelling around an erupting third molar. However, the chief complaint may be relatively involved, such as a lengthy history of a painful, nonhealing extraction site in a patient who received therapeutic irradiation. In this case a more detailed history of the chief complaint is necessary.

Medical History

Most dental practitioners find health history forms (questionnaires) to be an efficient means of initially collecting the medical history. When a credible patient completes a health history form, the dentist can use pertinent answers to direct the interview. Properly trained dental assistants can "red flag" important patient responses on the form (e.g., circling allergies to medications in red) to bring positive answers to the attention of the dentist.

Health questionnaires should be written clearly, be in lay language, and not be too lengthy. To lessen the chance of patients giving incomplete or inaccurate responses and to comply with Health Insurance Portability and Accountability Act regulations, the form should include a statement that assures the patient of the confidentiality of the information and a consent line identifying those individuals the patient approves of having access to the dental record, such as the primary care physician and other clinicians in the practice. The form should also include a place for the patient signature to verify that the patient has understood the questions and the accuracy of the answers. Numerous health questionnaires designed for dental patients are available from sources such as the American Dental Association, dental schools, and dental textbooks (Fig. 1-1). The dentist should choose a prepared form or formulate an individualized one.

The items listed in Box 1-2 (collected on a form or verbally) help establish a suitable health history database for patients; if the data are collected verbally, written documentation of the results of the inquiry is important.

In addition to this basic information, it is helpful to inquire specifically about common medical problems that are likely to alter dental management of the patient. These problems include angina, myocardial infarction (MI), heart murmurs, rheumatic heart disease, bleeding disorders (including anticoagulant use), asthma, lung disease, hepatitis, sexually transmitted disease, renal disease, diabetes, corticosteroid use, seizure disorder, stroke, and implanted prosthetic devices such as artificial joints or heart valves. Patients should be asked specifically about allergies to local anesthetics, aspirin, and penicillin. Female patients in the appropriate age group must also be asked at each visit whether they may be pregnant.

BOX 1-2

Baseline Health History Database

1. Past hospitalizations, operations, traumatic injuries, and serious illnesses
2. Recent minor illnesses or symptoms
3. Medications currently or recently in use and allergies (particularly drug allergies)
4. Description of health-related habits or addictions, such as the use of ethanol, tobacco, and illicit drugs and the amount and type of daily exercise
5. Date and result of last medical checkup or physician visit

MEDICAL HISTORY

Name ________________________ M _____ F _____ Date of Birth ____________

Address ____

Telephone: (Home) ______________ (Work) ______________ Height _______ Weight _______

Today's Date ________________ Occupation ______________________________

Answer all questions by circling either YES or NO and fill in all blank spaces where indicated. Answers to the following questions are for our records only and are confidential.

1. My last medical physical examination was on (approximate) ____________________

2. The name & address of my personal physician is ____________________

   ____

3. Are you now under the care of a physician . . . . YES NO
   If so, what is the condition being treated? ____________________

4. Have you had any serious illness or operation . . . . YES NO
   If so, what was the illness or operation? ____________________

5. Have you been hospitalized within the past 5 years . . . . YES NO
   If so, what was the problem? ____________________

6. Do you have or have you had any of the following diseases or problems:
   a. Rheumatic fever or rheumatic heart disease. . . . . YES NO
   b. Heart abnormalities present since birth . . . . YES NO
   c. Cardiovascular disease (heart trouble, heart attack, angina, stroke, high blood pressure, heart murmur). . . . . YES NO
      (1) Do you have pain or pressure in chest upon exertion . . . . YES NO
      (2) Are you ever short of breath after mild exercise. . . . . YES NO
      (3) Do your ankles swell . . . . YES NO
      (4) Do you get short of breath when you lie down, or do you require extra pillows when you sleep. . . . . YES NO
      (5) Have you been told you have a heart murmur . . . . YES NO
   d. Asthma or hay fever . . . . YES NO
   e. Hives or a skin rash . . . . YES NO
   f. Fainting spells or seizures. . . . . YES NO
   g. Diabetes. . . . . YES NO
      (1) Do you have to urinate (pass water) more than six times a day . . . . . . YES NO
      (2) Are you thirsty much of the time . . . . YES NO
      (3) Does your mouth usually feel dry. . . . . YES NO
   h. Hepatitis, jaundice or liver disease. . . . . YES NO
   i. Arthritis or other joint problems. . . . . YES NO
   j. Stomach ulcers. . . . . YES NO
   k. Kidney trouble. . . . . YES NO
   l. Tuberculosis. . . . . YES NO
   m. Do you have a persistent cough or cough up blood. . . . . YES NO
   n. Venereal disease . . . . YES NO
   o. Other (list) ____________________

   ____

   ____

7. Have you had abnormal bleeding associated with previous extractions, surgery, or trauma. . . . . YES NO
   a. Do you bruise easily . . . . YES NO
   b. Have you ever required a blood transfusion. . . . . YES NO
   c. If so, explain the circumstances ____________________

   ____

8. Do you have any blood disorder such as anemia, including sickle cell anemia. . . . . YES NO

9. Have you had surgery or radiation treatment for a tumor, cancer, or other condition of your head or neck . . . . YES NO

FIGURE 1-1 Example of health history questionnaire useful for screening dental patients. (Modified from a form provided by the American Dental Association.)

Continued

MEDICAL HISTORY—cont'd

10. Are you taking any drug or medicine or herb . . . . YES NO
    If so, what ____________________

11. Are you taking any of the following:
    a. Antibiotics or sulfa drugs . . . . YES NO
    b. Anticoagulants (blood thinners). . . . . YES NO
    c. Medicine for high blood pressure . . . . YES NO
    d. Cortisone (steroids) (including prednisone). . . . . YES NO
    e. Tranquilizers . . . . YES NO
    f. Aspirin. . . . . YES NO
    g. Insulin, tolbutamide (Orinase) or similar drug for diabetes . . . . YES NO
    h. Digitalis or drugs for heart trouble . . . . YES NO
    i. Nitroglycerin. . . . . YES NO
    j. Antihistamine . . . . YES NO
    k. Oral birth control drug or other hormonal therapy. . . . . YES NO
    l. Medicines for osteoporosis . . . . YES NO
    m. Other ____________________

12. Are you allergic or have you reacted adversely to:
    a. Local anesthetics (procaine [Novocain]). . . . . YES NO
    b. Penicillin or other antibiotics. . . . . YES NO
    c. Sulfa drugs . . . . YES NO
    d. Aspirin. . . . . YES NO
    e. Iodine or x-ray dyes . . . . YES NO
    f. Codeine or other narcotics. . . . . YES NO
    g. Other ____________________

13. Have you had any serious trouble associated with any previous dental treatment . . . . YES NO
    If so, explain ____________________

14. Do you have any disease, condition, or problem not listed above that you think I should know about. . . . . YES NO
    If so, explain ____________________

15. Are you employed in any situation which exposes you regularly to x-rays or other ionizing radiation . . . . YES NO

16. Are you wearing contact lenses . . . . YES NO

WOMEN:

17. Are you pregnant or have you recently missed a menstrual period. . . . . YES NO

18. Are you presently breast-feeding . . . . YES NO

Chief dental complaint (Why did you come to the office today?): ____________________

____
Signature of Patient (verifying accuracy of historical information)

____
Signature of Dentist

FIGURE 1-1, cont'd Example of health history questionnaire useful for screening dental patients. (Modified from a form provided by the American Dental Association.)

BOX 1-3

Common Health Conditions to Inquire About Verbally or on a Health Questionnaire

- Allergies to antibiotics or local anesthetics
- Angina
- Anticoagulant use
- Asthma
- Bleeding disorders
- Breast-feeding
- Corticosteroid use
- Diabetes
- Heart murmurs
- Hepatitis
- Hypertension
- Implanted prosthetic devices
- Lung disease
- Myocardial infarction (i.e., heart attack)
- Osteoporosis
- Pregnancy
- Renal disease
- Rheumatic heart disease
- Seizure disorder
- Sexually transmitted disease
- Tuberculosis

A brief family history can be useful and should focus on relevant inherited diseases, such as hemophilia (Box 1-3). The medical history should be updated periodically, at least annually. Many dentists have their assistants specifically ask each patient at checkup appointments whether there has been any change in health since the last dental visit. The dentist is alerted if a change has occurred, and changes are documented in the record.

Review of Systems

The review of systems is a sequential, comprehensive method of eliciting patient symptoms on an organ system basis. The review of systems may reveal undiagnosed medical conditions. This review can be extensive when performed by a physician for a patient with complicated medical problems. However, the review of systems conducted by the dentist before oral surgery should be guided by pertinent answers obtained from the history. For example, the review of the cardiovascular system in a patient with a history of ischemic heart disease includes questions concerning chest discomfort (during exertion, eating, or at rest), palpitations, fainting, and ankle swelling. Such questions help the dentist decide whether to perform surgery at all or to alter the surgical or anesthetic methods. If anxiety-controlling adjuncts such as intravenous (IV) and inhalation sedation are planned, the cardiovascular, respiratory, and nervous systems should always be reviewed; this can disclose previously undiagnosed problems that may jeopardize successful sedation. In the role of the oral health specialist, the dentist is expected to perform a quick review of the head, ears, eyes, nose, mouth, and throat on every patient, regardless of whether other systems are reviewed. Items to be reviewed are outlined in Box 1-4.

The need to review organ systems in addition to those in the maxillofacial region depends on clinical circumstances. The cardiovascular and respiratory systems commonly require evaluation before oral surgery or sedation (Box 1-5).

BOX 1-4

Routine Review of Head, Neck, and Maxillofacial Regions

Constitutional: Fever, chills, sweats, weight loss, fatigue, malaise, loss of appetite
Head: Headache, dizziness, fainting, insomnia
Ears: Decreased hearing, tinnitus (ringing), pain
Eyes: Blurring, double vision, excessive tearing, dryness, pain
Nose and sinuses: Rhinorrhea, epistaxis, problems breathing through nose, pain, change in sense of smell
Temporomandibular joint area: Pain, noise, limited jaw motion
Oral: Dental pain or sensitivity, lip or mucosal sores, problems chewing, problems speaking, bad breath, loose restorations, sore throat, loud snoring
Neck: Difficulty swallowing, change in voice, pain, stiffness

BOX 1-5

Review of Cardiovascular and Respiratory Systems

CARDIOVASCULAR REVIEW

Chest discomfort on exertion, when eating, or at rest; palpitations; fainting; ankle edema; shortness of breath (dyspnea) on exertion; dyspnea on assuming supine position (orthopnea or paroxysmal nocturnal dyspnea); postural hypotension; fatigue; leg muscle cramping

RESPIRATORY REVIEW

Dyspnea with exertion, wheezing, coughing, excessive sputum production, coughing up blood (hemoptysis)

PHYSICAL EXAMINATION

The physical examination of the dental patient focuses on the oral cavity and to a lesser degree on the entire maxillofacial region. Recording the results of the physical examination should be an exercise in accurate description rather than a listing of suspected medical diagnoses. For example, the clinician may find a mucosal lesion inside the lower lip that is 5 mm in diameter, raised and firm, and not painful to palpation. These physical findings should be recorded in a similarly descriptive manner; the dentist should not jump to a diagnosis and record only "fibroma on lip."

Any physical examination should begin with the measurement of vital signs. This serves as a screening device for unsuspected medical problems and as a baseline for future measurements. The techniques of measuring blood pressure and pulse rates are illustrated in Figures 1-2 and 1-3.

The physical evaluation of various parts of the body usually involves one or more of the following four primary means of evaluation: (1) inspection, (2) palpation, (3) percussion, and (4) auscultation. In the oral and maxillofacial regions, inspection should always be performed. The clinician should note hair distribution and texture, facial symmetry and proportion, eye movements and conjunctival color, nasal patency on each side, the presence or absence of skin lesions or discoloration, and neck or facial masses. A thorough inspection of the oral cavity is necessary, including the oropharynx, tongue, floor of the mouth, and oral mucosa (Fig. 1-4).

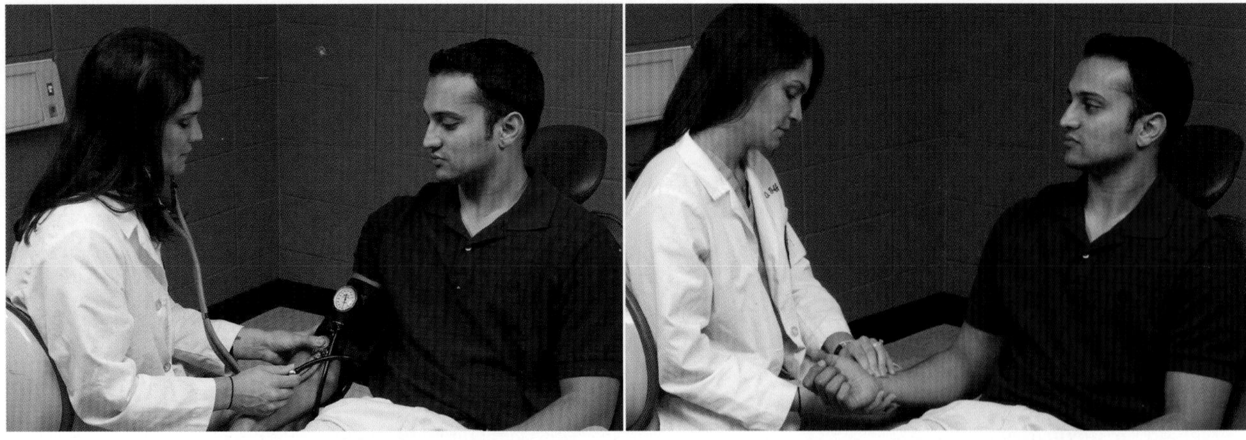

FIGURE 1-2 A, Measurement of systemic blood pressure. Cuff of proper size placed securely around upper arm so that lower edge of cuff lies 2 to 4 cm above antecubital fossa. Branchial artery is palpated in fossa, and stethoscope diaphragm is placed over artery and held in place with fingers of left hand. Squeeze bulb is held in palm of right hand, and valve is screwed closed with thumb and index finger of that hand. Bulb is then repeatedly squeezed until pressure gauge reads approximately 220 mm Hg. Air is allowed to escape slowly from cuff by partially opening valve while dentist listens through stethoscope. Gauge reading at point when faint blowing sound is first heard is systolic blood pressure. Gauge reading when sound from artery disappears is diastolic pressure. Once diastolic pressure reading is obtained, valve is opened to deflate cuff completely. B, Pulse rate and rhythm most commonly are evaluated by using tips of middle and index fingers of right hand to palpate radial artery at the wrist. Once rhythm has been determined to be regular, number of pulsations to occur during 30 seconds is multiplied by 2 to give number of pulses per minute. If weak pulse or irregular rhythm is discovered while palpating radial pulse, heart should be auscultated directly to determine heart rate and rhythm.

Palpation is important when examining temporomandibular joint function, salivary gland size and function, thyroid gland size, presence or absence of enlarged or tender lymph nodes, and induration of oral soft tissues, as well as for determining pain or the presence of fluctuance in areas of swelling.

Physicians commonly use percussion during thoracic and abdominal examinations, and the dentist can use it to test teeth and paranasal sinuses. The dentist uses auscultation primarily for temporomandibular joint evaluation, but it is also used for cardiac, pulmonary, and gastrointestinal systems evaluations (Box 1-6). A brief maxillofacial examination that all dentists should be able to perform is described in Box 1-7.

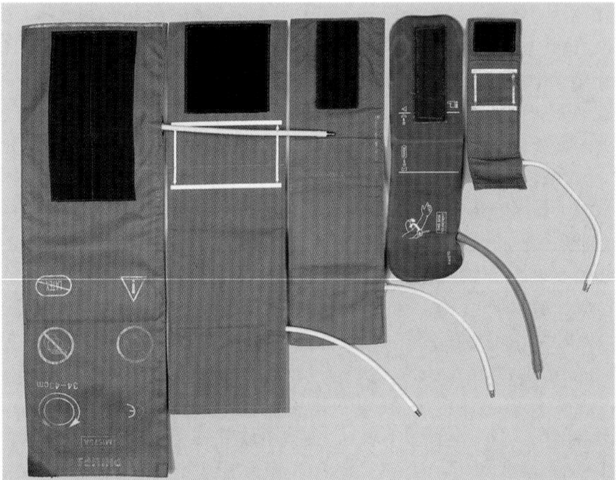

FIGURE 1-3 Blood pressure cuffs of varying sizes for patients with arms of different diameters (ranging from infant through obese patients). Use of an improper cuff size can jeopardize the accuracy of blood pressure results. Too small a cuff causes readings to be falsely high, and too large a cuff causes artificially low readings. Blood pressure cuffs typically are labeled as to the type and size of patient for whom they are designed.

BOX 1-6

Preoperative Physical Examination of the Oral and Maxillofacial Surgery Patient

INSPECTION

Head and face: General shape, symmetry, hair distribution
Ear: Normal reaction to sounds (otoscopic examination if indicated)
Eye: Symmetry, size, reactivity of pupil, color of sclera and conjunctiva, movement, test of vision
Nose: Septum, mucosa, patency
Mouth: Teeth, mucosa, pharynx, lips, tonsils
Neck: Size of thyroid gland, jugular venous distention

PALPATION

Temporomandibular joint: Crepitus, tenderness
Paranasal: Pain over sinuses
Mouth: Salivary glands, floor of mouth, lips, muscles of mastication
Neck: Thyroid gland size, lymph nodes

PERCUSSION

Paranasal: Resonance over sinuses (difficult to assess)
Mouth: Teeth

AUSCULTATION

Temporomandibular joint: Clicks, crepitus
Neck: Carotid bruits

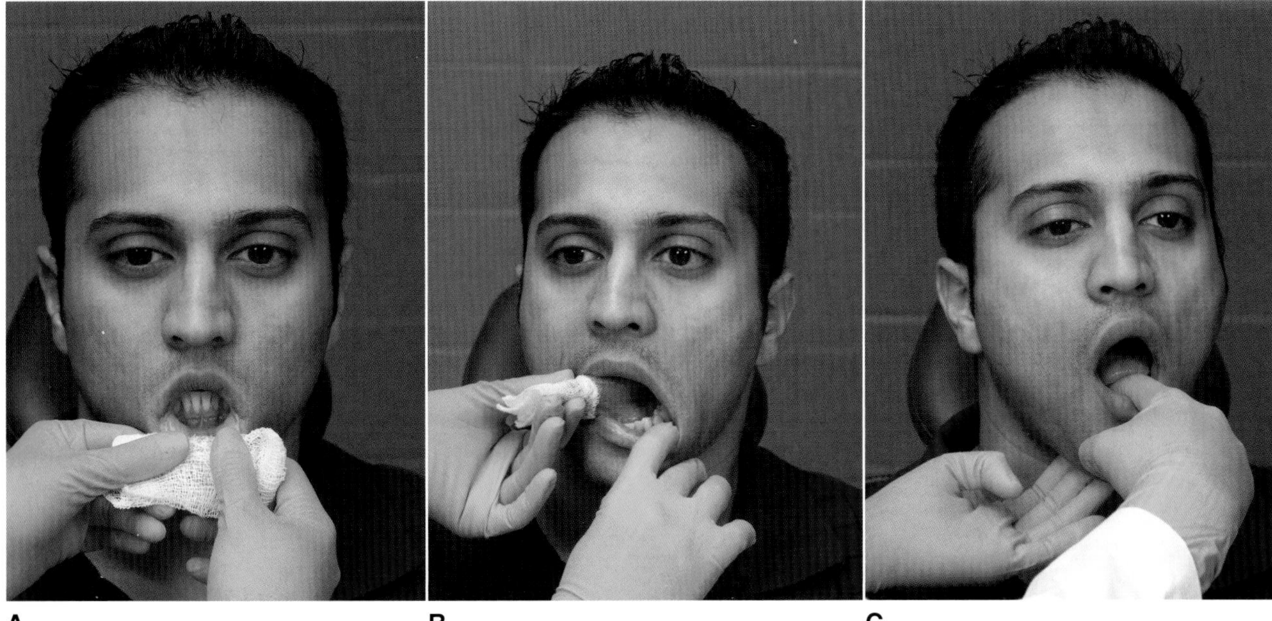

FIGURE 1-4 A, Lip mucosa examined by everting upper and lower lips. B, Tongue examined by having patient protrude it. Examiner then grasps tongue with cotton sponge and gently manipulates it to examine lateral borders. Patient also is asked to lift tongue to allow visualization of ventral surface and floor of mouth. C, Submandibular gland examined by bimanually feeling gland through floor of mouth and skin under floor of mouth.

The results of the medical evaluation are used to assign a physical status classification. A few classification systems exist, but the one most commonly used is the American Society of Anesthesiologists' (ASA) physical status classification system (Box 1-8).

BOX 1-7

Brief Maxillofacial Examination

While interviewing the patient, the dentist should visually examine the patient for general shape and symmetry of head and facial skeleton, eye movement, color of conjunctiva and sclera, and ability to hear. The clinician should listen for speech problems, temporomandibular joint sounds, and breathing ability.

ROUTINE EXAMINATION

Temporomandibular joint region:

- Palpate and auscultate joints.
- Measure range of motion of jaw and opening pattern.

Nose and paranasal region:

- Occlude nares individually to check for patency.
- Inspect anterior nasal mucosa.

Mouth:

- Take out all removable prostheses.
- Inspect oral cavity for dental, oral, and pharyngeal mucosal lesions; look at tonsils and uvula.
- Hold tongue out of mouth with dry gauze while inspecting lateral borders.
- Palpate tongue, lips, floor of mouth, and salivary glands (check for saliva).
- Palpate neck for lymph nodes and thyroid gland size. Inspect jugular veins.

Once an ASA physical status class has been determined, the dentist can decide whether required treatment can be safely and routinely performed in the dental office. If a patient is not ASA class I or a relatively healthy class II patient, the practitioner generally has the following four options: (1) modifying routine treatment plans by anxiety-reduction measures, pharmacologic anxiety-control techniques, more careful monitoring of the patient during treatment, or a combination of these methods (this is usually all that is necessary for ASA class II); (2) obtaining medical consultation for guidance in preparing patients to undergo ambulatory oral surgery (e.g., not fully reclining a patient with congestive heart failure); (3) refusing to treat the patient in the ambulatory setting; or (4) referring the patient to an oral-maxillofacial surgeon. Modifications to the ASA system designed to be more specific to dentistry are available but are not yet widely used among health care professionals.

BOX 1-8

American Society of Anesthesiologists (ASA) Classification of Physical Status

ASA I: A normal, healthy patient

ASA II: A patient with mild systemic disease or significant health risk factor

ASA III: A patient with severe systemic disease that is not incapacitating

ASA IV: A patient with severe systemic disease that is a constant threat to life

ASA V: A moribund patient who is not expected to survive without the operation

ASA VI: A declared brain-dead patient whose organs are being removed for donor purposes

MANAGEMENT OF PATIENTS WITH COMPROMISING MEDICAL CONDITIONS

Patients with medical conditions sometimes require modifications of their perioperative care when oral surgery is planned. This section discusses those considerations for the major categories of health problems.

Cardiovascular Problems

Ischemic Heart Disease

ANGINA PECTORIS. Obstruction of the arterial supply to the myocardium is one of the most common health problems dentists encounter. This condition occurs primarily in men over age 40 and is also prevalent in postmenopausal women. The basic disease process is a progressive narrowing or spasm (or both) of one or more of the coronary arteries. This leads to a discrepancy between the myocardial oxygen demand and the ability of the coronary arteries to supply oxygen-carrying blood. Myocardial oxygen demand can be increased, for example, by exertion, anxiety, or during digestion of a large meal. Angina is a symptom of ischemic heart disease produced when myocardial blood supply cannot be sufficiently increased to meet the increased oxygen requirements that result from coronary artery disease.* The myocardium becomes ischemic, producing a heavy pressure or squeezing sensation in the patient's substernal region that can radiate into the left shoulder and arm and into the mandibular region. The patient may complain of an intense sense of being unable to breathe adequately. Stimulation of vagal activity commonly occurs with nausea, sweating, and bradycardia. The discomfort typically disappears once the myocardial work requirements are lowered or the oxygen supply to the heart muscle is increased.

The practitioner's responsibility to a patient with a history of angina is to use all available preventive measures, thereby reducing the possibility that the surgical procedure will precipitate an anginal episode. Preventive measures begin with taking a careful history of the patient's angina. The patient should be questioned about the events that produce angina; the frequency, duration, and severity of angina; and the response to medications or diminished activity. The patient's physician can be consulted concerning the cardiac status.

If the patient's angina arises only during moderately vigorous exertion and responds readily to oral nitroglycerin administration, and if no recent increase in severity has occurred, ambulatory oral surgery procedures are usually safe when performed with proper precautions.

However, if anginal episodes occur with only minimal exertion, if several doses of nitroglycerin are needed to relieve chest discomfort, or if the patient has unstable angina (i.e., angina present at rest or worsening in frequency, severity, ease of precipitation, duration of attack, or predictability of response to medication), elective surgery should be deferred until a medical consultation is obtained. Alternatively, the patient can be referred to an oral-maxillofacial surgeon if emergency surgery is necessary.

Once the decision is made that ambulatory elective oral surgery can safely proceed, the patient should be prepared for surgery and the patient's myocardial oxygen demand should be lowered or prevented from rising. The increased oxygen demand during ambulatory oral surgery is the result primarily of patient anxiety. An anxiety-reduction protocol should therefore be used (Box 1-9). In addition, during surgery the patient can be given supplemental oxygen and can be premedicated with nitroglycerin (if the patient is extremely prone to angina). Profound local anesthesia is the best means of limiting patient anxiety. Although some controversy exists over the use of local anesthetics containing epinephrine in patients with angina, the benefits (e.g., prolonged and accentuated anesthesia) outweigh the risks. However, care should be taken to avoid excessive epinephrine administration by using proper injection techniques. Some clinicians also advise giving no more than 4 mL of a local anesthetic solution with a 1:100,000 concentration of epinephrine for a total adult dose of 0.04 mg in any 30-minute period.

Before and during surgery, vital signs should be monitored periodically. In addition, regular verbal contact with the patient should be maintained. The use of nitrous oxide or other conscious sedation methods for anxiety control in patients with ischemic heart disease should be considered. Fresh nitroglycerin should be nearby for use if necessary (Box 1-10).

The introduction of balloon-tipped catheters into narrowed coronary arteries for the purpose of reestablishing adequate

BOX 1-9

General Anxiety-Reduction Protocol

BEFORE APPOINTMENT
- Hypnotic agent to promote sleep on night before surgery (optional)
- Sedative agent to decrease anxiety on morning of surgery (optional)
- Morning appointment and schedule so that reception room time is minimized

DURING APPOINTMENT

Nonpharmacologic Means of Anxiety Control
- Frequent verbal reassurances
- Distracting conversation
- No surprises (clinician warns patient before doing anything that could cause anxiety)
- No unnecessary noise
- Surgical instruments out of patient's sight
- Relaxing background music

Pharmacologic Means of Anxiety Control
- Local anesthetics of sufficient intensity and duration
- Nitrous oxide
- Intravenous anxiolytics

AFTER SURGERY
- Succinct instructions for postoperative care
- Patient information on expected postsurgical sequelae (e.g., swelling or minor oozing of blood)
- Further reassurance
- Effective analgesics
- Patient information on who can be contacted if any problems arise
- Telephone call to patient at home during evening after surgery to check whether any problems exist

*The term *angina* is derived from the ancient Greek word for a choking sensation.

BOX 1-10

Management of Patient with History of Angina Pectoris

1. Consult patient's physician.
2. Use an anxiety-reduction protocol.
3. Have nitroglycerin tablets or spray readily available. Use nitroglycerin premedication if indicated.
4. Administer supplemental oxygen.
5. Ensure profound local anesthesia before starting surgery.
6. Consider use of nitrous oxide sedation.
7. Monitor vital signs closely.
8. Consider possible limitation of amount of epinephrine used (0.04 mg maximum).
9. Maintain verbal contact with patient throughout procedure to monitor status.

BOX 1-11

Management of Patient with a History of Myocardial Infarction

1. Consult patient's primary care physician.
2. Check with physcian if invasive dental care needed before 6 months since MI.
3. Check whether patient is using anticoagulants (including aspirin).
4. Use an anxiety-reduction protocol.
5. Have nitroglycerin available; use prophylactically if physician advises.
6. Administer supplemental oxygen.
7. Provide profound local anesthesia.
8. Consider nitrous oxide administration.
9. Monitor vital signs and maintain verbal contact.
10. Consider possible limitation of epinephrine used to 0.04 mg.
11. Consider referral to an oral and maxillofacial surgeon.

blood flow and stenting arteries open is becoming commonplace. If the angioplasty has been successful (based on cardiac stress testing), oral surgery can proceed soon thereafter, with the same precautions as those used for patients with angina.

MYOCARDIAL INFARCTION. MI occurs when ischemia (resulting from an oxygen demand and supply mismatch) causes cellular dysfunction and death. The infarcted area of myocardium becomes nonfunctional and eventually necrotic and is surrounded by an area of usually reversibly ischemic myocardium that is prone to serve as a nidus for dysrhythmias. During the early hours and weeks after an MI, treatment consists of limiting myocardial work requirements, increasing myocardial oxygen supply, and suppressing the production of dysrhythmias by irritable foci in ischemic tissue. In addition, if any of the primary conduction pathways are involved in the infarction, pacemaker insertion may be necessary. If the patient survives the early weeks after an MI, the variably sized necrotic area is gradually replaced with scar tissue, which is unable to contract or properly conduct electrical signals.

The management of an oral surgical problem in a patient who has had an MI begins with a consultation with the patient's physician. Generally, it is recommended that elective major surgical procedures be deferred until at least 6 months after an infarction. This delay is based on statistical evidence that the risk of reinfarction after an MI drops to as low as it will ever be by about 6 months, particularly if the patient is properly supervised medically. The advent of thrombolytic-based treatment strategies and improved MI care make an automatic 6-month wait to do dental work unnecessary. Straightforward oral surgical procedures typically performed in the dental office may be performed less than 6 months after an MI if the procedure is unlikely to provoke significant anxiety and the patient had an uneventful recovery from the MI. In addition, other dental procedures may proceed if cleared by the patient's physician via a medical consult.

Patients with a history of MI should be carefully questioned concerning their cardiovascular health. An attempt to elicit evidence of undiagnosed dysrhythmias or congestive heart failure (hypertrophic cardiomyopathy) should be made. Some patients who have had an MI take aspirin and other anticoagulants to decrease coronary thrombogenesis; this information should be sought because it can affect surgical decision making.

If more than 6 months have elapsed or physician clearance is obtained, the management of the patient who has had an MI is similar to care of the patient with angina. An anxiety-reduction program should be used. Supplemental oxygen can also be considered. Prophylactic nitroglycerin administration should be done only if directed by the patient's primary care physician, but nitroglycerin should be readily available. Local anesthetics containing epinephrine are safe to use if given in proper amounts using an aspiration technique. Vital signs should be monitored throughout the perioperative period (Box 1-11).

In general, with respect to major oral surgical care, patients who have had coronary artery bypass grafting (CABG) are treated in a manner similar to patients who have had an MI. Before major elective surgery is performed, 3 months are allowed to elapse. If major surgery is necessary before 3 months after the CABG, the patient's physician should be consulted. Patients who have had CABG usually have a history of angina, MI, or both and therefore should be managed as previously described. Routine office surgical procedures may be safely performed in patients less than 6 months after CABG surgery if their recovery has been uncomplicated and anxiety is kept to a minimum.

Cerebrovascular Accident (Stroke)

Patients who have had a cerebrovascular accident are always susceptible to further neurovascular accidents. These patients are generally prescribed anticoagulants and, if hypertensive, are taking blood pressure–lowering agents. If such a patient requires surgery, clearance by the patient's physician is desirable, as is a delay until significant hypertensive tendencies have been controlled. The patient's baseline neurologic status should be assessed and documented preoperatively. The patient should be treated by a nonpharmacologic anxiety-reduction protocol and have vital signs carefully monitored during surgery. If pharmacologic sedation is necessary, low concentrations of nitrous oxide can be used. Techniques to manage patients taking anticoagulants are discussed later in this chapter.

Dysrhythmias

Patients who are prone to or who have cardiac dysrhythmias usually have a history of ischemic heart disease requiring dental management modifications. Many advocate limiting the total amount of epinephrine administration to 0.04 mg. However, in addition, these patients may have been prescribed anticoagulants or have a permanent cardiac pacemaker. Pacemakers pose no contraindications to oral surgery, and no evidence exists that shows the need for antibiotic prophylaxis in patients with pacemakers. Electrical equipment, such as electrocautery and microwaves, should not be used near the patient. As with other medically compromised patients, vital signs should be carefully monitored.

Heart Abnormalities Predisposed Toward Infective Endocarditis

The internal cardiac surface, or endocardium, can be predisposed toward infection when abnormalities of its surface allow pathologic bacteria to attach and multiply. A complete description of this process and recommended means of possibly preventing it are discussed in Chapter 16.

Congestive Heart Failure (Hypertrophic Cardiomyopathy)

Congestive heart failure occurs when a diseased myocardium is unable to deliver the cardiac output demanded by the body or when excessive demands are placed on a normal myocardium. The heart begins to have an increased end-diastolic volume that, in the case of the normal myocardium, increases contractility through the Frank-Starling mechanism. However, as the normal or diseased myocardium further dilates, it becomes a less efficient pump, causing blood to back up into the pulmonary, hepatic, and mesenteric vascular beds. This eventually leads to pulmonary edema, hepatic dysfunction, and compromised intestinal nutrient absorption. The lowered cardiac output causes generalized weakness, and impaired renal clearance of excess fluid leads to vascular overload.

Symptoms of congestive heart failure include orthopnea, paroxysmal nocturnal dyspnea, and ankle edema. Orthopnea is a respiratory disorder that exhibits shortness of breath when the patient is in the supine position. Orthopnea usually occurs as a result of the redistribution of blood pooled in the lower extremity when a patient assumes the supine position (as when sleeping). The ability of the heart to handle the increased cardiac preload is overwhelmed, and blood backs up into the pulmonary circulation, producing pulmonary edema. Patients with orthopnea usually sleep with their upper body supported on several pillows.

Paroxysmal nocturnal dyspnea is a symptom of congestive heart failure that is similar to orthopnea. The patient has respiratory difficulty 1 or 2 hours after assuming a supine position. The disorder occurs when pooled blood and interstitial fluid reabsorbed into the vasculature from the legs are redistributed centrally, overwhelming the heart and producing pulmonary edema. Patients suddenly wake awhile after lying down to sleep feeling short of breath and are compelled to sit up to try to catch their breath.

Lower extremity edema usually appears as a swelling of the foot, the ankle, or both that is caused by an increase in interstitial fluid. Usually the fluid collects as a result of any problem that increases venous pressure or low serum protein, allowing increased amounts of plasma to remain in the tissue spaces of the feet. The edema is detected by pressing a finger into the swollen area for a few seconds; if an indentation in the soft tissue is left after the finger is removed, pedal edema is present.

BOX 1-12

Management of the Patient with Congestive Heart Failure (Hypertrophic Cardiomyopathy)

1. Defer treatment until heart function has been medically improved and physician believes treatment is possible.
2. Use an anxiety-reduction protocol.
3. Consider possible administration of supplemental oxygen.
4. Avoid supine position.
5. Consider referral to an oral and maxillofacial surgeon.

Other symptoms of congestive heart failure include weight gain and dyspnea on exertion.

Patients with congestive heart failure who are under a physician's care are usually following low-sodium diets to reduce fluid retention and are receiving diuretics to reduce intravascular volume; cardiac glycosides, such as digoxin, to improve cardiac efficiency; and sometimes afterload-reducing drugs, such as nitrates, β-adrenergic antagonists, or calcium channel antagonists, to control the amount of work the heart is required to do. In addition, patients with chronic atrial fibrillation caused by hypertrophic cardiomyopathy are usually prescribed anticoagulants to prevent atrial thrombus formation.

Patients with congestive heart failure that is well compensated through dietary and drug therapy can safely undergo ambulatory oral surgery. The anxiety-reduction protocol and supplemental oxygen are helpful. Patients with orthopnea should not be placed supine during any procedure. Surgery for patients with uncompensated hypertrophic cardiomyopathy is best deferred until compensation is achieved or procedures can be performed in the hospital setting (Box 1-12).

Pulmonary Problems

Asthma

When a patient relates a history of asthma, the dentist should first determine through further questioning whether the patient truly has asthma or has a respiratory problem such as allergic rhinitis that carries less significance for dental care. True asthma involves the episodic narrowing of small airways, which produces wheezing and dyspnea as a result of chemical, infectious, immunologic, or emotional stimulation, or a combination of these. Patients with asthma should be questioned concerning precipitating factors, frequency and severity of attacks, medications used, and response to medications. The severity of attacks can often be gauged by the need for emergency room visits and hospital admissions. Asthmatic patients should be questioned specifically about aspirin allergy because of the relatively high frequency of generalized nonsteroidal antiinflammatory drug (NSAID) allergy in asthmatic patients.

Physicians prescribe medications for patients with asthma according to the frequency, severity, and causes of their disease. Patients with severe asthma require xanthine-derived bronchodilators, such as theophylline, and corticosteroids. Cromolyn may be used to protect against acute attacks, but it is ineffective once bronchospasm occurs. Many patients carry sympathomimetic amines, such as epinephrine or metaproterenol, in an aerosol form that can be self-administered if wheezing begins.

Oral surgical management of the patient with asthma involves recognition of the role of anxiety in bronchospasm

BOX 1-13

Management of Asthmatic Patient

1. Defer dental treatment until asthma is well controlled and patient has no signs of a respiratory tract infection.
2. Listen to chest with stethoscope to detect wheezing before major oral surgical procedures or sedation.
3. Use an anxiety-reduction protocol, including nitrous oxide, but avoid use of respiratory depressants.
4. Consult physician about possible preoperative use of cromolyn sodium.
5. If patient is or has been chronically taking corticosteroids, provide prophylaxis for adrenal insufficiency (see p. 16).
6. Keep a bronchodilator-containing inhaler easily accessible.
7. Avoid use of nonsteroidal antiinflammatory drugs in susceptible patients.

initiation and of the potential adrenal suppression in patients receiving corticosteroid therapy (see previous discussion). Elective oral surgery should be deferred if a respiratory tract infection or wheezing is present. When surgery is performed, an anxiety-reduction protocol must be followed; if the patient takes steroids, the patient's primary care physician can be consulted concerning the possible need for corticosteroid augmentation during the perioperative period if a major surgical procedure is planned. Nitrous oxide is safe to administer to persons with asthma and is especially indicated for patients whose asthma is triggered by anxiety. The patient's own inhaler should be available during surgery, and drugs such as injectable epinephrine and theophylline should be kept in an emergency kit. The use of NSAIDs should be avoided because they often precipitate asthma attacks in susceptible individuals (Box 1-13).

Chronic Obstructive Pulmonary Disease

Obstructive and restrictive pulmonary diseases are usually grouped together under the heading of chronic obstructive pulmonary disease (COPD). In the past the terms *emphysema* and *bronchitis* were used to describe clinical manifestations of COPD, but COPD has been recognized to be a blend of pathologic pulmonary problems. COPD is usually caused by long-term exposure to pulmonary irritants, such as tobacco smoke, that cause metaplasia of pulmonary airway tissue. Airways are disrupted, lose their elastic properties, and become obstructed because of mucosal edema, excessive secretions, and bronchospasm, producing the clinical manifestations of COPD. Patients with COPD frequently become dyspneic during mild to moderate exertion. They have a chronic cough that produces large amounts of thick secretions, frequent respiratory tract infections, and barrel-shaped chests, and they may purse their lips to breathe and have audible wheezing during breathing.

Bronchodilators, such as theophylline, are usually prescribed for patients with significant COPD; in more severe cases, patients are given corticosteroids. Only in the most severe chronic cases is supplemental portable oxygen used.

When dentally managing patients with COPD who are receiving corticosteroids, the dentist should consider the use of additional supplementation before major surgery. Sedatives, hypnotics, and narcotics that depress respiration should be avoided. Patients may need to be kept in an upright sitting position in the dental chair to enable them to better handle their commonly copious pulmonary secretions. Finally, supplemental oxygen during surgery should not be used in patients with severe COPD unless the physician advises it. In contrast with healthy persons in whom an elevated arterial CO_2 level is the major stimulation to breathing, the patient with COPD becomes acclimated to elevated arterial CO_2 levels and comes to depend entirely on depressed arterial oxygen levels to stimulate breathing. If the arterial oxygen concentration is elevated by the administration of oxygen in a high concentration, the hypoxia-based respiratory stimulation is removed and the patient's respiratory rate may become critically slowed (Box 1-14).

BOX 1-14

Management of Patient with Chronic Obstructive Pulmonary Disease

1. Defer treatment until lung function has improved and treatment is possible.
2. Listen to the chest bilaterally with stethoscope to determine adequacy of breath sounds.
3. Use an anxiety-reduction protocol, but avoid use of respiratory depressants.
4. If patient requires chronic oxygen supplementation, continue at prescribed flow rate. If patient does not require supplemental oxygen therapy, consult physician before administering oxygen.
5. If patient chronically receives corticosteroid therapy, manage patient for adrenal insufficiency (see p. 16).
6. Avoid placing patient in supine position until confident that patient can tolerate it.
7. Keep a bronchodilator-containing inhaler accessible.
8. Closely monitor respiratory and heart rates.
9. Schedule afternoon appointments to allow for clearing of secretions.

Renal Problems

Renal Failure

Patients in renal failure require periodic renal dialysis. These patients need special consideration during oral surgical care. Chronic dialysis treatment typically requires the presence of an arteriovenous shunt (i.e., a large, surgically created junction between an artery and vein), which allows easy vascular access and heparin administration, allowing blood to move through the dialysis equipment without clotting. The dentist should not use the shunt for venous access except in an emergency.

Elective oral surgery is best undertaken the day after a dialysis treatment has been performed. This allows the heparin used during dialysis to disappear and the patient to be in the best physiologic status with respect to intravascular volume and metabolic by-products.

Drugs that depend on renal metabolism or excretion should be avoided or used in modified doses to prevent systemic toxicity. Drugs removed during dialysis will also necessitate special dosing regimens. Relatively nephrotoxic drugs, such as NSAIDs, should also be avoided in patients with seriously compromised kidneys.

Because of the higher incidence of hepatitis in renal dialysis patients, dentists should take the necessary precautions. The

BOX 1-15

Management of Patient with Renal Insufficiency and Patient Receiving Hemodialysis

1. Avoid the use of drugs that depend on renal metabolism or excretion. Modify the dose if such drugs are necessary.
2. Avoid the use of nephrotoxic drugs, such as nonsteroidal antiinflammatory drugs.
3. Defer dental care until the day after dialysis has been given.
4. Consult physician concerning prophylactic use of antibiotics.
5. Monitor blood pressure and heart rate.
6. Look for signs of secondary hyperparathyroidism.
7. Consider hepatitis B screening before dental treatment. Take hepatitis precautions if unable to screen for hepatitis.

altered appearance of bone caused by secondary hyperparathyroidism in patients with renal failure should also be noted. Metabolic radiolucencies should not be mistaken for dental disease (Box 1-15).

Renal Transplant and Transplant of Other Organs

The patient requiring surgery after renal or other major organ transplantation is usually receiving a variety of drugs to preserve the function of the transplanted tissue. These patients receive corticosteroids and may need supplemental corticosteroids in the perioperative period (see discussion on adrenal insufficiency later in this chapter).

Most of these patients also receive immunosuppressive agents that may cause otherwise self-limiting infections to become severe. Therefore a more aggressive use of antibiotics and early hospitalization for infections are warranted. The patient's primary care physician should be consulted concerning the need for prophylactic antibiotics.

Cyclosporine A, an immunosuppressive drug administered after organ transplantation, may cause gingival hyperplasia. The dentist performing oral surgery should recognize this so as not to wrongly attribute gingival hyperplasia entirely to hygiene problems.

Patients who have had renal transplants occasionally have problems with severe hypertension. Vital signs should be obtained before oral surgery is performed in these patients (Box 1-16).

Hypertension

Chronically elevated blood pressure for which the cause is unknown is called essential hypertension. Mild or moderate hypertension (i.e., systolic pressure of less than 200 mm Hg or diastolic pressure of less than 110 mm Hg) is usually not a problem in the performance of ambulatory oral surgical care.

Care of the poorly controlled hypertensive patient includes use of an anxiety-reduction protocol and monitoring of vital signs. Epinephrine-containing local anesthetics should be used cautiously; after surgery, patients should be advised to seek medical care for their hypertension.

Elective oral surgery for patients with severe hypertension (i.e., systolic pressure of 200 mm Hg or more or diastolic pressure of 110 mm Hg or more) should be postponed until the pressure is better controlled. Emergency oral surgery in severely hypertensive patients should be performed in a well-controlled environment or in the hospital to allow the patient to be carefully monitored during surgery and then to arrange for acute blood pressure control (Box 1-17).

BOX 1-16

Management of Patient with Renal Transplant*

1. Defer treatment until primary care physician or transplant surgeon clears patient for dental care.
2. Avoid use of nephrotoxic drugs†
3. Consider use of supplemental corticosteroids.
4. Monitor blood pressure.
5. Consider hepatitis B screening before dental care. Take hepatitis precautions if unable to screen for hepatitis.
6. Watch for presence of cyclosporine A–induced gingival hyperplasia. Emphasize importance of oral hygiene.
7. Consider prophylactic use of antibiotics, particularly for patients taking immunosuppressive agents.

*Most of these recommendations apply to patients with other transplanted organs.
†In patients with other transplanted organs, the clinician should avoid the use of drugs toxic to that organ.

BOX 1-17

Management of Hypertensive Patient

MILD TO MODERATE HYPERTENSION (SYSTOLIC >140 MM HG; DIASTOLIC >90 MM HG)

1. Recommend that the patient seek the primary care physician's guidance for medical therapy of hypertension.
2. Monitor the patient's blood pressure at each visit and whenever administration of epinephrine-containing local anesthetic surpasses 0.04 mg during a single visit.
3. Use an anxiety-reduction protocol.
4. Avoid rapid posture changes in patients taking drugs that cause vasodilation.
5. Avoid administration of sodium-containing intravenous solutions.

SEVERE HYPERTENSION (SYSTOLIC >200 MM HG; DIASTOLIC >110 MM HG)

1. Defer elective dental treatment until hypertension is better controlled.
2. Consider referral to an oral and maxillofacial surgeon for emergency problems.

Hepatic Disorders

The patient with severe liver damage resulting from infectious disease, ethanol abuse, or vascular or biliary congestion requires special consideration before oral surgery is performed. An alteration of dose or avoidance of drugs that require hepatic metabolism may be necessary.

The production of vitamin K–dependent coagulation factors (II, VII, IX, X) may be depressed in severe liver disease; therefore, obtaining an international normalized ratio (INR; prothrombin time [PT]) or partial thromboplastin time may be useful before surgery in patients with more severe liver disease. Portal hypertension caused by liver disease may also cause hypersplenism, a sequestering of platelets causing thrombocytopenia. Finding a prolonged Ivy's bleeding time reveals this

BOX 1-18

Management of Patient with Hepatic Insufficiency

1. Attempt to learn the cause of the liver problem; if the cause is hepatitis B, take usual precautions.
2. Avoid drugs requiring hepatic metabolism or excretion; if their use is necessary, modify the dose.
3. Screen patients with severe liver disease for bleeding disorders with platelet count, prothrombin time, partial thromboplastin time, and Ivy's bleeding time.
4. Attempt to avoid situations in which the patient might swallow large amounts of blood.

problem. Patients with severe liver dysfunction may require hospitalization for dental surgery because their decreased ability to metabolize the nitrogen in swallowed blood may cause encephalopathy. Finally, unless documented otherwise, a patient with liver disease should be presumed to carry hepatitis virus (Box 1-18).

Endocrine Disorders

Diabetes Mellitus

Diabetes mellitus is caused by an underproduction of insulin, a resistance of insulin receptors in end-organs to the effects of insulin, or both. Diabetes is commonly divided into insulin-dependent and non–insulin-dependent diabetes. Insulin-dependent diabetes usually begins during childhood or adolescence. The major problem in this form of diabetes is an underproduction of insulin, which results in the inability of the patient to use glucose properly. The serum glucose rises above the level at which renal reabsorption of all glucose can take place, causing glucosuria. The osmotic effect of the glucose solute results in polyuria, stimulating patient thirst and causing polydipsia (frequent consumption of liquids). In addition, carbohydrate metabolism is altered, leading to fat breakdown and the production of ketone bodies. This can produce ketoacidosis and the attendant tachypnea with somnolence and eventually coma.

Persons with insulin-dependent diabetes must strike a balance between caloric intake, exercise, and insulin dose. Any decrease in regular caloric intake or increase in activity, metabolic rate, or insulin dose can lead to hypoglycemia and vice versa.

Patients with non–insulin-dependent diabetes usually produce insulin but in insufficient amounts because of decreased insulin activity, insulin receptor resistance, or both. This form of diabetes typically begins in adulthood, is exacerbated by obesity, and does not usually require insulin therapy. This form of diabetes is treated by weight control, dietary restrictions, and the use of oral hypoglycemics. Insulin is required only if the patient is unable to maintain acceptable serum glucose levels using the usual therapeutic measures. Severe hyperglycemia in non–insulin-dependent diabetic patients rarely produces ketoacidosis but leads to a hyperosmolar state with altered levels of consciousness.

Short-term, mild to moderate hyperglycemia is usually not a significant problem for persons with diabetes. Therefore when an oral surgical procedure is planned, it is best to err on the side of hyperglycemia rather than hypoglycemia; that is, it is best to avoid an excessive insulin dose and to give a glucose source. Ambulatory oral surgery procedures should be performed early in the day, using an anxiety-reduction program. If IV sedation is not being used, the patient should be asked to eat a normal meal and take the usual morning amount of regular insulin and a half dose of neutral protamine hagedorn (NPH) insulin (Table 1-1). The patient's vital signs should be monitored; if signs of hypoglycemia, such as hypotension, hunger, drowsiness, nausea, diaphoresis, tachycardia, or a mood change, occur, an oral or IV supply of glucose should be administered. Ideally, offices have an electronic glucometer available with which the clinician or patient can readily determine serum glucose with a drop of the patient's blood. This device may avoid the need to steer the patient toward mild hyperglycemia. If the patient will be unable to eat temporarily after surgery, any delayed-action insulin (most commonly NPH) normally taken in the morning should be eliminated and restarted only after normal caloric intake resumes. The patient should be advised to monitor serum glucose closely for the first 24 hours postoperatively and adjust insulin accordingly.

TABLE 1-1

Types of Insulin*

Onset and Duration of Action	Name	Peak Effect of Action (Hours After Injection)	Duration of Action (Hours)
Fast (F)	Regular	2-3	6
	Semilente	3-6	12
Intermediate (I)	Globin zinc	6-8	18
	NPH	8-12	24
	Lente	8-12	24
Long (L)	Protamine zinc	16-24	36
	Ultralente	20-30	36

*Insulin sources are pork—F, I; beef—F, I, L; beef and pork—F, I, L; and recombinant DNA—F, I, L.

If a patient must miss a meal before a surgical procedure, the patient should be told to skip any morning insulin and only resume insulin once the patient is able to receive a supply of calories. Regular insulin should then be used, with the dose based on serum glucose monitoring and as directed by the patient's physician. Once the patient has resumed normal dietary habits and physical activity, the usual insulin regimen can be restarted.

Persons with well-controlled diabetes are no more susceptible to infections than persons without diabetes, but they have more difficulty containing infections. This is caused by altered leukocyte function or by other factors that affect the ability of the body to control an infection. Difficulty in containing infections is more significant in persons with poorly controlled diabetes. Therefore, elective oral surgery should be deferred in patients with poorly controlled diabetes until control is accomplished. However, if an emergency situation or a serious oral infection exists in any person with diabetes, consideration should be given to hospital admission to allow for acute control of the hyperglycemia and aggressive management of the infection. Many clinicians also believe that prophylactic antibiotics should be given routinely to patients with diabetes undergoing any surgical procedure. However, this position is controversial (Box 1-19).

BOX 1-19

Management of Patient with Diabetes

INSULIN-DEPENDENT DIABETES

1. Defer surgery until diabetes is well controlled; consult physician.
2. Schedule an early morning appointment; avoid lengthy appointments.
3. Use an anxiety-reduction protocol, but avoid deep sedation techniques in outpatients.
4. Monitor pulse, respiration, and blood pressure before, during, and after surgery.
5. Maintain verbal contact with patient during surgery.
6. If patient must not eat or drink before oral surgery and will have difficulty eating after surgery, instruct patient not to take the usual dose of regular or NPH insulin; start an IV with a 5% dextrose in water drip at 150 mL/h.
7. If allowed, have the patient eat a normal breakfast before surgery and take the usual dose of regular insulin, but only half the dose of NPH insulin.
8. Advise patients not to resume normal insulin doses until they are able to return to usual level of caloric intake and activity level.
9. Consult physician if any questions concerning modification of the insulin regimen arise.
10. Watch for signs of hypoglycemia.
11. Treat infections aggressively.

NON–INSULIN-DEPENDENT DIABETES

1. Defer surgery until diabetes is well controlled.
2. Schedule an early morning appointment; avoid lengthy appointments.
3 Use an anxiety-reduction protocol.
4. Monitor pulse, respiration, and blood pressure before, during, and after surgery.
5. Maintain verbal contact with the patient during surgery.
6. If patient must not eat or drink before oral surgery and will have difficulty eating after surgery, instruct patient to skip any oral hypoglycemic medications that day.
7. If patient can eat before and after surgery, instruct patient to eat a normal breakfast and to take the usual dose of hypoglycemic agent.
8. Watch for signs of hypoglycemia.
9. Treat infections aggressively.

NPH, Neutral protamine hagedorn.

Adrenal Insufficiency

Diseases of the adrenal cortex may cause adrenal insufficiency. Symptoms of primary adrenal insufficiency include weakness, weight loss, fatigue, and hyperpigmentation of skin and mucous membranes. However, the most common cause of adrenal insufficiency is chronic therapeutic corticosteroid administration (secondary adrenal insufficiency). Often, patients who regularly take corticosteroids have moon facies, buffalo humps, and thin, translucent skin. Their inability to increase endogenous corticosteroid levels in response to physiologic stress may cause them to become hypotensive, syncopal, nauseated, and feverish during complex, prolonged surgery.

If a patient with primary or secondary adrenal suppression requires complex oral surgery, the primary care physician should be consulted regarding the potential need for supplemental steroids. In general, minor procedures require only the use of an anxiety-reduction protocol. Thus supplemental steroids are not needed for most dental procedures. However, more complicated procedures, such as orthognathic surgery in an adrenally suppressed patient, usually necessitate steroid supplementation (Box 1-20).

BOX 1-20

Management of Patient with Adrenal Suppression Who Requires Major Oral Surgery*

If patient is currently taking corticosteroids,

1. Use an anxiety-reduction protocol.
2. Monitor pulse and blood pressure before, during, and after surgery.
3. Instruct patient to double usual daily dose on the day before, day of, and day after surgery.
4. On second postsurgical day, advise the patient to return to a usual steroid dose.

If the patient is not currently taking steroids but has received at least 20 mg of hydrocortisone (cortisol or equivalent) for more than 2 weeks within past year,

1. Use an anxiety-reduction protocol.
2. Monitor pulse and blood pressure before, during, and after surgery.
3. Instruct the patient to take 60 mg of hydrocortisone (or equivalent) the day before and the morning of surgery (or the dentist should administer 60 mg of hydrocortisone or equivalent intramuscularly or intravenously before complex surgery).
4. On the first 2 postsurgical days, the dose should be dropped to 40 mg and dropped to 20 mg for 3 days thereafter. The clinician can cease administration of supplemental steroids 6 days after surgery.

*If a major surgical procedure is planned, the clinician should strongly consider hospitalizing the patient. The clinician should consult the patient's physician if any questions arise concerning the need for or the dose of supplemental corticosteroids.

Hyperthyroidism

The thyroid gland problem of primary significance in oral surgery is thyrotoxicosis because thyrotoxicosis is the only thyroid gland disease in which an acute crisis can occur. Thyrotoxicosis is the result of an excess of circulating triiodothyronine and thyroxine, which is caused most frequently by Graves' disease, a multinodular goiter, or a thyroid adenoma. The early manifestations of excessive thyroid hormone production include fine, brittle hair, hyperpigmentation of skin, excessive sweating, tachycardia, palpitations, weight loss, and emotional lability. Patients frequently, although not invariably, have exophthalmos (a bulging forward of the globes caused by increases of fat in the orbit). If hyperthyroidism is not recognized early, the patient may have heart failure. The diagnosis is made by the demonstration of elevated circulating thyroid hormones, using direct or indirect laboratory techniques.

Thyrotoxic patients are usually treated with agents that block thyroid hormone synthesis and release, with a thyroidectomy, or with both. However, patients left untreated or incompletely treated can have a thyrotoxic crisis caused by the sudden release of large quantities of preformed thyroid hormones. Early symptoms of a thyrotoxic crisis include restlessness, nausea, and abdominal cramps. Later symptoms are a high fever, diaphoresis, tachycardia, and, eventually, cardiac

BOX 1-21

Management of Patient with Hyperthyroidism

1. Defer surgery until thyroid gland dysfunction is well controlled.
2. Monitor pulse and blood pressure before, during, and after surgery.
3. Limit amount of epinephrine used.

decompensation. The patient becomes stuporous and hypotensive, with death resulting if no intervention occurs.

The dentist may be able to diagnose previously unrecognized hyperthyroidism by taking a complete medical history and performing a careful examination of the patient, including thyroid gland inspection and palpation. If severe hyperthyroidism is suspected from the history and inspection, the gland should not be palpated because that manipulation alone can trigger a crisis. Patients suspected of being hyperthyroid should be referred for medical evaluation before oral surgery.

Patients with treated thyroid gland disease can safely undergo ambulatory oral surgery. However, if a patient is found to have an oral infection, the primary care physician should be notified, particularly if the patient shows signs of hyperthyroidism. Atropine and excessive amounts of epinephrine-containing solutions should be avoided if a patient is thought to have incompletely treated hyperthyroidism (Box 1-21).

Hypothyroidism

The dentist can play a role in the initial recognition of hypothyroidism. Early symptoms of hypothyroidism include fatigue, constipation, weight gain, hoarseness, headaches, arthralgia, menstrual disturbances, edema, dry skin, and brittle hair and fingernails. If the symptoms of hypothyroidism are mild, no modification of dental therapy is required.

Hematologic Problems

Hereditary Coagulopathies

Patients with inherited bleeding disorders are usually aware of their problem, allowing the clinician to take the necessary precautions before any surgical procedure. However, in many patients, prolonged bleeding after the extraction of a tooth may be the first evidence that a bleeding disorder exists. Therefore, all patients should be questioned concerning coagulation after previous injuries and surgery. A history of epistaxis (nosebleeds), easy bruising, hematuria, heavy menstrual bleeding, and spontaneous bleeding should alert the dentist to the possible need for a presurgical laboratory coagulation screening. A PT is used to test the extrinsic pathway factors (II, V, VII, and X), whereas a partial thromboplastin time is used to detect intrinsic pathway factors. To better standardize PT values within and between hospitals, the INR method has been developed. This technique adjusts the actual PT for variations in agents used to run the test, and the value is presented as a ratio between the patient's PT and a standardized value from the same laboratory.

Platelet inadequacy usually causes easy bruising and is evaluated by a bleeding time and platelet count. If a coagulopathy is suspected, the primary care physician or a hematologist should be consulted about more refined testing to better define the cause of the bleeding disorder and to help manage the patient in the perioperative period.

The management of patients with coagulopathies who require oral surgery depends on the nature of the bleeding disorder. Specific factor deficiencies—such as hemophilia A, B, or C or von Willebrand's disease—are usually managed by the perioperative administration of factor replacement and by the use of an antifibrinolytic agent such as aminocaproic acid (Amicar). The physician decides the form in which factor replacement is given, based on the degree of factor deficiency and on the patient's history of factor replacement. Patients who receive factor replacement sometimes contract hepatitis or human immunodeficiency virus. Therefore, appropriate staff protection measures should be taken during surgery.

Platelet problems may be quantitative or qualitative. Quantitative platelet deficiency may be a cyclic problem, and the hematologist can help determine the proper timing of elective surgery. Patients with a chronically low platelet count can be given platelet transfusions. Counts must usually dip below 50,000/mm^3 before abnormal postoperative bleeding occurs. If the platelet count is between 20,000/mm^3 and 50,000/mm^3, the hematologist may wish to withhold platelet transfusion until postoperative bleeding becomes a problem. However, platelet transfusions may be given to patients with counts higher than 50,000/mm^3 if a qualitative platelet problem exists. Platelet counts under 20,000/mm^3 usually require presurgical platelet transfusion or a delay in surgery until platelet numbers rise. Local anesthesia should be given by local infiltration rather than by field blocks to lessen the likelihood of damaging larger blood vessels, which can lead to prolonged postinjection bleeding and hematoma formation. Consideration should be given to the use of topical coagulation-promoting substances in oral wounds, and the patient should be carefully instructed in ways to avoid dislodging blood clots once they have formed (Box 1-22). See Chapter 11 for additional means of preventing or managing postextraction bleeding.

BOX 1-22

Management of Patient with a Coagulopathy*

1. Defer surgery until a hematologist is consulted about the patient's management.
2. Obtain baseline coagulation tests as indicated (prothrombin time, partial thromboplastin time, Ivy's bleeding time, platelet count) and a hepatitis screen.
3. Schedule the patient in a manner that allows surgery soon after any coagulation-correcting measures have been taken (after platelet transfusion, factor replacement, or aminocaproic acid administration).
4. Augment clotting during surgery with the use of topical coagulation-promoting substances, sutures, and well-placed pressure packs.
5. Monitor the wound for 2 hours to ensure that a good initial clot forms.
6. Instruct the patient in ways to prevent dislodgment of the clot and in what to do should bleeding restart.
7. Avoid prescribing nonsteriodal antiinflammatory drugs.
8. Take hepatitis precautions during surgery.

*Patients with severe coagulopathies who require major surgery should be hospitalized.

Therapeutic Anticoagulation

Therapeutic anticoagulation is administered to patients with thrombogenic implanted devices, such as prosthetic heart valves; with thrombogenic cardiovascular problems, such as atrial fibrillation or after MI; or with a need for extracorporeal blood flow, such as for hemodialysis. Patients may also take drugs with anticoagulant properties, such as aspirin, for secondary effect.

When elective oral surgery is necessary, the need for continuous anticoagulation must be weighed against the need for blood clotting after surgery. This decision should be made in consultation with the patient's primary care physician. Drugs such as aspirin do not usually need to be withdrawn to allow routine surgery. Patients taking heparin usually can have their surgery delayed until the circulating heparin is inactive (6 hours if heparin is given IV, 24 hours if given subcutaneously). Protamine sulfate, which reverses the effects of heparin, can also be used if emergency oral surgery cannot be deferred until heparin is naturally inactivated.

Patients requiring warfarin for anticoagulation but who also need elective oral surgery benefit from close cooperation between the patient's physician and dentist. Warfarin has a 2- to 3-day delay in the onset of action; therefore, alterations of warfarin anticoagulant effects appear several days after the dose is changed. The INR is used to gauge the anticoagulant action of warfarin. Most physicians will allow the INR to drop to about 2.0 during the perioperative period, which usually allows sufficient coagulation for safe surgery. Patients should stop taking warfarin 2 or 3 days before the planned surgery. On the morning of surgery, the INR value should be checked; if it is between 2 and 3 INR, routine oral surgery can be performed. If the PT is still greater than 3 INR, surgery should be delayed until the PT approaches 3 INR. Surgical wounds should be dressed with thrombogenic substances, and the patient should be given instruction in promoting clot retention. Warfarin therapy can be resumed the day of surgery (Box 1-23).

BOX 1-23

Management of Patient Whose Blood Is Therapeutically Anticoagulated

PATIENTS RECEIVING ASPIRIN OR OTHER PLATELET-INHIBITING DRUGS

1. Consult physician to determine the safety of stopping the anticoagulant drug for several days.
2. Defer surgery until the platelet-inhibiting drugs have been stopped for 5 days.
3. Take extra measures during and after surgery to help promote clot formation and retention.
4. Restart drug therapy on the day after surgery if no bleeding is present.

PATIENTS RECEIVING WARFARIN (COUMADIN)

1. Consult the patient's physician to determine the safety of allowing the prothrombin time (PT) to fall to 2.0 to 3.0 INR (international normalized ratio) for a few days.*
2. Obtain the baseline PT.
3. (a) If the PT is less than 3.1 INR, proceed with surgery and skip to step 6.
   (b) If the PT is more than 3.0 INR, go to step 4.
4. Stop warfarin approximately 2 days before surgery.
5. Check the PT daily, and proceed with surgery on the day when the PT falls to 3.0 INR.
6. Take extra measures during and after surgery to help promote clot formation and retention.
7. Restart warfarin on the day of surgery.

PATIENTS RECEIVING HEPARIN

1. Consult the patient's physician to determine the safety of stopping heparin for the perioperative period.
2. Defer surgery until at least 6 hours after the heparin is stopped or reverse heparin with protamine.
3. Restart heparin once a good clot has formed.

*If the patient's physician believes it is unsafe to allow the PT to fall, the patient must be hospitalized for conversion from warfarin to heparin anticoagulation during the perioperative period.

Neurologic Disorders

Seizure Disorders

Patients with a history of seizures should be questioned about the frequency, type, duration, and sequelae of seizures. Seizures can result from ethanol withdrawal, high fever, hypoglycemia, or traumatic brain damage, or they can be idiopathic. The dentist should inquire about medications used to control the seizure disorder, particularly about patient compliance and any recent measurement of serum levels. The patient's physician should be consulted concerning the seizure history and to establish whether oral surgery should be deferred for any reason. If the seizure disorder is well controlled, standard oral surgical care can be delivered without any further precautions (except for the use of an anxiety-reduction protocol; Box 1-24). If good control cannot be obtained, the patient should be referred to an oral-maxillofacial surgeon for treatment under deep sedation in the office or hospital.

BOX 1-24

Management of Patient with a Seizure Disorder

1. Defer surgery until the seizures are well controlled.
2. Consider having serum levels of antiseizure medications measured if patient compliance is questionable.
3. Use an anxiety-reduction protocol.
4. Avoid hypoglycemia and fatigue.

Ethanolism (Alcoholism)

Patients volunteering a history of ethanol abuse or in whom ethanolism is suspected and then confirmed through means other than history taking require special consideration before surgery. The primary problems ethanol abusers have in relation to dental care are hepatic insufficiency, ethanol and medication interaction, and withdrawal phenomena. Hepatic insufficiency has already been discussed (see p. 14). Ethanol interacts with many of the sedatives used for anxiety control during oral surgery. The interaction usually potentiates sedation and suppresses the gag reflex.

Finally, ethanol abusers may undergo withdrawal phenomenon in the perioperative period if they have acutely lowered their daily ethanol intake before seeking dental care. This phenomenon may exhibit mild agitation, tremors, seizure, diaphoresis, or rarely, delirium tremens with hallucinosis, considerable agitation, and circulatory collapse.

Patients requiring oral surgery who exhibit signs of severe alcoholic liver disease or signs of ethanol withdrawal should be treated in the hospital setting. Liver function tests, a coagulation profile, and medical consultation before surgery are desirable. In patients able to be treated on an ambulatory basis, the dose of drugs metabolized in the liver should be altered and the patients should be monitored closely for signs of oversedation.

MANAGEMENT OF PREGNANT AND POSTPARTUM PATIENTS

Pregnancy

Although not a disease state, pregnancy is still a situation in which special considerations are necessary when oral surgery is required. The primary concern when providing care for a pregnant patient is the prevention of genetic damage to the fetus. Two areas of oral surgical management with potential for creating fetal damage are (1) dental radiography and (2) drug administration. It is virtually impossible to perform an oral surgical procedure properly with neither radiographs nor the administration of medications; therefore, one option is to defer any elective oral surgery until after delivery to avoid fetal risk. Frequently, temporary measures can be used to delay surgery.

However, if surgery during pregnancy cannot be postponed, efforts should be made to lessen fetal exposure to teratogenic factors. In the case of imaging, use of protective aprons and taking digital periapical films of only the areas requiring surgery can accomplish this (Fig. 1-5). The list of drugs thought to pose little risk to the fetus is short. For purposes of oral surgery, the following drugs are believed least likely to harm a fetus when used in moderate amounts: lidocaine, bupivacaine, acetaminophen, codeine, penicillin, and cephalosporins. Although aspirin is otherwise safe to use, it should not be given late in the third trimester because of its anticoagulant property. All sedative drugs are best avoided in pregnant patients. Nitrous oxide should not be used during the first trimester but if necessary can be used in the second and third trimesters as long as it is delivered with at least 50% oxygen (Boxes 1-25 and 1-26). The Food and Drug Administration created a system of drug categorization based on the known degree of risk to the human fetus posed by particular drugs. When required to give a medication to a pregnant patient, the clinician should check that the drug falls into an acceptable risk category before administering it to the patient (Box 1-27).

Pregnancy can be emotionally and physiologically stressful; therefore an anxiety-reduction protocol is recommended. Patient vital signs should be obtained, with particular attention paid to any elevation in blood pressure (a possible sign of preeclampsia). A patient nearing delivery may need special positioning of the chair during care, because if the patient is placed in a nearly supine position, the uterine contents may cause compression of the inferior vena cava, compromising venous return to the heart and thereby cardiac output. The patient may need to be in a more upright position or have her torso turned slightly to one side during surgery. Frequent breaks to allow the patient to void are commonly necessary late in pregnancy because of fetal pressure on the urinary

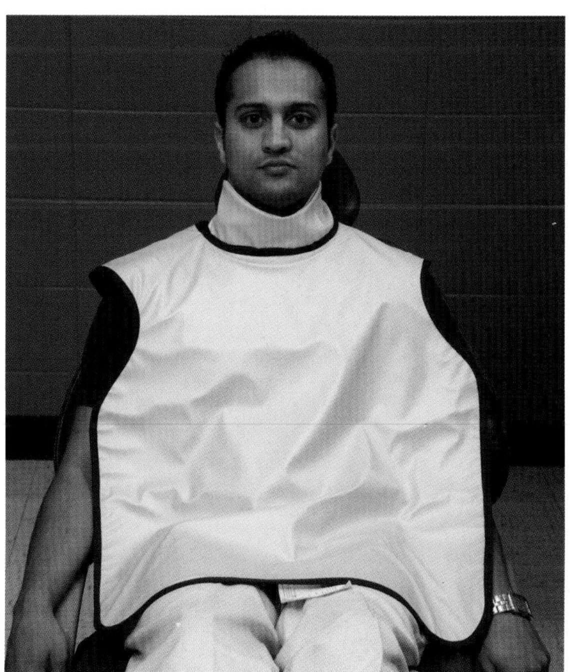

FIGURE 1-5 Proper lead apron shield is used during dental radiography.

BOX 1-25

Management of Patient Who Is Pregnant

1. Defer surgery until after delivery if possible.
2. Consult the patient's obstetrician if surgery cannot be delayed.
3. Avoid dental radiographs unless information about tooth roots or bone is necessary for proper dental care. If radiographs must be taken, use proper shielding.
4. Avoid the use of drugs with teratogenic potential. Use local anesthetics when anesthesia is necessary.
5. Use at least 50% oxygen if nitrous oxide sedation is used.
6. Avoid keeping the patient in the supine position for long periods, to prevent vena caval compression.
7. Allow the patient to take frequent trips to the restroom.

BOX 1-26

Dental Medications to Avoid in Pregnant Patients

ASPIRIN AND OTHER NONSTEROIDAL ANTIINFLAMMATORY DRUGS
- Carbamazepine
- Chloral hydrate (if chronically used)
- Chlordiazepoxide
- Corticosteroids
- Diazepam and other benzodiazepines
- Diphenhydramine hydrochloride (if chronically used)
- Morphine
- Nitrous oxide (if exposure is greater than 9 h/wk or O_2 is less than 50%)
- Pentazocine hydrochloride
- Phenobarbital
- Promethazine hydrochloride
- Propoxyphene
- Tetracyclines

BOX 1-27

Classification of Medications with Respect to Potential Fetal Risk

Category A: Controlled studies in women fail to demonstrate a fetal risk in the first trimester (and there is no evidence of risk in later trimesters), and the possibility of fetal harm appears remote.

Category B: Either animal reproduction studies have not demonstrated a fetal risk and there are no controlled studies in pregnant women, or animal reproduction studies have shown an adverse effect (other than decreased fertility) that was not confirmed in controlled studies on women in the first trimester (and there is no evidence of a risk in later trimesters).

Category C: Either studies in animals have revealed adverse fetal effects and there are no controlled studies in human beings, or studies in women and animals are not available. Drugs in this category should only be given if safer alternatives are not available and if the potential benefit justifies the known fetal risk or risks.

Category D: Positive evidence of human fetal risk exists, but benefits for pregnant women may be acceptable despite the risk, as in life-threatening or serious diseases for which safer drugs cannot be used or are ineffective. An appropriate statement must appear in the "warnings" section of the labeling of drugs in this category.

Category X: Either studies in animals or human beings have demonstrated fetal abnormalities, or there is evidence of fetal risk based on human experience (or both); and the risk of using the drug in pregnant women clearly outweighs any possible benefit. The drug is contraindicated in women who are or may become pregnant. An appropriate statement must appear in the "contraindications" section of the labeling of drugs in this category.

From: Ball KA: Endoscopic surgery, St Louis, 1997, Mosby; White RA, Klein SR: Endoscopic surgery, St Louis, 1991.

bladder. Before performing any oral surgery on a pregnant patient, the clinician should consult the patient's obstetrician.

Postpartum

Special considerations should be taken when providing oral surgical care for the postpartum patient who is breast-feeding a child. Avoiding drugs that are known to enter breast milk and to be potentially harmful to infants is prudent (the child's pediatrician can provide guidance). Information about some drugs is provided in Table 1-2. However, in general, all the drugs common in oral surgical care are safe to use in moderate doses, with the exception of corticosteroids, aminoglycosides, and tetracyclines, which should not be used.

TABLE 1-2

Effect of Dental Medications in Lactating Mothers

No Apparent Clinical Effects in Breast-Feeding Infants	Potentially Harmful Clinical Effects in Breast-Feeding Infants
Acetaminophen	Ampicillin
Antihistamines	Aspirin
Cephalexin	Atropine
Codeine	Barbiturates
Erythromycin	Chloral hydrate
Fluoride	Corticosteroids
Lidocaine	Diazepam
Meperidine	Metronidazole
Oxacillin	Penicillin
Pentazocine	Propoxyphene
	Tetracyclines

CHAPTER 2

Prevention and Management of Medical Emergencies

JAMES R. HUPP

CHAPTER OUTLINE

Serious medical emergencies in the dental office are, fortunately, rare. The primary reason for the limited frequency of emergencies in dental practice is the nature of dental education that prepares practitioners to recognize potential problems and manage them before they cause an emergency. However, when oral surgical procedures are necessary, the increased mental and physiological stress inherent in such interventions can push the patient with a poorly compensated medical condition into an emergency situation. Similarly, the advanced forms of pain and anxiety control frequently needed for oral surgery can predispose patients to emergency conditions. This chapter begins with a presentation of the various means of lowering the likelihood of medical emergencies in the dental office. The chapter also details ways to prepare for emergencies and discusses the clinical manifestations and initial management of the more common emergencies.

PREVENTION

An understanding of the relative frequency of emergencies and knowledge of those likely to produce serious morbidity and mortality is important when the dentist sets priorities for preventive measures. Malamed's study of patients in the dental school setting revealed that hyperventilation, seizures, and hypoglycemia were the three most common emergency situations occurring in patients before, during, or soon after general dental care. These were followed in frequency by vasovagal syncope, angina pectoris, orthostatic hypotension, and hypersensitivity (allergic) reactions. It is important to remember, though, that many of these diagnoses were presumptive and not completely verified, so the incidence of problems such as "hypoglycemia" may be overstated.

The incidence of medical emergencies is higher in patients receiving ambulatory oral surgery compared with those receiving nonsurgical care because of the following three factors: (1) surgery is more often stress provoking, (2) a greater number of medications are typically administered to perioperative patients, and (3) often longer appointments are necessary when performing surgery. These factors are known to increase the likelihood of medical emergencies. Other factors that increase the potential for emergencies are the age of the patient (very young and old patients being at greater risk), the increasing ability of the medical profession to keep relatively unhealthy persons ambulatory and able to seek dental care, and the increasing variety of drugs dentists administer in their offices.

Prevention is the cornerstone of management of medical emergencies. The first step is risk assessment. This begins with a careful medical evaluation that, in the dental office, requires accurately taking a medical history, including a review of systems guided by pertinent positive responses in the patient's history. Vital signs should be recorded, and a physical examination (tailored to the patient's medical history and present problems) should be performed. Techniques for this are described in Chapter 1.

BOX 2-1

Medical Emergencies Commonly Provoked by Anxiety

- Angina pectoris
- Thyroid storm
- Myocardial infarction
- Insulin shock
- Asthmatic bronchospasm
- Hyperventilation
- Adrenal insufficiency (acute)
- Epilepsy
- Severe hypertension

Although any patient can have a medical emergency at any time, certain medical conditions predispose patients to medical emergencies in the dental office. These conditions are more likely to turn into an emergency when the patient is physiologically or emotionally stressed. The most common conditions affected or precipitated by anxiety are listed in Box 2-1. Once those patients who are likely to have medical emergencies are recognized, the practitioner can prevent most problems from occurring by modifying the manner in which oral surgical care is delivered.

PREPARATION

Preparedness is the second most important factor (after prevention) in the management of medical emergencies. Preparation to handle emergencies includes four specific actions: (1) ensuring that the dentist's own education about emergency management is adequate and up to date, (2) having the auxiliary staff trained to assist in medical emergencies, (3) establishing a system to gain ready access to other health care providers able to assist during emergencies, and (4) equipping the office with equipment and supplies necessary to care initially for patients having serious problems (Box 2-2).

Continuing Education

In dental school, clinicians are trained in ways to assess patient risk and manage medical emergencies. However, because of the rarity of these problems, practitioners should seek continuing education in this area, not only to refresh their knowledge but also to learn new concepts concerning medical evaluation and management of emergencies. An important feature of continuing education should be to maintain certification in basic life support (BLS), including the use of automated external defibrillator units (Box 2-3). Many have recommended that continuing education in medical emergency management be obtained annually, with a BLS skills update and review obtained biannually. Dentists who deliver parenteral sedatives other than nitrous oxide are wise to become certified in advanced cardiac life support and to have the drugs and equipment necessary for advanced cardiac life support available.

BOX 2-2

Preparation for Medical Emergencies

1. Personal continuing education in emergency recognition and management
2. Auxiliary staff education in emergency recognition and management
3. Establishment and periodic testing of a system to access medical assistance readily when an emergency occurs
4. Equipping office with supplies necessary for emergency care

BOX 2-3

Basic Life Support

ABCs

- A—Airway
- B—Breathing
- C—Circulation

AIRWAY OBTAINED AND MAINTAINED BY COMBINATION OF THE FOLLOWING:

1. Extending head at the neck by pushing upward on the chin with one hand and pushing the forehead back with other hand
2. Pushing mandible forward by pressure on the mandibular angles
3. Pulling mandible forward by pulling on anterior mandible
4. Pulling tongue forward, using suture material or instrument to grasp anterior part of tongue

BREATHING PROVIDED BY ONE OF THE FOLLOWING:

1. Mouth-to-mouth or mouth-to-mask ventilation
2. Resuscitation bag ventilation

CIRCULATION PROVIDED BY EXTERNAL CARDIAC COMPRESSIONS

Office Staff Training

The dentist must ensure that all office personnel are trained to assist in the recognition and management of emergencies. This should include reinforcement by regular emergency drills in the office and by annual BLS skills renewal. The office staff should be preassigned specific responsibilities so that in the event of a problem, each person knows what will be expected of him or her during an emergency.

Access to Help

The ease of access to other health care providers varies from office to office. Seeking out individuals with training that would make them useful during a medical emergency is helpful. If the dental practice is located near other professional offices, prior arrangements should be made to obtain assistance in the event of an emergency. Not all physicians are well versed in the management of emergencies, and dentists must be selective in the physicians they contact for help during an emergency. Oral-maxillofacial surgeons are a good resource, as are most general surgeons, internists, and anesthesiologists. Ambulances carrying emergency medical technicians are useful to the dentist facing an emergency situation, and most communities now provide easy telephone access (911) to a rapid-response emergency medical technician team. Finally, it is important to identify a nearby hospital or freestanding emergency care facility with well-trained emergency care experts.

Once the dentist has established who can be of assistance in the event of an emergency, the appropriate telephone numbers should be kept readily available. Easily identified lists can be placed on each telephone, or numbers can be entered into the memory of an automatic-dial telephone. The numbers should be called periodically to test their accuracy.

Emergency Supplies and Equipment

The final means of preparing for emergencies is by ensuring that appropriate emergency drugs, supplies, and equipment are available in the office. One basic piece of equipment is the dental chair that should be capable of allowing the patient to be placed in a flat position or, even better, in a head-down, feet-raised position (Fig. 2-1, *A*). In addition, the chair must be capable of being lowered close to the floor to allow BLS to be performed properly, or standing stools should be kept in the office. Operatories should be large enough to allow a patient to be placed on the floor for BLS performance and should provide enough room for the dentist and others to deliver emergency care. If the operatory is too small to allow the patient to be placed on the floor, specially designed boards are available that can be placed under the patient's thorax to allow effective BLS administration in the dental chair.

Frequently, equipment used for respiratory assistance and the administration of injectable drugs is needed during office emergencies. Equipment for respiratory assistance includes oral and nasal airways, tonsil suction tips (Fig. 2-1, *B*), connector tubing that allows the use of high-volume suction, and resuscitation bags (e.g., air mask bag unit [AMBU bags]) with clear face masks (Fig. 2-1, *C*). Oral and nasal airways, and even laryngoscopes, and endotracheal tubes for trachea intubation may be helpful for dentists trained in their proper use or for others called into the office to assist during an emergency.

Useful drug administration equipment includes syringes and needles, tourniquets, intravenous (IV) solutions, indwelling catheters, and IV tubing (Table 2-1). Although emergency kits containing a variety of drugs are commercially available (Fig. 2-2), dentists may prefer to assemble their own kits. This allows properly educated dentists to choose only those agents they feel are likely to be most useful during an emergency. Custom kits also help the dentist to organize the kit in a manner that is easy to use during emergency situations. If dentists have made arrangements for help from nearby professionals, they may also want to include drugs in their kits that the assisting

A

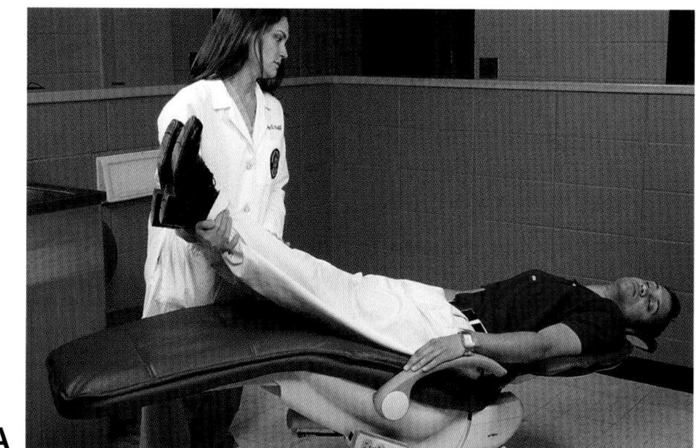

B

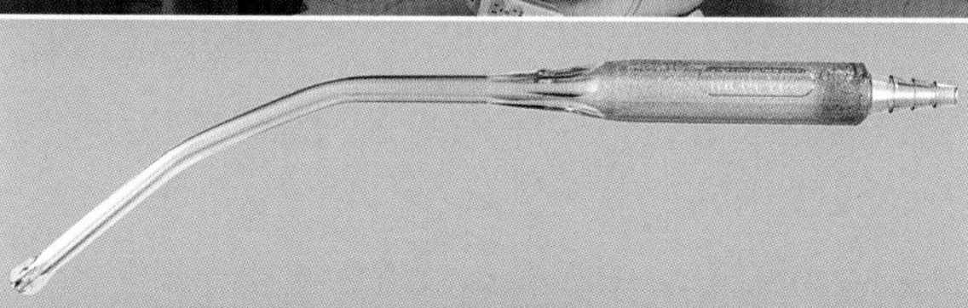

C

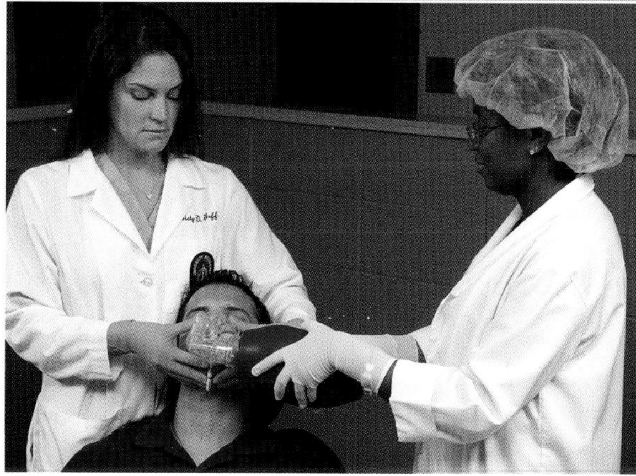

FIGURE 2-1 **A,** Dental chair placing patient in position such that the legs are raised above the level of the trunk. This position is useful for emergency conditions in which increased venous return to heart is necessary or when gastric contents or foreign body enters the upper airway. For fast and effective augmentation of venous return, the doctor or staff member can manually raise the patient's legs. **B,** Tonsil-type suction tip is useful for rapidly clearing large volumes of fluids out of the mouth and pharynx. **C,** Resuscitation (air mask bag unit [AMBU]) bag with clear face mask is properly positioned over the patient's nose and mouth. The doctor can use both hands to hold the mask in place while an assistant squeezes the bag. Oxygen-enriched air is provided by connecting the AMBU bag unit to an oxygen source at the other end of the bag.

TABLE 2-1

Emergency Supplies for the Dental Office

Use	Supplies
Establishment and maintenance of intravenous access	Plastic indwelling catheter Metal indwelling catheter Intravenous tubing with flow valve Tourniquet 1-inch wide plastic tape Crystalloid solution (normal saline, 5% dextrose in water)
High-volume suction	Large-diameter suction tip Tonsillar suction tip Extension tubing Connectors to adapt tubing to office suction
Drug administration	Plastic syringes (5 and 10 mL) Needles (18 and 21 gauge)
Oxygen administration	Clear face mask Resuscitation bag (air mask bag unit) Extension oxygen tubing (with and without nasal catheters) Oxygen cylinder with flow valve Oral and nasal airways* Endotracheal tube* Demand valve oxygen mask*

*For use by dentists with appropriate training or by those called to give medical assistance.

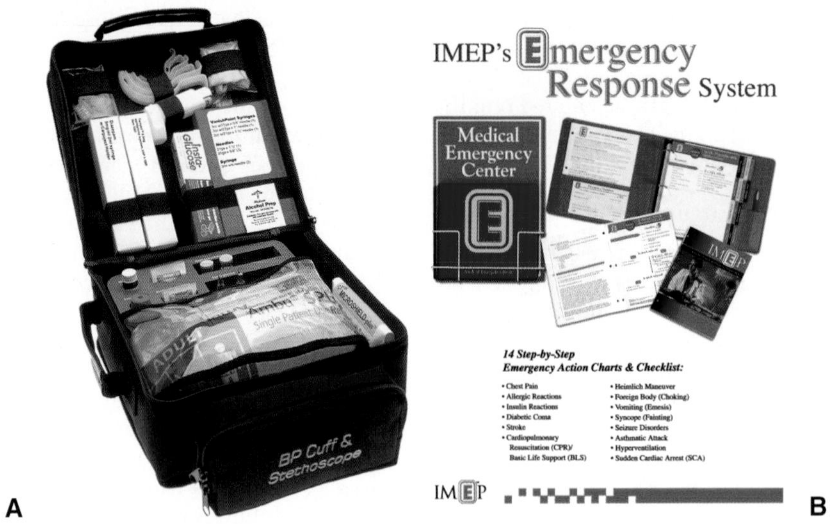

FIGURE 2-2 A, Example of commercially available emergency kit of appropriate size and complexity for dental office. B, Office emergency response systems are available to help guide the dentist and staff during emergencies and drills.

individuals suggest may be helpful. The drugs and any equipment in the kit must be well labeled and checked frequently for completeness and to ensure that no drugs have passed the expiration date. Labeling can include not only the drug name but also situations in which the drug is most commonly used. A list of drugs that should be considered for inclusion in a dental office emergency kit appears in Table 2-2.

TABLE 2-2

Emergency Drugs for the Dental Office

General Drug Group	Common Examples
PARENTERAL PREPARATIONS	
Analgesic	Morphine sulfate
Anticonvulsant	Diazepam, midazolam
Antihistamine	Diphenhydramine (Benadryl), chlorpheniramine (Chlor-Trimeton)
Antihypoglycemic	50% dextrose in water, glucagon
Corticosteroid	Methylprednisone (Solu-Medrol), dexamethasone (Decadron), hydrocortisone (Solu-Cortef)
Narcotic antagonist	Naloxone (Narcan)
Sympathomimetic	Epinephrine
Vagolytic	Atropine
ORAL PREPARATIONS	
Antihistamine	Diphenhydramine (Benadryl), chlorpheniramine (Chlor-Trimeton)
Antihypoglycemic	Candy, fruit juice, sugar
Vasodilator	Nitroglycerine (Nitrostat, Nitrolingual)
INHALED PREPARATIONS	
Bronchodilator	Metaproterenol (Alupent), epinephrine bitartrate (Medihaler-Epi)
Oxygen	—
Respiratory stimulant	Aromatic ammonia

One emergency item that must be available in dental offices is oxygen. Many dentists use oxygen supplied in a portable tank. If properly trained or assisted by a properly trained individual, the dentist needs to provide a means of delivering the oxygen *under positive pressure* to the patient. Establishing a system to check periodically that a sufficient supply of oxygen is always available is important. Dentists who use a central oxygen system also need to have oxygen available that is portable for use outside of the operatory, such as in the waiting room or during transport to an emergency facility.

MEDICAL EMERGENCIES

A brief description of the pathophysiology, clinical manifestations, and acute management of several emergency situations is presented in the following section. The section has been organized into a combination of *specific* problems, such as hypersensitivity reactions, and *symptom-oriented* problems, such as chest discomfort.

Hypersensitivity Reactions

Several of the drugs administered to patients undergoing oral surgery can act as antigenic stimuli, provoking allergic reactions. Of the four basic types of hypersensitivity reactions, only type I (immediate hypersensitivity) can cause an acute, life-threatening condition. Type I allergic reactions are mediated primarily by immunoglobulin E antibodies. As with all allergies, initiation of a type I response requires exposure to an antigen previously seen by the immune system. The reexposure to the antigen triggers a cascade of events that then are exhibited locally, systemically, or both in varying degrees of severity. Table 2-3 details the manifestations of type I hypersensitivity reactions and their management.

The least severe manifestation of type I hypersensitivity is dermatologic. Skin or mucosal reactions include localized areas of pruritus, erythema, urticaria (wheals consisting of slightly elevated areas of epithelial tissue that are erythematous and indurated), and angioedema (large areas of swollen tissue generally with little erythema or induration). Although skin

TABLE 2-3

Manifestations and Management of Hypersensitivity (Allergic) Reactions

Manifestations	Management
SKIN SIGNS	
◆ Delayed-onset skin signs: erythema, urticaria, pruritus, angioedema	◆ Stop administration of all drugs presently in use. ◆ Administer IV or IM Benadryl* 50 mg or Chlor-Trimeton[†] 10 mg. ◆ Refer to physician. ◆ Prescribe oral antihistamine, such as Benadryl 50 mg q6h or Chlor-Trimeton 10 mg q6h.
◆ Immediate-onset skin signs: erythema, urticaria, pruritus	◆ Stop administration of all drugs presently in use. Stop administration of all drugs presently in use. ◆ Administer epinephrine 0.3 mL 1:1000 SC, IM, or IV, or epinephrine 3 mL q5min if signs progress. ◆ Administer antihistamine IM or IV: Benadryl 50 mg or Chlor-Trimeton 10 mg. ◆ Monitor vital signs. ◆ Consult patient's physician. ◆ Observe in office for 1 hour. ◆ Prescribe Benadryl 50 mg q6h or Chlor-Trimeton 10 mg q6h.
RESPIRATORY TRACT SIGNS WITH OR WITHOUT CARDIOVASCULAR OR SKIN SIGNS	
◆ Wheezing, mild dyspnea	◆ Stop administration of all drugs presently in use. ◆ Place patient in sitting position. ◆ Administer epinephrine.[‡] ◆ Provide IV access. ◆ Consult patient's physician or emergency department physician. ◆ Observe in office for at least 1 hour. ◆ Prescribe antihistamine.
◆ Stridorous breathing (i.e., crowing sound), moderate to severe dyspnea	◆ Stop administration of all drugs presently in use. ◆ Sit the patient upright, and have someone summon medical assistance. ◆ Administer epinephrine.[‡] ◆ Give oxygen (6 L/min) by face mask or nasally. ◆ Monitor vital signs frequently. ◆ Administer antihistamine. ◆ Provide IV access; if signs worsen, treat as for anaphylaxis. ◆ Consult patient's physician or emergency room physician; prepare for transport to emergency room if signs do not improve rapidly.
◆ Anaphylaxis (with or without skin signs): malaise, wheezing, stridor, cyanosis, total airway obstruction, nausea and vomiting, abdominal cramps, urinary incontinence, tachycardia, hypotension, cardiac dysrhythmias, cardiac arrest	◆ Stop administration of all drugs. ◆ Position patient supine on back board or on floor and have someone summon assistance. ◆ Administer epinephrine.[‡] ◆ Initiate basic life support and monitor vital signs. ◆ Consider cricothyrotomy if trained to perform and if laryngospasm is not quickly relieved with epinephrine. ◆ Provide IV access. ◆ Give oxygen at 6 L/min. ◆ Administer antihistamine IV or IM. ◆ Prepare for transport.

*Brand of diphenhydramine.
[†]Brand of chlorpheniramine.
[‡]As described in "Immediate Onset" section.
IM, Intramuscular; *IV,* intravenous; *SC,* subcutaneous.

and mucosal reactions are not in themselves dangerous, they may be the first indication of more serious allergic manifestations that will soon follow. Skin lesions usually take anywhere from minutes to hours to appear; however, those appearing and progressing rapidly after administration of an antigenic drug are the most foreboding.

Allergic reactions affecting the respiratory tract are more serious and require more aggressive intervention. The involvement of small airways occurs with wheezing, as constriction of bronchial smooth muscle (bronchospasm) and airway mucosal inflammation occurs. The patient will complain of dyspnea and may eventually become cyanotic. Involvement of the larger airways usually first occurs at the narrowest portion of those air passages—the vocal cords in the larynx. Angioedema of the vocal cords causes partial or total airway obstruction. The patient is usually unable to speak and produces high-pitched crowing sounds (stridor) as air passes through constricted cords. As the edema worsens, total airway obstruction eventually occurs, which is an immediate threat to life.

Generalized anaphylaxis is the most dramatic hypersensitivity reaction, usually occurring within seconds or minutes after the parenteral administration of the antigenic medication; a more delayed onset occurs after oral or topical drug administration. A variety of signs and symptoms of anaphylaxis exist, but the most important with respect to early management are those resulting from cardiovascular and respiratory tract disturbances.

An anaphylactic reaction typically begins with a patient complaining of malaise or a feeling of impending doom. Skin manifestations soon appear, including flushing, urticaria, and pruritus on the face and trunk. Nausea and vomiting, abdominal cramping, and urinary incontinence may occur. Symptoms of respiratory embarrassment soon follow, with dyspnea and wheezing. Cyanosis of nail beds and mucosa appear next if air exchange becomes insufficient. Finally, total airway obstruction occurs, which causes the patient quickly to become unconscious. Disordered cardiovascular function initially occurs with tachycardia and palpitations. Blood pressure tends to fall because of falling cardiac output and peripheral vasodilation, and cardiac dysrhythmias appear. Cardiac output eventually may be compromised to a degree sufficient to cause loss of consciousness and cardiac arrest. Despite the potentially severe cardiovascular disturbances, the usual cause of death in patients having an anaphylactic reaction is laryngeal obstruction caused by vocal cord edema.

As with any potential emergency condition, prevention is the best strategy. During the initial interview and subsequent recall visits, patients should be questioned about drugs to which they have a history of allergy. In addition, dentists should ask patients specifically about medications they intend to use during the planned oral surgical care. If a patient claims to have an allergy to a particular drug, the clinician should question the patient further concerning the way in which the allergic reaction has exhibited and what was necessary to manage the problem. Many patients will claim an allergy to local anesthetics. However, before subjecting patients to alternative forms of anesthesia, the clinician should try to ensure that an allergy to the local anesthetic does indeed exist, because many patients have been told they had an allergic reaction when in fact they experienced a vasovagal hypotensive episode or mild palpitations. If an allergy is truly in question, the patient may require referral to a physician who can perform hypersensitivity testing. After it is determined that a patient does have a drug allergy, the information should be displayed prominently on the patient's record in a way to alert care providers but still protect patient confidentiality.

Management of allergic reactions depends on the severity of the signs and symptoms. The initial response to any sign of untoward reaction to a drug being given parenterally should be to cease its administration. If the allergic reaction is confined to the skin or mucosa, an antihistamine should be administered either IV or intramuscularly (IM). Diphenhydramine hydrochloride 50 mg or chlorpheniramine maleate 10 mg are commonly chosen antihistamines.[*] The antihistamine is then continued in an oral form (diphenhydramine [Benadryl] 50 mg or chlorpheniramine [Chlor-Trimeton] 8 mg) every 6 to 8 hours for 24 hours. Immediate, severe urticarial reactions warrant immediate parenteral (subcutaneous [SC] or IM) administration of 0.3 mL of a 1:1000 epinephrine solution, followed by an antihistamine. The patient's vital signs should be monitored frequently for 1 hour; if stable, the patient should be referred to a physician or an emergency care facility for further follow-up.

If a patient begins to show signs of lower respiratory tract involvement (i.e., wheezing during an allergic reaction), several actions should be initiated. Outside emergency assistance should be summoned. The patient should be placed in a semireclined position, and oxygen administration should be begun. Epinephrine should be administered by parenteral injection of 0.3 mL of a 1:1000 solution or with an aerosol inhaler (e.g., Medihaler-Epi, each inhalation of which delivers 0.3 mg). Epinephrine is short acting; if symptoms recur or continue, the dose can be repeated within 5 minutes. Antihistamines such as diphenhydramine or chlorpheniramine are then given. The patient should be transferred to the nearest emergency facility to allow further management as necessary.

If a patient shows signs of laryngeal obstruction (i.e., stridor), epinephrine (0.3 mL of 1:1000 solution) should be given as quickly as possible and oxygen should be administered. If a patient loses consciousness and attempts made to ventilate the patient's lungs fail, an emergency cricothyrotomy or tracheotomy may be required to bypass the laryngeal obstruction.[†] A description of the technique of cricothyrotomy or tracheotomy is beyond the scope of this book, but these techniques may be lifesaving in an anaphylactic reaction. Once an airway is reestablished, an antihistamine and further doses of epinephrine should be given. Vital signs should be monitored, and steps necessary to maintain the patient should be taken until emergency assistance is available.

Patients who show signs of cardiovascular system compromise should be closely monitored for the appearance of hypotension, which may necessitate initiation of BLS if cardiac output falls below the level necessary to maintain viability or if cardiac arrest occurs (Box 2-3).

Chest Discomfort

The appearance of chest discomfort in the perioperative period in a patient who may have ischemic heart disease calls for rapid identification of the cause so that appropriate measures can be taken (Box 2-4). Discomfort from cardiac ischemia is frequently described as a squeezing sensation, with a feeling of heaviness on the chest (Box 2-5). Discomfort usually begins in a retrosternal location, radiating to the left shoulder and arm. Patients with documented heart disease who have had such discomfort in the past will usually be able to confirm that the

*All doses given in this chapter are those recommended for an average adult. Doses will vary for children, for older adults, and for those with debilitating diseases. The clinician should consult a drug reference book for additional information.

†Cricothyrotomy is the surgical creation of an opening into the cricothyroid membrane just below the thyroid cartilage to create a path for ventilation that bypasses the vocal chords.

BOX 2-4

Clinical Characteristics of Chest Pain Caused by Myocardial Ischemia or Infarction

DISCOMFORT (PAIN) AS DESCRIBED BY PATIENTS

1. Squeezing, bursting, pressing, burning, choking, or crushing (not typically sharp or stabbing)
2. Substernally located, with variable radiation to left shoulder, arm, or left side (or a combination of these areas) of neck and mandible
3. Frequently associated at the onset with exertion, heavy meal, anxiety, or upon assuming horizontal posture
4. Relieved by vasodilators, such as nitroglycerin, or rest (in the case of angina)
5. Accompanied by dyspnea, nausea, weakness, palpitations, perspiration, or a feeling of impending doom (or a combination of these symptoms)

BOX 2-5

Differential Diagnosis of Acute-Onset Chest Pain

COMMON CAUSES

Cardiovascular system: Angina pectoris, myocardial infarction
Gastrointestinal tract: Dyspepsia (i.e., heartburn), hiatal hernia, reflux esophagitis, gastric ulcers
Musculoskeletal system: Intercostal muscle spasm, rib or chest muscle contusions
Psychological: Hyperventilation

UNCOMMON CAUSES

Cardiovascular system: Pericarditis, dissecting aortic aneurysm
Respiratory system: Pulmonary embolism, pleuritis, tracheobronchitis, mediastinitis, pneumothorax
Gastrointestinal tract: Esophageal rupture, achalasia
Musculoskeletal system: Osteochondritis, chondrosternitis
Psychological: Psychogenic chest pain (i.e., imagined chest pain)

discomfort is from the heart. For patients who are unable to remember such a sensation in the past or who have been assured by their physician that such discomfort does not represent heart disease, further information is useful before assuming a cardiac origin of the symptom. The patient should be asked to describe the exact location of the discomfort and any radiation, how the discomfort is changing with time, and if postural position affects the discomfort. Pain resulting from gastric reflux into the esophagus because of chair position should improve when the patient sits up and is given an antacid. Discomfort caused by costochondritis or pulmonary conditions should vary with respirations or be stimulated by manual pressure on the thorax. The only other common condition that can occur with chest discomfort is anxiety, which may be difficult to differentiate from cardiogenic problems without the use of monitoring devices not commonly present in the dental office.

If chest discomfort is suspected to be caused by myocardial ischemia or if that possibility cannot be ruled out, measures should be instituted that decrease myocardial work and increase myocardial oxygen supply. All dental care must be stopped, even if the surgery is only partially finished. The patient should be reassured that everything is under control while vital signs are being obtained, oxygen administration is started, and nitroglycerin is administered sublingually or by oral spray. The nitroglycerin dose should be 0.4 mg dissolved sublingually and repeated (if necessary) every 5 minutes as long as systolic blood pressure is at least 90 mm Hg, up to a maximum of three doses. If vital signs remain normal, the chest discomfort is relieved, and the amount of nitroglycerin that was required to relieve the discomfort was not more than normally necessary for that patient, the patient should be discharged with plans for future surgery to be done in an oral and maxillofacial surgery office or in a hospital after conferring with the patient's physician (Fig. 2-3).

Some circumstances do require transport to an emergency facility. If the pulse is irregular, rapid, or weak, or the blood pressure is found to be below baseline, outside emergency help should be summoned while the patient is placed in an almost supine position and oxygen and nitroglycerin therapy are started. Venous access should be initiated and a slow 5% dextrose in water drip should be begun, if possible, for use by emergency personnel. Another serious situation requiring transfer to a hospital is a case in which the patient's discomfort is not relieved after 20 minutes of appropriate therapy. In this case it should be presumed that a myocardial infarction is in progress. Such a patient is especially prone to the appearance of serious cardiac dysrhythmias or cardiac arrest; therefore, vital signs should be monitored frequently, and BLS should be instituted if indicated. Morphine sulfate (4 to 6 mg) may be administered IM or SC to help relieve the discomfort and reduce anxiety. Morphine also provides a beneficial effect for patients who are developing pulmonary edema (Fig. 2-3). Transfer to a hospital should be expedited because thrombolytic agents and/or an angioplasty plus stenting procedure may be able to preserve some or all of the ischemic myocardium.

Respiratory Difficulty

Many patients are predisposed to respiratory problems in the dental setting; these patients include patients with asthma or chronic obstructive pulmonary disease (COPD), extremely anxious patients, patients who are atopic, and those in whom a noninhalation sedative technique using respiratory depressant drugs is to be used. Special precautions should be taken to help prevent the occurrence of emergencies. If these patients are not treated promptly, the situation may become life threatening.

Asthma

Patients with a history of asthma can be a particular challenge to manage safely if emotional stress or many pharmacologic agents easily trigger their respiratory problems. Most patients with asthma are aware of the symptoms that signal the onset of bronchospasm. Patients will complain of shortness of breath and want to sit erect. Wheezing is usually audible, tachypnea and tachycardia begin, and patients start using their accessory muscles of respiration. As bronchospasm progresses, patients may become hypoxic and cyanotic, with eventual loss of consciousness (Box 2-6).

Management should start with placing patients in an erect or semierect position. Patients should then administer bronchodilators, using their own inhalers or one provided from the office emergency supply. The inhaler may contain epinephrine, isoproterenol, metaproterenol, or albuterol. Repeated doses should be administered cautiously to avoid

Patient experiencing chest discomfort

1. Terminate all dental treatment.
2. Position patient in semi-reclined posture.
3. Give nitroglycerin (TNG) (about 0.4 mg) tablet or spray.
4. Administer oxygen.
5. Check pulse and blood pressure.*

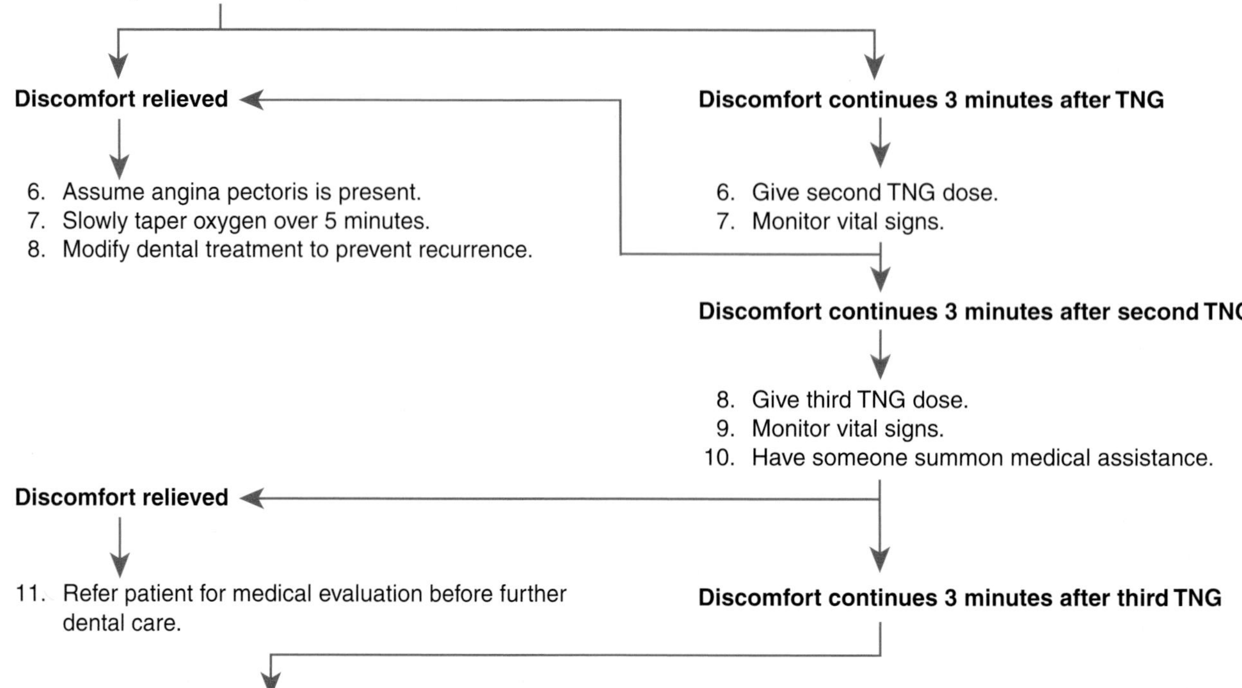

12. Assume myocardial infarction is in progress.
13. Administer 352 mg of aspirin
14. Start intravenous line with drip of a crystalloid solution at 30 mL/hr.
15. If severe discomfort, can titrate morphine sulfate (MS) 2 mg subcutaneously or intravenously every 3 minutes until relief is obtained.*
16. Prepare for transport to emergency care facility, administer Basic Life Support, if necessary.

*If blood pressure ever falls below 90 systolic or 50 diastolic, withhold TNG and MS, and call or wait for arrival of medical assistance.

FIGURE 2-3 Management of patient having chest discomfort while undergoing dental surgery.

BOX 2-6

Manifestations of an Acute Asthmatic Episode

MILD TO MODERATE
- Wheezing (audible with or without stethoscope)
- Dyspnea (i.e., labored breathing)
- Tachycardia
- Coughing
- Anxiety

SEVERE
- Intense dyspnea, with flaring of nostrils and use of accessory muscles of respiration
- Cyanosis of mucous membranes and nail beds
- Minimal breath sounds on auscultation
- Flushing of face
- Extreme anxiety
- Mental confusion
- Perspiration

overdosing the patient. Oxygen administration should follow, using nasal prongs or a face mask. In more severe asthmatic episodes or when aerosol therapy is ineffective, epinephrine (0.3 mL of a 1:1000 dilution) may be injected SC or IM. When patients have severe respiratory embarrassment, it may be necessary to obtain outside emergency medical assistance (Fig. 2-4).

Respiratory problems caused by drug allergy may be difficult to differentiate from those resulting from asthma. Management of the respiratory problems is the same in either case.

Hyperventilation

The most frequent cause of respiratory difficulty in the dental setting is anxiety that is expressed as hyperventilation, which is usually seen in patients in their teens, 20s, and 30s and can frequently be prevented through anxiety control. Dentists should be attuned to the signs of patient apprehension and, through the health interview, should encourage patients to express their concerns. Patients with extreme anxiety should be managed with an anxiety-reduction protocol. In addition, pharmacologic anxiolysis may be necessary.

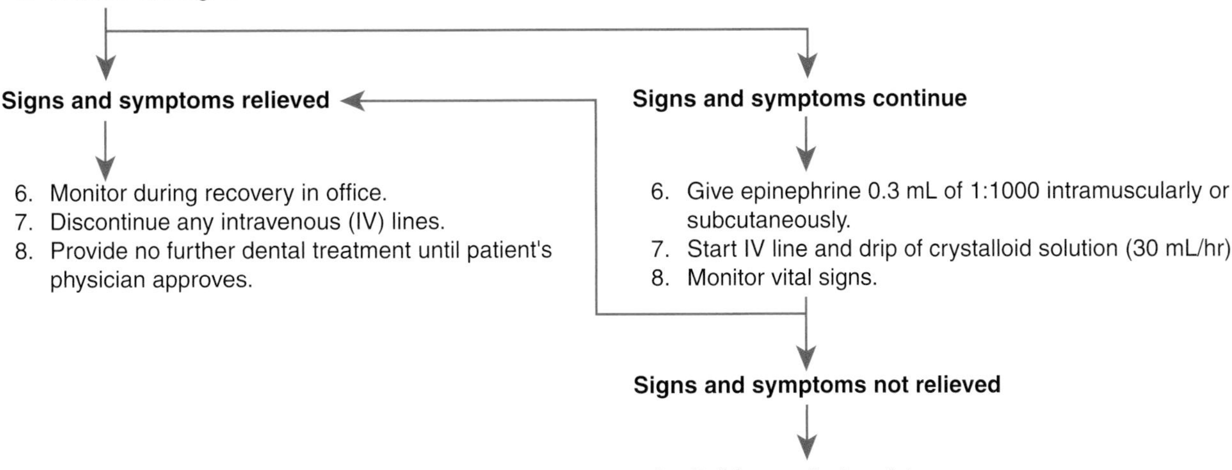

FIGURE 2-4 Management of acute asthmatic episode occurring during dental surgery.

The first manifestation of hyperventilation syndrome is frequently a complaint of an inability to get enough air. The patient breathes rapidly (tachypnea) and becomes agitated. The rapid ventilation increases elimination of CO_2 through the lungs. The patient soon becomes alkalotic; may complain of becoming light-headed and of having a tingling sensation in the fingers, toes, and perioral region; and may even develop muscle twitches or convulsions. Eventually loss of consciousness occurs (Box 2-7).

Management of a hyperventilating patient involves terminating the surgical procedure, positioning the patient in a semierect position, and providing reassurance. If symptoms of alkalosis occur, the patient should be forced to breathe into and out of a small bag. Oxygen-enriched air is not indicated. If hyperventilation continues, the clinician may have to administer a sedative such as midazolam, by giving 2 to 4 mg IM or by IV titration of the drug until hyperventilation ceases or the patient is sedated. Once hyperventilation stops, the patient should be rescheduled, with plans to use preoperative anxiolytics or intraoperative sedation (or both) in future visits (Box 2-8).

Chronic Obstructive Pulmonary Disease

Patients with well-compensated COPD can have difficulty during oral surgery. Many of these patients depend on maintaining an upright posture to breathe adequately. In addition, they become accustomed to having high arterial CO_2 levels and use a low level of blood oxygen as the primary stimulus to drive respirations. Many of these patients experience difficulty if placed in an almost supine position or given high-flow nasal oxygen. Patients with COPD often rely on their accessory muscles of respiration to breathe. Lying supine interferes with the use of these accessory muscles; therefore, patients will usually ask or struggle to sit up before problems resulting from positioning occur. Excessive lung secretions that are more difficult to clear when supine also accompany COPD.

If excessive oxygen is administered to a patient susceptible to COPD, the respiratory rate will fall, which produces cyanosis, and apnea may eventually occur. The treatment for such a problem is to discontinue oxygen administration before the

BOX 2-7

Manifestations of Hyperventilation Syndrome

NEUROLOGIC
- Dizziness
- Syncope
- Tingling or numbness of fingers, toes, or lips

RESPIRATORY
- Chest pain
- Feeling of shortness of breath
- Increased rate and depth of breaths
- Xerostomia

CARDIAC
- Palpitations
- Tachycardia

MUSCULOSKELETAL
- Muscle spasm
- Myalgia
- Tetany
- Tremor

PSYCHOLOGICAL
- Extreme anxiety

BOX 2-8

Management of Hyperventilation Syndrome

1. Terminate all dental treatment, and remove foreign bodies from mouth.
2. Position patient in chair in almost fully upright position.
3. Attempt to calm patient verbally.
4. Have patient breathe CO_2-enriched air, such as in and out of a small bag.
5. If symptoms persist or worsen, administer diazepam 10 mg IM or titrate slowly IV until anxiety is relieved, or administer midazolam 5 mg IM or titrate slowly IV until anxiety is relieved.
6. Monitor vital signs.
7. Perform all further dental surgery using anxiety-reducing measures.

patient becomes apneic. The respiratory rate should soon improve. If apnea occurs and the patient loses consciousness, artificial ventilation must be initiated and emergency assistance summoned.

Foreign-Body Aspiration

Aspiration of foreign bodies into the airway is always a potential problem during oral surgical and other dental procedures. This is especially true if the patient is positioned supine or semierect in the chair or is sufficiently sedated to dull the gag reflex. Objects that fall into the hypopharynx are frequently swallowed and usually pass harmlessly through the gastrointestinal tract. Even if the clinician feels confident that the material was swallowed, chest and abdominal radiographs should be obtained to eliminate the possibility of asymptomatic aspiration into the respiratory tract. Occasionally the foreign object is aspirated into the larynx, where in the lightly sedated or nonsedated patient, violent coughing will ensue that may expel the aspirated material. The patient can usually still talk and breathe. However, larger objects that are aspirated may obstruct the airway and become lodged in such a manner that coughing is ineffective because the lungs cannot be filled with air before the attempted cough. In this situation the patient usually cannot produce any vocalizations and becomes extremely anxious. Cyanosis soon appears, followed by loss of consciousness (Box 2-9).

BOX 2-9

Acute Manifestations of Aspiration into the Lower Respiratory Tract

LARGE FOREIGN BODY

- Coughing
- Choking sensation
- Stridorous breathing (i.e., crowing sounds)
- Severe dyspnea
- Feeling of something caught in throat
- Inability to breathe
- Cyanosis
- Loss of consciousness

GASTRIC CONTENTS

- Coughing
- Stridorous breathing
- Wheezing or rales (i.e., cracking sound) on chest auscultation
- Tachycardia
- Hypotension
- Dyspnea
- Cyanosis

The manner in which aspirated foreign bodies are managed depends primarily on the degree of airway obstruction. Patients with an intact gag reflex and a partially obstructed airway should be allowed to attempt to expel the foreign body by coughing. If the material will not come up, the patient should be given supplemental oxygen and transported to an emergency facility to allow laryngoscopy or bronchoscopy to be performed. The completely obstructed but awake patient should have abdominal thrusts (Fig. 2-5, *A*) or Heimlich maneuvers (Fig. 2-5, *B*) performed until successful expulsion of the object occurs or consciousness is lost. If a patient has a diminished gag reflex as a result of sedation or has a completely obstructed airway and loses consciousness, abdominal thrusts should be performed with the patient in a supine position. After each volley of thrusts, the patient should be quickly turned onto the side and the clinician should finger sweep the mouth to remove any object that may have been forced out. If the patient is not exchanging air, BLS should be started. If air cannot be blown into the lungs, additional abdominal thrusts should be attempted, followed by oral finger sweeps and BLS. Dentists trained in laryngoscopy can look into the larynx and use Magill forceps to try to remove any foreign material. If several attempts to relieve the obstruction fail, an emergency cricothyrotomy may be necessary (Fig. 2-6).

Gastric-Contents Aspiration

Aspiration of gastric contents into the lower respiratory tract presents another situation that frequently leads to serious respiratory difficulties. The particulate matter in gastric contents causes physical obstruction of pulmonary airways, but it is usually the high acidity of gastric material that produces more serious problems. The low pH of gastric juice quickly necrotizes the pulmonary tissue it contacts, and a respiratory distress syndrome soon follows, with transudation of fluid into pulmonary alveoli and a loss of functioning lung tissue. The patient with an intact gag reflex rarely aspirates gastric contents during vomiting. Rather, it is the patient with a diminished gag reflex caused by sedation, unconsciousness, or topical anesthesia in the oropharynx who is at greatest risk for gastric aspiration. The sedated or unconscious patient who aspirates a significant amount of gastric material will first show signs of respiratory difficulty, such as tachypnea and wheezing. Tachycardia and hypotension may soon occur, and as ventilatory capability worsens, cyanosis appears. Eventually respiratory failure occurs that is refractory to BLS and requires intubation and the delivery of high concentrations of oxygen.

Prevention of gastric aspiration involves instruction to patients to avoid eating or drinking for 8 hours before any oral surgery appointment during which they are to be moderately or deeply sedated.

A deeply sedated or unconscious patient who begins to vomit should be immediately placed into a head-down, feet-raised position and turned onto the right side to encourage oral drainage of vomitus. Box 2-10 lists several symptoms exhibited by patients preparing to vomit. High-volume suction

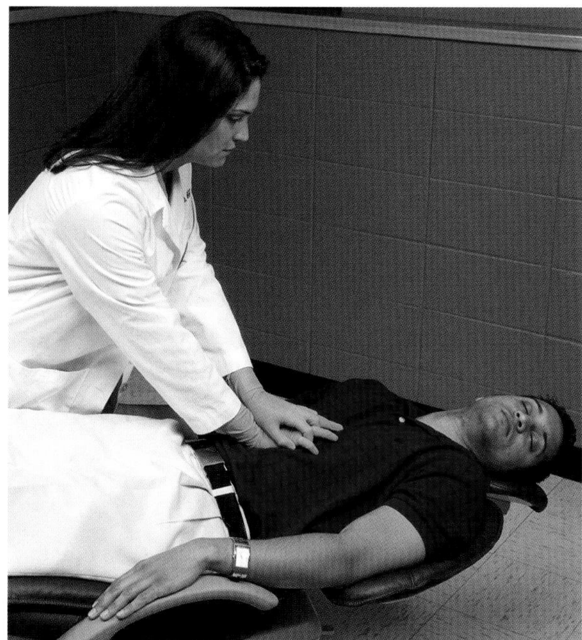

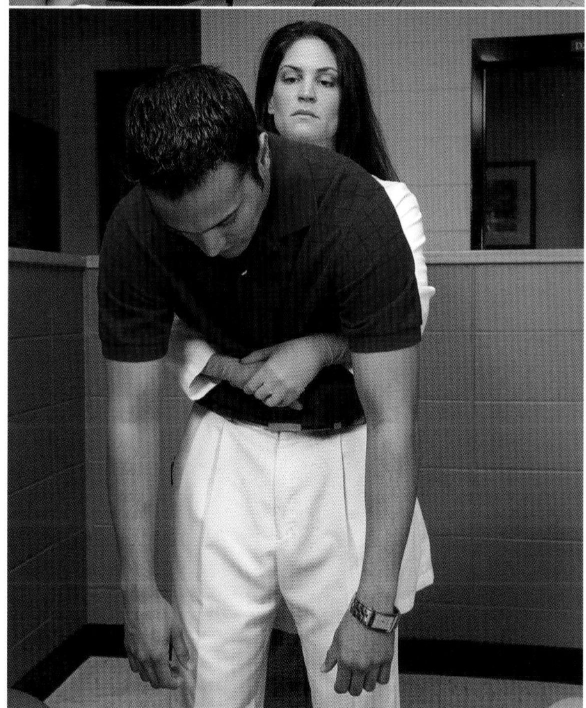

FIGURE 2-5 A, Method of performing abdominal thrusts for an unconscious patient with foreign body obstructing airway. Chair is first placed in recumbent position. The heel of the dentist's right palm is placed on the abdomen just below the xiphoid process, with the elbow kept locked and the left hand placed over the right for further delivery of force. Arms are quickly thrust into the patient's abdomen, directing force down and superiorly. B, Proper positioning for Heimlich maneuver is shown. Rescuer approaches the patient from behind and positions hands on the patient's abdomen, just below the rib cage. Rescuer's hands are then quickly pulled into the abdominal area, attempting to have any residual air in the lungs dislodge the obstruction from airway.

BOX 2-10

Manifestations of Patient Preparing to Vomit

- Nausea
- Feeling of warmth
- Frequent swallowing
- Feeling of anxiety
- Perspiration
- Gagging

should be used to assist removal of vomitus from the oral cavity. If the clinician suspects that gastric material may have entered the lower respiratory tract, a call should be placed for emergency assistance. The patient should be placed on supplemental oxygen and vital signs monitored. If possible, the dentist should gain venous access (i.e., start an IV line) and be prepared to administer crystalloid solution (e.g., normal saline or 5% dextrose in water) to help treat a falling blood pressure and allow emergency technicians to administer IV bronchodilators if necessary. Immediate transportation to an emergency facility is mandatory (Fig. 2-7).

Altered Consciousness

An alteration in a patient's level of consciousness may result from a large variety of medical problems. The altered state can range from mild light-headedness to a complete loss of consciousness. Without attempting to include all possible causes of altered consciousness, a discussion is presented of commonly occurring conditions that may lead to an acutely altered state of consciousness before or while patients are undergoing oral surgical procedures.

Vasovagal Syncope

The most common cause of a transient loss of consciousness in the dental office is vasovagal syncope. This generally occurs because of a series of cardiovascular events triggered by emotional stress brought on by the anticipation of or delivery of dental care. The initial event in a vasovagal syncopal episode is the stress-induced increase in amounts of catecholamines that cause a decrease in peripheral vascular resistance, tachycardia, and sweating. The patient may complain of feeling generalized warmth, nausea, and palpitations. As blood pools in the periphery, a drop in the arterial blood pressure appears, with a corresponding decrease in cerebral blood flow. The patient may then complain of feeling dizzy or weak. Compensatory mechanisms attempt to maintain adequate blood pressure, but they soon fade, leading to vagally mediated bradycardia. Once the blood pressure drops below levels necessary to sustain consciousness, syncope occurs (Fig. 2-8).

If cerebral ischemia is sufficiently slow to develop, the patient may first develop seizures. The syncopal episode and any accompanying seizure usually end rapidly once the patient assumes or is placed in a horizontal position with the feet elevated (Fig. 2-9). Once consciousness is regained, the patient may have pallor, nausea, and weakness for several minutes.

Prevention of vasovagal syncopal reactions involves proper patient preparation. The extremely anxious patient should be treated by using an anxiety-reduction protocol and, if necessary, should be given anxiolytic drugs before treatment. Oral

Large foreign body enters trachea or bronchus (e.g., tooth, dental instrument, crown)

1. Terminate all dental treatment.
2. Position patient in sitting posture.
3. Ask patient to try to cough object out.

Patient becomes unconscious

4. Have someone summon medical assistance.
5. Place patient in supine position.
6. Begin abdominal thrusts followed by turning patient on side and using finger to sweep oral cavity for foreign body.
7. Attempt to ventilate.

Able to ventilate

8. Start Basic Life Support.
9. Administer oxygen.
10. Transport.

Unable to ventilate

8. Repeat steps 6 and 7 twice, then
9. Perform laryngoscopy.*
10. Perform cricothyrotomy.*

Patient remains conscious

Symptoms persist

4. Heimlich maneuvers until effective.
5. Administer oxygen.
6. Have someone summon medical assistance.
7. Monitor vital signs.
8. Transport to emergency care facility.

Symptoms never occur or cease, and clinician is unsure where foreign body is

4. Administer oxygen.
5. Monitor vital signs.
6. Transport patient to emergency care facility for radiography and, possibly, perform bronchoscopy.

*For those dentists with appropriate training.

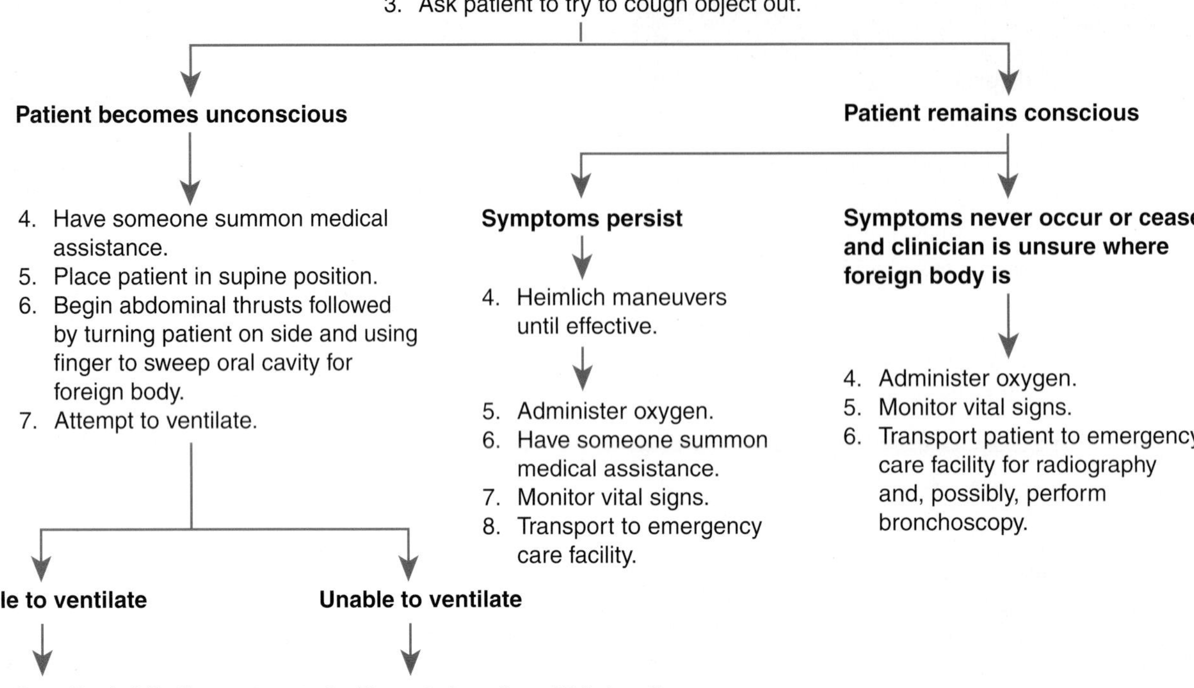

FIGURE 2-6 Management of respiratory tract foreign-body aspiration in patient undergoing dental surgery.

Management of vomiting patient with possible aspiration of gastric contents

1. Terminate all dental treatment.
2. Place patient on right side in horizontal position.
3. Suction oropharynx.

Once vomiting ceases, no symptoms of aspiration are present

4. Monitor vital signs for 30 minutes.
5. If any suspicion of aspiration occurs, transport to emergency care facility.

Once vomiting ceases, symptoms of aspiration are present

4. Have someone summon medical assistance.
5. Administer oxygen.
6. Start intravenous (IV) line, and run crystalloid solution at 150 mL/hr.
7. Monitor vital signs.

Signs of hypoxia

8. Perform endotracheal intubation; provide pulmonary lavage with normal saline and positive pressure oxygen.
9. Administer theophylline 250 mg IV slowly.
10. Start Basic Life Support, if breathing ceases.
11. Transport to emergency care facility.

No signs of hypoxia

8. Transport to emergency care facility.

FIGURE 2-7 Management of vomiting patient with possible aspiration of gastric contents.

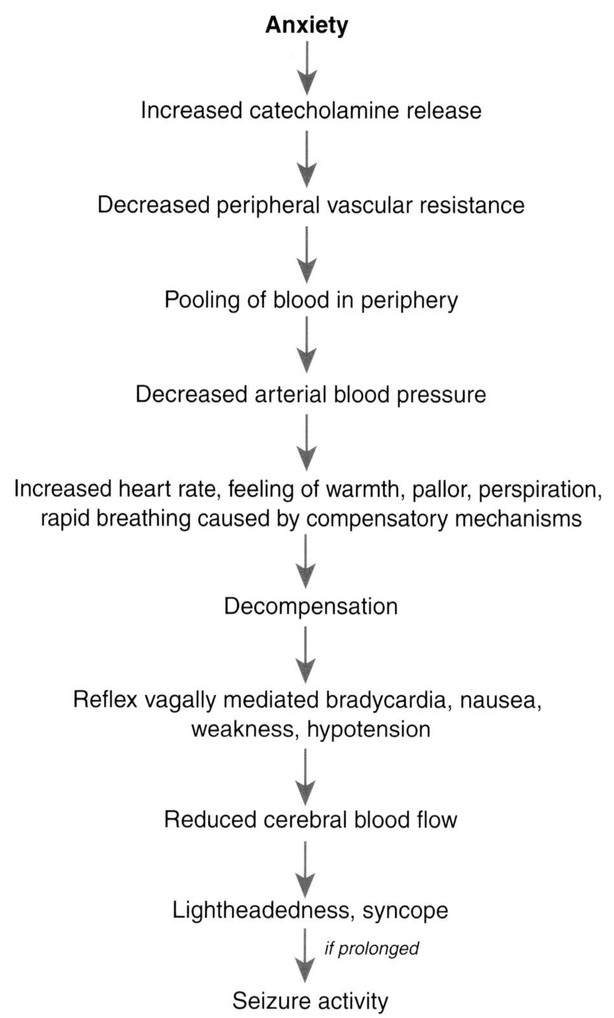

FIGURE 2-8 Pathophysiology and manifestations of vasovagal syncope.

surgical care should be provided while the patient is in a semisupine or fully supine position. Any signs of an impending syncopal episode should be quickly treated by placing the patient in a fully supine position or a position in which the legs are elevated above the level of the heart and by placing a cool, moist towel on the forehead. If the patient is hypoventilating and is slow to recover consciousness, a respiratory stimulant such as aromatic ammonia may be useful. If the return of consciousness is delayed for more than a minute, an alternative cause for depressed consciousness other than vasovagal syncope should be sought. After early recovery from the syncopal episode, the patient should be allowed to recover in the office and then be discharged with an escort. Future office visits by the patient will require preoperative sedation, additional anxiety-reducing measures, or both.

Orthostatic Hypotension

Another common cause of a transient altered state of consciousness in the dental setting is orthostatic (or postural) hypotension. This problem occurs because of pooling of blood in the periphery that is not remobilized quickly enough to prevent cerebral ischemia when a patient rapidly assumes an upright posture. The patient will therefore feel light-headed or become syncopal. Patients with orthostatic hypotension who remain conscious will usually complain of palpitations and generalized weakness. Most individuals who are not hypovolemic or have orthostatic hypotension resulting from the pharmacologic effects of drugs such as antihypertensive agents will quickly recover by reassuming the reclined position. Once symptoms disappear, the patient can generally sit up (although this should be done slowly) and sit on the edge of the chair for a few moments before standing. Blood pressure can be taken in each position and allowed to return to normal before a more upright posture is assumed (Box 2-11).

Some patients have a predisposition to orthostatic hypotension. In the ambulatory population, this is usually encountered in patients receiving the following medications: drugs that

Management of patient showing symptoms or signs of syncope

Prodrome:

1. Terminate all dental treatment.
2. Position patient in supine posture with legs raised above level of head.
3. Attempt to calm patient.
4. Place cool towel on patient's forehead.
5. Monitor vital signs.

Syncopal episode:

1. Terminate all dental treatment.
2. Position patient in supine posture with legs raised.
3. Check for breathing.

If absent:

4. Start Basic Life Support.
5. Have someone summon medical assistance.
6. Consider other causes of syncope, including hypoglycemia, cerebral vascular accident, or cardiac dysrhythmia.

If present:

4. Crush ammonia ampule under nose, administer O_2.
5. Monitor vital signs.
6. Have patient escorted home.
7. Plan anxiety control measures during future dental care.

FIGURE 2-9 Management of vasovagal syncope and its prodrome.

BOX 2-11

Management of Orthostatic Hypotension

1. Terminate all dental treatment.
2. Position patient in supine posture, with legs raised above the level of the head.
3. Monitor vital signs.
4. Once blood pressure improves, slowly return patient to sitting posture.
5. Discharge patient to home once vital signs are normal and stable.
6. Obtain medical consultation before any further dental care.

produce intravascular depletion, such as diuretics; drugs that produce peripheral vasodilation, such as most nondiuretic antihypertensives, narcotics, and many psychiatric drugs; and drugs that prevent the heart rate from increasing reflexively, such as β-sympathetic antagonist medications (e.g., propranolol). Patients with a predisposition to postural hypotension can usually be managed by allowing a much longer period to attain a standing position (i.e., by stopping at several increments while becoming upright to allow reflex cardiovascular compensation to occur). If the patient was sedated by using long-acting narcotics, an antagonist such as naloxone may be necessary. Patients with severe problems with postural hypotension as a result of drug therapy should be referred to their physician for possible modification of their drug regimen.

Seizure

Idiopathic seizure disorders are exhibited in many ways, ranging from grand mal seizures, with their frightening display of clonic contortions of the trunk and extremities, to petit mal seizures that may occur with only episodic absences (e.g., blank stare). Although rare, some seizure disorders, such as those resulting from injury-induced brain damage or damage from ethanol abuse, have a known cause. Usually the patient will have had the seizure disorder previously diagnosed and will be receiving antiseizure medications, such as phenytoin (Dilantin), phenobarbital, or valproic acid. Therefore the dentist should discover through the medical interview the degree of seizure control present to decide whether oral surgery can be safely performed. The patient should be asked to describe what witnesses have said occurs just before, during, and after the patient's seizures. Discovery of any factors that seem to precipitate the seizure, the patient's compliance with antiseizure drugs, and the recent frequency of seizure episodes is helpful. Patients with seizure disorders who appear to have good control of their disease, that is, infrequent episodes that are brief and are not easily precipitated by anxiety, are usually able to undergo oral surgery safely in the ambulatory setting. (See Chapter 1 for recommendations.)

The occurrence of a seizure while a patient is undergoing care in the dental office, although usually creating great concern among the office staff, is rarely an emergency that calls for actions other than simply protecting the patient from self-injury. However, management of the patient during and after a seizure varies, based on the type of seizure that occurs. The patient's ability to exchange air must be monitored by close observation. If it appears that the airway is obstructed, measures to reopen it must be taken, for example, by placing the head in moderate extension (chin pulled away from the chest) and moving the mandible away from the pharynx. If the patient vomits or seems to be having problems keeping secretions out of the airway, the patient's head must be positioned to the side to allow obstructing materials to drain out of the mouth. If possible, high-volume suction should be used to evacuate materials from the pharynx. Brief periods of apnea may occur, which require no treatment other than ensuring a patent airway. However, apnea for more than 30 seconds demands that BLS techniques be initiated. Although frequently described as being important, the placement of objects between the teeth in an attempt to prevent tongue biting is hazardous and therefore unwarranted.

Continuous or repeated seizures without periods of recovery between them are known as *status epilepticus*. This problem warrants notification of outside emergency assistance because it is the most common type of seizure disorder to cause mortality. Therapy includes instituting measures already described for self-limiting seizures; in addition, administration of a benzodiazepine is indicated. Injectable water-insoluble benzodiazepines such as diazepam must be given IV to allow predictability of results, which may be difficult in the patient having seizures if venous access is not already available. Injectable water-soluble benzodiazepines such as midazolam provide a better alternative, because IM injection will give a more rapid response. However, the doctor administering benzodiazepines for a seizure must be prepared to provide BLS because patients may experience a period of apnea after receiving a large, rapid dose of benzodiazepines.

After seizures have ceased, most patients will be left either somnolent or unconscious. Vital signs should be monitored carefully during this time, and the patient should not be allowed to leave the office until fully alert and in the company of an escort. The patient's primary care physician should be notified to decide whether medical evaluation is necessary and whether ambulatory dental care is advisable in the future (Fig. 2-10).

Tremors, palpitations, and extreme anxiety usually precede seizures caused by ethanol withdrawal. Therefore the appearance of these signs in a patient should warn the clinician to defer treatment until proper medical care for the patient's condition is instituted. Control is usually obtained by the use of benzodiazepines, which are used until the untoward effects of abstinence from ethanol cease. Seizures that occur in ethanol-abusing patients are treated in a similar manner to other seizures.

Local Anesthetic Toxicity

Local anesthetics, when properly used, are a safe and effective means of providing pain control when performing dentoalveolar surgery. However, as with all medications, toxicity reactions occur if the local anesthetic is given in an amount or in a manner that produces an excessive serum concentration.

Prevention of a toxicity reaction to local anesthetics generally involves several factors. First, the dose to be used should be the least amount of local anesthetic necessary to produce the intensity and duration of pain control required to successfully complete the planned surgical procedure. The patient's age, lean body mass, liver function, and history of problems with local anesthetics must be considered when choosing the dose of local anesthesia. The second factor to consider in preventing

Management of a seizing patient

Manifestations

Isolated, brief seizure

Tonic-clonic movements of trunk and extremities, loss of consciousness, vomiting, airway obstruction, loss of urinary and anal sphincter control

Acute management

1. Terminate all dental treatment.
2. Place in supine position.
3. Protect from nearby objects.

After seizure

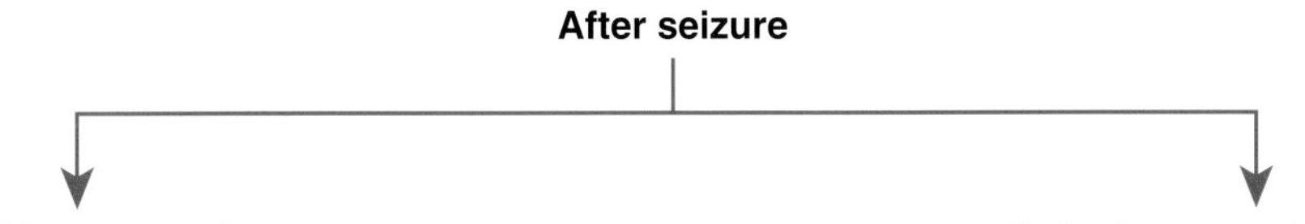

Patient is unconscious

4. Have someone summon medical assistance.
5. Place patient on side, and suction airway.
6. Monitor vital signs.
7. Initiate Basic Life Support (BLS), if necessary.
8. Administer oxygen.
9. Transport to emergency care facility.

Patient is conscious

4. Suction airway, if necessary.
5. Monitor vital signs.
6. Administer oxygen.
7. Consult physician.
8. Observe patient in office for 1 hour.
9. Have patient escorted home.

Repeated or sustained seizure (status epilepticus)

(as above)

1. Administer diazepam 5 mg/min intravenously (IV) up to 10 mg or midazolam 3 mg/min IV or intramuscularly up to 6 mg* titrated until seizures stop.
2. Have someone summon medical assistance.
3. Protect patient from nearby objects.

Once seizure ceases

4. Place patient on side, and suction airway.
5. Monitor vital signs.
6. Initiate BLS, if necessary.
7. Administer oxygen.
8. Transport to emergency care facility.

*Total dose can be doubled if no signs of respiratory depression occur. Total dose should be halved in children and older patients.

FIGURE 2-10 Manifestations and acute management of seizures.

a local anesthetic overdose reaction is the manner of drug administration. The dentist should give the required dose slowly, avoiding intravascular injection, and use vasoconstrictors to slow the entry of local anesthetics into the blood. One should remember that topical use of local anesthetics in wounds or on mucosal surfaces allows rapid entry of local anesthetics into the systemic circulation. The choice of local anesthetic agents is the third important factor to consider in attempting to lessen the risk of a toxicity reaction. Local anesthetics vary in their lipid solubility, vasodilatory properties, protein binding, and inherent toxicity. Therefore the dentist must be knowledgeable about the various local anesthetics available to make a rational decision when choosing which drug to administer and in what amounts (Table 2-4).

The clinical manifestations of a local anesthetic overdose vary depending on the severity of the overdose, how rapidly it occurs, and the duration of the excessive serum concentrations. Signs of a mild toxicity reaction may be limited to increased patient confusion, talkativeness, anxiety, and slurring of speech. As the severity of the overdose increases, the patient may display stuttering speech, nystagmus, and generalized tremors. Symptoms such as headache, dizziness, blurred vision, and drowsiness may also occur. The most serious manifestations of local anesthetic toxicity are the appearance of generalized tonic-clonic seizures and cardiac depression leading to cardiac arrest (Table 2-5).

Mild local anesthetic overdose reactions are managed by monitoring vital signs, instructing the patient to hyperventilate moderately with or without administering oxygen, and gaining venous access. If signs of anesthetic toxicity do not rapidly disappear, a slow IV 2.5- to 5-mg dose of diazepam should be given. Medical assistance should also be summoned if signs of toxicity do not rapidly resolve or progressively worsen.

If convulsions occur, patients should be protected from hurting themselves. Basic life support measures are instituted as needed, and venous access is gained, if possible, for administration of anticonvulsants. Medical assistance should be obtained. If venous access is available, diazepam should be slowly titrated until the seizures stop (5 to 25 mg is the usual effective range). Vital signs should be checked frequently.

Diabetes Mellitus

Diabetes mellitus is a metabolic disease in which the patient's long-term prognosis appears to depend on keeping serum glucose levels close to normal. An untreated insulin-dependent

TABLE 2-4

Suggested Maximum Dose of Local Anesthetics*

Drug	Common Brand	Concentration	Maximum dose (mg/kg)	Maximum Number of 1.8-mL Cartridges
Lidocaine	Xylocaine	2%	5	10
Lidocaine with epinephrine†	Xylocaine with epinephrine	2% lidocaine 1:100,000 epinephrine	5	10
Mepivacaine	Carbocaine	3%	5	6
Mepivacaine with levonordefrin	Carbocaine with Neo-Cobefrin	2% mepivacaine 1:20,000 levonordefrin	5	8
Prilocaine	Citanest	4%	5	6
Bupivacaine with epinephrine	Marcaine with epinephrine	0.5% bupivacaine 1:200,000 epinephrine	1.5	10
Etidocaine with epinephrine	Duranest with epinephrine	1.5% etidocaine 1:200,000 epinephrine	8	15

*Maximum doses are those for normal healthy individuals.
†Maximum dose of epinephrine is 0.2 mg per appointment.

TABLE 2-5

Manifestations and Management of Local Anesthetic Toxicity

Manifestations	Management
◆ Mild toxicity: talkativeness, anxiety, slurred speech, confusion	◆ Stop administration of local anesthetics ◆ Monitor all vital signs ◆ Observe in office for 1 hour
◆ Moderate toxicity: stuttering speech, nystagmus, tremors, headache, dizziness, blurred vision, drowsiness	◆ Stop administration of all local anesthetics ◆ Place in supine position ◆ Monitor vital signs ◆ Administer oxygen ◆ Observe in office for 1 hour
◆ Severe toxicity: seizure, cardiac dysrhythmia or arrest	◆ Place in supine position ◆ If seizure occurs, protect patient from nearby objects; suction contents of oral cavity if vomiting occurs ◆ Have someone summon medical assistance ◆ Monitor all vital signs ◆ Administer oxygen ◆ Start an IV ◆ Administer diazepam 5-10 mg slowly or midazolam 2-6 mg slowly ◆ Institute basic life support if necessary ◆ Transport to emergency care facility

diabetic person constantly runs the risk of developing ketoacidosis and its attendant alteration of consciousness, requiring emergency treatment. Although a compliant insulin-taking diabetic person may suffer long-term problems because of relatively high serum glucose levels, the more common emergency situation the person encounters is hypoglycemia resulting from a mismatch of insulin dose and serum glucose. Severe hypoglycemia is the emergency situation dentists are most likely to face when providing oral surgery for a diabetic patient.

Serum glucose concentration in the diabetic patient represents a balance between administered insulin, glucose placed into the serum from various sources, and glucose use. The two primary sources of glucose are dietary and gluconeogenesis from adipose tissue, muscle, and glycogen stores. Physical activity is the principal means by which serum glucose is lowered. Therefore, serum glucose levels can fall because of any or all of the following:

1. Increasing administered insulin
2. Decreasing dietary caloric intake
3. Increasing metabolic use of glucose (e.g., exercise, infection, or emotional stress)

Problems with hypoglycemia during dental care usually arise because the patient has acutely decreased caloric intake, an infection, or an increased metabolic rate caused by considerable anxiety. If the patient has not compensated for this diminution of available glucose by decreasing the usual dose of insulin, hypoglycemia results. Although patients taking oral

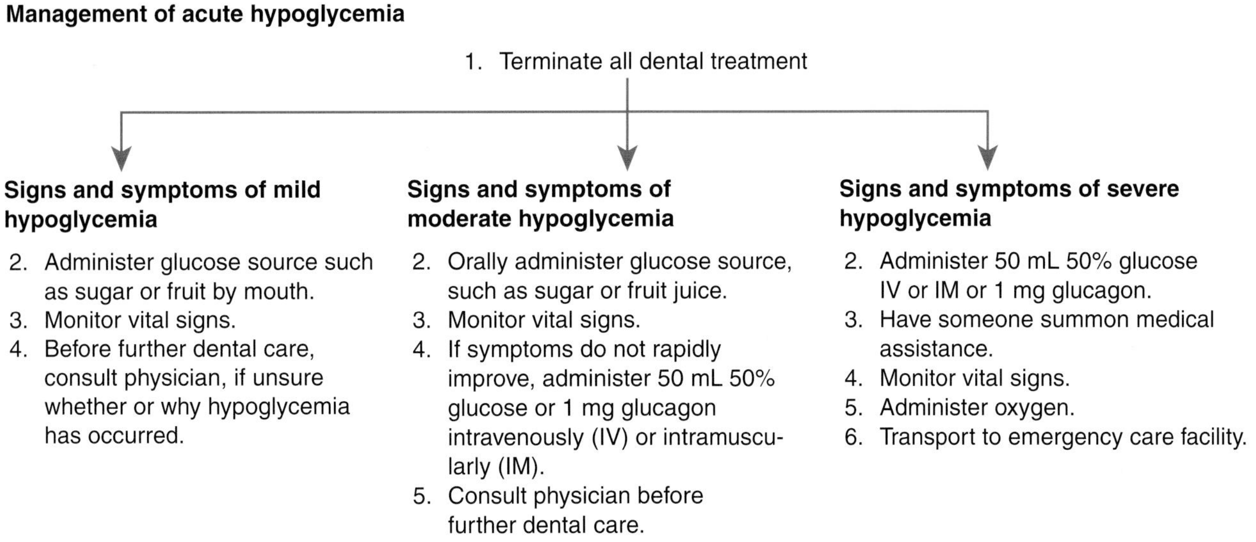

Management of acute hypoglycemia

1. Terminate all dental treatment

Signs and symptoms of mild hypoglycemia

2. Administer glucose source such as sugar or fruit by mouth.
3. Monitor vital signs.
4. Before further dental care, consult physician, if unsure whether or why hypoglycemia has occurred.

Signs and symptoms of moderate hypoglycemia

2. Orally administer glucose source, such as sugar or fruit juice.
3. Monitor vital signs.
4. If symptoms do not rapidly improve, administer 50 mL 50% glucose or 1 mg glucagon intravenously (IV) or intramuscularly (IM).
5. Consult physician before further dental care.

Signs and symptoms of severe hypoglycemia

2. Administer 50 mL 50% glucose IV or IM or 1 mg glucagon.
3. Have someone summon medical assistance.
4. Monitor vital signs.
5. Administer oxygen.
6. Transport to emergency care facility.

FIGURE 2-11 Management of acute hypoglycemia.

hypoglycemics can also have problems with hypoglycemia, their swings in serum glucose levels are usually less pronounced than those of insulin-dependent patients with diabetes, so they are much less likely to quickly become severely hypoglycemic.

Many patients with diabetes are well informed about their disease and are capable of diagnosing their own hypoglycemia before it becomes severe. The patient may feel hunger, nausea, or light-headedness or may develop a headache. The dentist may notice the patient becoming lethargic, with decreased spontaneity of conversation and ability to concentrate. As hypoglycemia worsens, the patient may become diaphoretic or have tachycardia, piloerection, or increased anxiety and exhibit unusual behavior. The patient may soon become stuporous or lose consciousness (Box 2-12).

Severe hypoglycemia in diabetic patients usually can be avoided through measures designed to keep serum glucose levels on the high side of normal or even temporarily above normal. During the health history interview, the dentist should get a clear idea of the degree of control of the patient's diabetes.

BOX 2-12

Manifestations of Acute Hypoglycemia

MILD
- Hunger
- Nausea
- Mood change
- Weakness

MODERATE
- Anxiety
- Behavior change: belligerence, confusion, uncooperativeness
- Pallor
- Perspiration
- Tachycardia

SEVERE
- Hypotension
- Seizures
- Unconsciousness

If patients do not regularly check their own urine or serum glucose, their physician should be contacted to determine whether routine dental care can be performed safely. Before any planned procedures, measures discussed in Chapter 1 concerning the diabetic patient should be taken.

If a diabetic patient indicates a feeling of low blood sugar or if signs or symptoms of hypoglycemia appear, the procedure being performed should be stopped and the patient should be allowed to consume a high-caloric carbohydrate, such as a few packets of sugar, a glass of fruit juice, or other sugar-containing beverages. If the patient fails to improve rapidly, becomes unconscious, or is otherwise unable to take a glucose source by mouth, venous access should be gained and an ampule (50 mL) of 50% glucose (dextrose) in water should be administered IV over 2 to 3 minutes. If venous access cannot be established, 1 mg of glucagon can be given IM. If 50% glucose and glucagon are unavailable, a 0.5-mL dose of 1:1000 epinephrine can be administered SC and repeated every 15 minutes as needed (Fig. 2-11).

A patient who seems to have recovered from a hypoglycemic episode should remain in the office for at least 1 hour, and further symptoms should be treated with oral glucose sources. The patient should be escorted home with instructions on how to avoid a hypoglycemic episode during the next dental appointment.

Thyroid Dysfunction

Hyperthyroidism and hypothyroidism are slowly developing disorders that can produce an altered state of consciousness but rarely cause emergencies. The most common circumstance in which an ambulatory, relatively healthy-appearing patient develops an emergency from thyroid dysfunction is when a thyroid storm (crisis) occurs.

Thyroid storm is sudden, severe exacerbation of hyperthyroidism that may or may not have been previously diagnosed. Thyroid storm can be precipitated by infection, surgery, trauma, pregnancy, or any other physiological or emotional stress. Patients predisposed to thyroid crisis frequently have signs of hyperthyroidism, such as tremor, tachycardia, weight loss, hypertension, irritability, intolerance to heat, and exophthalmos; they may have even received therapy for the thyroid disorder.

The clinician should consult the primary care physician of a patient with known hyperthyroidism before any oral surgical procedure. A determination of the adequacy of control of excessive thyroid hormone production should be obtained from the patient's physician, and if necessary, the patient should receive antithyroid drugs and iodide treatment preoperatively. If clearance for ambulatory surgery is given, the patient should be managed as shown in the outline in Chapter 1.

The first sign of a developing thyroid storm is an elevation of temperature and heart rate. Most of the usual signs and symptoms of untreated hyperthyroidism occur in an exaggerated form. The patient becomes irritable, delirious, or even comatose. Hypotension, vomiting, and diarrhea also occur.

Treatment of thyrotoxic crisis begins with termination of any procedure and notification of those outside the office able to give emergency assistance. Venous access should be obtained, crystalloid solution should be started at a moderate rate, and the patient should be kept as calm as possible. Attempts may be made to cool the patient until transported to a hospital, where antithyroid and sympathetic blocking drugs can be administered safely (Box 2-13).

BOX 2-13

Manifestations and Management of Acute Thyroid Storm

MANIFESTATIONS

- Abdominal pains
- Cardiac dysrhythmias
- Hyperpyrexia (i.e., fever)
- Nausea and vomiting
- Nervousness and agitation
- Palpitations
- Partial or complete loss of consciousness
- Tachycardia
- Tremor
- Weakness

MANAGEMENT

1. Terminate all dental treatment.
2. Have someone summon medical assistance.
3. Administer oxygen.
4. Monitor all vital signs.
5. Initiate basic life support if necessary.
6. Start an IV line with drip of crystalloid solution (150 mL/h).
7. Transport patient to emergency care facility.

Adrenal Insufficiency

Primary adrenocortical insufficiency (Addison's disease) or other medical conditions in which the adrenal cortex has been destroyed are rare. However, adrenal insufficiency resulting from exogenous corticosteroid administration is common because of the multitude of clinical conditions for which therapeutic corticosteroid administration is given. Patients with adrenal insufficiency are frequently not informed concerning their potential need for supplemental medication, and those with secondary adrenal insufficiency may fail to inform the dentist that they are taking corticosteroids. This is not a problem, provided the patient is not physiologically or emotionally stressed.

However, should the patient be stressed, adrenal suppression that results from exogenous corticosteroids may prevent the normal release of endogenous glucocorticoids in amounts needed to help the body meet the elevated metabolic demands. Patients at risk for acute adrenal insufficiency as a result of adrenal suppression are generally those who take at least 20 mg of cortisol (or its equivalent) daily for at least 2 weeks any time during the year preceding the planned major oral surgical procedure (Table 2-6). However, in most straightforward oral surgical procedures done under local anesthesia or nitrous oxide and local anesthesia, administration of supplemental corticosteroids is unnecessary. When significant adrenal suppression is suspected, the steps discussed in Chapter 1 should be followed.

Early clinical manifestations of acute adrenal insufficiency crisis include mental confusion, nausea, fatigue, and muscle weakness. As the condition worsens, the patient develops more severe mental confusion; pain in the back, abdomen, and legs; vomiting; and hypotension. Without treatment the patient will eventually begin to drift in and out of consciousness, with coma harkening the preterminal stage (Box 2-14).

Management of an adrenal crisis begins by stopping all dental treatment and taking vital signs. If the patient is found to be hypotensive, the patient must be placed immediately in a head-down, legs-elevated position. Medical assistance should be summoned. Oxygen should be administered and venous access gained. A 100-mg dose of hydrocortisone sodium succinate should be given IV (or IM, if necessary). IV fluids

TABLE 2-6

Equivalency of Commonly Used Glucocorticosteroids

Relative Duration of Action	Generic	Common Brand Name	Relative Glucocorticoid Potency	Relative Glucocorticoid Dose (mg)
Short	Cortisol (hydrocortisone)	Solu-Cortef	1	20
	Cortisone	—	0.8	25
	Prednisone	Deltasone	4	5
	Prednisolone	Delta-Cortef	4	5
	Methylprednisolone sodium succinate	Solu-Medrol	5	4
Intermediate	Triamcinolone	Kenalog	5	4
Long	Betamethasone	Celestone	25	0.6
	Dexamethasone	Decadron	30	0.75
	Methylprednisolone acetate	Depo-Medrol	5	4

BOX 2-14

Manifestations of Acute Adrenal Insufficiency

Abdominal pain
Confusion
Feeling of extreme fatigue
Hypotension
Myalgias
Nausea
Partial or total loss of consciousness
Weakness

should be rapidly administered until hypotension improves. Vital signs should be measured frequently while therapeutic measures are performed. Should the patient lose consciousness, the need for initiation of basic life support measures should be evaluated (Box 2-15).

Cerebrovascular Compromise

Alterations in cerebral blood flow can be compromised in three principal ways: (1) embolization of particulate matter from a distant site, (2) formation of a thrombus in a cerebral vessel, or (3) rupture of a vessel. Material that embolizes to the brain comes most frequently from thrombi in the left side of the heart, from the carotid artery, or from bacterial vegetations on infected heart surfaces. Cerebrovascular thrombi generally form in areas of atherosclerotic changes. Finally, vascular rupture can occur because of rare congenital defects in the vessel, that is, berry aneurysms.

The effect on the level of consciousness of a cerebrovascular problem depends on the severity of the cerebral lesion. If the problem rapidly resolves, such as happens with transient ischemic attacks, the symptoms of cerebral vascular compromise may last only a few seconds or minutes. However, if ischemia is severe enough, an infarction may occur in an area of the brain, leaving a neurologic deficit.

A transient ischemic attack that occurs during dental care requires that the procedure be terminated. However, little must be done for the patient other than reassurance, because most patients experience only a temporary numbness or weakness of both of the extremities on one side of the body or visual disturbance. Consciousness is usually unaltered. Transient ischemic attacks frequently precede a cerebral infarction, so immediate physician referral is important.

Cerebrovascular compromise that results from embolism usually occurs first with a mild headache, followed by the appearance of other neurologic symptoms, such as weakness in an extremity, vertigo, or dizziness. However, cerebral hemorrhage typically has the abrupt onset of a severe headache, followed in several hours by nausea, dizziness, vertigo, and diaphoresis. The patient may go on to lose consciousness (Box 2-16).

If signs or symptoms of a cerebrovascular compromise arise and are not transient, a major problem affecting the cerebral vasculature may be occurring. The procedure should be stopped, and frequent monitoring of vital signs should be begun. Medical help should be called to assist in the event the patient becomes hypotensive or unconscious and to transport the patient to a hospital where neurosurgical intervention or thrombolytic therapy can be initiated, as indicated. If the patient develops respiratory difficulty, oxygen should be administered. However, oxygen is otherwise contraindicated in patients with cerebrovascular insufficiency. Any narcotics that the patient has been administered should be reversed. If consciousness is lost, vital signs should be monitored frequently and cardiopulmonary resuscitation should be begun if necessary (Box 2-17).

BOX 2-15

Management of Acute Adrenal Insufficiency

1. Terminate all dental treatment.
2. Position patient in supine position, with legs raised above level of head.
3. Have someone summon medical assistance.
4. Administer corticosteroid (100 mg hydrocortisone IM or IV or its equivalent).
5. Administer oxygen.
6. Monitor vital signs.
7. Start an IV line and drip of crystalloid solution.
8. Start basic life support, if necessary.
9. Transport to emergency care facility.

BOX 2-16

Manifestations of Cerebrovascular Compromise in Progress

- Headache that can range from mild to the worst the patient has ever experienced
- Unilateral weakness or paralysis of extremities or facial muscles or both
- Slurring of speech or inability to speak
- Difficulty breathing or swallowing or both
- Loss of bladder and bowel control
- Seizures
- Visual disturbance
- Dizziness
- Partial or total loss of consciousness

BOX 2-17

Management of Cerebrovascular Compromise in Progress*

1. Terminate all dental treatment.
2. Have someone summon medical assistance.
3. Position patient in supine posture, with head slightly raised.
4. Monitor vital signs.
5. If loss of consciousness, administer oxygen and institute basic life support, as necessary.
6. Transport to emergency care facility.

*If symptoms are present only briefly (i.e., transient ischemic attacks), terminate dental treatment, monitor vital signs, and consult patient's physician concerning safety of further dental care.

CHAPTER 3

Principles of Surgery

JAMES R. HUPP

CHAPTER OUTLINE

Human tissues have genetically determined properties that make their responses to injury generally predictable. Depending on this predictability, principles of surgery that help to optimize the wound-healing environment have evolved through time and through basic and clinical research. This chapter presents the principles of surgical practice that clinicians and investigators have found most successful.

DEVELOPING A SURGICAL DIAGNOSIS

Most of the important decisions concerning a maxillofacial surgical procedure should be made long before the administration of anesthesia. The decision to perform surgery should be the culmination of several diagnostic steps. In the critical thinking analytic approach the surgeon first identifies the various signs and symptoms and relevant historical information; then, using available patient and scientific data and logical reasoning, the surgeon establishes the relationship between the individual problems.

The initial step in the presurgical evaluation is the collection of accurate and pertinent data. This is accomplished through patient interviews; physical, laboratory, and imaging examinations; and the use of consultants when necessary. Patient interviews and physical examinations should be performed in an unhurried, thoughtful fashion. The surgeon should not be willing to accept incomplete data, such as a poor-quality radiograph, especially when it is probable that additional data might change decisions concerning surgery.

For a good analysis, data must be organized into a form that allows for hypothesis testing; that is, the dentist should be able to consider a list of possible diseases and eliminate those unsupported by the patient data or evidence-based science. By using this method, along with the knowledge of which diseases have a probability of being present, the surgeon is usually able to reach a decision about whether surgery is indicated.

Clinicians must also be thoughtful observers. Whenever a procedure is performed, they should note all aspects of its outcome to advance their surgical knowledge and to improve future surgical results. This procedure should also be followed whenever a clinician is learning about a new technique. In addition, a clinician should practice evidence-based dentistry by evaluating the purported results of any new technique by weighing the scientific merit of studies used to investigate the technique. Frequently, scientific methods are violated by the unrecognized introduction of a placebo effect, observer bias, patient variability, or use of inadequate control groups.

BASIC NECESSITIES FOR SURGERY

Little difference exists between the basic necessities required for oral surgery and those required for the proper performance of other aspects of dentistry. The two principal requirements are (1) adequate visibility and (2) assistance.

Although visibility may seem too obvious to mention as a requirement for performing surgery, clinicians often underestimate its importance. Adequate visibility depends on the following three factors: (1) adequate access, (2) adequate light, and (3) a surgical field free of excess blood and other fluids.

Adequate access not only requires the patient's ability to open the mouth widely but also may require a surgically created exposure. Retraction of tissues away from the operative field provides much of the necessary access. (Proper retraction also protects tissues from being accidentally injured, for example, by cutting instruments.) Improved access is also gained by the creation of surgical flaps, which are discussed later in this chapter.

Adequate light is another obvious necessity for surgery. However, clinicians often forget that many surgical procedures place the surgeon or assistant in positions that block chair-based light sources. To correct this problem, the light source must continually be repositioned, or the surgeon or assistant must avoid obstructing the light or use a headlight.

A surgical field free of fluids is also necessary for adequate visibility. High-volume suctioning with a relatively small tip can quickly remove blood and other fluids from the field.

As in other types of dentistry, a properly trained assistant provides invaluable help during oral surgery. The assistant should be sufficiently familiar with the procedures being performed to anticipate the surgeon's needs. Performance of good surgery is extremely difficult with no or poor assistance.

ASEPTIC TECHNIQUE

Aseptic technique includes minimizing wound contamination by pathogenic microbes. This important surgical principle is discussed in detail in Chapter 5.

INCISIONS

Many oral and maxillofacial surgical procedures necessitate incisions. A few basic principles are important to remember when performing incisions.

The first principle is that a sharp blade of the proper size should be used. A sharp blade allows incisions to be made cleanly, without unnecessary damage caused by repeated strokes. The rate at which a blade dulls depends on the resistance of tissues through which the blade cuts. Bone and ligamental tissues dull blades more rapidly than does buccal mucosa. Therefore the surgeon should change blades whenever the knife does not seem to be incising easily.

The second principle is that a firm, continuous stroke should be used when incising. Repeated, tentative strokes increase the amount of damaged tissue within a wound and the amount of bleeding, thereby impairing wound healing. Long, continuous strokes are preferred to short, interrupted ones (Fig. 3-1, *A*).

The third principle is that the surgeon should carefully avoid cutting vital structures when incising. No patient's microanatomy is exactly the same. Therefore, to avoid unintentionally cutting large vessels or nerves, the surgeon must incise only deeply enough to define the next major layer when making incisions near to where major vessels and nerves run. Vessels can be more easily controlled before they are completely divided, and important nerves can usually be freed from adjacent tissue and retracted away from the area to be incised. In addition, when using a scalpel, the surgeon must remain focused on the blade to avoid accidentally cutting structures such as the lips when introducing and removing the blade to and from the mouth.

The fourth principle is that incisions through epithelial surfaces that the surgeon plans to reapproximate should be made with the blade held perpendicular to the epithelial surface. This angle produces squared wound edges that are easier to reorient properly during suturing and are less susceptible to necrosis of the wound edges as a result of ischemia (Fig. 3-1, *B*).

The fifth principle is that incisions in the oral cavity should be properly placed. Incisions through attached gingiva and over healthy bone are more desirable than those through unattached gingiva and over unhealthy or missing bone. Properly placed incisions allow the wound margins to be sutured over intact, healthy bone that is at least a few millimeters away from the damaged bone, thereby providing support for the healing wound. Incisions placed near the teeth for extractions should be made in the gingival sulcus, unless the clinician thinks that it is necessary to excise the marginal gingiva or to leave the marginal gingiva untouched.

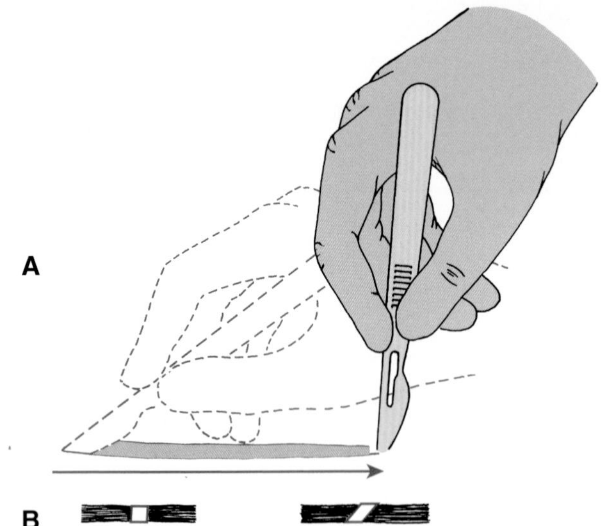

FIGURE 3-1 **A,** Proper method of making incision using No. 15 scalpel blade. Note scalpel motion made by moving hand at wrist and not by moving entire forearm. **B,** When creating tissue layer that is to be sutured closed, blade should be kept perpendicular to tissue surface to create squared wound edges. Holding blade at any angle other than 90 degrees to tissue surface creates an oblique cut that is difficult to close properly and that compromises blood supply to the wound edge. (Modified from Clark HB Jr: *Practical oral surgery,* ed 3, Philadelphia, 1965, Lea & Febiger.)

FLAP DESIGN

Surgical flaps are made to gain surgical access to an area or to move tissue from one place to another. Several basic principles of flap design must be followed to prevent the complications of flap surgery: necrosis, dehiscence, and tearing.

Prevention of Flap Necrosis

Flap necrosis can be prevented if the surgeon attends to four basic flap design principles. First, the apex (tip) of a flap should never be wider than the base, unless a major artery is present in the base. Flaps should have sides that run parallel to each other or, preferably, converge moving from the base to the apex of the flap. Second, generally the length of a flap should be no more than twice the width of the base. Preferably the width of the base should be greater than the length of the flap (Fig. 3-2). Strict adherence to this principle is less critical in the oral cavity, but in general the length of the flap should never exceed the width. Third, when possible, an axial blood supply should be included in the base of the flap. For example, a flap in the palate should be based toward the greater palatine artery. Fourth, the base of flaps should not be excessively twisted, stretched, or grasped with anything that might damage vessels, because these maneuvers can compromise the blood supply feeding and draining the flap.

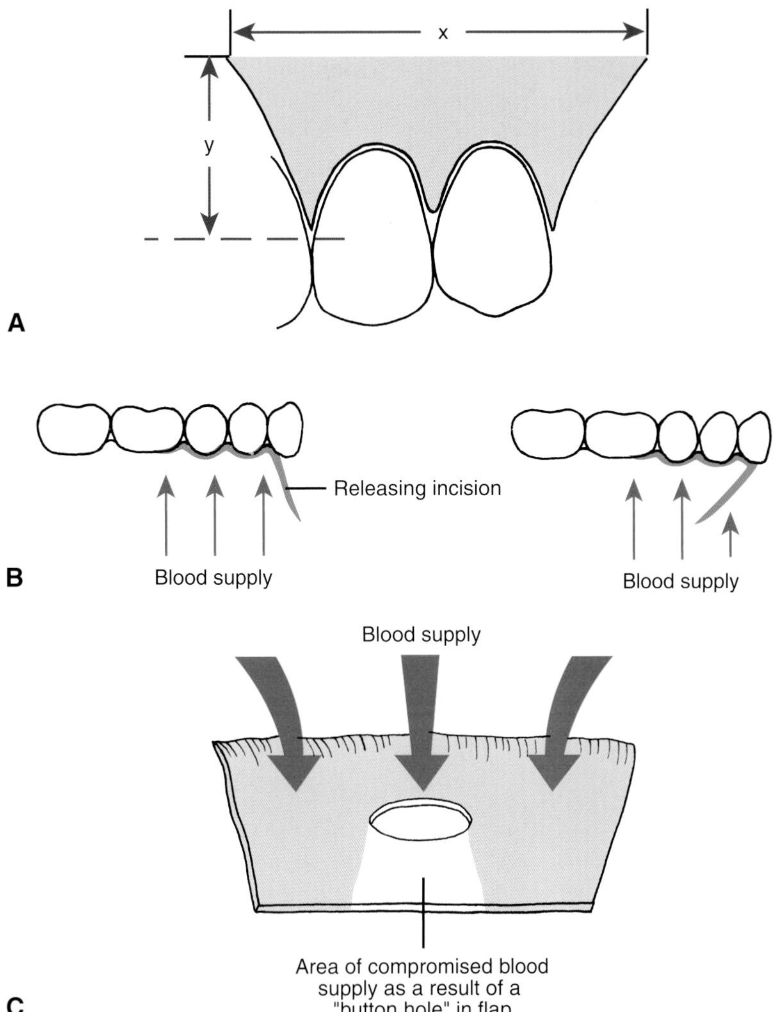

FIGURE 3-2 A, Principles of flap design. In general, flap base dimension (*x*) must not be less than height dimension (*y*), and preferably flap dimension should be $x = 2y$. B, When a releasing incision is used to reflect a two-sided flap, the incision should be designed to maximize flap blood supply by leaving wide base. Design on left is *correct;* design on right is *incorrect.* C, When a "buttonhole" occurs near free edge of flap, blood supply to flap tissue on side of hole away from flap base is compromised.

Prevention of Flap Dehiscence

Flap margin dehiscence (separation) is prevented by approximating the edges of the flap over healthy bone, by gently handling the edges of the flap, and by not placing the flap under tension. Dehiscence exposes underlying bone, producing pain, bone loss, and increased scarring.

Prevention of Flap Tearing

Tearing of a flap is a common complication of the inexperienced surgeon who attempts to perform a procedure using a flap that provides insufficient access. Because a properly repaired long incision heals just as quickly as a short one, it is preferable to create a flap at the onset of surgery that is large enough for the surgeon to avoid tearing it or interrupting surgery to enlarge it. Envelope flaps are those created by incisions that produce a one-sided flap. An example is an incision made around the necks of several teeth to expose the alveolar bone without any vertical releasing incisions. However, if an envelope flap does not provide sufficient access, another incision should be made to prevent it from tearing (Fig. 3-3). Vertical (oblique) releasing incisions should generally be placed one full tooth anterior to the area of any anticipated bone removal. The incision is generally started at the line angle of a tooth or in the adjacent interdental papilla and is carried obliquely apically into the unattached gingiva. A need for more than one releasing incision is uncommon when using a flap to gain oral surgical access.

TISSUE HANDLING

The difference between an acceptable and an excellent surgical outcome often rests on how the surgeon handles the tissues. The use of proper incision and flap design techniques plays a role; however, tissue also must be handled carefully. Excessive pulling or crushing, extremes of temperature, desiccation, or the use of unphysiologic chemicals easily damages tissue. Therefore the surgeon should use care whenever touching

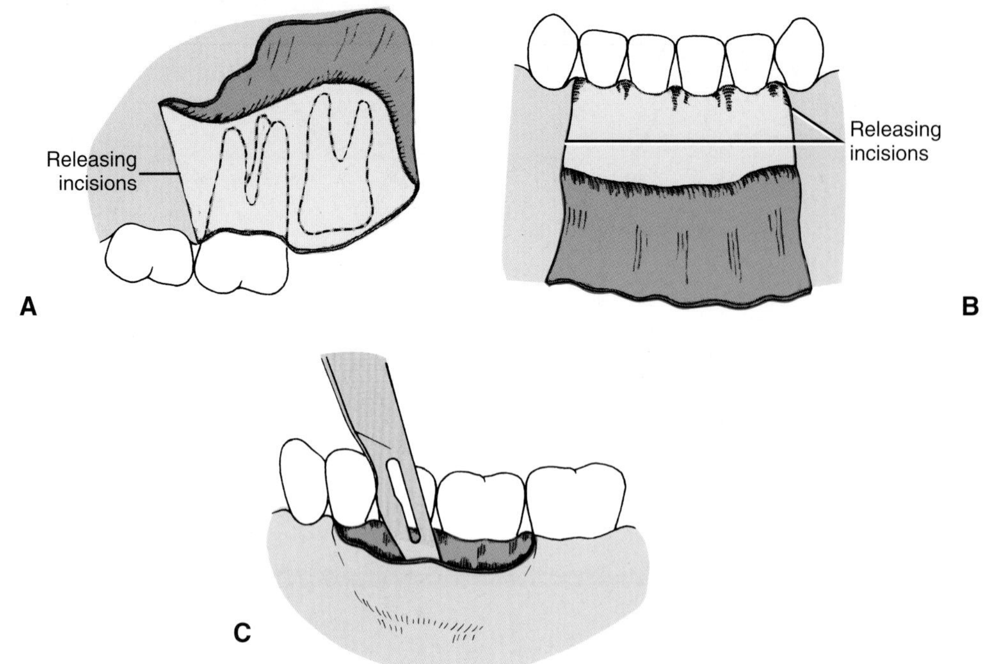

FIGURE 3-3 Three types of properly designed oral soft tissue flaps. A, Horizontal and single vertical incisions used to create two-sided flap. B, Horizontal and two vertical incisions used to create three-sided flap. C, Single horizontal incision used to create single-sided (envelope) flap.

tissue. When tissue forceps are used, they should not be pinched together too tightly; rather, they should be used delicately to hold the tissue. When possible, toothed forceps or tissue hooks should be used to hold tissue (Fig. 3-4). In addition, tissue should not be overaggressively retracted to gain greater surgical access. This includes not pulling excessively on the cheeks or tongue during surgery. When bone is cut, copious amounts of irrigation should be used to decrease the amount of bone damage from heat. Soft tissues should also be protected from frictional heat or direct trauma from drilling equipment. Tissues should not be allowed to desiccate; open wounds should be frequently moistened or covered with a damp sponge. Finally, only physiologic substances should come in contact with living tissue. For example, tissue forceps used to place a specimen into formalin during a biopsy procedure should not be returned to the wound until any contaminating formalin is thoroughly removed. The surgeon who handles tissue gently is rewarded with grateful patients whose wounds heal with fewer complications.

HEMOSTASIS

Prevention of excessive blood loss during surgery is important for preserving a patient's oxygen-carrying capacity. However, maintaining meticulous hemostasis during surgery is necessary for other important reasons. One is the decreased visibility that uncontrolled bleeding creates. Even high-volume suctioning cannot keep a surgical field completely dry, particularly in the well-vascularized oral and maxillofacial regions. Another problem bleeding causes is the formation of hematomas. Hematomas place pressure on wounds, decreasing vascularity; they increase tension on the wound edges; and they act as culture media, potentiating the development of a wound infection.

Means of Promoting Wound Hemostasis

Wound hemostasis can be obtained in four ways. The first is by assisting natural hemostatic mechanisms. This is usually accomplished by using a fabric sponge to place pressure on bleeding vessels or placing a hemostat on a vessel. Both methods cause stasis of blood in vessels, which promotes coagulation. A few

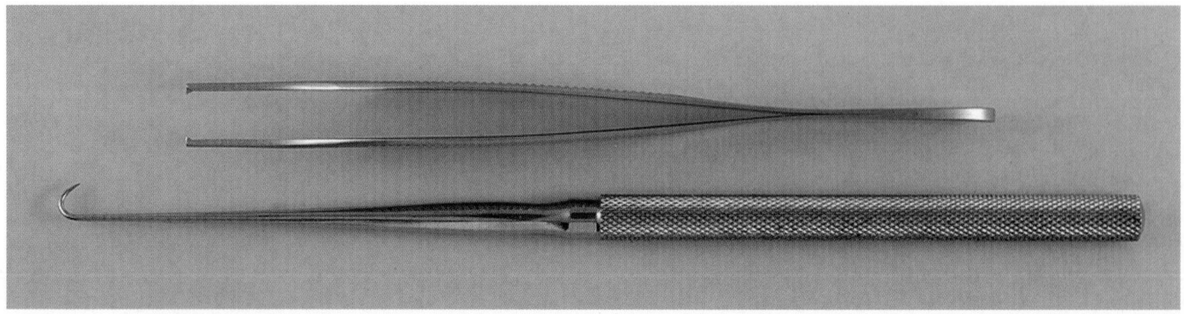

FIGURE 3-4 Instruments used to minimize damage while holding soft tissue. *Top,* Finely toothed tissue forceps (pickups); *bottom,* soft tissue (skin) hook.

small vessels generally require pressure for only 20 to 30 seconds, whereas larger vessels require 5 to 10 minutes of continuous pressure. The surgeon and assistants should dab rather than wipe the wound with sponges to remove extravasated blood. Wiping is more likely to reopen vessels that are already plugged by clotted blood.

A second means of obtaining hemostasis is by the use of heat to cause the ends of cut vessels to fuse (thermal coagulation). Heat is usually applied through an electrical current that the surgeon concentrates on the bleeding vessel by holding the vessel with a metal instrument, such as a hemostat, or by touching the vessel directly with an electrocautery tip. Three conditions should be created for proper use of thermal coagulation. First, the patient must be grounded, to allow the current to enter the body. Second, the cautery tip and any metal instrument the cautery tip contacts cannot touch the patient at any point other than the site of the bleeding vessel. Otherwise, the current may follow an undesirable path and create a burn. The third necessity for thermal coagulation is the removal of any blood or fluid that has accumulated around the vessel to be cauterized. Fluid acts as an energy sump and thus prevents a sufficient amount of heat from reaching the vessel to cause closure.

The third means of providing surgical hemostasis is by suture ligation. If a sizable vessel is already severed, each end is grasped with a hemostat. The surgeon then ties a nonresorbable suture around the vessel. If a vessel can be dissected free of surrounding connective tissue before it is cut, two hemostats can be placed on the vessel, with enough space left between them to cut the vessel. Once the vessel is severed, sutures are tied around each end and the hemostats are removed.

The fourth method of promoting hemostasis is by placing vasoconstrictive substances, such as epinephrine, in the wound or by applying procoagulants, such as commercial thrombin or collagen, on the wound. Epinephrine serves as a vasoconstrictor most effectively when placed in the site of desired vasoconstriction at least 7 minutes before surgery begins.

Dead Space Management

Dead space in a wound is any area that remains devoid of tissue after closure of the wound. Dead space is created by removing tissue in the depths of a wound or by not reapproximating all tissue planes during closure. Dead space in a wound usually fills with blood, which creates a hematoma with a high potential for infection.

Dead space can be eliminated in four ways. The first is by suturing tissue planes together to minimize the postoperative void. A second method is to place a pressure dressing over the repaired wound. The dressing compresses tissue planes together until they are bound by fibrin or pressed together by surgical edema (or both). This usually takes about 12 to 18 hours. The third way to eliminate dead space is to place packing into the void until bleeding has stopped and then to remove the packing. This technique is usually used when the surgeon is unable to tack tissue together or to place pressure dressings (e.g., when bony cavities are present). The packing material is usually impregnated with an antibacterial medication to lessen the chance of infection. The fourth means of preventing dead space is through the use of drains, by themselves or in addition to pressure dressings. Suction drains continually remove any blood that accumulates in a wound until the bleeding stops and the tissues bind together and eliminate dead space. Nonsuction drains allow any bleeding to drain to the surface rather than to form a hematoma (Fig. 3-5). In most routine oral surgical procedures performed by dentists, dead space creation is not a major problem.

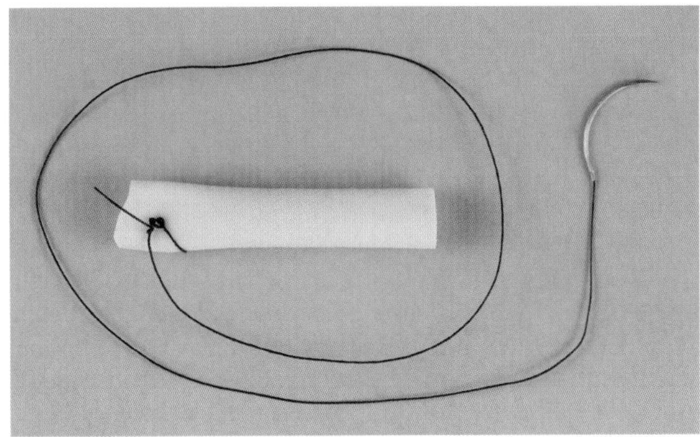

FIGURE 3-5 Example of nonsuction drain. This is a Penrose drain and is made of flexible, rubberized material that can be placed into wound during closure or after incision and drainage of abscess to prevent premature sealing of wound before blood or pus collections can drain to surface. Draining material runs along and through Penrose drain. In this illustration, a suture has been tied to drain and drain is ready for insertion into wound. Needled end of suture will be used to attach drain to wound edge to hold drain in place.

DECONTAMINATION AND DÉBRIDEMENT

Bacteria invariably contaminate all wounds that are open to the external or oral environment. Because the risk of infection rises with the increased size of an inoculum, one way to lessen the chance of wound infection is to decrease the bacterial count. This is easily accomplished by repeatedly irrigating the wound during surgery and closure. Irrigation dislodges bacteria and other foreign materials and rinses them out of the wound. Irrigation can be achieved by forcing *large volumes* of fluid under pressure on the wound. Although solutions containing antibiotics can be used, most surgeons simply use sterile saline or sterile water.

Wound débridement is the careful removal from injured tissue of necrotic and severely ischemic tissue and foreign material that would impede wound healing. In general, débridement is used only during care of traumatically incurred wounds or for severe tissue damage caused by a pathologic condition.

EDEMA CONTROL

Edema occurs after surgery as a result of tissue injury. Edema is an accumulation of fluid in the interstitial space because of transudation from damaged vessels and lymphatic obstruction by fibrin. Two variables help determine the degree of postsurgical edema. First, the greater the amount of tissue injury, the greater the amount of edema. Second, the more loose connective tissue that is contained in the injured region, the more edema is present. For example, attached gingiva has little loose connective tissue, so it exhibits little tendency toward edema; however, the lips and floor of the mouth contain large amounts of loose connective tissue and can swell significantly.

The dentist can control the amount of postsurgical edema by performing surgery in a manner that minimizes tissue damage. Some believe that ice applied to a freshly wounded area decreases vascularity and thereby diminishes transudation. However, no controlled study has verified the effectiveness of this practice. Patient positioning in the early postoperative period is also used to decrease edema by having the patient try to keep the head elevated above the rest of the body as much as possible during the first few postoperative days. Short-term, high-dose systemic corticosteroids can be administered to the patient and have an impressive ability to lessen inflammation and transudation (and thus edema). However, corticosteroids are useful for edema control only if administration is begun before tissue is damaged.

PATIENT GENERAL HEALTH AND NUTRITION

Proper wound healing depends on a patient's ability to resist infection, to provide essential nutrients for use as building materials, and to carry out reparative cellular processes. Numerous medical conditions impair a patient's ability to resist infection and heal wounds. These include conditions that establish a catabolic state of metabolism, that impede oxygen or nutrient delivery to tissues, or that require administration of drugs or physical agents that interfere with immunologic or wound-healing cells. Examples of diseases that induce a catabolic metabolic state include poorly controlled insulin-dependent diabetes mellitus, end-stage renal or hepatic disease, and malignant diseases. Conditions that interfere with the delivery of oxygen or nutrients to wounded tissues include severe chronic obstructive pulmonary disease, poorly compensated congestive heart failure, and drug addictions, such as ethanolism. Diseases requiring the administration of drugs that interfere with host defenses or wound-healing capabilities include autoimmune diseases for which long-term corticosteroid therapy is given and malignancies for which cytotoxic agents and irradiation are used.

The surgeon can help improve the patient's chances of having normal healing of an elective surgical wound by evaluating and optimizing the patient's general health status before surgery. For malnourished patients, this includes improving the nutritional status so that the patient is in a positive nitrogen balance and an anabolic metabolic state.

CHAPTER 4

Wound Repair

JAMES R. HUPP

CHAPTER OUTLINE

An important aspect of any surgical procedure is the preparation of the wound for healing. A thorough understanding of the biology of normal tissue repair is therefore mandatory for individuals intending to perform surgery.

Tissue injury can be caused by pathologic conditions or by traumatic events. The dental surgeon has some control over pathologic tissue damage such as the likelihood of a wound infection. However, the surgeon can favorably or unfavorably alter the amount and severity of traumatically induced tissue injury and therefore can contribute to promoting or impeding wound healing.

This chapter discusses the ways in which perioperative tissue injury occurs and the events normally present during the healing of soft and hard tissues.

CAUSES OF TISSUE DAMAGE

Traumatic injuries can be caused by physical or chemical insults (Box 4-1). Physical means of producing tissue damage include incision or crushing, extremes of temperature or irradiation, desiccation, and obstruction of arterial inflow or venous outflow. Chemicals able to cause injury include those with unphysiologic pH or tonicity, those that disrupt protein integrity, and those that cause ischemia by producing vascular constriction or thrombosis.

WOUND REPAIR

Epithelialization

Injured epithelium has a genetically programmed regenerative ability that allows it to reestablish its integrity through proliferation, migration, and a process known as *contact inhibition*. In general, any free edge of epithelium continues to migrate (by proliferation of germinal epithelial cells that advance the free edge forward) until it comes into contact with another free edge of epithelium, where it is signaled to stop growing laterally.

Although it is theorized that chemical mediators (released from epithelial cells that have lost contact with other epithelial cells circumferentially) regulate this process, no definitive evidence for this is yet available. Wounds in which only the surface epithelium is injured (i.e., abrasions) heal by proliferation of epithelium across the wound bed from the epithelium contained in rete pegs and adnexal tissues. Because epithelium does not normally contain blood vessels, the epithelium in wounds in which the subepithelial tissue is also damaged proliferates across whatever vascularized tissue bed is available and stays under the portion of the superficial blood clot that desiccates (i.e., forms a scab) until it reaches another epithelial margin. Once the wound is fully epithelialized, the scab loosens and is dislodged.

An example of the rarely detrimental effect of the process of contact inhibition controlling epithelialization occurs when an opening is accidentally made into a maxillary sinus during tooth extraction. If the epithelium of both the sinus wall and the oral mucosa is injured, it begins to proliferate in both areas. In this case the first free epithelial edge the sinus epithelium may contact is oral mucosa, thereby creating an oroantral fistula (i.e., an epithelialized tract between the oral cavity and the maxillary sinus).

The process of reepithelialization (i.e., secondary epithelialization) is sometimes used therapeutically by oral and maxillofacial surgeons during certain preprosthetic surgical procedures in which an area of oral mucosa is denuded of epithelium (i.e., unattached gingiva) and then left to epithelialize by adjacent epithelium (i.e., attached gingiva) creeping over the wound bed.

Stages of Wound Healing

Regardless of the cause of nonepithelial tissue injury, a stereotypic process is initiated that, if able to proceed unimpeded,

BOX 4-1

Causes of Tissue Damage

PHYSICAL
- Compromised blood flow
- Crushing
- Desiccation
- Incision
- Irradiation
- Overcooling
- Overheating

CHEMICAL
- Agents with unphysiologic pH
- Agents with unphysiologic tonicity
- Proteases
- Vasoconstrictors
- Thrombogenic agents

works to restore tissue integrity. This process is called wound healing. The process has been divided into basic stages that, although not mutually exclusive, take place in this sequence. These three basic stages are (1) inflammatory, (2) fibroplastic, and (3) remodeling.

Inflammatory Stage

The inflammatory stage begins the moment tissue injury occurs and, in the absence of factors that prolong inflammation, lasts 3 to 5 days. The inflammatory stage has two phases: vascular and cellular. The vascular events set in motion during inflammation begin with an initial vasoconstriction of disrupted vessels as a result of normal vascular tone. The vasoconstriction slows blood flow into the area of injury, promoting blood coagulation. Within minutes, histamine and prostaglandins E_1 and E_2, elaborated by white blood cells, cause vasodilation and open small spaces between endothelial cells, which allows plasma to leak and leukocytes to migrate into interstitial tissues. Fibrin from the transudated plasma causes lymphatic obstruction, and the transudated plasma—aided by obstructed lymphatic vessels—accumulates in the area of injury, functioning to dilute contaminants. This fluid collection is called edema (Fig. 4-1).

The cardinal signs of inflammation are redness (i.e., erythema) and swelling (i.e., edema), with warmth and pain—*rubor et tumour cum calore et dolore* (Celsius, 30 BC to AD 38)—and loss of function—*functio laesa* (Virchow, 1821-1902). Warmth and erythema are caused by vasodilation; swelling is caused by transudation of fluid; and pain and loss of function are caused by histamine, kinins, and prostaglandins released by leukocytes, as well as by pressure from edema.

The cellular phase of inflammation is triggered by the activation of serum complement by tissue trauma. Complement-split products, particularly C3a and C5a, act as chemotactic factors and cause polymorphonuclear leukocytes (neutrophils) to stick to the side of blood vessels (margination) and then migrate through the vessel walls (diapedesis). Once in contact with foreign materials (e.g., bacteria), the neutrophils release the contents of their lysosomes (degranulation). The lysosomal enzymes (consisting primarily of proteases) work to destroy bacteria and other foreign materials and to digest necrotic tissue. Clearance of debris is also aided by monocytes, such as macrophages, which phagocytize foreign and necrotic materials. With time, lymphocytes accumulate at the site of tissue injury. The lymphocytes are in the B or T groups: B lymphocytes are able to recognize antigenic material, produce antibodies that assist the remainder of the immune system in identifying foreign materials, and interact with complement to lyse foreign cells. T lymphocytes are divided into three principal subgroups: (1) helper T cells, which stimulate B cell proliferation and differentiation; (2) suppressor T cells, which work to regulate the function of helper T cells; and (3) cytotoxic (killer) T cells, which lyse cells bearing foreign antigens.

The inflammatory stage is sometimes referred to as the *lag phase,* because this is the period during which no significant gain in wound strength occurs (because little collagen deposition is taking place). The principal material holding a wound together during the inflammatory stage is fibrin, which possesses little tensile strength (Fig. 4-2).

Fibroplastic Stage

The strands of fibrin, which are derived from the blood coagulation, crisscross wounds to form a latticework on which fibroblasts can begin laying down ground substance and tropocollagen. This is the fibroplastic stage of wound repair. The ground substance consists of several mucopolysaccharides, which act to cement collagen fibers together. The fibroblasts transform local and circulating pluripotential mesenchymal cells that begin tropocollagen production on the third or fourth day after tissue injury. Fibroblasts also secrete fibronectin, a protein that performs several functions. Fibronectin helps stabilize fibrin, assists in recognizing foreign material that should be removed by the immune system, acts as a chemotactic factor for fibroblasts, and helps to guide macrophages along fibrin strands for eventual phagocytosis of fibrin by macrophages.

The fibrin network is also used by new capillaries, which bud from existing vessels along the margins of the wound and run along fibrin strands to cross the wound. As fibroplasia continues, with increasing ingrowth of new cells, fibrinolysis occurs, which is caused by plasmin brought in by the new capillaries to remove the fibrin strands that have become unnecessary (Fig. 4-3).

Fibroblasts deposit tropocollagen, which undergoes cross-linking to produce collagen. Initially, collagen is produced in excessive amounts and is laid down in a haphazard manner. The poor orientation of fibers decreases the effectiveness of a given amount of collagen to produce wound strength, so an overabundance of collagen is necessary to strengthen the healing wound initially. Despite the poor organization of collagen, wound strength rapidly increases during the fibroplastic stage, which normally lasts 2 to 3 weeks. If a wound is placed under tension at the beginning of fibroplasia, it tends to pull apart along the initial line of injury. However, if the wound were to be placed under tension near the end of fibroplasia, it would open along the junction between old collagen previously on the edges of the wound and newly deposited collagen. Clinically, the wound at the end of the fibroplastic stage will be stiff because of the excessive amount of collagen, erythematous because of the high degree of vascularization, and able to withstand 70% to 80% as much tension as uninjured tissue (Fig. 4-4).

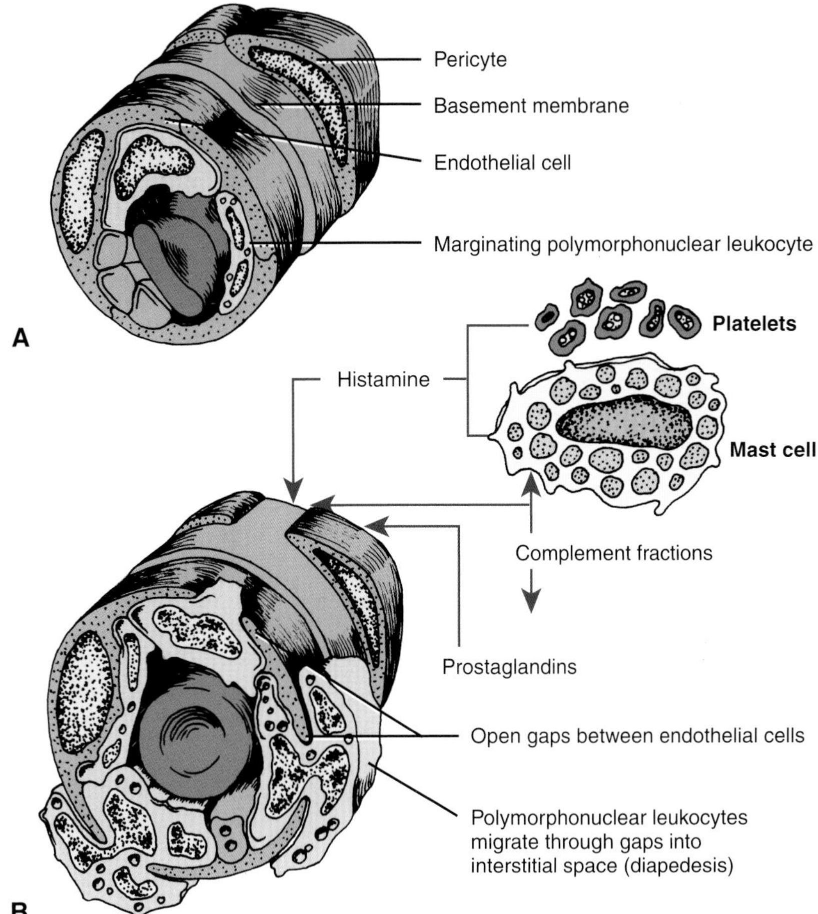

FIGURE 4-1 Early vascular responses to injury. Initial transient vasoconstriction (A) is soon followed by vasodilation (B). Vasodilation is caused by the actions of histamine, prostaglandins, and other vasodilatory substances. Dilation causes intercellular gaps to occur, which allows egress of plasma and emigration of leukocytes. (Copyright 1977 and 1981. Icon Learning Systems. Reprinted with permission from the *Clinical Symposia,* vol. 29/3 illustrated by John A. Craig, MD, and vol. 22/2 illustrated by Frank H. Netter, MD. All rights reserved.)

Remodeling Stage

The final stage of wound repair, which continues indefinitely, is known as the *remodeling stage,* although some use the term *wound maturation.* During this stage, many of the previous randomly laid collagen fibers are destroyed as they are replaced by new collagen fibers, which are oriented to better resist tensile forces on the wound. In addition, wound strength increases slowly but not with the same magnitude of increase seen during the fibroplastic stage. Wound strength never reaches more than 80% to 85% of the strength of uninjured tissue. Because of the more efficient orientation of the collagen fibers, fewer of them are necessary; the excess is removed, which allows the scar to soften. As wound metabolism lessens, vascularity is decreased, which diminishes wound erythema. Elastin found in normal skin and ligaments is not replaced during wound healing, so injuries in those tissues cause a loss of flexibility along the scarred area (Fig. 4-5).

A final process, which begins near the end of fibroplasia and continues during the early portion of remodeling, is wound contraction. In most cases wound contraction plays a beneficial role in wound repair, although the exact mechanism that contracts a wound is still unclear. During wound contraction the edges of a wound migrate toward each other. In a wound in which the edges are not or will not be placed in apposition, wound contraction diminishes the size of the wound. However, contraction can cause problems, such as those seen in victims of third-degree (full-thickness) burns of the skin, who develop deforming and debilitating contractures if wounds are not covered with skin grafts and aggressive physical therapy is not performed. Another example of detrimental contraction is seen in individuals suffering sharply curved lacerations, who frequently are left with a mound of tissue on the concave side of the scar because of wound contraction, even when the edges are well readapted. Contraction can be lessened by placement of a layer of epithelium between the free edges of a wound. Surgeons use this phenomenon when they place skin grafts on the bared periosteum during a vestibuloplasty or on full-thickness burn wounds.

SURGICAL SIGNIFICANCE OF WOUND HEALING CONCEPTS

The surgeon can create conditions that augment or impede the natural wound repair process. Adherence to surgical principles

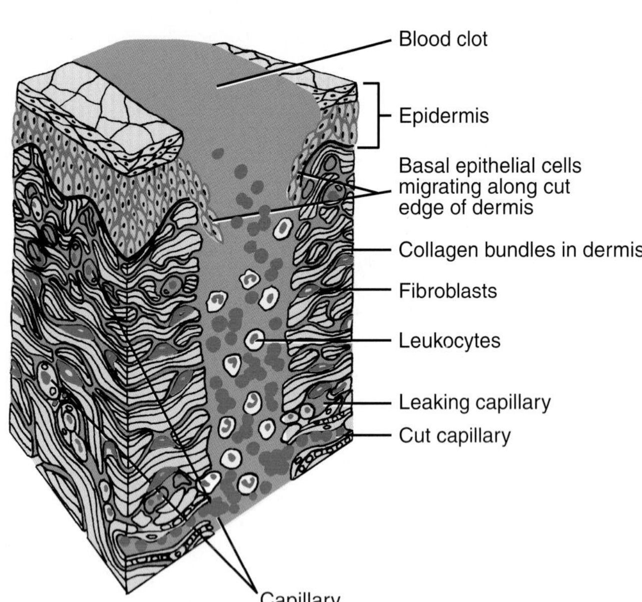

FIGURE 4-2 Inflammatory (lag) stage of wound repair. Wound fills with clotted blood, inflammatory cells, and plasma. Adjacent epithelium begins to migrate into wound, and undifferentiated mesenchymal cells begin to transform into fibroblasts. (Copyright 1977 and 1981. Icon Learning Systems. Reprinted with permission from the *Clinical Symposia,* vol. 29/3 illustrated by John A. Craig, MD, and vol. 22/2 illustrated by Frank H. Netter, MD. All rights reserved.)

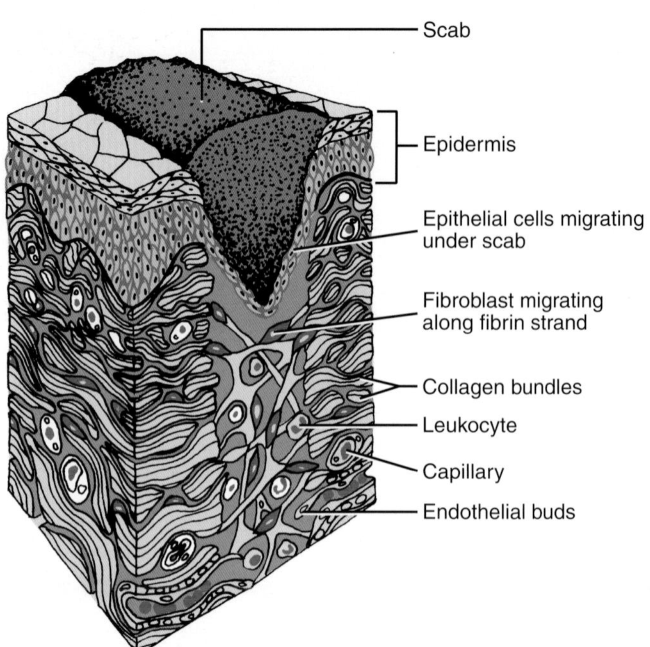

FIGURE 4-3 Migratory phase of fibroplastic stage of wound repair. Continued epithelial migration occurs, leukocytes dispose of foreign and necrotic materials, capillary ingrowth begins, and fibroblasts migrate into wound along fibrin strands. (Copyright 1977 and 1981. Icon Learning Systems. Reprinted with permission from the *Clinical Symposia,* vol. 29/3 illustrated by John A. Craig, MD, and vol. 22/2 illustrated by Frank H. Netter, MD. All rights reserved.)

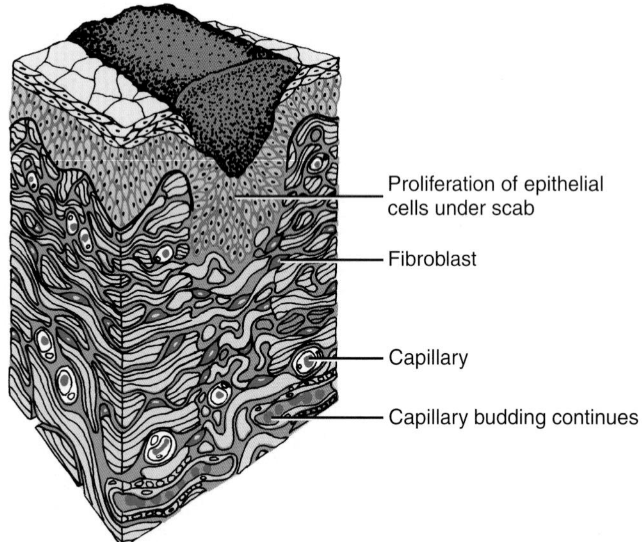

FIGURE 4-4 Proliferative phase of fibroplastic stage of wound repair. Proliferation increases epithelial thickness, collagen fibers are haphazardly laid down by fibroblasts, and budding capillaries begin to establish contact with their counterparts from other sites in wound. (Copyright 1977 and 1981. Icon Learning Systems. Reprinted with permission from the *Clinical Symposia,* vol. 29/3 illustrated by John A. Craig, MD, and vol. 22/2 illustrated by Frank H. Netter, MD. All rights reserved.)

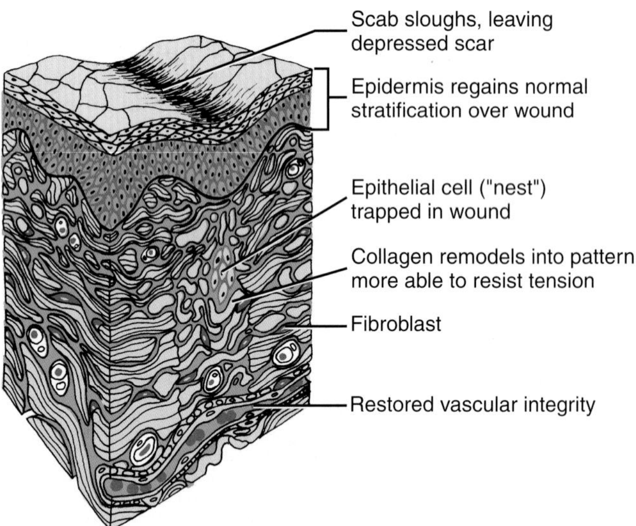

FIGURE 4-5 Remodeling stage of wound repair. Epithelial stratification is restored, collagen is remodeled into more efficiently organized patterns, fibroblasts slowly disappear, and vascular integrity is reestablished. (Copyright 1977 and 1981. Icon Learning Systems. Reprinted with permission from the *Clinical Symposia,* vol. 29/3 illustrated by John A. Craig, MD, and vol. 22/2 illustrated by Frank H. Netter, MD. All rights reserved.)

(see Chapter 3) facilitates optimal wound healing, with reestablishment of tissue continuity, minimization of scar size, and restoration of function. One should remember that no wound in skin, oral mucosa, or muscle heals without scar formation. The surgeon's goal with respect to scar formation is not to prevent a scar but rather to produce a scar that minimizes loss of function and looks as inconspicuous as possible.

Factors That Impair Wound Healing

Four factors can impair wound healing in an otherwise healthy individual: (1) foreign material, (2) necrotic tissue, (3) ischemia, and (4) wound tension.

Foreign Material

Foreign material is everything the host organism's immune system views as "nonself," including bacteria, dirt, and suture material. Foreign materials cause three basic problems. First, bacteria can proliferate and cause an infection in which bacterial proteins that destroy host tissue are released. Second, nonbacterial foreign material acts as a haven for bacteria by sheltering them from host defenses and thus promoting infection. Third, foreign material is often antigenic and can stimulate a chronic inflammatory reaction that decreases fibroplasia.

Necrotic Tissue

Necrotic tissue in a wound causes two problems. The first is that its presence serves as a barrier to the ingrowth of reparative cells. The inflammatory stage is then prolonged while white blood cells work to remove the necrotic debris through the processes of enzymatic lysis and phagocytosis. The second problem is that, similar to foreign material, necrotic tissue serves as a protected niche for bacteria. Necrotic tissue frequently includes blood that collects in a wound (hematoma), where it can serve as an excellent nutrient source for bacteria.

Ischemia

Decreased blood supply to a wound interferes with wound repair in several ways. Decreased blood supply can lead to further tissue necrosis and can lessen the delivery to a wound of antibodies, white blood cells, and antibiotics, which thereby increases the chances of wound infection. Wound ischemia decreases the delivery of oxygen and the nutrients necessary for proper healing. Ischemia can be caused by several things, including tight or incorrectly located sutures, improperly designed flaps, excessive external pressure on a wound, internal pressure on a wound (seen, for example, with hematomas), systemic hypotension, peripheral vascular disease, and anemia.

Tension

Tension on a wound is the final factor that can impede wound healing. Tension in this case is anything tending to hold wound edges apart. If sutures are used to pull tissues together forcefully, the tissue encompassed by the sutures will be strangulated, producing ischemia. If sutures are removed too early in the healing process, the wound under tension will probably reopen and then heal with excessive scar formation and wound contraction. If sutures are left in too long in an attempt to overcome wound tension, the wound will still tend to spread open during the remodeling stage of healing, and the tract into the epithelium through which the sutures ran will epithelialize and leave permanent disfiguring marks.

Healing by Primary, Secondary, and Tertiary Intention

Clinicians use the terms *primary intention* and *secondary intention* to describe the two basic methods of wound healing. In healing by primary intention, the edges of a wound in which there is no tissue loss are placed and stabilized in essentially the same anatomic position they held before injury and are allowed to heal. Wound repair then occurs with minimal scar tissue, because the tissues would not "perceive" that an injury had occurred. Strictly speaking, healing by primary intention is only a theoretic ideal, impossible to attain clinically; however, the term is generally used to designate wounds in which the edges are closely reapproximated. This method of wound repair lessens the amount of reepithelialization, collagen deposition, contraction, and remodeling necessary during healing. Therefore, healing occurs more rapidly, with a lower risk of infection and with less scar formation than in wounds allowed to heal by secondary intention. Examples of wounds that heal by primary intention include well-repaired lacerations or incisions, well-reduced bone fractures, and anatomic nerve reanastomoses of recently severed nerves. In contrast, healing by secondary intention implies that a gap is left between the edges of an incision or laceration or between bone or nerve ends after repair, or it implies that tissue loss has occurred in a wound that prevents approximation of wound edges. These situations require a large amount of epithelial migration, collagen deposition, contraction, and remodeling during healing. Healing is slower and produces more scar tissue than is the case with healing by primary intention. Examples of wounds allowed to heal by secondary intention include extraction sockets, poorly reduced fractures, deep ulcers, and large avulsive injuries of any soft tissue.

Some surgeons use the term *tertiary intention* to refer to the healing of wounds through the use of tissue grafts to cover large wounds and bridge the gap between wound edges.

Healing of Extraction Sockets

The removal of a tooth initiates the same sequence of inflammation, epithelialization, fibroplasia, and remodeling seen in prototypic skin or mucosal wounds. As previously mentioned, sockets heal by secondary intention, and many months must pass before a socket heals to the degree to which it becomes difficult to distinguish from the surrounding bone when viewed radiographically.

When a tooth is removed, the remaining empty socket consists of cortical bone (the radiographic lamina dura) covered by torn periodontal ligaments, with a rim of oral epithelium (gingiva) left at the coronal portion. The socket fills with blood, which coagulates and seals the socket from the oral environment.

The inflammatory stage occurs during the first week of healing. White blood cells enter the socket to remove contaminating bacteria from the area and begin to break down any debris, such as bone fragments, that are left in the socket. Fibroplasia also begins during the first week, with the ingrowth of fibroblasts and capillaries. The epithelium migrates down the socket wall until it reaches a level at which it contacts epithelium from the other side of the socket or it encounters the bed of granulation tissue (i.e., tissue filled with numerous immature capillaries and fibroblasts) under the blood clot over which the epithelium can migrate. Finally, during the first week of healing, osteoclasts accumulate along the crestal bone.

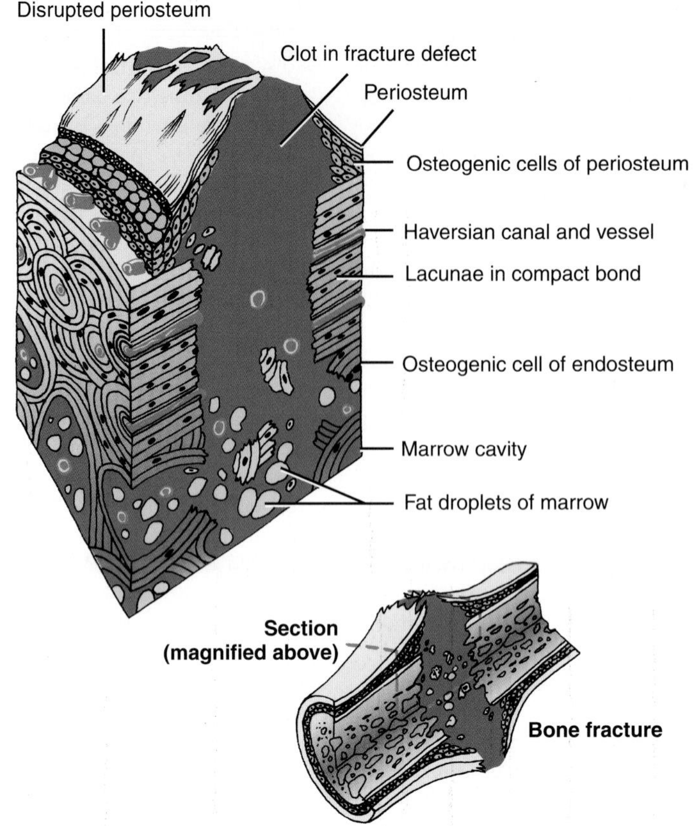

FIGURE 4-6 Early phase of fibroplastic stage of bone repair. Osteogenic cells from periosteum and marrow proliferate and differentiate into osteoblasts, osteoclasts, and chondroblasts, and capillary budding begins. (Copyright 1977 and 1981. Icon Learning Systems. Reprinted with permission from the *Clinical Symposia,* vol. 29/3 illustrated by John A. Craig, MD, and vol. 22/2 illustrated by Frank H. Netter, MD. All rights reserved.)

The second week is marked by the large amount of granulation tissue that fills the socket. Osteoid deposition has begun along the alveolar bone lining the socket. In smaller sockets the epithelium may have become fully intact by this point.

The processes begun during the second week continue during the third and fourth weeks of healing, with epithelialization of most sockets complete at this time. The cortical bone continues to be resorbed from the crest and walls of the socket, and new trabecular bone is laid down across the socket. Not until 4 to 6 months after extraction is the cortical bone lining a socket usually fully resorbed; this is recognized radiographically by a loss of a distinct lamina dura. As bone fills the socket, the epithelium moves toward the crest and eventually becomes level with adjacent crestal gingiva. The only visible remnant of the socket after 1 year is the rim of fibrous (scar) tissue that remains on the edentulous alveolar ridge.

Bone Healing

The events that occur during normal wound healing of soft tissue injuries (e.g., inflammation, fibroplasia, and remodeling) also take place during the repair of an injured bone. However, in contrast to soft tissues, osteoblasts and osteoclasts are also involved to reconstitute and remodel the damaged ossified tissue.

Osteogenic cells (osteoblasts) important to bone healing are derived from the following three sources: (1) periosteum, (2) endosteum, and (3) circulating pluripotential mesenchymal cells. Osteoclasts, derived from monocyte precursor cells, function to resorb necrotic bone and bone that needs to be remodeled. Osteoblasts then lay down osteoid, which if immobile during healing, usually goes on to calcify.

The terms *primary intention* and *secondary intention* are appropriate for descriptions of bone repair. If a bone is fractured* and the free ends of the bone are more than 1 mm or so apart, the bone heals by secondary intention; that is, during the fibroplastic stage of healing, a large amount of collagen must be laid down to bridge the bony gap (Fig. 4-6). The fibroblasts and osteoblasts actually produce so much fibrous matrix that the healing tissue extends circumferentially beyond the free ends of the bone and forms what is called a *callus* (Fig. 4-7). Under normal conditions the fibrous tissue, including the callus, ossifies. During the remodeling stage, bone that was haphazardly produced is resorbed by osteoclasts, and osteoblasts lay down new bone directed to resist low-grade tensions placed on the bone (Fig. 4-8).

*The term *fracture* used with respect to bone repair includes not only traumatically injured bone but also bone cuts purposely made by a surgeon during reconstructive surgery.

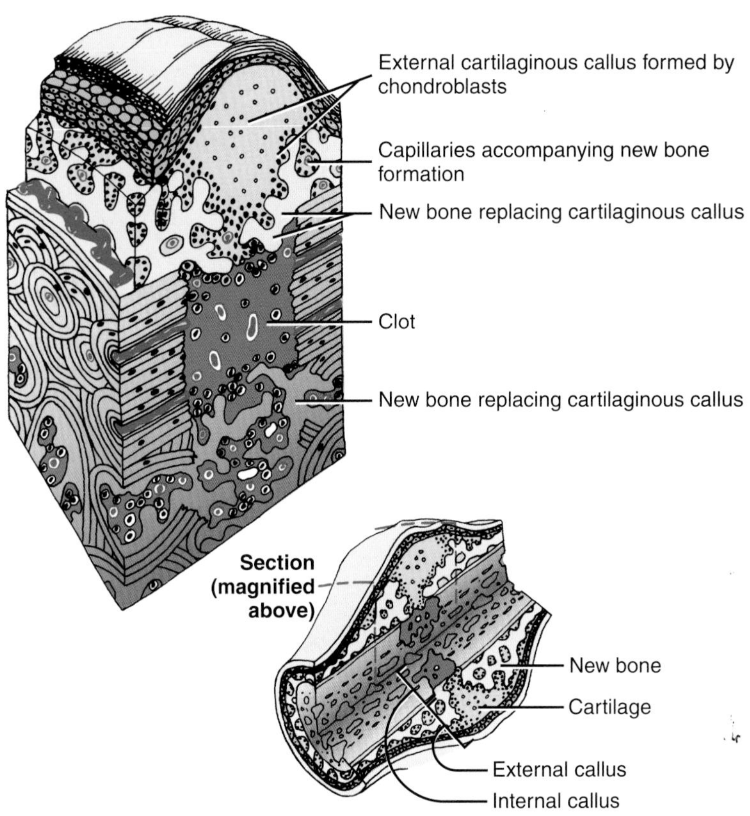

FIGURE 4-7 Late phase of fibroplastic stage of bone repair. Osteoclasts resorb necrotic bone. In areas of sufficient oxygen tension, osteoblasts lay down new bone; in areas of low oxygen tension, chondroblasts lay down cartilage. In addition, capillary ingrowth continues and internal and external calluses form. (Copyright 1977 and 1981. Icon Learning Systems. Reprinted with permission from the *Clinical Symposia,* vol. 29/3 illustrated by John A. Craig, MD, and vol. 22/2 illustrated by Frank H. Netter, MD. All rights reserved.)

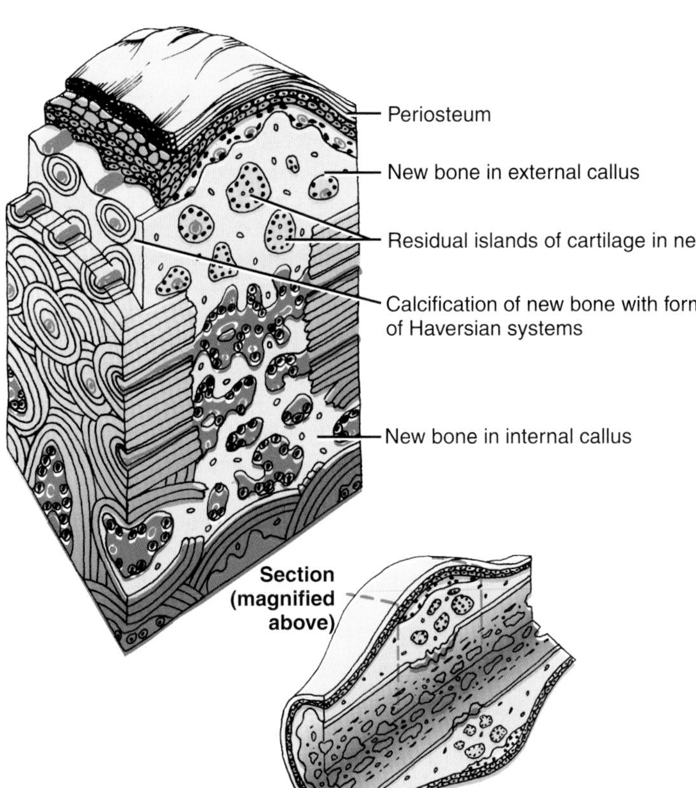

FIGURE 4-8 Remodeling stage of bone repair. Osteoclasts remove unnecessary bone, and osteoblasts lay new bone tissue in response to stresses placed on bone. New haversian systems develop as concentric layers of cortical bone are deposited along blood vessels. Calluses gradually decrease in size. (Copyright 1977 and 1981. Icon Learning Systems. Reprinted with permission from the *Clinical Symposia,* vol. 29/3 illustrated by John A. Craig, MD, and vol. 22/2 illustrated by Frank H. Netter, MD. All rights reserved.)

Healing of bone by primary intention occurs when the bone is incompletely fractured so that the fractured ends do not become separated from each other (greenstick fracture), or when a surgeon closely reapproximates and rigidly stabilizes the fractured ends of a bone (anatomic reduction of the fracture). In both of these situations, little fibrous tissue is produced and reossification of the tissue within the fracture area occurs quickly, with minimal callus formation. The surgical technique that comes closest to allowing bone to heal by primary intention is anatomic reduction of the application of bone plates that rigidly hold the ends of the bone together. This minimizes the distance between the ends of a fractured bone so that ossification across the fracture gap can occur with little intervening fibrous tissue formation.

Two factors are important to proper bone healing: (1) vascularity and (2) immobility. The fibrous connective tissue that forms in a bony fracture site requires a high degree of vascularity (which carries blood with a normal oxygen content) for eventual ossification. If vascularity or oxygen supplies are sufficiently compromised, cartilage forms instead of bone. Furthermore, if vascularity or oxygen supplies are poor, the fibrous tissue does not chondrify or ossify.

Placing bone under continuous or repeated cycles of some tension stimulates continued osteoblastic bone formation. Bone is formed perpendicular to lines of tension to help withstand the forces placed on it. This is the basis of the functional matrix concept of bone remodeling. However, excessive tension or torque placed on a healing fracture site produces mobility at the site. This mobility compromises vascularity of the wound and favors the formation of cartilage or fibrous tissue rather than bone along the fracture line; in a contaminated fracture it promotes wound infection (Fig. 4-8).

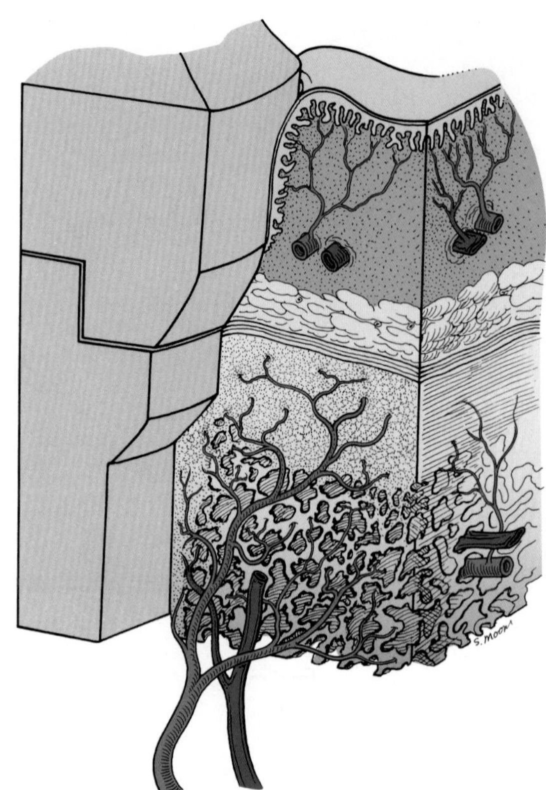

FIGURE 4-9 Osseointegrated implant with direct bone and implant contact. Surface epithelium migration along implant halted by the direct bone and implant integration.

Implant Osseointegration

The discovery of osseointegration in the 1960s forced a reexamination of traditional concepts of wound healing. Before acceptance of these findings it was thought that the body would eventually expel any foreign material placed through an epithelial surface. Expulsion would occur as the epithelium bordering the foreign material migrated down along the interface with the foreign material, finally fully surrounding the portion of the foreign body protruding into the body and causing the material to be completely external to the epithelial barrier. For a dental implant, this meant eventual loosening and loss of the implant.

The innate tendency of nonmalignant epithelium to surround and externalize foreign material was thought to be the result of the principle of contact inhibition (discussed previously), whereby any epithelial surface disrupted by any force or object triggers epithelial growth and migration. The epithelium continues to spread until it contacts other epithelial cells and is inhibited from further lateral growth. Investigators found that if an inert foreign material was placed through an epithelial barrier and allowed to develop a biologic bond with surrounding bone, epithelial migration down into the bone along the implant surface would be resisted. However, if instead, the implant had an intervening layer of connective tissue between itself and the bone, epithelium would migrate down the implant, externalizing it. Thus when an implant integrated with bone (osseointegration), lateral growth of epithelium stopped without contact inhibition, as it was classically conceived to function (Fig. 4-9).

The reasons why epithelium does not continue to migrate when it meets a bone and implant interface are still unclear. Nonetheless, dentistry has used this aberration in normal wound healing principles to provide integrated metal posts (implants) that are useful to stabilize dental prostheses. Surgeons use similar techniques to place implants through skin in other body sites to stabilize prosthetic ears, eyes, and noses.

Wound healing around dental implants involves the two basic factors: (1) healing of bone to the implant and (2) healing of alveolar soft tissue to the implant. Dental implants made of pure titanium are used in the discussion of healing around dental implants; similar healing occurs around properly placed implants made of other inert materials.

Bone healing onto the surface of an implant must occur before any soft tissue forms between the bone and implant surfaces. Maximizing the likelihood of bone winning this race with soft tissue to cover the implant requires the following four factors: (1) a short distance between the bone and implant, (2) viable bone at or near the surface of the bone along the implant, (3) no movement of the implant while bone is attaching to its surface, and (4) an implant surface free of contamination by organic or inorganic materials.

A short distance between the bone and implant depends on preparing a bony site into which the implant fits precisely. Minimizing bone damage during site preparation preserves the viability of bone near the implant surface. Much of the damage caused by preparing an implant site is the result of heat from friction during the cutting process.

Limiting heat production and rapidly dissipating the heat created at the site help protect the viability of bone along the cut surface. This is accomplished by using sharp bone-cutting instruments and limited cutting speeds to minimize frictional heat and by keeping the bone cool with irrigation during site preparation. Additional damage to the cut surface of bone may occur if the site becomes infected. This is addressed to some degree by using aseptic surgical techniques, systemic topical antibiotics, or both.

Keeping forces off the implant prevents movement along the healing bone and implant interface during the critical portion of the healing period. Countersinking implants and using low-profile healing screws decrease the ability of any forces to be delivered to the implant. Covering the top of the implant with gingiva during healing further protects it. Implants that are threaded or otherwise fit tightly into the prepared site are better protected from movement than nonthreaded or loose implants. Eventually, once initial integration has occurred, some limited daily pressure on the implant (1000 μm of strain) will actually hasten cortical bone deposition on the implant surface.

Finally, the surface to which bone is intended to attach must be free of surface contaminants. Such contaminants include bacteria, oil, glove powder, foreign metals, and foreign proteins. The surface of an implant intended to osseointegrate must not be handled with bare or gloved fingers or forceps made of a metal different from the implant and must not have retained machine oil or detergent.

The surface of pure titanium implants is completely covered by a 2000-Å-thick layer of titanium oxide. This stabilizes the surface, and it is to this oxidized surface that bone must attach for osseointegration to occur.

Regardless of how much care is taken to minimize damage to bone during implant site preparation, a superficial layer of bone along the surface of a prepared implant site becomes nonviable as a result of thermal and vascular trauma. Although the living cells in the bone die, the inorganic bone structure remains. Under the influence of local growth factors, bone cells directly underlying this bone structure and blood-borne undifferentiated mesenchymal cells repopulate and remodel the bony scaffold with osteoblasts, osteoclasts, and osteocytes. The nonviable bone is slowly replaced with new, viable cortical bone through the process of creeping substitution. Cutting cones move through the bone at a rate of 40 μm/d, removing dead bone and leaving new osteoid.

At the implant surface, glycosaminoglycans secreted by osteocytes coat the oxide layer. Soon osteoblasts begin to secrete a layer of osteoid over the proteoglycan layer. Bone then forms if proper conditions (e.g., no implant movement and good oxygen supply) continue during the months required for healing. The greater the amount of available implant surface, the greater the amount of implant osseointegration. Thus longer or wider-diameter implants and those with sandblasted rather than polished surfaces have more surface available for osseointegration.

The initial deposition of bone must occur before epithelium migrates onto or fibrous connective tissue forms on the implant surface. If soft tissue arrives first at any part of the implant surface, bone will never replace the soft tissue at that site. If too much of the implant surface becomes covered with soft tissue rather than bone, the implant will not become sufficiently osseointegrated to use for a dental prosthesis.

Clinicians have found that in some circumstances they can selectively aid the bone-forming process in its race to cover a surface before soft tissue fills the site. An example of this is the use of woven membranes that have a pore size adequate to allow oxygen and other nutrients to reach the bone grown beneath the membrane, while keeping fibroblasts and other tissue elements outside the membrane. By selectively excluding soft tissues, bone is "guided" into a desired position; thus *guided-tissue regeneration* is the term used to describe this process.

The component of an implant that extends through the oral mucosa also has the ability to alter the contact inhibition process that normally controls closure of openings through epithelium. In this case, once oral epithelium reaches the surface of a titanium abutment, it seems to stop migrating and secretes a ground substance that attaches the soft tissue to the metal. A hemidesmosomal, basal lamina system forms, further strengthening soft tissue attaching to the implant abutment.

Facial Neuropathology of Traumatic Origin

Injuries to sensory nerves of the maxillofacial region occasionally occur as the result of facial fractures, during the treatment of oral pathologic conditions, or when maxillofacial reconstructive surgery is performed. Fortunately, most injured nerves spontaneously recover. However, in the past little was done to treat persistent sensory nerve disorders. Recent advances in the understanding of how nerves heal and in the surgical means of repairing peripheral nerves provide patients with the possibility of partially or fully regaining normal nerve function.

The three branches of the trigeminal nerve injured most commonly, for which the altered sensation is clinically significant, are (1) the inferior alveolar-mental nerve, (2) the lingual nerve, and (3) the infraorbital nerve. When the inferior alveolar-mental nerve is injured, the usual causes are the following:

1. Mandibular (body) fractures
2. Preprosthetic surgical procedures
3. Sagittal split osteotomy surgery
4. Mandibular resection for oral neoplasms
5. Removal of impacted lower third molars

Lingual nerve damage occurs in the course of surgery to remove oral malignancies or impacted third molars. Injury to the infraorbital nerve is most common during zygomatico-maxillary complex or orbital blow-out fractures.

Classification

Research and clinical experience have shown that surgical intervention to repair damaged nerves is more successful when performed soon after the injury has occurred. Thus an understanding of the various types of nerve damage, especially their prognoses, is important because it enables the clinician to decide when referral for peripheral nerve surgery is warranted.

The three types of nerve injuries are (1) neurapraxia, (2) axonotmesis, and (3) neurotmesis (Fig. 4-10). Although a determination as to which type of nerve damage has occurred is usually made retrospectively, knowledge of the pathophysiology of each type is important for gaining an appreciation of nerve healing.

Neurapraxia, the least severe form of peripheral nerve injury, is a contusion of a nerve in which continuity of the

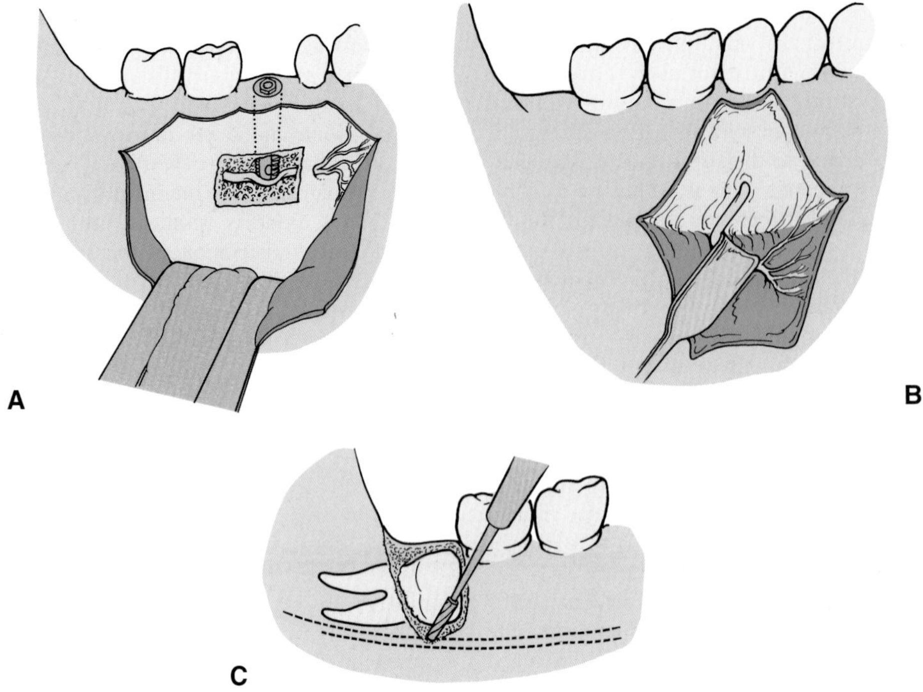

FIGURE 4-10 Three types of peripheral nerve injury. A, Neurapraxia. Injury to nerve causes no loss of continuity of axon or endoneurium. Example shown is implant placed in inferior alveolar canal, compressing the nerve. B, Axonotmesis. Injury to nerve causes loss of axonal continuity but preserves endoneurium. Example shown is overly aggressive retraction of mental nerve. C, Neurotmesis. Injury to nerve causes loss of axonal and endoneurium continuity. Example is cutting of inferior alveolar nerve during removal of deeply impacted third molar.

epineurial sheath and the axons is maintained. Blunt trauma or traction (i.e., stretching) of a nerve, inflammation around a nerve, or local ischemia of a nerve can produce a neurapraxia. Because there has been no loss in axonal continuity, spontaneous full recovery of nerve function usually occurs in a few days or weeks.

Axonotmesis has occurred when the continuity of the axons but not the epineurial sheath is disrupted. Severe blunt trauma, nerve crushing, or extreme traction of a nerve can produce this type of injury. Because the epineural sheath is still intact, axonal regeneration can (but does not always) occur with a resolution of nerve dysfunction in 2 to 6 months.

Neurotmesis, the most severe type of nerve injury, involves a complete loss of nerve continuity. This form of damage can be produced by badly displaced fractures, severance by bullets or knives during an assault, or by iatrogenic transection. Prognosis for spontaneous recovery of nerves that have undergone neurotmesis is poor, except if the ends of the affected nerve have somehow been left in approximation and properly oriented.

Nerve Healing

Nerve healing usually has two phases: (1) degeneration and (2) regeneration. Two types of degeneration can occur. The first is *segmental demyelination,* in which the myelin sheath is dissolved in isolated segments. This partial demyelination causes a slowing of conduction velocity and may prevent the transmission of some nerve impulses. Symptoms include paresthesia (a spontaneous and subjective altered sensation that a patient does not find painful), dysesthesia (a spontaneous and subjective altered sensation that a patient finds uncomfortable), hyperesthesia (excessive sensitivity of a nerve to stimulation), and hypoesthesia (decreased sensitivity of a nerve to stimulation). Segmental demyelination can occur after neurapraxic injuries or with vascular or connective tissue disorders (Fig. 4-11).

Wallerian degeneration is the second type of degeneration occurring after nerve trauma. In this process the axons and myelin sheath of the nerve distal to the site of nerve trunk interruption* (away from the central nervous system) undergo disintegration in their entirety. The axons proximal to the site of injury (toward the central nervous system) also undergo some degeneration, occasionally all the way to the cell body but generally just for a few nodes of Ranvier. Wallerian degeneration stops all nerve conduction distal to the proximal axonal stump. This type of degeneration follows nerve transsection and other destructive processes that affect peripheral nerves (Fig. 4-11).

Regeneration of a peripheral nerve can begin almost immediately after nerve injury. Normally the proximal nerve stump sends out a group of new fibers (the growth cone) that grow down the remnant Schwann cell tube. Growth progresses at a rate of 1 to 1.5 mm/d and continues until the site innervated by the nerve is reached or growth is blocked by fibrous connective tissue or bone. During regeneration, new myelin

*The terms *distal* and *proximal* used in the description of nerves and bones refer to positions farthest away from (i.e., distal) or nearest to (i.e., proximal) the central nervous system. In this case, distal is not used in the same sense as is common when referring to teeth and the dental arch.

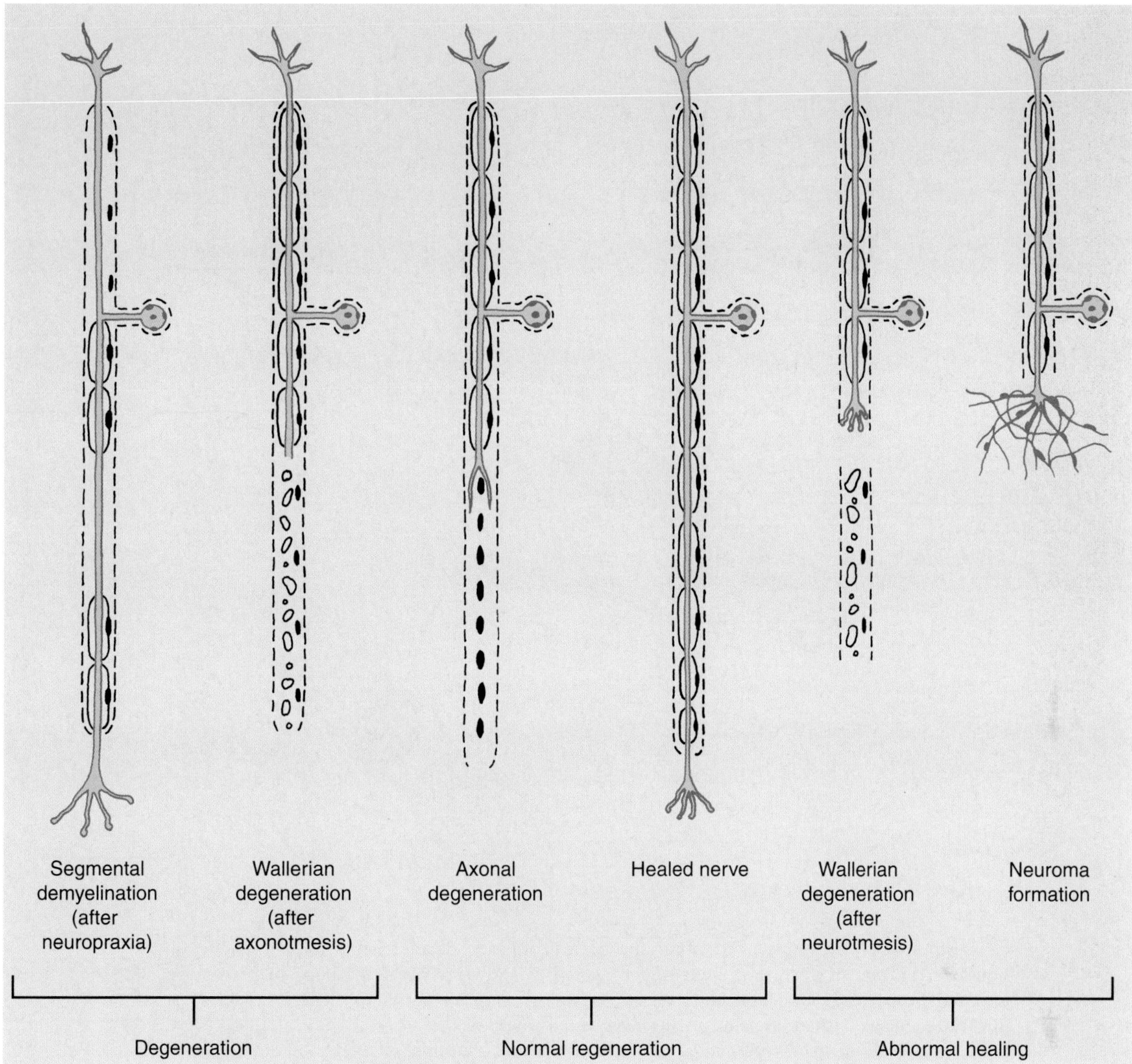

FIGURE 4-11 Diagram of normal and abnormal peripheral nerve response to injury.

sheaths may form as the axons increase in diameter. As functional contacts are made, the patient will experience altered sensations in the previously anesthetic area, which take the form of paresthesias or dysesthesias.

Problems can occur during regeneration that prevent normal nerve healing. If the continuity of the Schwann cell tube is disrupted, connective tissue may enter the tube while it is partially vacant. When the growth cone reaches the connective tissue obstruction, it may find a way around it and continue on, or it may form a mass of aimless nerve fibers that constitutes a traumatic *neuroma* subject to pain production when disturbed (Fig. 4-12).

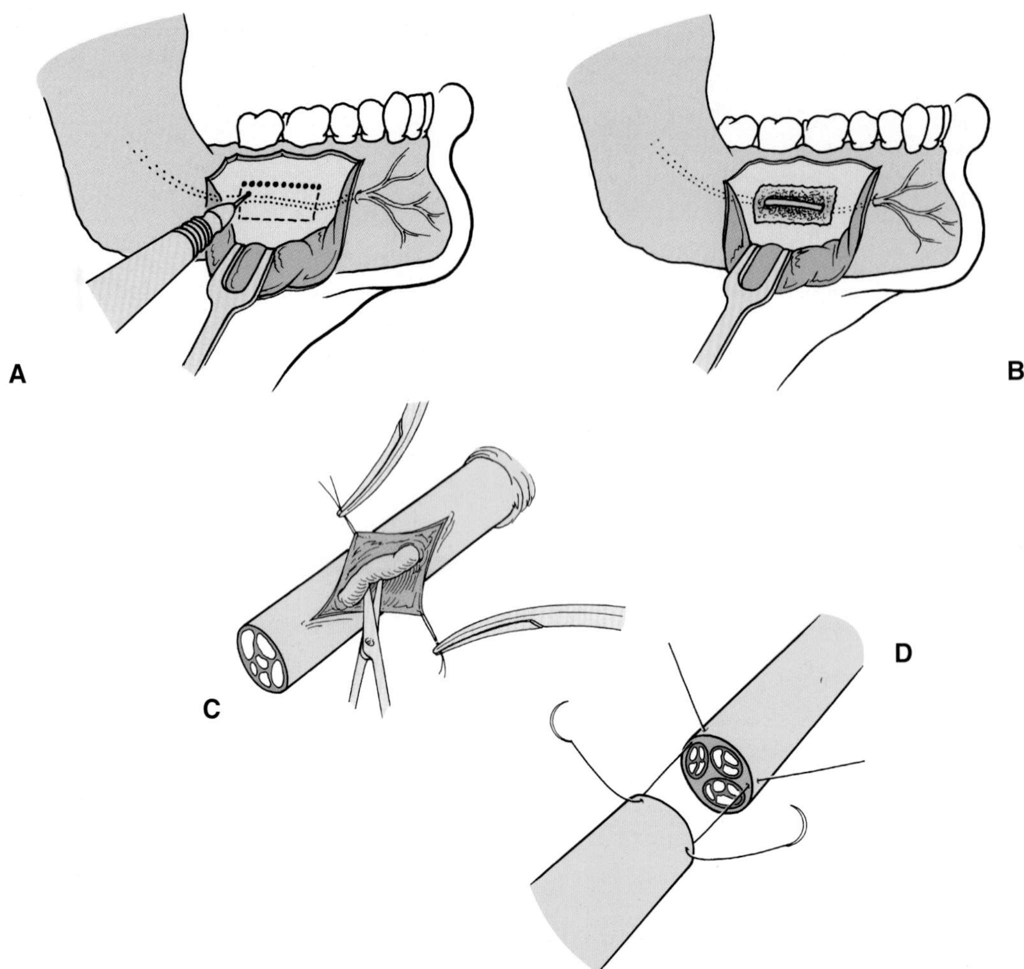

FIGURE 4-12 A, Example of intraoral approach to inferior alveolar nerve for microneurosurgery. Area over portion of nerve to be exposed is scored to allow the overlying bone to be removed. B, Exposed nerve ready for surgical repair. C, Opening of nerve trunk to expose fascicles. In this illustration an individual fascicle is being dissected away from the others as part of a decompression procedure. D, Epineurial repair of sectioned nerve trunk. Sutures are being placed to reestablish continuity of epineurium.

CHAPTER 5

Infection Control in Surgical Practice

JAMES R. HUPP

CHAPTER OUTLINE

It would be difficult for a person currently living in an industrialized society to have avoided being exposed to modern concepts of personal and public hygiene. Personal cleanliness and public sanitation have been ingrained in the culture of modern civilized societies through parental and public education and are reinforced by government regulations and media advertising. This awareness contrasts starkly with earlier centuries, when the importance of hygienic measures for the control of infectious diseases was not widely appreciated. The monumental work of Semmelweis, Koch, and Lister led to enlightenment about asepsis so that today the use of aseptic techniques seems instinctive.

Despite ongoing advancements in the area of infection control, health professionals must still learn and practice techniques that limit the spread of contagions. This is especially true for dentists performing surgery for two reasons: First, to perform surgery, the dentist typically violates an epithelial surface, the most important barrier against infection. Second, during most oral surgical procedures, the dentist, assistants, and equipment become contaminated with the patient's blood and saliva.

COMMUNICABLE PATHOGENIC ORGANISMS

Two of the most important pieces of knowledge in any conflict are the identity of the enemy and the enemy's strengths and weaknesses. In the case of oral surgery, the opposition includes virulent bacteria, mycobacteria, fungi, and viruses. The strengths of the opposition are the various means that organisms use to prevent their own destruction, and their weaknesses are their susceptibilities to chemical, biologic, and physical agents. By understanding the "enemy," the dentist can make rational decisions about infection control.

Bacteria

Upper Respiratory Tract Flora

Normal oral flora contains the microorganisms usually present in the saliva and on the surfaces of oral tissues in healthy, immunocompetent individuals who have not been exposed to agents that alter the composition of oral organisms. A complete description of this flora can be found in Chapter 15. In brief, normal oral flora consists of aerobic, gram-positive cocci (primarily streptococci), actinomycetes, anaerobic bacteria, and candidal species (Table 5-1). The total number of oral organisms is held in check by the following four main processes: (1) rapid epithelial turnover with desquamation; (2) host immunologic factors, such as salivary immunoglobulin A; (3) dilution by salivary flow; and (4) competition between oral organisms for available nutrients and attachment sites. Any agent—physical, biologic, or chemical—that alters any of the forces that keep oral microbes under control will permit poten-

TABLE 5-1

Normal Microbiologic Flora

Region	Bacteria
Oral cavity	Aerobic gram-positive organisms, primarily *Streptococcus* spp. *Actinomyces* spp. Anaerobic bacteria, including *Prevotella melaninogenica* *Candida* spp.
Nasal cavity	Aerobic gram-positive organisms, primarily *Streptococcus* spp. In children, *Haemophilus influenzae* frequently present In adults, *Staphylococcus aureus* frequently present
Facial skin	*Staphylococcus* spp., primarily *S. epidermidis*, occasionally *S. aureus* *Corynebacterium diphtheriae* *Propionibacterium acnes*
All areas below clavicles, including hands	*S. epidermidis* *C. diphtheriae* Gram-negative aerobes, such as *Escherichia coli*, *Klebsiella* spp., and *Proteus* spp. Anaerobic enteric organisms, including *Bacteroides fragilis*

tially pathologic organisms to overgrow and set the stage for a wound infection.

The flora of the nose and paranasal sinuses consists primarily of gram-positive aerobic streptococci and anaerobes. In addition, many children harbor *Haemophilus influenzae* bacteria in these areas, and many adults have *Staphylococcus aureus* as a part of their transient or resident nasal and paranasal sinus flora. The normal flora in this region of the body is limited by the presence of ciliated respiratory epithelium, secretory immunoglobulins, and epithelial desquamation. The epithelial cilia move organisms trapped in blankets of mucus into the alimentary tract.

Maxillofacial Skin Flora

The skin of the maxillofacial region has surprisingly few resident organisms in its normal flora. The bacteria *S. epidermidis* and *Corynebacterium diphtheriae* are the predominant species present. *Propionibacterium acnes* is found in pores and hair follicles, and many individuals carry *S. aureus*, spread from their nose, on their facial skin (Table 5-1).

The skin has several means of preventing surface organisms from entering. The most superficial layer of skin is composed of keratinized epithelial cells able to resist mild trauma. In addition, epithelial cells are joined by tight bonds that resist bacterial entrance.

Processes that alter skin flora are, for example, the application of occlusive dressings (which prevent skin desiccation and desquamation), dirt or dried blood (which provide increased nutrients for organisms), and antimicrobial agents (which disturb the balance between various organisms).

Nonmaxillofacial Flora

The flora below the region of the clavicles make up a gradually increasing number of aerobic gram-negative and anaerobic enteric organisms, especially moving toward the pelvic region and unwashed fingertips. General knowledge of these bacteria is important for dental surgeons when preparing themselves for surgery and when treating patients requiring venipuncture or other procedures away from the orofacial region.

Viral Organisms

Viruses are ubiquitous in the environment, but fortunately only a few pose a serious threat to the patient and the surgical team. The viral organisms that cause the most difficulty are the hepatitis B and C viruses and the human immunodeficiency virus (HIV). These viruses have differences in their susceptibility to inactivation that are important to understand when attempting to prevent their spread. Each virus is described with respect to hardiness and usual mode of transmission. In addition, the circumstances in which the clinician might suspect that an individual is carrying one of these viruses are briefly described, allowing the surgical team to take necessary precautions.

Hepatitis Viruses

Hepatitis A, B, C, and D viruses are responsible for most infectious hepatic diseases. Hepatitis A is spread primarily by contact with the feces of infected individuals. Hepatitis C may spread through contaminated feces or by contaminated blood. Hepatitis B and D are spread by contact with any human secretion.

The hepatitis B virus has the most serious risk of transmission for unvaccinated dentists, their staffs, and their patients. Hepatitis B virus is usually transmitted by the introduction of infected blood into the bloodstream of a susceptible person; however, infected individuals may also secrete large numbers of the virus in their saliva, which can enter an individual through any moist mucosal surface or epithelial (skin or mucosal) wound. Minute quantities of the virus have been found capable of transmitting disease (only 10^5 to 10^7 virions/mL blood). Unlike most viruses, the hepatitis virus is exceptionally resistant to desiccation and chemical disinfectants, including alcohols, phenols, and quaternary ammonium compounds. Therefore the hepatitis B virus is difficult to contain, particularly when oral surgery is being performed.

Fortunately, means of inactivating the virus include halogen-containing disinfectants (e.g., iodophor and hypochlorite), formaldehyde, ethylene oxide gas, all types of properly performed heat sterilization, and irradiation. These methods can be used to minimize the spread of hepatitis from one patient to another.

In addition to preventing patient-to-patient spread, the dentist and staff also need to take precautions to protect themselves from contamination, because several instances have occurred in which dentists have been the primary source of a hepatitis B epidemic. Dentists who perform oral surgical procedures are exposed to blood and saliva; therefore the dental surgery team should wear barriers to protect against contaminating any open wounds on the hands and any exposed mucosal surfaces. This includes wearing gloves, a face mask, and eyeglasses or goggles during surgery. The dental staff should continue to wear these protective devices when cleaning instruments and when handling impressions, casts, or specimens from patients. A common means of hepatitis inoculation is injury with a needle or blade that is contaminated with blood or saliva. In addition, members of the dental staff should receive hepatitis B

BOX 5-1

Methods Designed to Limit the Spread of Hepatitis Viruses

FROM INFECTED PATIENT TO OTHER PATIENTS

- Use disposable materials.
- Disinfect surfaces.
  - A. With halogen compounds
    1. Iodophors
    2. Hypochlorite (bleach)
  - B. With aldehydes
    1. Formaldehyde
    2. Glutaraldehyde
- Sterilize reusable instruments.
  - A. With heat
  - B. With ethylene oxide gas
- Use disposable materials.

FROM INFECTED PATIENT TO DENTAL STAFF

- Learn to recognize individuals likely to be carriers.
- Use barrier techniques (e.g., gloves, face mask, and eye protection) during surgery, when handling contaminated objects, and during cleanup.
- Promptly dispose of sharp objects into well-labeled protective containers.
- Dispose needles immediately after use or resheathing in-use instruments.
- Use an instrument to place a scalpel blade on or take one off a blade handle.
- Administer hepatitis B vaccine to dental staff.

vaccinations, which have been shown to effectively reduce an individual's susceptibility to hepatitis B infection, although the longevity of protection has not been definitively determined. Finally, office-cleaning personnel and commercial laboratory technicians can be protected by proper segregation and labeling of contaminated objects and by proper disposal of sharp objects (Box 5-1).

Recognition of all individuals known to be carriers of hepatitis B and C would aid in knowing when special precautions were necessary. However, only about half of the persons infected with hepatitis ever have clinical signs and symptoms of the infection, and some individuals who have completely recovered from the disease still shed intact virus particles in their secretions.

The concept of *universal precautions* was developed to address the inability of health care providers specifically to identify all patients with communicable diseases. The theory on which the universal precautions concept is based is that protection of self, staff, and patients from contamination by using barrier techniques when treating all patients as if they all had a communicable disease ensures that everyone is protected from those who do have an infectious process.

Universal precautions typically include having all doctors and staff who come in contact with patient blood or secretions, whether directly or in aerosol form, wear barrier devices, including a face mask, eye protection, and gloves. Universal precaution procedures go on to include decontaminating or disposing of all surfaces that are exposed to patient blood, tissue, and secretions. Finally, universal precautions mandate avoidance of touching, and thereby contaminating, surfaces (e.g., the dental record, uncovered light handles, and telephone) with contaminated gloves or instruments.

Human Immunodeficiency Virus

Because of its relative inability to survive outside the host organism, HIV (the cause of acquired immunodeficiency syndrome [AIDS]), acts in a fashion similar to other sexually transmitted infectious disease agents. That is, transfer of the virions from one individual to another requires direct contact between virus-laden blood or secretions from the infected host organism and a mucosal surface or epithelial wound of the potential host. Evidence has shown that the HIV loses its infectivity once desiccated. In addition, few persons carrying HIV secrete the virus in their saliva, and those who do tend to secrete extremely small amounts. No epidemiologic evidence supports the possibility of HIV infection by saliva alone. Even the blood of patients who are HIV-positive has low concentrations of infectious particles (10^6 particles/mL compared with 10^{13} particles/mL in hepatitis patients). This probably explains why professionals who are not in any of the known high-risk groups for HIV positivity have an extremely low probability of contracting it, even when exposed to the blood and secretions of large numbers of patients who are HIV-positive during the performance of surgery or if accidentally autoinoculated with contaminated blood or secretions. Nevertheless, until the transmission of HIV becomes fully understood, prudent surgeons will take steps to prevent the spread of infection from the HIV-carrying patient to themselves and their assistants through the use of universal precautions, including barrier techniques.

In general, the universal precautions used for bacterial, mycotic, and other viral processes protect the dentist, office staff, and other patients from the spread of the virus that causes AIDS (Box 5-1). Also important is that patients with depressed immune function be afforded extra care to prevent the spread of contagions to them. Thus all patients infected with HIV who have CD4+ T lymphocyte counts of less than 200/μL or category B or C HIV infection should be treated by doctors and staff free of clinically evident infectious diseases. These patients should not be put in a circumstance in which they are forced to be closely exposed to patients with clinically apparent symptoms of a communicable disease.

Mycobacterial Organisms

The only mycobacterial organism of significance to most dentists is *Mycobacterium tuberculosis*. Although tuberculosis (TB) is an uncommon disease in the United States and Canada, the frequent movement of persons between countries, including those where TB is common, continues to spread *M. tuberculosis* organisms worldwide. In addition, some newer strains of *M. tuberculosis* have become resistant to the drugs historically used to treat TB. Therefore it is important that measures be followed to prevent the spread of TB from patients to the dental team.

TB is transmitted primarily through exhaled aerosols that carry *M. tuberculosis* bacilli from the infected lungs of one individual to the lungs of another individual. Droplets are produced by those with untreated TB during breathing, coughing, sneezing, and speaking. *M. tuberculosis* is not a highly contagious microorganism. However, transmission can also occur via inadequately sterilized instruments, because although *M. tuberculosis* organisms do not form spores, they are highly resistant to desiccation and to most chemical disinfectants. To prevent transmission of TB from an infected individual to the dental staff, the staff should wear face masks whenever treating or in close contact with these patients. The organisms are sensitive to heat, ethylene oxide, and irradiation; therefore, to prevent their spread from patient to patient, all reusable instruments and supplies should be sterilized with heat or ethylene oxide gas. When safe to do so, patients with untreated TB should have their surgery postponed until they can begin treatment for their TB.

ASEPTIC TECHNIQUES AND UNIVERSAL PRECAUTIONS

Terminology

Different terms are used to describe various means of preventing infection. However, despite their differing definitions, terms such as *disinfection* and *sterilization* are often used interchangeably. This can lead to the misconception that a certain technique or chemical has sterilized an object when it has merely reduced the level of contamination. Therefore the dental team must be aware of the precise definition of words used for the various techniques of asepsis.

Sepsis is the breakdown of living tissue by the action of microorganisms and is usually accompanied by inflammation. Thus the mere presence of microorganisms, such as in bacteremia, does not constitute a septic state. *Asepsis* refers to the avoidance of sepsis. *Medical asepsis* is the attempt to keep patients, health care staff, and objects as free as possible of agents that cause infection. *Surgical asepsis* is the attempt to prevent microbes from gaining access to surgically created traumatic wounds.

Antiseptic and *disinfectant* are terms that are often misused. Both refer to substances that can prevent the multiplication of organisms capable of causing infection. The difference is that antiseptics are applied to living tissue, whereas disinfectants are designed for use on inanimate objects.

Sterility is the freedom from viable forms of microorganisms. Sterility represents an absolute state; there are no degrees of sterility. *Sanitization* is the reduction of the number of viable microorganisms to levels judged safe by public health standards. Sanitization should not be confused with sterilization. *Decontamination* is similar to sanitization, except that it is not connected with public health standards.

Concepts

Chemical and physical agents are the two principal means of reducing the number of microbes on a surface. Antiseptics, disinfectants, and ethylene oxide gas are the major chemical means of killing microorganisms on surfaces. Heat, irradiation, and mechanical dislodgment are the primary physical means of eliminating viable organisms (Box 5-2).

BOX 5-2

General Methods of Reducing the Number of Viable Organisms from a Surface

PHYSICAL
- Heat
- Mechanical dislodgment
- Radiation

CHEMICAL
- Antiseptics
- Disinfectants
- Ethylene oxide gas

The microbes that cause human disease include bacteria, viruses, mycobacteria, parasites, and fungi. The microbes within these groups have variable ability to resist chemical or physical agents. The microorganisms most resistant to elimination are bacterial endospores. Therefore in general, any method of sterilization or disinfection that kills endospores is also capable of eliminating bacteria, viruses, mycobacteria, fungi, mold, and parasites. This concept is used in monitoring the success of disinfection and sterilization techniques.

Techniques of Instrument Sterilization

Any means of instrument sterilization to be used in office-based dental and surgical care must be reliable, practical, and safe for the instruments. The three methods generally available for instrument sterilization are dry heat, moist heat, and ethylene oxide gas.

Sterilization with Heat

Heat is one of the oldest means of destroying microorganisms. Pasteur used heat to reduce the number of pathogens in liquids for preservation. Koch was the first to use heat for sterilization. He found that $1\frac{1}{2}$ hours of dry heat at 100° C would destroy all vegetative bacteria, but that 3 hours of dry heat at 140° C was necessary to eliminate the spores of anthrax bacilli. Koch then tested moist heat and found it a more efficient means of heat sterilization because it reduces the temperature and time necessary to kill spores. Moist heat is probably more effective because dry heat oxidizes cell proteins, a process requiring extremely high temperatures, whereas moist heat causes destructive protein coagulation quickly at relatively low temperatures.

Because spores are the most resistant forms of microbial life, they are used to monitor sterilization techniques. The spore of the bacteria *Bacillus stearothermophilus* is extremely resistant to heat and is therefore used to test the reliability of heat sterilization. These bacilli can be purchased by hospitals and private offices and run through the sterilizer with the instruments being sterilized. A laboratory then places the heat-treated spores into culture. If no growth occurs, the sterilization procedure was successful.

It has been shown that 6 months after sterilization the possibility of organisms entering sterilization bags increases, although some individuals think that an even longer period is acceptable as long as the bags are properly handled. Therefore, all sterilized items should be labeled with an expiration date that is no longer than 6 to 12 months in the future (Fig. 5-1).

A useful alternative technique for sterilely storing surgical instruments is to place them into cassettes that are double wrapped in specifically designed paper and sterilized as a set for use on a single patient.

DRY HEAT. Dry heat is a method of sterilization that can be provided in most dental offices because the necessary equipment is no more complicated than a thermostatically controlled oven and a timer. Dry heat is most commonly used to sterilize glassware and bulky items that can withstand heat but are susceptible to rust. The success of sterilization depends not only on attaining a certain temperature but also on maintaining the temperature for a sufficient time. Therefore the following three factors must be considered when using dry heat: (1) warm-up time for the oven and the materials to be sterilized, (2) heat conductivity of the materials, and (3) air-

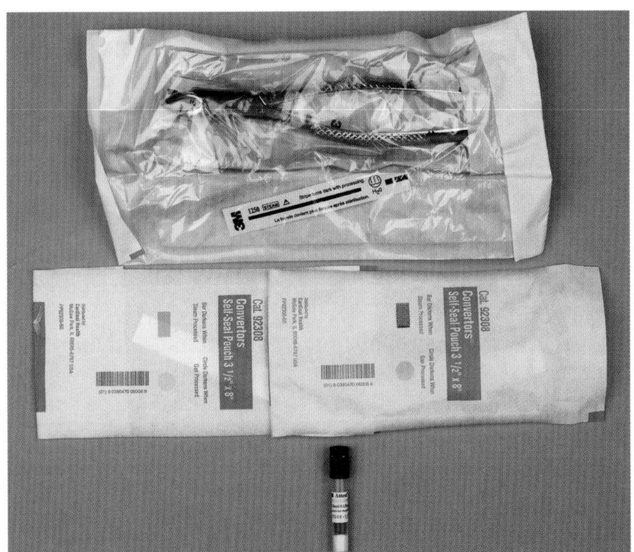

FIGURE 5-1 Tests of sterilization equipment. Color-coded packaging is made of paper and cellophane; test areas on package change color on exposure to sterilizing temperatures or to ethylene oxide gas (*top* and *center*). Vial contains spores of *Bacillus stearothermophilus*, which is used for testing efficiency of heat-sterilization equipment (*bottom*).

flow throughout the oven and through the objects being sterilized. In addition, time for the sterilized equipment to cool after heating must be taken into consideration. The time necessary for dry-heat sterilization limits its practicality in the ambulatory setting, because it lengthens the turnover time and forces the dentist to have many duplicate instruments.

The advantages of dry heat are the relative ease of use and the unlikelihood of damaging heat-resistant instruments. The disadvantages are the time necessary and the potential damage to heat-sensitive equipment. Guidelines for the use of dry-heat sterilization are provided in Table 5-2.

TABLE 5-2

Guidelines for Dry-Heat and Steam Sterilization

Temperature	Duration of Treatment or Exposure*
DRY HEAT	
121° C (250° F)	6-12 hours
140° C (285° F)	3 hours
150° C (300° F)	$2^1/_2$ hours
160° C (320° F)	2 hours
170° C (340° F)	1 hour
STEAM	
116° C (240° F)	60 minutes
118° C (245° F)	36 minutes
121° C (250° F)	24 minutes
125° C (257° F)	16 minutes
132° C (270° F)	4 minutes
138° C (280° F)	$1^1/_2$ minutes

*Times for dry-heat treatments do not begin until temperature of oven reaches goal. Use spore tests weekly to judge effectiveness of sterilization technique and equipment. Use temperature-sensitive monitors each time equipment is used to indicate that sterilization cycle was initiated.

MOIST HEAT. Moist heat is more efficient than dry heat for sterilization because it is effective at much lower temperatures and requires less time. The reason for this is based on several physical principles. First, water boiling at 100° C takes less time to kill organisms than does dry heat at the same temperature because water is better than air at transferring heat. Second, it takes approximately 7 times as much heat to convert boiling water to steam as it takes to cause the same amount of room temperature water to boil. When steam comes into contact with an object, the steam condenses and almost instantly releases that stored heat energy, which quickly denatures vital cell proteins. Saturated steam placed under pressure (autoclaving) is even more efficient than non-pressurized steam. This is because increasing pressure in a container of steam increases the boiling point of water so that the new steam entering a closed container gradually becomes hotter. Temperatures attainable by steam under pressure include 109° C at 5 psi, 115° C at 10 psi, 121° C at 15 psi, and 126° C at 20 psi (Table 5-2).

The container usually used for providing steam under pressure is known as an *autoclave* (Fig. 5-2). The autoclave works by creating steam and then, through a series of valves, increasing the pressure so that the steam becomes superheated. Instruments placed into an autoclave should be packaged to allow the free flow of steam to the equipment, such as by placing instruments in paper bags or wrapping them in cotton cloth.

Simply placing instruments in boiling water or free-flowing steam results in disinfection rather than sterilization, because at the temperature of 100° C, many spores and certain viruses survive.

The advantages of sterilization with moist heat are its effectiveness, speed, and the relative availability of office-proportioned autoclaving equipment. Disadvantages include the tendency of moist heat to dull and rust instruments and the cost of autoclaves (Table 5-3).

Gaseous Sterilization

Certain gases exert a lethal action on bacteria by destroying enzymes and other vital biochemical structures. Of the several gases available for sterilization, ethylene oxide is the most commonly used. Ethylene oxide is a highly flammable gas and

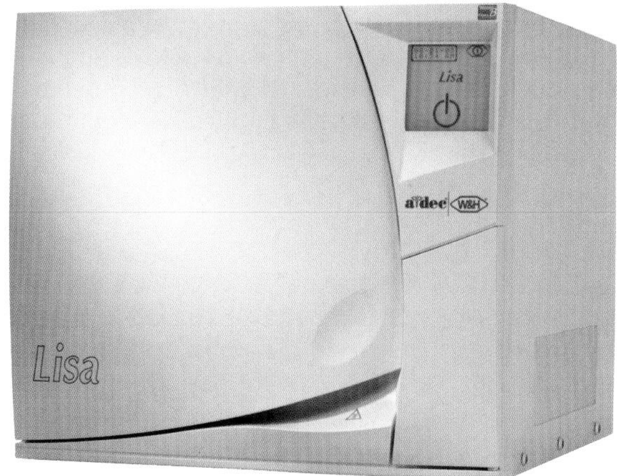

FIGURE 5-2 Office-proportioned autoclave that can be used as a steam and dry-heat sterilizer. (Lisa Sterilizer, Courtesy A-dec, Newburg, Ore.)

TABLE 5-3

Comparison of Dry-Heat Versus Moist-Heat Sterilization Techniques

	Dry Heat	Moist Heat
Principal antimicrobial effect	Oxidizes cell proteins	Denatures cell proteins
Time necessary to achieve sterilization	Long	Short
Equipment complexity and cost	Low	High
Tendency to dull or rust instruments	Low	High
Availability of equipment sized for office use	Good	Good

is mixed with carbon dioxide or nitrogen to make it safer to use. Because ethylene oxide gas is at room temperature, it can readily diffuse through porous materials, such as plastic and rubber. At 50° C ethylene oxide is effective for killing all organisms, including spores, within 3 hours. However, because it is highly toxic to animal tissue, equipment exposed to ethylene oxide must be aerated for 8 to 12 hours at 50° to 60° C or at ambient temperatures for 4 to 7 days.

The advantages of ethylene oxide for sterilization are its effectiveness for sterilizing porous materials, large equipment, and materials sensitive to heat or moisture. The disadvantages are the need for special equipment and the length of sterilization and aeration time necessary to reduce tissue toxicity. This technique is rarely practical for dental use, unless the dentist has easy access to a large facility willing to gas sterilize dental equipment (e.g., hospital or ambulatory surgery center).

Techniques of Instrument Disinfection

Many dental instruments cannot withstand the temperatures required for heat sterilization. Therefore if gaseous sterilization is not available and absolute sterility is not required, chemical disinfection can be performed. Chemical agents with potential disinfectant capabilities have been classified as being high, intermediate, or low in biocidal activity. The classification is based on the ability of the agent to inactivate vegetative bacteria, tubercle bacilli, bacterial spores, nonlipid viruses, and lipid viruses. Agents with low biocidal activity are effective only against vegetative bacteria and lipid viruses, intermediate disinfectants are effective against all microbes except bacterial spores, and agents with high activity are biocidal for all microbes. The classification depends not only on innate properties of the chemical but also, and just as important, on how the chemical is used (Table 5-4).

Substances acceptable for disinfecting dental instruments for surgery include glutaraldehyde, iodophors, chlorine compounds, and formaldehyde; glutaraldehyde-containing compounds are the most commonly used. Table 5-5 summarizes the biocidal activity of most of the acceptable disinfecting agents when used properly. Alcohols are not suitable for general dental disinfection, because they evaporate too rapidly; however, they can be used to disinfect local anesthetic cartridges.

Quaternary ammonium compounds are not recommended for dentistry because they are not effective against the hepatitis B virus and become inactivated by soap and anionic agents.

Certain procedures must be followed to ensure maximal disinfection, regardless of which disinfectant solution is used. The agent must be properly reformulated and discarded periodically, as specified by the manufacturer. Instruments must remain in contact with the solution for the designated period, and no new contaminated instruments should be added to the solution during that time. All instruments must be washed free of blood or other visible material before being placed in the solution.

Finally, after disinfection the instruments must be rinsed free of chemicals and used within a short time.

An outline of the preferred method of sterilization for selected dental instruments is presented in Table 5-6.

Maintenance of Sterility

Disposable Materials

Materials and drugs used during oral and maxillofacial surgery—such as sutures, local anesthetics, scalpel blades, and syringes with needles—are sterilized by the manufacturer with a variety of techniques, including gases, autoclaving, filtration, and irradiation. To maintain sterility, the dentist must only properly remove the material or drug from its container. Most surgical supplies are double wrapped (the only common exception is scalpel blades). The outer wrapper is designed to be handled in a nonsterile fashion and usually is sealed in a manner that allows an unsterile individual to unwrap it and discharge the material still wrapped in a sterile inner wrapper. The unsterile individual can allow the surgical material in the sterile inner wrapper to drop onto a sterile part of the surgical field or allow an individual gloved in a sterile fashion to remove the wrapped material in a sterile manner (Fig. 5-3). Scalpel blades are handled in a similar fashion; the unwrapped blade can be dropped onto the field or grasped in a sterile manner by another individual.

TABLE 5-4

Classification System for the Biocidal Effects of Chemical Disinfectants

Level of Biocidal Activity*	Vegetative Bacteria	Lipid Viruses	Nonlipid Viruses	Tubercle Bacilli	Bacterial Spores
Low	+	+	-	-	-
Intermediate	+	+	+	+	
High	+	+	+	+	+

*In absence of gross organic materials on surfaces being disinfected.

TABLE 5-5

Biocidal Activity of Various Chemical Disinfectants

Generic	Brand Names	Exposure Time	ACTIVITY LEVEL* Intermediate	High
Formaldehyde 3%				
8% or		≥ 30 minutes	+	
8% in 70% alcohol		10 hours		
Glutaraldehyde 2% with nonionic ethoxylates of linear alcohol	Wavicide, Sterall			
Room temperature		≥ 10 minutes	+	
40°-45° C		4 hours		+
60° C		4 hours		+
Glutaraldehyde 2% alkaline with phenolics buffer	Sporcidin			
Diluted 1:6		≥ 10 minutes	+	
Full strength		7 hours		+
Glutaraldehyde 2% alkaline	Cidex, Procide,	≥ 10 minutes	+	
	Glutarex, Omnicide	10 hours		+
1% Chlorine compound	Clorox			
Diluted 1:5		≥ 30 minutes	+	
O-phenylphenol 9% plus O-benzyl-p-chlorophenol 1%	Omni II			
Diluted 1:32		≥ 10 minutes	+	
Iodophors 1% iodine	Betadine, Isodine	≥ 30 minutes	+	

*Grossly visible contamination, such as blood, must be removed before chemical disinfection to maximize biocidal activity.

TABLE 5-6

Methods of Sterilization or Disinfection of Selected Dental Instruments

Items	Steam Autoclave (15-30 Minutes Required per Cycle)	Chemical Disinfection: Dry Heat Oven ($1\text{-}1\frac{1}{2}$ Hours Required per Cycle)	Sterilization*
Stainless instruments (loose) restorative burs	+ +	+ +	-
Instruments in packs	+ +	+ (Small packs)	-
Instrument tray setups, surgical or restorative	+ (Size limit)	+ +	-
Rustable instruments	(Only when coated with chemical protectant)	+ +	-
Handpiece (autoclave)	+ +	-	-
Handpiece (nonautoclave)		-	± (Iodophor disinfectant)
Angle attachments†	+	+	-
Rubber items	+ +	-	-
Rag wheels	+ +	+	-
Removable prosthetics	-	-	+‡
Heat-resistant plastic evacuators	+ +	+	-

*Chemical disinfecting/sterilizing solutions are not the method of choice for sterilization of any items used in the mouth. In some circumstances, they may be used when other, more suitable procedures have been precluded.

†Clinician should confirm with manufacturer that attachment is capable of withstanding heat sterilization.

‡Rinse prosthetic well, immerse in 1:10 household bleach solution (5%-6% sodium hypochlorite) for 5 minutes. Rinse the prosthetic (repeat disinfection procedure before returning to patient).

Surgical Field Maintenance

An absolutely sterile surgical field is impossible to attain. For oral procedures, even a relatively clean field is difficult to maintain because of oral and upper respiratory tract contamination. Therefore, during oral and maxillofacial surgery the goal is to prevent any organisms from the surgical staff or other patients from entering the patient's wound.

Once instruments are sterilized or disinfected, they should be set up for use during surgery in a manner that limits the likelihood of contamination by organisms foreign to the patient's maxillofacial flora. A flat platform, such as a Mayo stand, should be used, and two layers of sterile towels or waterproof paper should be placed on it. Then the clinician or assistant should lay the instrument pack on the platform and open out

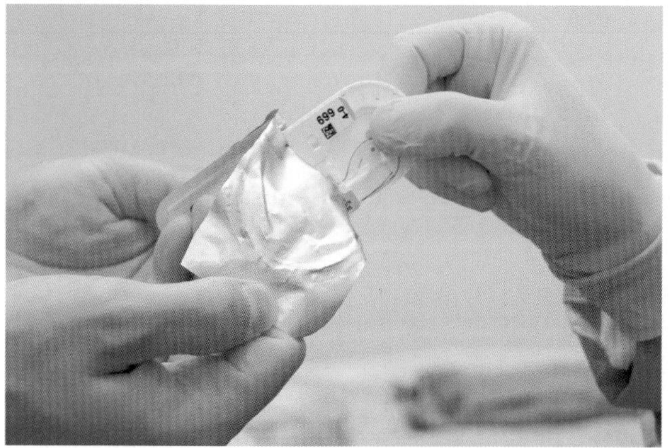

FIGURE 5-3 Method of sterilely transferring double-wrapped sterile supplies from clean individual (ungloved hands) to sterilely gowned individual (gloved hands). Package is designed to be peeled open from one end, without touching sterile interior of package. Sterile contents are then promptly presented to recipient.

the edges in a sterile fashion. Anything placed on the platform should be sterile or disinfected. Care should be taken not to allow excessive moisture to get on the towels or paper; if the towels become saturated, they can allow bacteria from the unsterile undersurface to wick up to the sterile instruments.

Operatory Disinfection

The various surfaces present in the dental operatory have different requirements concerning disinfection that depend on the potential for contamination and the degree of patient contact with the surface. Any surface that a patient or patient's secretions contact is a potential carrier of infectious organisms. In addition, when high-speed drilling equipment is used, patient blood and secretions are dispersed over much of the surfaces of the operatory. The operatory can be disinfected in two basic ways. The first is to wipe all surfaces with a hospital-grade disinfectant solution. The second is to cover surfaces with protective shields that are changed between each patient. Fortunately, many chemical disinfectants, including chlorine compounds and glutaraldehyde, can prevent transfer of the hepatitis viruses when used on surfaces in certain concentrations (0.2% for chlorine, 2% for glutaraldehyde). Headrests, tray tables, hosing and lines, nitrous oxide and chair controls, and light handles can be covered with commercially available, single-use, disposable covers; the rest of the dental chair can be quickly sprayed with a disinfectant. Countertops usually come into contact with patients only indirectly, so counters should be periodically disinfected, especially before surgical procedures. Limiting the number of objects left on counters in operatories will make periodic cleaning easier and more effective.

Soap dispensers and sink faucets are another source of contamination. Unless they can be activated without using the hands, they should be disinfected frequently because many bacteria survive—even thrive—in a soapy environment (discussed later in this section). This is one reason common soap is not the ideal agent when preparing hands for surgery.

Anesthetic equipment used to deliver gases, such as oxygen or nitrous oxide, may also spread infection patient to patient. Plastic nasal cannulas are designed to be discarded after one use. Nasal masks and the tubing leading to the mask from the source of the gases are available in disposable form or can be covered with disposable sleeves.

Surgical Staff Preparation

The preparation of the operating team for surgery differs according to the nature of the procedure being performed and the location of the surgery. The two basic types of personnel asepsis to be discussed are (1) the *clean* technique and (2) the *sterile* technique. Antiseptics are used during each of the techniques, so they are discussed first.

Hand and Arm Preparation

Antiseptics are used to prepare the surgical team's hands and arms before gloves are donned and to disinfect the surgical site. Because antiseptics are used on living tissue, they are designed to have low-tissue toxicity while maintaining disinfecting properties. The three antiseptics most commonly used in dentistry are (1) iodophors, (2) chlorhexidine, and (3) hexachlorophene.

Iodophors, such as polyvinylpyrrolidone-iodine (povidone-iodine) solution, have the broadest spectrum of antiseptic action, being effective for gram-positive and gram-negative bacteria, most viruses, *M. tuberculosis* organisms, spores, and fungi.

Iodophors are usually formulated in a 1% iodine solution. The scrub form has an added anionic detergent. Iodophors are preferred over noncompounded solutions of iodine because they are much less toxic to tissue than free iodine and more water soluble. However, iodophors are contraindicated for use on individuals sensitive to iodinated materials, those with untreated hypothyroidism, and pregnant women. Iodophors exert their effect over a period of several minutes, so the solution should remain in contact with the surface for at least a few minutes for maximal effect.

Chlorhexidine and hexachlorophene are other useful antiseptics. Chlorhexidine is used extensively worldwide and is available in the United States as a skin preparation solution and for internal use. The potential for systemic toxicity with repeated use of hexachlorophene has limited its use. Both agents are more effective against gram-positive than gram-negative bacteria, which makes them useful for maxillofacial prepping. Chlorhexidine and hexachlorophene are more effective when used repeatedly during the day because they accumulate on the skin and leave a residual antibacterial effect after each wash. However, their ineffectiveness against tubercle bacilli, spores, and many viruses makes them less effective than iodophors.

Clean Technique

The clean technique is generally used for office-based surgery that does not specifically require a sterile technique. Office oral surgical procedures that call for a sterile technique include any surgery in which skin is incised. The clean technique is designed as much to protect the dental staff and other patients from a particular patient as it is to protect the patient from pathogens that the dental staff may harbor.

When using a clean technique, the dental staff can wear clean street clothing covered by long-sleeved laboratory coats (Fig. 5-4). Another option is a dental uniform (e.g., surgical scrubs), with no further covering or covered by a long-sleeved surgical gown.

Dentists should wear gloves whenever they are providing dental care. When the clean technique is used, the hands can be washed with antiseptic soap and dried on a disposable towel

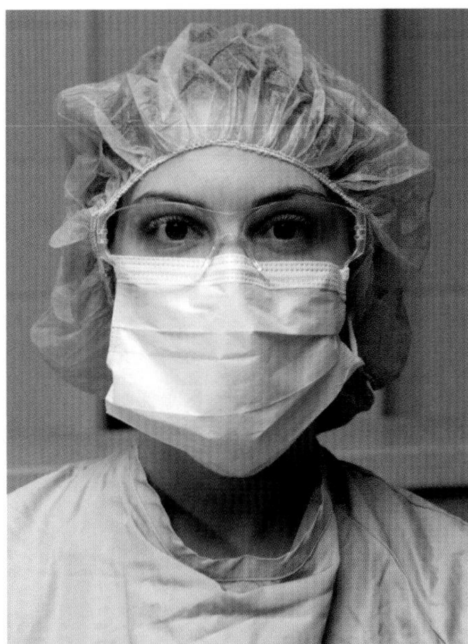

FIGURE 5-4 Surgeon ready for office oral surgery, wearing clean gown over street clothes, mask over nose and mouth, cap covering scalp hair, clean gloves, and shatter-resistant eye protection. Nondangling earrings are acceptable in clean technique.

before gloving. Gloves should be sterile and put on using an appropriate technique to maintain sterility of the external surfaces. The technique of sterile self-gloving is illustrated in Figure 5-5.

In general, eye protection should be worn when blood or saliva are dispersed, such as when high-speed cutting equipment is used (see Fig. 5-4). A mask should be used whenever aerosols are created or a surgical wound is to be made.

In most cases it is not absolutely necessary to prepare the operative site when using the clean technique. However, when surgery in the oral cavity is performed, the perioral skin may be decontaminated with the same solutions used to scrub the hands and the oral cavity may be prepared by brushing or rinsing with chlorhexidine gluconate (0.12%) or an alcohol-based mouthwash. These procedures reduce the amount of skin or oral mucosal contamination of the wound and decrease the microbial load of any aerosols made while using high-speed drills in the mouth. The dentist may desire to drape the patient to protect the patient's clothes, to keep objects from accidentally entering the patient's eyes, and to decrease suture contamination should it fall across an uncovered, unprepared part of the patient's body.

During an oral surgical procedure, only sterile water or sterile saline solution should be used to irrigate open wounds. A disposable injection syringe, a reusable bulb syringe, or an irrigation pump connected to a bag of intravenous solution can be used to deliver irrigation. Reservoirs feeding irrigation lines to handpieces are also available and can be filled with sterile irrigation fluids.

Sterile Technique

The sterile technique is used for office-based surgery when skin incisions are made or when surgery is performed in an operating room.* The purpose of sterile technique is to minimize the number of organisms that enter wounds created by the surgeon. The technique requires strict attention to detail and cooperation among the members of the surgical team.

The surgical hand and arm scrub is another means of lessening the chance of contaminating a patient's wound. Although sterile gloves are worn, gloves can be torn (especially when using high-speed drills or working around wires), thereby exposing the surgeon's skin. By proper scrubbing with antiseptic solutions, the surface bacterial level of the hands and arms is greatly reduced.

Most hospitals have a surgical scrub protocol that should be followed when performing surgery in those institutions. Although several acceptable methods can be used, standard to most techniques is the use of an antiseptic soap solution, a moderately stiff brush, and a fingernail cleaner. The hands and forearms are wetted in a scrub sink, and the hands are kept above the level of the elbows after wetting until the hands and arms are dried. A copious amount of antiseptic soap is applied to the hands and arms from either wall dispensers or antiseptic-impregnated scrub brushes. The antiseptic soap is allowed to remain on the arms while any dirt is removed from underneath each fingernail tip using a sharp-tipped fingernail cleaner.

Then more antiseptic soap is applied and scrubbing is begun, with repeated firm strokes of the scrub brush on every surface of the hands and forearms up to approximately 5 cm from the elbow. Scrub techniques based on the number of strokes to each surface are more reliable than a set time for scrubbing. An individual's scrub technique should follow a routine that has been designed to ensure that no forearm or hand surface is left improperly prepared. An example of an acceptable surgical scrub technique is shown in Chapter 31.

Postsurgical Asepsis

Wounds Management

A few principles of postsurgical care are useful to prevent the spread of pathogens. Wounds should be inspected or dressed by hands that are covered with fresh, clean gloves. When several patients are waiting, those without infectious problems should be seen first, and those with problems such as a draining abscess should be seen afterward.

Sharps Management

During and after any surgery, contaminated materials should be disposed of in such a way that the staff and other patients will not be infected. The most common risk for transmission of disease from infected patients to the staff is by accidental needle sticks or scalpel lacerations. Sharps injuries can be prevented by using the local anesthetic needle to scoop up the sheath after use using an instrument such as a hemostat to hold the cover while resheathing the needle or using automatically resheathing needles (Fig. 5-6, *A* and *B*); taking care never to apply or remove a blade from a scalpel handle without an instrument; and disposing of used blades, needles, and other sharp disposable items into rigid, well-marked receptacles specially designed for contaminated sharp objects (Fig. 5-6, *C*). For environmental protection, contaminated supplies should be discarded in properly labeled bags and removed by a reputable hazardous waste management company.

---

*A clean wound is made through intact skin that has been treated with an antiseptic.

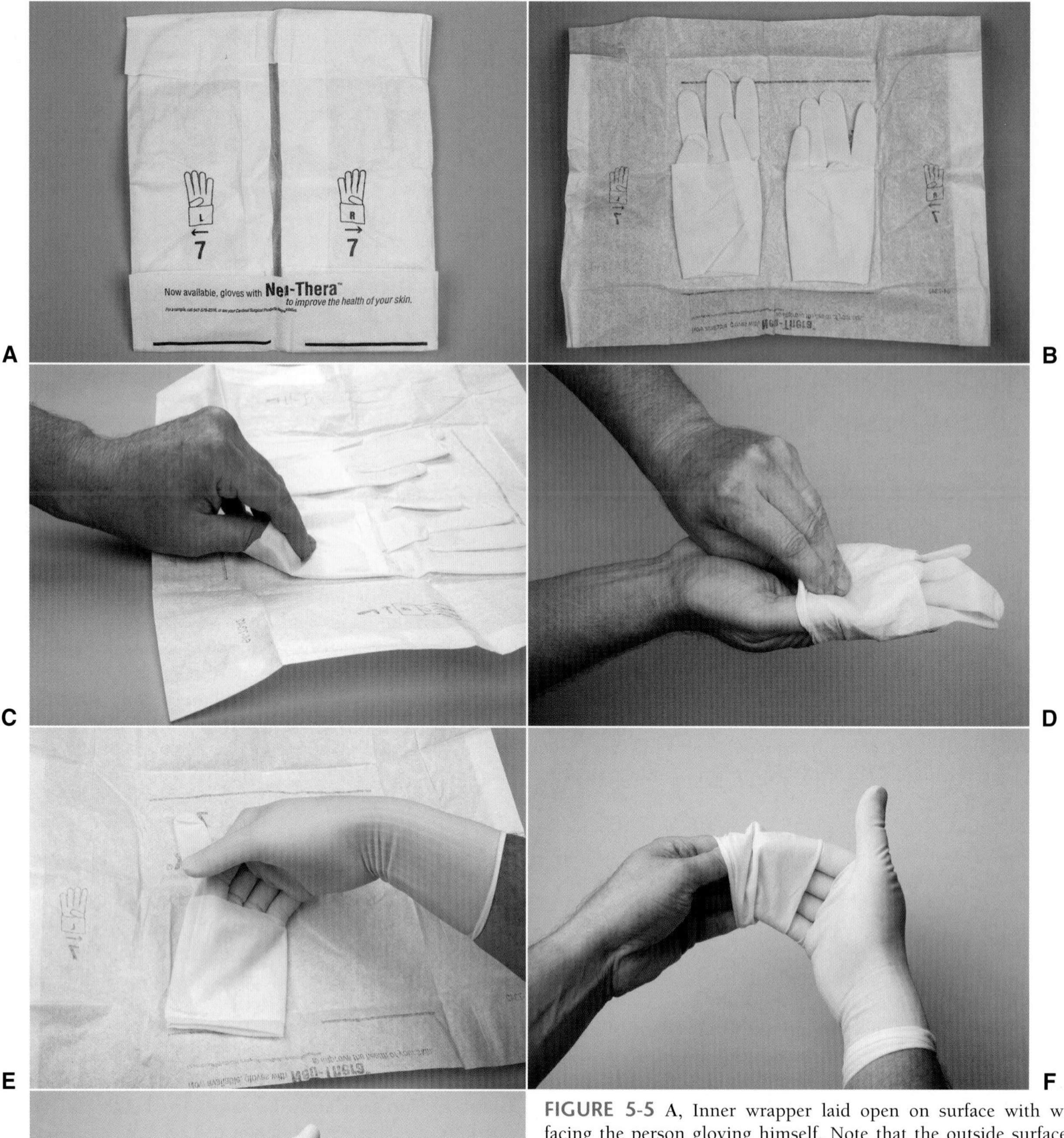

FIGURE 5-5 A, Inner wrapper laid open on surface with words facing the person gloving himself. Note that the outside surfaces of this wrapper considered are nonsterile, whereas the inner surface touching the gloves is sterile. B, While touching outside of wrapper, simultaneously pull the folds to each side exposing the gloves. C, Note that the open end of each glove is folded up to create a cuff; using the fingertip of the right hand, grasp the fold of the cuff of the left glove without touching anything else. Bring the glove to the outstretched fingers of the left hand and slide the finger into the glove while using the right hand to help pull the glove on. Release the glove's cuff without unfolding the cuff. D, Place the fingers of the left hand into the cuff of the right glove. Bring the glove to the outstretched fingers of the right hand. E, Slide the fingers of the right hand into the glove while continuing to hold the glove with the left fingers in the cuff to stabilize the glove. Once the glove is on unfurl the cuff using the fingers still within the cuff. F, Finally place the fingers of the right hand into the cuff of the left glove to unfurl the cuff. The gloves can now be used to ensure that the fingertips of each glove are fully into the glove fingertips while taking care to touch only the sterile glove surfaces (G).

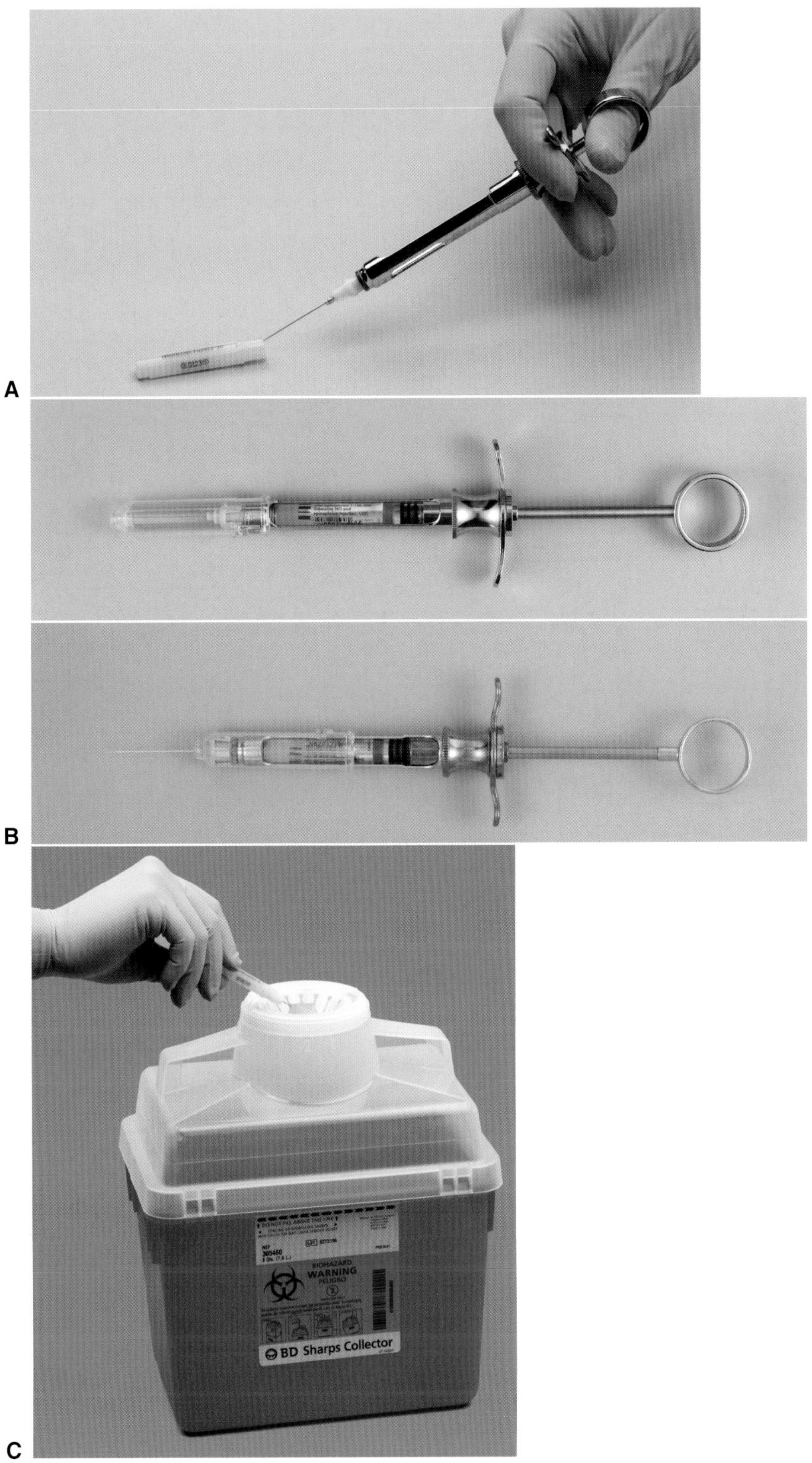

FIGURE 5-6 A, Scoop technique for resheathing needle. B, Self-resheathing needle. C, Proper disposal of sharp, disposable supplies into well-marked, rigid container to prevent accidental inoculation of office staff or cleaning workers with contaminated debris. (B, Courtesy Med Pro.)

PART II

Principles of Exodontia

For most persons, dentists and laypersons alike, the term oral surgery usually implies the removal of a tooth. The atraumatic extraction of a tooth is a procedure that requires finesse, knowledge, and skill on the part of the surgeon. The purpose of this section is to present the principles of exodontia, as well as the instrumentation, techniques, and management of patients who are undergoing extraction surgery.

Chapter 6 presents the armamentarium commonly used for office oral surgical procedures. The basic instrumentation and the fundamental applications of instruments to their surgical purposes are discussed. Many variations of the instruments presented are available.

Chapter 7 presents the basic aspects of how to remove an erupted tooth atraumatically. The preoperative assessment and preparation of the patient are briefly discussed. The position of the patient in the chair and the position of the surgeon, and the surgeon's hands for the removal of each tooth are discussed. The armamentarium and movements necessary to extract each type of tooth are discussed in detail.

Chapter 8 presents the basic aspects of managing complicated extractions. Complicated extractions primarily refer to retrieving tooth roots and teeth that are likely to fracture or, for some other reason, have an obstacle to extraction. In these situations, surgical removal of bone or surgical sectioning of the tooth is required.

Chapter 9 presents the fundamental aspects of management of impacted teeth. The rationale for timely removal of impacted teeth is presented in the initial portion of the chapter. Classification and determination of the degree of difficulty of the impaction follows. Last, a brief description of the basic surgical techniques required to remove impacted third molars is provided.

Chapter 10 presents the techniques for managing the patient during the postoperative period. This chapter discusses postoperative instructions that should be given to the patient, as well as postoperative medications.

Chapter 11 presents the common surgical complications that are encountered in the removal of teeth. Emphasis is placed on anticipating complications and taking measures to prevent or minimize them.

Last, Chapter 12 discusses the medical and legal considerations involved in basic exodontia. An important portion of this chapter discusses the concept of informed consent for the patient as it relates to exodontia.

CHAPTER 6

Instrumentation for Basic Oral Surgery

JAMES R. HUPP

CHAPTER OUTLINE

The purpose of this chapter is to introduce the instrumentation commonly required to perform routine dental extraction and other basic oral surgical operations. These instruments are used for a wide variety of purposes, including soft and hard tissue procedures. This chapter primarily deals with a description of the instruments.

INCISING TISSUE

Many surgical procedures begin with an incision. The primary instrument for making incisions is the scalpel, which is composed of a reusable handle and a disposable, sterile sharp blade. Scalpels are also available as a single-use scalpel with a plastic handle and fixed blade. The most commonly used handle for oral surgery is the No. 3 handle (Fig. 6-1). The tip of a scalpel handle is prepared to receive a variety of differently shaped scalpel blades to be inserted onto the slotted portion of the handle.

The most commonly used scalpel blade for intraoral surgery is the No. 15 blade (Fig. 6-2). The blade is small and is used to make incisions around teeth and through soft tissue. The blade is similar in shape to the larger No. 10 blade used for large skin incisions in other parts of the body. Other commonly used blades for intraoral surgery include the No. 11 and No. 12 blades. The No. 11 blade is a sharp-pointed blade that is used primarily for making small stab incisions, such as for incising into an abscess. The hooked No. 12 blade is useful for mucogingival procedures in which incisions are made on the posterior aspect of teeth or in the maxillary tuberosity area.

The scalpel blade is carefully loaded onto the handle holding the blade with a needle holder. This lessens the chance of injuring the fingers. The blade is held on the unsharpened edge, where it is reinforced with a small rib, and the handle is held so that the male portion of the fitting is pointing upward (Fig. 6-3 *A*). The scalpel blade is then slowly slid onto the handle along the grooves in the male portion until it clicks into position (Fig. 6-3, *B*). The scalpel is unloaded similarly. The needle holder grasps the end away from the blade (Fig. 6-3, *C*) and lifts it to disengage it from the male fitting. The scalpel is then slid off the handle (Fig. 6-3, *D*). The used blade is immediately discarded into a specifically designed, rigid-sided sharps container. These are usually red (see Fig. 5-6).

When using the scalpel to make an incision, the surgeon typically holds it in the pen grasp (Fig. 6-4) to allow maximal control of the blade as the incision is made. Mobile tissue should be held firmly in place under some tension so that as the incision is made, the blade will incise and not just push away the mucosa. When incising depressible soft tissue, an instrument such as a retractor should be used to hold the tissue taut during incision. When a mucoperiosteal incision is made, the blade should be pressed down firmly so that the incision penetrates the mucosa and periosteum with the same stroke.

Scalpel blades and blade-handle sets are designed for single-patient use. They are dulled easily when they come into

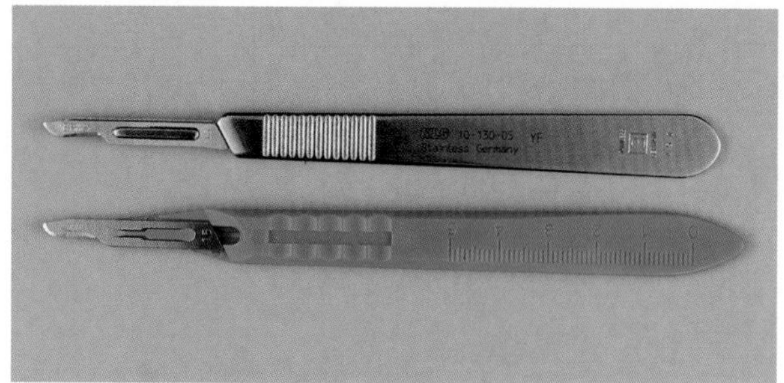

FIGURE 6-1 Scalpels are composed of handle and sharp, disposable blade. Scalpel No. 3 handle with No. 15 blade is most commonly used.

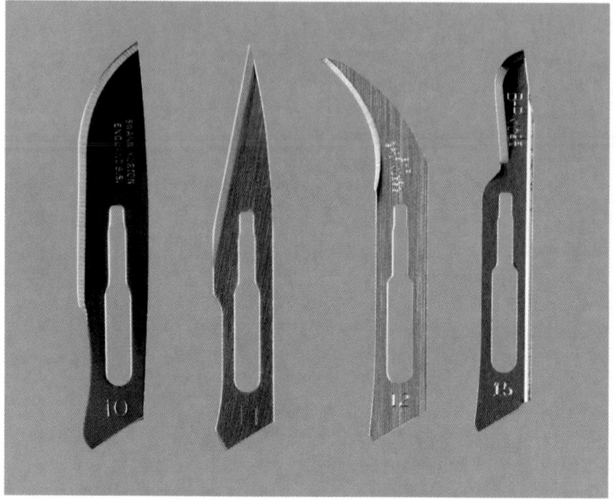

FIGURE 6-2 Scalpel blades used in oral surgery include No. 10, No. 11, No. 12, and No. 15, going from left to right.

contact with hard tissue such as bone or teeth, and even after repeated strokes through keratinized tissue. If several incisions through mucoperiosteum to bone are required, it may be necessary to use a second blade during a single operation. Dull blades do not make clean, sharp incisions in soft tissue and therefore should be replaced before they become overly dull.

ELEVATING MUCOPERIOSTEUM

When an incision through periosteum is made, ideally the periosteum should be reflected from the underlying cortical bone in a single layer with a periosteal elevator. The instrument that is most commonly used in oral surgery is the No. 9 Molt periosteal elevator (Fig. 6-5). This instrument has a sharp, pointed end and a broader, rounded end. The pointed end is used to begin periosteal reflection and to reflect dental papillae from between teeth, and the broad, rounded end is used to continue the elevation of periosteum from the bone.

Other types of periosteal elevators exist for use by periodontists, orthopedic surgeons, and other surgeons involved in work on bones.

The No. 9 Molt periosteal elevator can be used to reflect tissue by three methods: First, the pointed end can be used in a twisting, prying motion to elevate soft tissue. This is most commonly used when elevating a dental papilla from between teeth or the attached gingiva around a tooth to be extracted. The second method is the push stroke, in which the pointed or the broad end of the instrument is slid underneath the periosteum, separating it from the underlying bone. This is the most efficient stroke and results in the cleanest reflection of periosteum. The third method is a pull stroke. This method is occasionally useful but tends to shred or tear the periosteum unless it is done carefully.

RETRACTING SOFT TISSUE

Good access and vision are essential to performing excellent surgery. A variety of retractors have been designed to retract the cheeks, tongue, and mucoperiosteal flaps to provide access to visibility during surgery. Retractors also can help protect soft tissue from sharp cutting instruments.

The two most popular cheek retractors are (1) the right-angle Austin retractor (Fig. 6-6) and (2) the broad offset Minnesota retractor (Fig. 6-7). These retractors can also be used to retract the cheek and a mucoperiosteal flap simultaneously. Before the flap is created, the retractor is held loosely in the cheek, and once the flap is reflected, the retractor edge is placed on the bone and is then used to retract the flap.

The Seldin retractor is another type of instrument (Fig. 6-8) used to retract oral soft tissues. Although this retractor may look similar to a periosteal elevator, the leading edge is not sharp but instead is smooth; it should not be used to elevate mucoperiosteum. The No. 9 Molt periosteal elevator can also be used as a retractor. Once the periosteum has been elevated, the broad blade of the periosteal elevator is held firmly against the bone, with the mucoperiosteal flap elevated into a reflected position.

The instrument most commonly used to retract the tongue during routine exodontia is the mouth mirror. This is usually part of every basic setup, because it has the usual use for examining the mouth and doing indirect visualization for dental procedures. The mirror can also be used as a tongue or cheek retractor. The Weider tongue retractor is a broad, heart-shaped retractor that is serrated on one side so that it can more firmly engage the tongue and retract it medially and anteriorly (Fig. 6-9, *A*). When this retractor is used, care must be taken not to position it so far posteriorly that it causes gagging or pushes the tongue into the oropharynx (Fig. 6-9, *B*).

A towel clip (see Fig. 6-28) can also be used to hold the tongue. When a biopsy procedure is to be performed on the posterior aspect of the tongue, the most positive way to control the tongue is by holding the anterior tongue with a towel clip. Local anesthesia must be profound where the clip is placed, and it is wise to mention to the patient that this method of retraction may be used, if anticipated.

GRASPING SOFT TISSUE

Various oral surgical procedures require the surgeon to grasp soft tissue to incise it, stop bleeding or to pass a suture needle. The tissue forceps most commonly used for this purpose are the Adson forceps (pickup; Figure 6-10, *A*). These are delicate forceps with or without small teeth at the tips, which can be used to hold tissue gently and thereby stabilize it. When this instrument is used, care should be taken not to grasp the tissue too tightly, which will crush the tissue. Toothed forceps allow

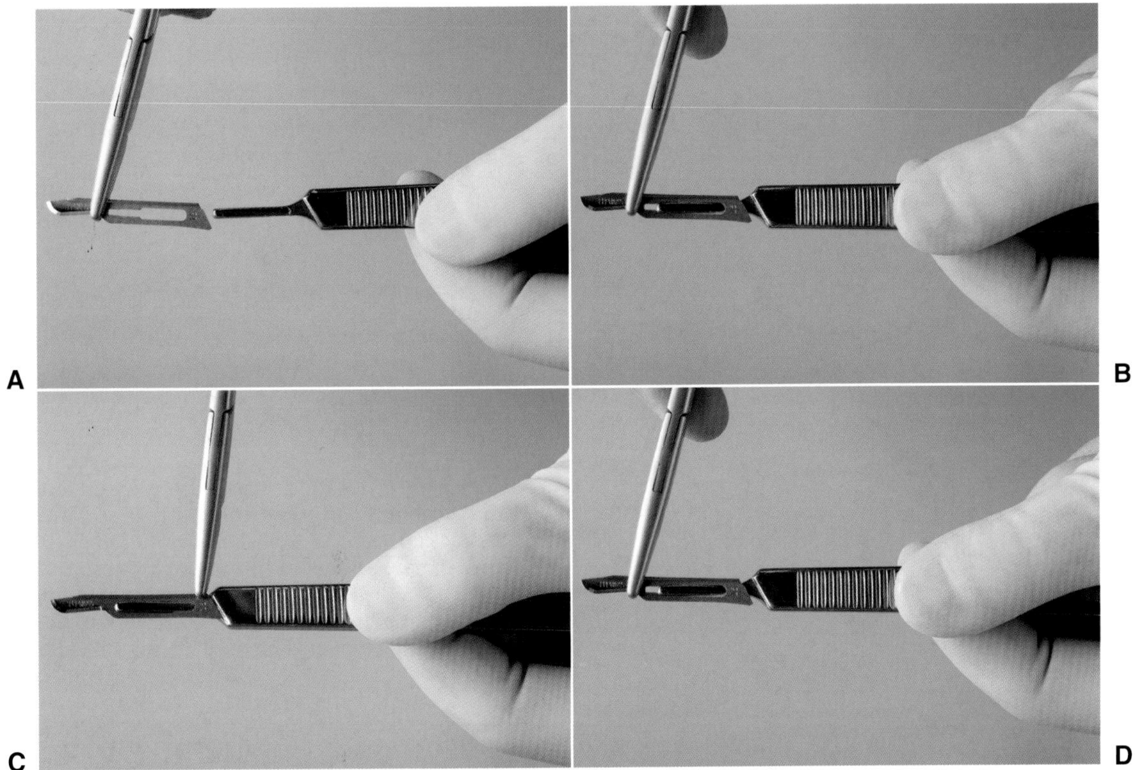

FIGURE 6-3 **A**, When loading scalpel blade, surgeon holds blade in needle holder and handle, with male portion of fitting pointing upward. **B**, Surgeon then slides blade into handle until it clicks into place. **C**, To remove blade, the surgeon uses needle holder to grasp end of blade next to the handle and lifts it to disengage it from the fitting. **D**, Surgeon then gently slides blade off the handle.

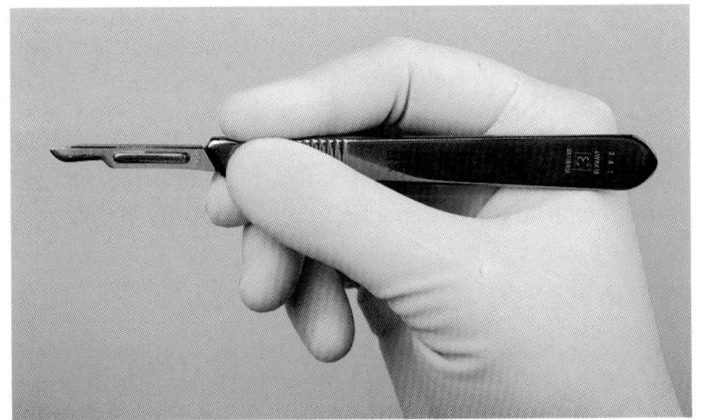

FIGURE 6-4 **A**, Scalpel is held in pen grasp to allow maximal control.

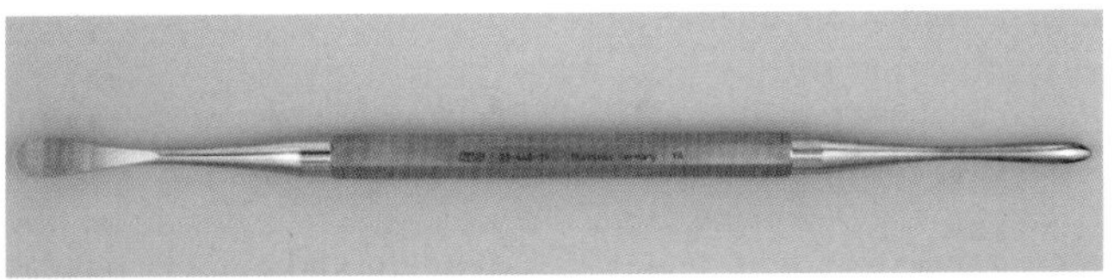

FIGURE 6-5 No. 9 Molt periosteal elevator is most commonly used in oral surgery.

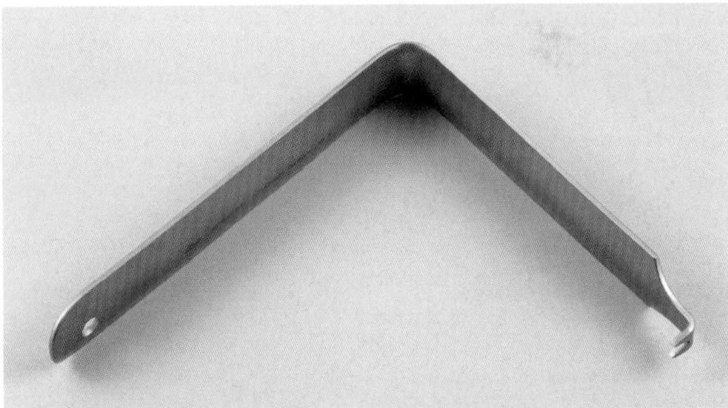

FIGURE 6-6 Austin retractor is a right-angle retractor that can be used to retract cheek, tongue, or flaps.

tissue to be held with a more delicate grip than untoothed forceps.

When working in the posterior part of the mouth, the Adson forceps may be too short. Longer forceps that have a similar shape are the Stillies forceps. These forceps are usually 7 to 9 inches long and can easily grasp tissue in the posterior part of the mouth and still leave enough of the instrument protruding beyond the lips for the surgeon to hold and control it easily (Fig. 6-10, *B*).

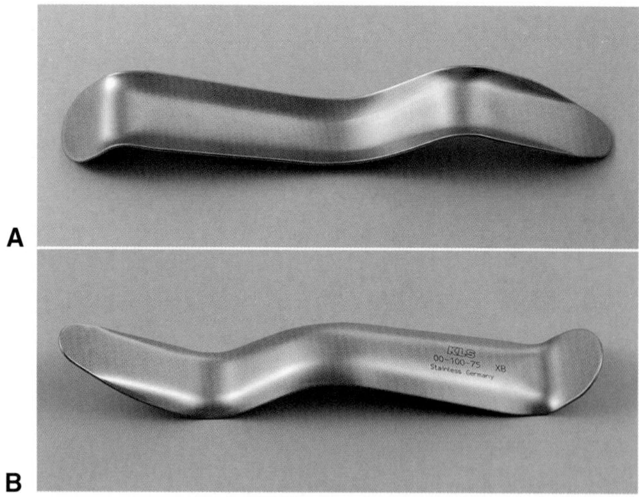

FIGURE 6-7 Minnesota retractor is an offset retractor used for retraction of cheeks and flaps. **A**, Front. **B**, Back.

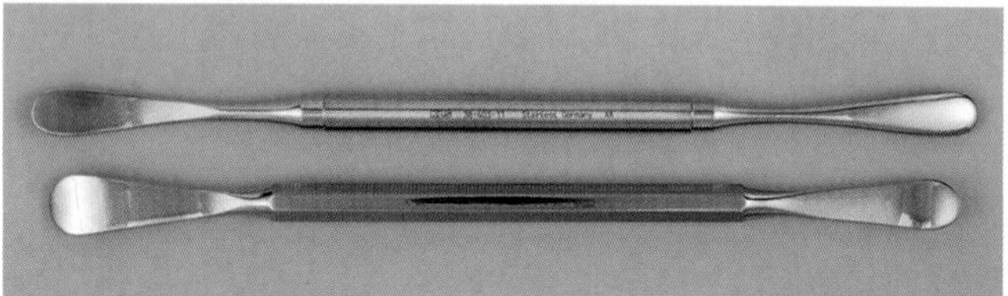

FIGURE 6-8 The Henahan (*top*) and Seldin (*bottom*) retractors are broader instruments that provide broader retraction and increased visualization.

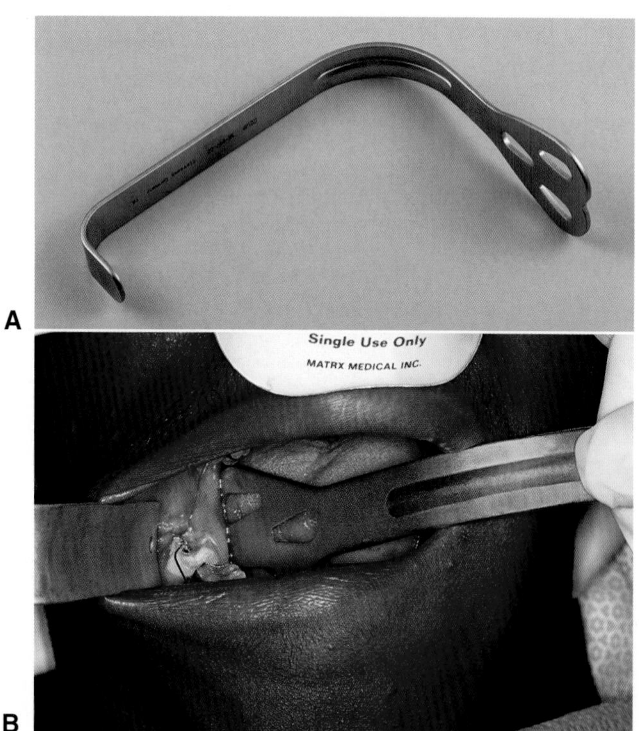

FIGURE 6-9 **A**, Weider retractor is a large retractor designed to retract tongue. Serrated surface helps to engage tongue so that it can be held securely. **B**, Weider retractor is used to hold tongue away from surgical field. Austin retractor is used to retract cheek.

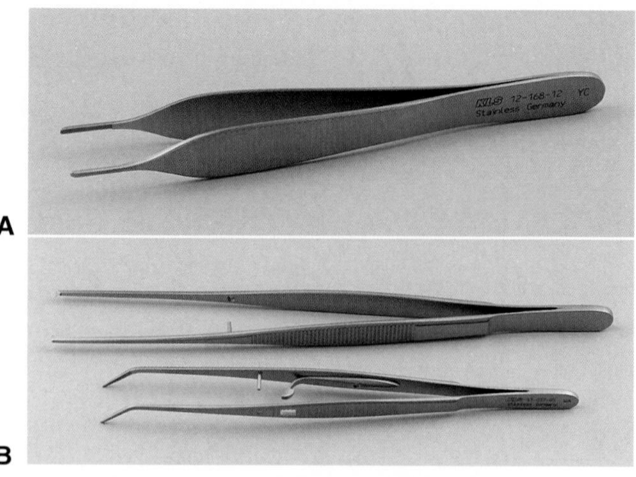

FIGURE 6-10 **A**, Small, delicate Adson tissue forceps are used to gently stabilize soft tissue for suturing or dissection. **B**, The Stillies pickup (*top*) is longer than the Adson pickup and is used to handle tissue in the more posterior aspect of the mouth. The college pliers (*bottom*) are angled forceps that are used for picking up small objects in the mouth or from the tray stand. The college pliers shown here are the locking version.

Occasionally, it is more convenient to have an angled forceps. Such a forceps is the college, or cotton, forceps (see Fig. 6-10, *B*). Although these forceps are not especially useful for handling tissue, they are an excellent instrument for picking up loose fragments of tooth, amalgam, or other foreign material and for placing or removing gauze packs.

In some types of surgery, especially when removing larger amounts of tissue or doing biopsies, such as in an epulis fissurata, forceps with locking handles and teeth that will grip the tissue firmly are necessary. In this situation the Allis tissue forceps are used (Fig. 6-11, *A* and *B*). The locking handle allows the forceps to be placed in the proper position and then to be held by an assistant to provide the necessary tension for proper dissection of the tissue. The Allis forceps should never be used on tissue that is to be left in the mouth because they cause a relatively large amount of tissue destruction as a result of crushing injury (Fig. 6-11, *C*). However, the forceps can be used to grasp the tongue in a manner similar to a towel clamp.

CONTROLLING HEMORRHAGES

When incisions are made through tissue, small arteries and veins are incised, causing bleeding. For most dentoalveolar surgery, pressure on the wound is usually sufficient to control bleeding. Occasionally, pressure does not stop bleeding from a larger artery or vein. When this occurs, an instrument called a hemostat is useful (Fig. 6-12, *A*). Hemostats come in a variety of shapes, may be small and delicate or larger, and are straight or curved. The hemostat most commonly used in surgery is a curved hemostat (Fig. 6-12, *B*).

A hemostat has long, delicate beaks used to grasp tissue and a locking handle. The locking mechanism allows the surgeon to clamp the hemostat onto a vessel and then let go of the instrument, which will remain clamped onto the tissue. This is useful when the surgeon plans to place a suture around the vessel or cauterize it (use heat to sear the vessel closed).

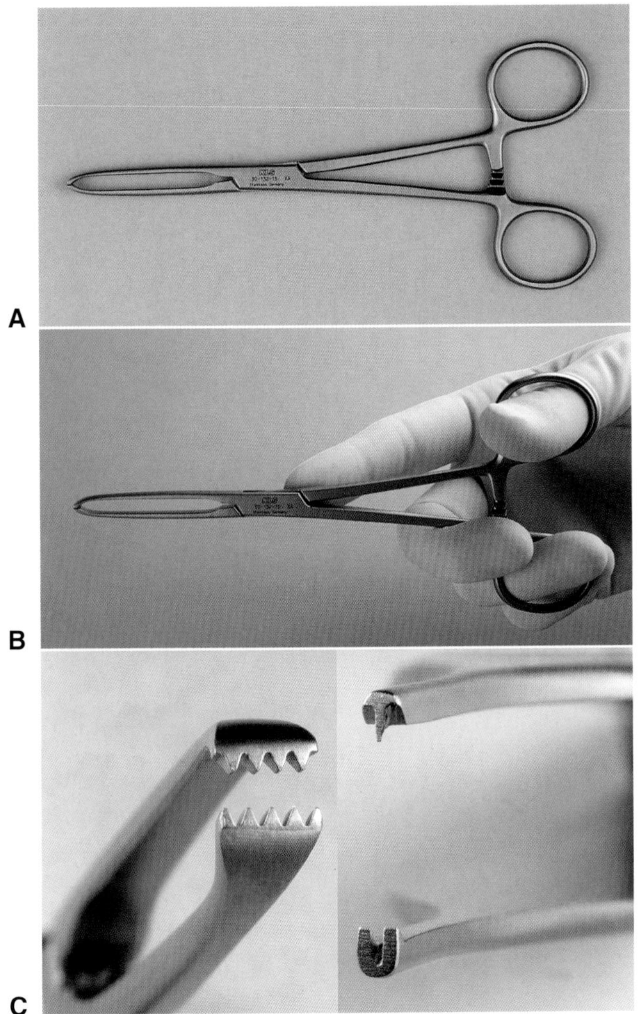

FIGURE 6-11 A, Allis tissue forceps are useful for grasping and holding tissue that will be excised. B, Allis forceps are held in same fashion as needle holder. C, Comparison of Adson beaks (*right*) with Allis beaks (*left*) shows difference in their design and use.

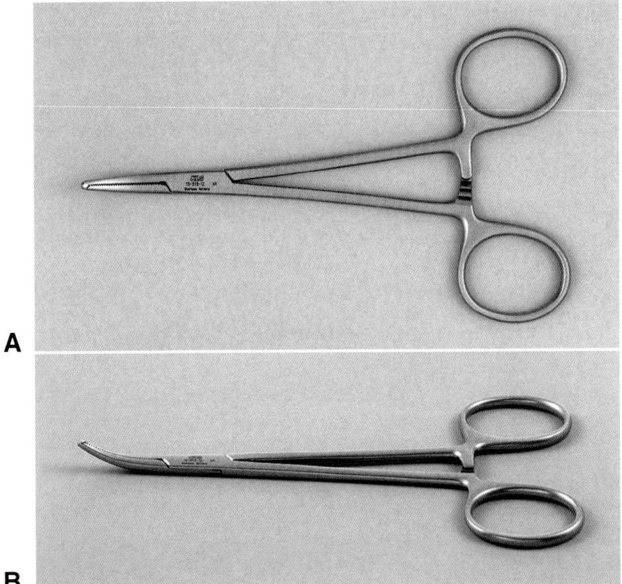

FIGURE 6-12 A, Superior view of hemostat used for oral surgery. B, Oblique view of curved hemostat. Straight hemostats are also available.

In addition to its use as an instrument for controlling bleeding, the hemostat is especially useful in oral surgery to remove granulation tissue from tooth sockets and to pick up small root tips, pieces of calculus, amalgam, fragments, and any other small particles that have dropped into the wound or adjacent areas.

REMOVING BONE

Rongeurs

The instrument most commonly used for removing bone in dentoalveolar surgery is the rongeur forceps. This instrument has sharp blades that are squeezed together by the handles, cutting or pinching through the bone. Rongeur forceps have a mechanism incorporated so that when hand pressure is released, the instrument reopens. This allows the surgeon to make repeated bone trimming actions without manually reopening the instrument (Fig. 6-13, *A*). The two major designs for rongeur forceps are (1) a side-cutting forceps and (2) the side- and end-cutting forceps (Figure 6-13, *B*).

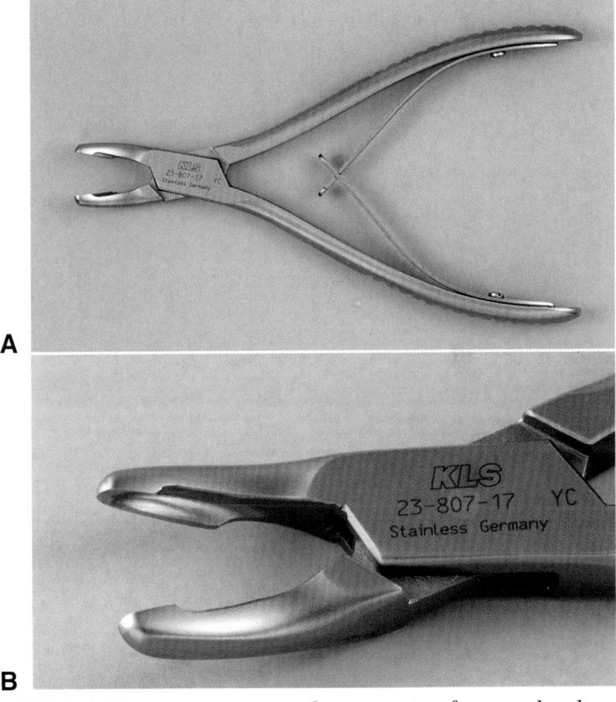

FIGURE 6-13 A, Rongeurs are bone-cutting forceps that have spring-loaded handles. B, Blumenthal rongeurs are combination end-cutting and side-cutting blades. They are preferred for oral surgery procedures.

The side- and end-cutting forceps (Blumenthal rongeurs) are more practical for most dentoalveolar surgical procedures that require bone removal. Because these forceps are end-cutting, they can be inserted into sockets for removal of interradicular bone, and they can also be used to remove sharp edges of bone. Rongeurs can be used to remove large amounts of bone efficiently and quickly. Because rongeurs are delicate instruments, the surgeon should not use the rongeurs to remove large amounts of bone in single bites. Rather, smaller amounts of bone should be removed in multiple bites. Likewise, the rongeurs should never be used to remove teeth, because this practice will quickly dull and destroy the instrument and risks losing the tooth into the throat because rongeurs are not well designed to hold firmly onto an extracted tooth. Rongeurs are usually expensive, so care should be taken to keep them sharp and in working order.

Bur and Handpiece

Another method for removing bone is with a bur in a handpiece. This is the technique that most surgeons use when removing bone for surgical removal of teeth. High-speed, high-torque handpieces with sharp carbide burs remove cortical bone efficiently. Burs such as a No. 557 or No. 703 fissure bur or a No. 8 round burs are used. When large amounts of bone must be removed, such as in torus reduction, a large bone bur that resembles an acrylic bur is used.

The handpiece that is used must be completely sterilizable. When a handpiece is purchased, the manufacturer's specifications must be checked carefully to ensure that this is possible. The handpiece should have high speed and torque (Fig. 6-14). This allows the bone removal to be done rapidly and allows efficient sectioning of teeth. The handpiece must not exhaust air into the operative field, making it unwise to use typical high-speed turbine drills for routine restorative dentistry. The reason is that the air exhausted into the wound may be forced into deeper tissue planes and produce tissue emphysema, a dangerous occurrence.

Mallet and Chisel

Occasionally, bone removal is performed using a mallet and chisel (Fig. 6-15). The mallet and chisel are often used when removing lingual tori. The edge of the chisel must be kept sharp to function properly. (See Chapter 13.)

Bone File

Final smoothing of bone before suturing a mucoperiosteal flap back into position is usually performed with a small bone file (Fig. 6-16, *A*). The bone file is usually a double-ended instrument with a small and large end. The bone file cannot be used efficiently for removal of large amounts of bone; therefore, it is used only for final smoothing. The teeth of many bone files are arranged in such a fashion that they remove bone only on a *pull* stroke (Fig. 6-16, *B*). Pushing this type of bone file against bone results only in burnishing and crushing the bone, and should be avoided.

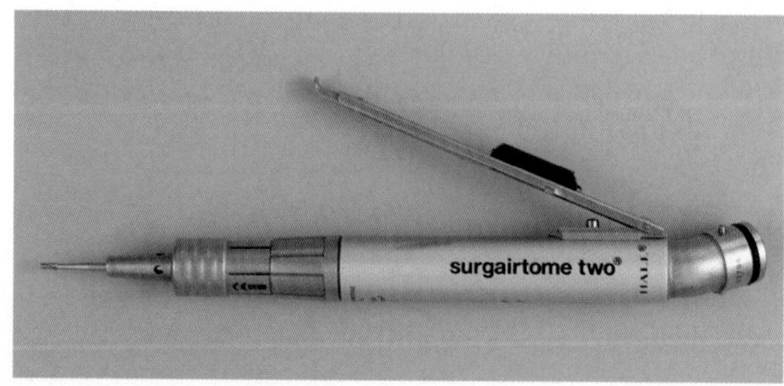

FIGURE 6-14 Typical moderate-speed, high-torque, sterilizable handpiece with No. 703 bur.

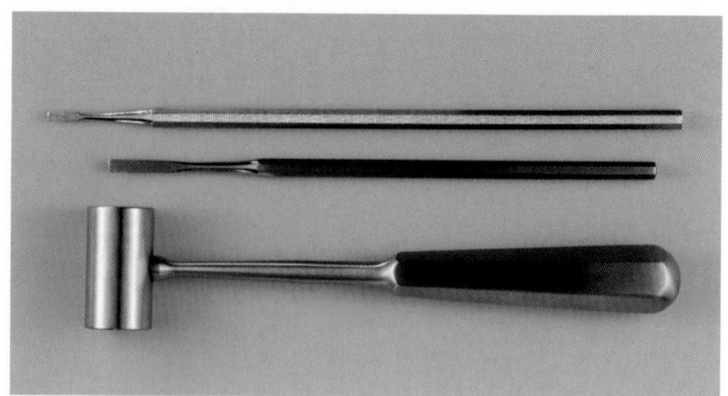

FIGURE 6-15 Surgical mallet and chisel can be used for removing bone.

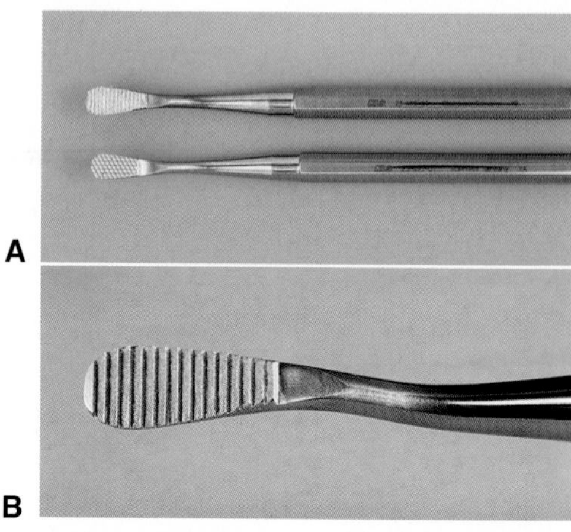

FIGURE 6-16 **A**, Double-ended bone file is used for smoothing small, sharp edges or spicules of bone. **B**, Teeth of bone file are effective only in pull stroke.

REMOVING SOFT TISSUE FROM BONY CAVITIES

The curette commonly used for oral surgery is an angled, double-ended instrument used to remove soft tissue from bony defects (Fig. 6-17). The principal use is to remove granulomas or small cysts from periapical lesions, but the curette is also used to remove small amounts of granulation tissue debris from a tooth socket. Note that the periapical curette is distinctly different from the periodontal curette in design and function.

SUTURING SOFT TISSUE

Once a surgical procedure has been completed, the mucoperiosteal flap is returned to its original position and is held in place by sutures. The needle holder is the instrument used to place the sutures.

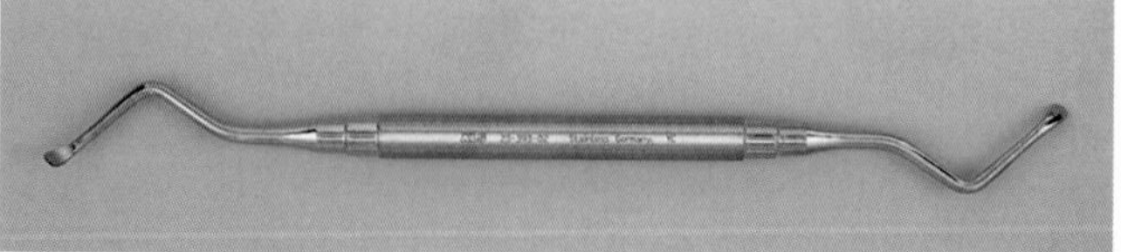

FIGURE 6-17 Periapical curette is a double-ended, spoon-shaped instrument used to remove soft tissue from bony cavities.

Needle Holder

The needle holder is an instrument with a locking handle and a short, blunt beak. For intraoral placement of sutures, a 6-inch (15-cm) needle holder is usually recommended (Fig. 6-18). The beaks of a needle holder are shorter and stronger than the beaks of a hemostat (Fig. 6-19). The face of a beak of the needle holder is crosshatched to permit a positive grasp of the suture needle. The hemostat has parallel grooves on the face of the beaks, thereby decreasing the control over needle and suture. Therefore the hemostat is a poor instrument for suturing.

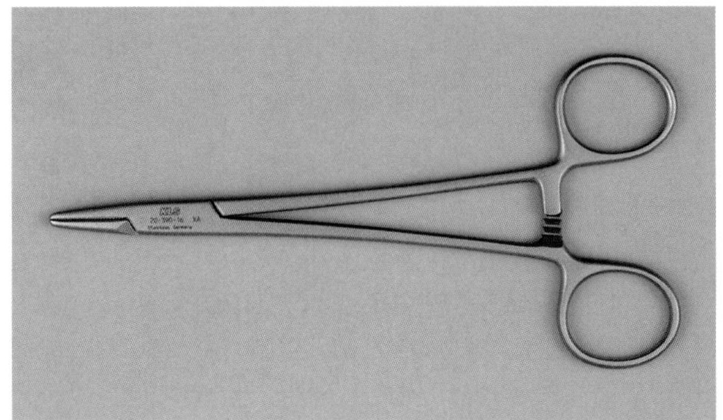

FIGURE 6-18 A needle holder has locking handle and short, stout beak.

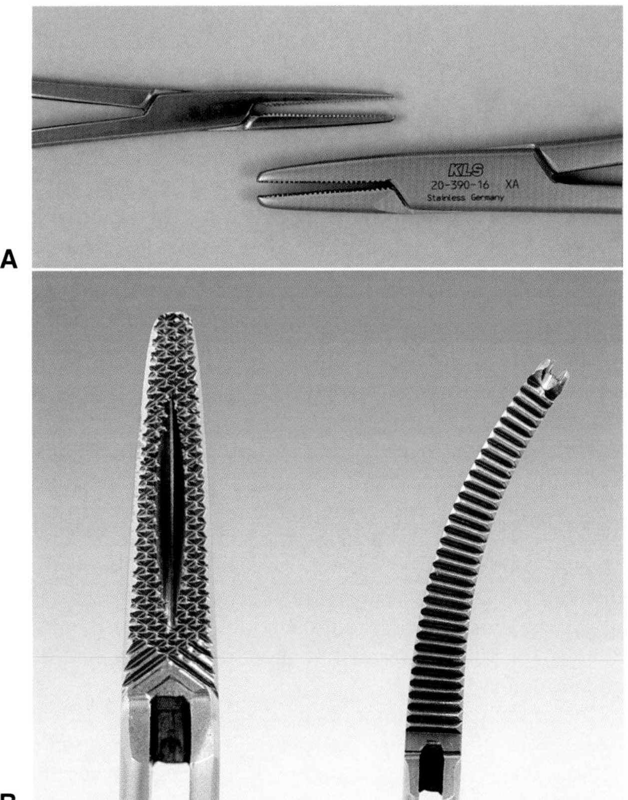

FIGURE 6-19 **A**, Hemostat (*top*) has longer, thinner beak compared with needle holder (*bottom*) and therefore should not be used for suturing. **B**, Face of shorter beak of needle holder is crosshatched to ensure positive grip on needle (*left*). Face of hemostat has parallel grooves that do not allow a firm grip on needle (*right*).

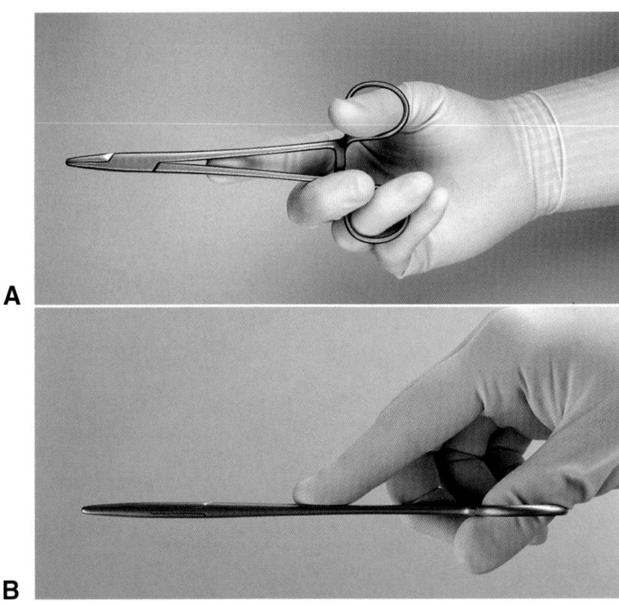

FIGURE 6-20 Needle holder is held by using thumb and ring finger in rings (**A**) and first and second finger to control instrument (**B**).

To control the locking handles properly and to direct the long needle holder, the surgeon must hold the instrument in the proper fashion (Fig. 6-20). The thumb and ring finger are inserted through the rings. The index finger is held along the length of the needle holder to steady and direct it. The second finger aids in controlling the locking mechanism. The index finger should not be put through the finger ring because this will result in dramatic decrease in control.

Suture Needle

The needle used in closing mucosal incisions is usually a small half-circle or three-eighths–circle suture needle. The needle is curved to allow it to pass through a limited space, where a straight needle cannot reach, and passage can be done with a twist of the wrist. Suture needles come in a large variety of shapes, from very small to very large (Fig. 6-21, *A*). The tips of suture needles are either tapered, such as a sewing needle, or they have triangular tips that allow them to be cutting needles. A cutting needle will pass through mucoperiosteum more easily than a tapered needle (Fig. 6-21, *B*). The cutting portion of the needle extends about one third the length of the needle, and the remaining portion of the needle is round. Tapered needles are used for more delicate tissues such as for ocular or vascular surgery. Care must be taken with cutting needles because they can cut through tissues lateral to the track of the needle if not used carefully and correctly. The suture material is usually purchased already swaged on by the manufacturer.

The curved needle is held approximately two thirds of the distance between the tip and the base of the needle (Fig. 6-22). This allows enough of the needle to be exposed to pass through the tissue, while allowing the needle holder to grasp the needle in its strong portion to prevent bending of the needle. Techniques for placing sutures are further discussed in Chapter 8.

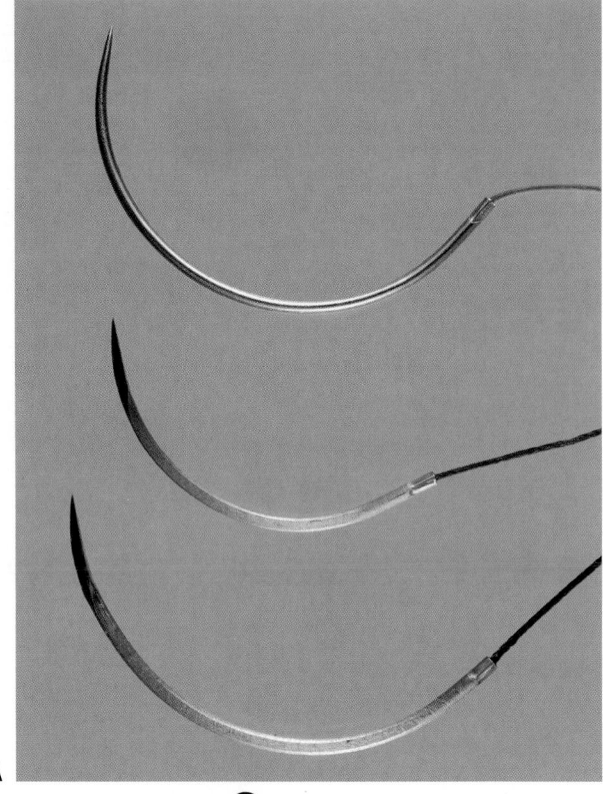

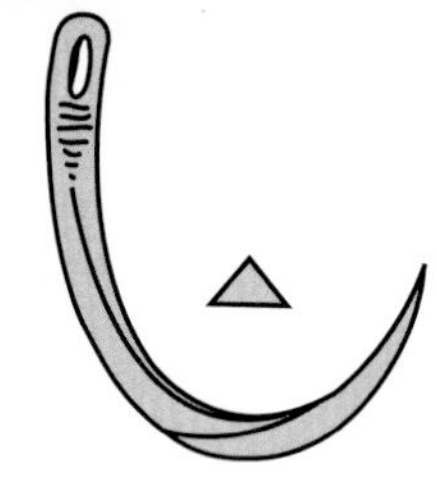

FIGURE 6-21 A, Comparison of needles used in oral surgery. Top is C-17 needle, which is usually 4-0 size suture. Middle is PS-2 needle, and bottom is SH. All are cutting needles, and suture material is swagged onto the needle. B, Tip of needle used to suture mucoperiosteum is triangular in cross section to make it a cutting needle.

Suture Material

Many types of suture materials are available. The materials are classified by diameter, resorbability, and whether they are monofilament or polyfilament.

The size of suture relates to its diameter and is designated by a series of zeros. The diameter most commonly used in the suturing of oral mucosa is 3-0 (000). A larger size suture is 2-0, or 0. Smaller sizes are designated, for example, 4-0, 5-0, and 6-0. Sutures of very fine size, such as 6-0, are usually used in conspicuous places on the skin, such as the face, because properly placed smaller sutures usually cause less scarring. Sutures of size 3-0 are large enough to withstand the tension placed on them intraorally and strong enough for easier knot tying with a needle holder compared with smaller-diameter sutures.

Sutures may be resorbable or nonresorbable. Nonresorbable suture materials include types such as silk, nylon, vinyl, and stainless steel. The most commonly used nonresorbable suture in the oral cavity is silk. Nylon, vinyl, and stainless steel are rarely used in the mouth. Resorbable sutures are primarily made of gut. Although the term *catgut* is often used to designate this type of suture, gut actually is derived from the serosal surface of sheep intestines. Plain catgut resorbs quickly in the oral cavity, rarely lasting longer than 3 to 5 days. Gut that has been treated by tanning solutions (chromic acid) and is therefore called *chromic gut* lasts longer—up to 7 to 10 days. Several synthetic resorbable sutures are also available. These are materials that are long chains of polymers braided into suture material. Examples are polyglycolic acid and polylactic acid. These materials are slowly resorbed, taking up to 4 weeks before they are resorbed. Such long-lasting resorbable sutures are rarely indicated in the oral cavity for basic oral surgery.

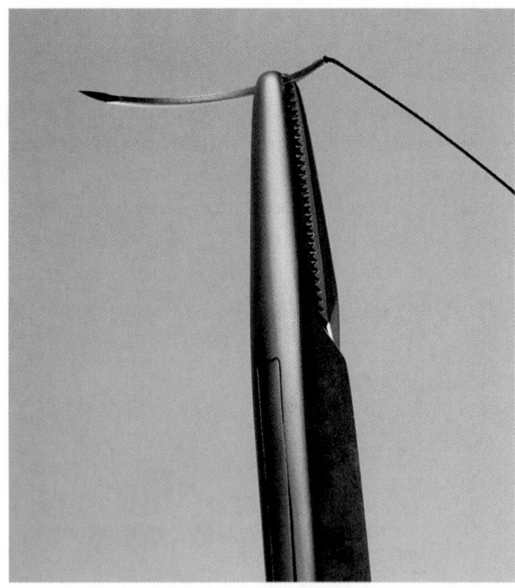

FIGURE 6-22 Needle holder grasps curved needle two thirds of the distance from tip of needle.

Finally, sutures are classified based on whether they are monofilament or polyfilament. Monofilament sutures are sutures such as plain and chromic gut, nylon, and stainless steel. Polyfilament sutures are silk, polyglycolic acid, and polylactic acid. Sutures that are made of braided material are easy to handle and tie and rarely come untied. The cut ends are usually soft and nonirritating to the tongue and surrounding soft tissues. However, because of the multiple filaments, they tend to "wick" oral fluids along the suture to the underlying tissues. This wicking action may carry bacteria along with the saliva. Monofilament sutures do not cause this wicking action but may be more difficult to tie, tend to come untied, and the cut ends are stiffer and therefore more irritating to the tongue and soft tissues.

One of the most commonly used suture for the oral cavity is 3-0 black silk. The size 3-0 has the appropriate amount of strength; the polyfilament nature of the silk makes it easy to tie and well tolerated by the patient's soft tissues. The color makes the suture easy to see when the patient returns for suture removal. Sutures that are holding mucosa together usually stay no longer than 5 to 7 days, so the wicking action is of little clinical importance. Many surgeons prefer 3-0 chromic suture to avoid the need to later remove it. (Techniques for suturing and knot tying are presented in Chapter 8.)

Scissors

The final instruments necessary for placing sutures are suture scissors (Fig. 6-23). The suture scissors usually have short cutting edges because their sole purpose is to cut sutures. The most commonly used suture scissors for oral surgery are the Dean scissors. These scissors have slightly curved handles and serrated blades that make cutting sutures easier. Suture scissors usually have long handles and thumb and finger rings. The scissors are held in the same way as the needle holder.

Other types of scissors are designed for cutting soft tissue. The two major types of tissue scissors are the Iris scissors and the Metzenbaum scissors (Fig. 6-24, *A*). These scissors can have straight or curved blades. The Iris scissors are small, sharp-pointed, delicate tools used for fine work. The Metzenbaum scissors are used for undermining soft tissue and for cutting. They can have either sharp or blunt (rounded) tips. Tissue scissors such as the Iris or Metzenbaum scissors should not be used to cut sutures because the suture material will dull the edges of the blades and make them less effective and more traumatic when cutting tissue. The exception is when removing very fine sutures placed in skin incisions in the face. Scissors with thin, pointed tips such as an Iris may be useful.

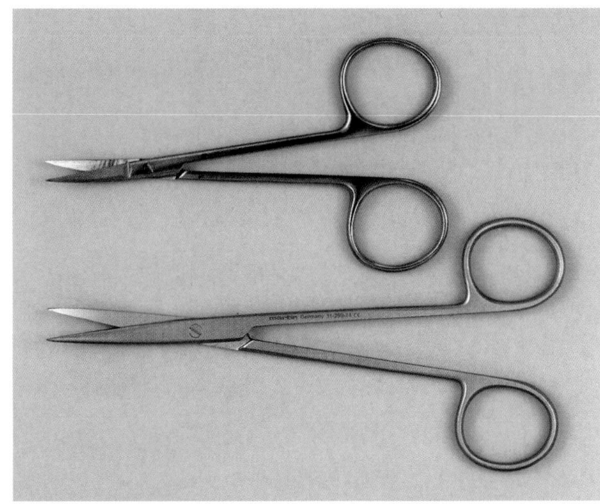

FIGURE 6-24 Soft tissue scissors are of two designs: Iris scissors (*top*) are small, sharp-pointed scissors. Metzenbaum scissors (*bottom*) are longer, delicate scissors. Metzenbaum scissors are available as either sharp tipped (shown here) or blunt-tipped.

HOLDING THE MOUTH OPEN

When performing extractions of mandibular teeth, it is necessary to support the mandible to prevent stress on the temporomandibular joints. Supporting the patient's jaw on a bite block will protect the joints. The bite block is just what the name implies (Fig. 6-25, *A* and *B*). The bite block is a soft, rubberlike block on which the patient can rest the teeth. The patient opens the mouth to a comfortably wide position, and the rubber bite block is inserted, which holds the mouth in the desired position. Bite blocks come in several sizes to fit variously sized patients and produce varying degrees of opening. Should the surgeon need the mouth to open wider using any size of bite block, the patient must open more widely and the bite block must be positioned more to the posterior of the mouth. For most adult patients a pediatric-sized bite block is adequate when placed over the molar teeth.

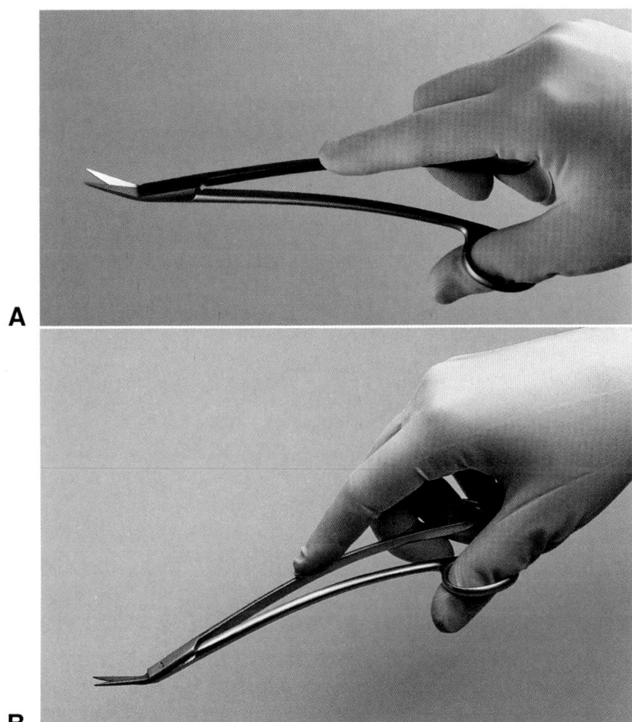

FIGURE 6-23 A and B, Suture scissors should be held in same fashion as needle holder.

The side-action mouth prop or Molt mouth prop (Fig. 6-26) can be used by the operator to open the mouth wider if necessary. This mouth prop has a ratchet-type action, opening the mouth wider as the handle is closed. This type of mouth prop should be used with caution because great pressure can be applied to the teeth and temporomandibular joint, and injury may occur with injudicious use. This type of mouth prop is useful in patients who are deeply sedated or have mild forms of trismus.

Whenever a bite block or side-action mouth prop is used, the surgeon should take care to avoid opening the mouth too widely because it may cause stress on the jaw joint. Occasionally, this may result in stretch injury to the joint, necessitating additional treatment. When long procedures are being performed, it is a good idea periodically to remove the prop and allow the patient to move the jaw and rest the muscles for a short time.

SUCTIONING

To provide adequate visualization, blood, saliva, and irrigating solutions must be suctioned from the operative site. The surgical suction is one that has a smaller orifice than the type used in general dentistry to more rapidly evacuate fluids from the surgical site to maintain adequate visualization. Many of these suctions are designed with several orifices so that the soft tissue will not become aspirated into the suction hole and cause tissue injury (Fig. 6-27, *A*).

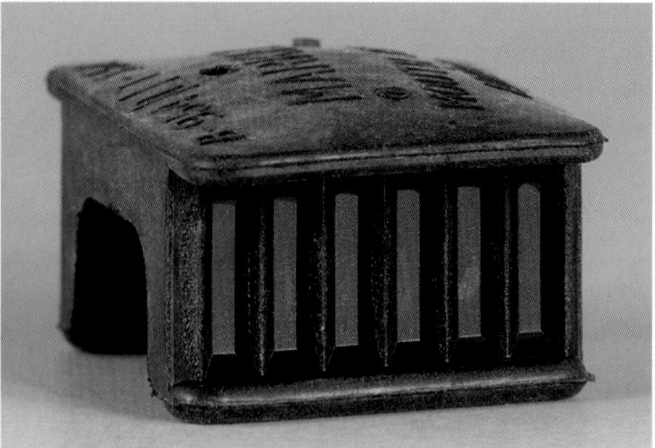

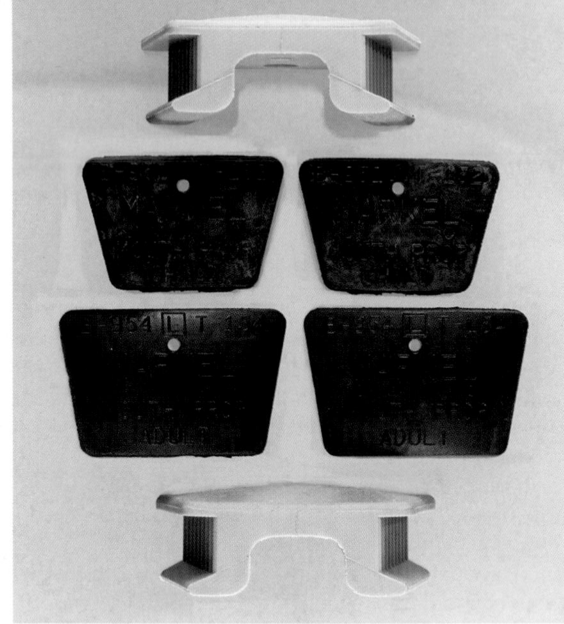

FIGURE 6-25 **A**, Silicone bite block is used to hold mouth open in position chosen by patient. **B**, The sides of the bite block are corrugated to provide a surface for the teeth to engage. **C**, The blocks come in a variety of sizes.

The Fraser suction has a hole in the handle portion that can be covered as needed. When hard tissue is being cut under copious irrigation, the hole is covered so that the solution is removed rapidly. When soft tissue is being suctioned, the hole can be left uncovered to prevent tissue injury or soft tissue obstruction of the suction tip (Fig. 6-27, *B*).

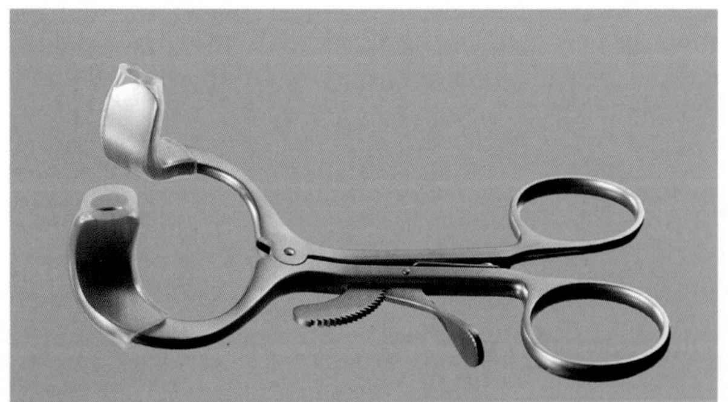

FIGURE 6-26 Side-action, or Molt, mouth prop can be used to open patient's mouth when patient is unable to cooperate, such as during sedation or has some degree of trismus.

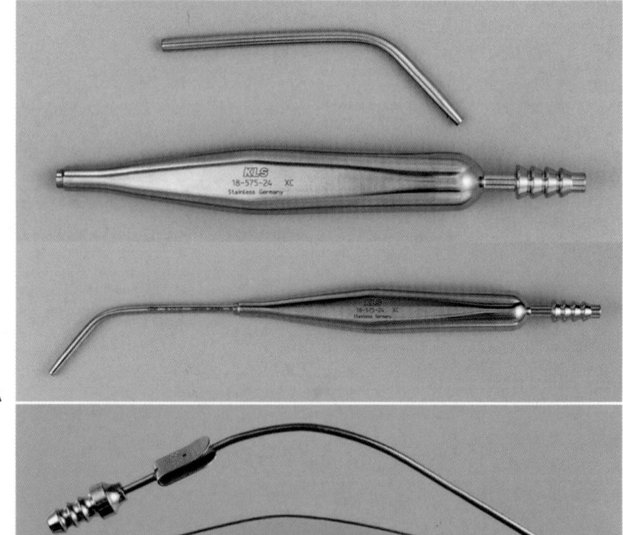

FIGURE 6-27 **A**, Typical surgical suction has small-diameter tip. Suction tips usually have a hole to prevent tissue injury caused by excess suction pressure. Top is unassembled for cleaning; bottom is assembled for use. **B**, Fraser suction tip has blade in handle to allow operator more control over amount of suction power. Holding the thumb over the hole increases suction at the tip. Wire stylet is used to clean tip when bone or tooth particles plug suction.

HOLDING TOWELS AND DRAPES IN POSITION

When drapes are placed around a patient, they can be held together with a towel clip (Fig. 6-28). This instrument has a locking handle and finger and thumb rings. The action ends of the towel clip can be sharp or blunt. Those with curved points penetrate the towels and drapes. When this instrument is used, the operator must exercise extreme caution not to pinch the patient's underlying skin.

IRRIGATING

When a handpiece and bur are used to remove bone, it is essential that the area be irrigated with a steady stream of irrigating solution, usually sterile saline or sterile water. The irrigation cools the bur and prevents bone-damaging heat buildup. The irrigation also increases the efficiency of the bur by washing away bone chips from the flutes of the bur and by providing a certain amount of lubrication. In addition, once a surgical procedure is completed and before the mucoperiosteal flap is sutured back into position, the surgical field should be thoroughly irrigated. A large plastic syringe with a blunt 18-gauge needle is commonly used for irrigation. Although the syringe is disposable, it can be sterilized multiple times before it must be discarded. The needle should be blunt and smooth so that it does not damage soft tissue, and it should be angled for more efficient direction of the irrigating stream (Fig. 6-29).

EXTRACTING TEETH

One of the most important instruments used in the extraction procedure is the dental elevator. These instruments are used to luxate teeth (loosen them) from the surrounding bone. Loosening teeth before the application of the dental forceps makes extractions easier. By elevating the teeth before the application of the forceps, the clinician can minimize the incidence of broken roots, teeth, and bone. Finally, luxation of teeth before forceps application facilitates the removal of a broken root should it occur, because the prior elevator use is likely to loosen the root in the dental socket. In addition to their role in loosening teeth from the surrounding bone, dental elevators are also used to expand alveolar bone. By expanding the buccocervical plate of bone, the surgeon facilitates the removal of a tooth that has a limited and obstructed path for removal. Finally, elevators are used to remove broken or surgically sectioned roots from their sockets.

Dental Elevators

The three major components of the elevator are the handle, shank, and blade (Fig. 6-30). The handle of the elevator is usually of generous size, so it can be held comfortably in the hand to apply substantial but controlled force. The application of specifically applied force is critical in the proper use of dental elevators. In some situations, cross bar or T-bar handles are used. These instruments must be used with great caution because they can generate an excessive amount of force (Fig. 6-31).

The shank of the elevator simply connects the handle to the working end, or blade, of the elevator. The shank is generally of substantial size and is strong enough to transmit the force from the handle to the blade. The blade of the elevator is the working tip of the elevator and is used to transmit the force to the tooth, bone, or both.

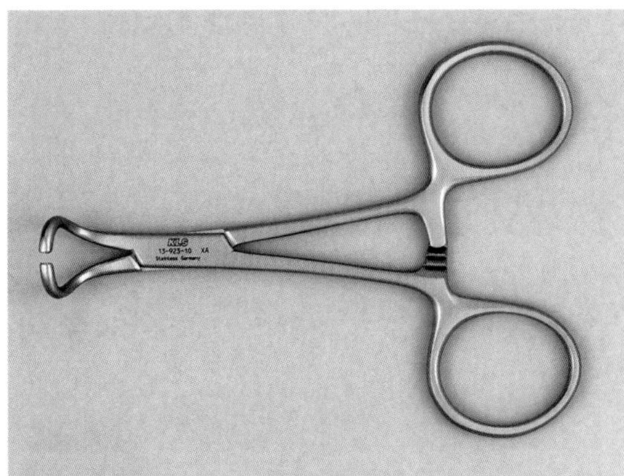

FIGURE 6-28 Towel clip is used to hold drapes in position. Tips clasp towels, and locking handles maintain drape in position. The clip shown has nonpenetrating blunt tips. Towel clamps with sharp penetrating tips are also available.

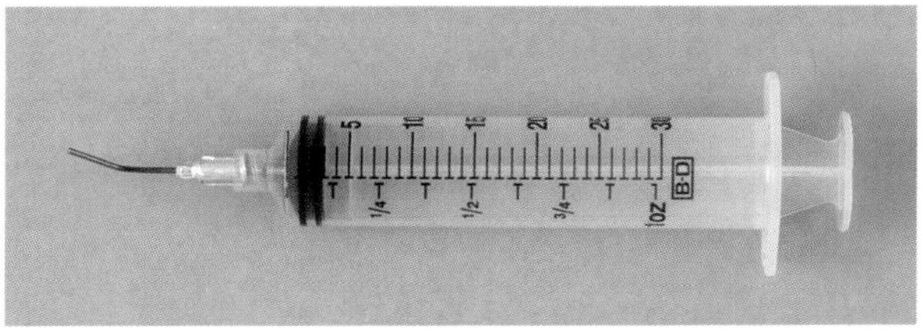

FIGURE 6-29 Large plastic syringes may be used to deliver irrigation solution to operative site using an angled blunt tip.

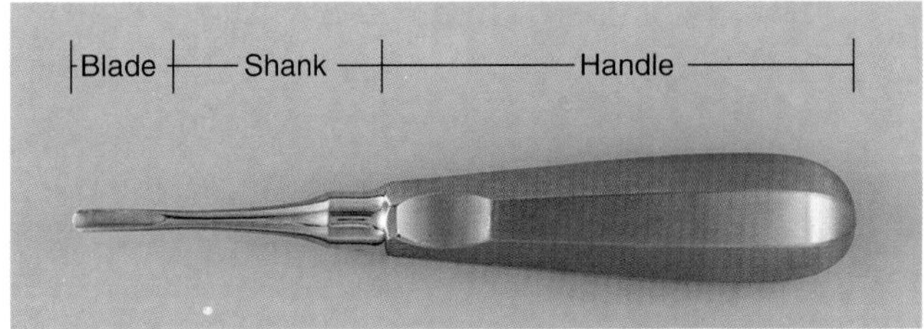

FIGURE 6-30 The major components of an elevator are the handle, shank, and blade.

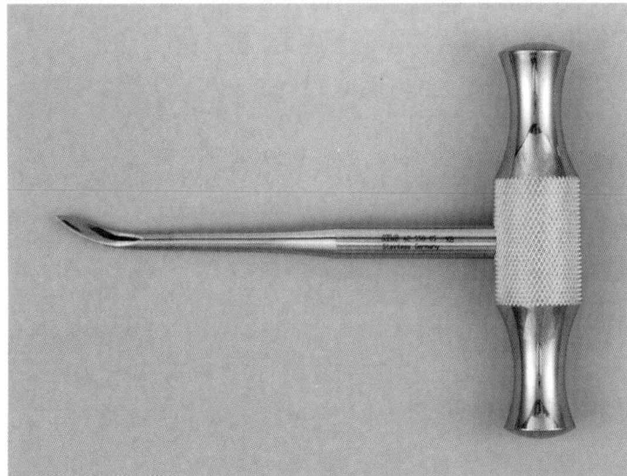

FIGURE 6-31 Cross bar handle is used on certain elevators. This type of handle can generate large amounts of force and therefore must be used with great caution.

Types of Elevators

The biggest variation in the type of elevator is in the shape and size of the blade. The three basic types of elevators are (1) the straight type; (2) the triangle or pennant-shape type; and (3) the pick type. The straight elevator is the most commonly used elevator to luxate teeth (Fig. 6-32, *A*). The blade of the straight elevator has a concave surface on one side that is placed toward the tooth to be elevated (Fig. 6-32, *B*). The small straight elevator, No. 301, is frequently used for beginning the luxation of an erupted tooth, before application of the forceps (Fig. 6-33). Larger straight elevators are used to displace roots from their sockets and are also used to luxate teeth that are more widely spaced or once a smaller-sized straight elevator becomes less effective. The most commonly used large straight elevator is the No. 34S, but the No. 46 and No. 77R are also used occasionally.

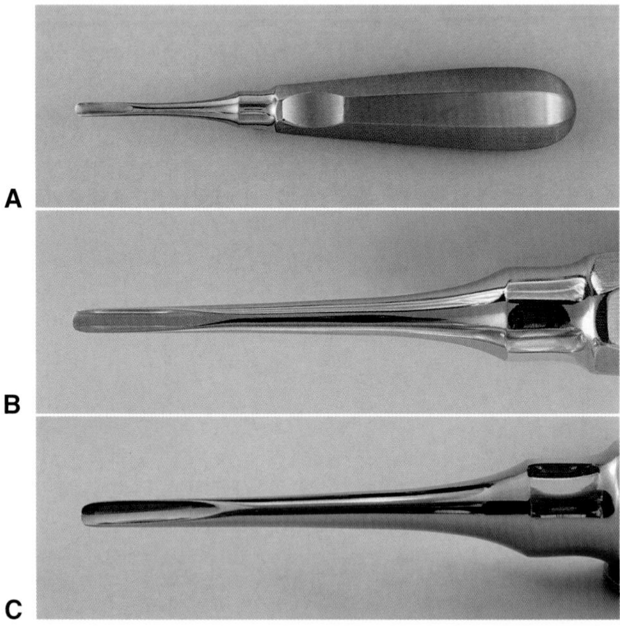

FIGURE 6-32 A, Straight elevators are most commonly used elevators. **B** and **C**, Blade of straight elevator is concave on its working side.

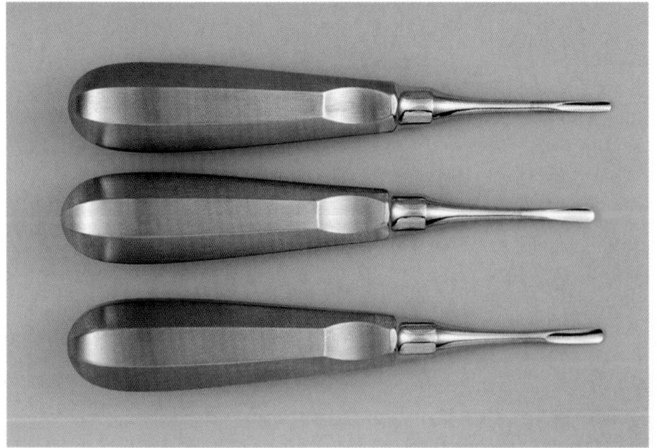

FIGURE 6-33 Variety of sizes of straight elevators, which vary based on width of the blade.

The shape of the blade of the straight elevator can be angled from the shank, allowing this instrument to be used in the more posterior aspects of the mouth. Two examples of the angled-shank elevator with a blade similar to the straight elevator are the Miller elevator and the Potts elevator.

The second most commonly used type of elevator is the triangular elevator (Fig. 6-34). These elevators are provided in pairs: a left and a right. The triangular elevator is most useful when a broken root remains in the tooth socket and the adjacent socket is empty. A typical example would be when a mandibular first molar is fractured, leaving the distal root in the socket but the mesial root removed with the crown. The tip of the triangular elevator is placed into the socket, with the shank of the elevator resting on the buccal plate of bone. The elevator is then turned in a wheel-and-axle rotation, with the sharp tip of the elevator engaging the cementum of the remaining distal root; the elevator is then turned and the root is delivered. Triangular elevators come in a variety of types and angulations, but the Cryer is the most common type.

The third type of elevator that is used with some frequency is the pick-type elevator. This type of elevator is used to remove roots. The heavy version of the pick is the Crane pick (Fig. 6-35). This instrument is used as a lever to elevate a broken root from the tooth socket. Usually it is necessary to drill a hole with a bur (purchase point) approximately 3 mm deep into the root just at the bony crest. The tip of the pick is then inserted into the hole, and with the buccal plate of bone as a fulcrum, the root is elevated from the tooth socket. Occasionally the sharp point can be used without preparing a purchase point by engaging the cementum or furcation of the tooth.

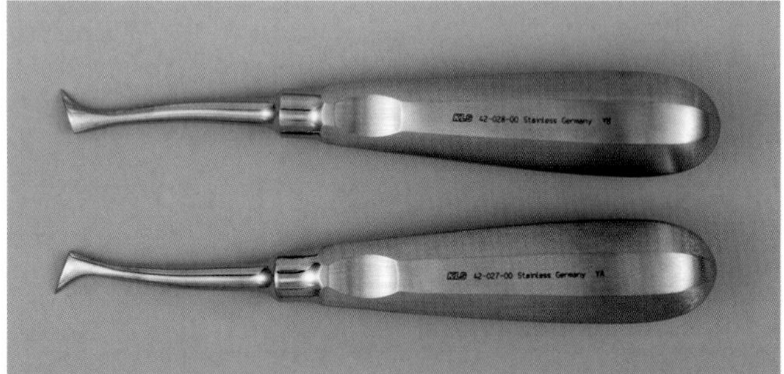

FIGURE 6-34 Triangular elevators (Cryer) are pairs of instruments and are therefore used for mesial or distal roots.

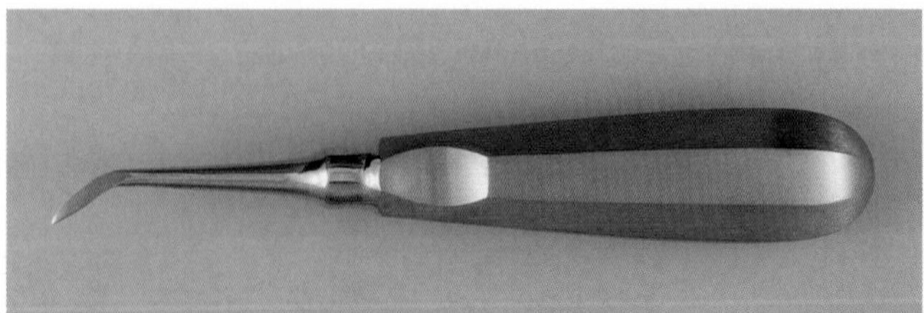

FIGURE 6-35 Crane pick is a heavy instrument used to elevate whole roots or even teeth after purchase point has been prepared with bur.

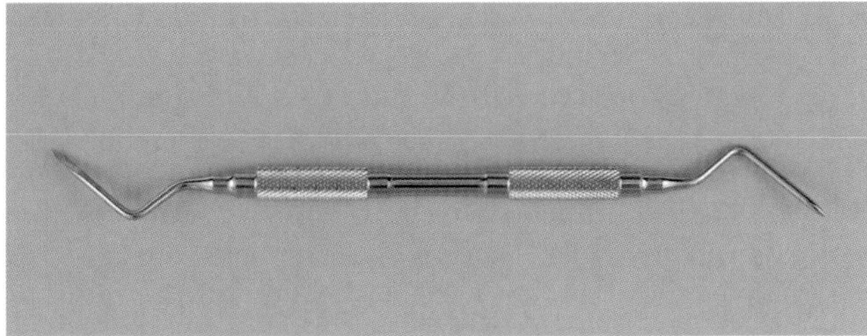

FIGURE 6-36 Delicate root tip pick is used to tease root tip fragments from socket. The fine tip can be broken off or bent if instrument is used improperly.

The second type of pick is the root tip pick or apex elevator (Fig. 6-36). The root tip pick is a delicate instrument that is used to tease small root tips from their sockets. It must be emphasized that this is a thin instrument and should not be used as a wheel-and-axle or lever type of elevator like the Cryer elevator or the Crane pick. The root tip pick is used to tease the very small root end of a tooth by inserting the tip into the periodontal ligament space between the root tip and socket wall.

Extraction Forceps

The extraction forceps are instruments used for removing the tooth from the alveolar bone. These forceps are designed in many styles and configurations to adapt to the variety of teeth for which they are used. Each basic design offers a multiplicity of variations to coincide with individual operator preferences. This section deals with the basic fundamental designs and touches on several of the variations.

Forceps Components

The basic components of dental extraction forceps are the handle, hinge, and beaks (Fig. 6-37). The handles are usually of adequate size to be handled comfortably and deliver sufficient pressure and leverage to remove the required tooth. The handles have a serrated surface to allow a positive grip and to prevent slippage.

The handles of the forceps are held differently, depending on the position of the tooth to be removed. Maxillary forceps are held with the palm underneath the forceps so that the beak is directed in a superior direction (Fig. 6-38). The forceps used for removal of mandibular teeth are held with the palm on top of the forceps so that the beak is pointed down toward the teeth (Fig. 6-39). The handles of the forceps are usually straight but may be curved. This provides the operator with a sense of better fit (Fig. 6-40).

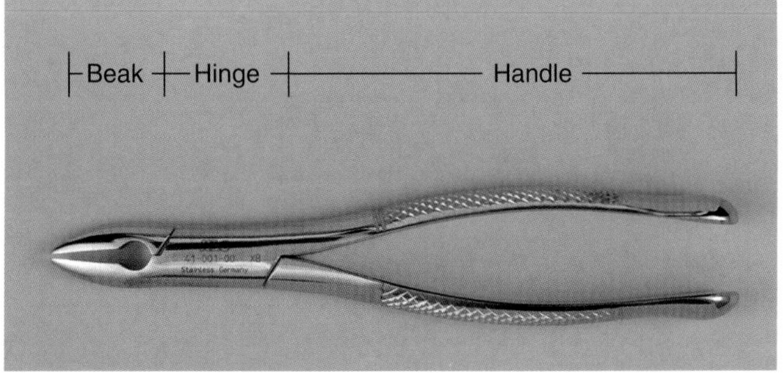

FIGURE 6-37 Basic components of extraction forceps.

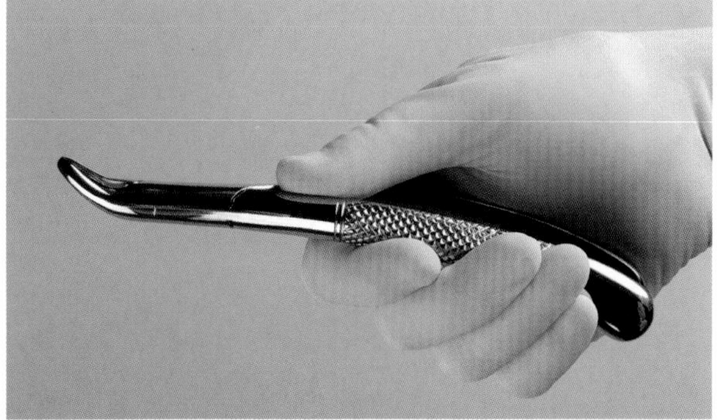

FIGURE 6-38 Forceps used to remove maxillary teeth are held with palm under handle.

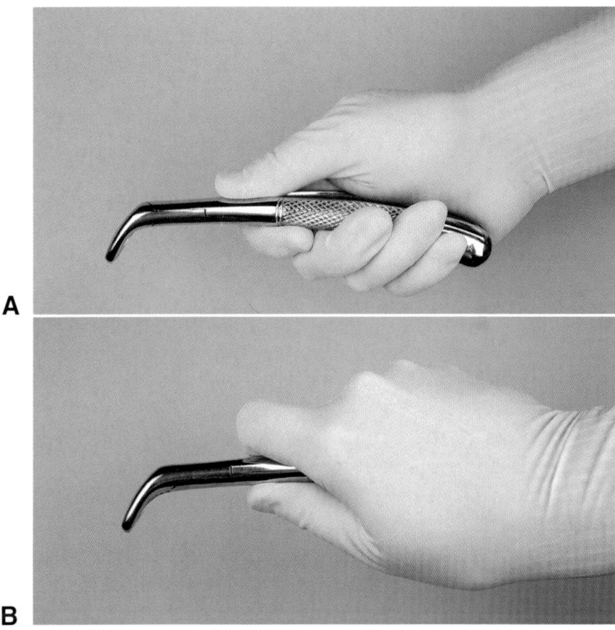

FIGURE 6-39 A, Forceps used to remove mandibular teeth are held with palm on top of forceps. B, Firmer grip for delivering greater amounts of rotational force can be achieved by moving thumb around and under handle.

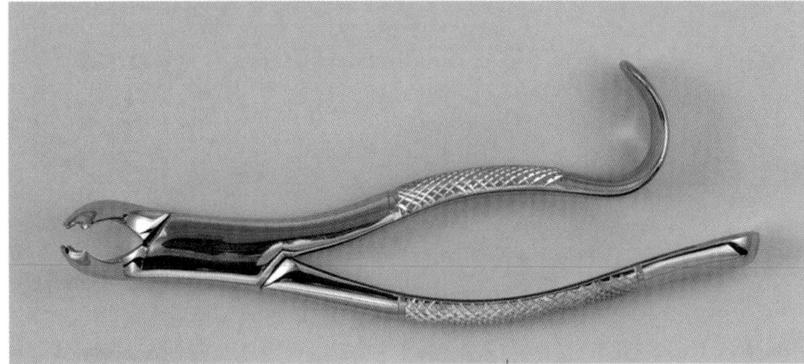

FIGURE 6-40 Straight handles are usually preferred, but curved handles are preferred by some surgeons.

The hinge of the forceps, like the shank of the elevator, is merely a mechanism for connecting the handle to the beak. The hinge transfers and concentrates the force applied to the handles to the beak. One distinct difference in styles does exist: The usual American type of forceps has a hinge in a

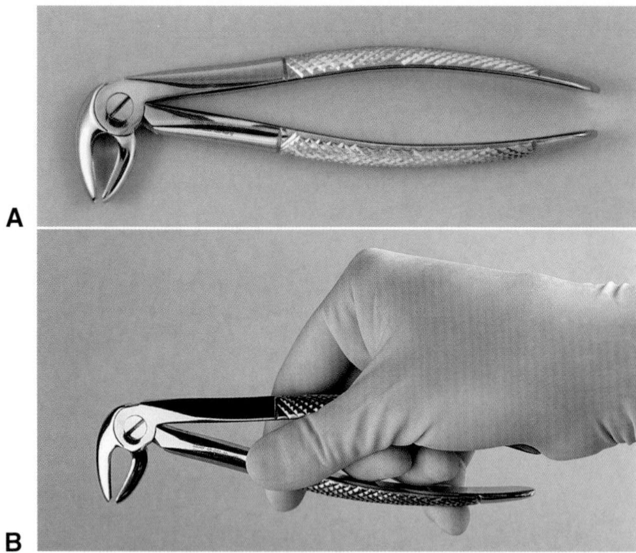

FIGURE 6-41 A, English style of forceps has hinge in vertical direction. B, English style of forceps is held in vertical direction.

horizontal direction and is used as has been described (see Fig. 6-37). The English preference is for a vertical hinge and corresponding vertically positioned handle (Fig. 6-41, *A*). Thus the English-style handle and hinge are used with the hand held in a vertical direction as opposed to a horizontal direction (Fig. 6-41, *B*).

The beaks of the extraction forceps are the source of the greatest variation among forceps. The beak is designed to adapt to the tooth root near the junction of the crown and root. One must remember that the beaks of the forceps are designed to be adapted to the *root structure* of the tooth and not to the crown of the tooth. In a sense then, different beaks are designed for single-rooted teeth, two-rooted teeth, and three-rooted teeth. The design variation is such that the tips of the beaks will adapt closely to the various root formations, improving the surgeon's control of forces on the root and decreasing the chance for root fracture. The more closely the beaks of the forceps adapt to the tooth roots, the more efficient the extraction and the less chance for undesired outcomes.

A final design variation is in the width of the beak. Some forceps beaks are narrow because their primary use is to remove narrow teeth, such as incisor teeth. Other forceps beaks are broader because the teeth they are designed to remove are substantially wider, such as lower molar teeth. Forceps designed to remove a lower incisor can theoretically be used to remove a lower molar, but the beaks are so narrow that they will be inefficient for that application. Similarly, the broader molar forceps will not adapt to the narrow space occupied by the lower incisor and therefore cannot be used in that situation without damage to adjacent teeth.

The beaks of forceps are angled so that they can be placed parallel to the long axis of the tooth, with the handle in a comfortable position. Therefore the beaks of maxillary forceps are usually parallel to the handles. Maxillary molar forceps are offset in a bayonet fashion to allow the operator to reach the posterior aspect of the mouth comfortably and yet keep the beaks parallel to the long axis of the tooth. The beaks of mandibular forceps are usually set perpendicular to the handles, which allows the surgeon to reach the lower teeth and maintain a comfortable, controlled position.

Maxillary Forceps

The removal of maxillary teeth requires the use of instruments designed for single-rooted teeth and for teeth with three roots. The maxillary incisors, canine teeth, and premolar teeth are considered to be single-rooted teeth. The maxillary first premolar frequently has a bifurcated root, but because this occurs in the apical one third, it has no influence on the design of the forceps. The maxillary molars have trifurcated roots, and there are extraction forceps that will adapt to that configuration.

After some elevation, the single-rooted maxillary teeth are usually removed with *maxillary universal forceps,* usually No. 150 (Fig. 6-42). The No. 150 forceps are slightly S-shaped when viewed from the side and are essentially straight when viewed from above. The beaks of the forceps curve to meet only at the tip. The slight curve of the No. 150 allows the operator to reach not only the incisors but also the premolars comfortably. The beak of the No. 150 forceps comes in a style

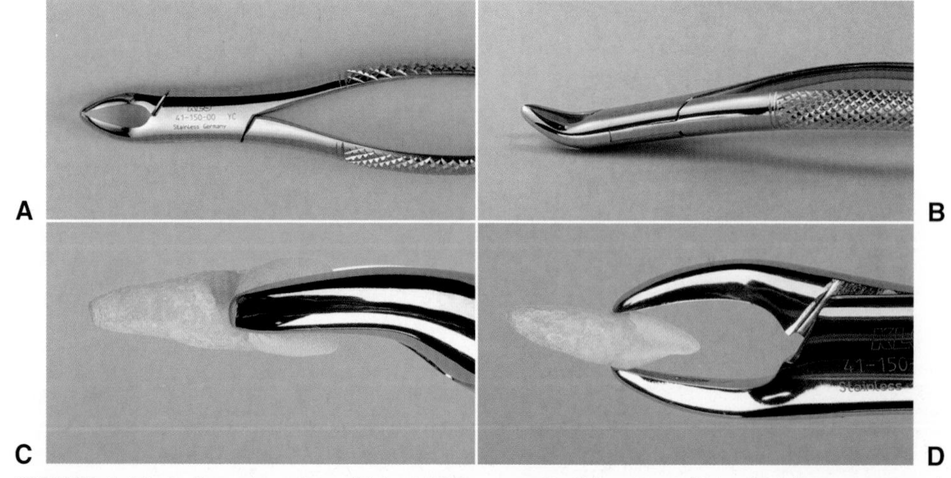

FIGURE 6-42 A, Superior view of No. 150 forceps. B, Side view of No. 150 forceps. C and D, No. 150 forceps adapted to maxillary central incisor.

that has been modified slightly to form the No. 150A forceps (Fig. 6-43). The No. 150A is useful for the maxillary premolar teeth and should not be used for the incisors because its adaptation to the roots of the incisors is poor.

In addition to the No. 150 forceps, *straight forceps* are also available. The No. 1 forceps (Fig. 6-44), which can be used for maxillary incisors and canines, are easier to use than the No. 150 for upper incisors.

The maxillary molar teeth are three-rooted teeth with a single palatal root and a buccal bifurcation. Therefore, forceps that are specifically adapted to fit the maxillary molars must have a smooth, concave surface for the palatal root and a beak with a pointed design that will fit into the buccal bifurcation. This requires that the molar forceps come in pairs: a left and a right. Additionally, the molar forceps should be offset so that the surgeon can reach the posterior aspect of the mouth and remain in the correct position. The most commonly used molar forceps are the No. 53 right and left (Fig. 6-45). These forceps are designed to fit anatomically around the palatal beak, and the pointed buccal beak fits into the buccal bifurcation. The beak is offset to allow for good surgeon positioning.

A design variation is shown in the No. 88 right and left forceps, which have a longer, more accentuated, pointed beak formation (Fig. 6-46). These forceps are known as *upper cowhorn forceps*. They are particularly useful for maxillary molars with crowns that are severely carious. The sharply pointed beaks may reach deeper into the trifurcation to sound

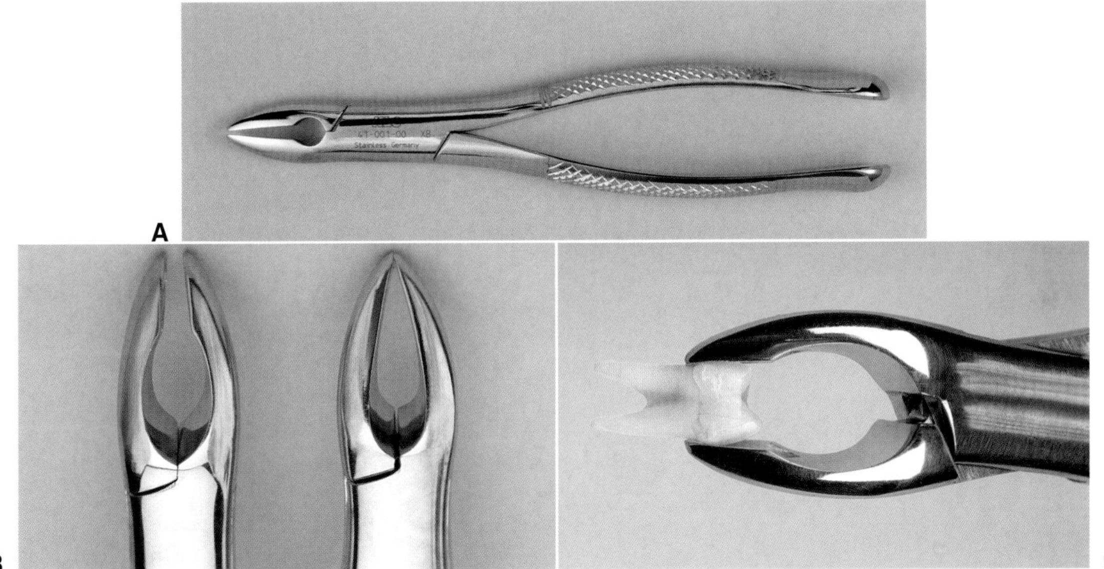

FIGURE 6-43 **A**, Superior view of No. 150A forceps. **B**, No. 150A forceps have parallel beaks that do not touch in distinction from 150 forceps beak. **C**, Adaptation of No. 150A forceps to maxillary premolar.

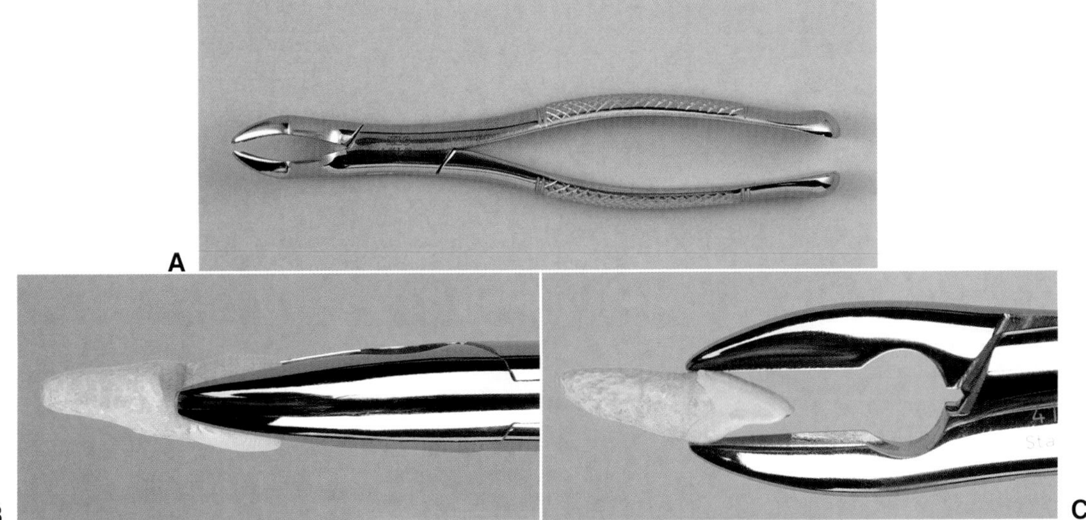

FIGURE 6-44 **A**, Superior view of the No. 1 forceps. **B** and **C** No. 1 forceps adapted to incisor.

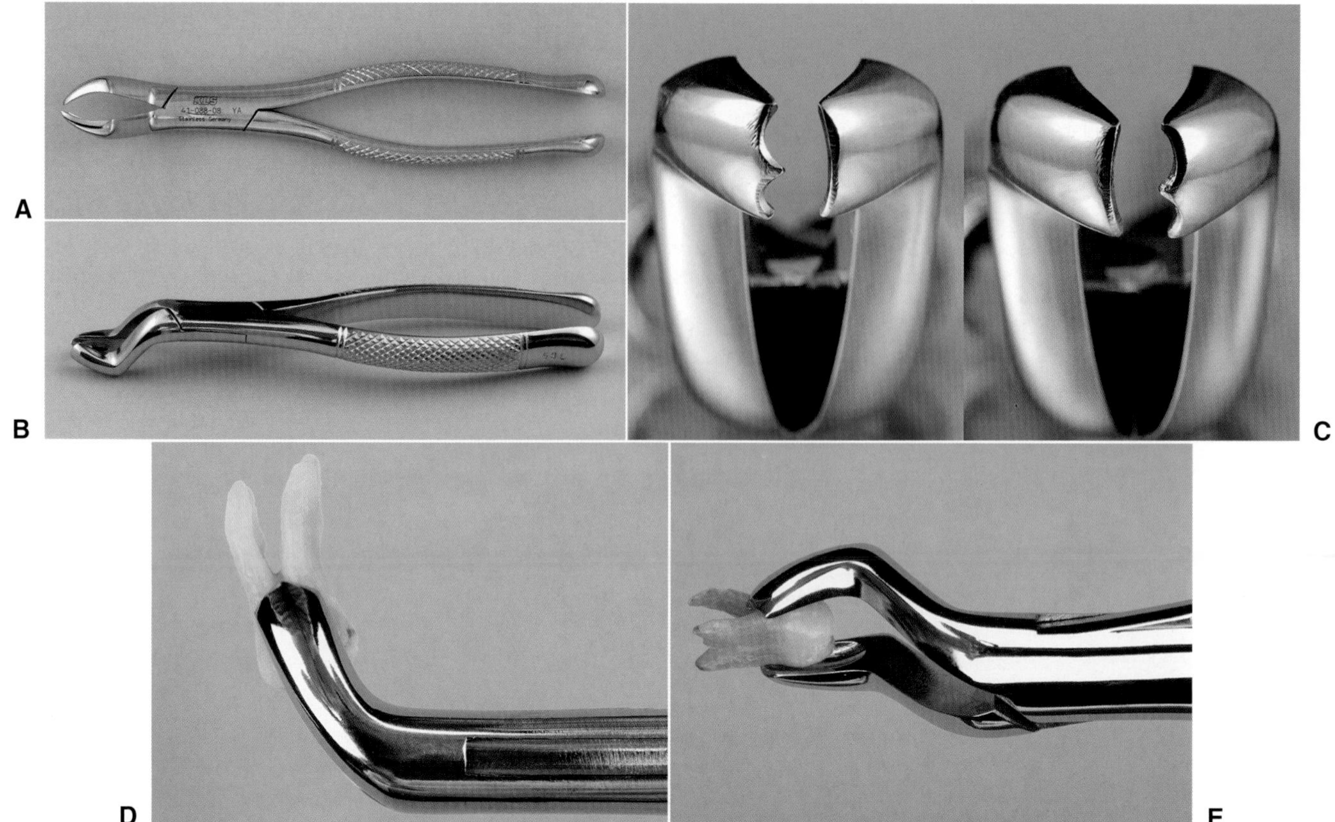

FIGURE 6-45 A, Superior view of the No. 53L forceps. B, Oblique view of No. 53L forceps. C, *Right*, No. 53L; *left*, No. 53R. D and E, No. 53L adapted to maxillary molar.

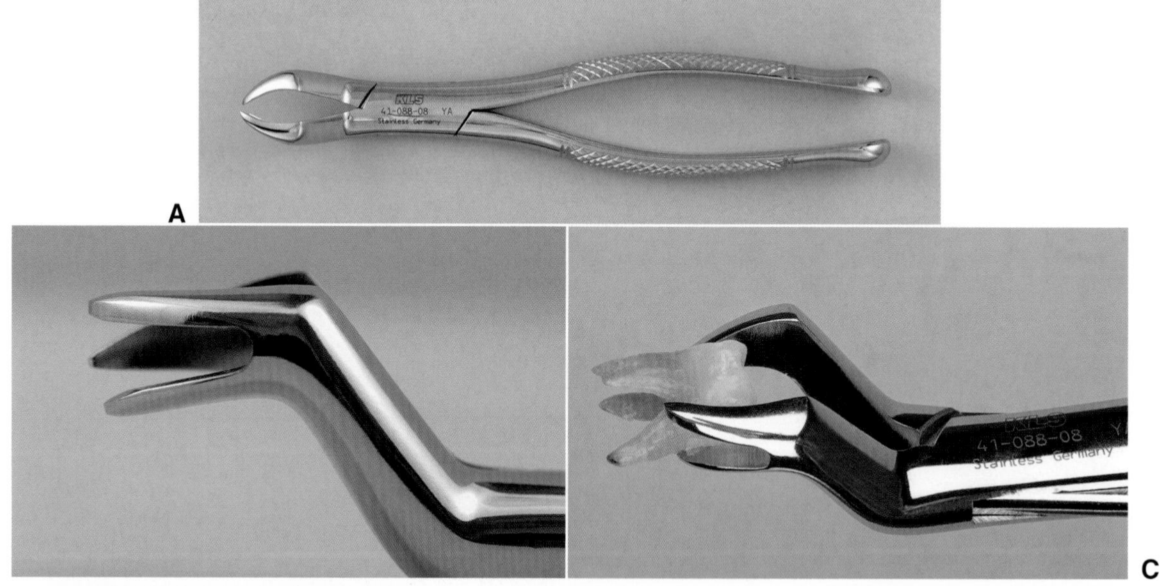

FIGURE 6-46 A, Superior view of No. 88L forceps. B, Side view of No. 88L forceps. C, No. 88R adapted to maxillary molar.

dentin. The major disadvantage is that they crush crestal alveolar bone, and when used on intact teeth without due caution, fracture of large amounts of buccal alveolar bone may occur.

On occasion, maxillary second molars and erupted third molars have a single conical root. In this situation, forceps with broad, smooth beaks that are offset from the handle can be useful. The No. 210S forceps exemplify this design (Fig. 6-47). Another design variation is shown in the offset molar forceps with very narrow beaks. These forceps are used primarily to remove broken maxillary molar roots but can be used for

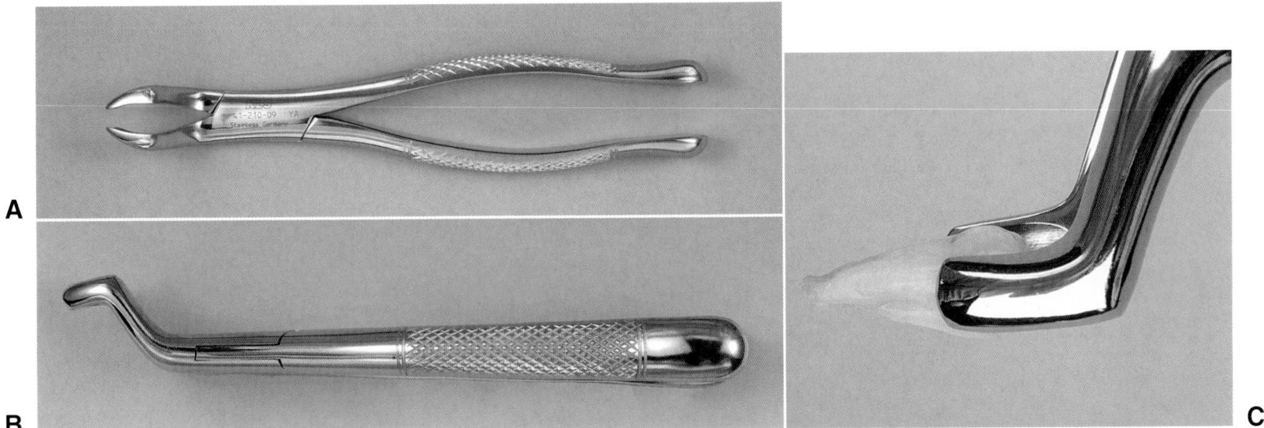

FIGURE 6-47 A, Superior view of No. 210S forceps. B, Side view of No. 210S forceps. C, No. 210S adapted to maxillary molar.

removal of narrow premolars and for lower incisors. These forceps, the No. 65, are also known as root tip forceps (Fig. 6-48).

A smaller version of the No. 150, the No. 150S, is useful for removing primary teeth (Fig. 6-49). These forceps adapt well to all maxillary primary teeth and can be used as universal primary tooth forceps.

Mandibular Forceps

Extraction of mandibular teeth requires forceps that can be used for single-rooted teeth for the incisors, canines, and premolars, as well as for two-rooted teeth for the molars. The forceps most commonly used for the single-rooted teeth are the *lower universal forceps,* or the No. 151 (Fig. 6-50). These forceps have handles similar in shape to the No. 150, but the beaks are pointed inferiorly for the lower teeth. The beaks are smooth and narrow and meet only at the tip. This allows the beaks to fit near the cervical line of the tooth and to grasp the root.

The No. 151A forceps have been modified slightly for mandibular premolar teeth (Fig. 6-51). These forceps should not be used for other lower teeth because their form prevents adaptation to the roots of the teeth.

The English style of vertical-hinge forceps can be used for the single-rooted teeth in the mandible (Fig. 6-52). Great force can be generated with these forceps. Unless great care is used, the incidence of root fracture is high with this instrument. Therefore, it is rarely used by the inexperienced, beginning surgeon.

The mandibular molars are bifurcated, two-rooted teeth that allow the use of forceps that anatomically adapt to the tooth. Because the bifurcation is on the buccal and the lingual sides, only a single molar forceps are necessary for the both sides, in contradistinction to the maxilla, for which a right- and left-paired molar forceps set is required.

A useful lower molar forceps are the No. 17 (Fig. 6-53). These forceps are usually straight-handled, and the beaks are set obliquely downward. The beaks have pointed tips in the center to be set into the bifurcation of lower molar teeth. The remainder of the beak adapts well to the sides of the furcation. Because of the pointed tips, the No. 17 forceps cannot be used for molar teeth, which have fused, conical roots. For this purpose the No. 151 forceps are used.

A major design variation in lower molar forceps is the No. 87, the so-called *cowhorn forceps* (Fig. 6-54). These instruments

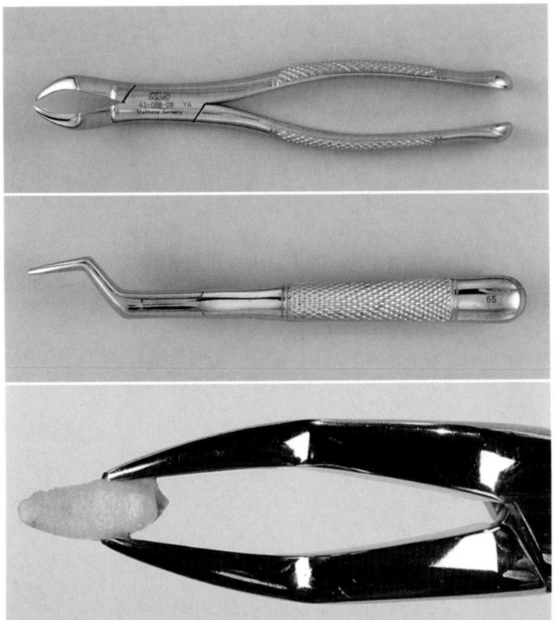

FIGURE 6-48 A, Superior view of No. 65 forceps. B, Side view of No. 65 forceps. C, No. 65 adapted to broken root.

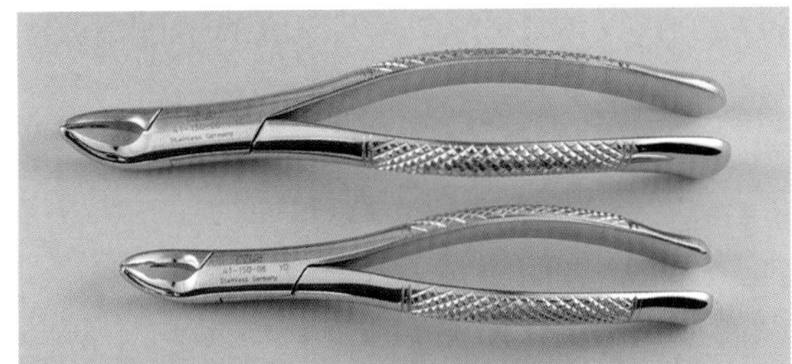

FIGURE 6-49 No. 150S (*bottom*) is smaller version of No. 150 forceps (*top*) and is used for primary teeth.

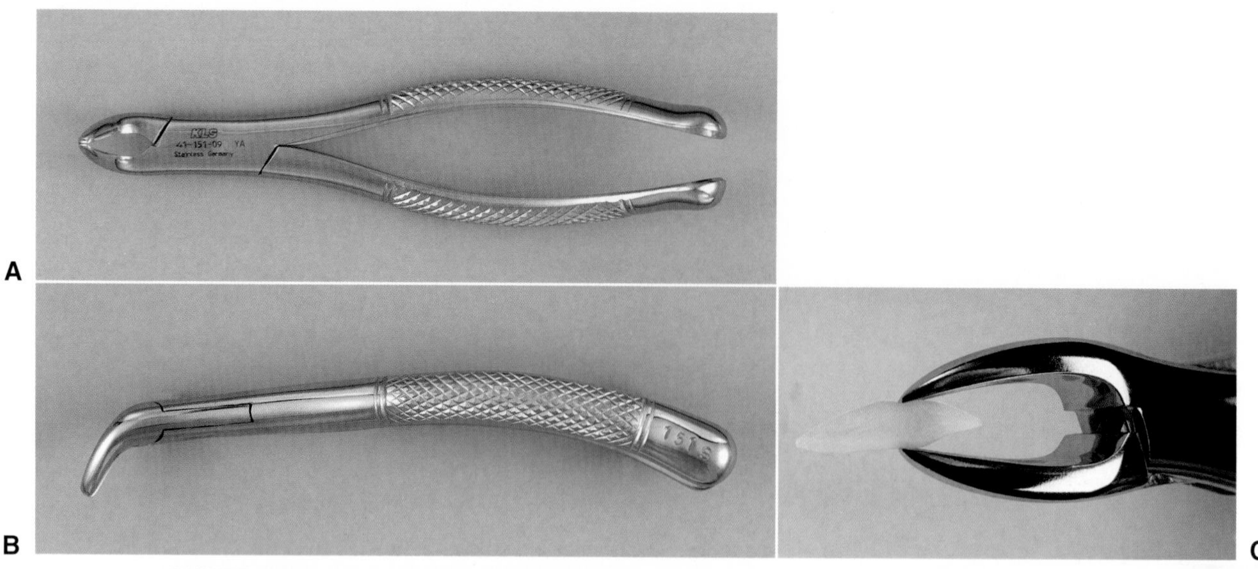

FIGURE 6-50 A, Superior view of No. 151 forceps. B, Side view of No. 151 forceps. C, No. 151 forceps adapted to mandibular incisor.

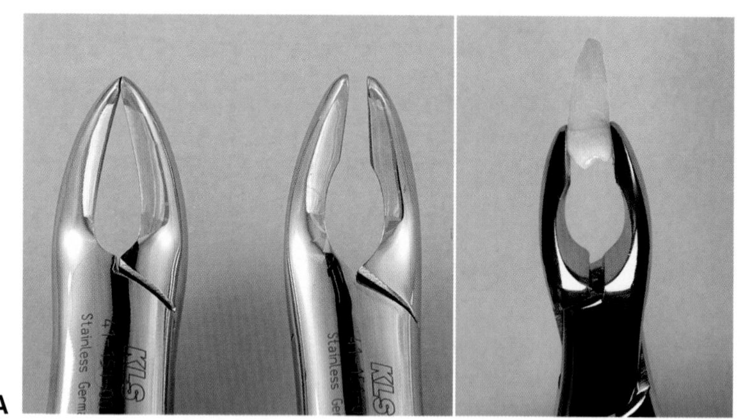

FIGURE 6-51 A, No. 151A forceps have beaks that are parallel and do not adapt well to roots of most teeth in contradistinction to the No. 151 forceps beaks. B, No. 151A forceps adapted to a lower premolar tooth. The lack of close adaptation of tips of beak to root of tooth is visualized.

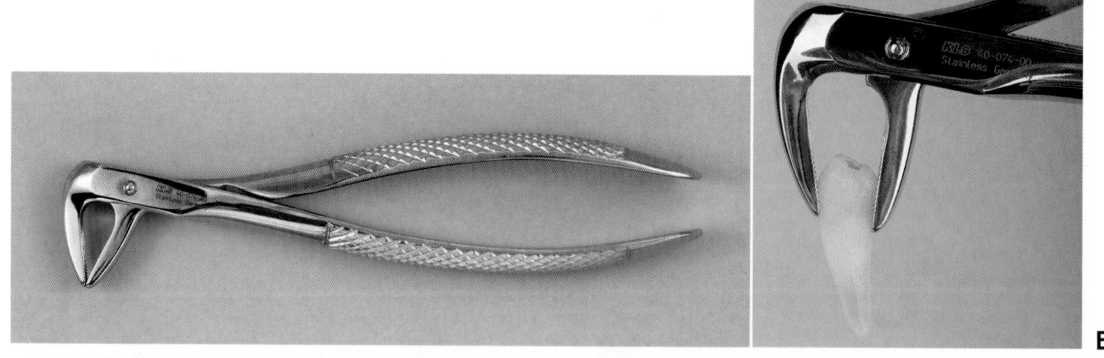

FIGURE 6-52 A, Side view of English style of forceps. B, Forceps adapted to lower premolar.

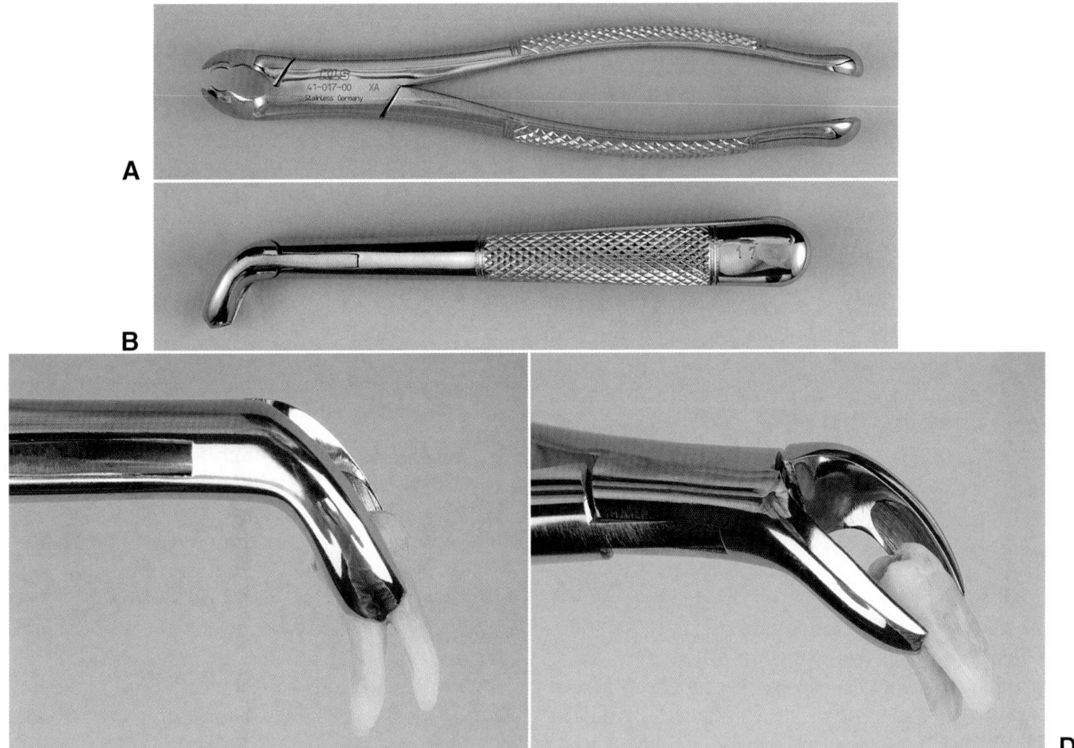

FIGURE 6-53 A, Superior view of No. 17 molar forceps. B, Side view of No. 17 molar forceps. C and D, No. 17 forceps adapted to lower molar.

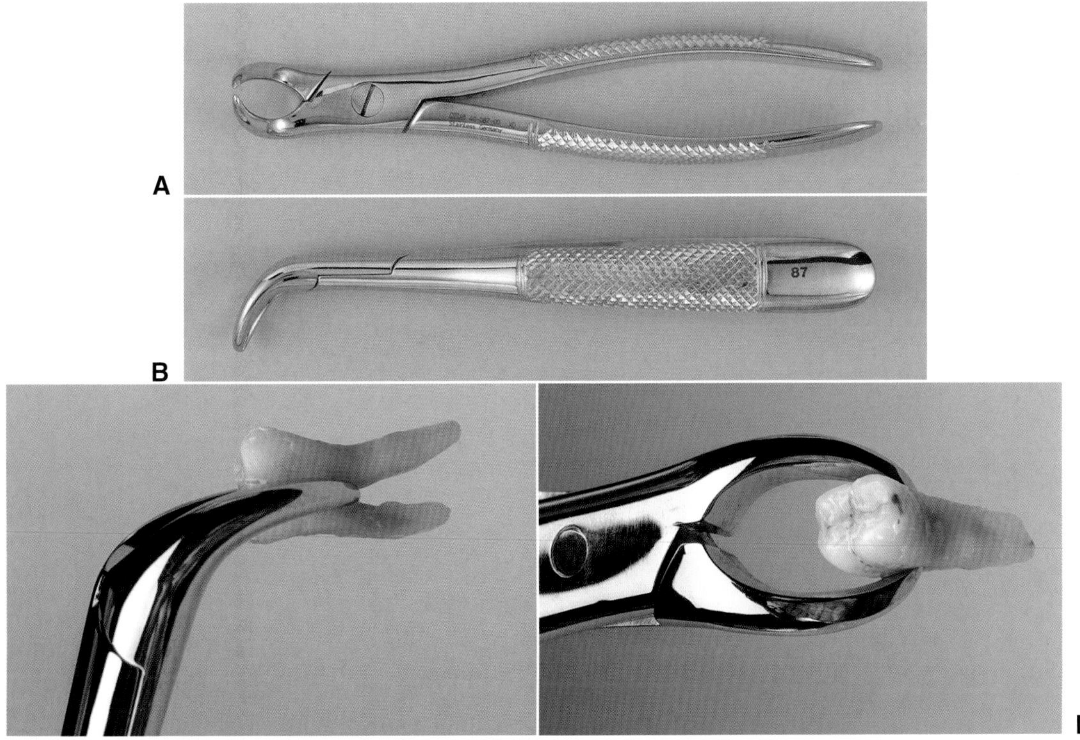

FIGURE 6-54 A, Superior view of cowhorn No. 87 forceps. B, Side view of cowhorn forceps. C and D, Cowhorn forceps adapted to lower molar tooth.

are designed with two pointed, heavy beaks that enter into the bifurcation of lower molars. After the forceps are seated into the correct position, usually while pumping the handles up and down, the tooth is actually elevated by squeezing the handles of the forceps together tightly. As beaks are squeezed into the bifurcation, they use the buccal and lingual cortical plates as fulcrums, and the tooth can be literally squeezed out of the socket. As with the English style of forceps, improper use of cowhorn forceps can result in an increase in the incidence of untoward effects, such as fractures of the alveolar bone or damage to maxillary teeth if the forceps are not properly controlled by the surgeon as the molar exits the socket. The beginning surgeon should therefore use cowhorn forceps with caution.

The No. 151 is also adapted for primary teeth. The No. 151S is the same general design as the No. 151 but is scaled down to adapt to the primary teeth. These forceps are adequate for removal of all primary mandibular teeth (Fig. 6-55).

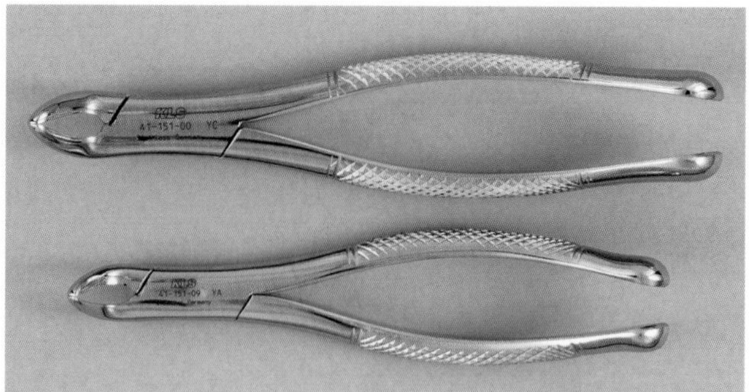

FIGURE 6-55 No. 151S (*bottom*) is the smaller version of No. 151 (*top*) and is used to extract primary teeth.

INSTRUMENT TRAY SYSTEMS

Many dentists find it practical to use the tray method to assemble instruments. Standard sets of instruments are packaged together, sterilized, and then unwrapped at surgery. The typical basic extraction pack includes a local anesthesia syringe, a needle, a local anesthesia cartridge, a No. 9 periosteal elevator, a periapical curette, a small and large straight elevator, a pair of college pliers, a curved hemostat, a towel clip, an Austin or Minnesota retractor, a suction tip, and 2 × 2-inch or 4 × 4-inch gauze (Fig. 6-56). The required forceps would be added to this tray.

A tray used for surgical extractions would include the items from the basic extraction tray plus a needle holder and suture, a pair of suture scissors, a blade handle and blade, Adson tissue forceps, a bone file, a tongue retractor, a pair of Cryer elevators, a rongeur, and a handpiece and bur (Fig. 6-57). These instruments permit incision and reflection of soft tissue, removal of bone, sectioning of teeth, retrieval of roots, débridement of the wound, and suturing of the soft tissue.

The biopsy tray includes the basic tray minus the elevators, plus a blade handle and blade, needle holder and suture, suture scissors, Metzenbaum scissors, Allis tissue forceps, Adson tissue forceps, and curved hemostat (Fig. 6-58). These instruments permit incision and dissection of a soft tissue specimen and closure of the wound with sutures.

The postoperative tray has the necessary instruments to irrigate the surgical site and remove sutures (Fig. 6-59). The tray usually includes scissors, college pliers, an irrigation syringe, cotton applicator sticks, gauze, and suction tip.

The instruments may be placed on a flat tray, wrapped with sterilization paper, and sterilized. When ready for use, the tray is taken to the operatory and opened in a manner to preserve instrument sterility, and the instruments are used from the tray. This system requires a large autoclave to accommodate the tray.

Alternately, metal cassettes can be used instead of a tray. Cassettes are more compact but must also be wrapped in sterilization paper.

The appendix includes prices for the instruments listed for these trays. A casual review of the cost of the surgical instruments will reflect why the surgeon and staff should make every effort to take good care of instruments.

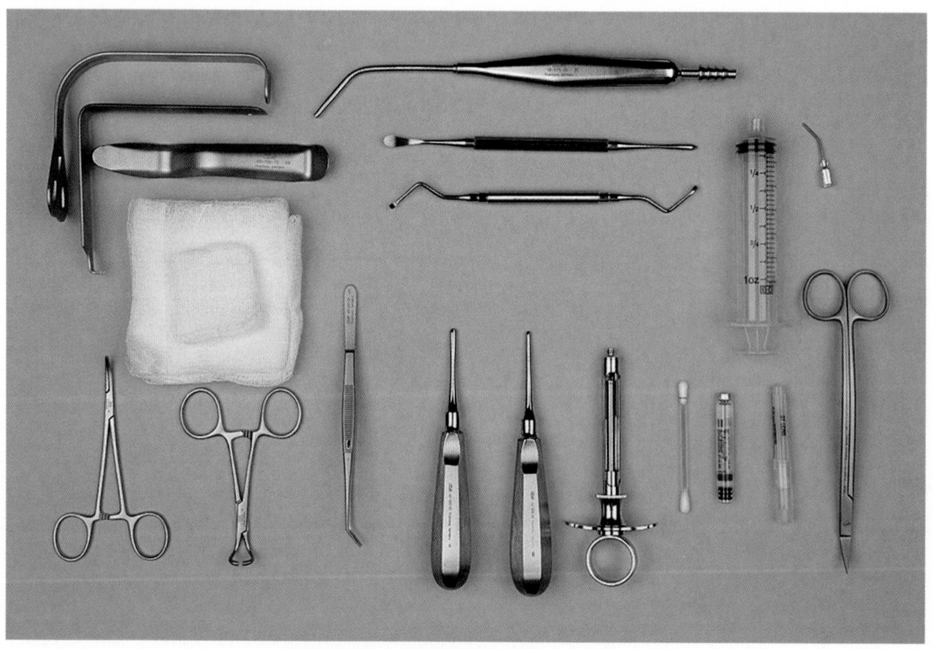

FIGURE 6-56 Basic extraction tray.

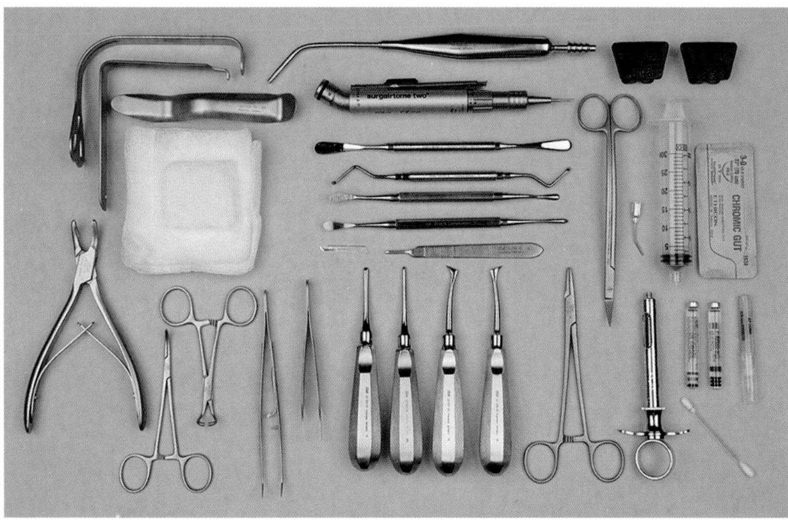

FIGURE 6-57 Surgical extraction tray adds necessary instrumentation to reflect soft tissue flaps, remove bone, section teeth, retrieve roots, and suture flaps back into position.

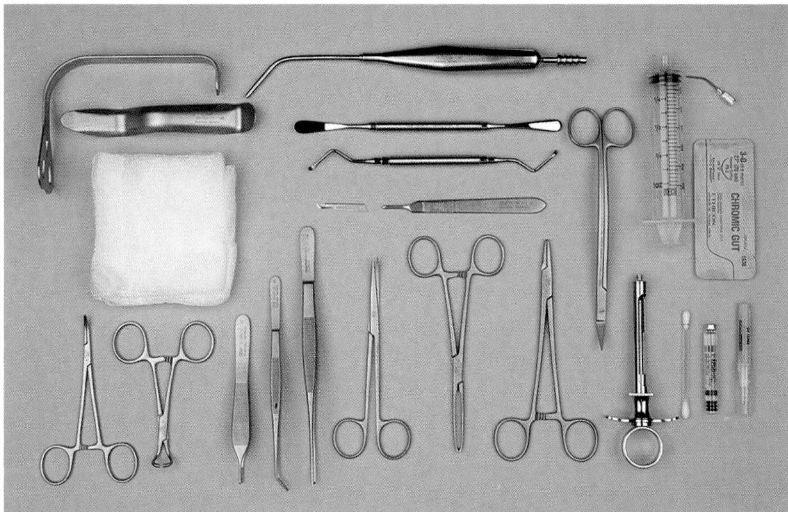

FIGURE 6-58 Biopsy tray adds equipment necessary to remove soft tissue specimen and suture wound closed.

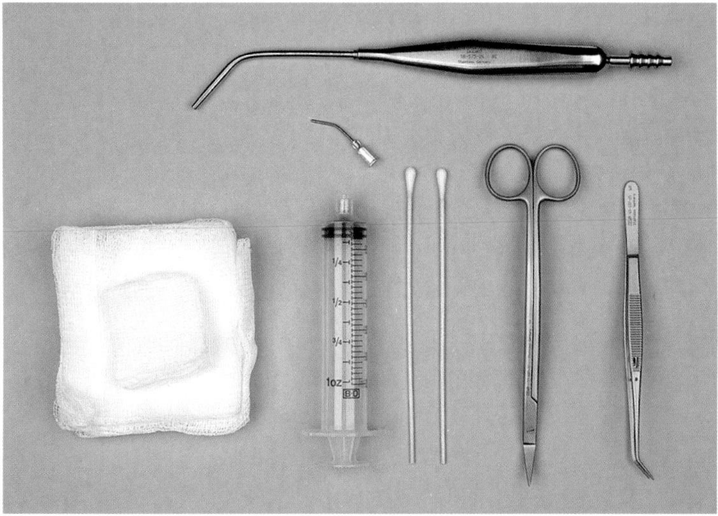

FIGURE 6-59 Postoperative tray includes instruments necessary to remove sutures and irrigate mouth.

CHAPTER 7

Principles of Uncomplicated Exodontia

JAMES R. HUPP

CHAPTER OUTLINE

Extraction of a tooth is a procedure that combines the principles of surgery and principles from physics and mechanics. When these principles are applied correctly, a tooth can usually be removed from the alveolar process without untoward force or sequelae. This chapter presents the principles of surgery and mechanics related to uncomplicated tooth extraction. In addition, there is a detailed description of techniques for removal of specific teeth with specific instruments.

Proper tooth removal does not require a large amount of surgeon strength but rather should be accomplished with finesse. Removal of an erupted tooth involves the use of controlled force in a manner such that the tooth is not pulled from the bone, but instead is gently lifted from the alveolar process. During preextraction planning the degree of difficulty anticipated for removing a particular tooth is assessed. If that assessment leads the surgeon to believe that the degree of difficulty will be high or if initial attempts at tooth removal confirm this, a deliberate surgical approach—not an application of excessive force—should be taken. Excessive force may injure local soft tissues and damage surrounding bone and teeth. Moreover, excessive force and haste during an extraction heightens the intraoperative and postoperative discomfort and patient anxiety.

PAIN AND ANXIETY CONTROL

Removal of even a loose tooth causes pain. Thus profound local anesthesia is required to prevent pain during extractions. Local anesthesia must be absolutely profound to eliminate sensation from the pulp, periodontal ligament, and adjacent soft tissues. However, even with profound local anesthesia, patients will still experience discomfort from pressure placed on a tooth and surrounding tissues during most extractions.

Equally important is for the dentist to recognize the anxiety that usually exists in patients about to undergo tooth extraction. Few patients face this procedure with tranquility, and even stoic patients with no overt signs of anxiety are likely to have internal feelings of distress.

Local Anesthesia

Profound local anesthesia is needed if the tooth is to be removed without pain for the patient; therefore, it is essential that the surgeon remember the precise innervations of all teeth and surrounding soft tissue and the kinds of injection necessary to anesthetize those nerves completely. Table 7-1 summarizes the sensory innervation of the teeth and surrounding tissue. An important point to remember is that, in areas of nerve transition, cross-innervation exists. For example, in the region of the mandibular second premolar, the buccal soft tissues are innervated primarily by the mental branch of the inferior alveolar nerve but also by terminal branches of the long buccal nerve. Therefore, it is appropriate to supplement an inferior alveolar nerve block with a long buccal nerve block to achieve adequate anesthesia of the buccal soft tissue when extracting a lower second premolar.

When anesthetizing a maxillary tooth for extraction, the surgeon should anesthetize the adjacent teeth as well. During the extraction process the adjacent teeth are usually subjected to some pressure, which may be sufficient to cause pain. This is also true for mandibular extractions, but the mandibular block injection usually produces sufficient anesthesia to adjacent teeth.

Dense local anesthesia results in the loss of all pain, temperature, and touch sensations, but it does not anesthetize the proprioceptive fibers of the involved nerves. Thus during an extraction the patient feels a sensation of pressure, especially when the force is intense. The surgeon must therefore remember that the patient will need to distinguish between sharp pain and the dull, albeit intense, feeling of pressure when determining the adequacy of anesthesia.

Even with profound soft tissue anesthesia and apparent pulpal anesthesia, a patient may continue to have sharp pain as a tooth is luxated. This is especially likely when the teeth have a pulpitis or the surrounding soft and hard tissues are inflamed or infected. A technique that should be used in these situations is the periodontal ligament injection. When this injection is delivered properly and the local anesthetic solution is injected under pressure, immediate profound local anesthesia occurs in almost all situations. The anesthesia is short-lived, so the surgical procedure should be one that can be accomplished within 15 to 20 minutes.

One must keep in mind the pharmacology of the various local anesthetic solutions that are used so that they can be used properly. Table 7-2 summarizes the commonly used local anesthetics and the amount of time they can be expected to provide complete anesthesia. The surgeon must remember that pulpal anesthesia of maxillary teeth after local infiltration lasts a much shorter time than pulpal anesthesia of mandibular teeth after block anesthesia. In addition, pulpal anesthesia disappears 60 to 90 minutes before soft tissue anesthesia. Therefore, it is common that a patient has lip anesthesia but has lost pulpal anesthesia and may be experiencing pain.

Only a certain amount of local anesthetic can be safely used in a given patient. To provide anesthesia for multiple tooth extractions, it may be necessary to inject multiple cartridges of local anesthetic. Thus it is important to know how many cartridges of a given local anesthetic solution can be administered safely. Table 7-3 summarizes (in two different ways) the maximum amounts of local anesthetic that can be used. First, each local anesthetic has a recommended maximum dose based on

TABLE 7-1

Sensory Innervation of Jaws

Nerve	Teeth	Soft Tissue
Inferior alveolar nerve	All mandibular teeth	Buccal soft tissue of premolars, canine, and incisors
Lingual nerve	None	Lingual soft tissue of all teeth
Long buccal nerve	None	Buccal soft tissue of molars and second premolar
Anterior superior alveolar nerve	Maxillary incisors and canine tooth	Buccal soft tissue of incisors and canine
Middle superior alveolar nerve	Maxillary premolars and portion of first molar tooth	Buccal soft tissue of premolars
Posterior superior alveolar nerve	Maxillary molars except for portion of first molar tooth	Buccal soft tissue of molars
Anterior palatine nerve	None	Lingual soft tissue of molars and premolars
Nasopalatine nerve	None	Lingual soft tissue of incisors and canine

TABLE 7-2

Duration of Anesthesia

Local Anesthetic	Maxillary Teeth	Mandibular Teeth	Soft Tissue
Group 1*	10-20 minutes	40-60 minutes	2-3 hours
Group 2†	50-60 minutes	90-100 minutes	3-4 hours
Group 3‡	60-90 minutes	3 hours	4-9 hours

*Group 1—local anesthetics without vasoconstrictors:
Mepivacaine 3%
Prilocaine 4%

†Group 2—local anesthetics with vasoconstrictors:
Lidocaine 2% with 1:50,000 or 1:100,000 epinephrine
Mepivacaine 2% with 1:20,000 levonordefrin
Prilocaine 4% with 1:400,000 epinephrine
Articaine 4% with 1:100,000 epinephrine

‡Group 3—long-acting local anesthetics:
Bupivacaine 0.5% with 1:200,000 epinephrine
Etidocaine 1.5% with 1:200,000 epinephrine

TABLE 7-3

Recommended Maximum Local Anesthetic Doses

Drug/Solution	Maximum Amount (mg/kg)	Number of Cartridges for 70-kg (154-lb) Adult	Number of Cartridges for 20-kg (44-lb) Child
Lidocaine 2% with 1:100,000 epinephrine	5.0	10	3.0
Mepivacaine 2% with 1:20,000 levonordefrin	5.0	10	3.0
Mepivacaine 3% (no vasoconstrictor)	5.0	6	2.0
Prilocaine 4% with 1:200,000 epinephrine	5.0	6	2.0
Articaine 4% with 1:100,000 epinephrine	7.0	6	1.5
Bupivacaine 0.5% with 1:200,000 epinephrine	1.5	10	3.0
Etidocaine 1.5% with 1:200,000 epinephrine	8.0	15	5.0

milligrams per kilogram. The second column in Table 7-3 indicates the number of cartridges that can safely be used on a healthy 154-lb (70-kg) adult. Rarely is it necessary to exceed this dose, even in patients larger than 154 lb. Patients who are smaller, especially children, should be given proportionally less local anesthetic. A common risky situation involving local anesthetic overdose is the small child to whom 3% mepivacaine (Carbocaine) is administered. For a child who weighs 44 lb (20 kg), the recommended maximum amount of mepivacaine is 100 mg. If the child is given two cartridges of 1.8 mL each, the dose totals 108 mg. Therefore, a third cartridge of 3% mepivacaine should not be administered. As with any drug, the smallest amount of local anesthetic solution sufficient to provide profound anesthesia is the proper amount.

Although it is self-evident that local anesthesia is necessary for intraoperative pain control, the surgeon should also acknowledge its role in postoperative pain control. For routine extractions where only mild to moderate analgesics will be necessary, usually no additional local anesthetic is necessary. After procedures that have been more traumatic (e.g., the removal of impacted teeth) and where stronger analgesics are likely to be necessary, many surgeons use a long-lasting local anesthetic (e.g., bupivacaine) instead of or in addition to their usual local anesthetic. By doing this, the clinician provides the patient with 4 to 8 hours of local anesthesia with no pain. This method also allows adequate time for the patient to take the oral analgesics and for the analgesics to take effect before any discomfort begins.

Sedation

Management of patient anxiety must be a major consideration in oral surgical procedures. Anxiety is a more important factor in oral surgical procedures than in most other areas of dentistry. Patients are frequently already in pain and may be agitated and fatigued, both of which lower the patient's ability to handle pain or pain-producing situations. Patients who are to have extractions may have preconceived notions or prior experiences of how painful such a procedure will be; they may have seen other patients, including family members, who have reported how painful it is to have a tooth extraction. Many are convinced that the procedure they are about to undergo will be very unpleasant. In addition, patients may experience certain psychological complications when oral surgical procedures are being performed. The removal of teeth causes a variety of reactions; a patient may mourn for lost body parts or perceive the extraction as a confirmation that youth has passed. This then adds to the presurgical anxiety present because of fear of pain.

Finally, anxiety is normal even in patients with positive past experiences with extractions because the procedure is truly uncomfortable. As noted previously, although the sharp pain is eliminated by local anesthetic, a considerable amount of pressure sensation still exists. Other noxious stimuli are present during an extraction procedure, such as the sounds of cracking of bone and clinking of instruments. For these reasons, prudent dentists use a planned method of anxiety control to prepare themselves and their patients for the anxiety associated with tooth extraction.

Anxiety control begins in most cases with a proper explanation of the planned procedure, including assurance that there will be no sharp pain and an expression of concern and empathy from the dentist. For the mildly anxious patient with a caring dentist, no pharmacologic assistance is typically necessary for routine extractions.

As patient anxiety increases, it often becomes necessary to use pharmacologic assistance. Fundamental to all anxiety-control techniques are a thorough explanation of the procedure and an expression of concern. These are augmented with drugs given in a variety of ways. Preoperatively orally administered drugs, such as diazepam, may provide a patient with rest the night before the surgery and some relief of anxiety in the morning. However, orally administered drugs are usually not profound enough to control moderate to severe anxiety once the patient enters the operative suite and are difficult to titrate.

Sedation by the inhalation of nitrous oxide is frequently the technique of choice for anxious patients and may be the only technique required for many patients who have mild to moderate anxiety. An extremely anxious patient who is to have several uncomplicated extractions may require deeper sedation, usually by the intravenous route. Sedation with anxiolytic drugs, such as using diazepam or midazolam with or without a narcotic, allows patients with moderate severe anxiety to undergo surgical procedures with minimal psychological stress. If the dentist is not skilled at using this modality, the patient should be referred to a surgeon who is trained to provide it.

PRESURGICAL MEDICAL ASSESSMENT

When evaluating a patient preoperatively, it is critical that the surgeon examine the patient's medical status. Patients can have a variety of maladies that require treatment modification or medical management before the surgery can be performed safely. Special measures may be needed to control bleeding, lessen the chance of infection, and prevent worsening of the patient's preexisting disease state. This information is discussed in detail in Chapter 1. The reader should refer to that chapter for information regarding the specifics of altering surgical treatment for medical management reasons.

INDICATIONS FOR REMOVAL OF TEETH

Teeth are extracted for a variety of reasons. This section discusses a variety of general indications for removing teeth. One must remember that these indications are guidelines and not absolute rules.

Caries

Perhaps the most common and widely accepted reason to remove a tooth is that it is so severely carious that it cannot be restored. The extent to which the tooth is carious and is considered to be nonrestorable is a judgment call to be made between the dentist and the patient. Sometimes the complexity and cost of steps required to salvage a severely carious tooth also makes extraction a reasonable choice. This is particularly true with the availability of reliable implant-supported prostheses.

Pulpal Necrosis

A second, closely aligned rationale for removing a tooth is the presence of pulp necrosis or irreversible pulpitis that is not amenable to endodontics. This may be the result of a patient declining endodontic treatment or of a root canal that is tortuous, calcified, and untreatable by standard endodontic techniques. Also included in this general indication category is the case in which endodontic treatment has been done but has failed to relieve pain or provide drainage, and the patient does not desire retreatment.

Periodontal Disease

A common reason for tooth removal is severe and extensive periodontal disease. If severe adult periodontitis has existed for some time, excessive bone loss and irreversible tooth mobility will be found. In these situations the hypermobile teeth should be extracted. Also ongoing periodontal bone loss may jeopardize the chance for straightforward implant placement, making extraction a sensible step before a tooth becomes mobile.

Orthodontic Reasons

Patients who are about to undergo orthodontic correction of crowded dentition frequently require the extraction of teeth to provide space for tooth alignment. The most commonly extracted teeth are the maxillary and mandibular premolars, but a mandibular incisor may occasionally need to be extracted for this same reason. Great care should be taken to ensure that extraction is indeed necessary and that the proper tooth or teeth are removed if someone other than the surgeon doing the extraction has asked for the extractions.

Malposed Teeth

Teeth that are malposed or malpositioned may be indicated for removal in several situations. If they traumatize soft tissue and cannot be repositioned by orthodontic treatment, they should be extracted. A common example of this is the maxillary third molar, which erupts in severe buccal version and causes ulceration and soft tissue trauma of the cheek. Another example is malposed teeth that are hypererupted because of the loss of teeth in the opposing arch. If prosthetic rehabilitation is to be carried out in the opposing arch, the hypererupted teeth may interfere with construction of an adequate prosthesis. In this situation the malposed teeth should be considered for extraction.

Cracked Teeth

An uncommon indication for extraction of teeth is a tooth with a cracked crown or a fractured root. The cracked tooth can be painful and is unmanageable by a more conservative technique. Even endodontic and complex restorative procedures cannot relieve the pain of a cracked tooth.

Impacted Teeth

Impacted teeth should be considered for removal. If it is clear that a partially impacted tooth is unable to erupt into a functional occlusion because of inadequate space, interference from adjacent teeth, or some other reason, it should be considered for surgical removal. See Chapter 9 for a more thorough discussion of this topic.

Supernumerary Teeth

Supernumerary teeth are usually impacted and should be removed. A supernumerary tooth may interfere with eruption of succedaneous teeth and has the potential for causing their resorption and displacement.

Teeth Associated with Pathologic Lesions

Teeth that are involved in pathologic lesions may require removal. In some situations the teeth can be retained and endodontic therapy performed. However, if maintaining the tooth compromises the complete surgical removal of the lesion when complete removal is critical, the tooth should be removed.

Radiation Therapy

Patients who are to receive radiation therapy for oral, head, or neck cancer should consider having teeth removed in the line of radiation therapy. However, many of these teeth can be retained with proper care. See Chapter 18 for a more thorough discussion of the effects of radiation therapy on the teeth and jaws.

Teeth Involved with Jaw Fractures

Patients who sustain fractures of the mandible or the alveolar process sometimes must have teeth removed. In some situations the tooth involved in the line of fracture can be maintained, but if the tooth is injured, infected, or severely luxated from the surrounding bony tissue or interferes with proper reduction and fixation of the fracture, its removal may be necessary.

Financial Issues

A final indication for removal of teeth relates to the financial status of the patient. All of the indications for extraction already mentioned may become stronger if the patient is unwilling or unable financially to support the decision to maintain the tooth. The inability of the patient to pay for the procedure or to take enough time from work to allow it to be performed may require that the tooth be removed. Also implant dentistry may be more cost-effective for a patient than maintaining a questionable tooth.

CONTRAINDICATIONS FOR THE REMOVAL OF TEETH

Even if a given tooth meets one of the requirements for removal, in some situations the tooth should not be removed because of other factors or contraindications to extraction. These factors, like the indications, are relative in their strength. In some situations the contraindication can be modified by the use of additional care or treatment, and the indicated extraction can be performed. In other situations, however, the contraindication may be so significant that the tooth should not be removed until the severity of the problem has been resolved. Generally the contraindications are divided into two groups: systemic and local.

Systemic Contraindications

Systemic contraindications preclude extraction because the patient's systemic health is such that the ability to withstand the surgical insult may be compromised (see Chapter 1). One systemic contraindication is a group of conditions called severe uncontrolled metabolic diseases. Brittle diabetes and end-stage renal disease with severe uremia are part of this group. Patients with mild diabetes or well-controlled severe diabetes can be treated as reasonably normal patients. Only when the disease process becomes uncontrolled should the patient not have a tooth removed in a routine manner.

Patients who have uncontrolled leukemia and lymphoma should not have teeth removed until the malignancy can be brought under control. The potential complications are infection as a result of nonfunctioning white cells and excessive bleeding as a result of an inadequate number of platelets. Patients with any of a variety of severe uncontrolled cardiac diseases should also have their extractions deferred until the disease can be brought under control. Patients with severe myocardial ischemia, such as unstable angina pectoris, and patients who have had a recent significant myocardial infarction should not have a tooth extracted except as an emergency in the hospital setting. Patients who have malignant hypertension should also have extractions deferred, because persistent bleeding, acute myocardial insufficiency, and cerebrovascular accidents are more likely to occur as a result of stress caused by the extraction. Patients who have severe, uncontrolled cardiac dysrhythmias should have their extraction procedures deferred as well.

Pregnancy is a relative contraindication to extractions; patients who are in the first or third trimester should have their extractions deferred if possible. The latter part of the first trimester and the first month of the last trimester may be as safe as the middle trimester for a routine uncomplicated extraction, but more extensive surgical procedures requiring drugs other than local anesthetics should be deferred until after the child has been delivered.

Patients who have a severe bleeding diathesis, such as hemophilia, or severe platelet disorders should not have teeth extracted until the coagulopathy has been corrected. Most severe bleeding disorders can be controlled by the administration of coagulation factors or platelet transfusions. Close coordination with the patient's hematologist can result in an uncomplicated recovery from the extraction procedure in most situations. Similarly, patients who take anticoagulants can have routine extractions performed when care is taken to manage the patient appropriately.

Finally, patients who take or have taken a variety of medications should have surgery performed with caution. Drugs to watch for include corticosteroids, immunosuppressive agents, bisphosphonates, and cancer chemotherapeutic agents.

Local Contraindications

Extractions of indicated teeth have several local contraindications. The most important and most critical is a history of therapeutic radiation for cancer. Extractions performed in an area of radiation may result in osteoradionecrosis and therefore must be done with extreme caution. Chapter 18 discusses this in detail.

Teeth that are located within an area of tumor, especially a malignant tumor, should not be extracted. The surgical procedure for extraction could disseminate malignant cells and thereby seed metastases.

Patients who have severe pericoronitis around an impacted mandibular third molar should not have the tooth extracted until the pericoronitis has been treated. Nonsurgical treatment should include irrigations, antibiotics, and removal of the maxillary third molar if necessary to relieve impingement on the edematous soft tissue overlying the mandibular impaction. If the mandibular third molar is removed in the face of severe pericoronitis, the incidence of complications increases. If the pericoronitis is mild and the tooth can be removed easily, then immediate extraction may be performed.

Finally, the acute dentoalveolar abscess must be mentioned. Many prospective studies make it abundantly clear that the most rapid resolution of an infection resulting from pulpal necrosis is obtained when the tooth is removed as early as possible. Therefore, acute infection is not a contraindication to extraction. However, it may be difficult to extract such a tooth because the patient may not be able to open the mouth sufficiently wide, or it may be difficult to reach a state of profound local anesthesia. If access and anesthesia considerations can be met, the tooth should be removed as early as possible. Otherwise, antibiotic therapy should be started and extraction planned as soon as possible.

CLINICAL EVALUATION OF TEETH FOR REMOVAL

In the preoperative assessment period, the tooth to be extracted should be examined carefully to assess the difficulty of the extraction. A variety of factors must be specifically examined to make the appropriate assessment.

Access to the Tooth

The first factor to be examined in preoperative assessment is the extent to which the patient can open the mouth. Any limitation of opening may compromise the ability of the surgeon to do a routine uncomplicated extraction. If the patient's opening is substantially compromised, the surgeon should plan for a surgical approach to the tooth instead of an elevator or forceps extraction. Additionally the surgeon should look for the cause of the reduction of opening. The most likely causes are trismus associated with infection around or in the muscles of

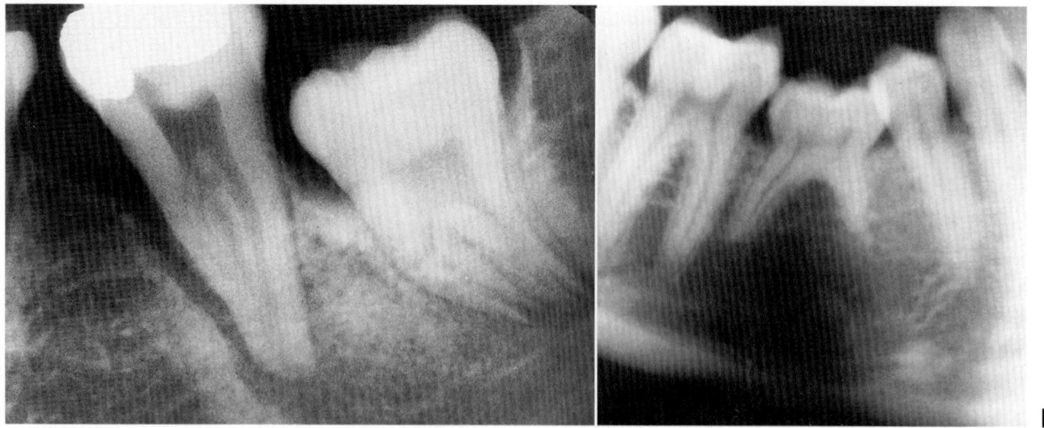

FIGURE 7-1 **A**, Tooth with severe periodontal disease with bone loss and wide periodontal ligament space. This kind of tooth is easy to remove. **B**, Retained mandibular second primary molar with an absent succedaneous tooth. The molar is partially submerged, and likelihood for ankylosed roots is high.

mastication, temporomandibular joint (TMJ) dysfunction (especially internal joint derangement with displacement of the disk without reduction or TMJ ankylosis), and muscle fibrosis.

The location and position of the tooth to be extracted within a dental arch should be examined. A properly aligned tooth has a normal access for placement of elevators and forceps. However, crowded or otherwise malposed teeth may present difficulty in positioning the proper forceps onto the tooth for extraction. When access is a problem, a compromise forceps must be chosen or a surgical approach may be indicated.

Mobility of the Tooth

The mobility of the tooth to be extracted should be assessed preoperatively. Greater-than-normal mobility is frequently seen with severe periodontal disease. If the teeth are excessively mobile, an uncomplicated tooth removal should be expected, but there may be more complicated soft tissue management after the extraction (Fig. 7-1, *A*).

Teeth that have less-than-normal mobility should be carefully assessed for the presence of hypercementosis or ankylosis of the roots. Ankylosis is often seen with primary molars that are retained and have become submerged (Fig. 7-1, *B*); in addition, ankylosis is seen occasionally in nonvital teeth that have had endodontic therapy many years before the extraction. If the clinician believes that the tooth is ankylosed, it is wise to plan for a surgical removal of the tooth as opposed to a forceps extraction.

Condition of the Crown

The assessment of the crown of the tooth before the extraction should be related to the presence of large caries or restorations in the crown. If large portions of the crown have been destroyed by caries, the likelihood of crushing the crown during the extraction is increased, thus causing more difficulty in removing the tooth (Fig. 7-2). Similarly, the presence of large amalgam restorations produces a weakness in the crown, and the restoration will probably fracture during the extraction process (Fig. 7-3). In addition, a tooth that has been endodontically treated becomes desiccated and crumbles easily when force is applied. In these three situations it is critical that

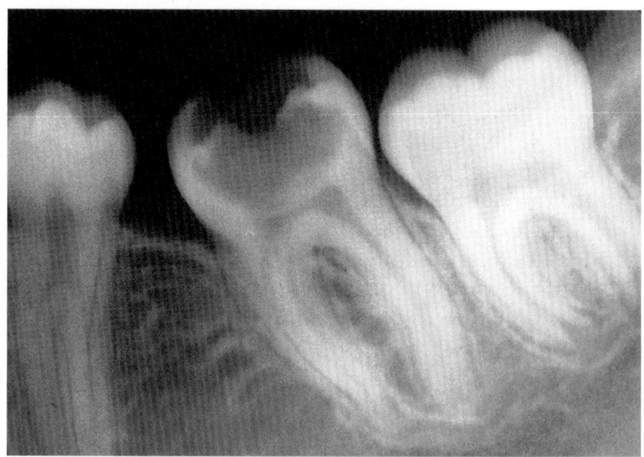

FIGURE 7-2 Teeth with large carious lesions are likely to fracture during extraction, making extraction more difficult.

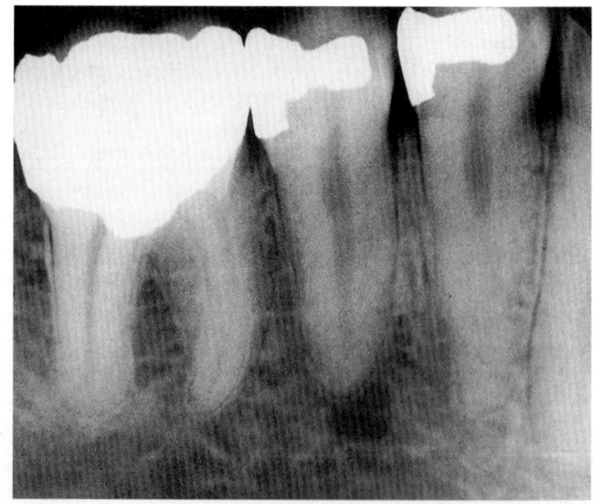

FIGURE 7-3 Teeth with large amalgam restorations are likely to be fragile and to fracture when extraction forces are applied.

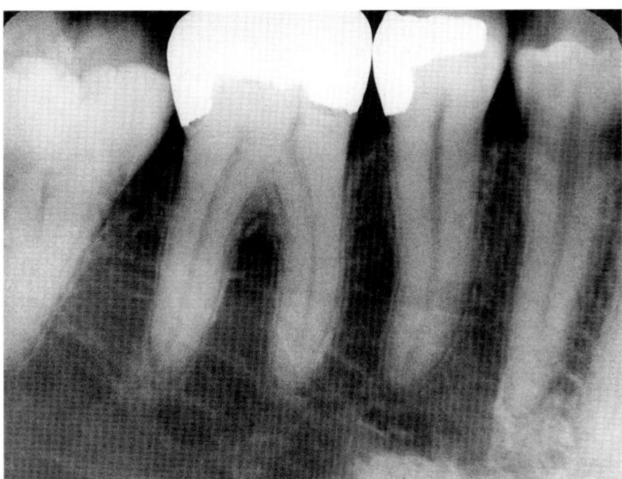

FIGURE 7-4 Mandibular first molar. If the molar is to be removed, surgeon must take care not to fracture amalgam in second premolar with elevators or forceps.

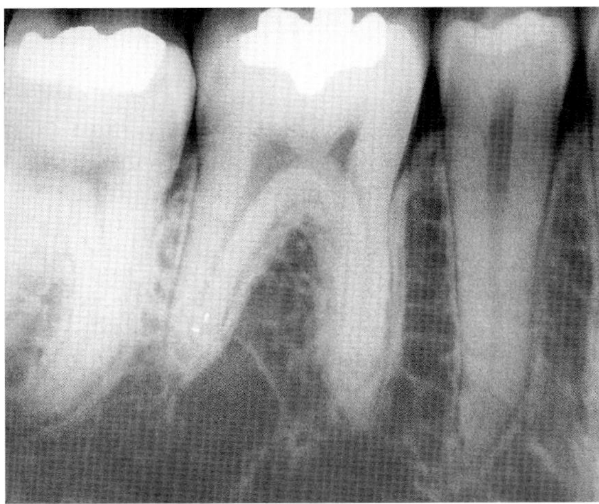

FIGURE 7-5 Properly exposed radiographs for extraction of mandibular first molar.

the tooth be elevated as much as possible and that the forceps then be applied as far apically as possible so as to grasp the root portion of the tooth instead of the crown.

If the tooth to be extracted has a large accumulation of calculus, the gross accumulation should be removed with a scaler or ultrasonic cleaner before extraction. The reasons for this are that calculus interferes with the placement of the forceps in the appropriate fashion, and fractured calculus may contaminate the empty tooth socket once the tooth is extracted.

The surgeon should also assess the condition of the adjacent teeth. If the adjacent teeth have large amalgams or crowns or have had endodontic therapy, it is important to keep this in mind when elevators and forceps are used to mobilize and remove the indicated tooth. If the adjacent teeth have large restorations, the surgeon should use elevators with extreme caution because fracture or displacement of the restorations may occur (Fig. 7-4). The patient should be informed before the surgical procedure about possible damage to these restorations during the informed consent process.

RADIOGRAPHIC EXAMINATION OF TOOTH FOR REMOVAL

It is essential that proper radiographs be taken of any tooth to be removed. In general, periapical radiographs provide the most accurate and detailed information concerning the tooth, its roots, and the surrounding tissue. Panoramic radiographs are used frequently, but their greatest usefulness is for impacted teeth as opposed to erupted teeth.

For radiographs to have their maximal value, they must meet certain criteria. First of all, radiographs must be properly exposed, with adequate penetration and good contrast. The radiographic film or sensor should have been properly positioned so that it shows all portions of the crown and roots of the tooth under consideration without distortion (Fig. 7-5). If not using digital imaging, the radiograph must be properly processed, with good fixation, drying, and mounting. The mounting should be labeled with the patient's name and the date on which the film was exposed. The radiograph should be mounted in the American Dental Association standardized method, which is to view the radiograph as if looking at the patient; the raised dot on the film faces the observer. The radiograph should be reasonably current so as to depict the presently existing situation. Radiographs older than 1 year should probably be retaken before surgery. Finally, nondigital radiographs must be mounted on a view box that is visible to the surgeon during the operation, and digital images should be displayed so the surgeon can easily look at them during extractions. Radiographs that are taken but not available during surgery are of limited value.

The relationship of the tooth to be extracted to adjacent erupted and unerupted teeth should be noted. If the tooth is a primary tooth, the relationship of its roots to the underlying succedaneous tooth should be carefully considered. The extraction of the primary teeth possibly can injure or dislodge the underlying tooth. If surgical removal of a root or part of a root is necessary, the relationship of the root structures of adjacent teeth must be known. Bone removal should be performed judiciously whenever it is necessary, but it is particularly important to be careful if adjacent roots are close to the root being removed.

Relationship to Vital Structures

When performing extractions of the maxillary molars, it is essential to be aware of the proximity of the roots of the molars to the floor of the maxillary sinus. If only a thin layer of bone exists between the sinus and the roots of the molar teeth, the potential for perforation of the maxillary sinus during the extraction increases. Thus the surgical treatment plan may be altered to an open surgical technique, with division of the maxillary molar roots into individual roots before the extraction proceeds (Fig. 7-6).

The inferior alveolar canal may approximate the roots of the mandibular molars. Although the removal of an erupted tooth rarely impinges on the inferior alveolar canal, if an impacted tooth is to be removed, it is important that the relationship between the molar roots and the canal be assessed. Such an extraction may lead to injury of the canal and cause consequent damage to the inferior alveolar nerve (Fig. 7-7).

Radiographs taken before the removal of mandibular premolar teeth should include the mental foramen. Should a

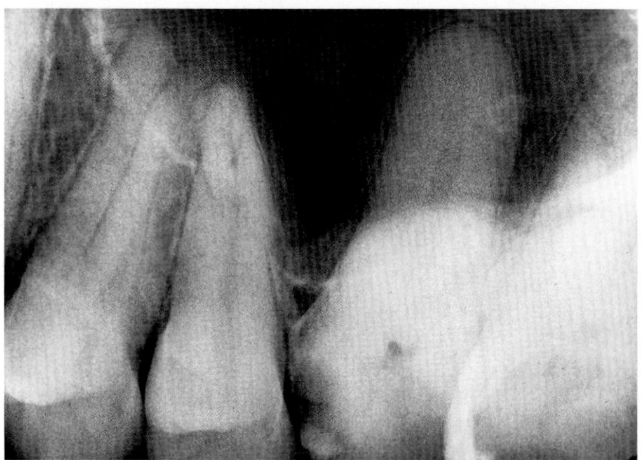

FIGURE 7-6 Maxillary molar teeth immediately adjacent to sinus present increased danger of sinus exposure.

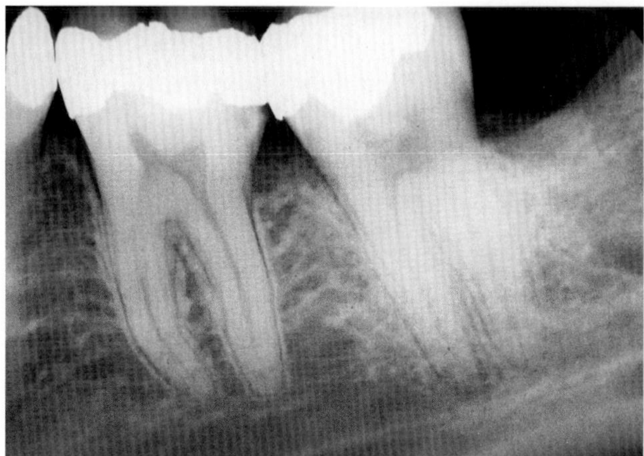

FIGURE 7-7 Mandibular molar teeth that are close to inferior alveolar canal. Third molar removal is a procedure most likely to result in injury to nerve.

surgical flap be required to retrieve a premolar root, it is essential that the surgeon know where the mental foramen is to avoid injuring the mental nerve during flap development (Fig. 7-3; Fig. 7-8).

Configuration of Roots

Radiographic assessment of the tooth to be extracted probably contributes most to the determination of difficulty of the extraction. The first factor to evaluate is the number of roots on the tooth to be extracted. Most teeth have the typical number of roots, in which case the surgical plan can be carried out in the usual fashion, but many teeth do have an abnormal number of roots. If the number of roots is known before the tooth is extracted, an alteration in the plan can be made to prevent fracture of the additional roots (Fig. 7-9).

The surgeon must know the curvature of the roots and the degree of root divergence to plan the extraction procedure. Roots of the usual number and of average size may still diverge substantially and thus make the total root width so wide that it prevents extraction with forceps. In situations of excess curvature with wide divergence, surgical extraction may be required with planned division of the crown (Fig. 7-10).

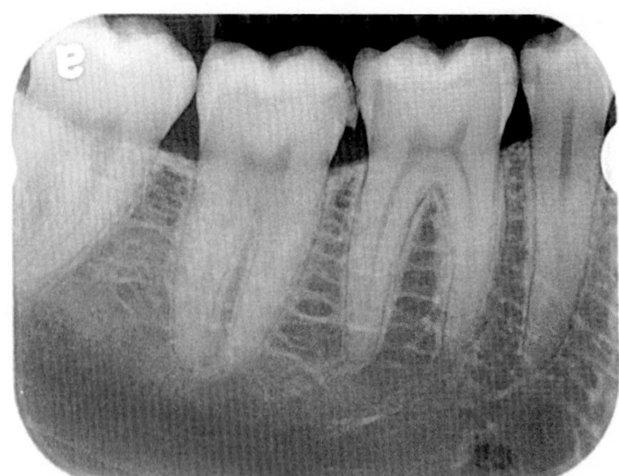

FIGURE 7-8 Before premolar extractions that require a surgical flap are performed, it is essential to know the relationship of the mental foramen to root apices. Note radiolucent area at apex of second premolar, which represents mental foramen.

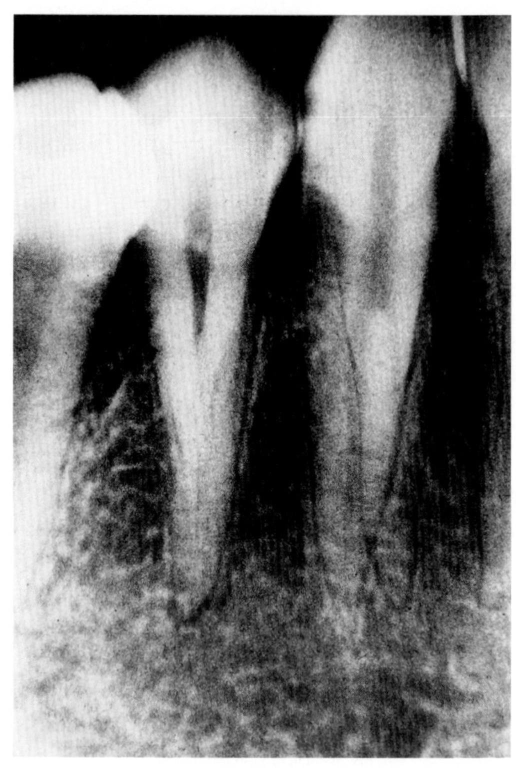

FIGURE 7-9 Mandibular canine tooth with two roots. Knowledge of this fact preoperatively may result in less traumatic extraction.

The shape of the individual root must be taken into consideration. Roots may have short, conic shapes that make them easy to remove. However, long roots with severe and abrupt curves or hooks at their apical end are more difficult to remove. The surgeon must have knowledge of the shapes of the roots before surgery to plan adequately (Fig. 7-11).

The size of the root must be assessed. Teeth with short roots are easier to remove than teeth with long roots. A long root that is bulbous as a result of hypercementosis is even more difficult to remove. The periapical radiographs of older patients should be examined carefully for evidence of hypercementosis because this process seems to be a result of aging (Fig. 7-12).

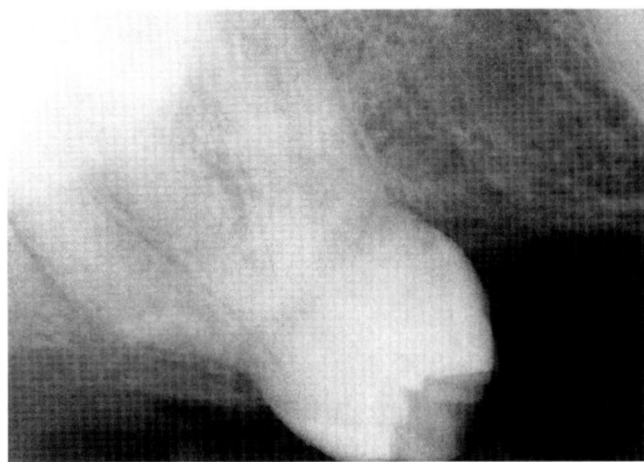

FIGURE 7-10 Widely divergent roots of this maxillary first molar make extraction more difficult.

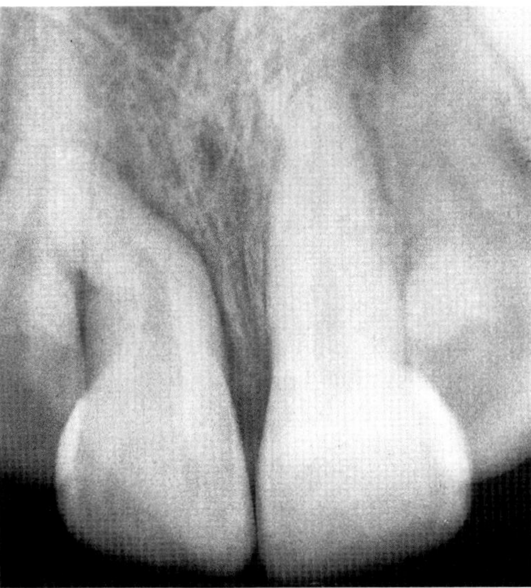

FIGURE 7-11 Curvature of roots of this tooth is unexpected. Preoperative radiographs allow surgeon to plan extraction more carefully.

The surgeon should look for evidence of caries extending into the roots. Root caries may substantially weaken the root and make it more liable to fracture when the force of the forceps is applied (Fig. 7-13).

Root resorption, internal or external, should be assessed on examination of the radiograph. Like root caries, root resorption weakens the root structure and renders it more likely to be fractured. Surgical extraction may be considered in situations of extensive root resorption (Fig. 7-14).

The tooth should be evaluated for previous endodontic therapy. If there was endodontic therapy many years before the extraction process, there may be ankylosis or the tooth root may be more brittle. In both situations, surgical extraction may be indicated (Fig. 7-15).

Condition of Surrounding Bone

Careful examination of the periapical radiograph indicates the density of the bone surrounding the tooth to be extracted. Bone that is more radiolucent is likely to be less dense, which makes the extraction easier. However, if the bone appears to be radiographically opaque (indicating increased density) with evidence of condensing osteitis or other sclerosis-like processes, it will be more difficult to extract.

The surrounding bone should also be examined carefully for evidence of an apical pathologic condition. Teeth that have nonvital pulps may have periapical radiolucencies that represent granulomas or cysts. Awareness of the presence of such lesions is important because these teeth should be removed at the time of surgery (Fig. 7-16).

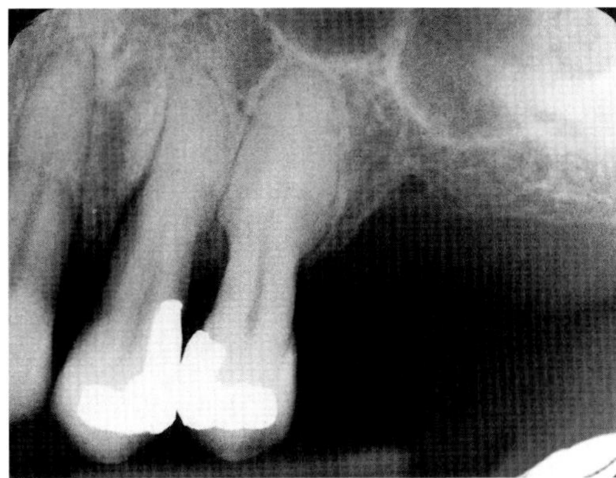

FIGURE 7-12 Hypercementosis increases difficulty of these extractions because roots are larger at apical end than at cervical end. Surgical extraction will probably be required.

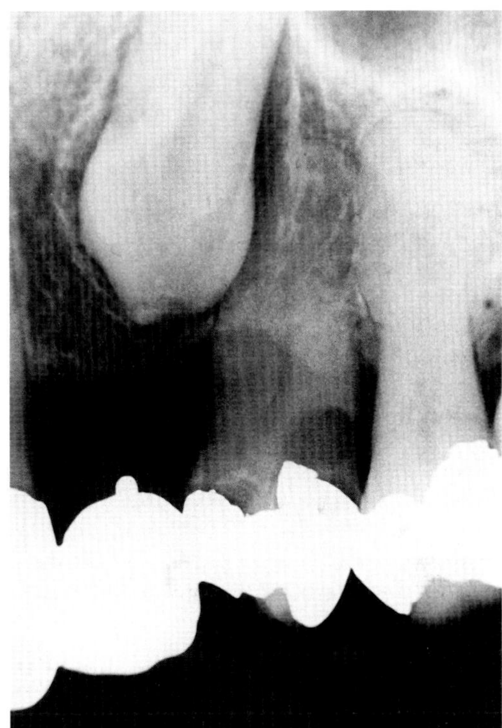

FIGURE 7-13 Root caries in first premolar tooth make extraction more difficult because fracture of tooth is likely. Note hypercementosis of second premolar.

PATIENT AND SURGEON PREPARATION

Surgeons must prevent inadvertent injury or transmission of infection to their patients or to themselves. The concept of

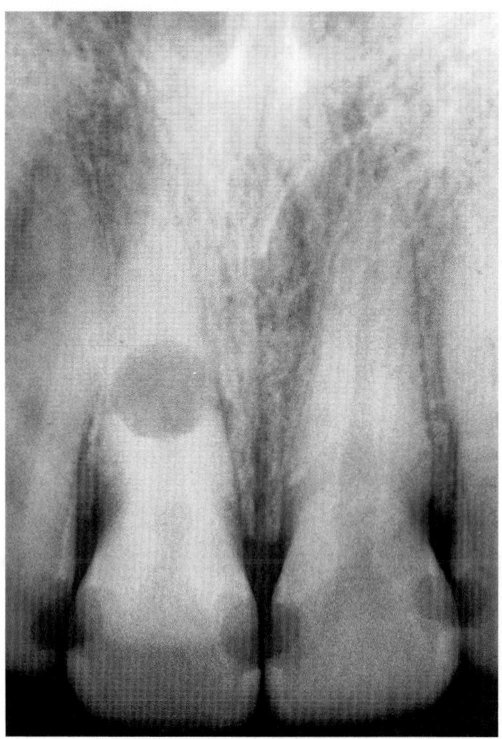

FIGURE 7-14 Internal resorption of root makes closed extraction almost impossible because fracture of root will almost surely occur.

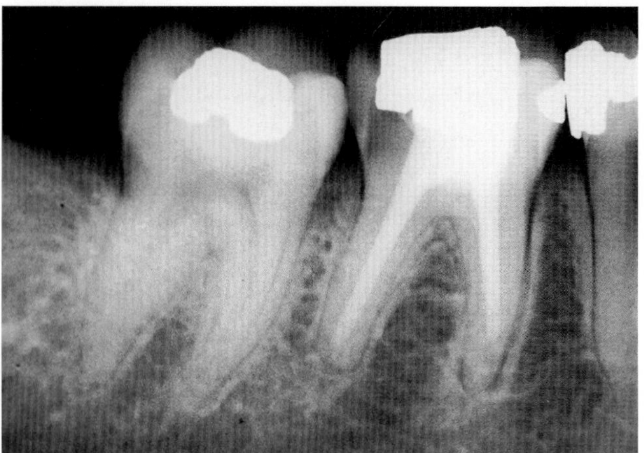

FIGURE 7-15 Tooth made brittle by previous endodontic therapy. Tooth is thus more difficult to remove.

universal precautions states that all patients must be viewed as having blood-borne diseases that can be transmitted to the surgical team and other patients. To prevent this transmission, surgical gloves, surgical mask, and eyewear with side-shields are required. (See Chapter 5 for a detailed discussion of this topic.) Additionally, most authorities recommend that the surgical team wear long-sleeved gowns that can be changed when they become visibly soiled (Fig. 7-17).

If the surgeon has long hair, it is essential that the hair be held in position with barrettes or other holding devices and be covered with a surgical cap. A major breach in aseptic technique is to allow the surgeon's hair to hang over the patient's face.

Before the patient undergoes the surgical procedure, a minimal amount of draping is necessary. A sterile drape should be put across the patient's chest to decrease the risk of contamination (Fig. 7-17).

Before the extraction, patients can be advised to rinse their mouths vigorously with an antiseptic mouth rinse such as chlorhexidine. This reduces the bacterial contamination in the patient's mouth to some degree, which may help to reduce the incidence of postoperative infection.

To prevent teeth or fragments of teeth from falling into the mouth and potentially being swallowed or aspirated into the lungs, many surgeons prefer to place a partially unfolded 4 × 4-inch gauze loosely into the back of the mouth. This oral partition serves as a barrier so that, should a tooth slip from the forceps or shatter under the pressure of the forceps, it will be caught in the gauze rather than be swallowed or aspirated. The surgeon must take care that the gauze is not positioned so far posteriorly that it makes the patient gag. The surgeon

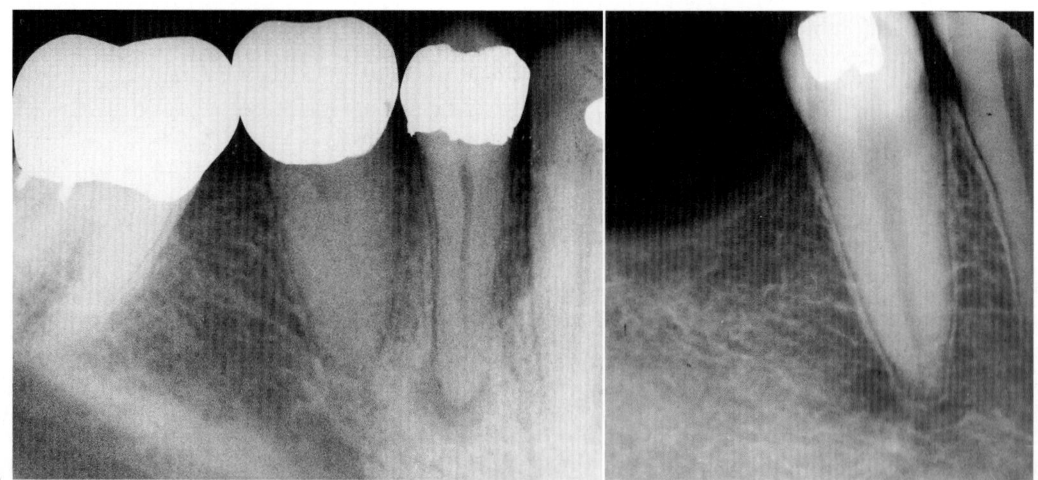

FIGURE 7-16 A, Periapical radiolucency. Surgeon must be aware of this before extraction to allow proper management. B, Periapical radiolucency around mandibular premolar represents mental foramen. Surgeon must be aware that this is not a pathologic condition. Intact lamina dura is noted in B but not in A.

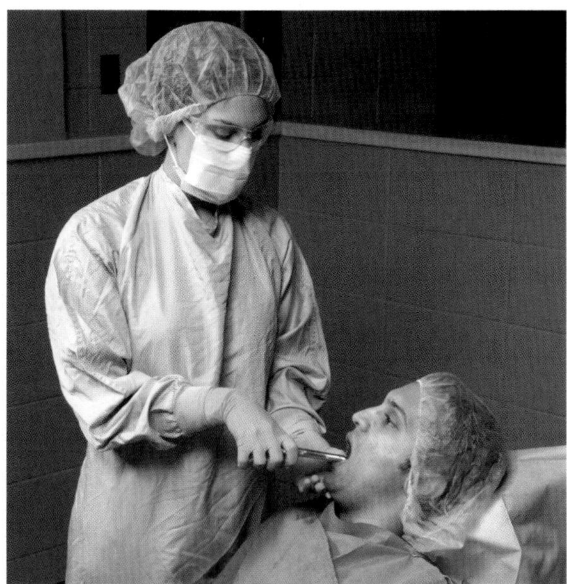

FIGURE 7-17 Surgeon, prepared by wearing protective eyeglasses, mask, and gloves. Surgeons should have short or pinned-back hair and should wear long-sleeved smocks that are changed daily or sooner if they become soiled. Patient should have waterproof drape.

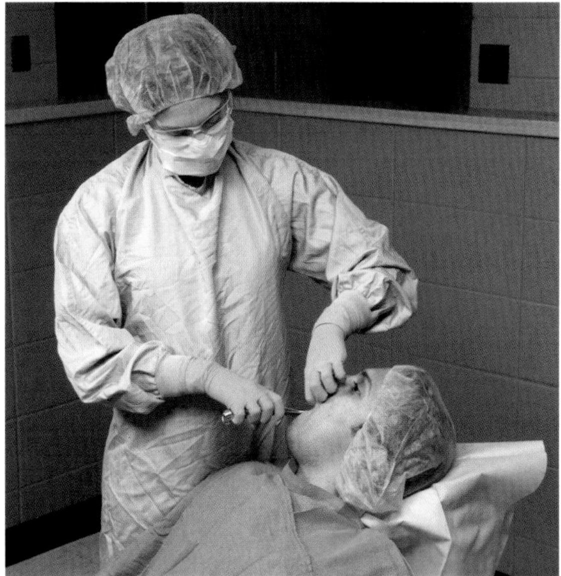

FIGURE 7-18 Patient positioned for maxillary extraction: tilted back so that maxillary occlusal plane is at about 60-degree angle to floor. Height of chair should put patient's mouth slightly below surgeon's elbow.

should explain the purpose of the partition to gain the patient's acceptance and cooperation for allowing the gauze to be placed.

CHAIR POSITION FOR EXTRACTIONS

The positions of the patient, chair, and operator are critical for successful completion of the extraction. The best position is one that is comfortable for the patient and surgeon and that allows the surgeon to have maximal control of the force that is being delivered to the patient's tooth through the elevators and forceps. The correct position allows the surgeon to keep the arms close to the body and provides stability and support; it also allows the surgeon to keep the wrists straight enough to deliver the force with the arm and shoulder and not with the hand. The force delivered can thus be controlled in the face of sudden loss of resistance from a root or fracture of the bone.

Dentists usually stand during extractions, so the positions for a standing surgeon will be described first. Modifications that are necessary to operate in a seated position will be presented later. Also descriptions of techniques are for the right-handed operator. Left-handed surgeons should reverse the instructions when working on various quadrants.

For a maxillary extraction the chair should be tipped backward so that the maxillary occlusal plane is at an angle of about 60 degrees to the floor. Raising the patient's legs at the same time helps improve the patient's comfort. The height of the chair should be such that the height of the patient's mouth is at or slightly below the operator's elbow level (Fig. 7-18). Novices commonly have the chair too high. During an operation on the maxillary right quadrant, the patient's head should be turned *substantially* toward the operator so that adequate access and visualization can be achieved (Fig. 7-19). For extraction of teeth in the maxillary anterior portion of the arch, the patient should be looking straight ahead (Fig. 7-20). The

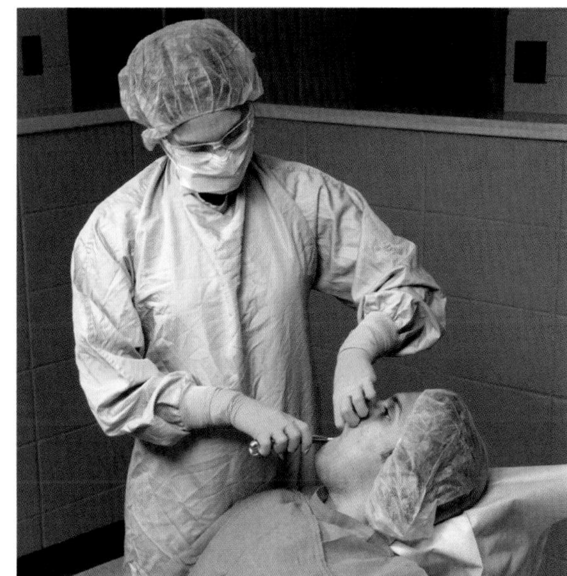

FIGURE 7-19 Extraction of teeth in maxillary right quadrant. Note that surgeon turns patient's head toward self.

position for the maxillary left portion of the arch is similar, except that the patient's head is turned *slightly* toward the operator (Fig. 7-21).

For the extraction of mandibular teeth, the patient should be positioned in a more upright position so that when the mouth is opened widely, the occlusal plane is parallel to the floor. A properly sized bite block should be used to stabilize the mandible when the extraction forceps are used. Even though the surgeon will support the jaw, the additional support provided by the bite block will result in less stress being transmitted to the jaws. Care should be taken to avoid using too

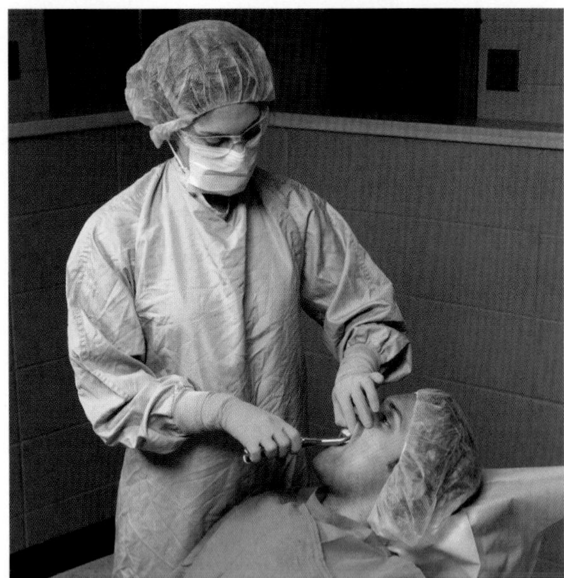

FIGURE 7-20 Extraction of anterior maxillary teeth. Patient looks straight ahead.

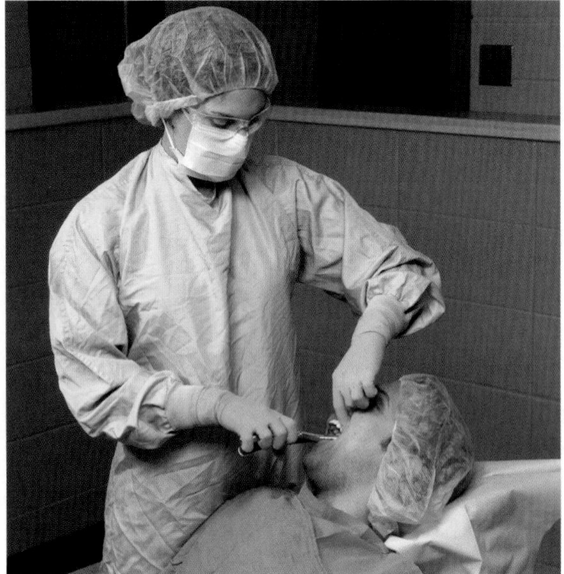

FIGURE 7-21 Patient with head turned slightly toward surgeon for extraction of maxillary left posterior teeth.

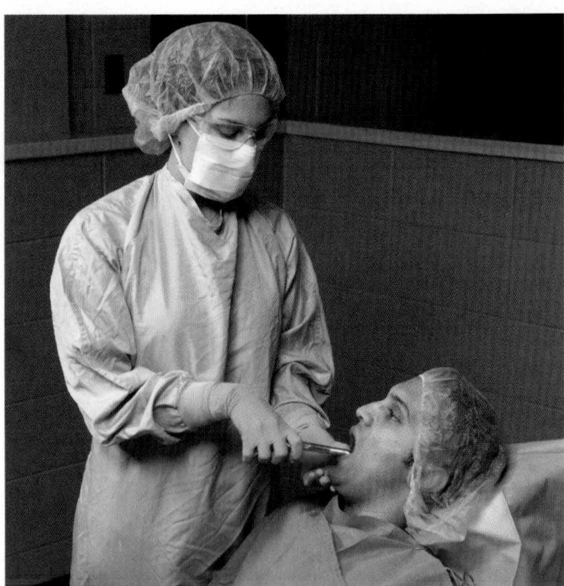

FIGURE 7-22 For mandibular extractions, patient is more upright so that mandibular occlusal plane of opened mouth is parallel to floor. Height of chair is also lower to allow operator's arm to be straighter.

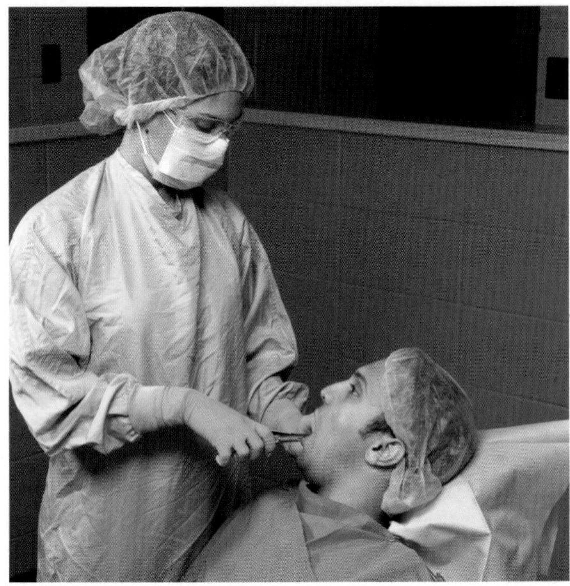

FIGURE 7-23 Patient with head turned toward surgeon for removal of mandibular right teeth.

large of a bite block because large ones can overstretch the TMJ ligaments and cause patient discomfort. The chair should be lower than for extraction of maxillary teeth, and the surgeon's arm should be inclined downward to approximately a 120-degree angle at the elbow (Fig. 7-22), which provides a comfortable, stable position that is more controllable than the higher position. During removal of the mandibular right posterior teeth, the patient's head should be turned severely toward the surgeon to allow adequate access to the jaw, and the surgeon should maintain the proper arm and hand position (Fig. 7-23). When removing teeth in the anterior region of the mandible, the surgeon should rotate around to the side of the patient (Figs. 7-24 and 7-25). When operating on the left posterior mandibular region, the surgeon should stand in front of the patient, but the patient's head should not turn so severely toward the surgeon (Fig. 7-26).

Some surgeons prefer to approach the mandibular teeth from a posterior position. This allows the left hand of the surgeon to support the mandible better, but it requires that the forceps be held opposite the usual method and that the surgeon views the field with an upside-down perspective. The left hand of the surgeon goes around the patient's head and supports the mandible. The usual behind-the-patient approach is seen in Figures 7-27 and 7-28.

If the surgeon chooses to sit while performing extractions, several modifications must be made. For maxillary extractions, the patient is positioned in a reclining position similar to that

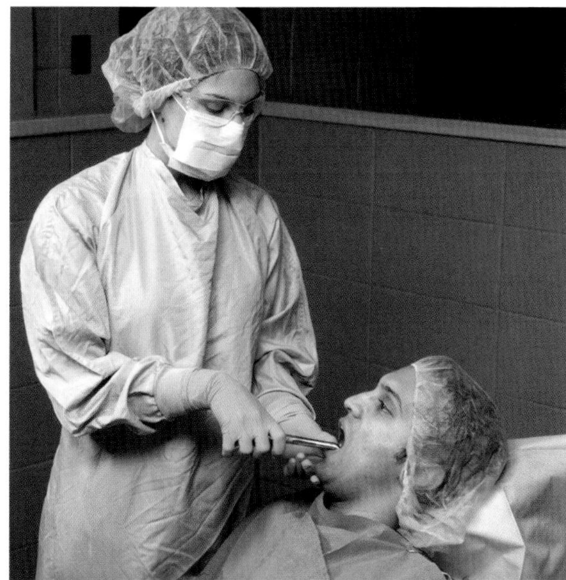

FIGURE 7-24 For extraction of mandibular anterior teeth, surgeon stands at side of patient, who looks straight ahead.

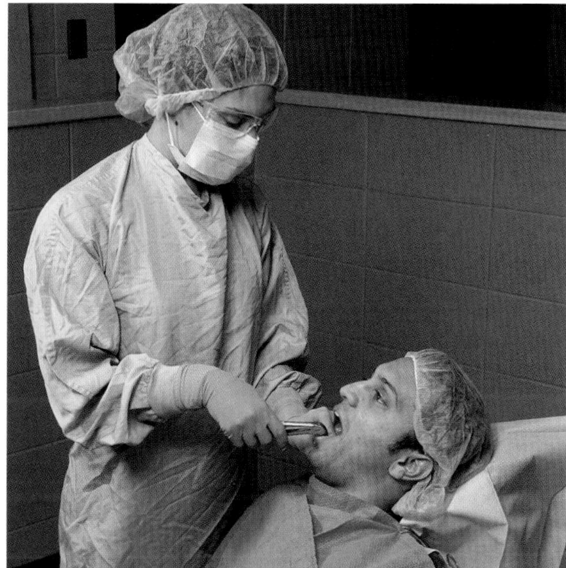

FIGURE 7-25 When English style of forceps is used for anterior mandibular teeth, patient's head is positioned straight.

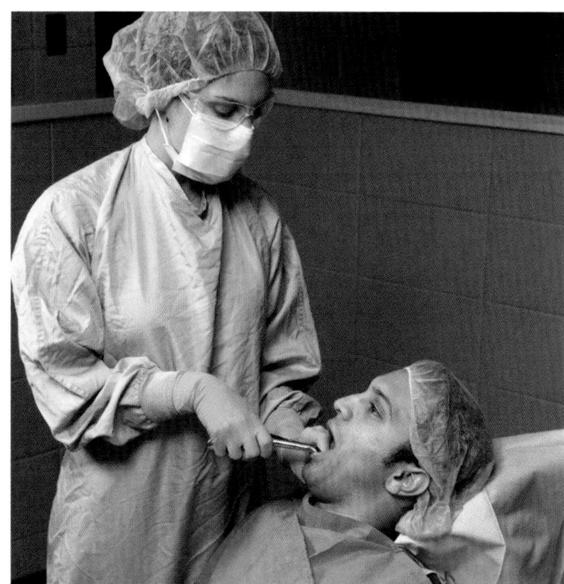

FIGURE 7-26 For extraction of mandibular posterior teeth, patient turns slightly toward surgeon.

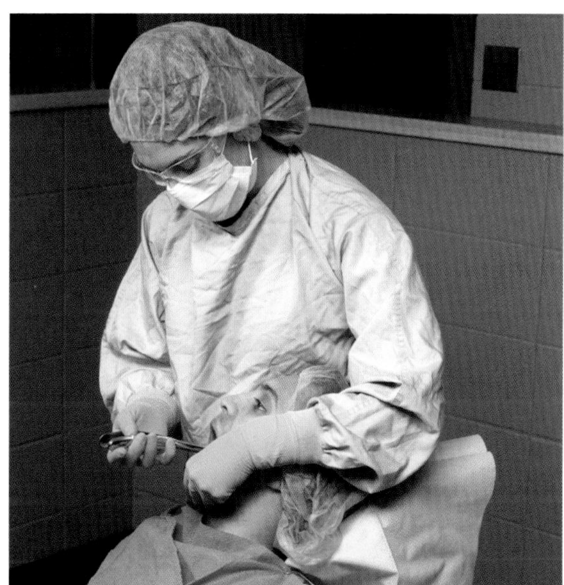

FIGURE 7-27 Behind-the-patient approach for extraction of posterior right mandibular teeth. This allows surgeon to be in comfortable, stable position.

used when the surgeon is standing. However, the patient is not reclined as much; therefore the maxillary occlusal plane is not perpendicular to the floor as it is when the surgeon is standing. The patient should be lowered as far as possible so that the level of the patient's mouth is as near as possible to the surgeon's elbow (Fig. 7-29). The arm and hand position for extraction of the maxillary anterior and posterior teeth is similar to the position used for the same extractions performed while standing (Fig. 7-30).

As when the surgeon is standing, for extraction of teeth in the lower arch, the patient is a bit more upright than for extraction of maxillary teeth. The surgeon can work from the front of the patient (Figs. 7-31 and 7-32) or from behind the patient (Figs. 7-33 and 7-34). When the English style of forceps is used, the surgeon's position is usually behind the patient (Fig. 7-35). It should be noted that the surgeon and the assistant have hand and arm positions similar to those used when the surgeon is in the standing position.

MECHANICAL PRINCIPLES INVOLVED IN TOOTH EXTRACTION

The removal of teeth from the alveolar process requires the use of the following mechanical principles and simple machines: the lever, wedge, and wheel and axle.

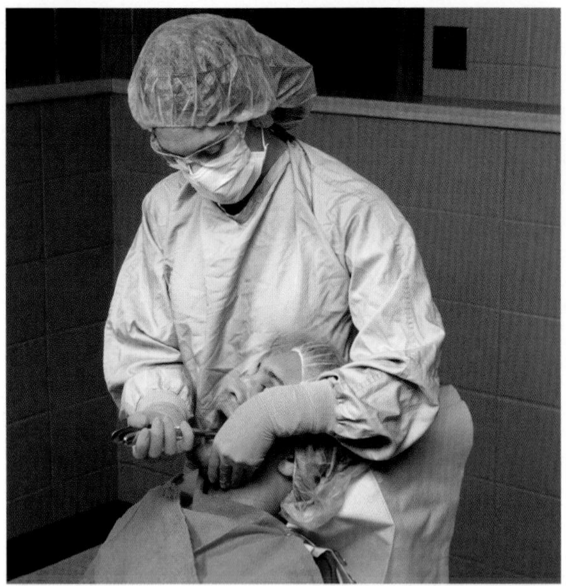

FIGURE 7-28 Behind-the-patient approach for extraction of posterior left mandibular teeth. Hand is positioned under forceps.

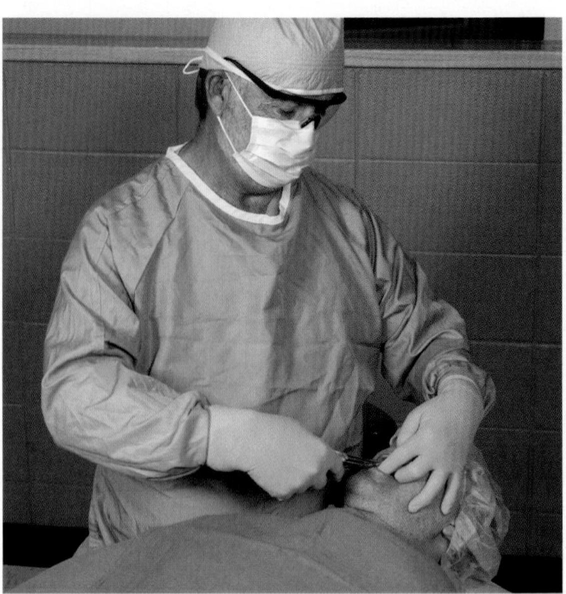

FIGURE 7-30 For extraction of maxillary teeth, patient is reclined back approximately 60 degrees. Hand and forceps positions are same as for standing position.

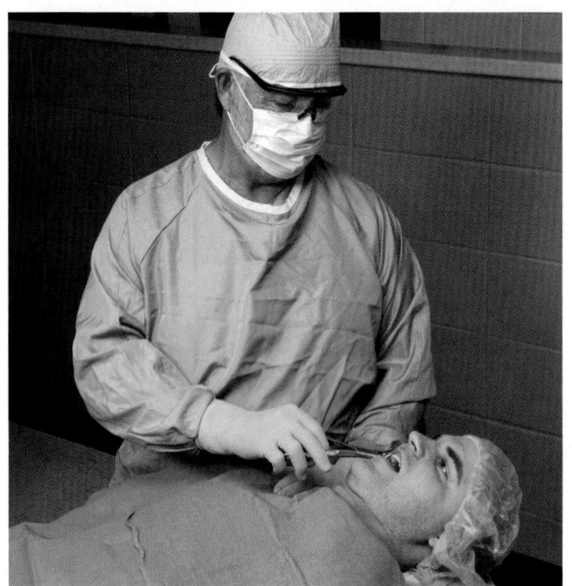

FIGURE 7-29 In seated position, patient is positioned as low as possible so that mouth is level with surgeon's elbow.

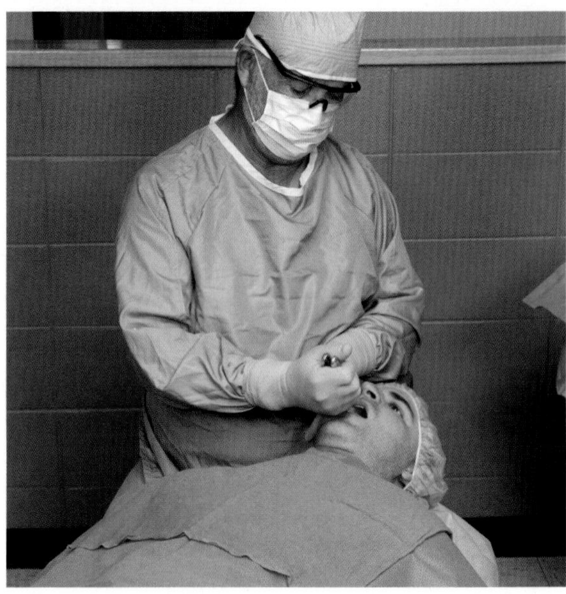

FIGURE 7-31 For extraction of mandibular teeth, operator holds forceps underhanded.

Elevators are used primarily as levers. A lever is a mechanism for transmitting a modest force—with the mechanical advantages of a long lever arm and a short effector arm—into a small movement against great resistance (Fig. 7-36). An example of the use of a level is when a Crane pick is inserted into a purchase point of a tooth and then is used to elevate the tooth (Fig. 7-37).

The second machine that is useful is the wedge (Fig. 7-38). The wedge is useful in several different ways for the extraction of teeth. First, the beaks of the extraction forceps are usually narrow at their tips; they broaden as they go superiorly. When the forceps are used, there should be a conscious effort made to force the tips of the forceps into the periodontal ligament space at the bony crest to expand the bone and force the tooth out of the socket (Fig. 7-39). The wedge principle is also useful when a straight elevator is used to luxate a tooth from its socket. A small elevator is forced into the periodontal ligament space, which displaces the root toward the occlusion and therefore out of the socket (Fig. 7-40).

The third machine used in tooth extraction is the wheel and axle, which is most closely identified with the triangular, or pennant-shaped, elevator. When one root of a multiple-rooted tooth is left in the alveolar process, the pennant-shaped elevator, like a Cryer, is positioned into the socket and turned. The handle then serves as the axle and the tip of the triangular elevator acts as a wheel and engages and elevates the tooth root from the socket (Fig. 7-41).

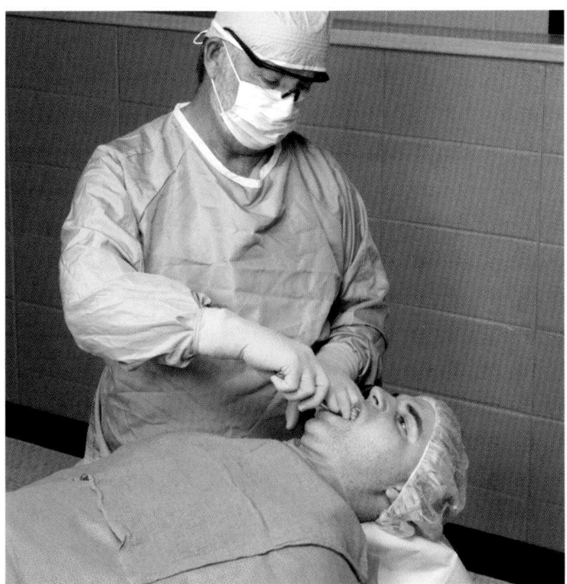

FIGURE 7-32 For removal of mandibular posterior teeth, surgeon's hand can hold forceps from above.

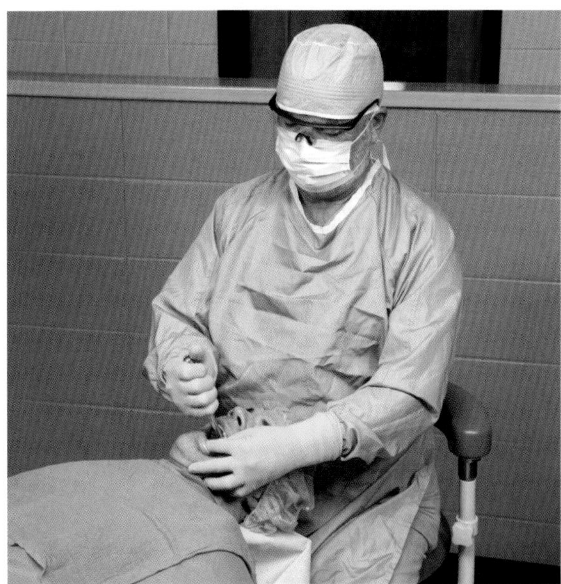

FIGURE 7-34 The behind-the-patient position can be used for removal of mandibular posterior teeth. Hand is positioned under forceps for maximum control.

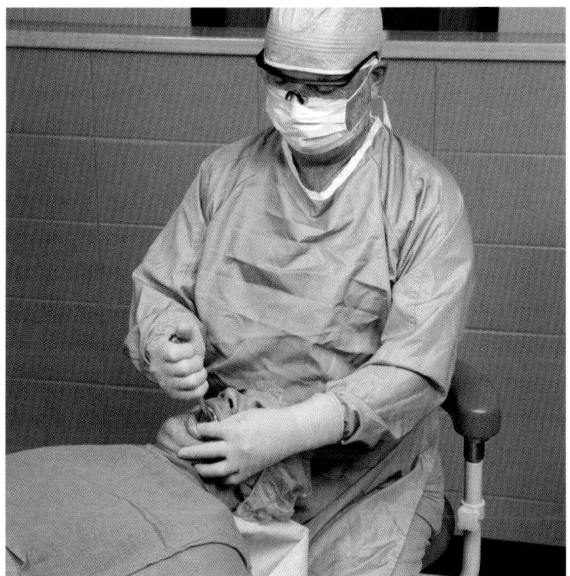

FIGURE 7-33 For removal of anterior teeth, surgeon moves to position behind patient so that mandible and alveolar process can be supported by surgeon's other hand.

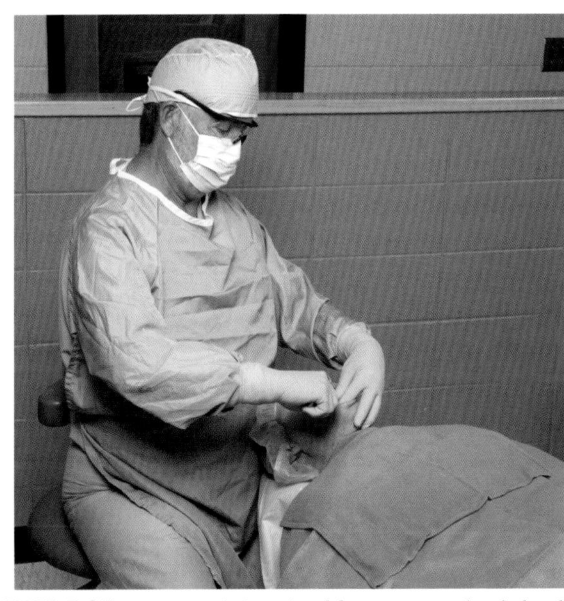

FIGURE 7-35 When English style of forceps is used, a behind-the-patient position is preferred.

PRINCIPLES OF ELEVATOR AND FORCEPS USE

The primary instruments used to remove a tooth from the alveolar process are the elevator and extraction forceps. Elevators help in the luxation of a tooth, and forceps continue that process through bone expansion and disruption of periodontal attachments. The goal of forceps use is twofold: (1) expansion of the bony socket by use of the wedge-shaped beaks of the forceps and the movements of the tooth itself with the forceps, and (2) removal of the tooth from the socket.

The dental elevator consists of a handle, shank, and blade. The handle of the elevator is usually in line with the shank and is enlarged to allow it to be grasped in the palm of the hand.

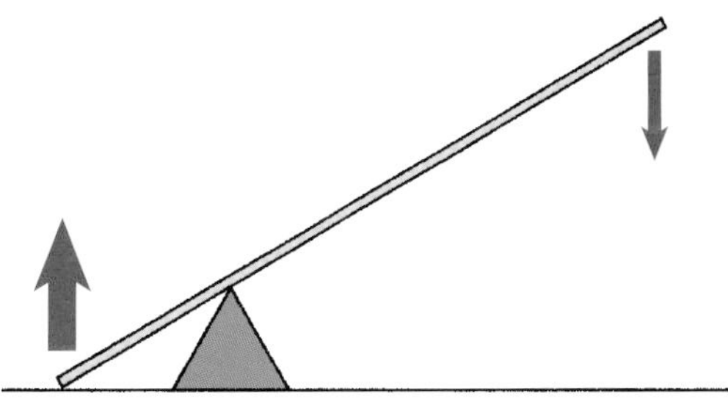

FIGURE 7-36 First-class lever transforms small force and large movement to small movement and large force.

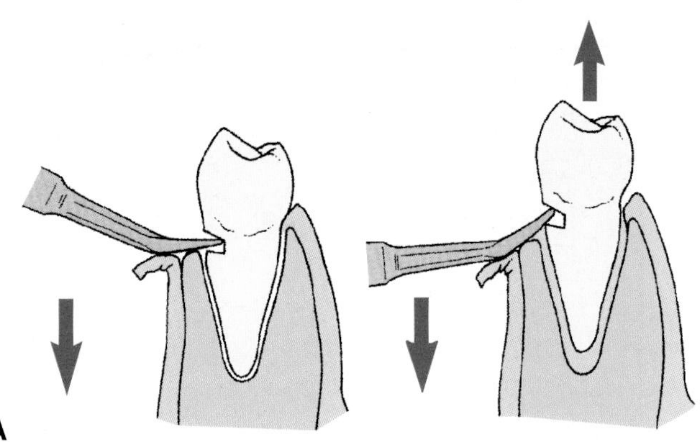

FIGURE 7-37 In removal of this mandibular premolar tooth, purchase point has been placed in tooth, which creates first-class lever situation. When Crane pick is inserted into purchase point and handle forces apically (A), tooth is elevated occlusally out of socket with buccoalveolar bone used as fulcrum (B).

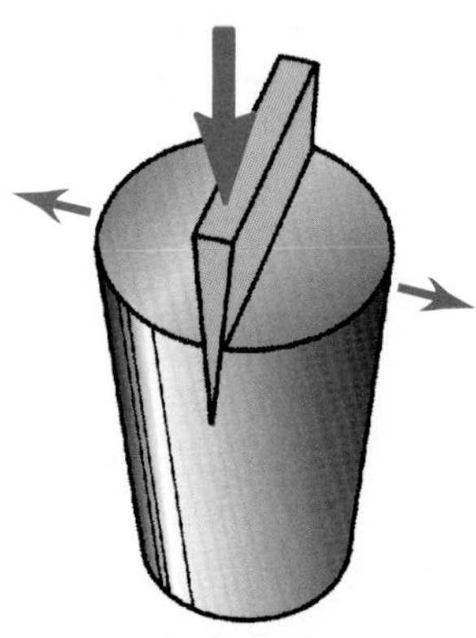

FIGURE 7-38 Wedge can be used to expand, split, and displace portions of substance that receives it.

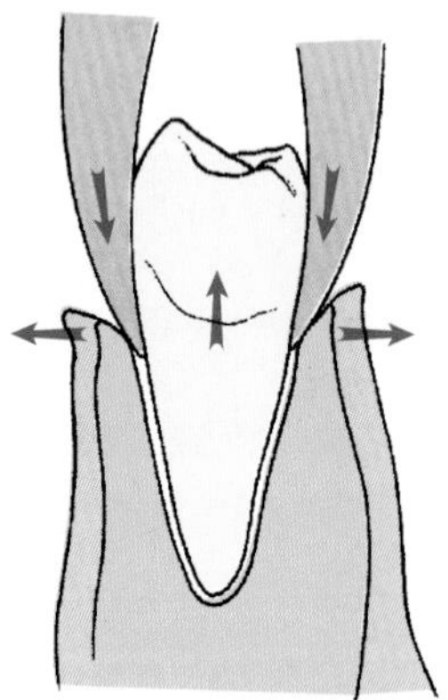

FIGURE 7-39 Beaks of forceps act as wedge to expand alveolar bone and displace tooth in occlusal direction.

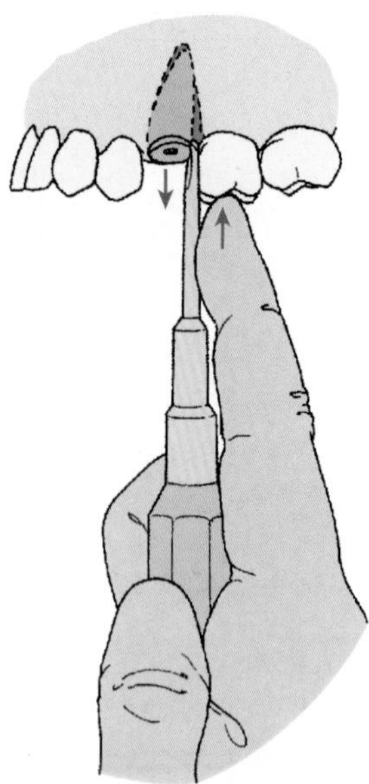

FIGURE 7-40 Small, straight elevator, used as wedge to displace tooth root from its socket.

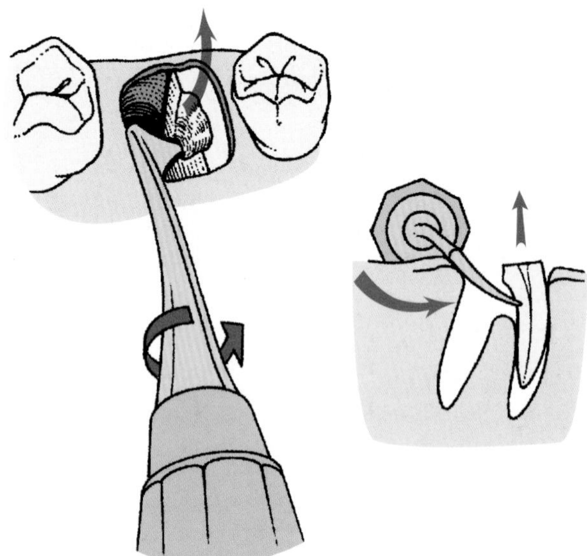

FIGURE 7-41 Triangular elevator in role of wheel-and-axle machine used to retrieve root from socket.

The elevator may also have flattened areas for fingers to grasp to help direct the elevator. The handle can also be set perpendicular to the shank (cross bar–type elevators). The shank connects the handle to the blade. Blades can be straight, triangular (Cryer), curved (Potts), or pointed (Crane pick).

The forceps can apply five major motions to luxate the teeth and expand the bony socket: The first is apical pressure, which accomplishes two goals. Although the tooth moves in an apical direction minimally, the tooth socket is expanded by the insertion of the beaks down into the periodontal ligament space (Fig. 7-42). Thus apical pressure of the forceps on the tooth causes bony expansion. A second accomplishment of apical pressure is that the center of rotation of the tooth is displaced apically. Because the tooth is moving in response to the force placed on it by the forceps, the forceps become the instrument of expansion. If the fulcrum is high (Fig. 7-43), a larger amount of force is placed on the apical region of the tooth, which increases the chance of fracturing the root end. If the beaks of the forceps are forced into the periodontal ligament space, the center of rotation is moved apically, which results in greater movement of the expansion forces at the crest

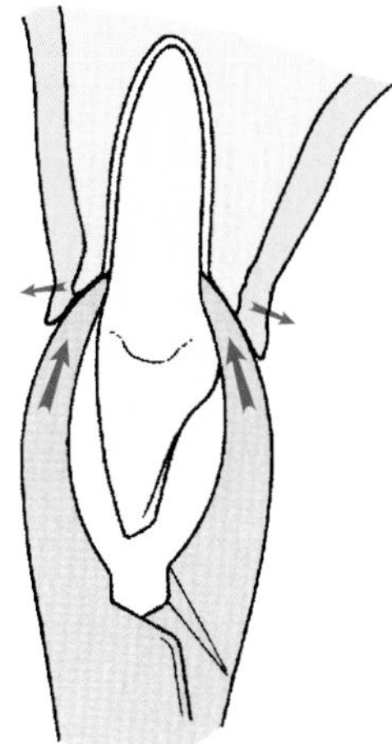

FIGURE 7-42 Extraction forceps should be seated with strong apical pressure to expand crestal bone and to displace center of rotation as far apically as possible.

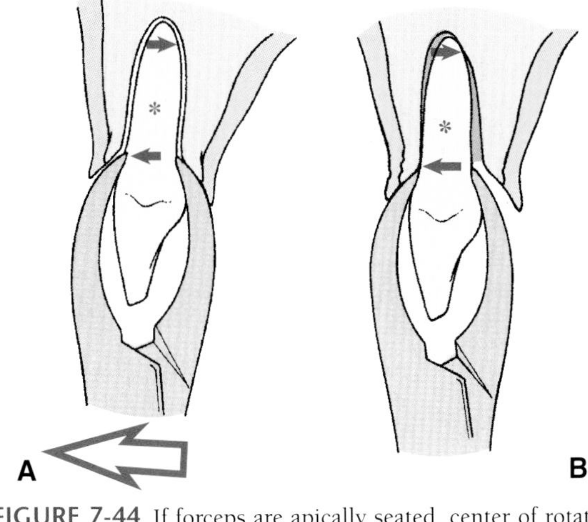

FIGURE 7-44 If forceps are apically seated, center of rotation (*) is displaced apically and less apical pressures are generated (**A**). This results in greater expansion of buccal cortex, less movement of apex of tooth, and therefore less chance of fracture of root (**B**).

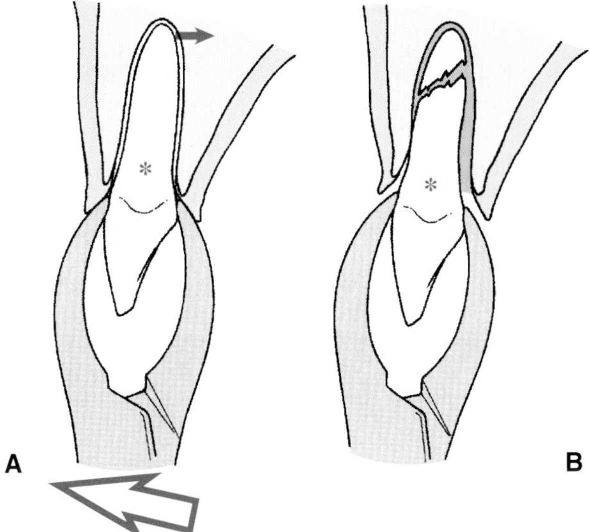

FIGURE 7-43 If center of rotation (*) is not far enough apically, it is too far occlusally, which results in excess movement of tooth apex (**A**). **B**, Excess motion of root apex caused by high center of rotation results in fracture of root apex.

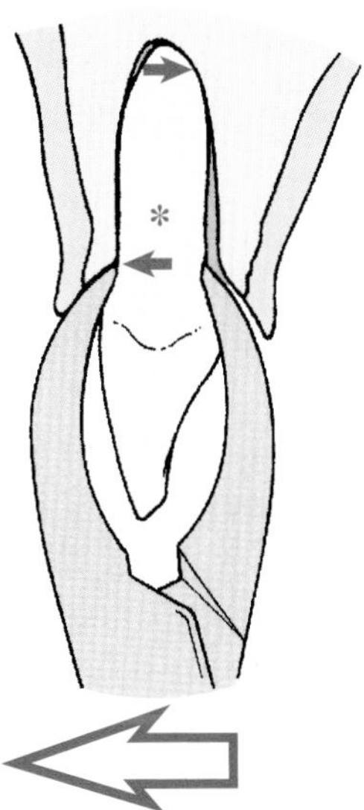

FIGURE 7-45 Buccal pressure applied to tooth will expand buccocortical plate toward crestal bone, with some lingual expansion at apical end of root. *Asterisk,* Center of rotation.

of the ridge and less force moving the apex of the tooth lingually (Fig. 7-44). This process decreases the chance for apical root fracture.

The second major pressure or movement applied by forceps is the buccal force. Buccal pressures result in expansion of the buccal plate, particularly at the crest of the ridge (Fig. 7-45). Although buccal pressure causes expansion forces at the crest of the ridge, it is important to remember that it also causes lingual apical pressure. Thus, excessive force can fracture buccal bone or cause a fracture of the apical portion of the root.

Third, lingual or palatal pressure is similar to the concept of buccal pressure but is aimed at expanding the linguocrestal bone and, at the same time, avoiding excessive pressures on the buccal apical bone (Fig. 7-46).

Fourth, rotational pressure, as the name implies, rotates the tooth, which causes some internal expansion of the tooth socket. Teeth with single, conical roots (such as the maxillary incisors and mandibular premolars) and with roots that are not curved are most amenable to luxation by this technique (Fig. 7-47). Teeth that have other than conical roots or that have multiple roots—especially if those roots are curved—are more likely to fracture under this type of pressure.

Finally, tractional forces are useful for delivering the tooth from the socket once adequate bony expansion is achieved. Tractional forces should be limited to the final portion of the extraction process and should be gentle (Fig. 7-48). If excessive force is needed, other maneuvers should be redone to improve root luxation.

In summary, a variety of forces can be used to remove teeth. A strong apical force is always useful and should be applied whenever the forceps are adapted to the tooth. Most teeth are removed by a combination of buccal and lingual (palatal)

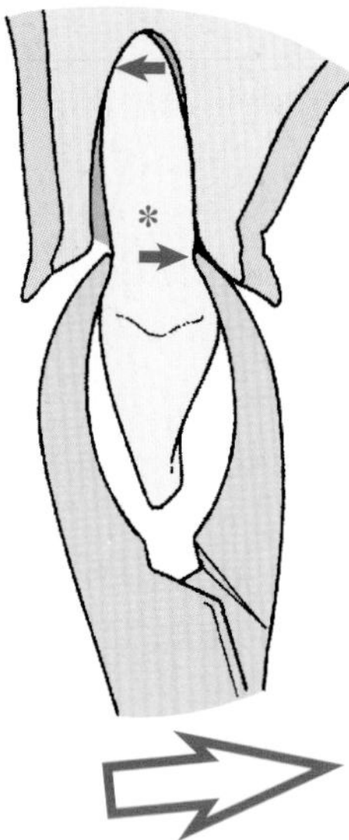

FIGURE 7-46 Lingual pressure will expand linguocortical plate at crestal area and slightly expand buccal bone at apical area. *Asterisk*, Center of rotation.

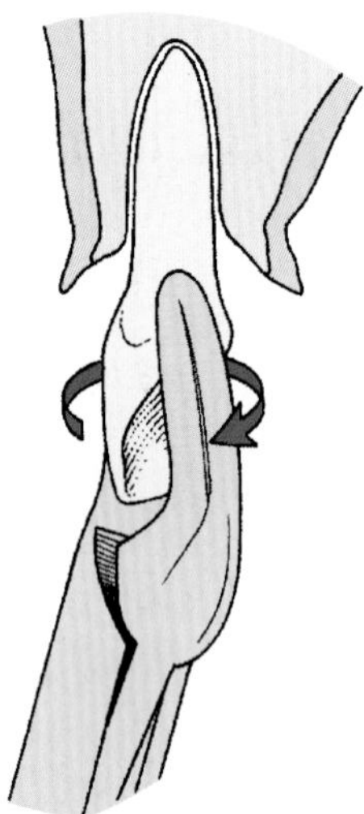

FIGURE 7-47 Rotational forces, useful for teeth with conical roots, such as maxillary incisors and mandibular premolars.

forces. Because maxillary buccal bone is usually thinner and the palatal bone is a thicker cortical bone, maxillary teeth are usually removed by strong buccal forces and less vigorous palatal forces. In the mandible the buccal bone is thinner from the midline posteriorly to the area of the molars. Therefore the incisors, canines, and premolars are removed primarily as a result of strong buccal force and less vigorous lingual pressures. The mandibular molar teeth have thicker buccal bone and usually require a stronger lingual pressure than the other teeth in the mouth. As mentioned before, rotational forces are useful for single-rooted teeth that have conic roots and no severe curvatures at the root end. The maxillary incisors, particularly the central incisor and mandibular premolars (especially the second premolar) are most amenable to rotational forces.

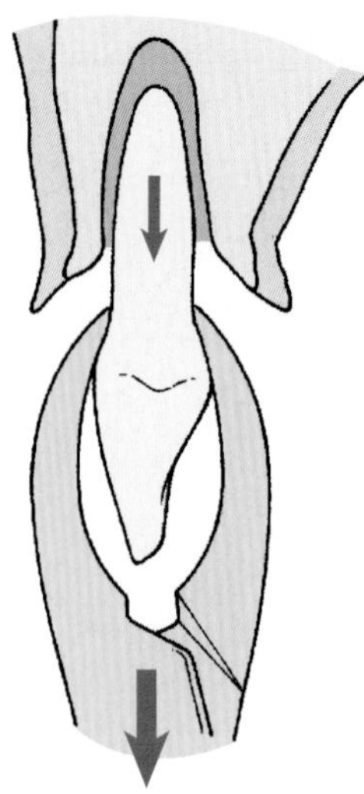

FIGURE 7-48 Tractional forces are useful for final removal of tooth from socket. They should always be small forces because teeth are not pulled.

PROCEDURE FOR CLOSED EXTRACTION

An erupted root can be extracted using one of two major techniques: closed or open. The closed technique is also known as the routine technique. The open technique is also known as the surgical, or flap, technique. This section discusses the closed extraction technique; the open technique is discussed in Chapter 8.

The closed technique is the most frequently used technique and is given primary consideration for almost every extraction. The open technique is used when the clinician believes that excessive force would be necessary to remove the tooth, when a substantial amount of the crown is missing or covered by tissue, or when access to the root of a tooth is difficult, such as when a fragile crown is present.

The correct technique for any situation should lead to an atraumatic extraction; the wrong technique may result in an excessively traumatic and lengthy extraction.

Whatever technique is chosen, the three fundamental requirements for a good extraction remain the same: (1) adequate access and visualization of the field of surgery, (2) an unimpeded pathway for the removal of the tooth, and (3) the use of controlled force to luxate and remove the tooth.

For the tooth to be removed from the bony socket, it is usually necessary to expand the alveolar bony walls to allow the tooth root an unimpeded pathway, and it is necessary to tear the periodontal ligament fibers that hold the tooth in the bony socket. The use of elevators and forceps as levers and wedges with steadily increasing force can accomplish these two objectives.

Five general steps make up the closed extraction procedure:

Step 1: Loosening of soft tissue attachment from the cervical portion of the tooth. The first step in removing a tooth by the closed extraction technique is to loosen the soft tissue from around the tooth with a sharp instrument, such as a scalpel blade or the sharp end of the No. 9 periosteal elevator (Fig. 7-49). The purpose of loosening the soft tissue from the tooth is twofold. First, it allows the surgeon to ensure that profound anesthesia has been achieved.

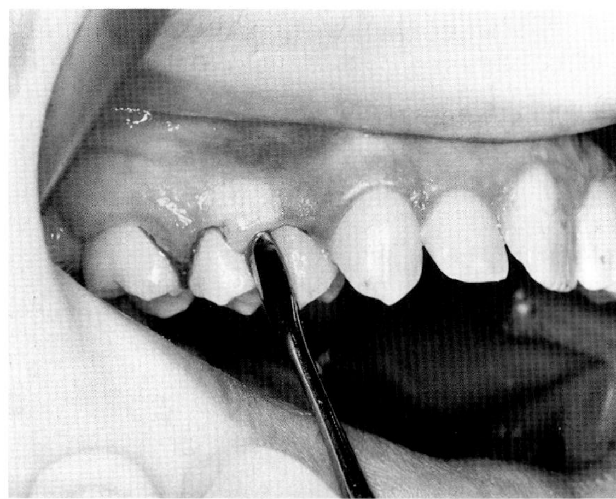

FIGURE 7-49 Periosteal elevator, used to loosen gingival attachment from tooth and the interdental papilla.

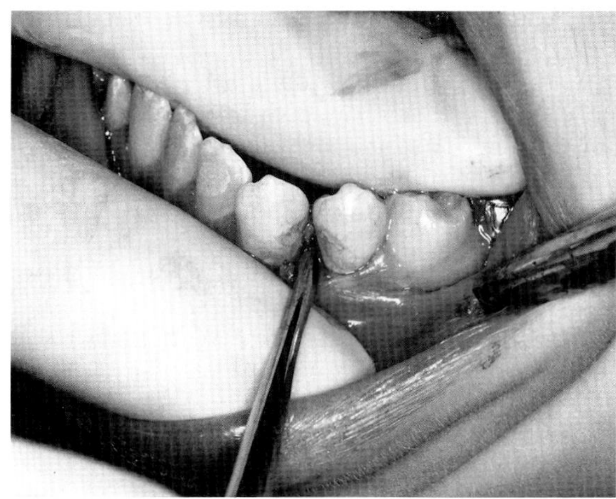

FIGURE 7-50 Small, straight elevator, inserted perpendicular to tooth after papilla has been reflected.

When this step has been performed, the dentist informs the patient that the surgery is about to begin and that the first step will be to push the soft tissue away from the tooth. A small amount of pressure is felt at this step, but no sensation of sharpness or discomfort. The surgeon then begins the soft tissue loosening procedure, gently at first and then with increasing force.

The second reason that the soft tissue is loosened is to allow the elevator and tooth extraction forceps to be positioned more apically, without interference from or impingement on the soft tissue of the gingiva. As the soft tissue is loosened away from the tooth, it is slightly reflected, which thereby increases the width of the gingival sulcus and allows easy entrance of the beveled wedge tip of the forceps beaks. The adjacent gingival papilla of the tooth should also be reflected to avoid damage by the insertion of the straight elevator.

Step 2: Luxation of the tooth with a dental elevator. The next step is to begin the luxation of the tooth with a dental elevator, usually the straight elevator. Expansion and dilation of the alveolar bone and tearing of the periodontal ligament require that the tooth be luxated in several ways. The straight elevator is inserted perpendicular to the tooth into the interdental space, after reflection of the interdental papilla (Fig. 7-50). The elevator is then turned in such a way that the inferior portion of the blade rests on the alveolar bone and the superior, or occlusal, portion of the blade is turned toward the tooth being extracted (Fig. 7-51). Strong, slow, forceful turning of the handle moves the tooth in a posterior direction, which results in some expansion of the alveolar bone and tearing of the periodontal ligament. If the tooth is intact and in contact with stable teeth anterior and posterior to it, the amount of movement achieved with the straight elevator will be minimal. The usefulness of this step is greater if the patient does not have a tooth posterior to the tooth being extracted or if it is broken down to an extent that the crowns do not inhibit movement of the tooth.

In certain situations the elevator can be turned in the opposite direction and more vertical displacement of the tooth will be achieved, which can possibly result in complete removal of the tooth (Fig. 7-52).

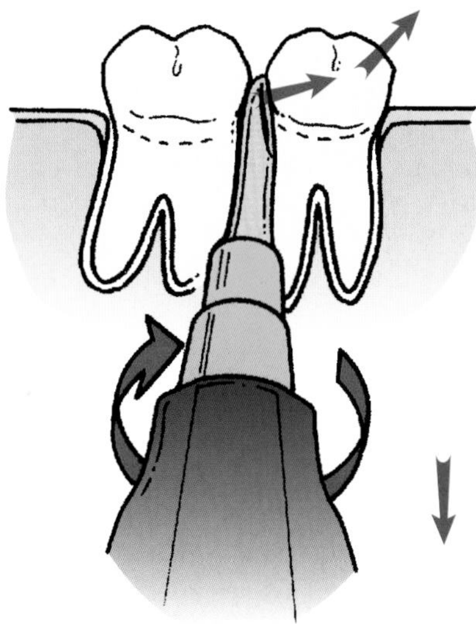

FIGURE 7-51 Handle of small, straight elevator, turned so that occlusal side of elevator blade is turned toward tooth. The handle is also moved apically to help elevate the tooth.

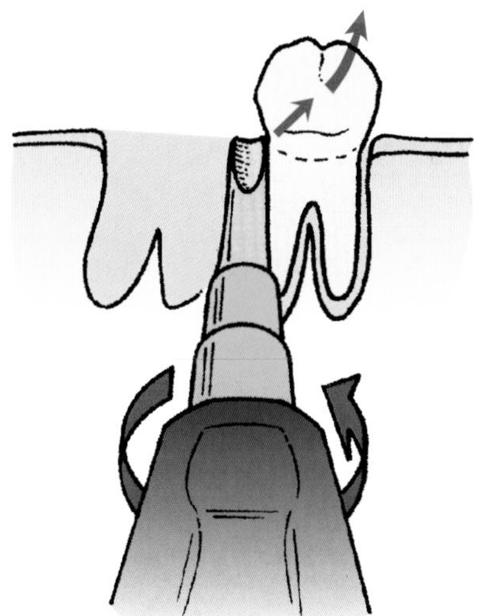

FIGURE 7-52 Handle of elevator, which may be turned in opposite direction to displace tooth further from socket. This can be accomplished only if no tooth is adjacent posteriorly.

Luxation of teeth with a straight elevator should be performed with caution. Excessive forces can damage and even displace the teeth adjacent to those being extracted. This is especially true if the adjacent tooth has a large restoration or carious lesion. This is only the initial step in the elevation process. Next, the small, straight elevator is inserted into the periodontal ligament space at the mesial-buccal line angle. The elevator is advanced apically while being rotated back and forth, helping luxate the tooth with its wedge action as it is advanced apically. A similar action with the elevator can then be done at the distal-buccal line angle. When a small, straight elevator becomes too easy to twist, a larger-sized elevator is used to do the same apical advancement. Often the tooth will loosen sufficiently to be removed easily with the forceps.

Step 3: Adaptation of the forceps to the tooth. The proper forceps are then chosen for the tooth to be extracted. The beaks of the forceps should be shaped to adapt anatomically to the tooth, apical to the cervical line, that is, to the root surface. The forceps are then seated onto the tooth so that the tips of the forceps beaks grasp the root underneath the loosened soft tissue (Fig. 7-53). The lingual beak is usually seated first and then the buccal beak. Care must be taken to confirm that the tips of the forceps beaks are beneath the soft tissue and not engaging an adjacent tooth. Once the forceps have been positioned on the tooth, the surgeon grasps the handles of the forceps at the ends to maximize mechanical advantage and control (Fig. 7-54).

If the tooth is malposed in such a fashion that the usual forceps cannot grasp the tooth without injury to adjacent teeth, another forceps with narrower beaks should be used. The maxillary root forceps can often be useful for crowded lower anterior teeth (Fig. 7-55).

The beaks of the forceps must be held parallel to the long axis of the tooth so that the forces generated by the application of pressure to the forceps handle can be delivered along the long axis of the tooth for maximal effectiveness in dilating and expanding the alveolar bone. If the beaks are not parallel to the long axis of the tooth, it is increasingly likely that the tooth root will fracture.

The forceps are then forced apically as far as possible to grasp the root of the tooth as apically as possible. This

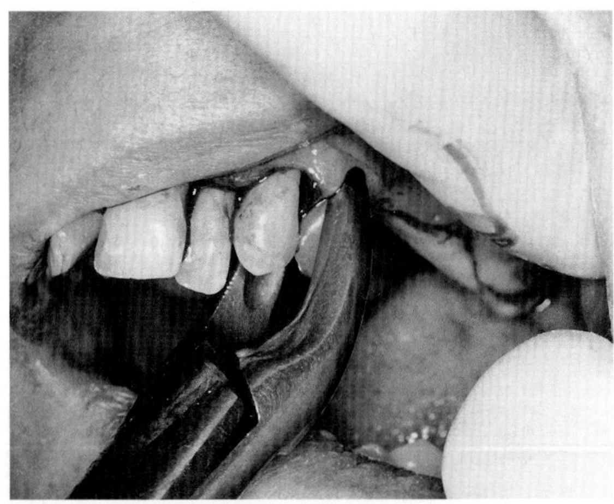

FIGURE 7-53 Tips of forceps beak, forced apically under soft tissue.

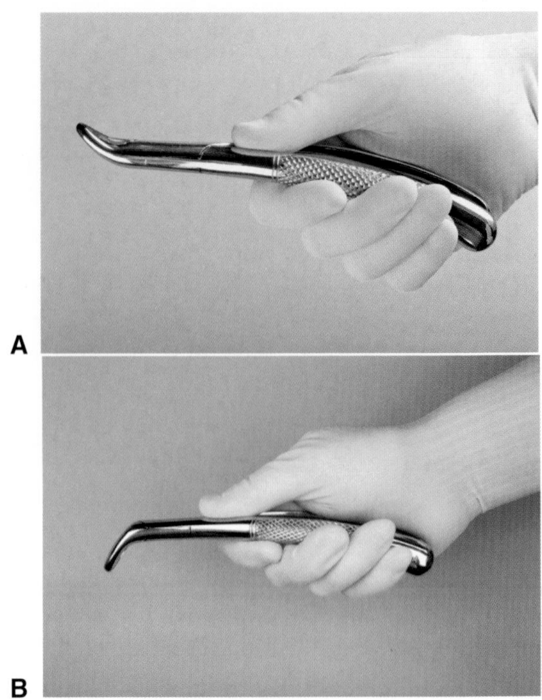

FIGURE 7-54 Forceps handles, held at very ends to maximize mechanical advantage and control. **A**, Maxillary universal forceps. **B**, Mandibular universal forceps.

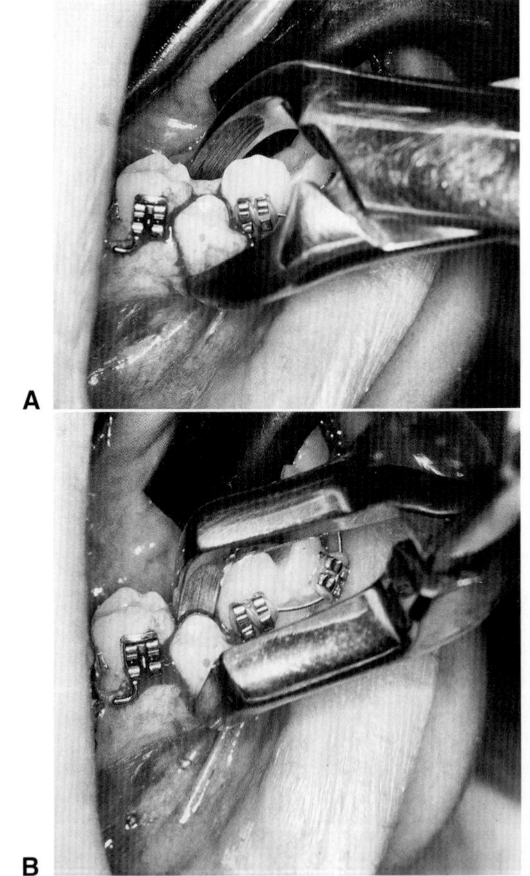

FIGURE 7-55 **A**, No. 151 forceps, too wide to grasp premolar to be extracted without luxating adjacent teeth. **B**, Maxillary root forceps, which can be adapted easily to tooth for extraction.

accomplishes two things: First, the beaks of the forceps act as wedges to dilate the crestal bone on the buccal and lingual aspects. Second, by forcing the beaks apically, the center of rotation (or fulcrum) of the forces applied to the tooth is displaced toward the apex of the tooth, which results in greater effectiveness of bone expansion and less likelihood of fracturing the apical end of the tooth.

At this point the surgeon's hand should be grasping the forceps firmly, with the wrist locked and the arm held against the body; the surgeon should be prepared to apply force with the shoulder and upper arm without any wrist pressure. The surgeon should be standing straight, with the feet comfortably apart.

Step 4: Luxation of the tooth with the forceps. The surgeon begins to luxate the tooth by using the motions discussed earlier. The major portion of the force is directed toward the thinnest and therefore weakest bone. Thus in the maxilla and all but the molar teeth in the mandible, the major movement is labial and buccal (i.e., toward the thinner layer of bone). The surgeon uses slow, steady force to displace the tooth buccally rather than a series of rapid, small movements that do little to expand bone. The motion is deliberate and slow, and it gradually increases in force. The tooth is then moved again toward the opposite direction with slow, deliberate, strong pressure. As the alveolar bone begins to expand, the forceps are reseated apically with a strong, deliberate motion, which causes additional expansion of the alveolar bone and further displaces the center of the rotation apically. Buccal and lingual pressures continue to expand the alveolar socket. For some teeth, rotational motions are then used to help expand the tooth socket and tear the periodontal ligament attachments.

Beginning surgeons have a tendency to apply inadequate pressure for insufficient amounts of time. The following three factors must be reemphasized: (1) The forceps must be apically seated as far as possible and reseated periodically during the extraction; (2) the forces applied in the buccal and lingual directions should be slow, deliberate pressures and not jerky wiggles; and (3) the force should be held for several seconds to allow the bone time to expand. One must remember that teeth are not pulled; rather, they are gently lifted from the socket once the alveolar process has been sufficiently expanded.

Step 5: Removal of the tooth from the socket. Once the alveolar bone has expanded sufficiently and the tooth has been luxated, a slight tractional force, usually directed buccally, can be used. Tractional forces should be minimized, because this is the last motion that is used once the alveolar process is sufficiently expanded and the periodontal ligament is completely severed.

One should remember that luxation of the tooth with the forceps and removal of the tooth from the bone are separate steps in the extraction. Luxation is directed toward expansion of the bone and disruption of the periodontal ligament. The tooth is not removed from the bone until these two goals are accomplished. The novice surgeon should realize that the major role of the forceps is not to remove the tooth but rather to expand the bone so that the tooth can be removed.

For teeth that are malposed or have unusual positions in the alveolar process, the luxation with the forceps and removal from the alveolar process will be in unusual directions. The surgeon must develop a sense for the direction the tooth wants to move and then be able to move it in that direction. Careful preoperative assessment and planning help to guide this determination during the extraction.

Role of Opposite Hand

During use of the forceps and elevators to luxate and remove teeth, it is important that the surgeon's opposite hand play an active role in the procedure. For the right-handed operator, the left hand has a variety of functions. The left hand is responsible for reflecting the soft tissues of the cheeks, lips, and tongue to provide adequate visualization of the area of surgery. The left hand helps to protect other teeth from the forceps, should it release suddenly from the tooth socket. The left hand helps to stabilize the patient's head during the extraction process. In some situations, greater amounts of force are required to expand heavy alveolar bone; therefore the patient's head requires active assistance to be held steady. The opposite hand plays an important role in supporting and stabilizing the jaw when mandibular teeth are being extracted. The opposite hand is often necessary to apply considerable pressure to expand heavy mandibular bone, and such forces can cause discomfort and even injury to the TMJ unless a steady hand counteracts them. A bite block placed on the contralateral side is also used to help support the jaw in this situation. Finally, the opposite hand supports the alveolar process and provides tactile information to the operator concerning the expansion of the alveolar process during the luxation period. In some situations, it is impossible for the opposite hand to perform all of these functions at the same time, so the surgeon requires an assistant to help with some of them.

Role of Assistant During Extraction

For a successful outcome in any surgical procedure, it is essential to have a skilled assistant. During the extraction the assistant plays a variety of important roles that contribute to making the surgical experience atraumatic. The assistant helps the surgeon visualize and gain access to the operative area by reflecting the soft tissue of the cheeks and tongue so that the surgeon can have an unobstructed view of the surgical field. Even during a closed extraction, the assistant can reflect the soft tissue so that the surgeon can apply the instruments to loosen the soft tissue attachment and adapt the forceps to the tooth in the most effective manner.

Another major activity of the assistant is to suction away blood, saliva, and the irrigating solutions used during the surgical procedure. This prevents fluids from accumulating and makes proper visualization of the surgical field possible. Suctioning is also important for patient comfort, because most patients are unable to tolerate an accumulation of blood or other fluids in their throats.

During the extraction the assistant should also help to protect the teeth of the opposite arch, which is especially important when removing lower posterior teeth. If traction forces are necessary to remove a lower tooth, occasionally the tooth releases suddenly and the forceps strike the maxillary teeth and may fracture a tooth cusp. The assistant should hold a suction tip or a finger against the maxillary teeth to protect them from an unexpected blow.

During the extraction of mandibular teeth, the assistant may play an important role by supporting the mandible during the application of the extraction forces. A surgeon who uses the hand to reflect the soft tissue may not be able to support the mandible. If this is the case, the assistant plays an important role in stabilizing the mandible to prevent TMJ discomfort. Most often the surgeon stabilizes the mandible, which makes this role less important for the assistant.

The assistant also provides psychological and emotional support for the patient by helping alleviate patient anxiety during the surgery. The assistant is important in gaining the patient's confidence and cooperation by using positive language and physical contact with the patient during the preparation and performance of the surgery. The assistant should avoid making casual, offhand comments that may increase the patients' anxiety and lessen their cooperation.

SPECIFIC TECHNIQUES FOR REMOVAL OF EACH TOOTH

This section describes specific techniques for the removal of each tooth in the mouth. In some situations, several teeth are grouped together (e.g., the maxillary anterior teeth) because the technique for their removal is essentially the same.

Maxillary Teeth

In the correct position for extraction of maxillary left or anterior teeth, the left index finger of the surgeon should reflect the lip and cheek tissue; the thumb should rest on the palatal alveolar process (Fig. 7-56). In this way the left hand is able to reflect the soft tissue of the cheek, stabilize the patient's head, support the alveolar process, and provide tactile information to the surgeon regarding the progress of the extraction. When such a position is used during the extraction of a maxillary molar, the surgeon can frequently feel with the left hand the palatal root of the molar becoming free in the alveolar process before realizing it with the forceps or extracting hand. For the right side, the index finger is positioned on the palate and the thumb on the buccal aspect.

Incisor Teeth

The maxillary incisor teeth are extracted with the upper universal forceps (No. 150), although other forceps can be used.

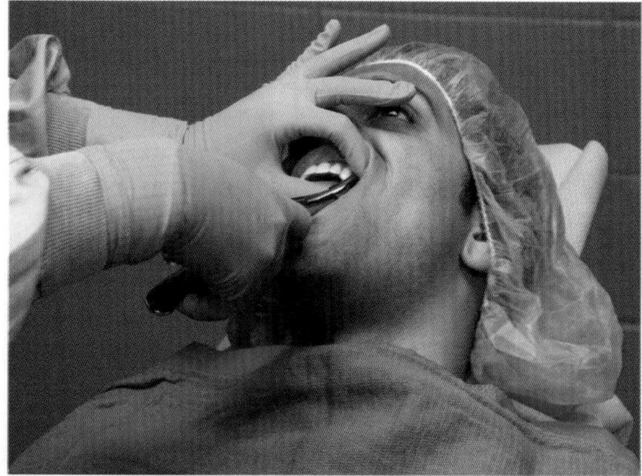

FIGURE 7-56 Extraction of maxillary left posterior teeth. Left index finger reflects lip and cheek and supports alveolar process on buccal aspect. Thumb is positioned on palatal aspect of alveolar process and supports alveolar process. Head is steadied by this grip, and tactile information is gained regarding tooth and bone movement.

The maxillary incisors generally have conic roots, with the lateral ones being slightly longer and more slender. The lateral incisor is more likely also to have a distal curvature on the apical one third of the root, so this must be checked radiographically before the tooth is extracted. The alveolar bone is thin on the labial side and heavier on the palatal side, which indicates that the major expansion of the alveolar process will be in the labial direction. The initial movement is slow, steady, and firm in the labial direction, which expands the crestal buccal bone. A less vigorous palatal force is then used, followed by a slow, firm, rotational force. Rotational movement should be minimized for the lateral incisor, especially if a curvature exists on the tooth. The tooth is delivered in the labial-incisal direction with a small amount of tractional force (Fig. 7-57).

Canine

The maxillary canine is usually the longest tooth in the mouth. The root is oblong in cross section and usually produces a bulge called the canine eminence on the anterior surface of the maxilla. The result is that the bone over the labial aspect of the maxillary canine is usually thin. In spite of the thin labial bone, this tooth can be difficult to extract simply because of its long root. Additionally, it is not uncommon for a segment of labial alveolar bone to fracture from the labial plate and be removed with the tooth.

The upper universal (No. 150) forceps are the preferred instrument for removing the maxillary canine. As with all extractions the initial placement of the beaks of the forceps on the canine tooth should be as far apically as possible. The initial movement is apical and then to the buccal aspect, with return pressure to the palatal. As the bone is expanded and the tooth mobilized, the forceps should be repositioned apically. A small amount of rotational force may be useful in expanding the tooth socket, especially if the adjacent teeth are missing or have just been extracted. After the tooth has been well luxated, it is delivered from the socket in a labial-incisal direction with labial tractional forces (Fig. 7-58).

If, during the luxation process with the forceps, the surgeon feels a portion of the labial bone fracture, the surgeon must make a decision concerning the next step. If the palpating finger indicates that a small amount of bone has fractured free and is attached to the canine tooth, the extraction should continue in the usual manner, with caution taken not to tear the soft tissue. However, if the palpating finger indicates that a large portion of labial alveolar plate has fractured, the surgeon should stop the surgical procedure. Usually the fractured portion of bone is attached to periosteum and therefore is viable. The surgeon should use a thin periosteal elevator to raise a small amount of mucosa from around the tooth, down to the level of the fractured bone.

The canine tooth should then be stabilized with the extraction forceps, and the surgeon should attempt to free the fractured bone from the tooth, with the periosteal elevator as a lever to separate the bone from the tooth root. If this can be accomplished, the tooth can be removed and the bone left in place attached to the periosteum. Normal healing should occur. If the bone becomes detached from the periosteum during these attempts, it should be removed, because it is probably nonvital and may actually prolong wound healing. This same procedure can be used whenever alveolar bone is fractured during extraction.

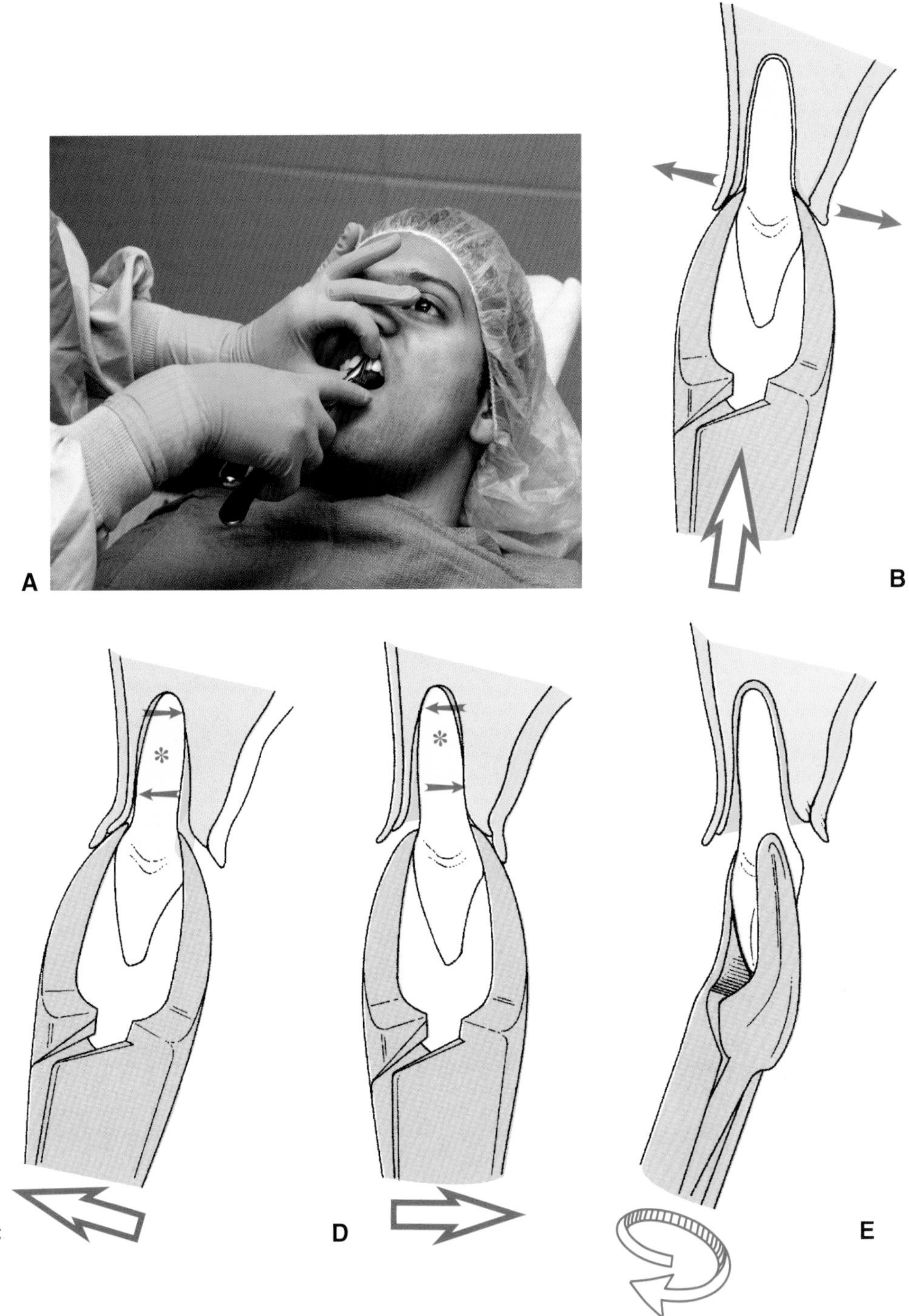

FIGURE 7-57 A, Maxillary incisors are extracted with No. 150 forceps. Left hand grasps alveolar process. B, Forceps are seated as far apically as possible. C, Luxation is begun with labial force. D, Slight lingual force is used. E, Tooth is delivered to labial incisor with rotational, tractional movement.

Prevention of fractured labial plate is important. If during the luxation process with the forceps a normal amount of pressure has not resulted in any movement of the tooth, the surgeon should seriously consider doing an open extraction. By reflecting a soft tissue flap and removing a small amount of bone, the surgeon may be able to remove the stubborn canine tooth without fracturing a larger amount of labial bone. By using the open technique, there will be an overall reduction in bone loss and in postoperative healing time.

First Premolar

The maxillary first premolar is a single-rooted tooth in its first two thirds, with a bifurcation into a buccolingual root usually occurring in the apical one third to one half. These roots may

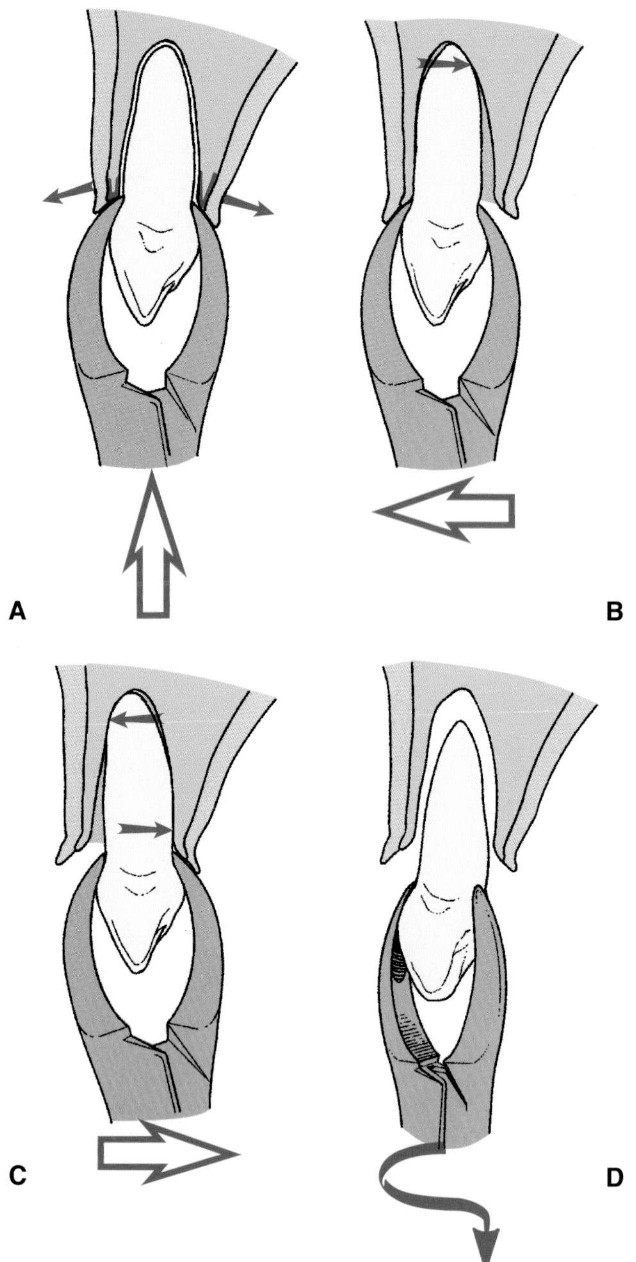

FIGURE 7-58 A, Hand and forceps position for removal of maxillary canine is similar to that for incisors. Forceps are seated as far apically as possible. B, Initial movement is buccally. C, Small amounts of lingual force are applied. D, Tooth is delivered in labial-incisal direction with slight rotational force.

be extremely thin and are subject to fracture, especially in older patients in whom bone density is great and bone elasticity is diminished. Perhaps the most common root fracture when extracting teeth in adults occurs with this tooth. As with other maxillary teeth, the buccal bone is thin compared with the palatal bone.

The upper universal (No. 150) forceps are the instrument of choice. Alternatively, the No. 150A forceps can be used for removal of the maxillary first premolar.

Because of the high likelihood of root fracture, the tooth should be luxated as much as possible with the straight elevator. If root fracture does occur, a mobile root tip can be removed more easily than one that has not been well luxated.

Because of the bifurcation of the tooth into two thin root tips, extraction forces should be carefully controlled during removal of the maxillary first premolar. Initial movements should be buccal. Palatal movements are made with small amounts of force to prevent fracture of the palatal root tip, which is harder to retrieve. When the tooth is luxated buccally, the most likely tooth root to break is the labial. When the tooth is luxated in the palatal direction, the most likely root to break is the palatal root. Of the two root tips, the labial is easier to retrieve because of the thin, overlying bone. Therefore, buccal pressures should be greater than palatal pressures. Any rotational force should be avoided. Final delivery of the tooth from the tooth socket is with tractional force in the occlusal direction and slightly buccal (Fig. 7-59).

Second Premolar

The maxillary second premolar is a single-rooted tooth for the entire length of the root. The root is thick and has a blunt end. Consequently, the root of the second premolar rarely fractures. The overlying alveolar bone is similar to that of other maxillary teeth in that it is thin toward the bucca, with a heavy palatal alveolar palate.

The recommended forceps are the maxillary universal forceps, or No. 150; some surgeons prefer the No. 150A. The forceps are forced as far apically as possible so as to gain maximal mechanical advantage in removing this tooth. Because the tooth root is strong and blunt, the extraction requires strong movements to the buccal, back to the palate, and then in the buccoocclusal direction with a rotational, tractional force (Fig. 7-60).

Molar

The maxillary first molar has three large and strong roots. The buccal roots are usually close together, and the palatal root diverges widely toward the palate. If the two buccal roots are also widely divergent, it becomes difficult to remove this tooth by closed extraction. Once again the overlying alveolar bone is similar to that of other teeth in the maxilla; the buccal plate is thin and the palatal cortical plate is thick and heavy. When evaluating this tooth radiographically, the dentist should note the size, curvature, and apparent divergence of the three roots. Additionally the dentist should look carefully at the relationship of the tooth roots to the maxillary sinus. If the sinus is in proximity to the roots and the roots are widely divergent, sinus perforation caused by removal of a portion of the sinus floor during tooth removal is increasingly likely. If this appears to be likely after preoperative evaluation, the surgeon should strongly consider a surgical extraction.

The paired forceps No. 53R and No. 53L are usually used for extraction of the maxillary molars. These two forceps have tip projections on the buccal beaks to fit into the buccal bifurcation. Some surgeons prefer to use the No. 89 and No. 90 forceps. These two forceps are especially useful if the crown of the molar tooth has serious caries or large restorations.

The upper molar forceps are adapted to the tooth and are apically seated as far as possible in the usual fashion (Fig. 7-61). The basic extraction movement is to use strong buccal and palatal pressures, with stronger forces toward the buccal than toward the palate. Rotational forces are not useful for extrac-

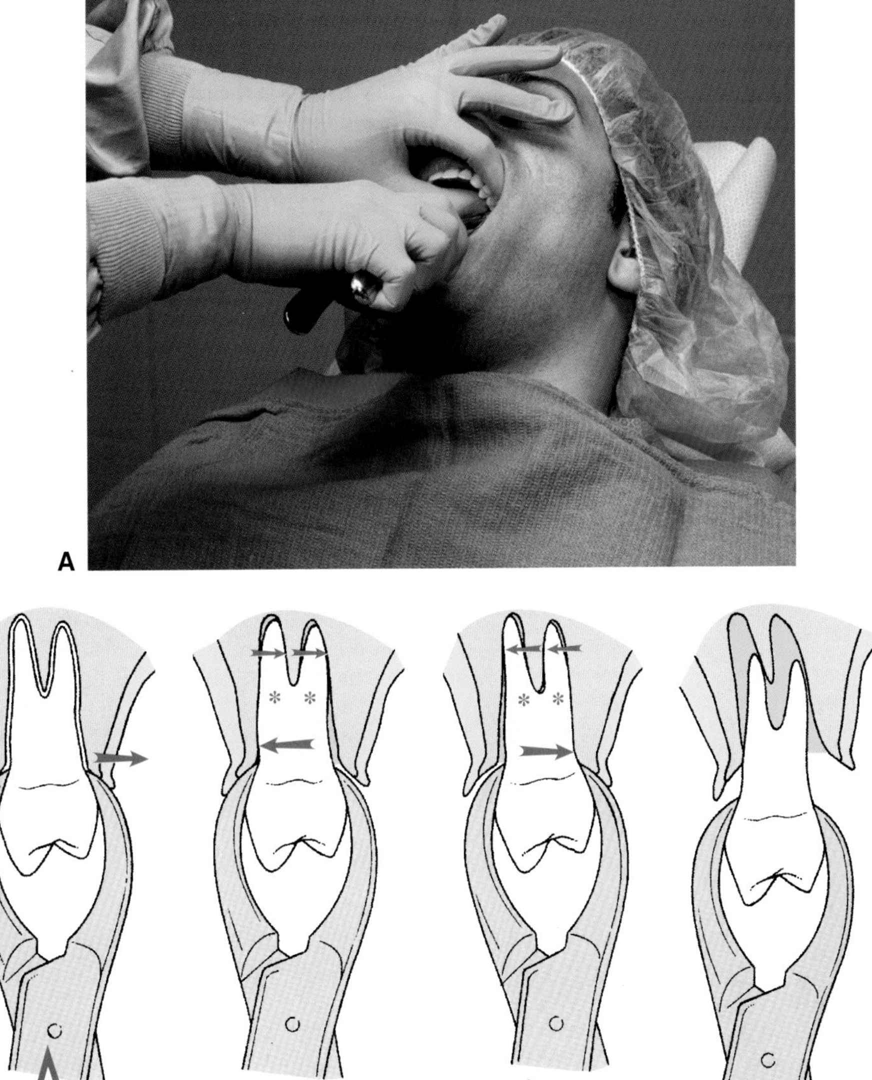

FIGURE 7-59 A, Maxillary premolars are removed with No. 150 forceps. Hand position is similar to that used for anterior teeth. B, Firm apical pressure is applied first to lower center of rotation as far as possible and to expand crestal bone. C, Buccal pressure is applied initially to expand buccocortical plate. Apices of roots are pushed lingually and are therefore subject to fracture. D, Palatal pressure is applied but less vigorously than buccal pressure. E, Tooth is delivered in buccoocclusal direction with combination of buccal and tractional forces.

tion of this tooth because of its three roots. As mentioned in the discussion of the extraction of the maxillary first premolar, it is preferable to fracture a buccal root than a palatal root (because it is easier to retrieve the buccal roots). Therefore, if the tooth has widely divergent roots and the dentist suspects that one root may be fractured, the tooth should be luxated in such a way as to prevent fracturing the palatal root. The dentist must minimize palatal force, because this is the force that fractures the palatal root. Strong, slow, steady, buccal pressure expands the buccocortical plate and tears the periodontal ligament fibers that hold the palatal root in its position. Palatal forces should be used but kept to a minimum.

The anatomy of the maxillary second molar is similar to that of the maxillary first molar except that the roots tend to be shorter and less divergent, with the buccal roots more commonly fused into a single root. This means that the tooth is more easily extracted by the same technique described for the first molar.

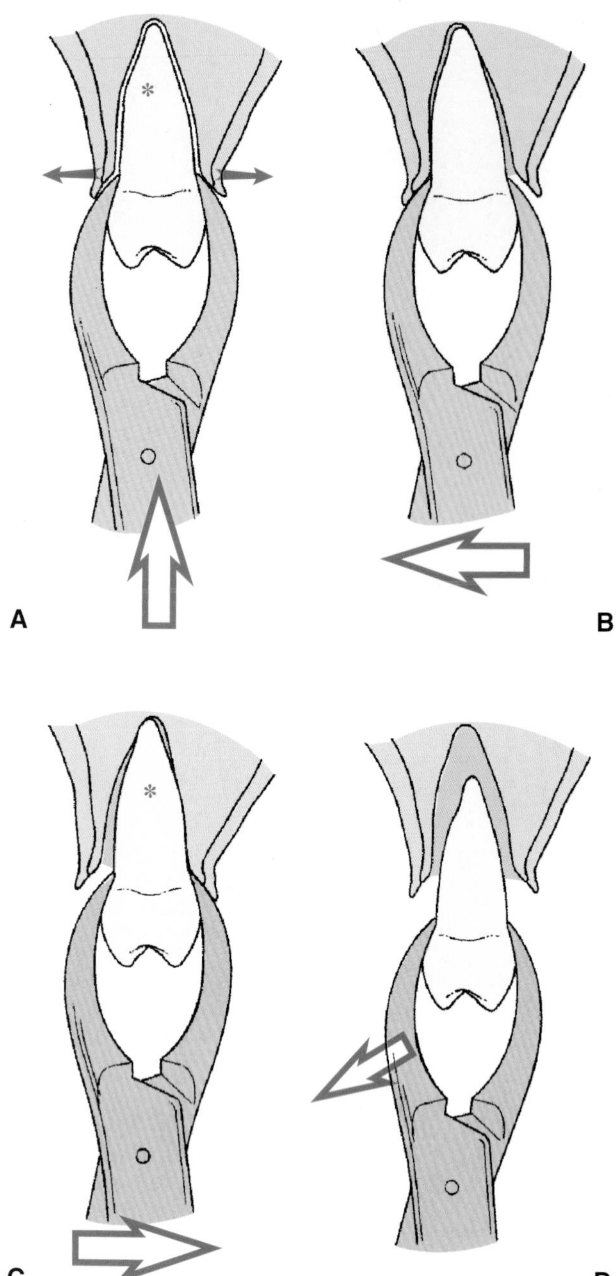

FIGURE 7-60 A, When extracting maxillary second premolar, forceps are seated as far apically as possible. B, Luxation is begun with buccal pressure. C, Very slight lingual pressure is used. D, Tooth is delivered in buccoocclusal direction.

The erupted maxillary third molar frequently has conic roots and is usually extracted with the No. 210S forceps, which are universal forceps used for the left and right sides. The tooth is usually easily removed, because the buccal bone is thin and the roots are usually fused and conic. The erupted third molar is also frequently extracted by the use of elevators alone. Clear visualization of the maxillary third molar on the preoperative radiograph is important because the root anatomy of this tooth is variable and often small, dilacerated, hooked roots exist in this area. Retrieval of fractured roots in this area is difficult.

Mandibular Teeth

When removing lower molar teeth, the index finger of the left hand is in the buccal vestibule and the second finger is in the lingual vestibule, reflecting the lip, cheek, and tongue (Fig. 7-62). The thumb of the left hand is placed below the chin so that the mandible is held between the fingers and thumb, which support the mandible and minimize TMJ pressures. This technique provides less tactile information, but during extraction of mandibular teeth the need to support the mandible supersedes the need to support the alveolar process. A useful alternative is to place a bite block between the teeth on the contralateral side (Fig. 7-63). The bite block allows the patient to help provide stabilizing forces to limit the pressure on the TMJs. The surgeon's hand should continue to provide additional support to the jaw.

Anterior Teeth

The mandibular incisors and canines are similar in shape, with the incisors being shorter and slightly thinner and the canine roots being longer and heavier. The incisor roots are more likely to be fractured because they are thin and therefore should be removed only after adequate preextraction luxation. The alveolar bone that overlies the incisors and canines is thin on the labial and lingual sides. The bone over the canine may be thicker, especially on the lingual aspect.

The lower universal (No. 151) forceps are usually used to remove these teeth. Alternative choices include the No. 151A or the English style of Ashe forceps. The forceps beaks are positioned on the teeth and seated apically with strong force. The extraction movements are generally in the labial and lingual directions, with equal pressures both ways. Once the tooth has become luxated and mobile, rotational movement may be used to expand the alveolar bone further. The tooth is removed from the socket with tractional forces in a labial-incisal direction (Fig. 7-64).

Premolars

The mandibular premolars are among the easiest teeth to remove. The roots tend to be straight and conic, albeit sometimes slender. The overlying alveolar bone is thin on the buccal aspect and heavier on the lingual side.

The lower universal (No. 151) forceps are usually chosen for the extraction of the mandibular premolars. The No. 151A forceps and the English style of forceps are popular alternatives for extraction of these teeth.

The forceps are apically forced as far as possible, with the basic movements being toward the buccal aspect, returning to the lingual aspect, and finally, rotating. Rotational movement is used more when extracting these teeth than for any others, except perhaps the maxillary central incisor. The tooth is then delivered in the occlusobuccal direction (Fig. 7-65). Careful preoperative radiographic assessment must be performed to assure the operator that no root curvature exists in the apical third of the tooth. If such a curvature does exist, the rotational movements should be reduced or eliminated from the extraction procedure (Fig. 7-66).

Molars

The mandibular molars usually have two roots, with roots of the first molar more widely divergent than those of the second molar. Additionally, the roots may converge at the apical one

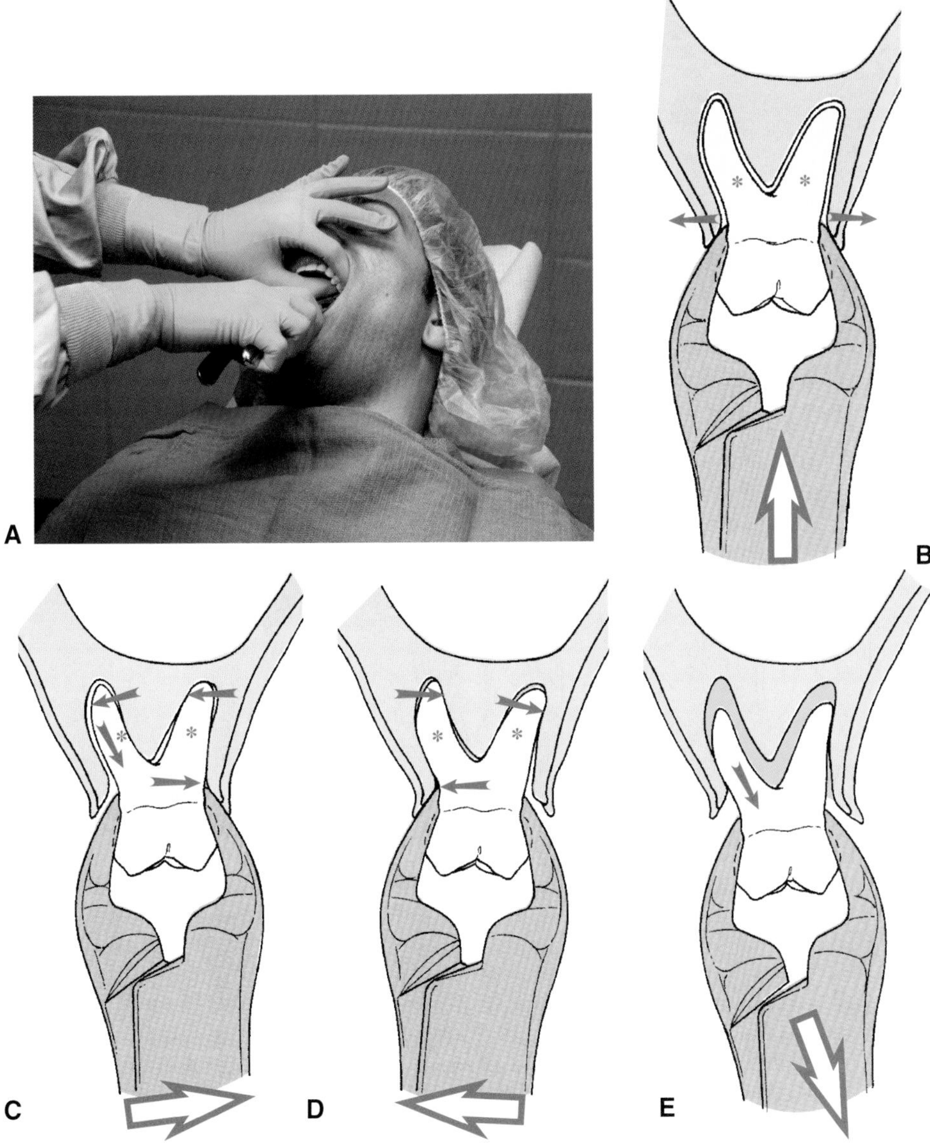

FIGURE 7-61 A, Extraction of maxillary molars. Soft tissue of lips and cheek is reflected, and alveolar process is grasped with opposite hand. B, Forceps beaks are seated apically as far as possible. C, Luxation is begun with strong buccal force. D, Lingual pressures are used only moderately. E, Tooth is delivered in buccoocclusal direction.

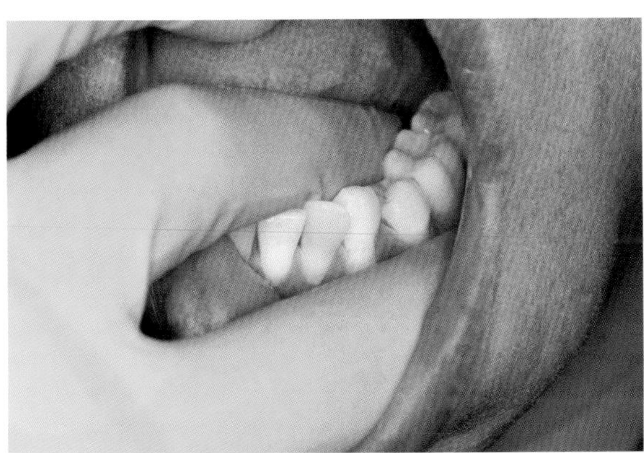

FIGURE 7-62 Extraction of mandibular left posterior teeth. Surgeon's left index finger is positioned in buccal vestibule, reflecting cheek, and second finger is positioned in lingual vestibule, reflecting tongue. Thumb is positioned under chin. Mandible is grasped between fingers and thumb to provide support during extraction.

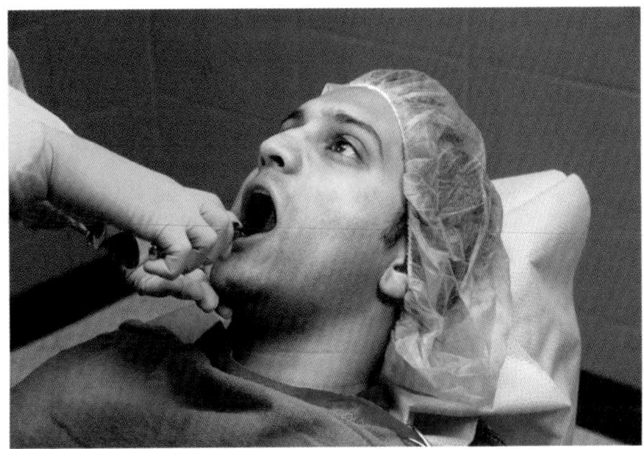

FIGURE 7-63 To provide support for the mandible to prevent excessive temporomandibular joint pressures, a rubber bite block can be placed between the teeth on the contralateral side.

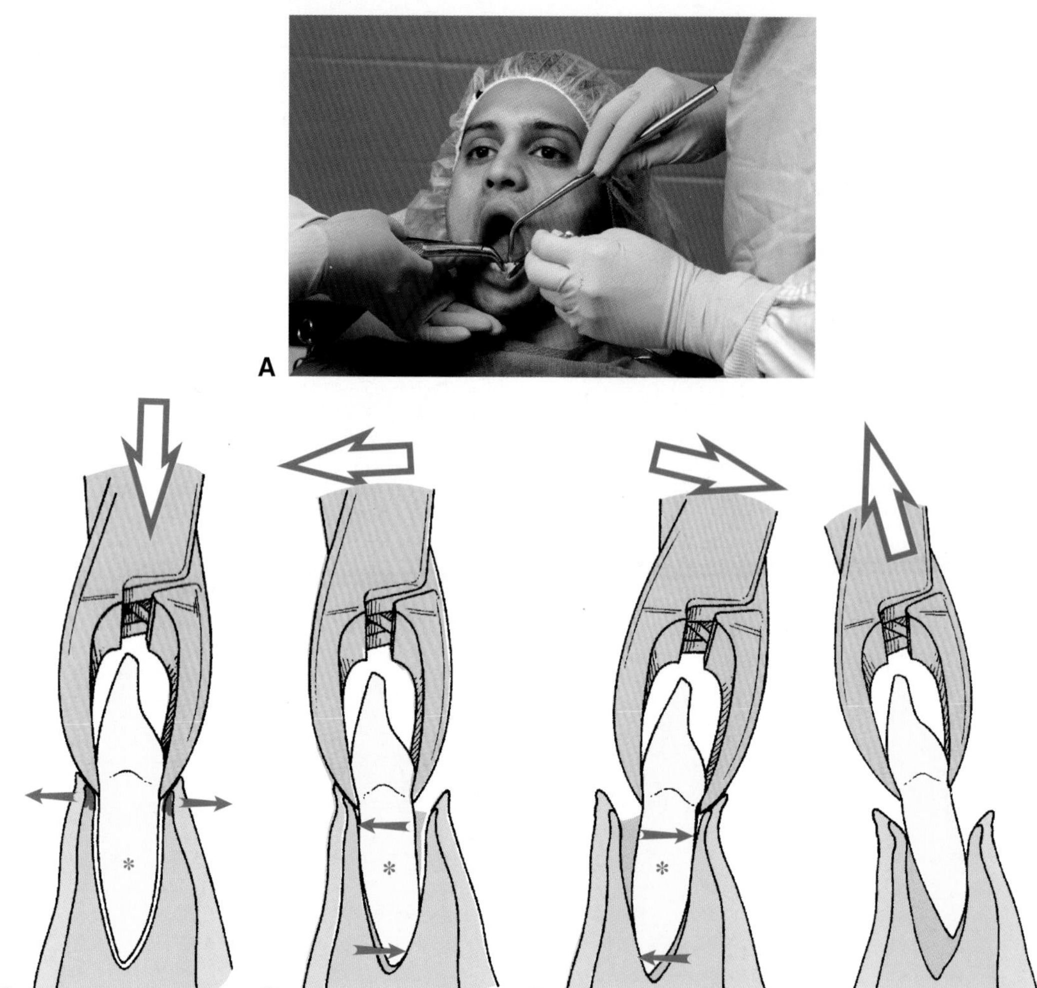

FIGURE 7-64 A, When extracting mandibular anterior teeth, No. 151 forceps are used. Assistant retracts cheek and provides suction. B, Forceps are seated apically as far as possible. C, Moderate labial pressure is used to initiate luxation process. D, Lingual force is used to continue expansion of bone. E, Tooth is delivered in labial-incisal direction.

third, which increases the difficulty of extraction. The roots are generally heavy and strong. The overlying alveolar bone is heavier than the bone on any other teeth in the mouth. The combination of long, strong, divergent roots with heavy overlying buccolingual bone makes the mandibular first molar the most difficult of all teeth to extract.

The No. 17 forceps are usually used for extraction of the mandibular molars; they have small tip projections on both beaks to fit into the bifurcation of the tooth roots. The forceps are adapted to the root of the tooth in the usual fashion, and strong apical pressure is applied to set the beaks of the forceps apically as far as possible. Strong buccolingual motion is then used to expand the tooth socket and allow the tooth to be delivered in the buccoocclusal direction. The linguoalveolar bone around the second molar is thinner than the buccal plate, so the second molar can be removed more easily with stronger lingual than buccal pressures (Fig. 7-67).

If the tooth roots are clearly bifurcated, the No. 23, or cowhorn, forceps can be used. This instrument is designed to be closed forcefully with the handles, thereby squeezing the beaks of the forceps into the bifurcation. This creates force against the crest of the alveolar ridge on the buccolingual aspects and literally forces the tooth superiorly directly out of the tooth socket (Fig. 7-68). If initially this is not successful, the forceps are given buccolingual movements to expand the alveolar bone, and the forceps handles are moved up and down to seat the beaks more fully into the furcation. More squeezing of the handles is performed. Care must be taken with these forceps to prevent damaging the maxillary teeth because the lower molar may actually pop out of the socket and thus release the forceps to strike the upper teeth.

Erupted mandibular third molars usually have fused conic roots. Because a bifurcation is not likely, the No. 222 forceps—a short-beaked, right-angled forceps—are used to extract this tooth. The lingual plate of bone is definitely thinner than the buccocortical plate, so most of the extraction forces should be delivered to the lingual aspect. The third molar is delivered in the linguoocclusal direction. The erupted mandibular third molar that is in function can be a deceptively difficult tooth to extract. The dentist should give serious consideration to using the straight elevator to achieve a moderate degree of luxation before applying the forceps. Pressure should be gradually

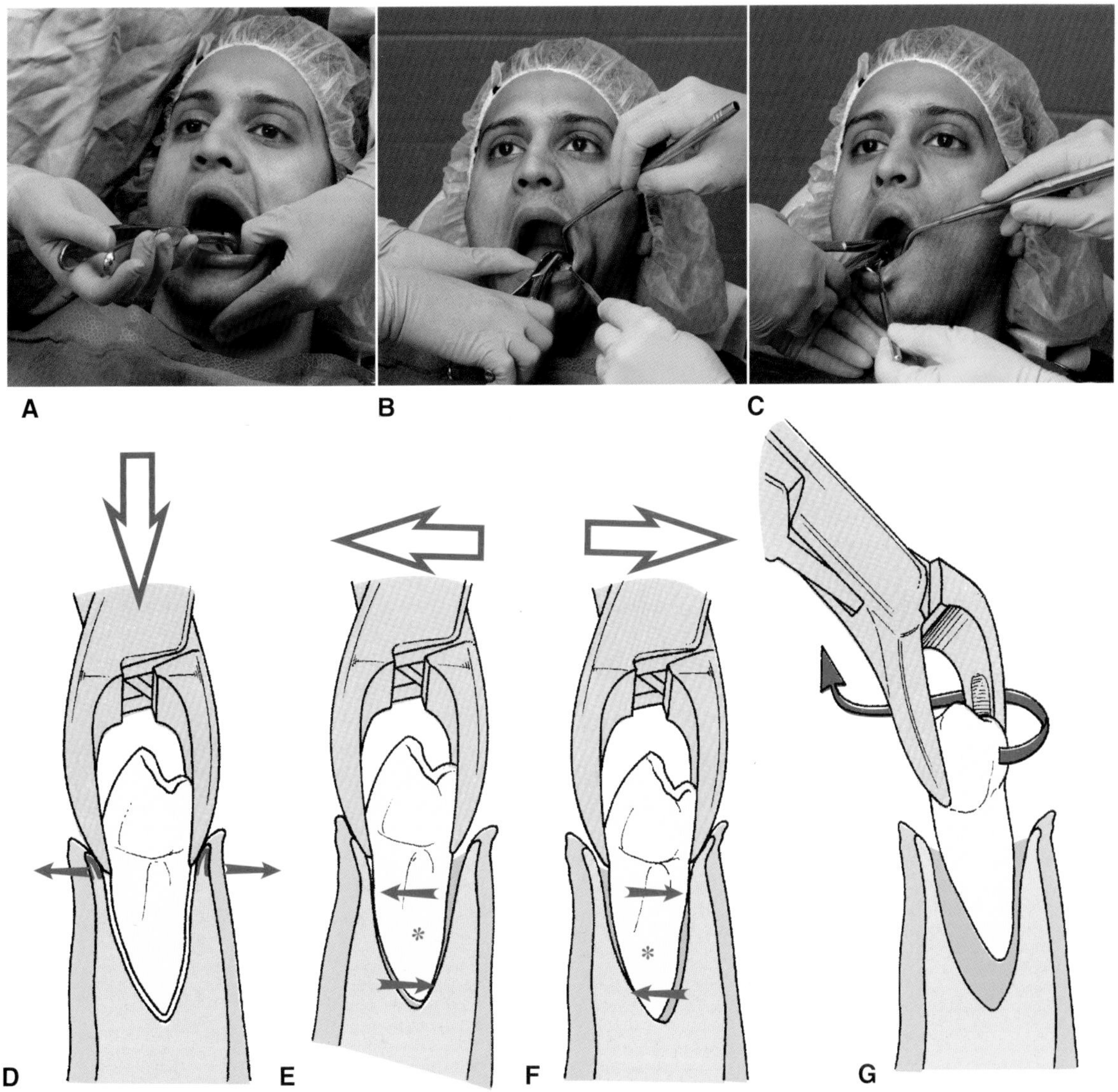

FIGURE 7-65 A, Extraction of mandibular premolar. Mandible is stabilized, soft tissue is reflected, and No. 151 forceps are positioned. B, Hand position is modified slightly for behind-the-patient technique. C, English style of forceps can also be used. D, Forceps are seated apically as far as possible to displace center of rotation and to begin expansion of crestal bone. E, Buccal forceps are applied to begin luxation process. F, Slight lingual pressure is used. G, Tooth is delivered with rotational, tractional force.

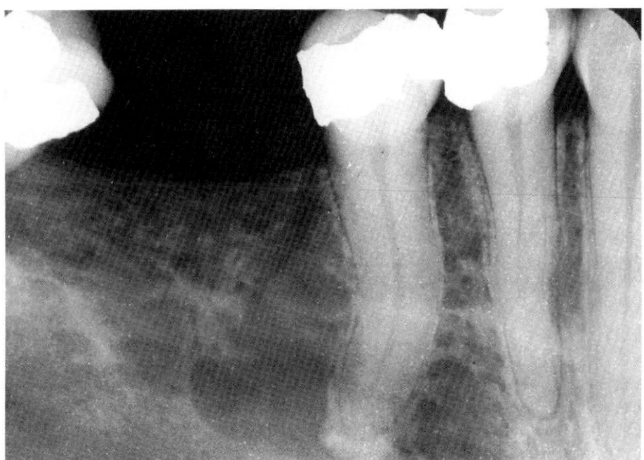

FIGURE 7-66 If curvature of premolar root exists, rotational extraction forces will result in fracture of curved portion of root, and therefore such forces should be minimized.

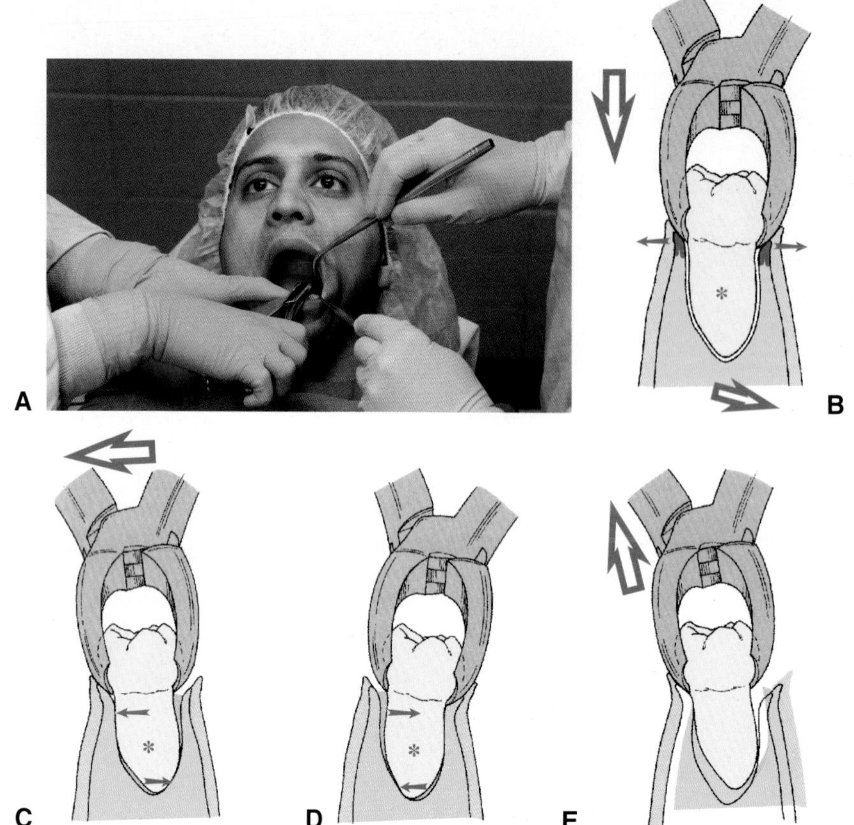

FIGURE 7-67 A, Mandibular molars are extracted with No. 17 or No. 23 forceps. Hand positions of surgeon and assistant are same for both forceps. B, No. 17 forceps are seated as far apically as possible. C, Luxation of molar is begun with strong buccal movement. D, Strong lingual pressure is used to continue luxation. E, Tooth is delivered in buccoocclusal direction.

increased, and attempts to mobilize the tooth should be made before final strong pressures are delivered.

Modifications for Extraction of Primary Teeth

Rarely is it necessary to remove primary teeth before substantial root resorption has occurred. However, when removal is required, it must be done with a great deal of care because the roots of the primary teeth are long and delicate and are subject to fracture. This is especially true because the succedaneous tooth causes resorption of coronal portions of the root structure and thereby weakens it. The forceps usually used are an adaptation of the upper and lower universal forceps, the No. 150S and the No. 151S. They are adapted and forced apically in the usual fashion, with slow, steady pressures toward the buccal aspect and return movements toward the lingual aspect.

Rotational motions may be used but should be minimal and should be used judiciously with multirooted teeth. The dentist should pay careful attention to the direction of least resistance and deliver the tooth into that path. If the roots of the primary molar tooth embrace the crown of the permanent premolar, the surgeon should consider sectioning the tooth. Rarely, the roots hold the crown of the permanent premolar firmly enough in their grasp to cause it to be extracted also.

POSTEXTRACTION TOOTH SOCKET CARE

Once the tooth has been removed, the socket requires proper care. The socket should be débrided only if necessary. If a periapical lesion is visible on the preoperative radiograph and there was no granuloma attached to the tooth when it was removed, the periapical region should be carefully curetted with a periapical curette to remove the granuloma or cyst. If any debris is obvious, such as calculus, amalgam, or tooth fragment remaining in the socket, it should be gently removed with a curette or suction tip (Fig. 7-69). However, if neither a periapical lesion nor debris is present, the socket *should not be curetted.* The remnants of the periodontal ligament and the bleeding bony walls are in the best condition to provide for rapid healing. Vigorous curettage of the socket wall merely produces additional injury and may delay healing.

The expanded buccolingual plates should be compressed back to their original configuration. Finger pressure should be applied to the buccolingual cortical plate to compress the plates gently but firmly to their original position. This helps prevent bony undercuts that may have been caused by excessive expansion of the buccocortical plate, especially after first molar extraction. Care should be taken to not overreduce the socket if implant placement is planned or possible in the future.

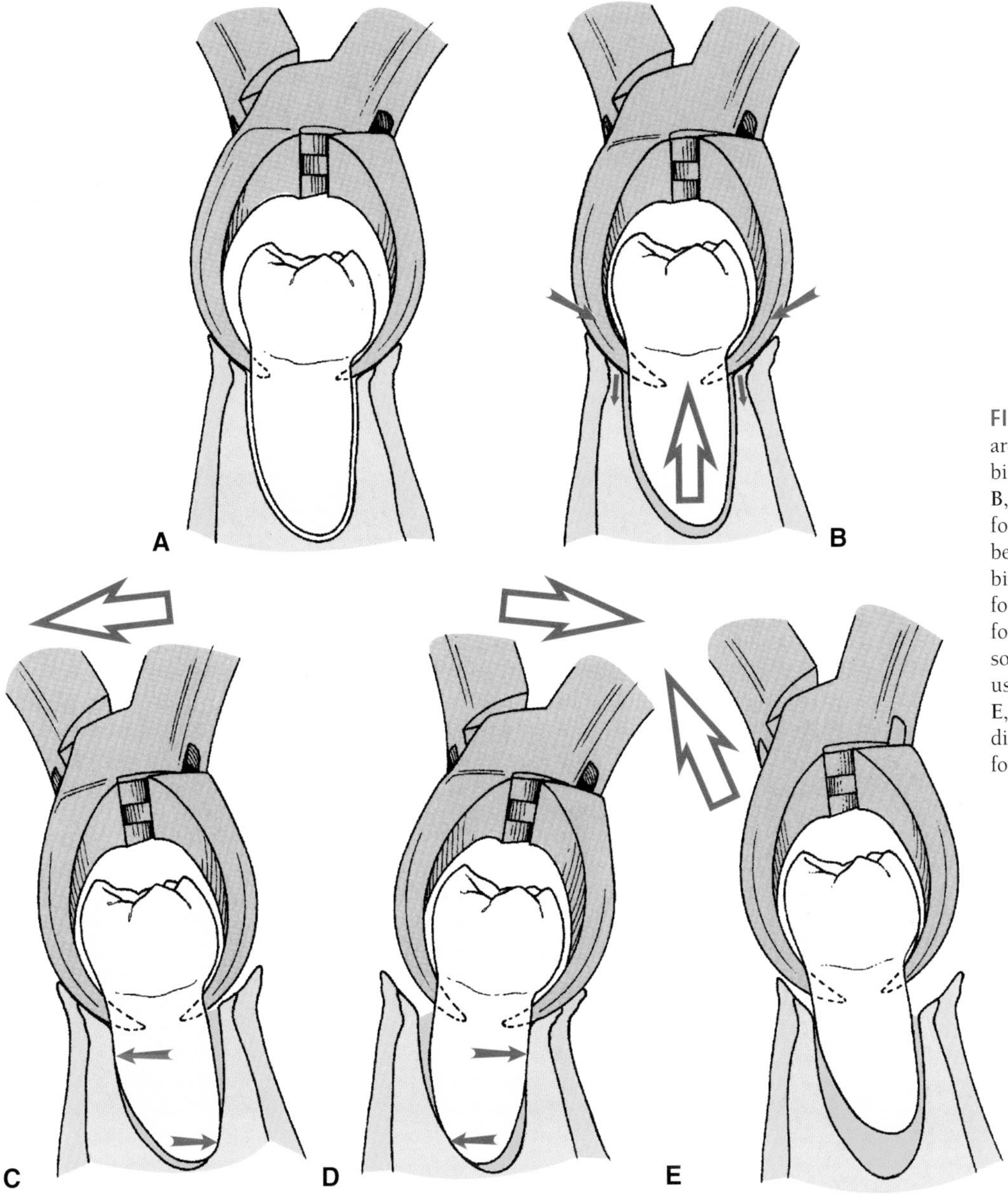

FIGURE 7-68 A, No. 23 forceps are carefully positioned to engage bifurcation area of lower molar. B, Handles of forceps are squeezed forcibly together, which causes beaks of forceps to be forced into bifurcation and exerts tractional forces on tooth. C, Strong buccal forces are then used to expand socket. D, Strong lingual forces are used to luxate tooth further. E, Tooth is delivered in buccoocclusal direction with buccal and tractional forces.

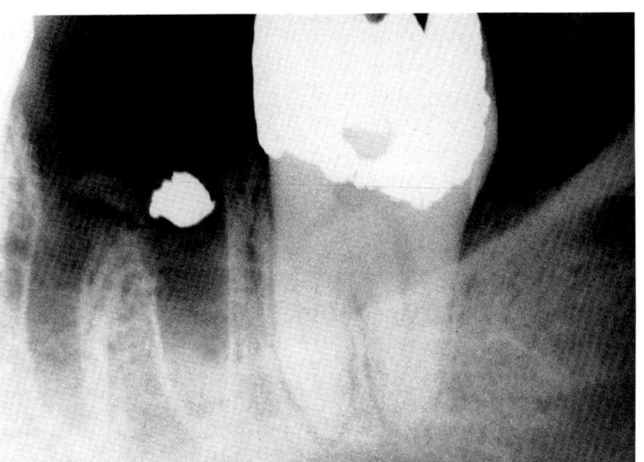

FIGURE 7-69 Amalgam fragment left in this tooth socket after extraction because surgeon failed to inspect and débride surgical field.

If the teeth were removed because of periodontal disease, there may be an accumulation of excess granulation tissue around the gingival cuff. If this is the case, special attention should be given to removing this granulation tissue with a curette, tissue scissors, or hemostat. The arterioles of granulation tissue have little or no capacity to retract and constrict, which leads to bothersome bleeding if excessive granulation tissue is left in place.

Finally, the bone should be palpated through the overlying mucosa to check for any sharp, bony projections. If any exist, the mucosa should be reflected and the sharp edges smoothed judiciously with a bone file or trimmed with a rongeur.

Initial control of hemorrhage is achieved by use of a moistened 2 × 2-inch gauze placed over the extraction socket. The gauze should be positioned so that when the patient closes the teeth together, it fits into the space previously occupied by the crown of the tooth. The pressure of biting the teeth together is placed on the gauze and is transmitted to the socket. This pressure results in hemostasis. If the gauze is simply placed on the occlusal table, the pressure applied to the bleeding socket is insufficient to achieve adequate hemostasis (Fig. 7-70). A larger gauze sponge (4 × 4 inches) may be required if multiple teeth have been extracted or if the opposing arch is edentulous.

The extraction of multiple teeth at one sitting is a more involved and complex procedure and is discussed in Chapter 8.

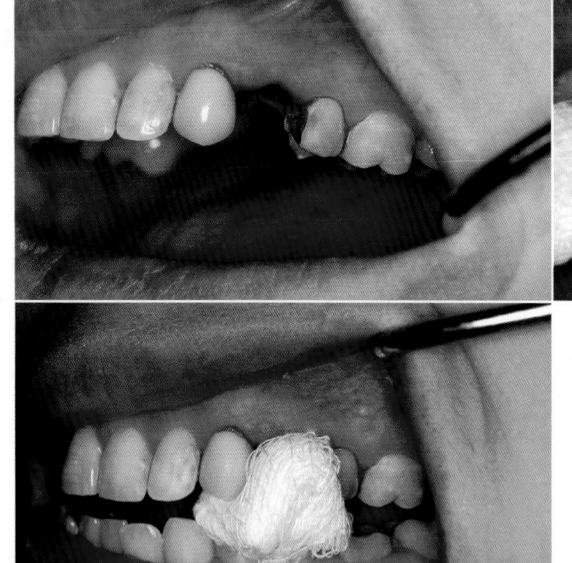

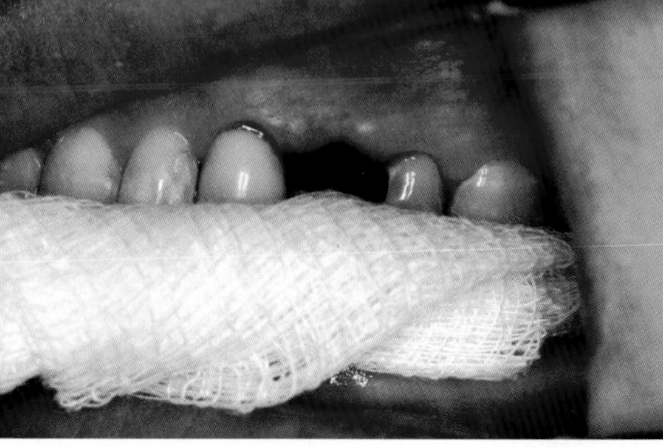

FIGURE 7-70 **A**, After extraction of single tooth, small space exists where crown of tooth was located. **B**, Gauze pad (2 × 2-inch pad) is folded in half twice and placed into space. When patient bites on gauze, pressure is transmitted to gingiva and socket. **C**, If large gauze is used, pressure goes on teeth, not on gingiva or socket.

CHAPTER 8

Principles of More Complex Exodontia

JAMES R. HUPP

CHAPTER OUTLINE

The removal of most erupted teeth can be achieved by closed delivery, but occasionally these techniques do not suffice. The open or surgical extraction technique is the method used for removing roots that were fractured during routine extraction of teeth and cannot be extracted by the routine closed methods for a variety of reasons. In addition, removal of multiple teeth during one surgical session requires more than the routine removal of teeth as described in Chapter 7. Flaps are commonly required for recontouring and smoothing bone.

This chapter discusses techniques for surgical tooth extraction. The principles of flap design, development, management, and suturing are explained, as are the principles of open extraction of single-rooted and multirooted teeth. Also discussed are the principles involved in multiple extractions and concomitant alveoloplasty.

PRINCIPLES OF FLAP DESIGN, DEVELOPMENT, AND MANAGEMENT

The term *flap* used in this chapter indicates a section of soft tissue that (1) is outlined by a surgical incision, (2) carries its own blood supply, (3) allows surgical access to underlying tissues, (4) can be replaced in the original position, and (5) can be maintained with sutures and is expected to heal. Soft tissue flaps are frequently used in oral surgical, periodontal, and endodontic procedures to gain access to underlying tooth and bone structures. To perform a tooth extraction properly, the dental surgeon must have a clear understanding of the principles of design, development, and management of soft tissue flaps.

Design Parameters for Soft Tissue Flaps

To provide adequate exposure and promote proper healing, the flap must be correctly designed. The surgeon must remember that several parameters exist when designing a flap for a specific situation.

When the flap is outlined, the base of the flap must usually be broader than the free margin to preserve an adequate blood supply. This means that all areas of the flap must have a source of uninterrupted vasculature to prevent ischemic necrosis of the entire flap or portions of it (Fig. 8-1).

The flap must be of adequate size for several reasons. Sufficient soft tissue reflection is required to provide necessary visualization of the area. Adequate access also must exist for the insertion of instruments required to perform the surgery. In addition, the flap must be held out of the operative field by a retractor that must rest on intact bone. There must be enough flap reflection to permit the retractor to hold the flap without tension. Furthermore, soft tissue heals across the incision, not along the length of the incision, and sharp incisions heal more rapidly than torn tissue. Therefore a long, straight incision with adequate flap reflection heals more rapidly than a short, torn incision, which heals slowly by secondary intention. For an envelope flap to be of adequate size, the length of the flap in the anteroposterior dimension usually extends two teeth anterior and one tooth posterior to the area of surgery (Fig. 8-2, *A*). If a relaxing incision is to be made, the incision should extend one tooth anterior and one tooth posterior to the area of surgery (Fig. 8-2, *B*).

Flaps for tooth removal should be full-thickness mucoperiosteal flaps. This means that the flap includes the surface mucosa, submucosa, and periosteum. Because the goal of the

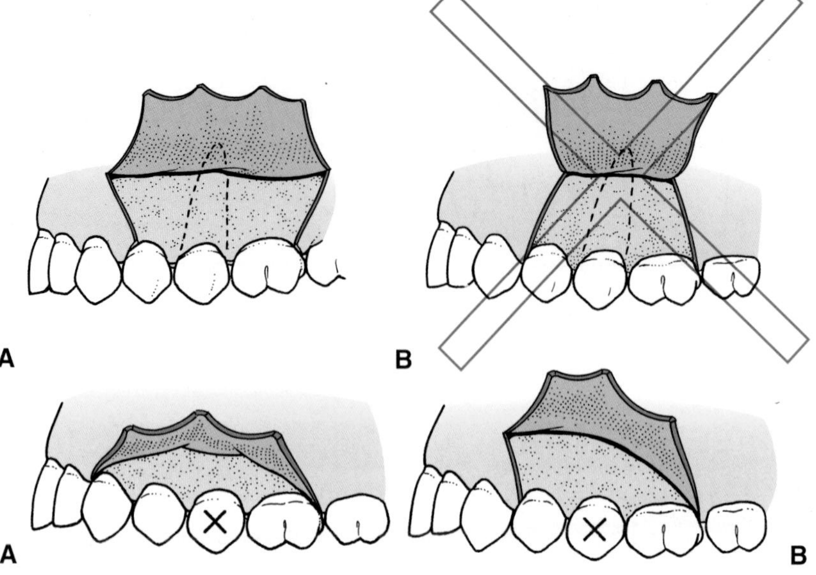

FIGURE 8-1 **A**, Flap must have base that is broader than free gingival margin. **B**, If flap is too narrow at its base, the blood supply may be inadequate, which can lead to flap necrosis.

FIGURE 8-2 **A**, To have sufficient access to root of second premolar, envelope flap should extend anteriorly, mesial to canine, and posteriorly, distal to first molar. **B**, If releasing incision (i.e., three-cornered flap) is used, flap extends mesial to first premolar.

surgery is to remove or reshape the bone, all overlying tissue must be reflected from it. In addition, full-thickness flaps are necessary because the periosteum is the primary tissue responsible for bone healing, and replacement of the periosteum in its original position hastens that healing process. In addition, torn, split, and macerated tissue heals more slowly than a cleanly reflected, full-thickness flap. And the tissue plane between bone and periosteum is relatively avascular, so less bleeding is produced when a full-thickness flap is elevated.

The incisions that outline the flap must be made over intact bone that will be present after the surgical procedure is complete. If the pathologic condition has eroded the buccocortical plate, the incision must be at least 6 or 8 mm away from it. In addition, if bone is to be removed over a particular tooth, the incision must be sufficiently distant from it so that after the bone is removed, the incision is 6 to 8 mm away from the bony defect created by surgery. If the incision line is unsupported by sound bone, it tends to collapse into the bony defect, which results in wound dehiscence and delayed healing (Fig. 8-3).

The flap should be designed to avoid injury to local vital structures in the area of the surgery. The two most important structures that can be damaged are located in the mandible; these are the lingual nerve and the mental nerve. When making incisions in the posterior mandible, especially in the region of the third molar, incisions should be well away from the lingual aspect of the mandible. In this area the lingual nerve may closely adhere to the lingual aspect of the mandible, and incisions in this area may result in damaging or even severing that nerve, with consequent prolonged temporary or permanent anesthesia of the tongue. In the same way, surgery in the apical area of the mandibular premolar teeth should be carefully planned and executed to avoid injury to the mental nerve. Envelope incisions should be used if at all possible, and releasing incisions should be well anterior or posterior to the area of the exit of the mental nerve from the mandible.

Flaps in the maxilla rarely endanger any vital structures. On the facial aspect of the maxillary alveolar process, no nerves or arteries exist that are likely to be damaged. When reflecting a palatal flap, the surgeon must remember that the major blood supply to the palatal soft tissue comes through the greater palatine artery, which emerges from the greater palatine foramen at the posterior lateral aspect of the hard palate. This artery courses forward and has an anastomosis with the nasopalatine artery. The nasopalatine nerves and arteries exit the incisive foramen to supply the anterior palatal gingiva. If the anterior palatal tissue must be reflected, the artery and the nerve can be incised at the level of the foramen without much risk. The likelihood of bothersome bleeding is small, and the nerve regenerates quickly. The temporary numbness usually does not bother the patient. However, vertical-releasing incisions in the posterior aspect of the palate should be avoided because they usually sever the greater palatine artery within the tissue, which results in bleeding that may be difficult to control.

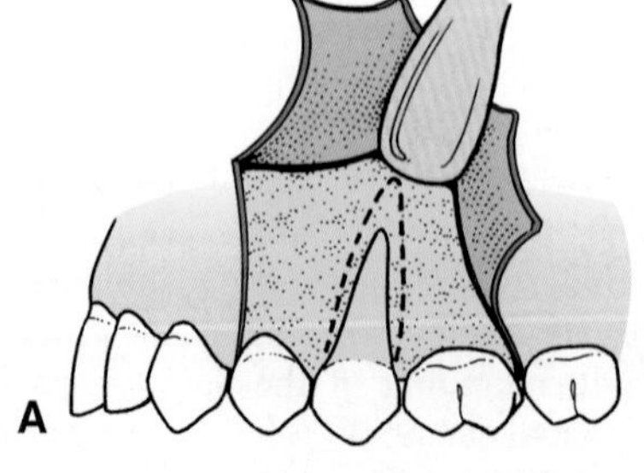

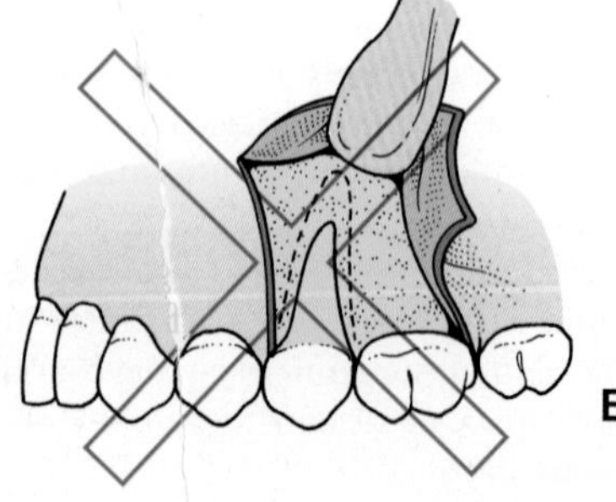

FIGURE 8-3 **A**, When designing flap, it is necessary to anticipate how much bone will be removed so that after surgery is complete, the incision rests over sound bone. In this situation, the vertical release was one tooth anterior to bone removal and left an adequate margin of sound bone. **B**, When releasing incision is made too close to bone removal, delayed healing results.

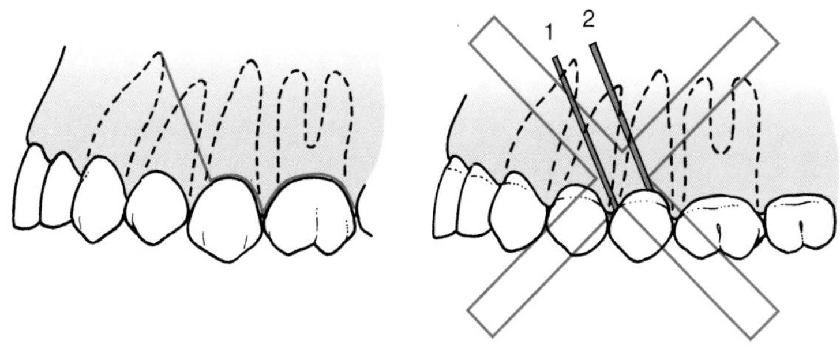

FIGURE 8-4 A, Correct position for end of vertical-releasing incision is at line angle (mesiobuccal angle in this figure) of tooth. Likewise, incision does not cross canine eminence. Crossing such bony prominences results in increased chance for wound dehiscence. B, These two incisions are made incorrectly: *(1)* incision crosses prominence over canine tooth, which increases risk of delayed healing; incision through papilla results in unnecessary damage; *(2)* incision crosses attached gingiva directly over facial aspect of tooth, which is likely to result in soft tissue defect and periodontal and aesthetic deformities.

Releasing incisions are used only when necessary and not routinely. Envelope incisions usually provide the adequate visualization required for tooth extraction in most areas. When vertical-releasing incisions are necessary, only a single vertical incision is used, which is usually at the anterior end of the envelope component. The vertical-releasing incision is not a straight vertical incision but is oblique, to allow the base of the flap to be broader than the free gingival margin. A vertical-releasing incision is made so that it does not cross bony prominences, such as the canine eminence; to do so would increase the likelihood of tension in the suture line, which would result in wound dehiscence.

Vertical-releasing incisions should cross the free gingival margin at the line angle of a tooth and should not be directly on the facial aspect of the tooth nor directly in the papilla (Fig. 8-4). Incisions that cross the free margin of the gingiva directly over the facial aspect of the tooth do not heal properly because of tension; the result is a defect in the attached gingiva. Because the facial bone is frequently thin, such incisions also result in vertical clefting of the bone. Incisions that cross the gingival papilla damage the papilla unnecessarily and increase the chances for localized periodontal problems; such incisions should be avoided.

Types of Mucoperiosteal Flaps

A variety of intraoral tissue flaps can be used. The most common incision is the sulcular incision which, when not combined with a releasing incision, produces the envelope flap. In the dentulous patient the incision is made in the gingival sulcus to the crestal bone, through the periosteum, and the full-thickness mucoperiosteal flap is reflected apically (Fig. 8-2, *A*). This flap usually provides sufficient access to perform the necessary surgery.

If the patient is edentulous, the envelope incision is usually made along the scar at the crest of the ridge. No vital structures are found in this area, and the envelope incision can be as long as is required to provide adequate access. The only exception occurs in extremely atrophic mandibles where the inferior alveolar nerve may rest on top of the residual alveolar ridge. Once the incision is made tissue can be reflected buccally or lingually as necessary for recontouring of the ridge or the removal of a mandibular torus.

If the sulcular incision has a vertical-releasing incision, it is a three-cornered flap, with corners at the posterior end of the envelope incision, at the inferior aspect of the vertical incision, and at the superior aspect of the vertical-releasing incision (Fig. 8-5). This incision provides for greater access with a shorter sulcular incision. When greater access is necessary in an apical direction, especially in the posterior aspect of the mouth, this incision is frequently necessary. The vertical component is more difficult to close and may cause some mildly prolonged healing, but if care is taken when suturing, the healing period is not noticeably lengthened.

The four-cornered flap is an envelope incision with two releasing incisions. Two corners are at the superior aspect of the releasing incision, and two corners are at either end of the envelope component of the incision (Fig. 8-6). Although this flap provides substantial access in areas that have limited anteroposterior dimension, it is rarely indicated. When releasing incisions are necessary, a three-cornered flap usually suffices.

An incision that is used occasionally to approach the root apex is a semilunar incision (Fig. 8-7). This incision avoids trauma to the papillae and gingival margin but provides limited access because the entire root of the tooth is not visible. This incision is most useful for periapical surgery of a limited extent.

An incision useful on the palate is the Y incision, which is named for its shape. This incision is useful for surgical access to the bony palate for removal of a palatal torus. The tissue overlying a torus is usually thin and must be carefully reflected. The anterolateral extensions of the midline incision are anterior to the region of the canine tooth. The extensions are anterior enough in this position that they do not sever

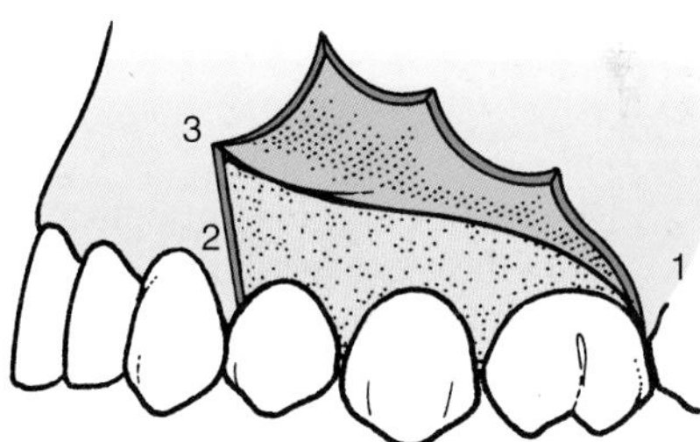

FIGURE 8-5 Vertical-releasing incision converts envelope incision into three-cornered flap (corners numbered).

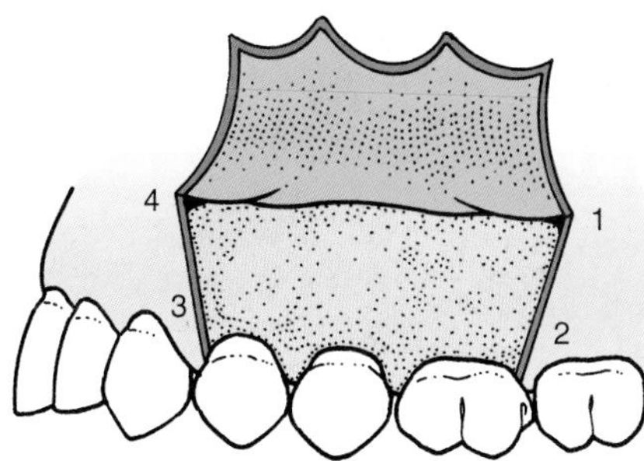

FIGURE 8-6 Vertical-releasing incisions at other end of envelope incision converts envelope incision into four-cornered flap (corners numbered).

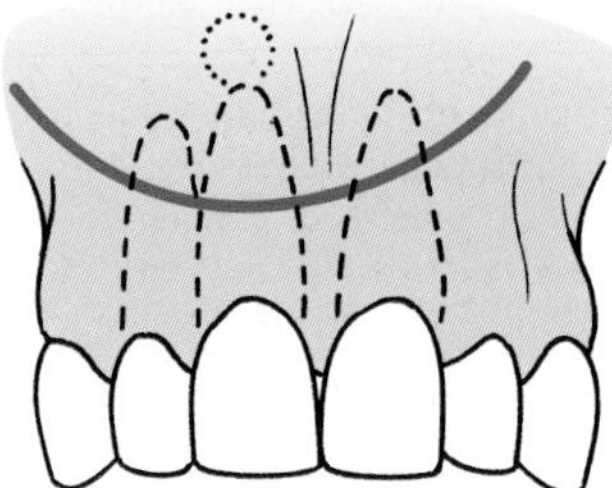

FIGURE 8-7 Semilunar incision, designed to avoid marginal attached gingiva when working on a root apex. Incision is most useful when only a limited amount of access is necessary.

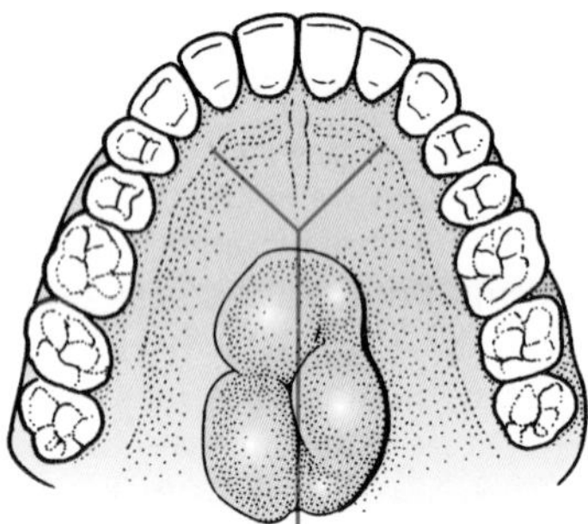

FIGURE 8-8 Y incision is useful on palate for adequate access to remove a palatal torus. Two anterior limbs serve as releasing incisions to provide for greater access.

major branches of the greater palatine artery; therefore, bleeding is not usually a problem (Fig. 8-8).

Developing a Mucoperiosteal Flap

Several specific considerations are involved in developing flaps for surgical tooth extraction. The first step is to incise the soft tissue to allow reflection of the flap. The No. 15 blade is used on a No. 3 scalpel handle, and it is held in the pen grasp (Fig. 8-9). The blade is held at a slight angle to the teeth, and the incision is made posteriorly to anteriorly in the gingival sulcus by drawing the knife toward the operator. One smooth continuous stroke is used while keeping the knife blade in contact with bone throughout the entire incision (Figs. 8-10 and 8-11).

The scalpel blade is an extremely sharp instrument, but it dulls rapidly when it is pressed against bone, such as when making a mucoperiosteal incision. If more than one flap is to be reflected, the surgeon should change blades between incisions.

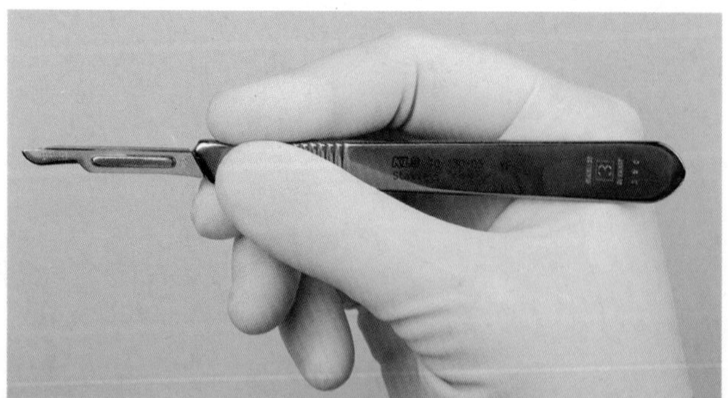

FIGURE 8-9 Scalpel handle is held in pen grasp for maximal control and tactile sensitivity.

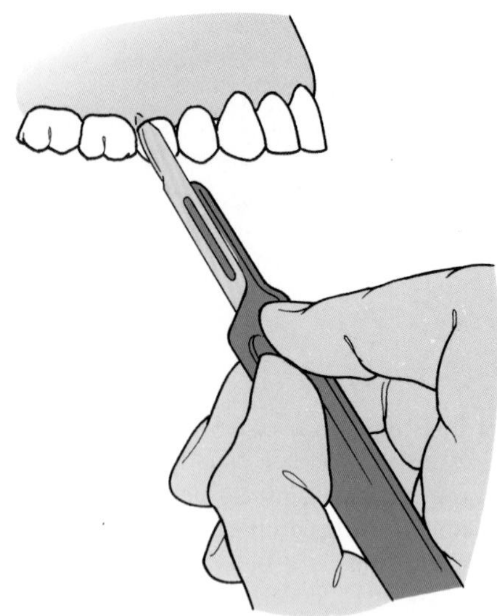

FIGURE 8-10 No. 15 blade is used to incise gingival sulcus.

If a vertical-releasing incision is made, the tissue is apically reflected, with the opposite hand tensing the alveolar mucosa so that the incision can be made cleanly through it. If the alveolar mucosa is not tensed, the knife will not incise cleanly through the mucosa, and a jagged incision will result.

Reflection of the flap begins at a papilla. The sharp end of the No. 9 periosteal elevator begins a reflection (Fig. 8-12). The sharp end is slipped underneath the papilla in the area of the incision and is turned laterally to pry the papilla away from the underlying bone. This technique is used along the entire extent of the free gingival incision. If it is difficult to elevate the tissue at any one spot, the incision is probably incomplete, and that area should be reincised. Once the entire free edge of the flap has been reflected with the sharp end of the elevator, the broad end is used to reflect the mucoperiosteal flap to the extent desired.

If a three-cornered flap is used, the initial reflection is accomplished with the sharp end of the No. 9 elevator on the first papilla only. Once the flap reflection is started, the broad end of the periosteal elevator is inserted at the middle corner of the flap, and the dissection is carried out with a pushing stroke, posteriorly and apically. This facilitates the rapid and atraumatic reflection of the soft tissue flap (Fig. 8-13).

Once the flap has been reflected the desired amount, the periosteal elevator can be used as a retractor to hold the flap in its proper reflected position. To accomplish this effectively, the retractor is held perpendicular to the bone tissue while resting on sound bone and not trapping soft tissue between the retractor and bone. The periosteal elevator therefore is maintained in its proper position, and the soft tissue flap is held without tension (Fig. 8-14). The Seldin elevator or the Minnesota or Austin retractors can be used similarly when broader exposure is necessary. The retractor should not be forced against the soft tissue in an attempt to pull the tissue out of the field. Instead, the retractor is positioned in the proper place and held firmly against the bone. By retracting in this fashion, the surgeon primarily focuses on the surgical field rather than on the retractor; thereby the chance of inadvertently tearing the flap is lessened.

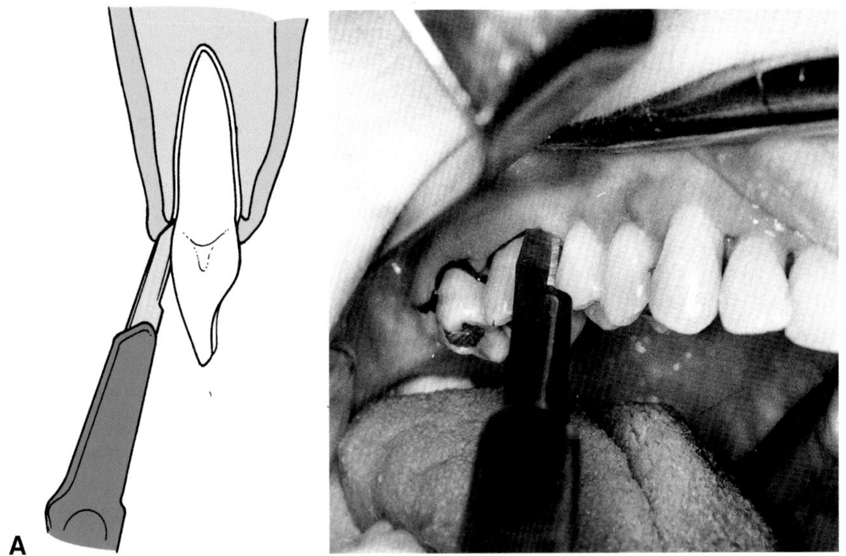

FIGURE 8-11 A, Knife is angled slightly away from tooth and incises soft tissue, including periosteum, at crestal bone. B, Incision is started posteriorly and is carried anteriorly, with care taken to incise completely through interdental papilla.

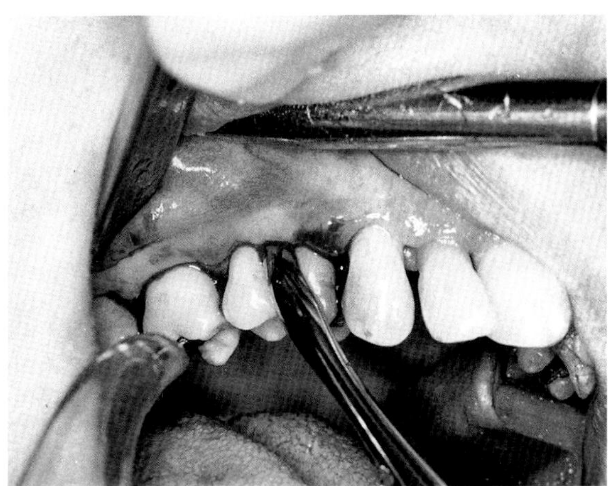

FIGURE 8-12 Reflection of flap is begun by using sharp end of periosteal elevator to pry away interdental papilla.

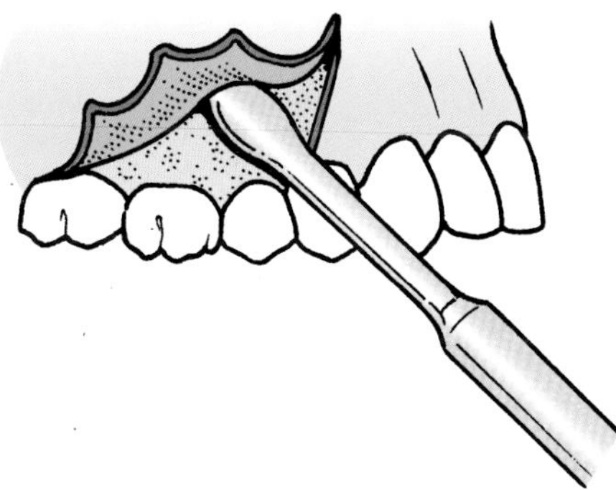

FIGURE 8-13 When three-cornered flap is used, only anterior papilla is reflected with sharp end of elevator. Broad end is then used with push stroke to elevate posterosuperiorly.

Principles of Suturing

Once the surgical procedure is completed and the wound is properly irrigated and débrided, the surgeon must return the flap to its original position or, if necessary, arrange it in a new position; the flap should be held in place with sutures. Sutures perform multiple functions. The most obvious and important function that sutures perform is to coapt wound margins; that is, to hold the flap in position and approximate the two wound edges. The sharper the incision and the less trauma inflicted on the wound margin, the more probable is healing by primary intention. If the space between the two wound edges is minimal, wound healing will be rapid and complete. If tears or excessive

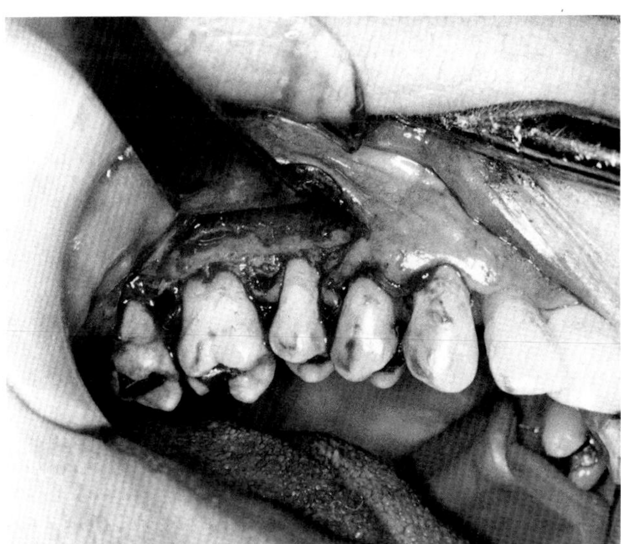

FIGURE 8-14 Periosteal elevator (Seldin elevator) is used to reflect mucoperiosteal flap. Elevator placed perpendicular to bone and held in place by pushing firmly against bone, not by pushing it apically against soft tissue.

trauma to the wound edges occur, wound healing will be by secondary intention.

Sutures also aid in hemostasis. If the underlying tissue is bleeding, the surface mucosa or skin should not be closed, because the bleeding in the underlying tissues may continue and result in the formation of a hematoma. Surface sutures aid in hemostasis but only as a tamponade in a generally oozing area, such as a tooth socket. Overlying tissue should never be sutured tightly in an attempt to gain hemostasis in a bleeding tooth socket.

Sutures help hold a soft tissue flap over bone. This is an important function because bone that is not covered with soft tissue becomes nonvital and requires an excessively long time to heal. When mucoperiosteal flaps are reflected from alveolar bone, it is important that the extent of the bone be recovered with the soft tissue flaps. Unless appropriate suture techniques are used, the flap may retract away from the bone, which exposes it and results in delayed healing.

Sutures may aid in maintaining a blood clot in the alveolar socket. A special suture, such as a figure-of-eight suture, can provide a barrier to clot displacement (Fig. 8-15). However, it should be emphasized that suturing across an open wound socket plays a minor role in maintaining the blood clot in the tooth socket.

The armamentarium includes a needle holder, a suture needle, and suture material. The needle holder of choice is 15 cm (about 6 inches) in length and has a locking handle. The needle holder is held with the thumb and ring finger through the rings and with the index finger along the length of the needle holder to provide stability and control (Fig. 8-16).

The suture needle usually used in the mouth is a small three-eighths to one-half circle with a reverse cutting edge. The cutting edge helps the needle pass through the tough mucoperiosteal flap tissue. Needle sizes and shapes have been assigned numbers. The most common needle shapes used for oral surgery are the three-eighths and half-circle cutting needles (Fig. 8-17).

The technique used for suturing is deceptively difficult. The use of the needle holder and the technique that is necessary to pass the curved needle through the tissue are difficult to learn. The following discussion presents the technique used in suturing; practice is necessary before suturing can be performed with skill and finesse.

When the envelope flap is repositioned into its correct location, it is held in place with sutures that are placed through the papillae only. Sutures are not placed across the empty tooth socket because the edges of the wound would not be supported over sound bone (Fig. 8-18). When reapproximating the flap, the suture is passed first through the mobile (usually facial) tissue; the needle is regrasped with the needle holder and is passed through the attached tissue of the lingual papilla. If the two margins of the wound are close together, the experienced surgeon may be able to insert the needle through both sides of the wound in a single pass. However, for better precision it is best to use two passes in most situations (Fig. 8-19).

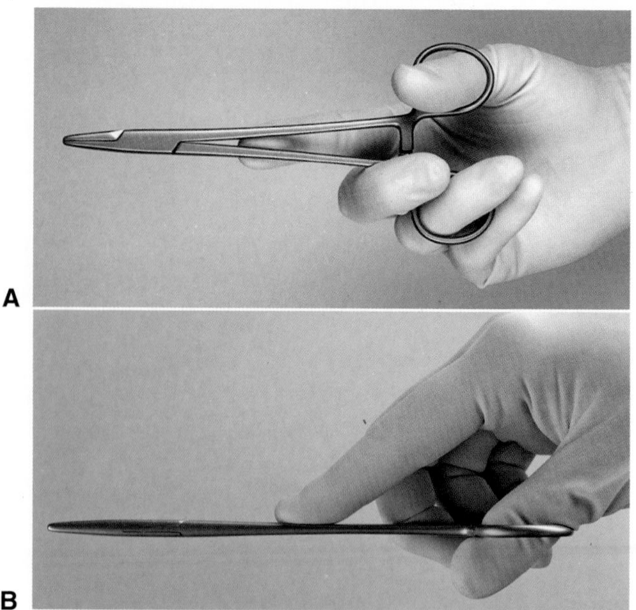

FIGURE 8-16 Needle holder is held with thumb and ring finger (A). Index finger extends along instrument for stability and control (B).

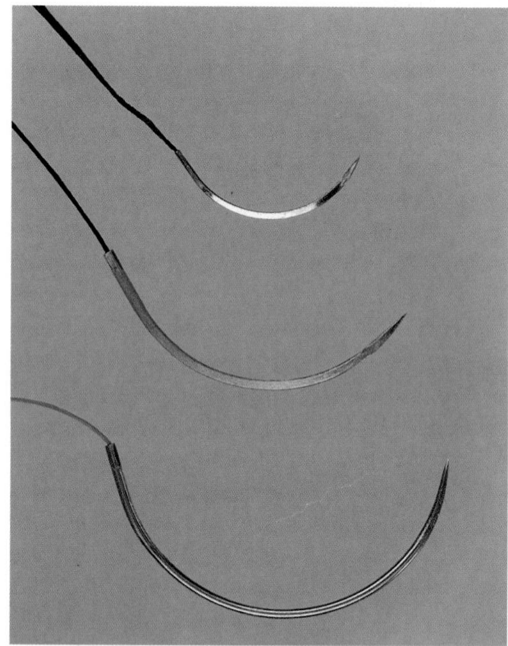

FIGURE 8-17 The shapes and types of needles most commonly used in oral surgery are the three-eighths-circle and half-circle cutting needles shown here. Top is PS-2, middle is FS-2, and lower is X-1.

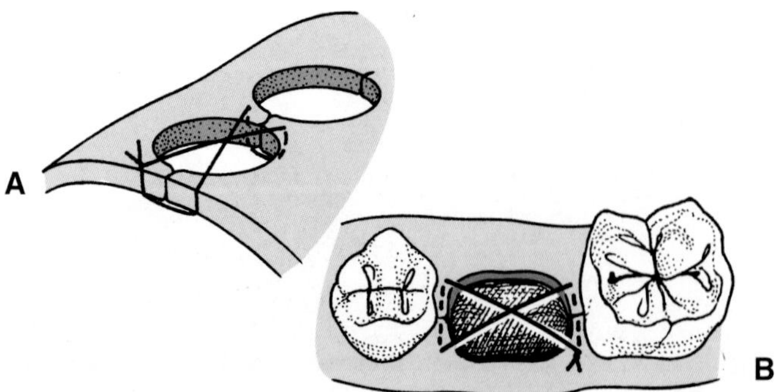

FIGURE 8-15 A, Figure-of-eight suture, occasionally placed over top of socket to aid in hemostasis. B, This suture is usually performed to help maintain piece of oxidized cellulose in tooth socket.

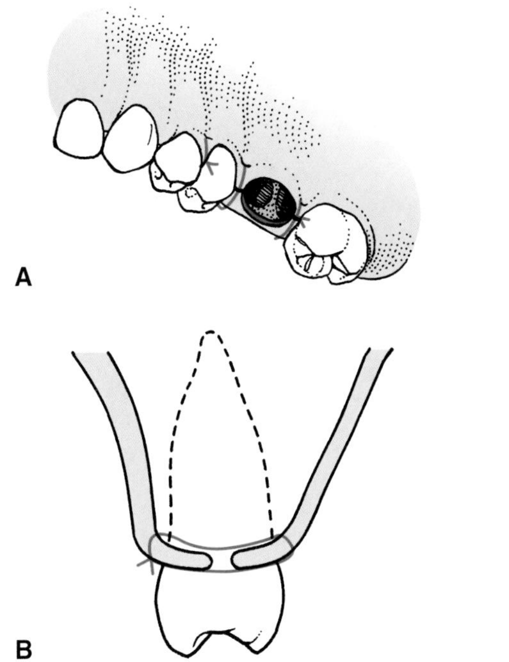

FIGURE 8-18 A, Flap held in place with sutures in papillae. B, Cross-sectional view of suture.

When passing the needle through the tissue, the needle should enter the surface of the mucosa at a right angle, to make the smallest possible hole in the mucosal flap (Fig. 8-20). If the needle passes through the tissue obliquely, the suture will tear through the surface layers of the flap when the suture knot is tied, which results in greater injury to the soft tissue.

When passing the needle through the flap, the surgeon must ensure that an adequate amount of tissue is taken, to prevent the needle or suture from pulling through the soft tissue flap. Because the flap that is being sutured is a mucoperiosteal flap and should not be tied tightly, a small amount of tissue is necessary. The minimal amount of tissue between the suture and the edge of the flap should be 3 mm. Once the sutures are passed through the mobile flap and the immobile lingual tissue, they are tied with an instrument tie (Fig. 8-21).

The surgeon must remember that the purpose of the suture is merely to reapproximate the tissue, and therefore the suture should not be tied too tightly. Sutures that are too tight cause ischemia of the flap margin and result in tissue necrosis, with eventual tearing of the suture through the tissue. Thus sutures that are too tightly tied result in wound dehiscence more frequently than sutures that are loosely tied. As a clinical guideline, there should be no blanching or obvious ischemia of the wound edges. If this occurs the suture should be removed and replaced. The knot should be positioned so that it does not fall directly over the incision line, because this causes

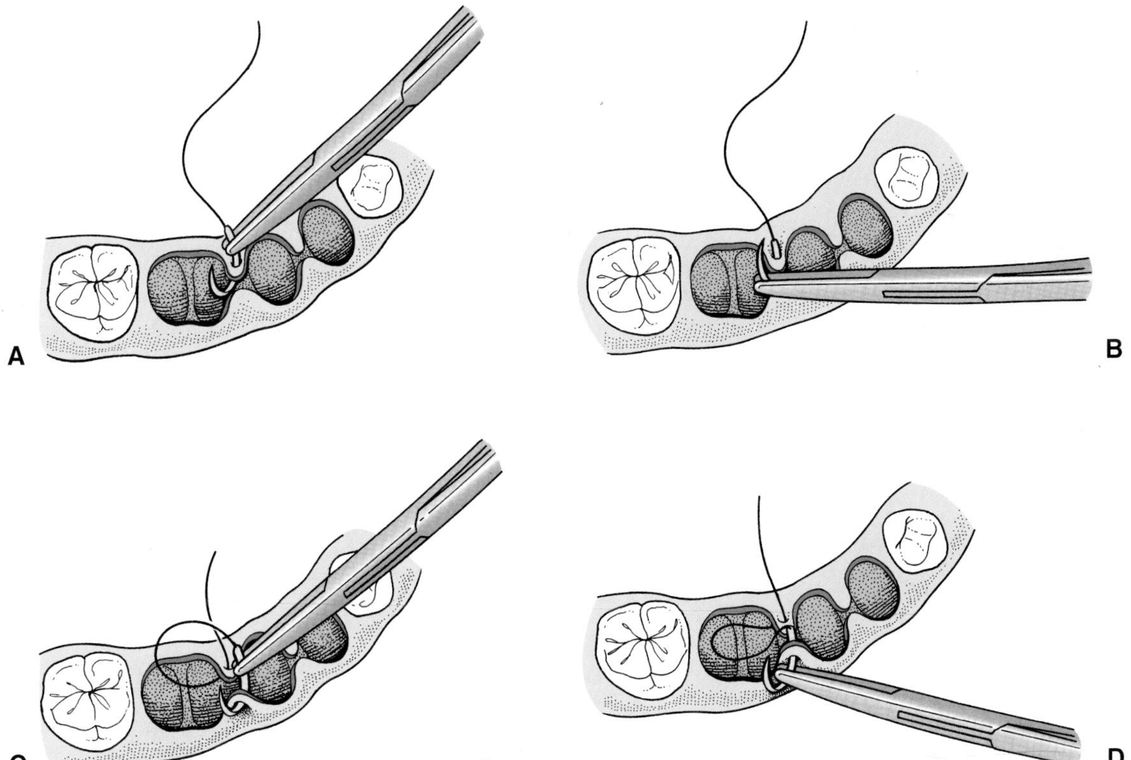

FIGURE 8-19 When mucosal flap is back in position, suture is passed through two sides of socket in separate passes of needle. A, Needle is held by needle holder and passed through papilla, usually of mobile tissue first. B, Needle holder is then released from needle; it regrasps needle on underside of tissue and is turned through flap. C, Needle is then passed through opposite side of soft tissue papilla in similar fashion. D, Finally, needle holder grasps needle on opposite side to complete passing of suture through both sides of mucosa.

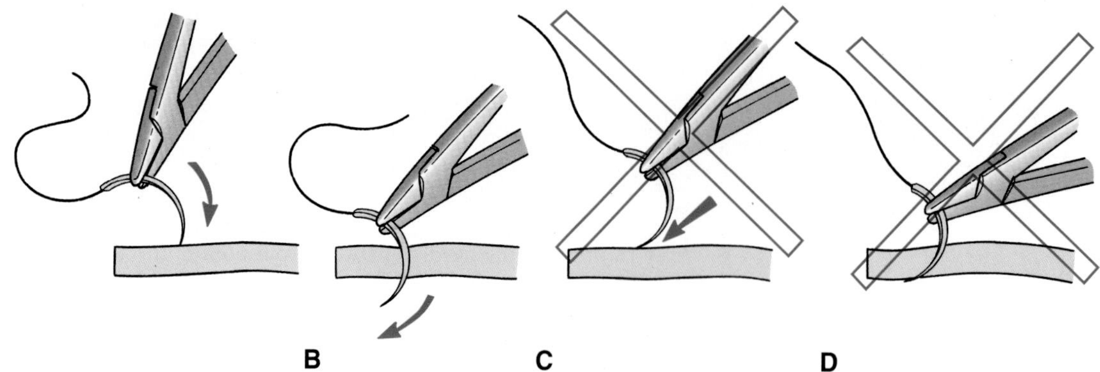

FIGURE 8-20 A, When passing through soft tissue of mucosa, needle should enter surface of tissue at right angle. B, Needle holder should be turned so that needle passes easily through tissue at right angles. C, If needle enters soft tissue at acute angle and is pushed (rather than turned) through tissue, tearing of mucosa with needle or with suture is likely to occur (D).

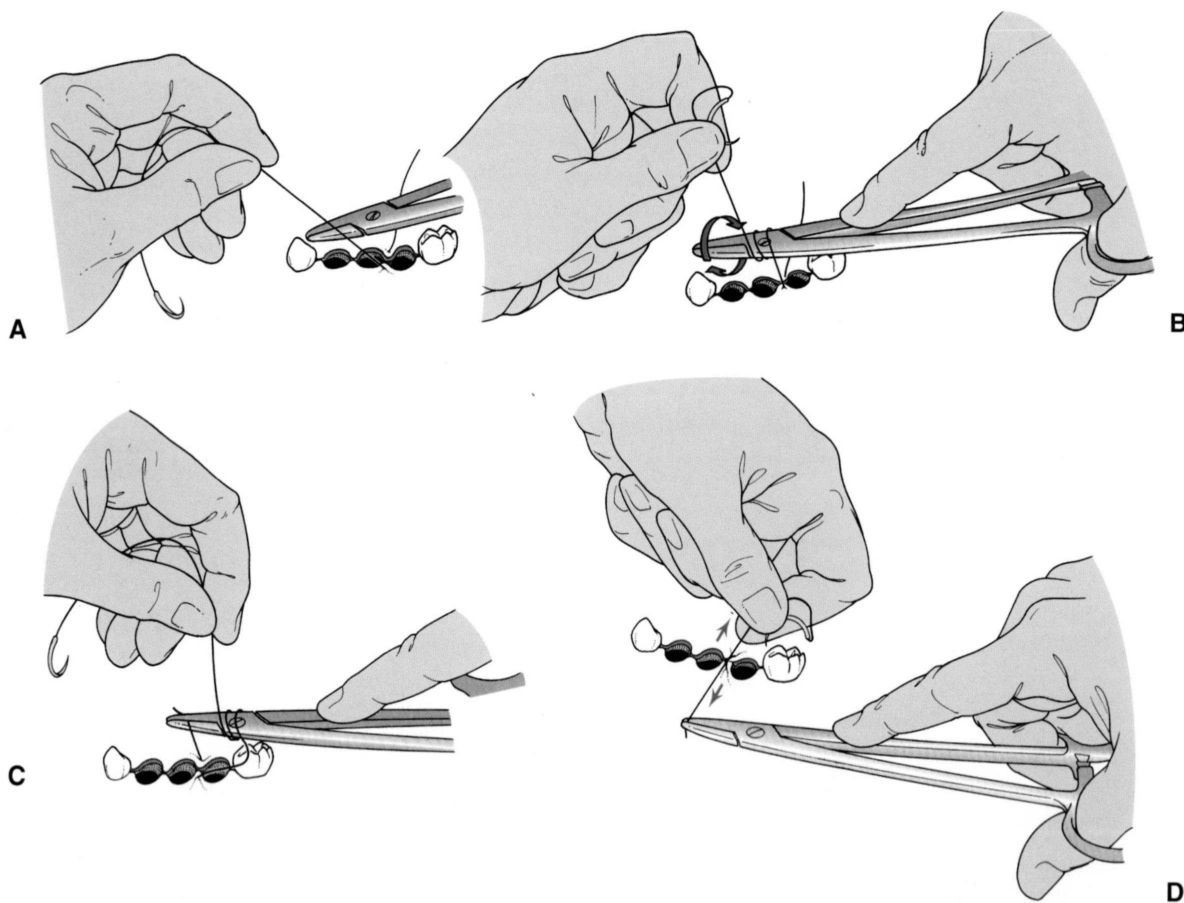

FIGURE 8-21 Most intraoral sutures are tied with an instrument tie. A, Suture is pulled through tissue until short tail of suture (approximately 15 to 20 mm long) remains. Needle holder is held horizontally by right hand in preparation for knot-tying procedure. B, Left hand then wraps long end of suture around needle holder twice in clockwise direction to make two loops of suture around needle holder. C, Surgeon then opens needle holder and grasps short end of suture near its end. D, Ends of suture are then pulled to tighten knot. Needle holder should not pull suture at all until knot is nearly tied, to avoid lengthening that portion of suture.

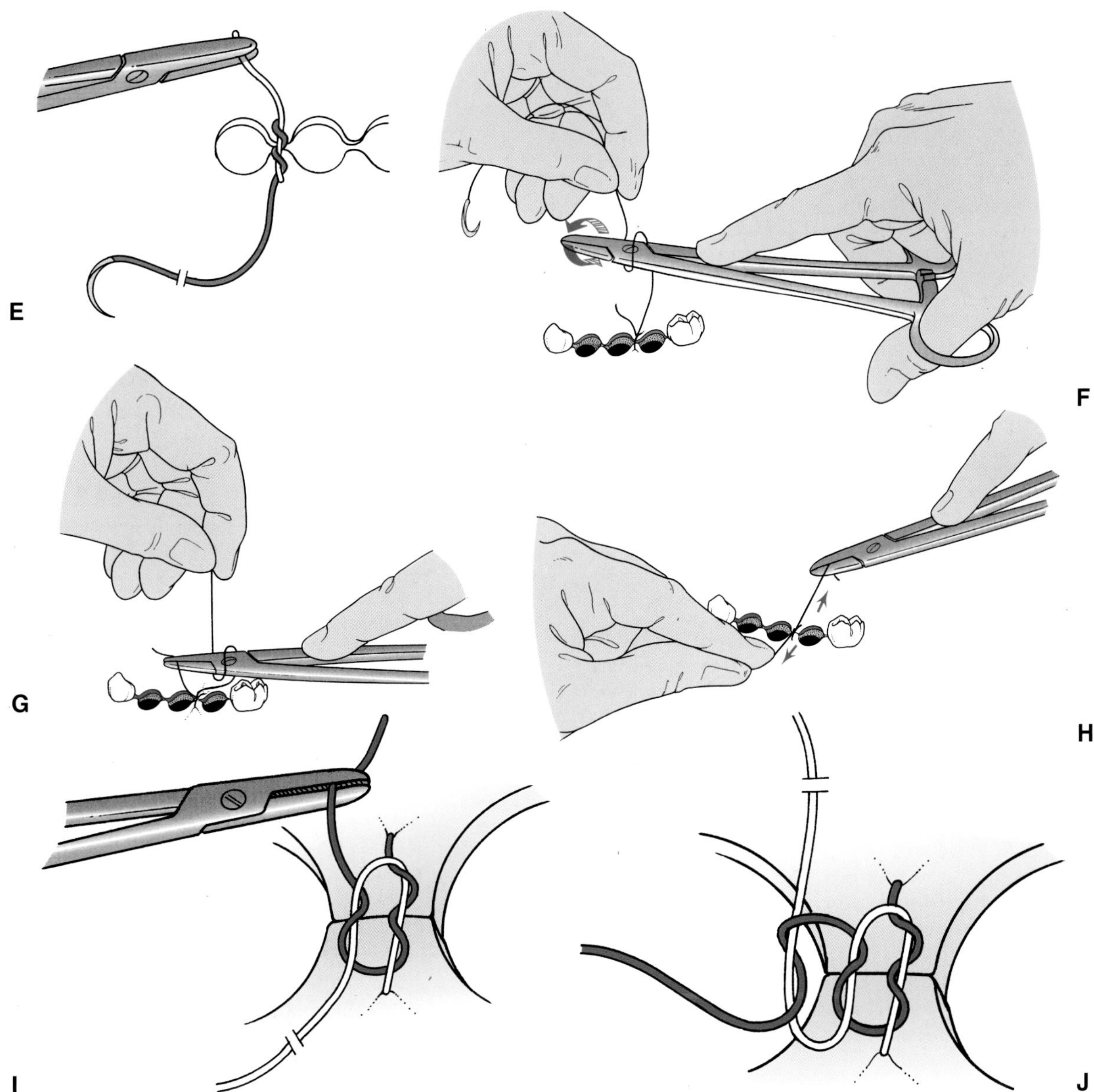

FIGURE 8-21, cont'd Most intraoral sutures are tied with an instrument tie. E, End of first step of surgeon's knot. The double wrap has resulted in double overhand knot. This increases friction in knot and will keep wound edges together until second portion of knot is tied. F, Needle holder is then released from short end of suture and held in same position as when knot-tying procedure began. Left hand then makes single wrap in counterclockwise direction. G, Needle holder then grasps short end of suture at its end. H, This portion of knot is completed by pulling this loop firmly down against previous portion of knot. I, This completes surgeon's knot. Double loop of first pass holds tissue together until second portion of square knot can be tied. J, Most surgeons add third throw to their instrument tie when using a resorbable material. Needle holder is repositioned in original position, and one wrap is placed around needle holder in original clockwise direction. Short end of suture is grasped and tightened down firmly to form second square knot. Final throw of three knots is tightened firmly. (Note: for demonstration purposes, first knot left loose here, but in actual knot tying, first knot is tightened before creating second knot.)

additional pressure on the incision. Therefore the knot should be positioned to the side of the incision.

If a three-cornered flap is used, the vertical end of the incision must be closed separately. Two sutures usually are required to close the vertical end properly. Before the sutures are inserted, the No. 9 periosteal elevator should be used to slightly elevate the nonflap side of the incision, freeing the margin to facilitate passage of the needle through the tissue (Fig. 8-22). The first suture is placed across the papilla, where the vertical release incision was made. This is a known, easily identifiable landmark that is most important when repositioning a three-cornered flap. The remainder of the envelope portion of the

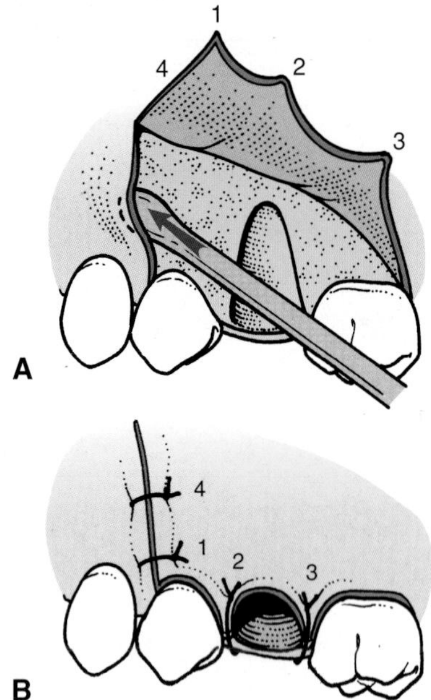

FIGURE 8-22 A, To make the suturing of three-cornered flap easier, periosteal elevator is used to elevate small amount of fixed tissue so that suture can be passed through entire thickness of mucoperiosteum. B, When three-cornered flap is repositioned, first suture is placed at occlusal end of vertical-releasing incision (1). Papillae are then sutured sequentially (2, 3), and finally, if necessary, superior aspect of releasing incision is sutured (4).

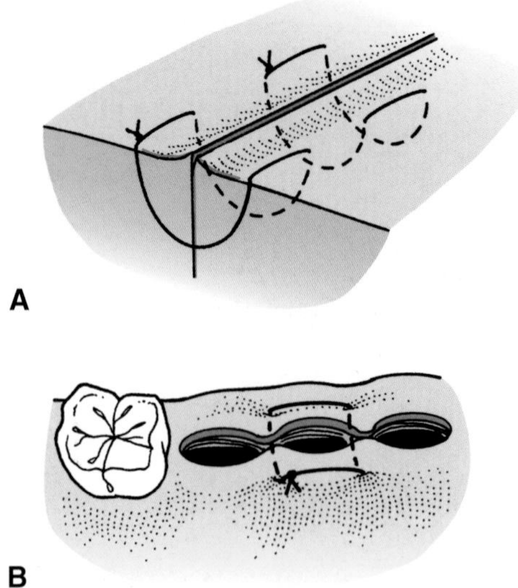

FIGURE 8-23 A, Horizontal mattress suture is sometimes used to close soft tissue wounds. Use of this suture decreases number of individual sutures that have to be placed; however, more importantly, it compresses wound together slightly and everts wound edges. B, Single horizontal mattress suture can be placed across both papillae of tooth socket and serves in similar way as do two individual sutures.

incision is then closed, after which the vertical component is closed. The slight reflection of the nonflap side of the incision greatly eases the placing of sutures.

Sutures may be configured in several different ways. The simple interrupted suture is the one most commonly used in the oral cavity. This suture simply goes through one side of the wound, comes up through the other side of the wound, and is tied in a knot at the top. These sutures can be placed quickly, and the tension on each suture can be adjusted individually. If one suture is lost, the remaining sutures stay in position.

A suture technique that is useful for suturing two adjacent papillae with a single suture is the horizontal mattress suture (Fig. 8-23). A slight variation of that suture is the figure-of-eight suture, which holds the two papilla in position and puts a cross over the top of the socket that may help hold the blood clot in position (Fig. 8-15).

If the incision is long, continuous sutures can be used efficiently. When using this technique, a knot does not have to be made for each suture, which makes it quicker to suture a long-span incision and leaves fewer knots to collect debris. The continuous simple suture can be locking or nonlocking (Fig. 8-24). The horizontal mattress suture also can be used in a running fashion. A disadvantage of the continuous suture is that if one suture pulls through, the entire suture line becomes loose.

Nonresorbable sutures are left in place for approximately 5 to 7 days. After this time, sutures play no useful role and probably increase the contamination of the underlying submucosa. The suture is cut using the tips of a sharp, pointed pair of suture scissors and is removed by pulling it toward the incision line (not away from the suture line).

PRINCIPLES AND TECHNIQUES FOR OPEN EXTRACTIONS

Surgical or open extraction of an erupted tooth is a technique that should not be reserved for the extreme situation. A prudently used open extraction technique may be more conservative and cause less operative morbidity than a closed extraction. Forceps extraction techniques that require great force may result not only in removal of the tooth but also of large amounts of associated bone and occasionally the floor of the maxillary sinus (Fig. 8-25). The bone loss may be less if a soft tissue flap is reflected and a proper amount of bone is removed; it may also be less if the tooth is sectioned. The morbidity of fragments of bone that may be literally torn from the jaw by the "conservative" closed technique greatly exceeds the morbidity of controlled surgical extraction.

Indications for Open Extraction

It is prudent for the surgeon to evaluate carefully each patient and each tooth to be removed for the possibility of an open extraction. Although the vast majority of decisions are to perform a closed extraction, the surgeon must be aware continually that open extraction may be the less traumatic of the two.

As a general guideline, surgeons should consider performing an elective surgical extraction when they perceive a possible need for excessive force to extract a tooth. The term *excessive* means that the force will probably result in a fracture of bone, a tooth root, or both. In any case, the excessive bone loss, the need for additional surgery to retrieve the root, or both can cause undue morbidity. The following are examples of situations in which closed extraction may require excessive force.

The surgeon should strongly consider performing an open extraction after initial attempts at forceps extraction have

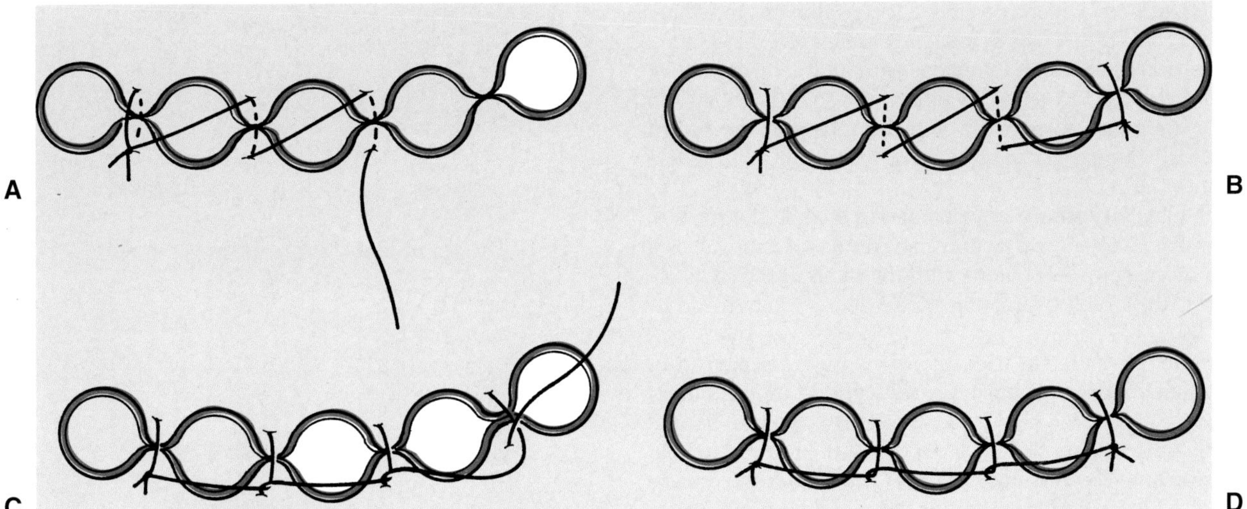

FIGURE 8-24 When multiple sutures are to be placed, incision can be closed with running or continuous suture. **A**, First papilla is closed and knot tied in usual way. Long end of suture is held, and adjacent papilla is sutured, without knot being tied but just with suture being pulled firmly through tissue. **B**, Succeeding papillae are then sutured until final one is sutured and final knot is tied. Final appearance is with suture going across each empty socket. **C**, Continuous locking suture can be made by passing long end of suture underneath loop before it is pulled through tissue. **D**, This puts suture on deep periosteal and mucosal surfaces directly across papilla and may aid in more direct apposition of tissues.

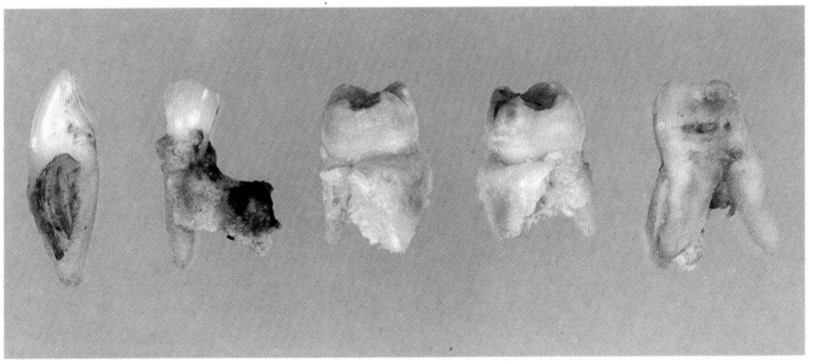

FIGURE 8-25 Forceps extraction of these teeth resulted in removal of bone and tooth, instead of just the tooth.

failed. Instead of applying greater amounts of force that may not be controlled, the surgeon should simply reflect a soft tissue flap, section the tooth, remove some bone, and extract the tooth in sections. In these situations the philosophy of "divide and conquer" results in the most efficient extraction.

If the preoperative assessment reveals that the patient has thick or especially dense bone, particularly on the buccocortical plate, surgical extraction should be considered. The extraction of most teeth depends on the expansion of the buccocortical plate. If this bone is especially thick, then adequate expansion is less likely to occur and fracture of the root is more likely. Whereas young patients have bone that is more elastic and more likely to expand with controlled force, older patients usually have denser, more highly calcified bone that is less likely to provide adequate expansion during luxation of the tooth. Dense bone in the older patient warrants even more caution.

Occasionally, the dentist treats a patient who has very short clinical crowns with evidence of severe attrition. If such attrition is the result of bruxism, it is likely that the teeth are surrounded by dense, thick bone with strong periodontal ligament attachments (Fig. 8-26). The surgeon should exercise extreme caution if removal of such teeth is attempted with a closed technique. An open technique usually results in a quicker, more straightforward extraction.

Careful review of the preoperative radiographs may reveal tooth roots that are likely to cause difficulty if the tooth is extracted by the standard forceps technique. One condition commonly seen among older patients is hypercementosis. In this situation, cementum has continued to be deposited on the tooth and has formed a large bulbous root that is difficult to remove through the available tooth socket opening. Great force used to expand the bone may result in fracture of the root or buccocortical bone (Fig. 8-27).

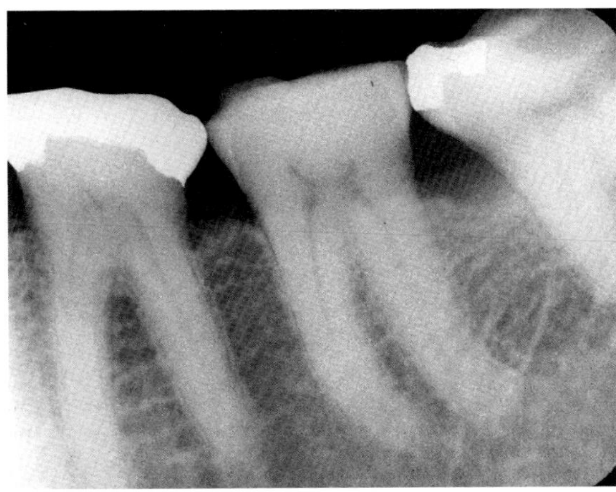

FIGURE 8-26 Teeth that exhibit evidence of bruxism may have denser bone and stronger periodontal ligament attachment, which make them more difficult to extract.

Roots that are widely divergent, especially the maxillary first molar roots (Fig. 8-28) or roots that have severe dilaceration or hooks, are also difficult to remove without fracturing one or more of the roots (Fig. 8-29). By reflecting a soft tissue flap and dividing the roots prospectively with a bur, a more controlled and planned extraction can be performed and will result in less damage overall.

If the maxillary sinus has expanded to include the roots of the maxillary molars, extraction may result in removal of a portion of the sinus floor along with the tooth. If the roots are divergent, then such a situation is even more likely to occur (Fig. 8-30).

Teeth that have crowns with extensive caries, especially root caries, or that have large amalgam restorations are candidates for open extraction (Fig. 8-31). Although forceps should primarily grasp the tooth root, a portion of the force is applied to the crown. Such pressures can crush and shatter the crowns of teeth with extensive caries or large restorations. Open extraction can circumvent the need for extensive force and result in a quicker, less traumatic extraction. Teeth with crowns that have already been lost to caries and that present as retained roots should also be considered for open extraction. If extensive periodontal disease is found around such teeth, it may be possible to deliver them easily with straight elevators or Cryer elevators. However, if the bone is firm around the tooth and no periodontal disease exists, the surgeon should consider an open extraction.

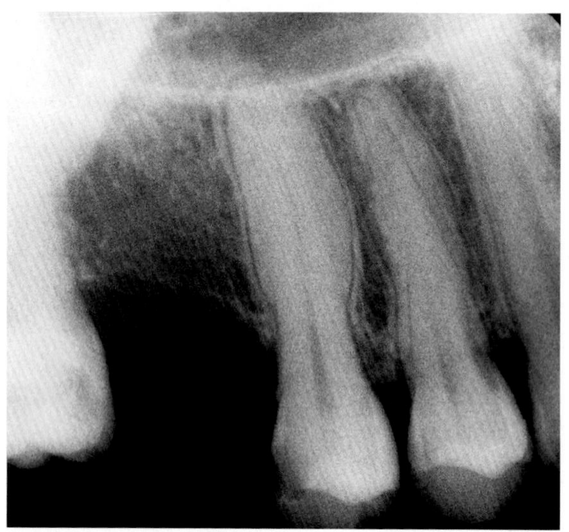

FIGURE 8-27 Hypercementosis of root makes forceps delivery difficult.

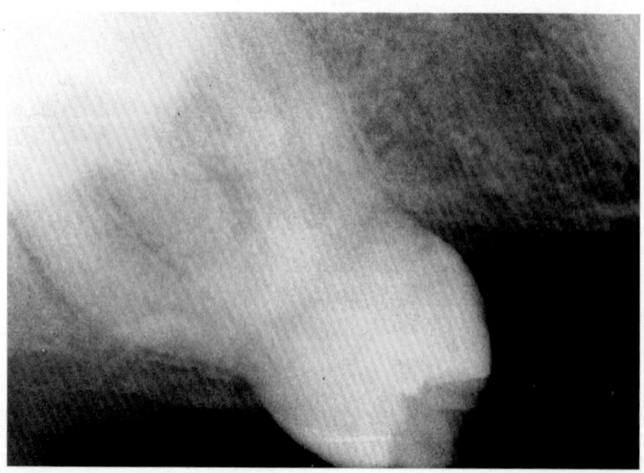

FIGURE 8-28 Widely divergent roots increase likelihood of fracture of bone, tooth root, or both.

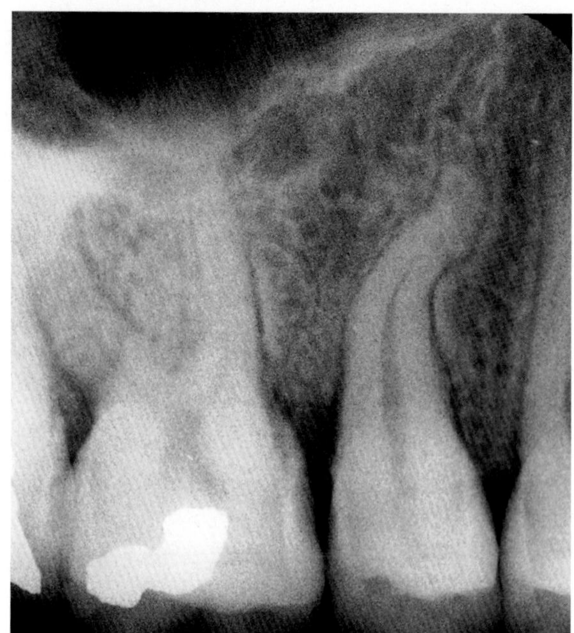

FIGURE 8-29 Severe dilaceration of roots may result in fracture of root unless surgical extraction is performed.

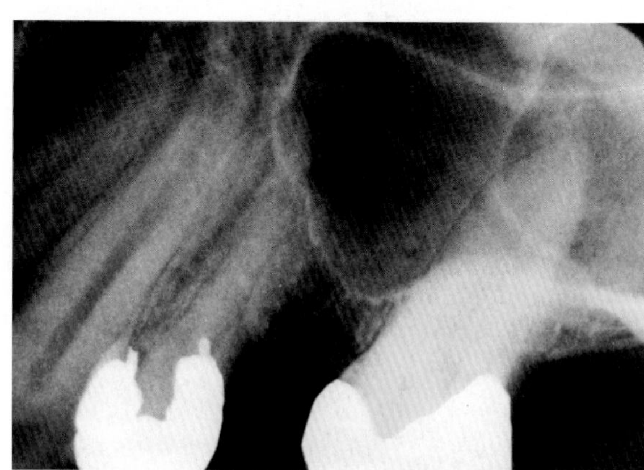

FIGURE 8-30 Maxillary molar teeth "in" the floor of maxillary sinus increase chance of fracture of sinus floor, with resulting sinus perforation.

Technique for Open Extraction of Single-Rooted Tooth

The technique for open extraction of a single-rooted tooth is straightforward but requires attention to detail because several decisions must be made during the operation. Single-rooted teeth are those that have resisted attempts at closed extraction or that have fractured at the cervical line and therefore exist only as a root. The technique is essentially the same for both.

The first step is to provide adequate visualization and access by reflecting a sufficiently large mucoperiosteal flap. In most situations an envelope flap that is extended two teeth anterior

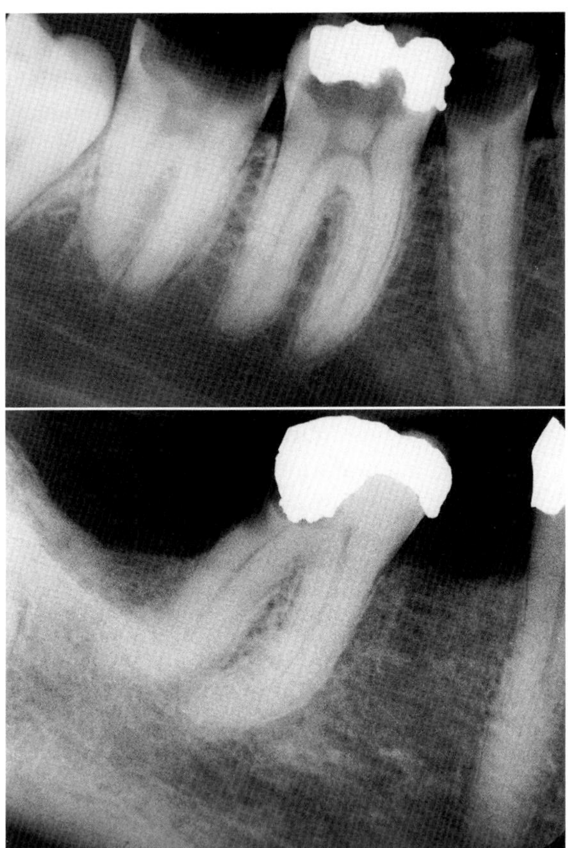

FIGURE 8-31 Large caries or large restorations may lead to fracture of crown of tooth and therefore to more difficult extraction.

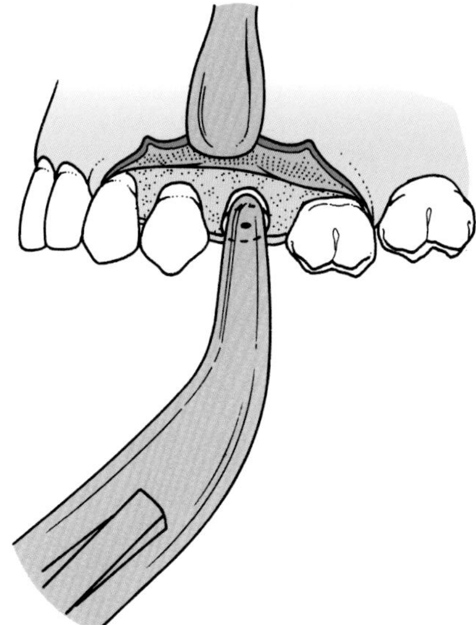

FIGURE 8-32 Small envelope flap can be reflected to expose fractured root. Under direct visualization, forceps can be seated more apically into periodontal ligament space, which eliminates need for bone removal.

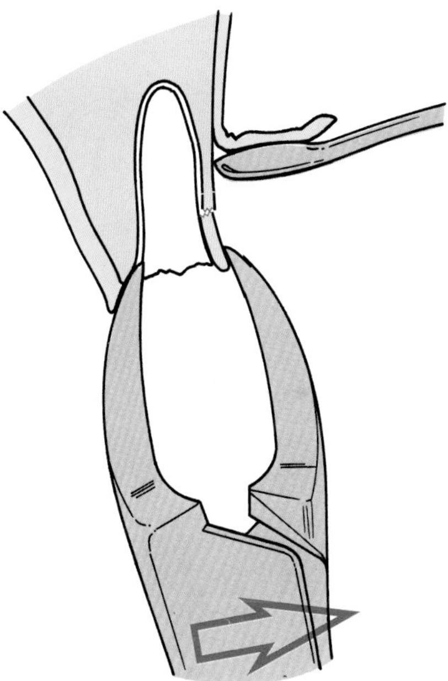

FIGURE 8-33 If root is fractured at level of bone, buccal beak of forceps can be used to remove small portion of bone at same time that root is grasped.

and one tooth posterior to the tooth to be removed is sufficient. If a releasing incision is necessary, it should be placed at least one tooth anterior to the extraction site (Fig. 8-2).

Once an adequate flap has been reflected and is held in its proper position by a periosteal elevator, the surgeon must determine the need for bone removal. Several options are available: First, the surgeon may attempt to reseat the extraction forceps under direct visualization and therefore achieve a better mechanical advantage and remove the tooth with no bone removal at all (Fig. 8-32).

The second option is to grasp a bit of buccal bone under the buccal beak of the forceps to obtain a better mechanical advantage and grasp of the tooth root. This may allow the surgeon to luxate the tooth sufficiently to remove it without any additional bone removal (Fig. 8-33). A small amount of buccal bone is pinched off and removed with the tooth.

The third option is to use the straight elevator, pushing it down the periodontal ligament space of the tooth (Fig. 8-34). The index finger of the surgeon's hand must support the force of the elevator so that the total movement is controlled and no slippage of the elevator occurs. A small wiggling motion should be used to help expand the periodontal ligament space, which allows the small straight elevator to enter the space and act as a wedge to displace the root occlusally. This approach continues with the use of larger straight elevators until the tooth is successfully luxated.

The fourth and final option is to proceed with bone removal over the area of the tooth. Most surgeons currently prefer a bur to remove the bone. The width of buccal bone that is removed is essentially the same width as the tooth in a mesiodistal direction (Fig. 8-35). In a vertical dimension, bone should be removed approximately one half to two thirds the length of the tooth root (Fig. 8-36). This amount of bone removal sufficiently reduces the amount of force necessary to displace the tooth and makes removal relatively easy. A small straight elevator (Fig. 8-37) or forceps can be used to remove the tooth (Fig. 8-38).

If the tooth is still difficult to extract after removal of bone, a purchase point can be made in the root with the bur at the

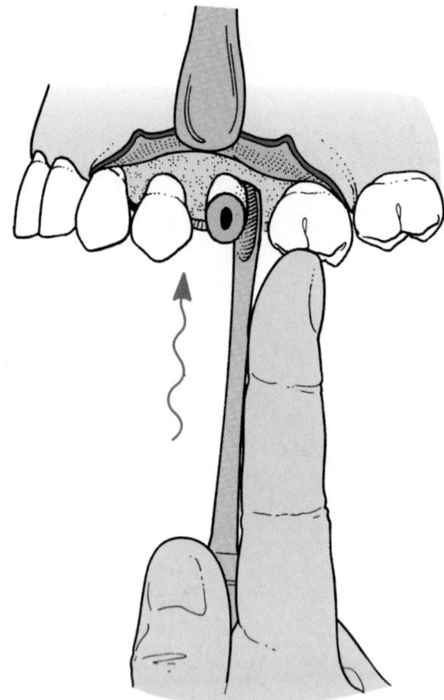

FIGURE 8-34 Small straight elevator can be used as shoehorn to luxate broken root. When straight elevator is used in this position, hand must be securely supported on adjacent teeth to prevent inadvertent slippage of instrument from tooth and subsequent injury to adjacent tissue.

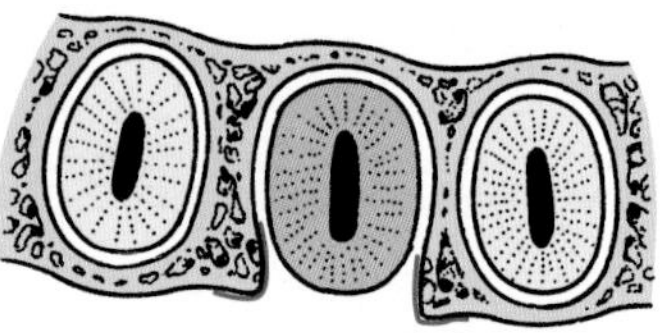

FIGURE 8-35 When removing bone from buccal surface of tooth or tooth root to facilitate removal of that root, mesiodistal width of bone removal should be approximately same as mesiodistal dimension of tooth root itself. This allows unimpeded path for removal of root in buccal direction.

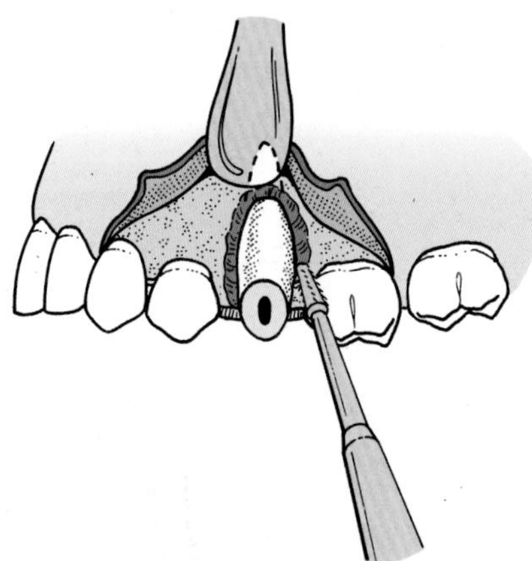

FIGURE 8-36 Bone is removed with bone-cutting bur after reflection of standard envelope flap. Bone should be removed approximately one half to two thirds the length of tooth root.

most apical portion of the area of bone removal (Fig. 8-39). Care should be taken to limit bone removal to only that needed to remove the root to preserve bone for possible implant placement. This hole should be about 3 mm in diameter and deep enough to allow the insertion of an instrument. A heavy elevator, such as a Crane pick, can be used to elevate or lever the tooth from its socket (Fig. 8-40, *A*). The soft tissue is repositioned and sutured (Fig. 8-40, *B*).

The bone edges should be checked; if sharp, they should be smoothed with a bone file. By replacing the soft tissue flap and gently palpating it with a finger, the clinician can check edge sharpness. Removal of bone with a rongeur is rarely indicated because the rongeur tends to remove too much bone.

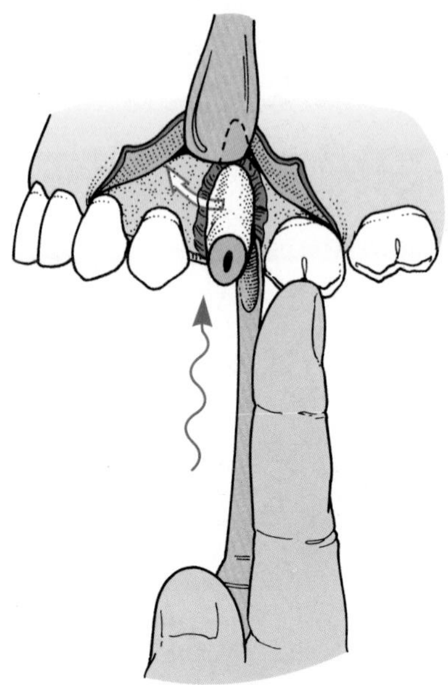

FIGURE 8-37 Once appropriate amount of buccal bone has been removed, straight elevator can be used down palatal aspect of tooth to displace tooth root in buccal direction. One must remember that when elevator is used in this direction, surgeon's hand must be firmly supported on adjacent teeth to prevent slippage of instrument and injury to adjacent soft tissues.

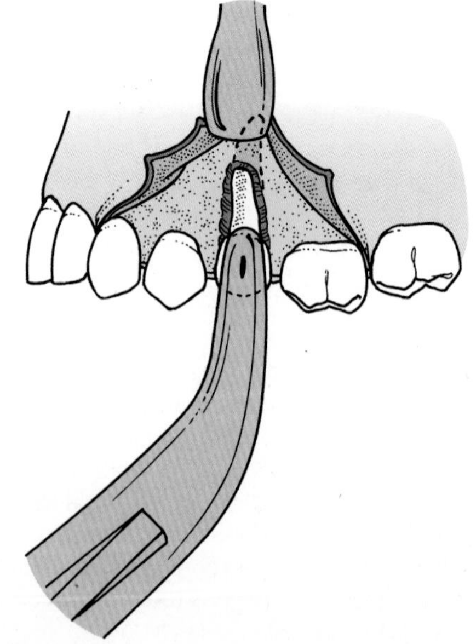

FIGURE 8-38 After bone has been removed and tooth root luxated with straight elevator, forceps can be used to remove root.

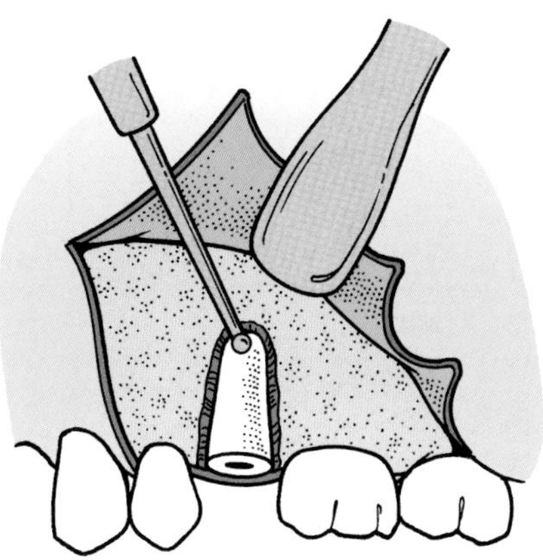

FIGURE 8-39 If tooth root is solid in bone, buccal bone can be removed and purchase point can be made for insertion of elevator.

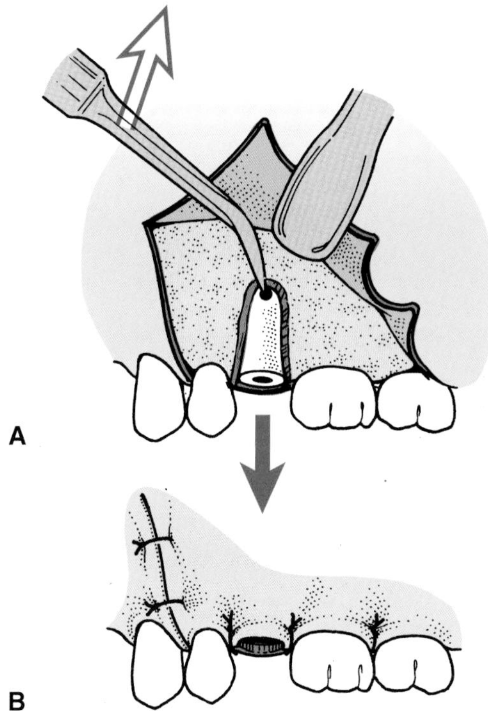

FIGURE 8-40 A, Triangular elevator, such as Crane pick, is then inserted into purchase point, and tooth is elevated from its socket. B, The flap is repositioned and sutured over intact bone.

Once the tooth is delivered, the entire surgical field should be thoroughly irrigated with copious amounts of saline. Special attention should be directed toward the most inferior portion of the flap (where it joins the bone), because this is a common place for debris to settle, especially in mandibular extractions. If the debris is not removed carefully by curettage or irrigation, it can cause delayed healing or even a small subperiosteal abscess in the ensuing 3 to 4 weeks. The flap is then set in its original position and sutured into place with 3-0 black silk or chromic sutures. If the incision were properly planned and executed, the suture line will be supported on sound, intact bone.

Technique for Open Extraction of Multirooted Teeth

If the decision is made to perform an open extraction of a multirooted tooth, such as a mandibular or maxillary molar, the same surgical technique used for the single-rooted tooth is generally used. The major difference is that the tooth may be divided with a bur to convert a multirooted tooth into two or three single-rooted teeth. If the crown of the tooth remains intact, the crown portion is sectioned in such a way as to facilitate removal of roots. However, if the crown portion of the tooth is missing and only the roots remain, the goal is to separate the roots to make them easier to remove with elevators.

Removal of the lower first molar with an intact crown is usually done by sectioning the tooth buccolingually and thereby dividing the tooth into a mesial half (with mesial root and half of the crown) and a distal half. An envelope incision is also made, and a small amount of crestal bone is removed. Once the tooth is sectioned, it is luxated with straight elevators to begin the mobilization process. The sectioned tooth is treated as a lower premolar tooth and is removed with a lower universal forceps (Fig. 8-41). The flap is repositioned and sutured.

The surgical technique begins with the reflection of an adequate flap (Fig. 8-42, *A* and *B*). The surgeon selects an envelope or three-cornered flap as the requirement for access and personal preference dictate. Evaluation of the need for sectioning roots and removing bone is made at this stage, as it was with the single-rooted tooth. Occasionally, forceps, elevators, or both are positioned with direct visualization to achieve better mechanical advantage and to remove the tooth without removing the bone.

However, in most situations a small amount of crestal bone should be removed, and the tooth should be divided. Tooth sectioning is usually accomplished with a straight handpiece with a straight bur, such as the No. 8 round bur, or with a fissure bur, such as the No. 557 or No. 703 bur (Fig. 8-42, *C*). Once the tooth is sectioned, the small straight elevator is used to luxate and mobilize the sectioned roots (Fig. 8-42, *D*). The straight elevator may be used to deliver the mobilized sectioned tooth (Fig. 8-42, *E*). If the crown of the tooth is sectioned, upper or lower universal forceps are used to remove the individual portions of the sectioned tooth (Fig. 8-42, *F*). If the crown is missing, then straight and triangular elevators are used to elevate the tooth roots from the sockets.

Sometimes, a remaining root may be difficult to remove, and additional bone removal (as is described for a single-rooted tooth) may be necessary. Occasionally, it is necessary to prepare a purchase point with the bur and to use an elevator, such as the Crane pick, to elevate the remaining root.

After the tooth and all the root fragments have been removed, the flap is repositioned and the surgical area is palpated for sharp bony edges. If any sharp edges are present, they are smoothed with a bone file. The wound is thoroughly irrigated and débrided of loose fragments of tooth, bone, calculus, and other debris. The flap is repositioned again and sutured in the usual fashion (Fig. 8-42, *G*).

An alternative method for removing the lower first molar is to reflect the soft tissue flap and remove sufficient buccal bone to expose the bifurcation. Then the bur is used to section the mesial root from the tooth and convert the molar into a single-rooted tooth (Fig. 8-43). The crown with the mesial root intact is extracted with No. 17 lower molar forceps. The remaining

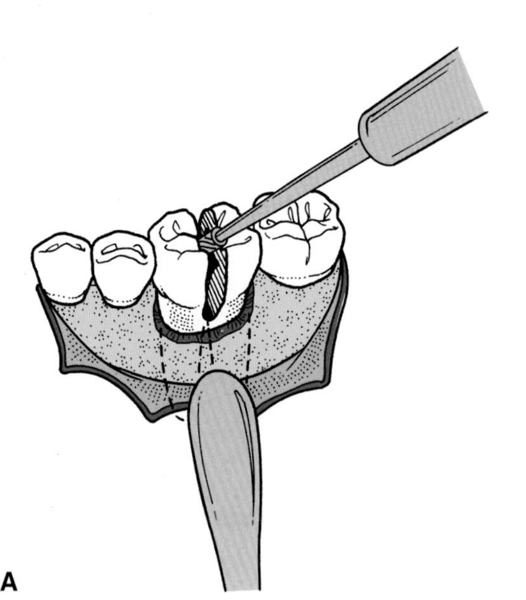

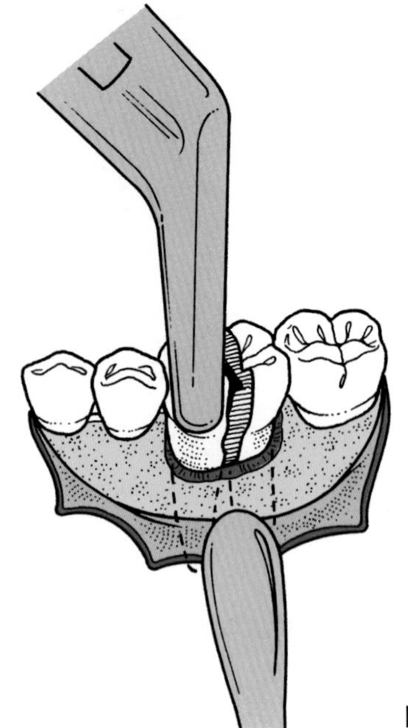

FIGURE 8-41 If lower molar is difficult to extract, it can be sectioned into single-rooted teeth. **A**, Envelope incision is reflected, and small amount of crestal bone is removed to expose bifurcation. Drill is then used to section the tooth into mesial and distal halves. **B**, Lower universal forceps are used to remove two crown and root portions separately.

mesial root is elevated from the socket with a Cryer elevator. The elevator is inserted into the empty tooth socket and rotated, using the wheel-and-axle principle. The sharp tip of the elevator engages the cementum of the remaining root, which is elevated occlusally from the socket. If the interradicular bone is heavy, the first rotation or two of the Cryer elevator removes the bone, which allows the elevator to engage the cementum of the tooth on the second or third rotation.

If the crown of the mandibular molar has been lost, the procedure again begins with the reflection of an envelope flap and removal of a small amount of crestal bone. The bur is used to section the two roots into mesial and distal components (Fig. 8-44, *A*). The small straight elevator is used to mobilize and luxate the mesial root, which is delivered from its socket by insertion of the Cryer elevator into the slot prepared by the dental bur (Fig. 8-44, *B*). The Cryer elevator is rotated in the wheel-and-axle manner, and the mesial root is delivered occlusally from the tooth socket. The opposite member of the paired Cryer instruments is inserted into the empty root socket and rotated through the interradicular bone to engage and deliver the remaining root (Fig. 8-44, *C*).

Extraction of maxillary molars with widely divergent buccal and palatal roots that require excessive force to extract can be done more prudently by dividing the root into several sections. This three-rooted tooth must be divided in a pattern different from that of the two-rooted mandibular molar. If the crown of the tooth is intact, the two buccal roots are sectioned from the tooth and the crown is removed along with the palatal root.

The standard envelope flap is reflected, and a small portion of crestal bone is removed to expose the trifurcation area. The bur is used to section off the mesiobuccal and distobuccal roots (Fig. 8-45, *A*). With gentle but firm buccoocclusal pressure, the upper molar forceps deliver the crown and palatal root along the long axis of the root (Fig. 8-45, *B*). No palatal force should be delivered with the forceps to the crown portion because this results in fracture of the palatal root. The entire delivery force should be in the buccal direction. A small straight elevator is then used to luxate the buccal roots (Fig. 8-45, *C*), which can then be delivered with a Cryer elevator used in the usual fashion (Fig. 8-45, *D*) or with a straight elevator. If straight elevators are used, the surgeon should remember that the maxillary sinus might be close to these roots, so apically directed forces must be kept to a minimum and carefully controlled. The entire force of the straight elevator should be in a mesiodistal direction or toward the palate, and only slight pressure should be applied apically.

If the crown of the maxillary molar is missing or fractured, the roots should be divided into two buccal roots and a palatal root. The same general approach as before is used. An envelope flap is reflected and retracted with a periosteal elevator. A moderate amount of buccal bone is removed to expose the tooth for sectioning (Fig. 8-46, *A*). The roots are sectioned into the two buccal roots and a single palatal root. Next, the roots are luxated with a straight elevator and delivered with Cryer elevators, according to the preference of the surgeon (Fig. 8-46, *B* and *C*). Occasionally, enough access to the roots exists so that a maxillary root forceps or upper universal forceps can be used to deliver the roots independently (Fig. 8-46, *D*). Finally, the palatal root is delivered after the two buccal roots have been removed. Often much of the interradicular bone is lost by this time; therefore the small straight elevator can be used efficiently. The elevator is forced down the periodontal ligament space on the palatal aspect with gentle, controlled wiggling motions, which causes displacement of the tooth in the buccoocclusal direction (Fig. 8-46, *E*).

Removal of Root Fragments and Tips

If fracture of the apical one third (3 to 4 mm) of the root occurs during a closed extraction, an orderly procedure should be used to remove the root tip from the socket. Initial attempts should be made to extract the root fragment by a closed technique, but the surgeon should begin a surgical technique if the closed technique is not immediately successful. Whichever technique is chosen, two requirements for extraction are

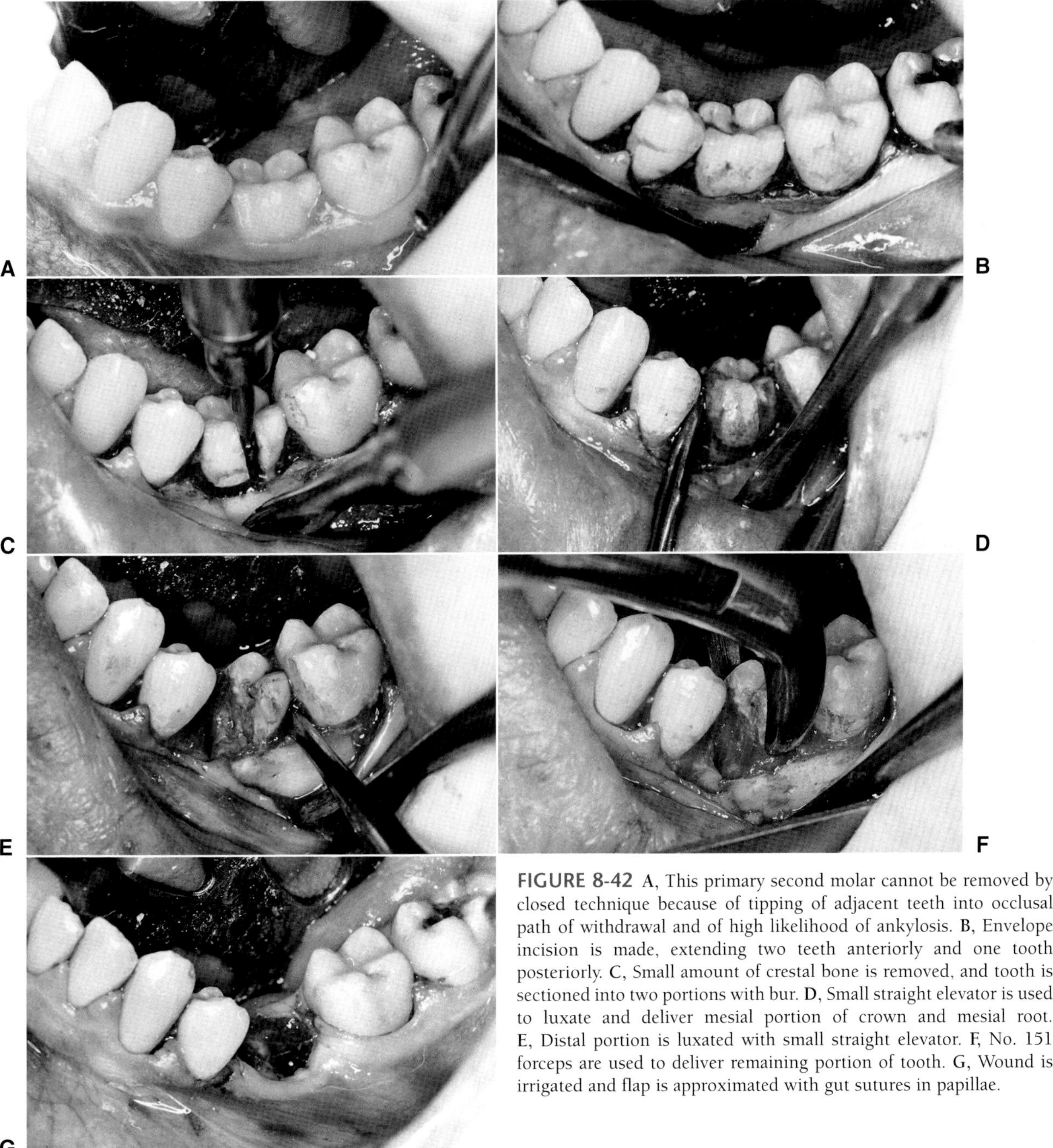

FIGURE 8-42 A, This primary second molar cannot be removed by closed technique because of tipping of adjacent teeth into occlusal path of withdrawal and of high likelihood of ankylosis. B, Envelope incision is made, extending two teeth anteriorly and one tooth posteriorly. C, Small amount of crestal bone is removed, and tooth is sectioned into two portions with bur. D, Small straight elevator is used to luxate and deliver mesial portion of crown and mesial root. E, Distal portion is luxated with small straight elevator. F, No. 151 forceps are used to deliver remaining portion of tooth. G, Wound is irrigated and flap is approximated with gut sutures in papillae.

critically important: excellent light and excellent suction, preferably with a suction tip of small diameter. Removal of a small root tip fragment is difficult unless the surgeon can clearly visualize it. Also important is that an irrigation syringe be available to flush blood and debris from around the root tip so that it can be clearly seen.

The closed technique for root tip retrieval is defined as *any technique that does not require reflection of soft tissue flaps and removal of bone.* Closed techniques are most useful when the tooth was well luxated and mobile before the root tip fractured. If sufficient luxation occurred before the fracture, the root tip often is mobile and can be removed with the closed technique. However, if the tooth was not well mobilized before the fracture, the closed technique is less likely to be successful. The closed technique is also less likely to be successful if the clinician finds a bulbous hypercementosed root with bony interferences that prevent extraction of the root tip fragment. In addition, severe dilaceration of the root end may prevent the use of the closed technique.

Once the fracture has occurred, the patient should be repositioned so that adequate visualization (with proper lighting), irrigation, and suction are achieved. The tooth socket should be irrigated vigorously and suctioned with a small suction tip because the loose tooth fragment occasionally can be irrigated from the socket. Once irrigation and suction are completed, the surgeon should inspect the tooth socket

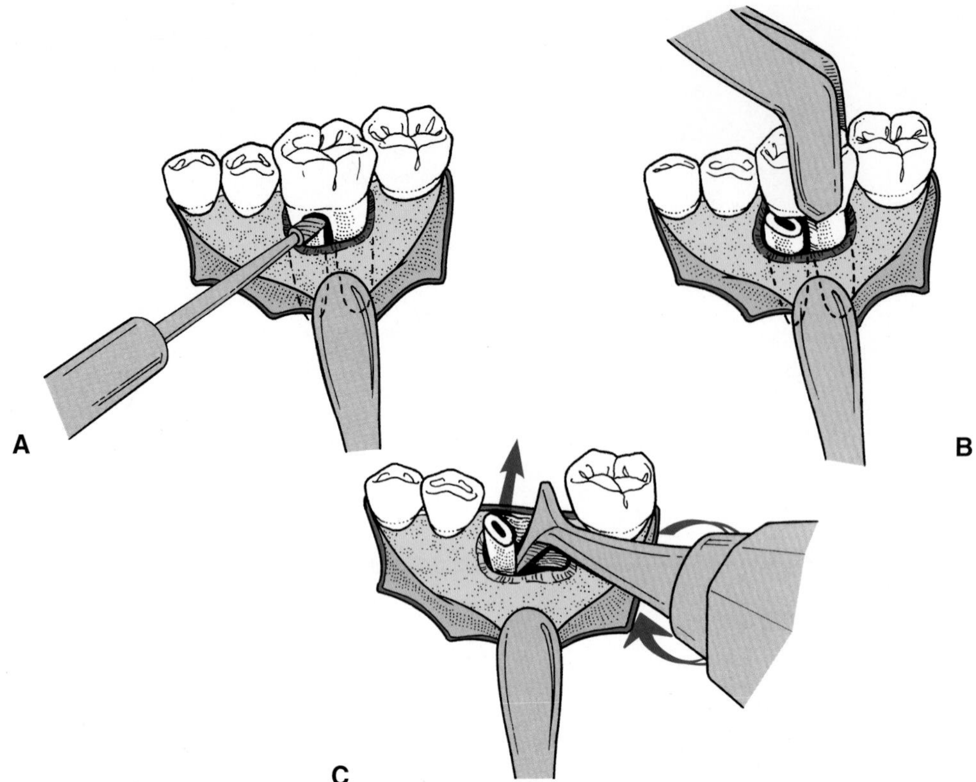

FIGURE 8-43 **A**, Alternative method of sectioning is to use bur to remove mesial root from first molar. **B**, No. 178 forceps are then used to grasp crown of tooth and remove the crown and distal root. **C**, Cryer elevator is then used to remove mesial root. Point of Cryer elevator is inserted into empty socket of distal root and turned in wheel-and-axle fashion, with sharp point engaging interseptal bone and root and elevating mesial root from its socket.

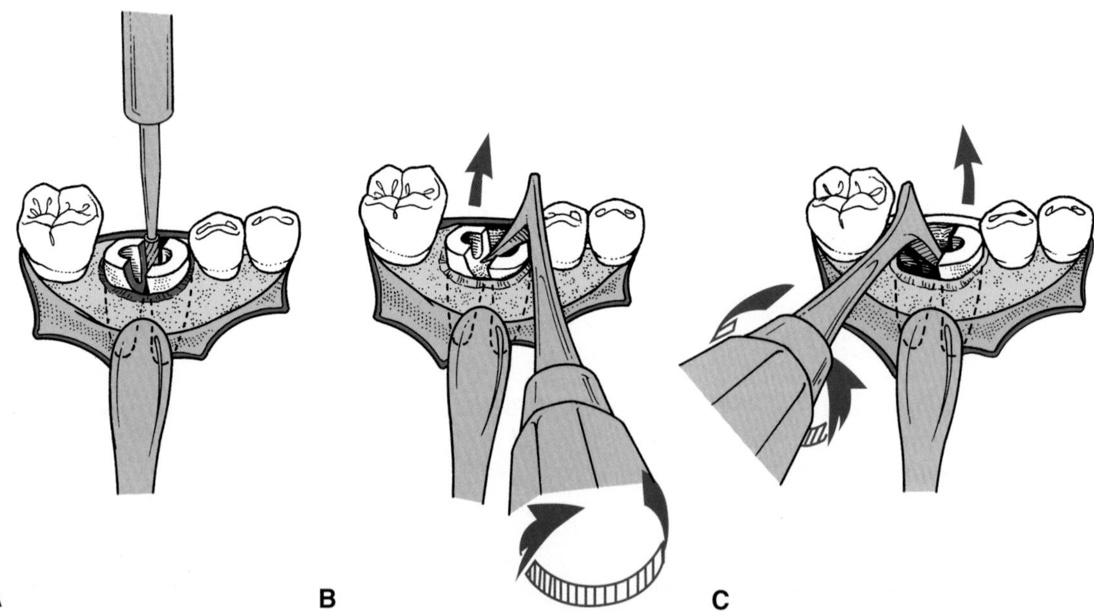

FIGURE 8-44 **A**, When crown of lower molar is lost because of fracture or caries, small envelope flap is reflected and small amount of crestal bone is removed. Bur is then used to section tooth into two individual roots. **B**, After small straight elevator has been used to mobilize roots, Cryer elevator is used to elevate distal root. Tip of elevator is placed into slot prepared by bur, and elevator is turned to deliver the root. **C**, Opposite member of paired Cryer elevators is then used to deliver remaining tooth root with same type of rotational movement.

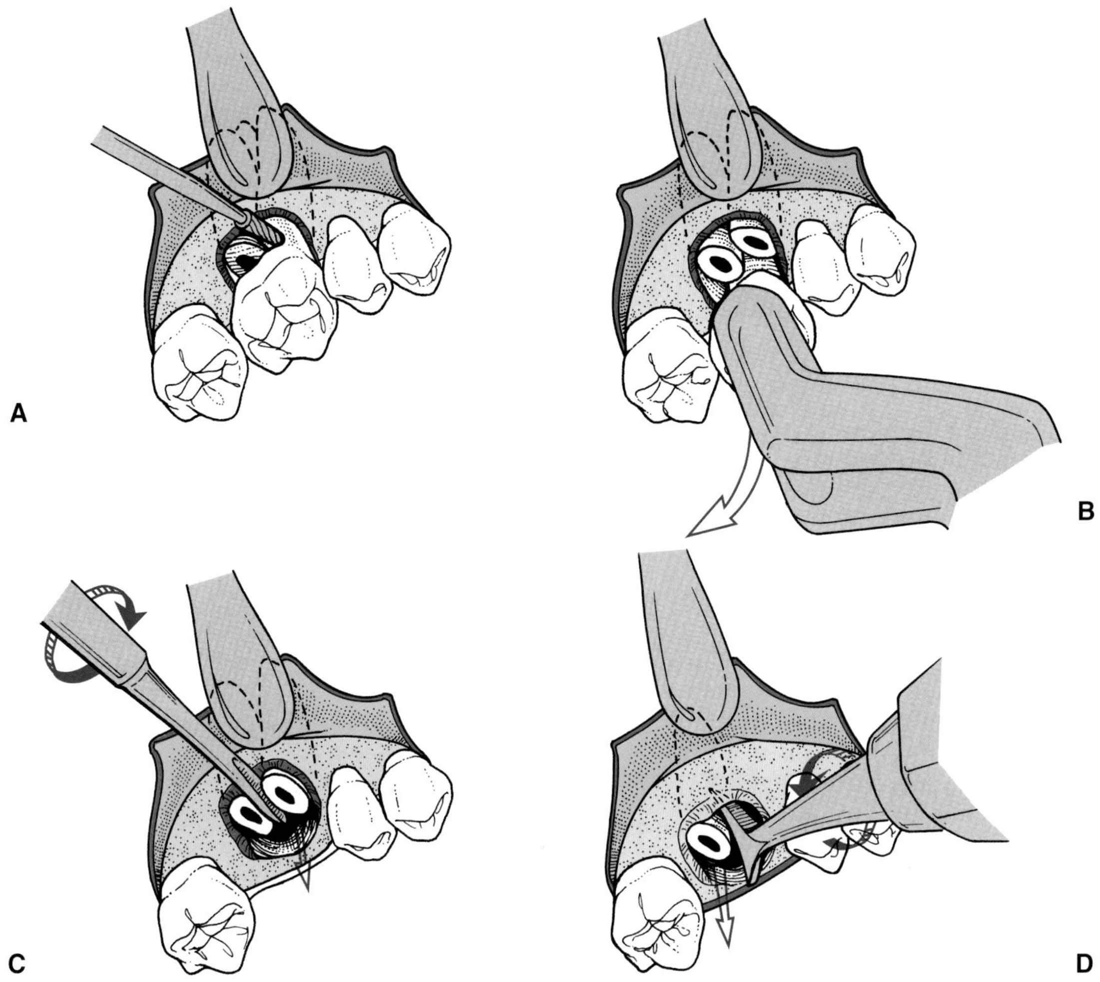

FIGURE 8-45 A, When intact maxillary molar must be divided for judicious removal (as when extreme divergence of roots is found), small envelope incision is made and small amount of crestal bone is removed. This allows bur to be used to section buccal roots from crown portion of tooth. B, Upper molar forceps are then used to remove crown portion of tooth along with palatal root. Tooth is delivered in buccoocclusal direction, and no palatal pressure is used, because it would probably cause fracture of palatal root from crown portion. C, Straight elevator is then used to mobilize buccal roots and can occasionally be used to deliver these roots. D, Cryer elevator can be used in usual fashion by placing tip of elevator into empty socket and rotating it to deliver remaining root.

carefully to assess whether the root has been removed from the socket. The extracted tooth can also be examined to see whether and how much of a root remains.

If the irrigation-suction technique is unsuccessful, the next step is to tease the root apex from the socket with a root tip pick. A root tip pick is a delicate instrument and cannot be used as the Cryer elevator can to remove bone and elevate entire roots. The root tip pick is inserted into the periodontal ligament space, and the root is teased out of the socket (Fig. 8-47). Neither excessive apical or lateral force should be applied to the root tip pick. Excessive apical force could result in displacement of the root tip into other anatomic locations, such as the maxillary sinus. Excessive lateral force could result in the bending or fracture of the end of the root tip pick.

The root tip also can be removed with the small straight elevator. This technique is indicated more often for the removal of larger root fragments. The technique is similar to that of the root tip pick because the small straight elevator is wedged into the periodontal ligament space, where it acts like a wedge to deliver the tooth fragment toward the occlusal plane (Fig. 8-48). Strong apical pressure should be avoided because it may force the root into the underlying tissues.

Displacement of root tips into the maxillary sinus can occur in the maxillary premolar and molar areas. When the straight elevator is used to remove small root tips in this fashion, the surgeon's hand must always be supported on an adjacent tooth or a solid bony prominence. This support allows the surgeon to deliver carefully controlled force and to decrease the possibility of displacing tooth fragments or the instrument into an unwanted place. The surgeon must be able to visualize the top of the fractured root clearly to see the periodontal ligament space. The straight elevator must be inserted into this space and not blindly pushed down into the socket.

If the closed technique is unsuccessful, the surgeon should switch without delay to the open technique. It is important for the surgeon to recognize that a smooth, efficient, properly per-

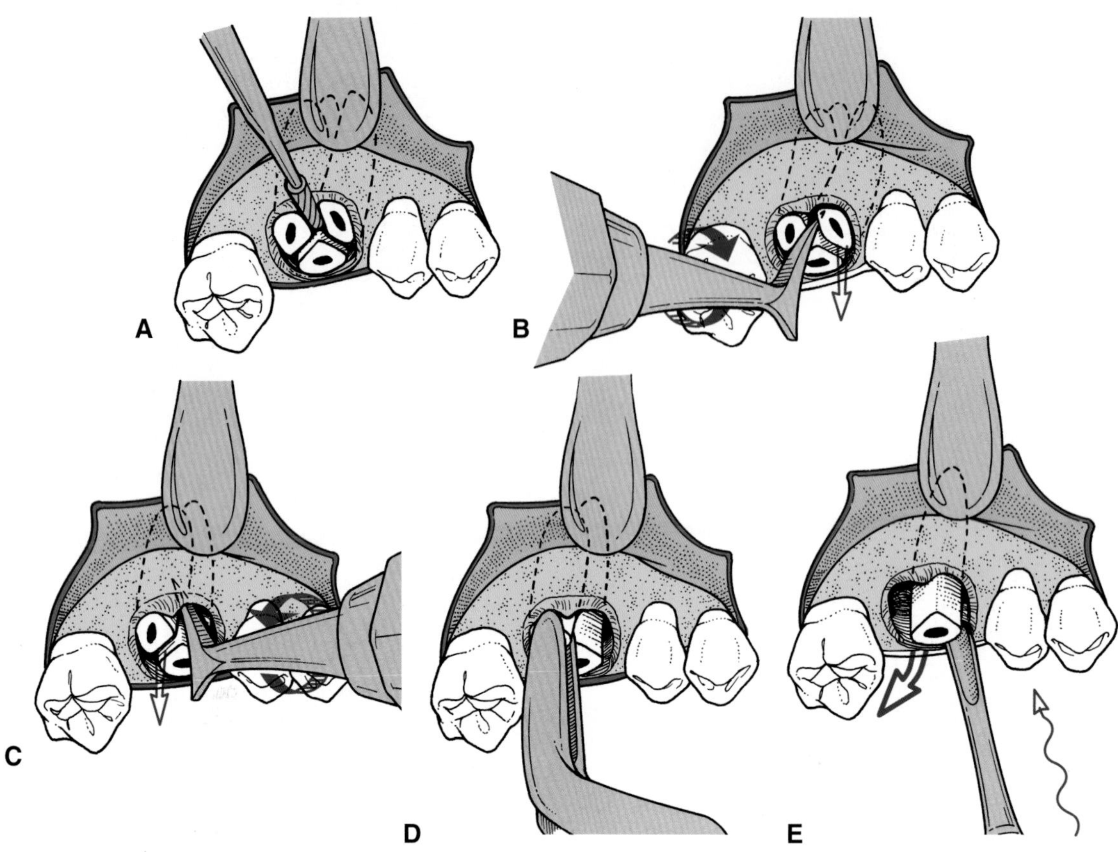

FIGURE 8-46 A, If crown of upper molar has been lost to caries or has been fractured from roots, small envelope incision is reflected and small amount of crestal bone is removed. Bur is then used to section three roots into independent portions. B, After roots have been luxated with small straight elevator, mesiobuccal root is delivered with Cryer elevator placed into slot prepared by bur. C, Once mesiobuccal root has been removed, Cryer elevator is again used to deliver distal buccal root. Tip of Cryer elevator is placed into empty socket of mesiobuccal root and turned in usual fashion to deliver tooth root. D, Maxillary root forceps occasionally can be used to grasp and deliver remaining root. Palatal root can then be delivered with straight elevator or with Cryer elevator. If straight elevator is used, it is placed between root and palatal bone and gently wiggled in effort to displace palatal root in buccoocclusal direction. E, Small straight elevator can be used to elevate and displace remaining root of maxillary third molar in buccoocclusal direction with gentle wiggling pressures.

FIGURE 8-47 A, When small (2 to 4 mm) portion of root apex is fractured from tooth, root tip pick can be used to retrieve it. B, Root tip pick is teased into periodontal ligament space and used to luxate root tip gently from its socket.

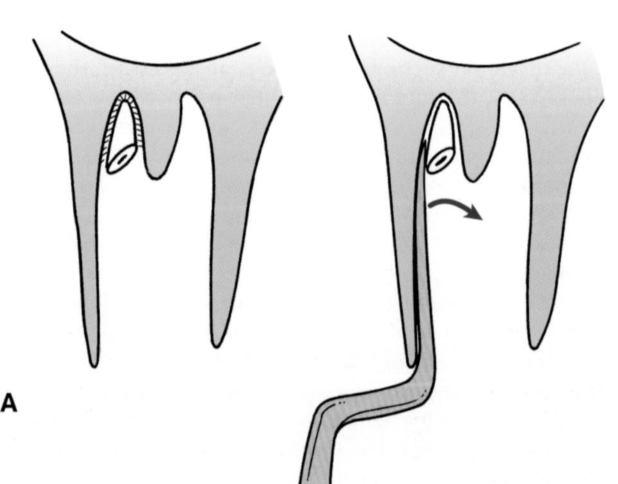

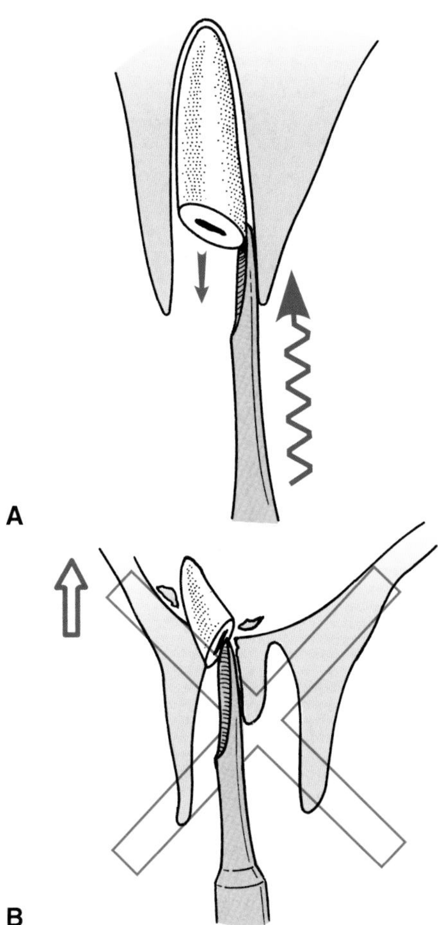

FIGURE 8-48 A, When larger portion of tooth root is left behind after extraction of tooth, small straight elevator can sometimes be used as wedge to displace tooth in occlusal direction. One must remember that pressure applied in such fashion should be in gentle wiggling motions; excessive pressure should not be applied. B, Excessive pressure in apical direction results in displacement of tooth root into undesirable places, such as maxillary sinus.

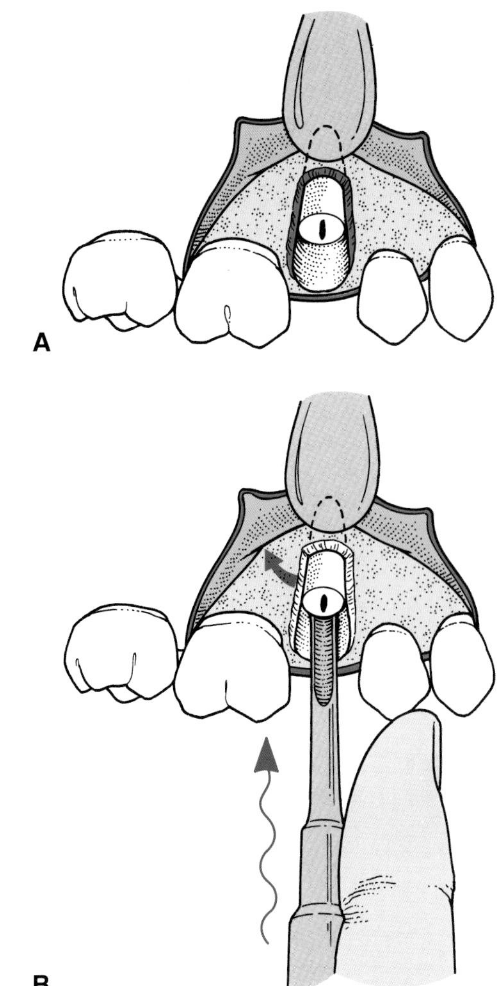

FIGURE 8-49 A, If root cannot be retrieved by closed techniques, soft tissue flap is reflected and bone overlying root is removed with bur. B, Small straight elevator is then used to luxate root buccally by wedging straight elevator into palatal periodontal ligament space.

formed open retrieval of a root fragment is less traumatic than a prolonged, time-consuming, frustrating attempt at closed retrieval.

Two main open techniques are used to remove root tips. The first is simply an extension of the technique described for surgical removal of single-rooted teeth. A soft tissue flap with a releasing incision is reflected and retracted with a periosteal elevator. Bone is removed with a bur to expose the buccal surface of the tooth root. The root is buccally delivered through the opening with a small straight elevator. The wound is irrigated and the flap is repositioned and sutured (Fig. 8-49).

A modification of the open technique just described can be performed to deliver the root fragment without removal of too much of the buccal plate overlying the tooth. This technique is known as the open-window technique. A soft tissue flap is reflected in the same fashion as for the approach just covered, and the apex area of the tooth fragment is located. A dental bur is used to remove the bone overlying the apex of the tooth, exposing the root fragment. A root tip pick or small elevator is then inserted into the window, and the tooth is displaced out of the socket (Fig. 8-50).

The preferred flap technique is the three-cornered flap because of a need for more extensive exposure of the apical areas. The open-window approach is especially indicated when the buccocrestal bone must be left intact such as in the removal of maxillary premolars for orthodontic purposes, especially in adults.

Justification for Leaving Root Fragments

When a root tip has fractured and closed approaches of removal have been unsuccessful, and when the open approach may be excessively traumatic, the surgeon may consider leaving the root in place. As with any surgical approach, the surgeon must balance the benefits of surgery against the risks of surgery. In some situations the risks of removing a small root tip may outweigh the benefits.

Three conditions must exist for a tooth root to be left in the alveolar process. First, the root fragment must be small, usually no more than 4 to 5 mm in length. Second, the root must be deeply embedded in bone and not superficial, to prevent subsequent bone resorption from exposing the tooth root and interfering with any prosthesis that will be constructed over

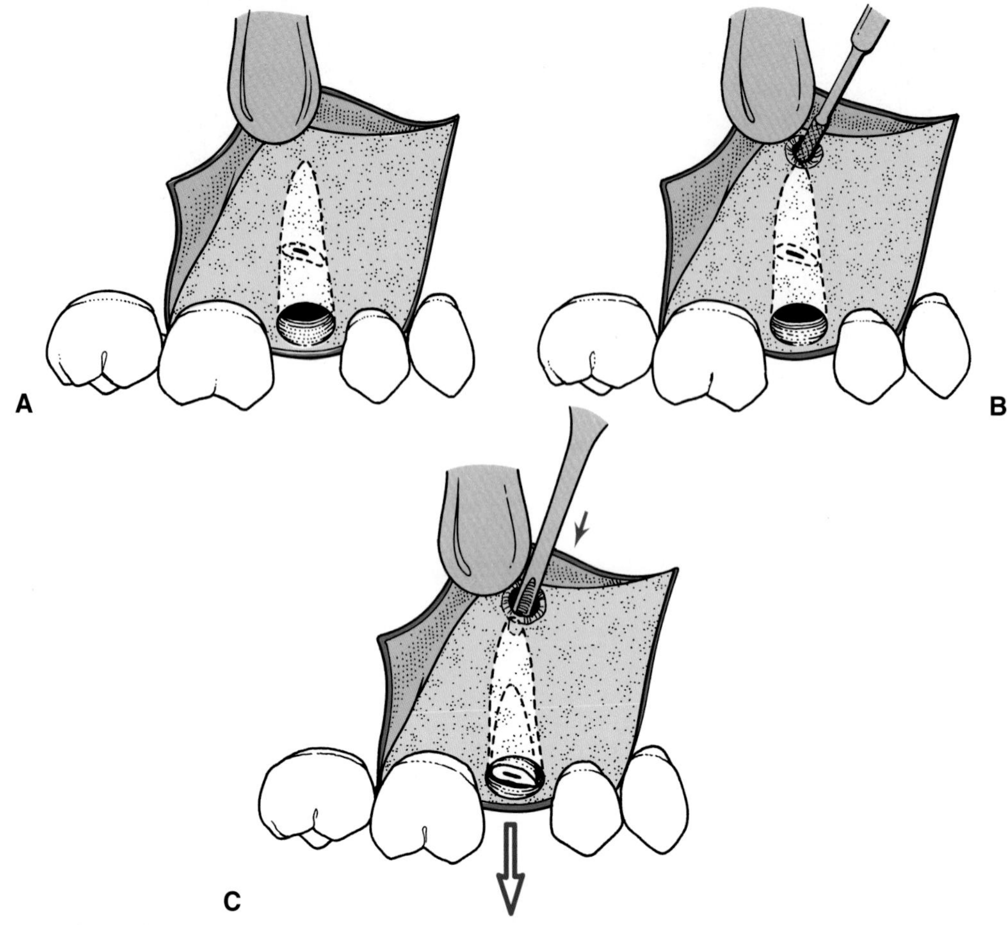

FIGURE 8-50 A, Open-window approach for retrieving root is indicated when buccocrestal bone must be maintained. Three-cornered flap is reflected to expose area overlying apex of root fragment being recovered. B, Bur is used to uncover apex of root and allow sufficient access for insertion of straight elevator. C, Small straight elevator is then used to displace tooth out of tooth socket.

the edentulous area. Third, the tooth involved must not be infected, and there must be no radiolucency around the root apex. This lessens the likelihood that subsequent infections will result from leaving the root in position. If these three conditions exist, then consideration can be given to leaving the root.

For the surgeon to leave a small, deeply embedded, noninfected root tip in place, the risk of surgery must be greater than the benefit. This risk is considered to be greater if one of the following three conditions exists: First, the risk is too great if removal of the root will cause excessive destruction of surrounding tissue, that is, if excessive amounts of bony tissue must be removed to retrieve the root. For example, reaching a small palatal root tip of a maxillary first molar may require the removal of large amounts of bone.

Second, the risk is too great if removal of the root endangers important structures, most commonly the inferior alveolar nerve, at the mental foramen or along the course of the inferior alveolar canal. If surgical retrieval of a root runs a high risk of permanent or even a prolonged temporary anesthesia of the inferior alveolar nerve, the surgeon should seriously consider leaving the root tip in place.

Finally, the risks outweigh the benefits if attempts at recovering the root tip are at high risk of displacing the root tip into tissue spaces or into the maxillary sinus. The roots most often displaced into the maxillary sinus are those of the maxillary molars. If the preoperative radiograph shows that the bone is thin over the roots of the teeth and that the separation between the teeth and maxillary sinus is small, the prudent surgeon may choose to leave a small root fragment rather than risk displacing it into the maxillary sinus. Likewise, roots of the mandibular second and third molars can be displaced into the submandibular space during attempts to remove them. During retrieval of any root tip, apical pressure by an elevator may displace teeth into tissue spaces or into the sinus.

If the surgeon elects to leave a root tip in place, a strict protocol should be observed. The patient must be informed that, in the surgeon's judgment, leaving the root in its position will do less harm than surgery. In addition, radiographic documentation of the presence and position of the root tip must be obtained and retained in the patient's record. The fact that the patient was informed of the decision to leave the root tip in position must be recorded in the patient's chart. In addition, the patient should be recalled for several routine periodic follow-ups over the ensuing year to track the fate of this root. The patient should be instructed to contact the surgeon immediately should any problems develop in the area of the retained root.

MULTIPLE EXTRACTIONS

If multiple adjacent teeth are to be extracted at a single sitting, slight modifications of the routine extraction procedure must be made to facilitate a smooth transition from a dentulous to an edentulous state that allows for proper rehabilitation with a fixed or removable prosthesis. This section discusses those modifications.

Treatment Planning

In most situations where multiple teeth are to be removed, preextraction planning regarding replacement of the teeth to be removed is necessary. This may be a full or removable partial denture or placement of a single or multiple implants. Before the teeth are extracted, the surgeon and restorative dentist should communicate and make a determination of the need for items such as interim partial immediate dentures. The discussion should also include a consideration of the need for any other type of soft tissue surgery, such as tuberosity reduction or the removal of undercuts or tori in critical areas. If dental implants are to be placed at a later time, it may also be desirable to limit bone trimming and socket compression. In some situations, dental implants may be placed at the same time as the teeth are removed, which would require the preparation of a surgical guide stent to assist in aligning the implants appropriately.

Extraction Sequencing

The order in which multiple teeth are extracted deserves some discussion. Maxillary teeth should usually be removed first for several reasons. First, an infiltration anesthetic has a more rapid onset and also disappears more rapidly. This means that the surgeon can begin the surgical procedure sooner after the injections have been given; in addition, surgery should not be delayed because profound anesthesia is lost more quickly in the maxilla. In addition, maxillary teeth should be removed first because during the extraction process, debris such as portions of amalgams, fractured crowns, and bone chips may fall into the empty sockets of the lower teeth if the lower surgery is performed first. In addition, maxillary teeth are removed with a major component of buccal force. Little or no vertical traction force is used in removal of these teeth, as is commonly required with mandibular teeth. A single minor disadvantage for extracting maxillary teeth first is that if hemorrhage is not controlled in the maxilla before mandibular teeth are extracted, the hemorrhage may interfere with visualization during mandibular surgery. Hemorrhage is usually not a major problem because hemostasis should be achieved in one area before the surgeon turns attention to another area of surgery, and the surgical assistant should be able to keep the surgical field free from blood with adequate suction.

Tooth removal usually begins with extraction of the most posterior teeth first. This allows for the more effective use of dental elevators to luxate and mobilize teeth before the forceps are used to extract the tooth. The two teeth that are the most difficult to remove, the first molar and canine, should be extracted last. Removal of the teeth on either side weakens the bony socket on the mesial and distal side of these teeth, and their subsequent extraction is made more straightforward.

Thus, for example, if teeth in the maxillary and mandibular left quadrants are to be extracted, the following order is recommended: (1) maxillary posterior teeth, leaving the first molar; (2) maxillary anterior teeth, leaving the canine; (3) maxillary first molar; (4) maxillary canine; (5) mandibular posterior teeth, leaving the first molar; (6) mandibular anterior teeth, leaving the canine; (7) mandibular first molar; and (8) mandibular canine.

Technique for Multiple Extractions

The surgical procedure for removing multiple adjacent teeth is modified slightly. The first step in removing a single tooth is to loosen the soft tissue attachment from around the tooth. When performing multiple extractions, the soft tissue reflection is extended slightly to form a small envelope flap to expose the crestal bone only (Fig. 8-51, *A* to *C*). The teeth are luxated with the straight elevator (Fig. 8-51, *D*) and are delivered with forceps in the usual fashion. If removing any of the teeth is likely to require excessive force, the surgeon should remove a small amount of buccal bone to prevent fracture and excessive bone loss.

After the extractions are completed, the buccolingual plates are pressed into their preexisting position with firm pressure unless implants are planned. The soft tissue is repositioned, and the surgeon palpates the ridge to determine whether any areas of sharp bony spicules can be found. If a removable partial or complete denture is planned, undercuts should be identified. If any sharp spicules or undercuts exist, the bone rongeur is used to remove the larger areas of interference, and a bone file used to smooth any sharp spicules (Fig. 8-51, *E* and *F*). The area is irrigated thoroughly with sterile saline. The soft tissue is inspected for the presence of excess granulation tissue. If any granulation tissue is present, it should be removed because it may prolong postoperative hemorrhage. The soft tissue is then reapproximated and inspected for excess gingiva. If the teeth are being removed because of severe periodontitis with bone loss, it is common for the soft tissue flaps to overlap and cause redundant tissue. If this is the situation, the gingiva should be trimmed so that no overlap occurs when the soft tissue is apposed. However, if no redundant tissue exists, the surgeon must not try to gain primary closure over the extraction sockets. If this is done, the depth of the vestibule decreases, which may interfere with denture construction and wear. Finally, the papillae are sutured into position (Fig. 8-51, *G*). Interrupted or continuous sutures are used, depending on the preference of the surgeon, planning removal in about a week (Fig. 8-51, *H* and *I*).

In some patients a more extensive alveoloplasty after multiple extractions is necessary. Chapter 13 has an in-depth discussion of this technique.

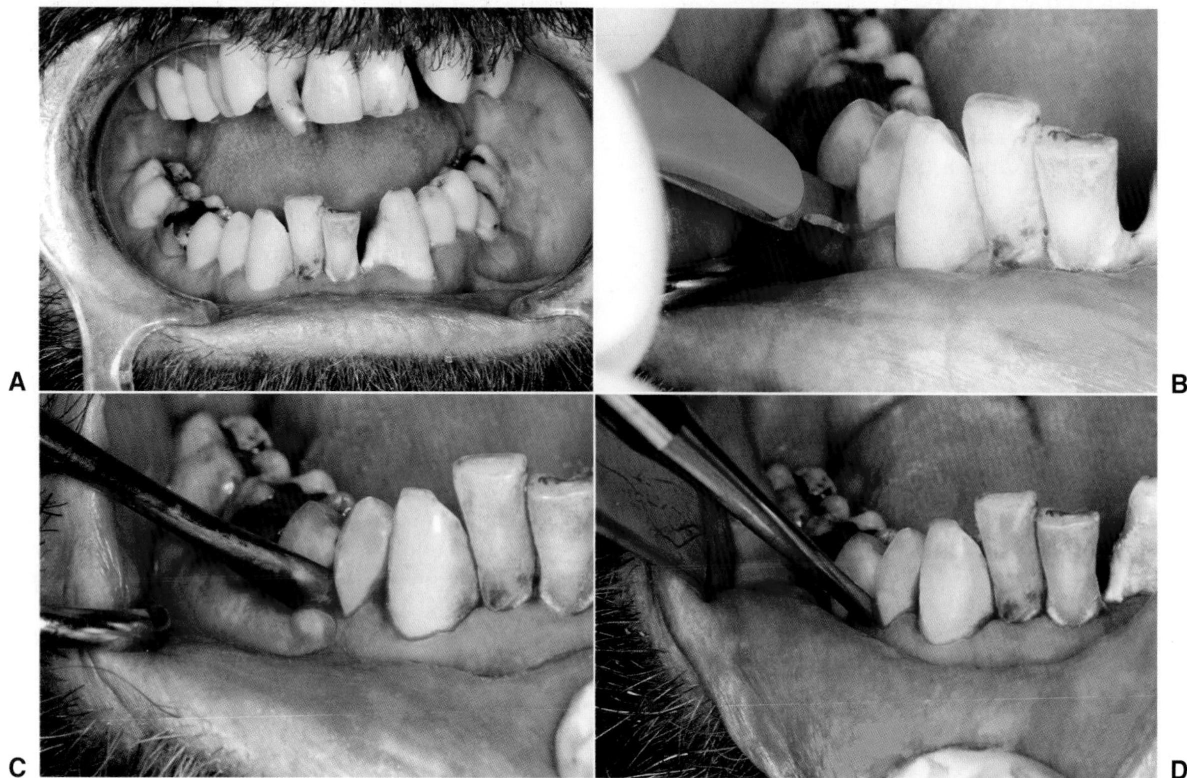

FIGURE 8-51 **A**, This patient's remaining mandibular teeth are to be extracted. The broad zone of attached gingiva is demonstrated in adequate vestibular depth. **B**, After adequate anesthesia is achieved, soft tissue attachment to teeth is incised with No. 15 blade. Incision is carried around necks of teeth and through interdental papilla. **C**, Periosteal elevator is used to reflect labial soft tissue just to crest of labioalveolar bone. **D**, Small straight elevator is used to luxate teeth before forceps are used. Surgeon's opposite hand is reflecting soft tissue and stabilizing mandible. Teeth adjacent to mandibular canine are extracted first, which makes extraction of remaining canine tooth easier to accomplish.

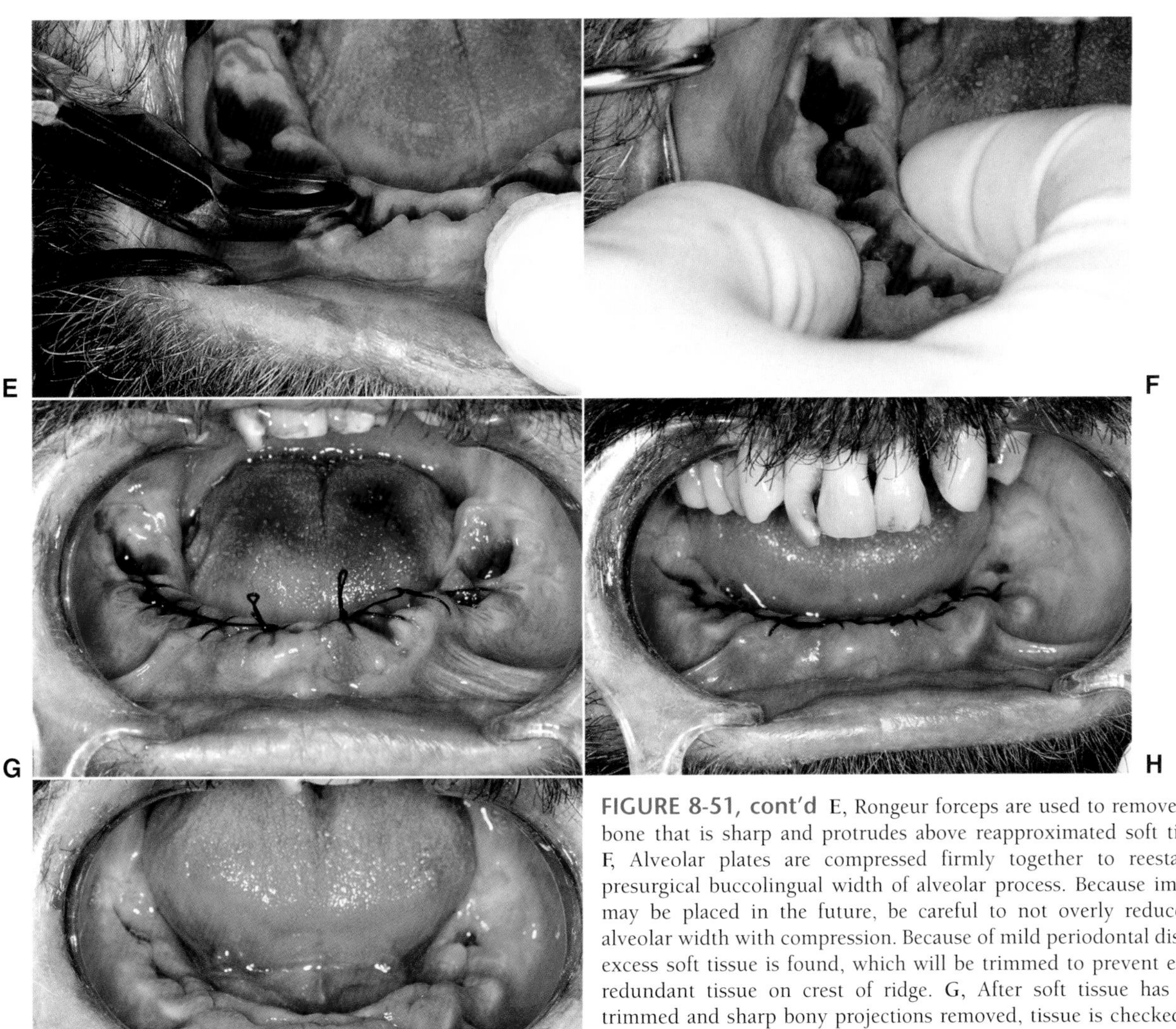

FIGURE 8-51, cont'd E, Rongeur forceps are used to remove only bone that is sharp and protrudes above reapproximated soft tissue. F, Alveolar plates are compressed firmly together to reestablish presurgical buccolingual width of alveolar process. Because implant may be placed in the future, be careful to not overly reduce the alveolar width with compression. Because of mild periodontal disease, excess soft tissue is found, which will be trimmed to prevent excess redundant tissue on crest of ridge. G, After soft tissue has been trimmed and sharp bony projections removed, tissue is checked one final time for completeness of soft tissue surgery. Tissue is closed with interrupted black silk sutures across papilla. This approximates soft tissue at papilla but leaves tooth socket open. Soft tissue is not mobilized to achieve primary closure because this would tend to reduce vestibular height. H and I, Patient returns for suture removal 1 week later. Normal healing has occurred, and sutures are ready for removal. The broad band of attached tissue remains on ridge, similar to what existed in preoperative situation (see *A*).

CHAPTER 9

Principles of Management of Impacted Teeth

JAMES R. HUPP

CHAPTER OUTLINE

An impacted tooth is one that fails to erupt into the dental arch within the expected time. The tooth becomes impacted because adjacent teeth, dense overlying bone, excessive soft tissue, or a genetic abnormality prevents eruption. Because impacted teeth do not erupt, they are retained for the patient's lifetime unless surgically removed or exposed because of resorption of overlying tissues. The term *unerupted* includes impacted teeth and teeth that are in the process of erupting.

Teeth most often become impacted because of inadequate dental arch length and space in which to erupt; that is, the total length of the alveolar bone arch is smaller than the total length of the tooth arch. The most common impacted teeth are the maxillary and mandibular third molars, followed by the maxillary canines and mandibular premolars. The third molars are the most frequently impacted because they are the last teeth to erupt; therefore, they are the most likely to have inadequate space for eruption.

In the anterior maxilla, the canine is also commonly prevented from erupting by crowding of other teeth. The canine usually erupts after the maxillary lateral incisor and maxillary first premolar. If space is inadequate to allow eruption, the canine becomes impacted or erupts labial to the dental arch. In the anterior mandible a similar situation affects the mandibular premolars because they erupt after the mandibular first molar and mandibular canine. Therefore if room for eruption is inadequate, one of the premolars, usually the second premolar, remains unerupted and becomes impacted or erupts into a buccal or lingual position in relation to the dental arch.

As a general rule, all impacted teeth should be removed unless removal is contraindicated. Extraction should be performed as soon as the dentist determines that the tooth is impacted. Removal of impacted teeth becomes more difficult with advancing age. The dentist should typically *not* recommend that impacted teeth be left in place until they cause difficulty. If the tooth is left in place until problems arise, the patient may experience an increased incidence of local tissue morbidity, loss of or damage to adjacent teeth and bone, and potential injury to adjacent vital structures. Additionally, if removal of impacted teeth is deferred until they cause problems later in life, surgery is more likely to be complicated and hazardous because the patient may have compromising systemic diseases and the surrounding bone becomes more dense. A fundamental precept of the philosophy of dentistry is that problems should be prevented. Preventive dentistry dictates that impacted teeth are to be removed before complications arise unless removal will cause more serious problems.

This chapter discusses the management of impacted teeth. The chapter is not a thorough or in-depth discussion of the technical aspects of surgical impaction removal. Instead, the goal is to provide the information necessary for proper management and a basis for predicting the difficulty of surgery.

INDICATIONS FOR REMOVAL OF IMPACTED TEETH

All impacted teeth should be considered for removal as soon as the diagnosis is made. The average age for completion of the eruption of the third molar is age 20, although eruption may continue in some patients until age 25. During normal development the lower third molar begins in a horizontal angulation, and as the tooth develops and the jaw grows, the angulation changes from horizontal to mesioangular to vertical. Failure of rotation from the mesioangular to the vertical direction is the most common cause of lower third molars becoming impacted. The second major factor is that the mesiodistal dimension of the teeth versus the length of the jaw is such that inadequate room exists in the alveolar process anterior to the anterior border of the ramus to allow the tooth to erupt into position.

As noted before, some third molars continue to erupt after age 20 particularly in males, coming into final position by age 25. Multiple factors are associated with continued eruption. When late eruption occurs, the unerupted tooth is usually covered with only soft tissue or slightly with bone. These teeth are almost always in a vertical position and are relatively superficially positioned with respect to the occlusal plane of the adjacent second molar, and completion of root development is late.

Finally and perhaps most importantly, sufficient space needs to exist between the anterior border of the ramus and the second molar to allow eruption.[1,2] Likewise, if the tooth does not erupt after age 20, it is most likely covered with bone. In addition, the tooth is likely a mesioangular impaction and is located lower in the alveolar process near the cervical level of the adjacent second molar. Therefore the dentist can use these parameters to predict whether a tooth will erupt into the arch or remain impacted.

Early removal reduces the postoperative morbidity and allows for the best healing.[3-6] Younger patients tolerate the procedure better, recovering more quickly and with less interference to their daily lives. Periodontal healing is better in the younger patient because of better and more complete regeneration of the periodontal tissues on the distal of the second molar. Also, nerve recovery is better if injured in younger patients. Moreover, the procedure is easier to perform in younger patients because the bone is less dense and root formation is incomplete. The ideal time for removal of impacted third molars is when the roots of the teeth are one third formed and before they are two thirds formed, usually during the late teenage years, between ages 17 and 20.

If impacted teeth are left in the alveolar process, it is highly probable that one or more of several problems will result.[7,8]

Prevention of Periodontal Disease

Erupted teeth adjacent to impacted teeth are predisposed to periodontal disease (Figs. 9-1 and 9-2). The mere presence of an impacted mandibular third molar decreases the amount of bone on the distal aspect of an adjacent second molar. Because the most difficult tooth surface to keep clean is the distal aspect of the last tooth in the arch, patients commonly have gingival inflammation with apical migration of the gingival

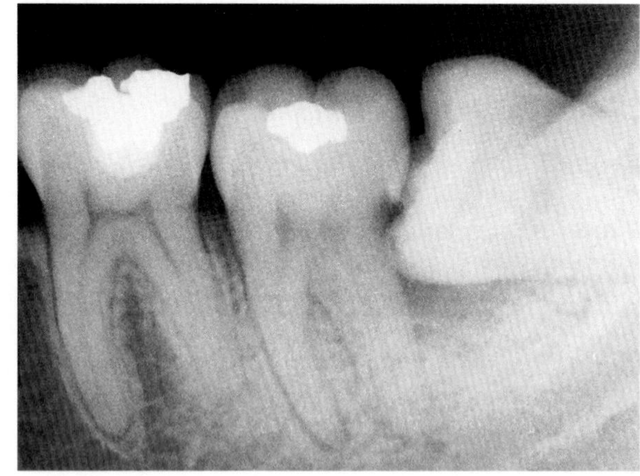

FIGURE 9-1 Radiograph of mandibular third molar impacted against second molar, with bone loss resulting from presence of third molar.

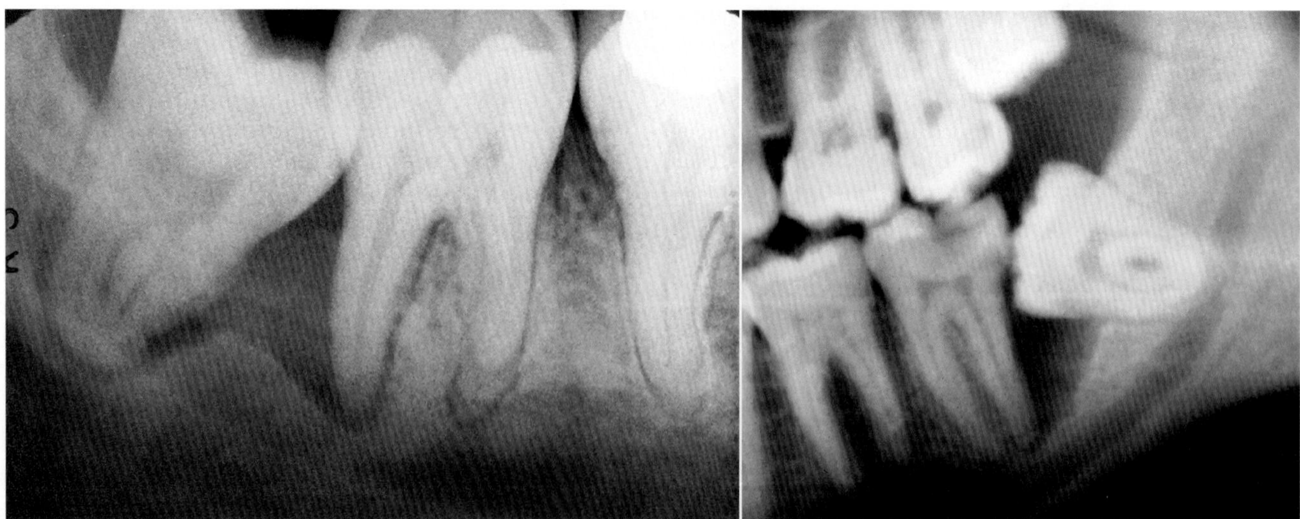

FIGURE 9-2 Radiographs show variations of mandibular third molar impacted against second molar, with severe bone loss resulting from periodontal disease and third molar.

attachment on the distal aspect of the second molar. With even minor gingivitis the causative bacteria have access to a large portion of the root surface, which results in the early formation of tooth-compromising periodontitis. Patients with impacted mandibular third molars often have deep periodontal pockets on the distal aspect of the second molars even though they have normal sulcular depth in the remainder of the mouth.

The accelerated periodontal problem resulting from an impacted third molar is especially serious in the maxilla. As a periodontal pocket expands apically, it comes to involve the distal furcation of the maxillary second molar. This occurs relatively early, which makes advancement of the periodontal disease more rapid and severe. In addition, treatment of the localized periodontal disease around the maxillary second molar is more difficult because of the distal furcation involvement.

By removing the impacted third molars early, periodontal disease can be prevented and the likelihood of bony healing and optimal bone fill into the area previously occupied by the crown of the third molar is increased.[4-6]

Prevention of Dental Caries

When a third molar is impacted or partially impacted, the bacteria that cause dental caries can be exposed to the distal aspect of the second molar, as well as to the third molar. Even in situations in which no obvious communication between the mouth and the impacted third molar exists, there may be enough communication to allow for caries initiation (Figs. 9-3 to 9-5).

Prevention of Pericoronitis

When a tooth is partially impacted with a large amount of soft tissue over the axial and occlusal surfaces, the patient frequently has one or more episodes of pericoronitis.[9] Pericoronitis is an infection of the soft tissue around the crown of a partially impacted tooth and is usually caused by normal oral flora. For most patients the bacteria and host defenses maintain a delicate balance, but even normal host defenses cannot eliminate the bacteria (Fig. 9-6).

If the host defenses are compromised (e.g., during minor illnesses, such as influenza or an upper respiratory infection, or because of immune-compromising drugs) infection can occur. Thus although the impacted tooth has been present for

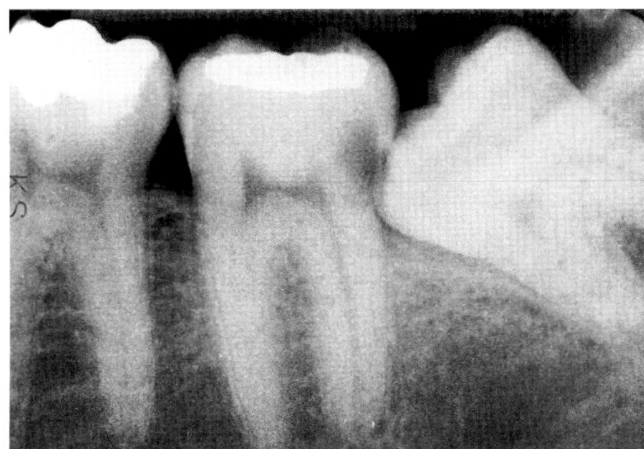

FIGURE 9-3 Radiograph of caries in mandibular second molar resulting from presence of impacted third molar.

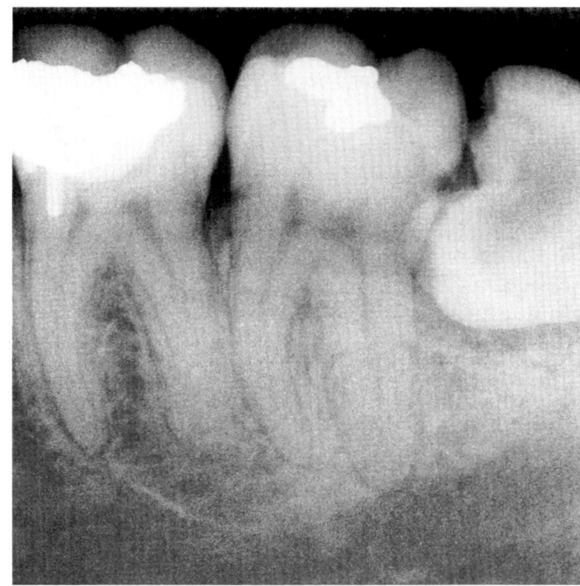

FIGURE 9-4 Radiograph of caries in mandibular impacted molar.

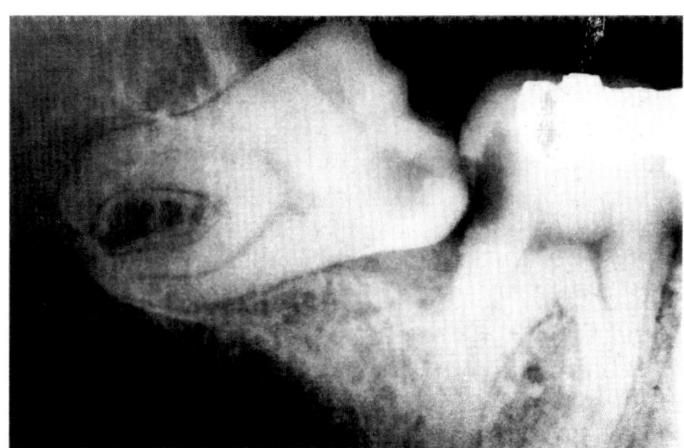

FIGURE 9-5 Radiograph of caries in impacted third molar and second molar.

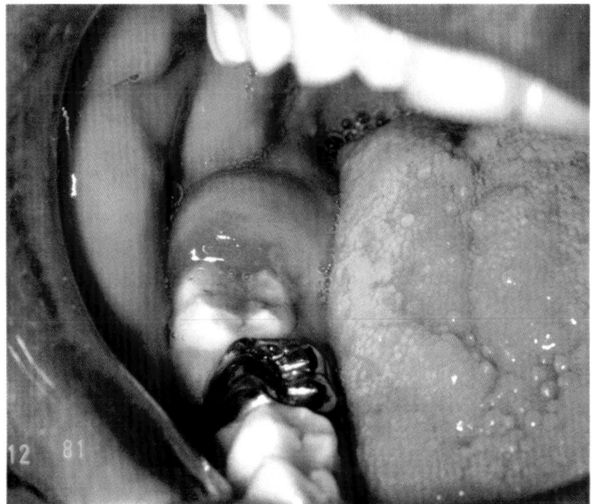

FIGURE 9-6 Pericoronitis in area of impacted tooth #32 exhibiting classic signs of inflammation with erythema and swelling. If opposing tooth #1 is erupted, it commonly impinges on this area of swelling when teeth brought are into occlusion, causing even more pain and swelling.

some time without infection, if the patient experiences even a mild, transient decrease in host defenses, pericoronitis commonly results and may result even without any immunologic problems.

Pericoronitis can also arise following minor trauma from a maxillary third molar. The soft tissue that covers the occlusal surface of the partially erupted mandibular third molar (known as the *operculum*) can be traumatized and become swollen. Often the maxillary third molar further traumatizes the already swollen operculum, which causes a further increase in swelling that is now traumatized more easily. This spiraling cycle of trauma and swelling is often interrupted only by removal of the maxillary third molar.

Another common cause of pericoronitis is entrapment of food under the operculum. During eating, food debris may become lodged into the pocket between the operculum and the impacted tooth. Because this pocket cannot be cleaned, bacteria colonize it and pericoronitis results.

Streptococci and a large variety of anaerobic bacteria (the usual bacteria that inhabit the gingival sulcus) cause pericoronitis. Pericoronitis can be treated initially by mechanically débriding the large periodontal pocket that exists under the operculum by using hydrogen peroxide as an irrigating solution. Hydrogen peroxide not only mechanically removes bacteria with its foaming action, it also reduces the number of anaerobic bacteria by releasing oxygen into the usually anaerobic environment of the pocket. Other irrigants, such as chlorhexidine or iodophors, can also reduce the bacterial counts of the pocket. Even saline solutions, if delivered with pressure via a syringe can reduce the bacterial numbers and flush away food debris.

Pericoronitis can present as a mild infection or as a severe infection that requires hospitalization of the patient. Just as the severity of the infection varies, the treatment and management of this problem vary from mild to aggressive.

In its mildest form, pericoronitis is a localized tissue swelling and soreness. For patients with a mild infection, irrigation and curettage by the dentist and home irrigations by the patient usually suffice.

If the infection is slightly more severe with a large amount of local soft tissue swelling being traumatized by a maxillary third molar, the dentist should consider immediately extracting the maxillary third molar in addition to local irrigation.

For patients who have (in addition to local swelling and pain) mild facial swelling, mild trismus resulting from inflammation extending into the muscles of mastication, or a low-grade fever, the dentist should consider administering an antibiotic along with irrigation delivered under pressure and extraction. The antibiotic of choice is penicillin or, in the case of penicillin allergy, clindamycin.

Pericoronitis can lead to serious fascial space infections. Because the infection begins in the posterior mouth, it can spread rapidly into the fascial spaces of the mandibular ramus and the lateral neck. If a patient has trismus (with an inability to open the mouth more than 20 mm), a temperature of greater than 101.2° F, facial swelling, pain, and malaise, the patient should be referred to an oral-maxillofacial surgeon, who is likely to admit the patient to the hospital for parenteral antibiotic administration and careful monitoring.

Patients who have had one episode of pericoronitis, although managed successfully by these methods, are highly likely to continue to have episodes of pericoronitis unless the offending mandibular third molar is removed. The patient should be informed that the tooth should be removed at the earliest possible time to prevent recurrent infections. However, the mandibular third molar should not be removed until the signs and symptoms of pericoronitis have completely resolved. The incidence of postoperative complications, specifically dry socket and postoperative infection, increases if the tooth is removed during the time of active soft tissue infection. More bleeding and slower healing also occur when a tooth is removed in the face of pericoronitis.

Prevention of pericoronitis can be achieved by removing the impacted third molars before they penetrate the oral mucosa and are visible. Although excision of the surrounding soft tissue, or operculectomy, has been advocated as a method for preventing pericoronitis without removal of the impacted tooth, it is painful and is usually ineffective. The soft tissue excess tends to recur because it drapes over the impacted tooth and causes regrowth of the operculum. The gingival pocket on the distal also remains deep after operculectomy. The overwhelming majority of cases of pericoronitis can be prevented only by extraction of the tooth.

Prevention of Root Resorption

Occasionally, an impacted tooth causes sufficient pressure on the root of an adjacent tooth to cause root resorption (Fig. 9-7). Although the process by which root resorption occurs is not well defined, it appears to be similar to the resorption process primary teeth undergo during the eruptive process of the succedaneous teeth. Removal of the impacted tooth may result in salvage of the adjacent tooth by cemental repair. Endodontic therapy may be required to save these teeth.

Impacted Teeth Under a Dental Prosthesis

When a patient has an edentulous area restored, there are several reasons that impacted teeth in the area should be removed before the prosthetic appliance is constructed. After teeth are extracted, the alveolar process slowly undergoes resorption. This is particularly true with tissue-borne prostheses. Thus the impacted tooth becomes closer to the surface of the bone, giving the appearance of erupting. The denture may compress the soft tissue onto the impacted tooth, which is no longer covered with bone; the result is ulceration of the overlying soft tissue and initiation of an odontogenic infection (Fig. 9-8).

Impacted teeth should be removed before a prosthesis is constructed because if the impacted tooth must be removed after construction, the alveolar ridge may be so altered by the extraction that the prosthesis becomes unattractive and less functional (Fig. 9-9). In addition, if removal of impacted teeth in edentulous areas is achieved before the prosthesis is made, the patient is probably in good physical condition. Waiting until the overlying bone has resorbed and ulceration with infection occurs does not produce a favorable situation for extraction. If extraction is postponed, the patient will be older and more likely to be in poorer health.

Furthermore, the mandible may have become atrophic, which increases the likelihood of fracture during tooth removal (Fig. 9-10). And if implants are planned near the position of impacted teeth, removal is warranted to eliminate the risk of interference with the implantation procedure.

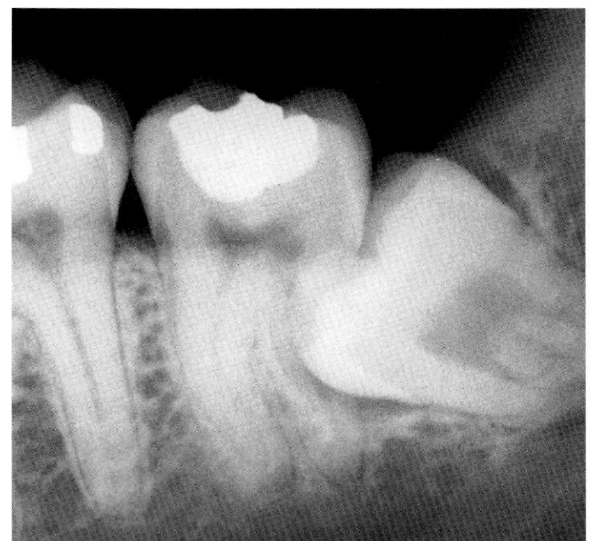

A

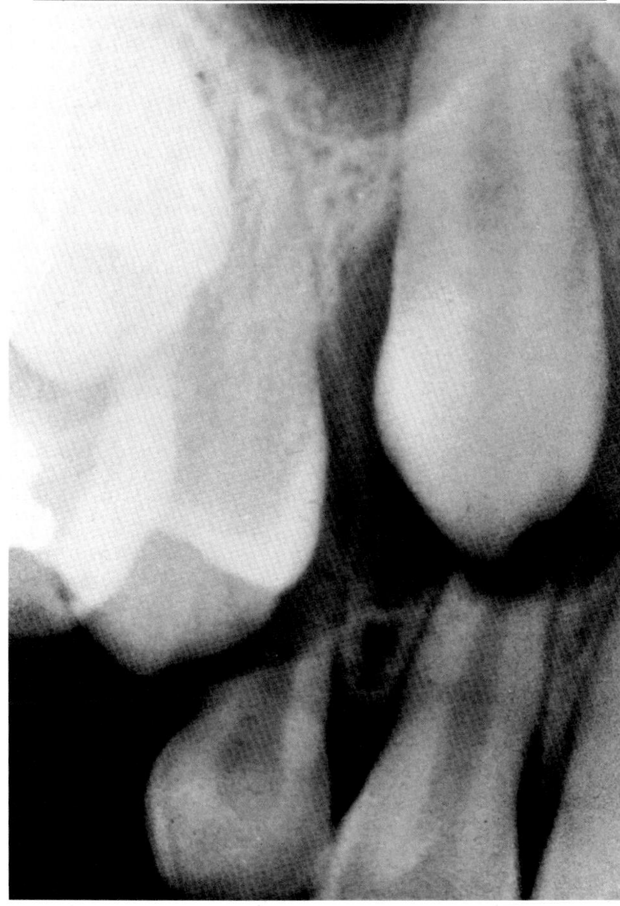

B

FIGURE 9-7 A, Root resorption of second molar as result of impacted third molar. B, Root resorption of maxillary lateral incisors as result of impacted canine.

Prevention of Odontogenic Cysts and Tumors

When impacted teeth are retained completely within the alveolar process, the associated follicular sac is also frequently retained. Although in most patients the dental follicle maintains its original size, it may undergo cystic degeneration and become a dentigerous cyst or keratocyst. If the patient is closely followed, the dentist can diagnose the cyst before it reaches large proportions (Fig. 9-11). However, unmonitored cysts can reach enormous sizes (Fig. 9-12). As a general guideline, if the follicular space around the crown of the tooth is greater than 3 mm, the preoperative diagnosis of a dentigerous cyst is reasonable.

In the same way that odontogenic cysts can occur around impacted teeth, odontogenic tumors can arise from the epithelium contained within the dental follicle. The most common odontogenic tumor to occur in this region is the ameloblastoma. Usually, ameloblastomas in this area must be treated aggressively by excision of the overlying soft tissue and of at least a portion of the mandible. Occasionally, other odontogenic tumors may occur in conjunction with impacted teeth (Fig. 9-13).

Although the overall incidence of odontogenic cysts and tumors around impacted teeth is not high,[10] the overwhelming majority of pathologic conditions of the mandibular third molar are associated with unerupted teeth. It is therefore recommended that impacted teeth be removed to prevent the occurrence of cysts and tumors.

Treatment of Pain of Unexplained Origin

Occasionally, patients come to the dentist complaining of pain in the retromolar region of the mandible for no obvious reasons. If conditions such as myofascial pain dysfunction syndrome and other facial pain disorders are excluded and if the patient has an unerupted tooth, removal of the tooth sometimes results in resolution of the pain.

Prevention of Jaw Fractures

An impacted third molar in the mandible occupies space that is usually filled with bone. This weakens the mandible and renders the jaw more susceptible to fracture at the site of the impacted tooth (Fig. 9-14). If the jaw fractures through the area of an impacted third molar, the impacted third molar is frequently removed before the fracture is reduced, and intermaxillary fixation is applied (see Chapter 24).

Facilitation of Orthodontic Treatment

When patients require retraction of first and second molars by orthodontic techniques, the presence of impacted third molars may interfere with the treatment. It is therefore recommended that impacted third molars be removed before orthodontic therapy is begun.[11,12]

Some orthodontic approaches to a malocclusion might benefit from the placement of retromolar implants to provide distal anchorage. When this is planned, removal of impacted lower third molars is necessary.

Optimal Periodontal Healing

As noted before, one of the most important indications for removal of impacted third molars is to preserve the periodontal health of the adjacent second molar. A great deal of attention has been given to the two primary parameters of periodontal health after third molar surgery, that is, bone height and periodontal attachment level on the distal aspect of the second molar.

Recent studies have provided information on which to base the likelihood of optimal periodontal tissue healing.[13-15] The two most important factors have been shown to be the extent of the preoperative infrabony defect on the distal aspect of the second molar and the patient's age at the time of surgery. If a large amount of distal bone is missing because of the presence

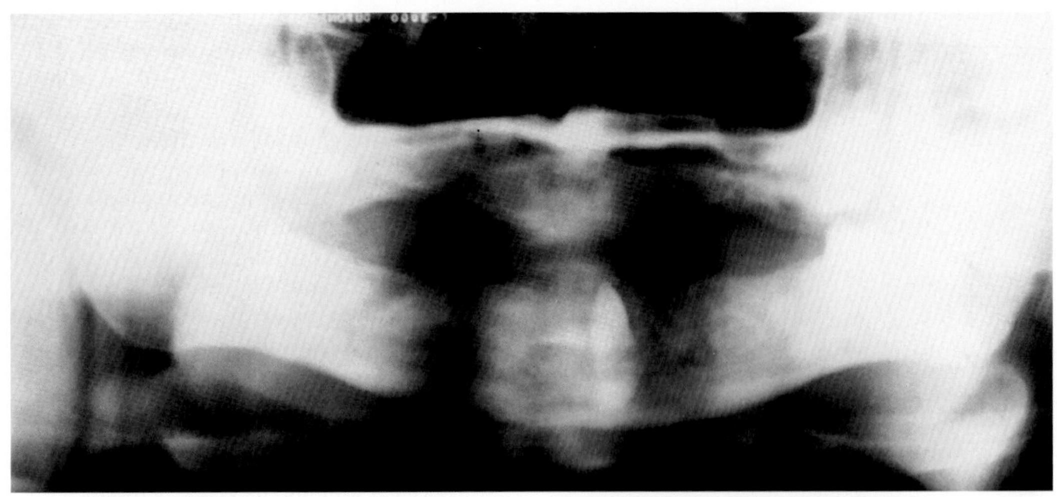

FIGURE 9-8 Impacted tooth retained under denture. Tooth is now at surface and is causing infection.

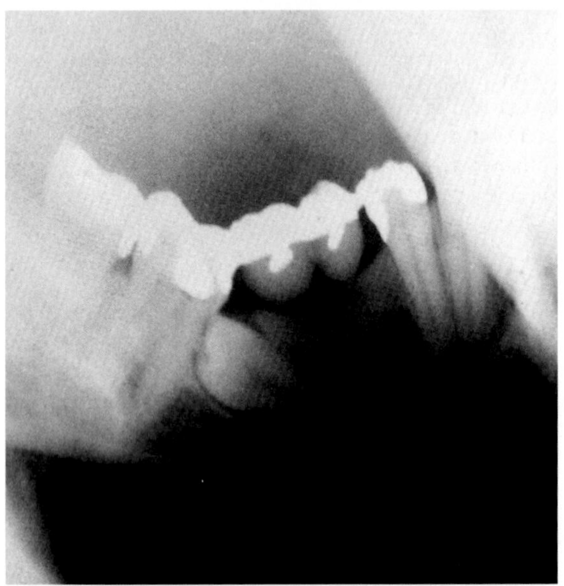

FIGURE 9-9 Impacted tooth under fixed bridge. Tooth must be removed and therefore may jeopardize bridge.

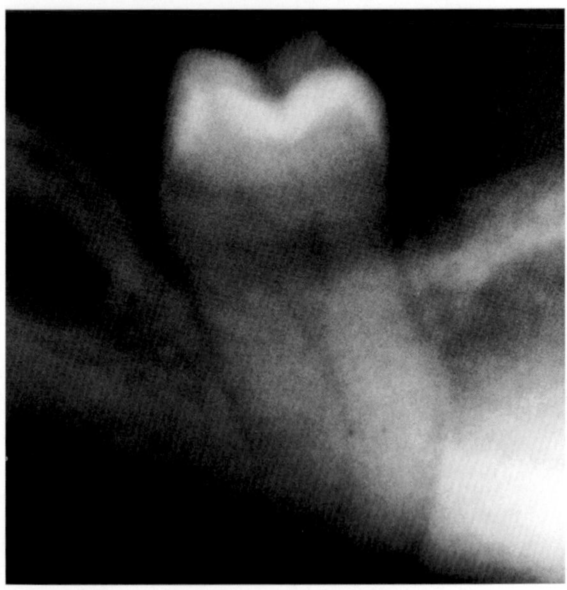

FIGURE 9-10 Impaction in atrophic mandible, which may result in jaw fracture during extraction.

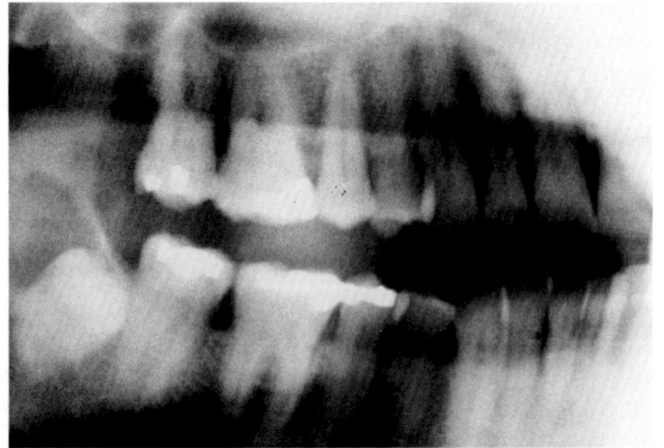

FIGURE 9-11 Small dentigerous cyst arising around impacted tooth.

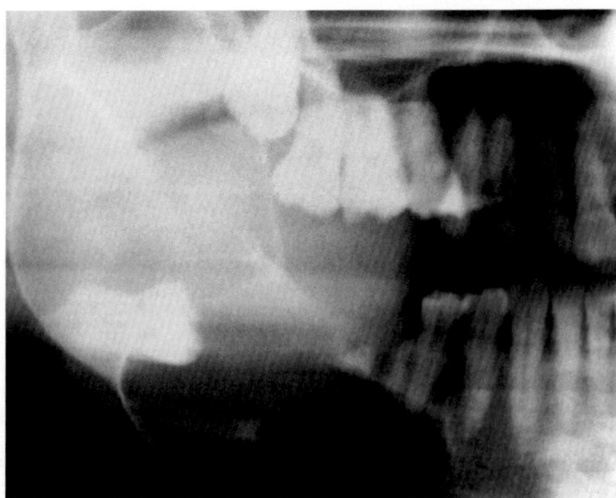

FIGURE 9-12 Large dentigerous cyst that extends from coronoid process to mental foramen. Cyst has displaced impacted third molar to inferior border of mandible.

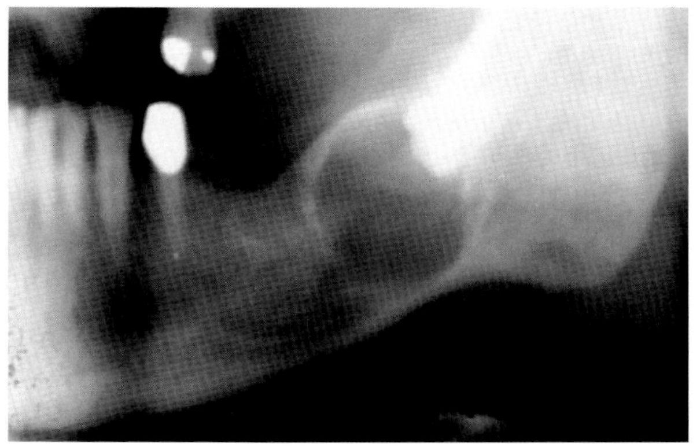

FIGURE 9-13 Ameloblastoma associated with crown of impacted third molar. (Courtesy Dr. Frances Gordy.)

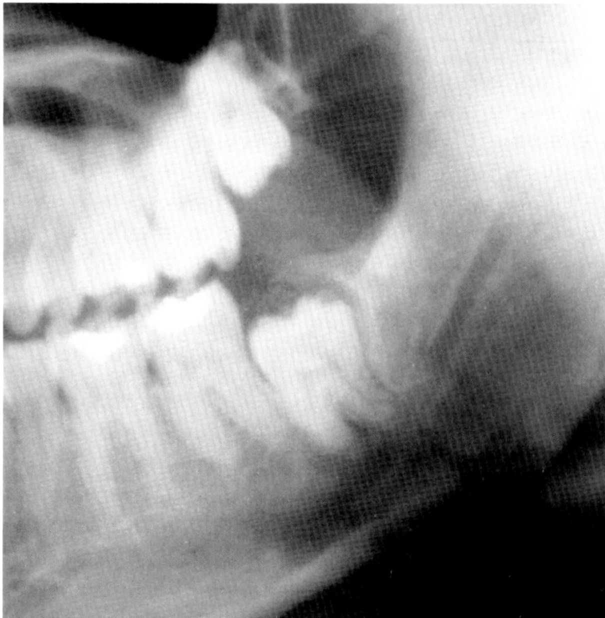

FIGURE 9-14 Fracture of mandible that occurred through location of impacted third molar.

of the impacted tooth and its associated follicle, it is less likely that the infrabony pocket can be decreased. Likewise, if the patient is older, then the likelihood of optimal bony healing is decreased. Patients whose third molars are removed before age 25 are more likely to have better bone healing than those whose impacted teeth are removed after age 25. In the younger patient, not only is the initial periodontal healing better, but the long-term continued regeneration of the periodontium is clearly better.[14]

As mentioned previously, unerupted teeth may continue to erupt until age 25. Because the terminal portion of the eruption process occurs slowly, the chance of developing pericoronitis increases, and so does the amount of contact between the third molar and second molar. Both of these factors decrease the possibility for optimal periodontal healing. However, it should be noted that the asymptomatic completely bony impacted third molar in a patient older than age 30 should probably be left in place unless some specific pathologic condition develops. Removal of such asymptomatic completely impacted third molars in older patients clearly results in pocket depths and alveolar bone loss, which are greater than if the tooth were left in place.

CONTRAINDICATIONS FOR REMOVAL OF IMPACTED TEETH

All impacted teeth should be removed unless specific contraindications justify leaving them in position. When the potential benefits outweigh the potential complications and risks, the procedure should be performed. Similarly, when the risks are greater than the potential benefits, the procedure should be deferred.

Contraindications for the removal of impacted teeth primarily involve the patient's physical status.

Extremes of Age

The third molar tooth bud can be radiographically visualized by age 6. Some surgeons think that removal of the tooth bud at age 7 to 9 can be accomplished with minimal surgical morbidity and therefore should be performed at this age. However, most surgeons believe that it is not possible to predict accurately if the forming third molar will be impacted. The consensus is that very early removal of third molars should be deferred until an accurate diagnosis of impaction can be made.

The most common contraindication for the removal of impacted teeth is advanced age. As a patient ages, the bone becomes highly calcified and therefore less flexible and less likely to bend under the forces of tooth extraction. The result is that more bone must be surgically removed to displace the tooth from its socket.

Similarly, as patients age, they respond less favorably and with more postoperative sequelae. An 18-year-old patient may have 1 or 2 days of discomfort and swelling after the removal of an impacted tooth, whereas a similar procedure may result in a 4- or 5-day recovery period for a 50-year-old patient.

Finally, if a tooth has been retained in the alveolar process for many years without periodontal disease, caries, or cystic degeneration, it is unlikely that these unfavorable sequelae will occur. Therefore in an older patient (usually over age 35) with an impacted tooth that shows no signs of disease and that has a radiographically detectable layer of overlying bone, the tooth should not be removed (Fig. 9-15). The dentist caring for the patient should check the impacted tooth radiographically every 1 or 2 years to ensure that no adverse sequelae occur.

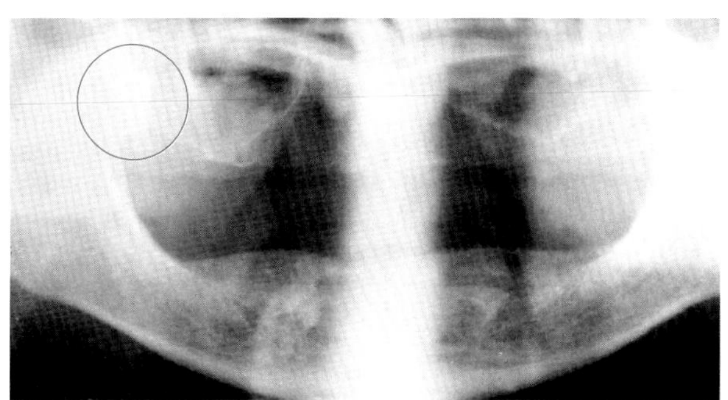

FIGURE 9-15 Impacted maxillary right third molar in 63-year-old patient. This molar should not be extracted because it is deeply embedded and no signs of disease are present.

If the impacted tooth shows signs of cystic formation or periodontal disease involving the adjacent tooth or the impacted tooth, if it is a single impacted tooth underneath a prosthesis with thin overlying bone, or if it becomes symptomatic as the result of infection, the tooth should be removed.

Compromised Medical Status

A compromised medical status may contraindicate the removal of an impacted tooth. Frequently, compromised medical status and advancing age go hand in hand. If the impacted tooth is asymptomatic, its surgical removal must be viewed as elective. If the patient's cardiovascular or respiratory function or host defenses for combating infection are seriously compromised or if the patient has a serious acquired or congenital coagulopathy, the surgeon should consider leaving the tooth in the alveolar process. However, if the tooth becomes symptomatic, the surgeon should consider working with the patient's physician to plan removal of the tooth with the least operative and post-operative medical sequelae.

Probable Excessive Damage to Adjacent Structures

If the impacted tooth lies in an area in which its removal may seriously jeopardize adjacent nerves, teeth, or previously constructed bridges, it may be prudent to leave the tooth in place. When the dentist makes the decision not to remove a tooth, the reasons must be weighed against potential future complications. For younger patients who may have the sequelae of impacted teeth, it may be wise to remove the tooth while taking special measures to prevent damage to adjacent structures. However, for the older patient with no signs of impending complications and for whom the probability of such complications is low, the impacted tooth should not be removed. A classic example of such a case is the older patient with a potentially severe periodontal defect on the distal aspect of the second molar but in whom removal of the third molar would almost surely result in the loss of the second molar. In this situation the impacted tooth should not be removed.

Summary

The preceding discussion of indications and contraindications for the removal of impacted third molars has been designed to point out that there are various risks and benefits for removing impacted teeth in patients. Patients who have one or more pathologic symptoms or problems should have their impacted teeth removed. Most of the symptomatic, pathologic problems that result from impacted third molars occur because of partially erupted teeth and occur less commonly with a complete bony impaction.

Less clear is what should be done with impacted teeth before they cause symptoms or problems. In making a decision as to whether an impacted third molar should be removed, one must consider a variety of factors. First, the available room in the arch into which the tooth can erupt must be considered. If adequate room exists, then the clinician may choose to defer removal of the tooth until eruption is complete. A second consideration is the status of the impacted tooth and the age of the patient. It is critical to remember that the average age of complete eruption is 20 but that eruption may continue to occur up to age 25. A tooth that appears to be a mesioangular impaction at age 17 may eventually become more vertical and erupt into the mouth. If insufficient room exists to accommodate the tooth and a soft tissue operculum exists over the posterior aspect, then pathologic sequelae are likely to occur.

Although there have been some attempts at making very early predictions of whether a tooth is going to be impacted, these efforts have not yet resulted in a reliable predictive model. However, by the time the patient reaches age 18, the dentist can reasonably predict whether there will be adequate room into which the tooth can erupt with sufficient clearance of the anterior ramus to prevent soft tissue operculum formation. At this time, if surgical removal is chosen, soft tissue and bone tissue healing will occur at its maximal level. At age 18 or 19, if the diagnosis for inadequate room for functional eruption can be made, then the asymptomatic third molar can be removed and the long-term periodontal health of the second molar will be maximized.

CLASSIFICATION SYSTEMS OF IMPACTED TEETH

Removal of impacted teeth can be relatively straightforward or extremely difficult, even for the experienced surgeon. To determine the degree of difficulty preoperatively, the surgeon should examine the clinical circumstances methodically. The primary factor determining the difficulty of the removal is accessibility. Accessibility is determined by adjacent teeth or other structures impairing access or delivery pathway, and the ease of exposing the tooth, of preparing a pathway for its delivery, and of preparing or taking advantage of a preexisting purchase point. With careful classification of the impacted teeth using a variety of systems, the surgeon can approach the proposed surgery in an orderly fashion and predict whether any extraordinary surgical approaches will be necessary or if the patient will encounter certain postoperative problems.

The majority of classification schemes are based on analysis of a radiograph. The panoramic radiograph shows the most accurate picture of the total anatomy of the region and is the radiograph of choice for planning removal of impacted third molars. In some circumstances a well-positioned periapical radiograph is adequate as long as all parts of the impacted tooth are visible along with important adjacent anatomy. When the roots of a lower third molar appear very close to or superimpose over the inferior alveolar canal on a panoramic radiograph, a cone-beam CT scan may be useful. This imaging technique can actually show the relationship of the roots to the canal.

For each patient the surgeon should carefully analyze the factors discussed in this section. By combining these factors, the dentist can assess the difficulty of the surgery and elect to extract the impacted teeth that are within his or her skill level. However, for the patient's well-being and the dentist's peace of mind, the patient should be referred to a specialist if a tooth presents a difficult surgical situation or the dentist cannot offer optimal pain and anxiety control.

Angulation

The most commonly used classification system with respect to treatment planning uses a determination of the angulation of the long axis of the impacted third molar with respect to the long axis of the adjacent second molar. Teeth at certain inclinations have ready-made pathways for removal, whereas pathways for teeth of other inclinations require the removal of substantial amounts of bone. This classification system provides an initial useful evaluation of the difficulty of extractions but is not sufficient by itself to define difficulty of molar removal fully.

The impaction generally acknowledged as the least difficult impaction to remove is the mesioangular, particularly when only partially impacted (Fig. 9-16). The mesioangular-impacted tooth is tilted toward the second molar in a mesial direction. This type of impaction is the most commonly seen, making up approximately 43% of all impacted teeth.

When the long axis of the third molar is perpendicular to the second molar, the impacted tooth is considered horizontal (Fig. 9-17). This type of impaction is usually considered more difficult to remove than the mesioangular impaction. Horizontal impactions occur less frequently, being seen in approximately 3% of all mandibular impactions.

In the vertical impaction the long axis of the impacted tooth runs parallel to the long axis of the second molar. This impaction occurs with the second greatest frequency, accounting for approximately 38% of all impactions, and is third in difficulty of removal (Fig. 9-18).

Finally, the distoangular impaction is the tooth with the most difficult angulation for removal (Fig. 9-19). In the distoangular impaction the long axis of the third molar is distally or posteriorly angled away from the second molar. This impaction is the most difficult to remove because the tooth has a withdrawal pathway that runs into the mandibular ramus, and its removal requires significant surgical intervention. Distoangular impactions occur uncommonly and account for only approximately 6% of all impacted third molars. Erupted third molars may be in a distoangular position. When this occurs, they are much more difficult to remove than other erupted teeth. The reason is that the third molar's mesial root is very close to the root of the second molar.

In addition to the relationship between the angulation of the long axes of the second and third molars, the teeth can also be angled in buccal, lingual, or palatal directions. When approaching lower third molars, the possible presence of a high-riding lingual nerve still makes a buccal approach appropriate even when the tooth is inclined toward the lingual.

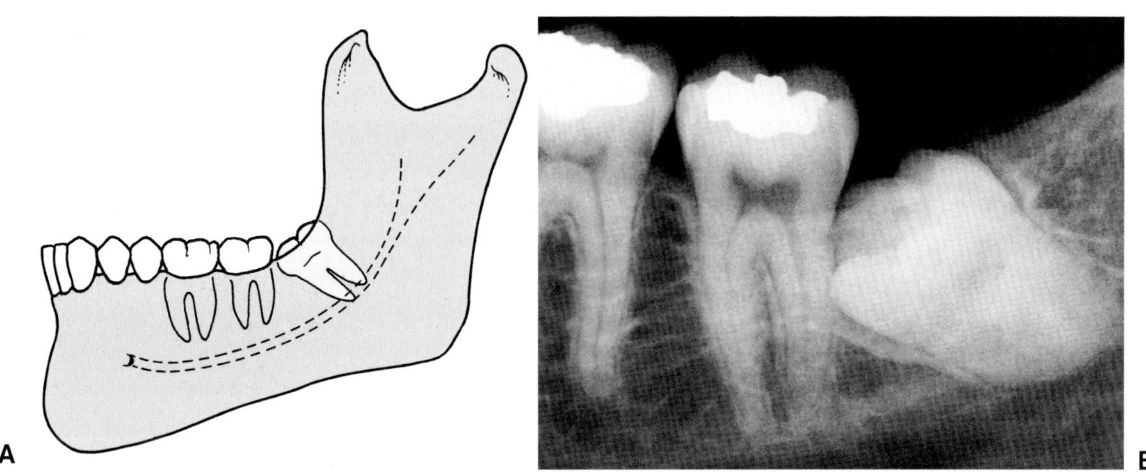

FIGURE 9-16 A, Mesioangular impaction—most common and easiest impaction to remove. B, Mesioangular impaction is usually in proximity to second molar.

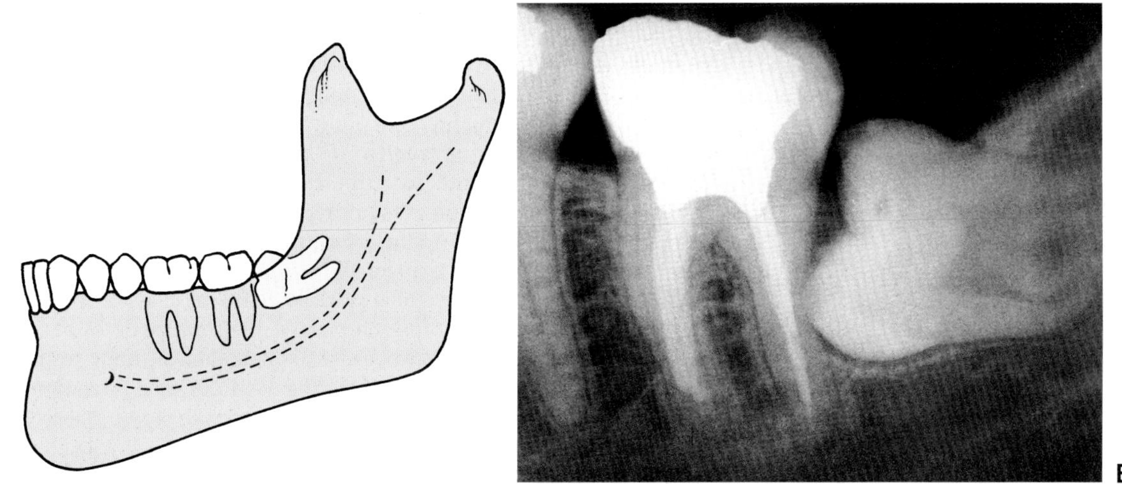

FIGURE 9-17 A, Horizontal impaction—uncommon and more difficult to remove than mesioangular impaction. B, Occlusal surface of horizontal impacted third molar is usually immediately adjacent to root of second molar, which often produces early severe periodontal disease.

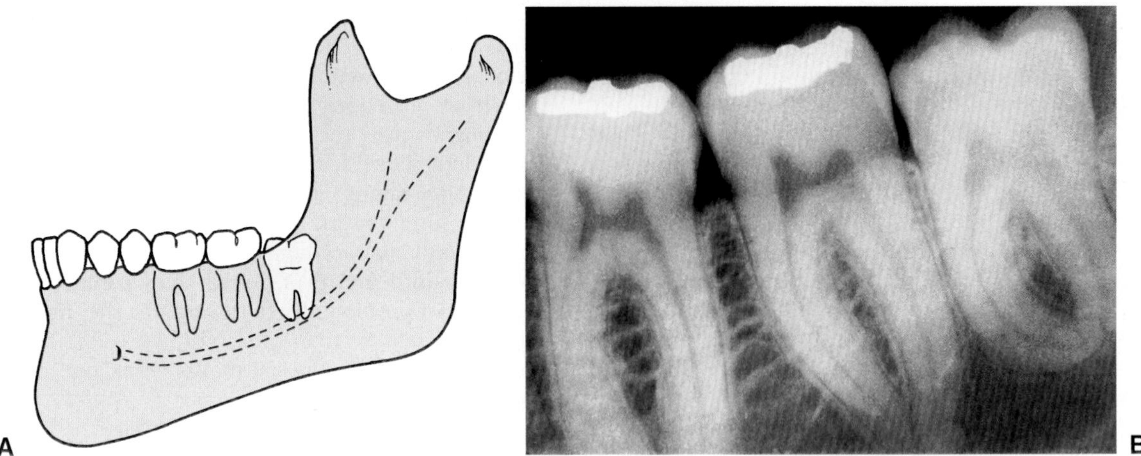

FIGURE 9-18 A, Vertical impaction—second most common impaction and second most difficult to remove. B, Vertical impaction is frequently covered on its posterior aspect with bone of anterior ramus of mandible.

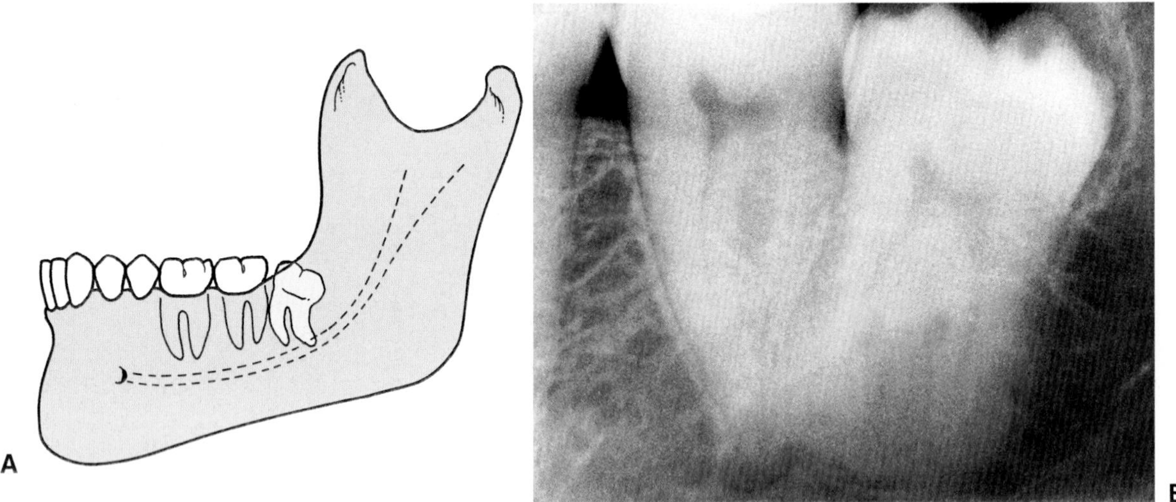

FIGURE 9-19 A, Distoangular impaction—uncommon and most difficult of the four types to remove. B, Occlusal surface of distoangular impaction is usually embedded in ramus of mandible and requires significant bone removal for extraction.

Rarely, a tooth is a transverse impaction, that is, in an absolutely horizontal position in a buccolingual direction. The occlusal surface of the tooth can face the buccal or lingual direction. To determine buccal or lingual version accurately, the dentist must take a perpendicular occlusal film. However, this determination is usually not necessary because the surgeon can make this identification early in the operation, and the buccal or lingual position of the tooth does not greatly influence the approach to the surgery.

Relationship to Anterior Border of Ramus

Another method for classifying impacted mandibular third molars is based on the amount of impacted tooth that is covered with the bone of the mandibular ramus. This classification is known as the *Pell and Gregory classification* and is sometimes referred to as the *Pell and Gregory classes 1, 2,* and *3*. For this classification it is important that the surgeon carefully examine the relationship between the tooth and the anterior part of the ramus. If the mesiodistal diameter of the crown is completely anterior to the anterior border of the mandibular ramus, it is in a class 1 relationship. If the tooth is angled in a vertical direction, the chances for the tooth to erupt into a normal position are good if root formation is incomplete (Fig. 9-20).

If the tooth is positioned posteriorly so that approximately one half is covered by the ramus, the relationship of the tooth with the ramus is class 2. In the class 2 situation the tooth cannot erupt completely free from bone over the crown and distal aspect because a small shelf of bone overlies the distal portion of the tooth (Fig. 9-21). A class 3 relationship between the tooth and ramus occurs when the tooth is located completely within the mandibular ramus (Fig. 9-22). Obviously, the class 1 relationship provides the greatest accessibility to the impacted tooth and therefore such a tooth is the easiest to remove. The class 3 relationship provides the least accessibility and therefore presents the greatest difficulty.

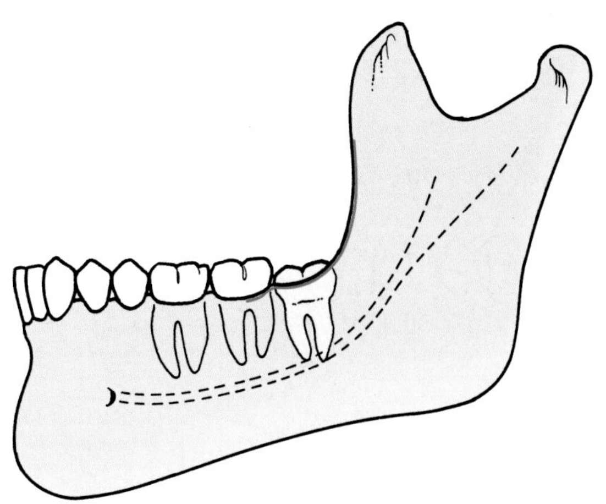

FIGURE 9-20 Pell and Gregory class 1 impaction. Mandibular third molar has sufficient anteroposterior room (i.e., anterior-to-anterior border of ramus) to erupt.

Relationship to Occlusal Plane

The depth of the impacted tooth compared with the height of the adjacent second molar provides the next classification system for determining the difficulty of impaction removal. This classification system was also suggested by Pell and Gregory and is called *Pell and Gregory A, B,* and *C* classification. In this classification the degree of difficulty is measured by the thickness of the overlying bone; that is, the degree of difficulty increases as the depth of the impacted tooth increases. As the tooth becomes less accessible and it becomes more difficult to section the tooth and to prepare purchase points, the overall difficulty of the operation substantially increases.

A class A impaction is one in which the occlusal surface of the impacted tooth is level or nearly level with the occlusal plane of the second molar (Fig. 9-23). A class B impaction is an impacted tooth with an occlusal surface between the occlusal plane and the cervical line of the second molar (Fig. 9-24). Finally, the class C impaction is one in which the occlusal surface of the impacted tooth is below the cervical line of the second molar (Fig. 9-25).

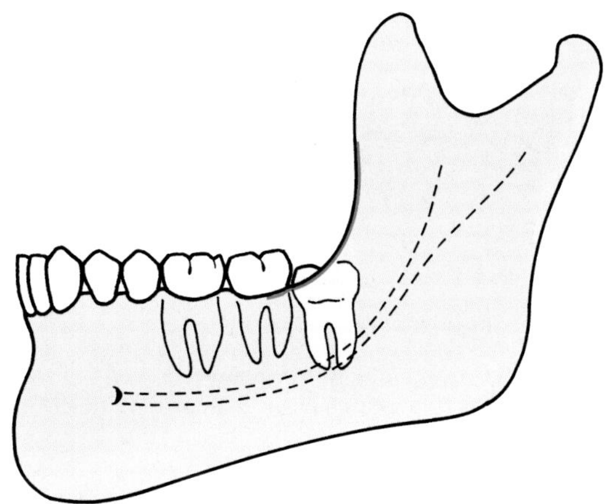

FIGURE 9-21 Pell and Gregory class 2 impaction. Approximately half is covered by anterior portion of ramus of mandible.

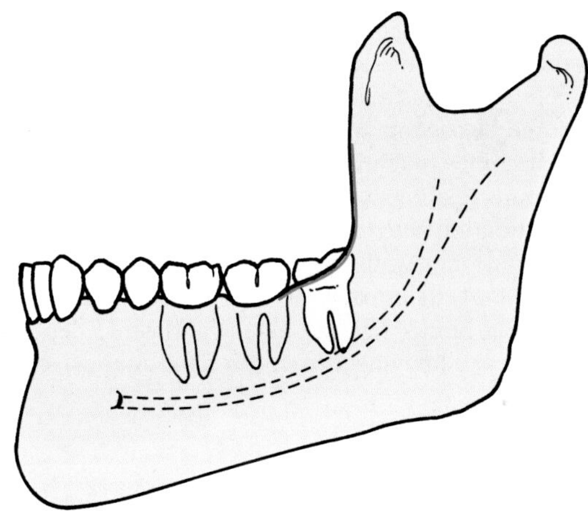

FIGURE 9-23 Pell and Gregory class A impaction. Occlusal plane of impacted tooth is at same level as occlusal plane of second molar.

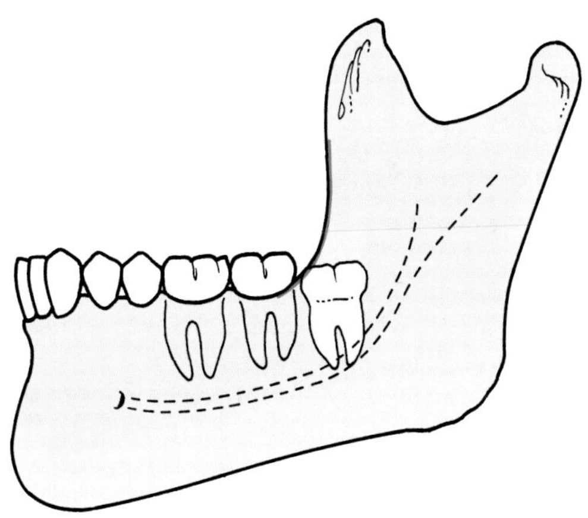

FIGURE 9-22 Pell and Gregory class 3 impaction. Impacted third molar is completely embedded in bone of ramus of mandible.

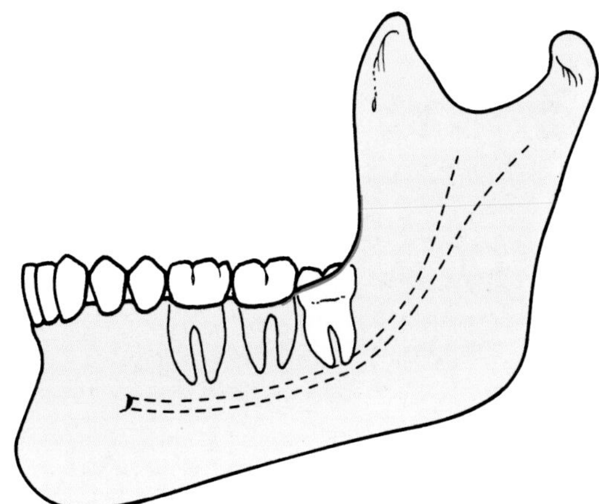

FIGURE 9-24 Pell and Gregory class B impaction. Occlusal plane of impacted tooth is between occlusal plane and cervical line of second molar.

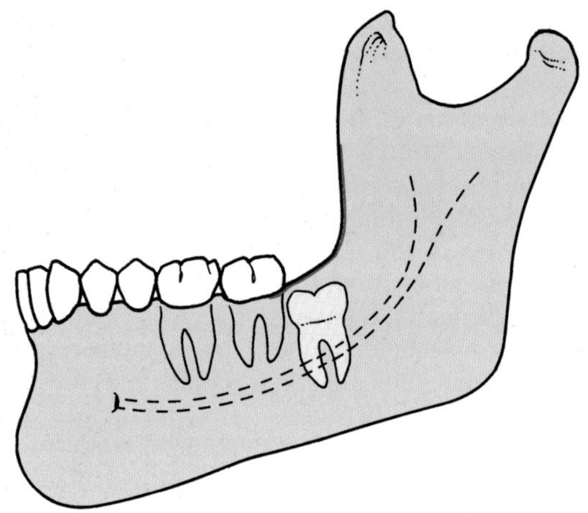

FIGURE 9-25 Pell and Gregory class C impaction. Impacted tooth is below cervical line of second molar.

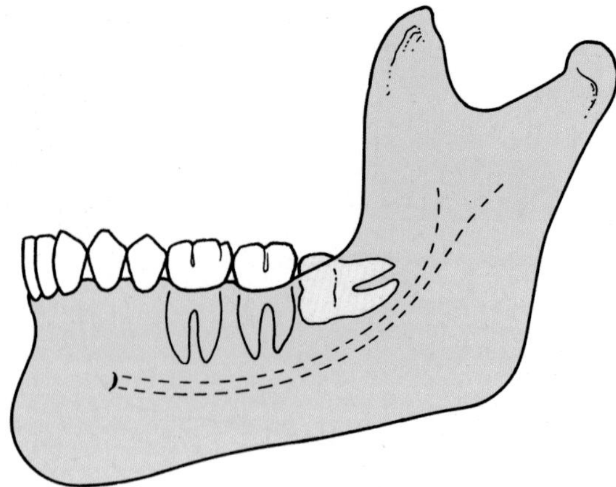

FIGURE 9-27 Horizontal impaction with class 2 ramus relationship and class B depth makes it moderately difficult to extract.

Summary

The three classification systems discussed so far are used in conjunction to determine the difficulty of an extraction. For example, a mesioangular impaction with a class 1 ramus and a class A depth is usually straightforward to remove (Fig. 9-26). However, as the ramus relationship changes to a class 2 and the depth of the impaction increases to a class B, the degree of difficulty becomes much greater. A horizontal impaction with a class 2 ramus relationship and a class B depth is a moderately difficult extraction and one that most experienced general practitioners do not want to attempt (Fig. 9-27). Finally, the most difficult of all impactions is a distoangular impaction with a class 3 ramus relationship at a class C depth. Even specialists view removing this tooth as a surgical challenge (Fig. 9-28).

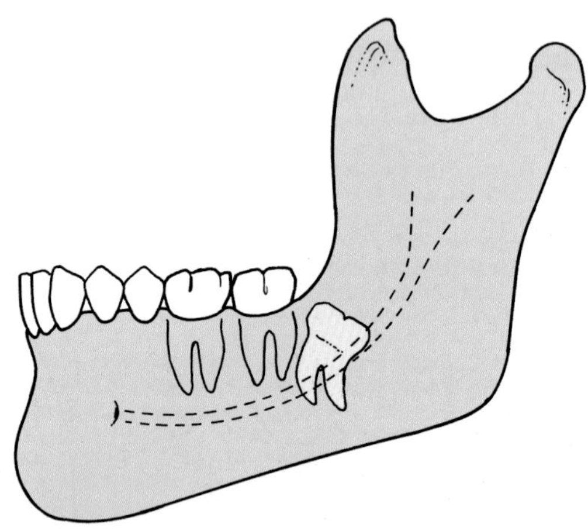

FIGURE 9-28 Impaction with distoangular, class 3 ramus relationship and class C depth makes it extremely difficult to remove safely.

ROOT MORPHOLOGY

Just as the root morphology of the erupted tooth has a major influence on the degree of difficulty of a closed extraction, root morphology plays a major role in determining the degree of difficulty of the removal of an impacted tooth. Several factors must be considered when assessing the morphologic structure of the root.

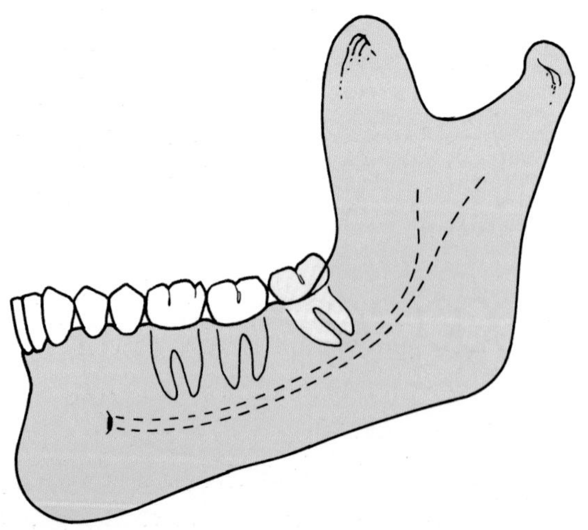

FIGURE 9-26 Mesioangular impaction with class 1 ramus relationship and class A depth. All three classifications make it easiest type of impaction to remove.

The first consideration is the length of the root. As discussed before, the optimal time for removal of an impacted tooth is when the root is one third to two thirds formed. When this is the case, the ends of the roots are blunt (Fig. 9-29). If the tooth is not removed during a formative stage and the entire length of the root develops, the possibility increases for abnormal root morphology and for fracture of the root tips during extraction or the root tips impeding root delivery. If the root development is limited (i.e., less than one third complete), the tooth is often more difficult to remove because it tends to roll in its socket like a marble, which prevents routine elevation (Fig. 9-30). The next factor to be assessed is whether the roots are fused into a single, conical root (Fig. 9-31) or whether they are separate and distinct roots. The fused, conical roots are more straightforward to remove than widely separated roots (Fig. 9-32).

The curvature of the tooth roots also plays a role in the difficulty of the extraction. Severely curved or dilacerated roots are more difficult to remove than straight or slightly curved

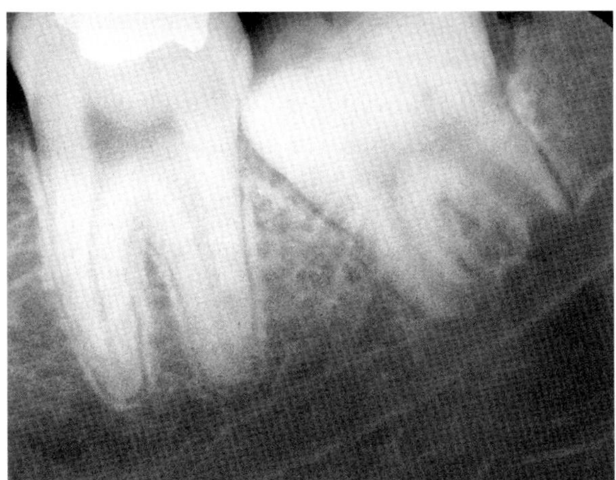

FIGURE 9-29 Roots that are two thirds formed, which are less difficult to remove.

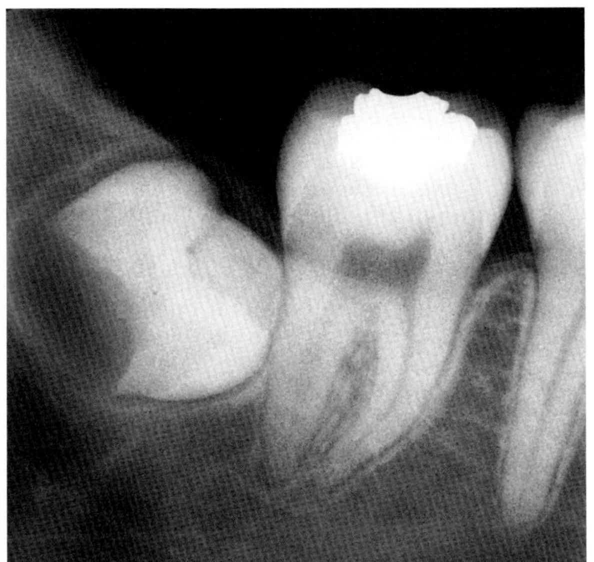

FIGURE 9-30 Lack of root development. If extraction is attempted, crown will often roll around in crypt, making it difficult to remove.

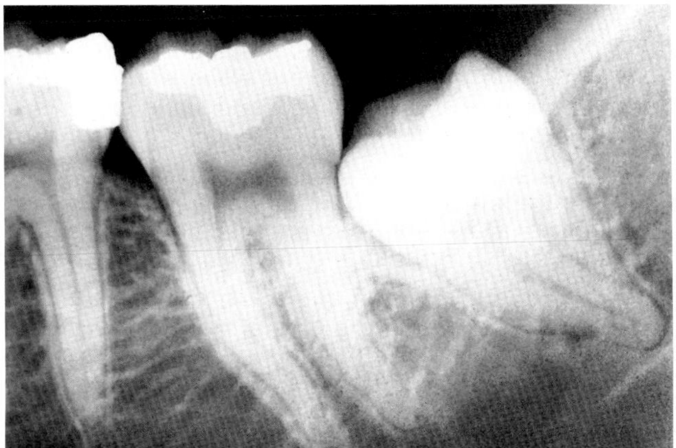

FIGURE 9-31 Fused roots with conical shape.

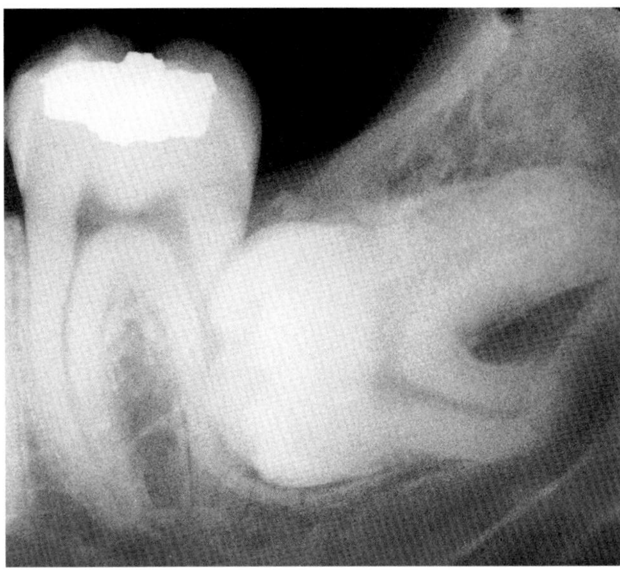

FIGURE 9-32 Divergent roots with severe curvature. Such roots are more difficult to remove.

roots (Fig. 9-32). The surgeon should carefully examine the apical area of impacted teeth on the radiograph to assess the presence of small, abnormal, and sharply hooked roots that will probably fracture if the surgeon does not give them special consideration.

The direction of the tooth root curvature is also important to examine preoperatively. During removal of a mesioangular impaction, roots that are curved gently in the distal direction (following along the pathway of extraction) can be removed without the force that can fracture the roots. However, if the roots of a mesioangular impaction are straight or curved mesially, the roots commonly fracture if the tooth is not sectioned before being delivered.

The total width of the roots in the mesiodistal direction should be compared with the width of the tooth at the cervical line. If the tooth root width is greater, the extraction will be more difficult. More bone must be removed, or the tooth should be sectioned before extraction.

Finally, the surgeon should assess the periodontal ligament space. Although in most patients the periodontal ligament space is of normal dimensions, it sometimes is wider or narrower. The wider the periodontal ligament space, typically the easier the tooth is to remove (Fig. 9-33). However, older patients, especially those over age 40, tend to have a much narrower periodontal ligament space that increases the difficulty of the extraction.

Size of Follicular Sac

The size of the follicle around the impacted tooth can help determine the difficulty of the extraction. If the follicular sac is wide (almost cystic in size), much less bone must be removed, which makes the tooth more straightforward to extract (Fig. 9-34). (Young patients are more likely to have large follicles, which is another factor that makes extractions less complex in younger patients.) However, if the follicular space around the crown of the tooth is narrow or nonexistent, the surgeon must create space around the crown, increasing the difficulty of the procedure and usually the time required to remove the tooth.

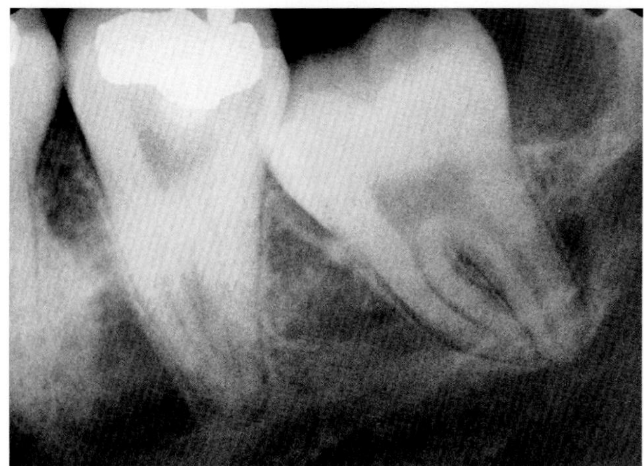

FIGURE 9-33 Wide periodontal ligament space. The widened space makes extraction process less difficult.

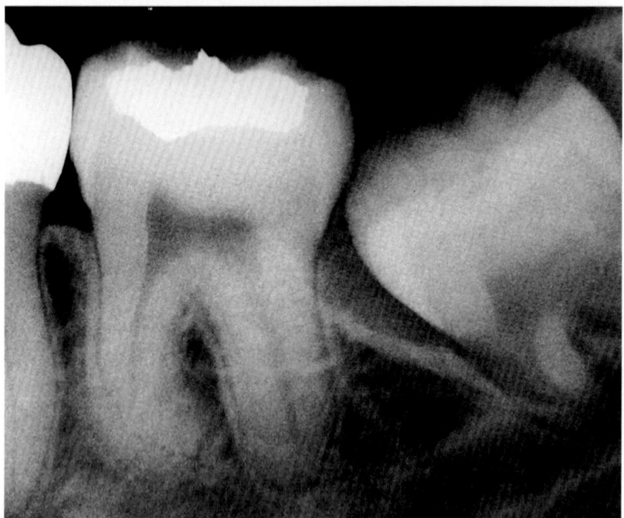

FIGURE 9-34 Large follicular sac. When space of sac is large, amount of bone removal required is decreased.

Density of Surrounding Bone

The density of the bone surrounding the tooth plays a role in determining the difficulty of the extraction. Although some clues can be seen on the radiographs, variations in radiographic density and angulation render bone density interpretations based on radiographs unreliable. Bone density is best determined by the patient's age. Patients who are 18 years of age or younger have bone densities favorable for tooth removal. The bone is less dense, is more likely to be pliable, and expands and bends somewhat, which allows the socket to be expanded by elevators or by luxation forces applied to the tooth itself. Additionally, the less dense bone is easier to cut with a dental bur and can be removed more rapidly than denser bone.

Conversely, patients who are older than age 35 have much denser bone and thus decreased flexibility and ability to expand. In these patients the surgeon must remove all interfering bone, because it is not possible to expand the bony socket. In addition, as the bone increases in density, it becomes more difficult to remove with a dental bur, and the bone removal process takes longer. Also, excessive force is more likely to fracture very dense bone compared with less dense bone of a similar cross section.

Contact with Mandibular Second Molar

If space exists between the second molar and the impacted third molar, the extraction will be easier to approach because damage to the second molar is less likely. However, if the tooth is a distoangular or horizontal impaction, it is frequently in direct contact with the adjacent second molar. To remove the third molar safely without injuring the second molar, the surgeon must be cautious with pressure from elevators or with the bur when removing bone. If the second molar has caries or a large restoration or has been endodontically treated, the surgeon must take special care not to fracture the restoration or a portion of the carious crown. The patient should still be forewarned of this possibility (see Fig. 9-17, *B*).

Relationship to Inferior Alveolar Nerve

Impacted mandibular third molars frequently have roots that are superimposed on the inferior alveolar canal on radiographs. Although the canal is usually on the buccal aspect of the tooth, it is still in proximity to the roots. Therefore, one of the potential sequelae of impacted third molar removal is damage to the inferior alveolar nerve. This commonly results in some altered sensation (paresthesia or anesthesia) of the lower lip and chin on the injured side. Although this altered sensation is usually brief (lasting only a few days), it may extend for weeks or months; on rare occasions it can be permanent. The duration depends on the extent of nerve damage. If the root ends of the tooth appear to be close to the inferior alveolar canal on a radiograph, the surgeon must take special care to avoid injuring the nerve (Fig. 9-35), which greatly increases the difficulty of the procedure. The increasing availability of cone-beam computerized tomographic scans will make preoperative assessment of the root and canal relationship easier to view, helping guide surgical decisions.

Nature of Overlying Tissue

The preceding systems classify factors that make third molar extraction more straightforward or difficult. The classification system discussed now does not fit into these categories. However, this classification is the system used by most dental insurance companies and is the one by which the surgeon charges for the services.

The dental insurance companies separate types of third molar impactions into three categories. The three types of impactions are (1) soft tissue, (2) partial bony, and (3) full bony. An impaction is defined as a *soft tissue impaction* when the height of the contour of the tooth is above the level of the alveolar bone, and the superficial portion of the tooth is covered only by soft tissue (Fig. 9-36). To remove the soft tissue impaction, the surgeon must incise the soft tissue and reflect a soft tissue flap to obtain access to the tooth to elevate it from its socket. The soft tissue impaction is usually the easiest of the three extractions but can be complex based on factors discussed in the preceding sections.

The *partial bony impaction* occurs when the superficial portion of the tooth is covered by soft tissue but at least a portion of the height of the contour of the tooth is below the level of the surrounding alveolar bone (Fig. 9-37). To remove the tooth, the surgeon must incise the soft tissue, reflect a soft tissue flap, and remove the bone above the height of the

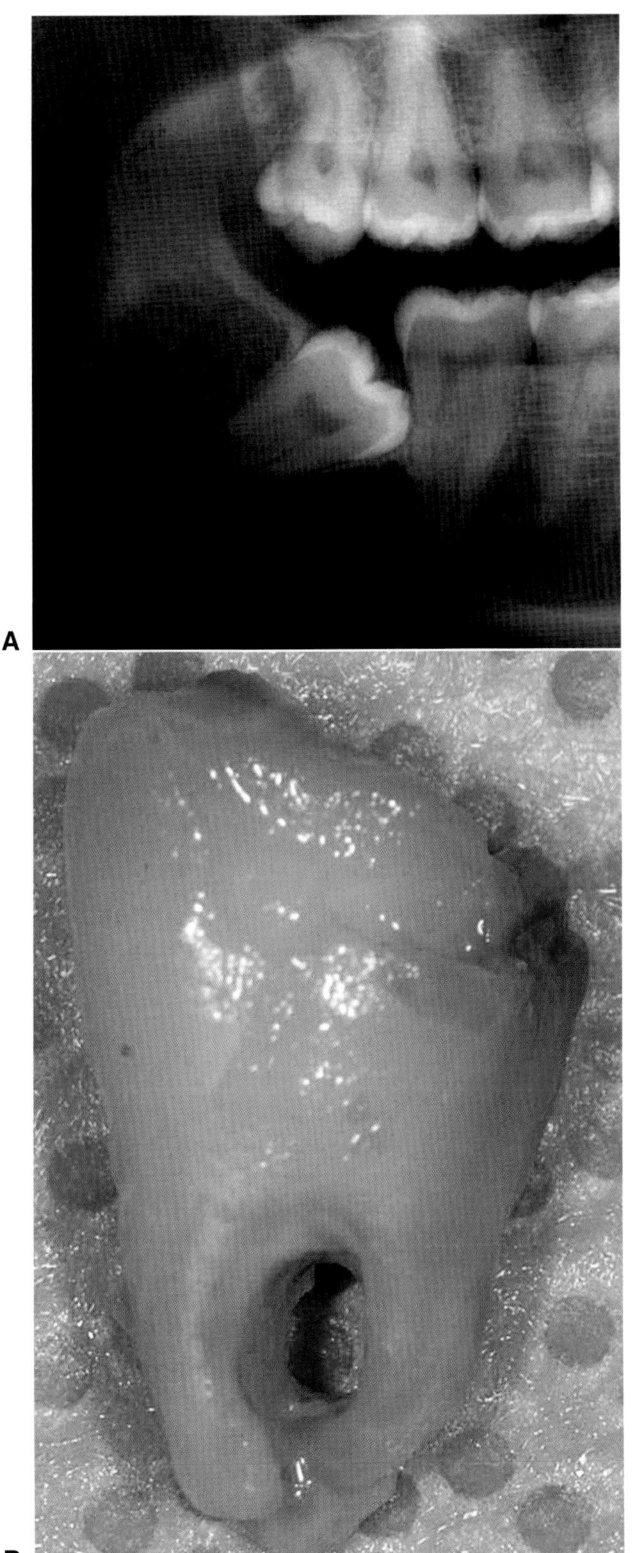

FIGURE 9-35 A, Radiographic view of mandibular third molar that suggests proximity to the inferior alveolar nerve. B, Hole through the root of the third molar seen in the radiograph after removal. During removal, inferior alveolar neurovascular bundle was severed. (Courtesy Dr. Edward Ellis III.)

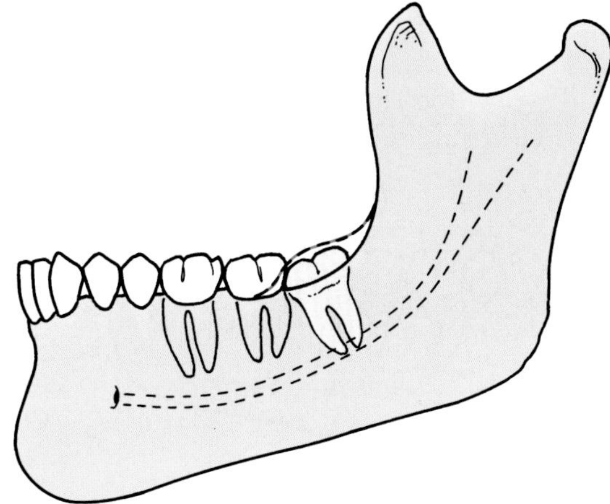

FIGURE 9-36 Soft tissue impaction in which crown of tooth is covered by soft tissue only and can be removed without bone removal.

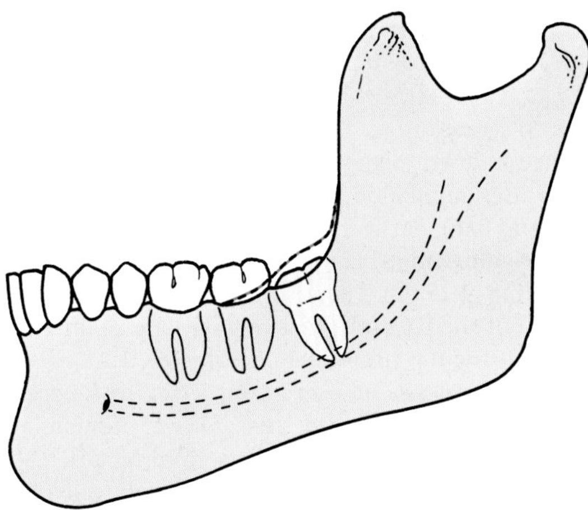

FIGURE 9-37 Partial bony impaction in which part of tooth, usually posterior aspect, is covered with bone and requires bone removal or tooth sectioning for extraction.

contour. The surgeon may need to divide the tooth in addition to removing bone. A partial bony impacted tooth is commonly more difficult to remove than a full bony impacted third molar.

The *complete bony impaction* is an impacted tooth that is completely encased in bone so that, when the surgeon reflects the soft tissue flap, no tooth is visible (Fig. 9-38). To remove the tooth, extensive amounts of bone must be removed, and the tooth almost always requires sectioning.

Although this classification is extensively used, it frequently has no relationship to the difficulty of the extraction or the likelihood of complications (Boxes 9-1 and 9-2). The parameters of angulation, ramus relationship, root morphology, and patient age are more relevant to treatment planning than the system used by third-party dental insurers. The surgeon must use all of the information available to determine the difficulty of the proposed surgery.

MODIFICATION OF CLASSIFICATION SYSTEMS FOR MAXILLARY IMPACTED TEETH

The classification systems for the maxillary impacted third molar are essentially the same as for the impacted mandibular

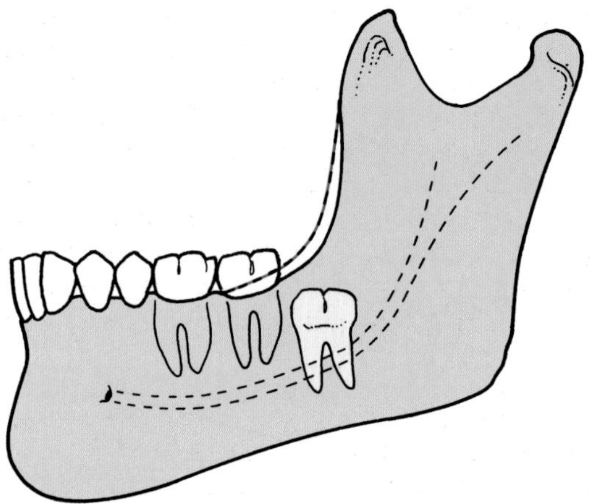

FIGURE 9-38 Complete bony impaction in which tooth is completely covered with bone and requires extensive removal of bone for extraction.

third molar. However, several distinctions and additions must be made to assess more accurately the difficulty of removal during the treatment planning phase of the procedure.

Concerning angulation, the three types of maxillary third molars are (1) the vertical impaction (Fig. 9-39, *A*), (2) the distoangular impaction (Fig. 9-39, *B*), and (3) the mesioangular impaction (Fig. 9-39, *C*). The vertical impaction occurs approximately 63% of the time, the distoangular approximately 25%, and the mesioangular position approximately 12% of the time. Rarely, other positions, such as a transverse, inverted, or horizontal position, are encountered; these unusual positions account for less than 1% of impacted maxillary third molars.

The same angulations in mandibular third molar extractions cause opposite degrees of difficulty for maxillary third molar extractions. Vertical and distoangular impactions are the less complex to remove, whereas mesioangular impactions are the most difficult (exactly the opposite of impacted mandibular third molars). Mesioangular impactions are more difficult to remove because the bone that overlies the impaction and requires removal or expansion is on the posterior aspect of the tooth, and is much thicker than in the vertical or distoangular impaction. In addition, access to the mesioangularly positioned tooth is more difficult if an erupted second molar is in place.

BOX 9-1

Factors That Make Impaction Surgery Less Difficult

1. Mesioangular position
2. Class 1 ramus
3. Class A depth
4. Roots one third to two thirds formed*
5. Fused conical roots
6. Wide periodontal ligament*
7. Large follicle*
8. Elastic bone*
9. Separated from second molar
10. Separated from inferior alveolar nerve*
11. Soft tissue impaction

*Present in the young patient.

BOX 9-2

Factors That Make Impaction Surgery More Difficult

1. Distoangular
2. Class 3 ramus
3. Class C depth
4. Long, thin roots*
5. Divergent curved roots
6. Narrow periodontal ligament
7. Thin follicle*
8. Dense, inelastic bone*
9. Contact with second molar
10. Close to inferior alveolar canal
11. Complete bony impaction*

*Present in older patients.

The position of the maxillary third molar in a buccopalatal direction is also important for determining the difficulty of the removal. Most maxillary third molars are angled toward the buccal aspect of the alveolar process; this makes the overlying bone in that area thin and therefore easy to remove or expand. Occasionally, the impacted maxillary third molar is positioned toward the palatal aspect of the alveolar process. This makes the tooth much more difficult to extract because greater amounts

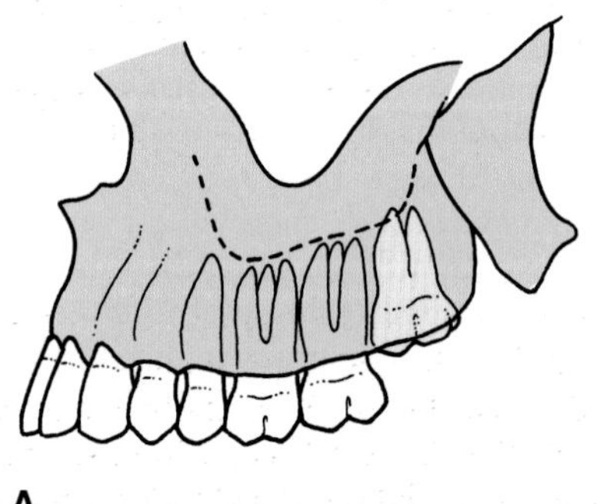

A

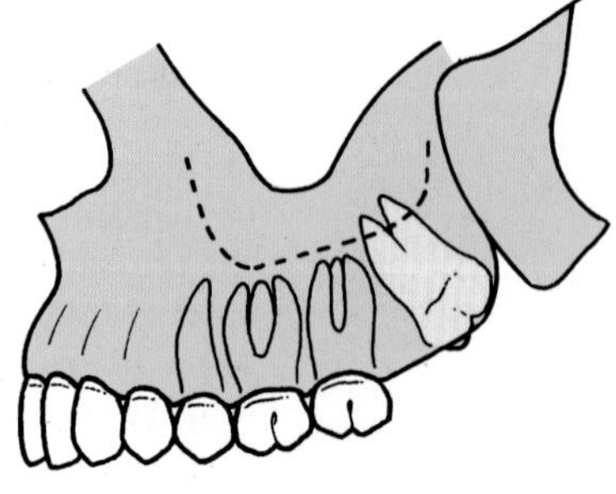

B

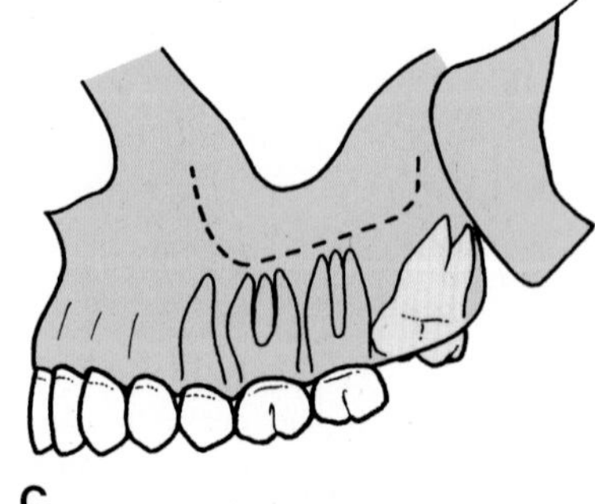

C

FIGURE 9-39 A, Vertical impaction of maxillary third molar. This angle accounts for 63% of impactions. B, Distoangular impaction of maxillary third molar. This angle accounts for 25% of impactions. C, Mesioangular impaction of maxillary third molar. This angle accounts for 12% of impactions.

of bone must be removed to gain access to the underlying tooth and an approach from the palatal aspect risks injury to nerves and vessels of the palatine foramina. A combination of radiographic assessment and clinical digital palpation of the tuberosity area can usually help determine whether the maxillary third molar is in the buccopalatal position. If the tooth is positioned toward the buccal, a palpable bulge is found in the area; if the tooth is palatally positioned, a bony deficit is found in that region. If a more palatal position is determined by clinical examination, the surgeon must anticipate a longer, more involved procedure.

The most common factor that causes difficulty with maxillary third molar removal is a thin, nonfused root with erratic curvature (Fig. 9-40). The majority of maxillary third molars have fused roots that are conical. However, the surgeon should examine the preoperative radiograph carefully to ensure that an unusual root pattern is not present. The surgeon should also check the periodontal ligament, because the wider the ligament space, the less difficult the tooth is to remove. In addition, similar to mandibular third molars, the periodontal ligament space tends to decrease as the patient ages.

The follicle surrounding the crown of the impacted tooth also has an influence on the difficulty of the extraction. If the follicular space is broad, the tooth will be easier to remove than if the follicular space is thin or nonexistent.

Bone density is also an important factor in maxillary impaction removal and is related closely to the age of the patient. The younger the patient, the more elastic and expandable the bone surrounding the impacted third molar.

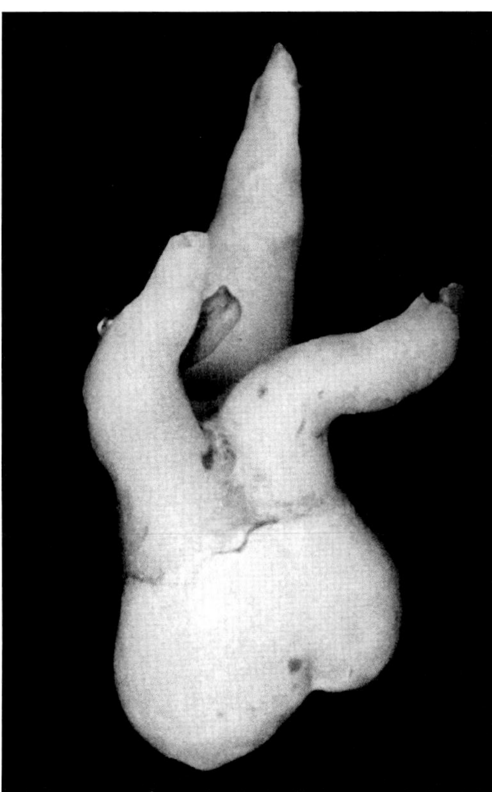

FIGURE 9-40 The maxillary third molar has the most erratic and variable root formation of all teeth.

The relationship to the adjacent second molar tooth also influences the difficulty of the extraction. Extraction may require that additional bone be removed to displace the tooth tucked under the height of contour of the closely adjacent second molar. In addition, because the use of elevators is common in the removal of maxillary third molars, the surgeon must be aware of the existence of large restorations or caries in the adjacent second molar. Injudicious use of elevators can result in the fracture of restorations or brittle crowns of teeth.

The type of impaction, with respect to overlying tissue, must also be considered for maxillary third molars. The insurance industry classification system used for maxillary teeth is the same as the system that is used for mandibular teeth: soft tissue impaction, partial bony impaction, and complete bony impaction. The definitions of these types of impactions are precisely the same as those used for the mandibular third molars.

Two additional factors influence the difficulty of maxillary third molar removal but do not exist for the mandibular third molars. Both factors are related to the structure and position of the maxillary sinus. First, the maxillary sinus is in intimate contact with the roots of the molars; and, frequently, the maxillary third molar actually forms a portion of the posterior sinus wall. If this is the case, removal of the maxillary third molar may result in maxillary sinus complications, such as sinusitis or an oroantral fistula. The presence of the maxillary sinus does not necessarily make the removal of the impacted tooth more difficult, but it increases the likelihood of postoperative complications and morbidity.

Finally, in maxillary third molar removal the tuberosity of the posterior maxilla can be fractured. This is true even when the third molar is erupted or if an erupted second molar is the most distal remaining tooth. Such fractures are possible, especially when dense and nonelastic bone exists, such as in older patients. In addition, a large maxillary sinus makes the surrounding alveolar bone thin and more susceptible to fracture when excessive force is applied. A root morphology that has divergent roots requires greater force to remove and can make bone fracture more likely. In addition, mesioangular impactions increase the possibility of fractures (see Fig. 9-39, *C*). In these situations the overlying tuberosity is heavier, but the surrounding bone is usually thinner. When the surgeon prepares a purchase point at the mesiocervical line, fracture of the tuberosity becomes a greater risk if (1) the bone is nonelastic (as in older patients), (2) the tooth is multirooted with large bulbous roots (as in older patients), (3) the maxillary sinus is large and greatly pneumatized to include the roots of the impacted third molar, or (4) the surgeon uses excessive force to elevate the tooth. Management of the fractured tuberosity is discussed in Chapter 11.

REMOVAL OF OTHER IMPACTED TEETH

After the mandibular and maxillary third molars, the next most commonly impacted tooth is the maxillary canine.

If the dentist decides that the tooth should be removed, it must be determined whether the tooth is positioned labially, toward the palate, or in the middle of the alveolar process. If the tooth is on the labial aspect, a soft tissue flap can be reflected to allow removal of the overlying bone and the tooth. However, if the tooth is on the palatal aspect or in the intermediate buccolingual position, it is much more difficult to remove. Therefore, when assessing the impacted maxillary canine for removal, the surgeon's most important assessment is of the buccolingual position of the tooth.

Similar considerations are necessary for other impactions, such as mandibular premolars and supernumerary teeth. The supernumerary tooth in the midline of the maxilla, called a *mesiodens,* is almost always found on the palate and should be approached from the palatal direction for removal.

When a buried canine is positioned in such a way that orthodontic manipulation can assist the proper positioning, the tooth can be exposed and bracketed. A flap is created to allow the soft tissue to be repositioned apically should this be required for maximum keratinized tissue management. The overlying bone tissue is then removed with burs as is necessary. Once the area is débrided, the surface of the tooth is prepared by the usual standard procedures of etching and applying primer. The bracket is then luted onto the surface of the tooth. A wire can be used to connect the bracket to the orthodontic appliance or, more commonly, a gold chain is attached from the orthodontic bracket to the orthodontic arch wire. The gold chain provides a greater degree of flexibility, and the incidence of breakage of the chain is much less than breakage of a wire. The soft tissue is then sutured in such a way as to provide the maximum coverage of the exposed tissue with keratinized tissue. As the tooth is pulled into place with the orthodontic appliances, the soft tissue surrounding the newly positioned tooth should have adequate keratinized tissue, and the tooth should be in an ideal position.

If the tooth is positioned toward the palatal aspect, the tooth may be repositioned or removed. If the tooth is repositioned, it is surgically exposed and guided into position orthodontically. In this procedure the overlying soft tissue is excised; flaps are not needed to gain attached tissue. Because the bone in the palate is thicker, a bur is usually necessary to remove the overlying bone. The exposed tooth then is managed in the same manner as is the labially positioned tooth (Fig. 9-41).

SURGICAL PROCEDURE

The principles and steps for removing impacted teeth are the same as for other surgical extractions. Five basic steps make up the technique: The first step is to have adequate exposure of

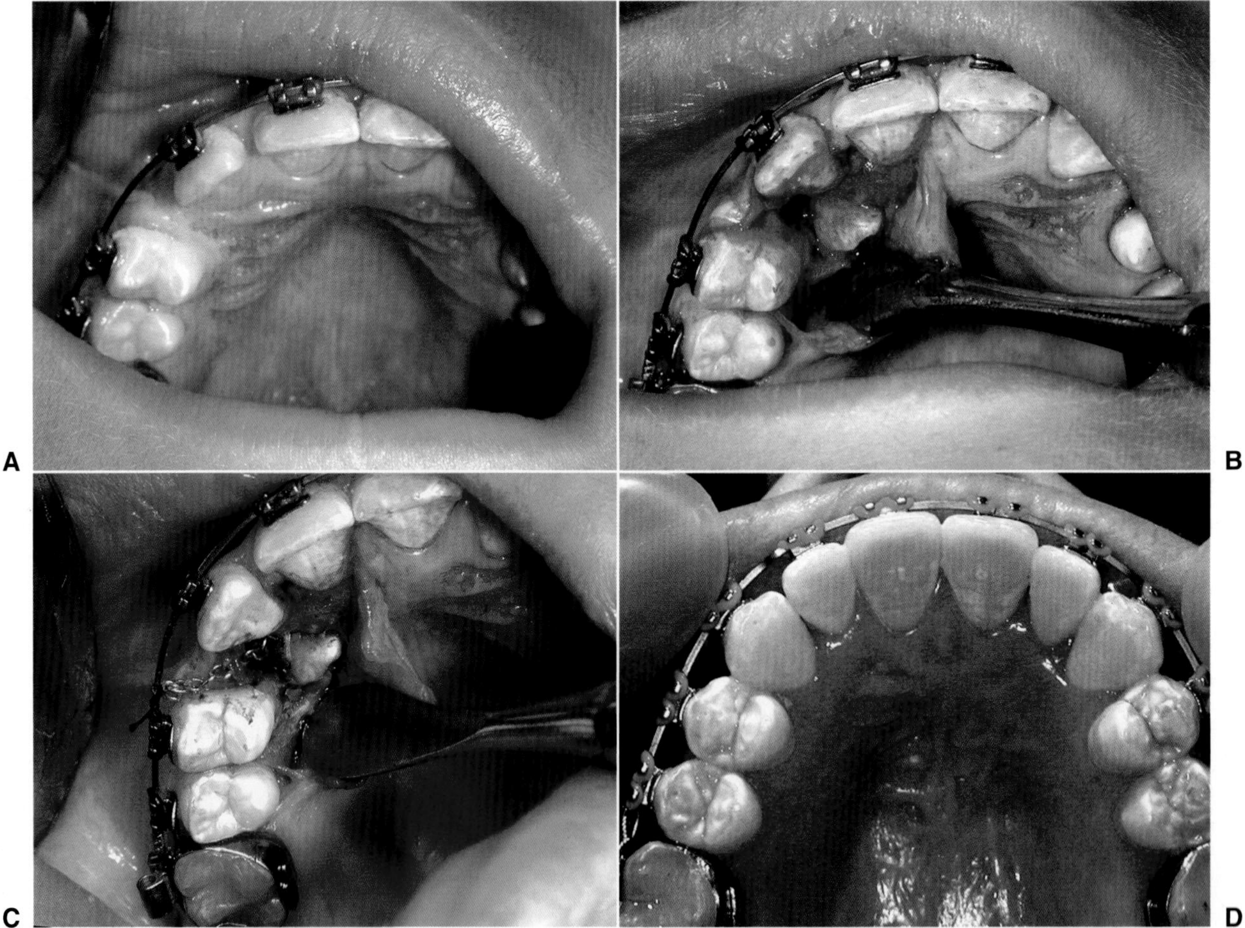

FIGURE 9-41 A, Labially positioned impacted maxillary canine. Tooth should be uncovered with apically positioned flap procedure to preserve attached gingiva. B, Mucoperiosteal flap is outlined, allowing for repositioning of keratinized mucosa over exposed tooth. When flap is reflected, thin overlying bone is removed. C, Tissue is retracted and bonded to tooth with a wire or a gold chain. Flap is apically sutured to tooth. D, After 6 months, exposed tooth is in desired position, with broad zone of attached gingiva. (Courtesy Dr. Myron Tucker.)

the area of the impacted tooth. This means that the reflected soft tissue flap must be of an adequate dimension to allow the surgeon to retract the soft tissue and perform the necessary surgery without seriously damaging the flap. The second step is to assess the need for bone removal and to remove a sufficient amount of bone to expose the tooth for any needed sectioning and delivery. The third step, if needed, is to divide the tooth with a bur to allow the tooth to be extracted without removing unnecessarily large amounts of bone. Purchase points may also be placed at this step. In the fourth step the sectioned or unsectioned tooth is delivered from the alveolar process with the appropriate elevators. Finally, in the fifth step the bone in areas of elevation is smoothed with a bone file; the wound is thoroughly irrigated with a sterile, physiologic solution; and the flap is reapproximated with sutures. The following discussion elaborates on these steps for the removal of impacted third molars.

Although the surgical approach to the removal of impacted teeth is similar to other surgical tooth extractions, it is important to keep in mind several distinct differences. For instance, the typical surgical extraction of a tooth or tooth root requires the removal of a relatively small amount of bone. However, when an impacted tooth (especially a mandibular third molar) is extracted, the amount of bone that must be removed to deliver the tooth is substantially greater. This bone is also much denser than it is for typical surgical extractions, and its removal requires better instrumentation and a higher degree of surgical skill.

Impacted teeth also frequently require sectioning, whereas other types of tooth extractions do not. Although erupted maxillary and mandibular molars are occasionally divided for removal, it is not a routine step in the extraction of these teeth. However, with impacted mandibular third molars, the surgeon is required to divide the tooth in a substantial majority of patients. The surgeon must therefore have the necessary equipment for such sectioning and the necessary skills and experience for dividing the tooth along the proper planes.

Unlike most other types of surgical tooth extractions, for an impacted tooth removal the surgeon must be able to balance the degree of bone removal and sectioning. Essentially, all impacted teeth can be removed without sectioning if a large amount of bone is removed. However, the removal of excessive amounts of bone unnecessarily prolongs the healing period and may result in a weakened jaw. Therefore the surgeon should remove most bony impacted mandibular third molars only after sectioning them. However, removal of a small amount of bone with multiple divisions of the tooth may cause the tooth sectioning process to take an excessively long time, thus unnecessarily prolonging the operation. The surgeon must remove an adequate amount of bone and section the tooth into a reasonable number of pieces, both to hasten healing and to minimize the time of the surgical procedure.

Step 1: Reflecting adequate flaps for accessibility. The difficulty of removing an impacted tooth depends on its accessibility. To gain access to the area and to visualize the overlying bone that must be removed, the surgeon must reflect an adequate mucoperiosteal flap. The reflection must be of a dimension adequate to allow the placement and stabilization of retractors and instruments for the removal of bone.

In most situations the envelope flap is the preferred technique. The envelope flap is quicker to close and heals better than the three-cornered flap (envelope flap with a releasing incision). However, if the surgeon requires greater access to the more apical areas of the tooth, which might stretch and tear the envelope flap, the surgeon should consider using a three-cornered flap.

The preferred incision for the removal of an impacted mandibular third molar is an envelope incision that extends from the mesial papilla of the mandibular first molar, around the necks of the teeth to the distobuccal line angle of the second molar, and then posteriorly to and *laterally* up the anterior border of the mandibular ramus (Fig. 9-42, *A*).

The incision must not continue posteriorly in a straight line because the mandible diverges laterally. An incision that extends straight posteriorly falls off the bone and into the sublingual space and may damage the lingual nerve, which is in proximity to the mandible in the area of the third molar. If this nerve is traumatized, the patient will probably have lingual nerve anesthesia, which is extremely disturbing to patients. The incision must always be kept over bone; therefore the surgeon should carefully palpate the retromolar area before beginning the incision.

The flap is reflected laterally to expose the external oblique ridge with a periosteal elevator (Fig. 9-42, *B*). The surgeon should not reflect more than a few millimeters beyond the external oblique ridge because this results in increased morbidity and an increased number of complications after surgery. The retractor is placed on the buccal shelf, just lateral to the external oblique ridge, and it is stabilized by applying pressure toward the bone. This results in a retractor that is stable and does not continually traumatize the soft tissue. The Austin and the Minnesota retractors are the most commonly used for flap retraction when removing mandibular third molars.

If the impacted third molar is deeply embedded in bone and requires more extensive bone removal, a releasing incision may be useful (Fig. 9-42, *C* and *D*). The flap created by this incision can be reflected farther apically, without risk of tearing the tissue.

The recommended incision for the maxillary third molar is also an envelope incision. The incision extends posteriorly over the tuberosity from the distal of the second molar and anteriorly to the mesial aspect of the first molar (Fig. 9-43, *A* and *B*). In situations in which greater access is required (e.g., in a deeply embedded impaction), a release incision extending from the mesial aspect of the second molar can be used (Fig. 9-43, *C* and *D*).

In the removal of third molars it is vital that the flap be large enough for adequate access and visibility of the surgical site. The flap must have a broad base if a releasing incision is used. The incision must be made with a smooth stroke of the scalpel, which is kept in contact with bone throughout the entire incision so that the mucosa and periosteum are completely incised. This allows a full-thickness mucoperiosteal flap to be reflected. The incision should be designed so that it can be closed over solid bone (rather than over a bony defect). This is achieved by extending the incision at least one tooth anterior to the surgical site when a vertical-releasing incision is used. The incision should avoid vital anatomic structures. Only a single releasing incision should be used.

Step 2: Removal of overlying bone. Once the soft tissue is elevated and retracted so that the surgical field can be visualized, the surgeon must make a judgment concerning the amount of bone to be removed. In some situations the

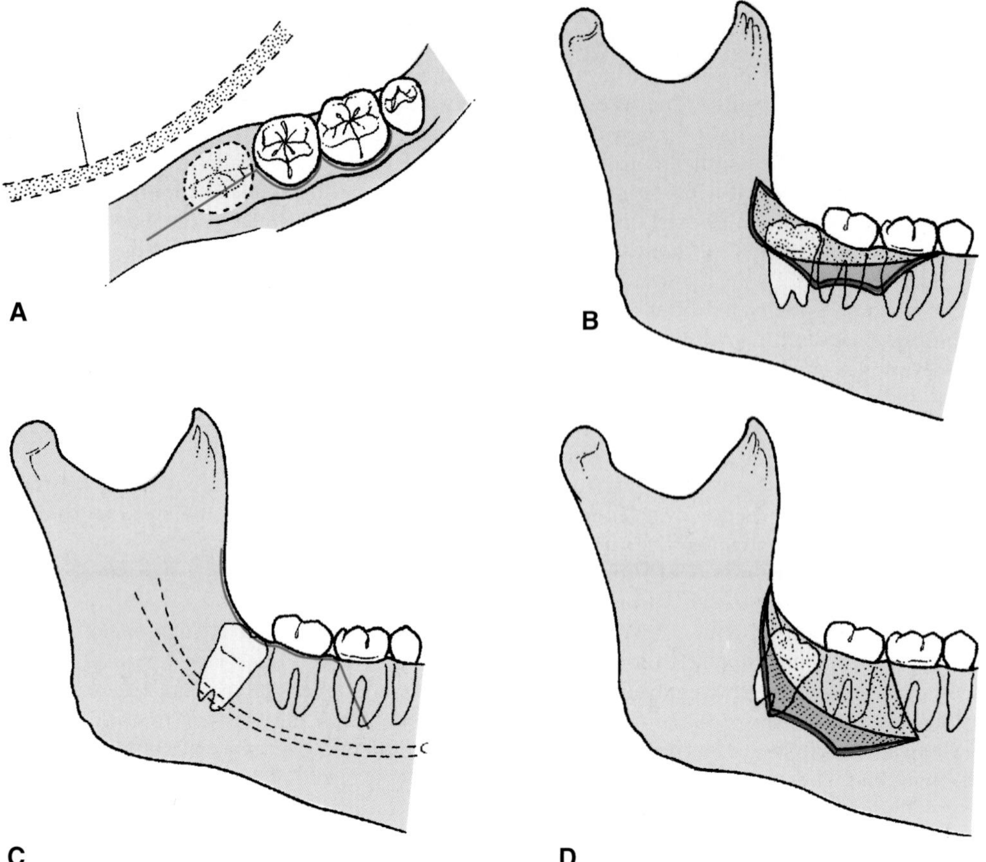

FIGURE 9-42 A, Envelope incision is most commonly used to reflect soft tissue for removal of impacted third molar. Posterior extension of incision should laterally diverge to avoid injury to lingual nerve. B, Envelope incision is laterally reflected to expose bone overlying impacted tooth. C, When three-cornered flap is made, a releasing incision is made at mesial aspect of second molar. D, When soft tissue flap is reflected by means of a releasing incision, greater visibility is possible, especially at apical aspect of surgical field.

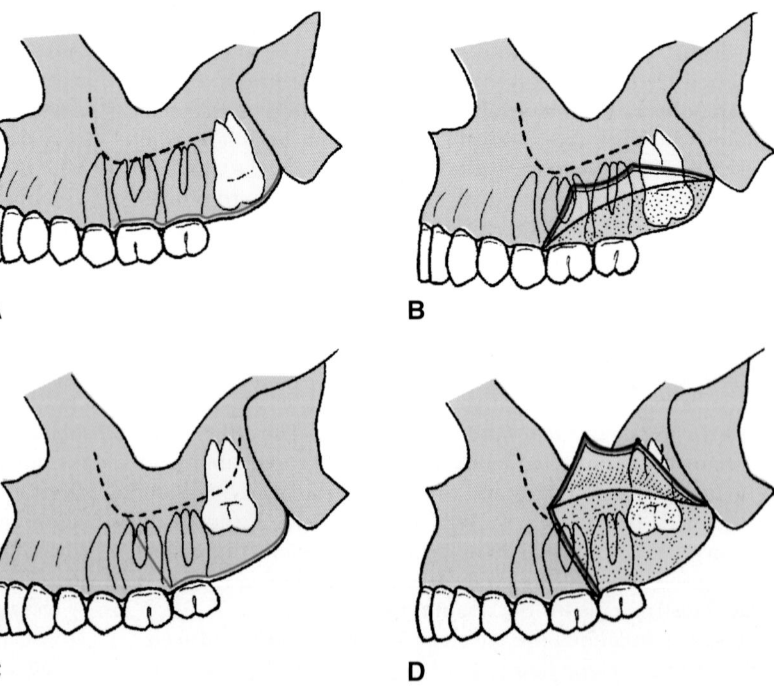

FIGURE 9-43 A, Envelope flap is most commonly used flap for removal of maxillary impacted teeth. B, When soft tissue is reflected, bone overlying third molar is easily visualized. C, If tooth is deeply impacted, a releasing incision into the vestibule can be used to gain greater access. D, When three-cornered flap is reflected, the more apical portions become more visible.

tooth can be sectioned with a bur and delivered without bone removal. In most cases, however, some bone removal is required.

The bone on the occlusal aspect and on the buccal and distal aspects down to the cervical line of the impacted tooth should be removed initially. The amount of bone that must be removed varies with the depth of the impaction, the morphology of the roots, and the angulation of the tooth. Bone should not be removed from the lingual aspect of the mandible because of the likelihood of damaging the lingual nerve.

The burs that are used to remove the bone overlying the impacted tooth vary with surgeons' preferences. A large round bur, such as a No. 8, is desirable, because it is an end-cutting bur and can be used effectively for drilling with a pushing motion. The tip of a fissure bur, such as a No. 703 bur, does not cut well, but the edge rapidly removes bone and quickly sections teeth when used in a lateral direction. Note that a dental handpiece such as used for restorative dentistry should never be used to remove bone around third molars to section them.

The typical bone removal for the extraction of an impacted mandibular tooth is illustrated in Figure 9-44. The bone on the occlusal aspect of the tooth is removed first to expose the crown of the tooth. Then the cortical bone on the buccal aspect of the tooth is removed down to the cervical line. Next, the bur can be used to remove bone between the tooth and the cortical bone in the cancellous area of the bone with a maneuver called *ditching*. This provides access for elevators to gain purchase points and a pathway for delivery of the tooth. No bone is removed from the lingual aspect so as to protect the lingual nerve from injury.

For maxillary teeth, bone removal is usually unnecessary, but when it is, bone is removed primarily on the buccal aspect of the tooth, down to the cervical line to expose the entire clinical crown. Usually bone removal can be accomplished

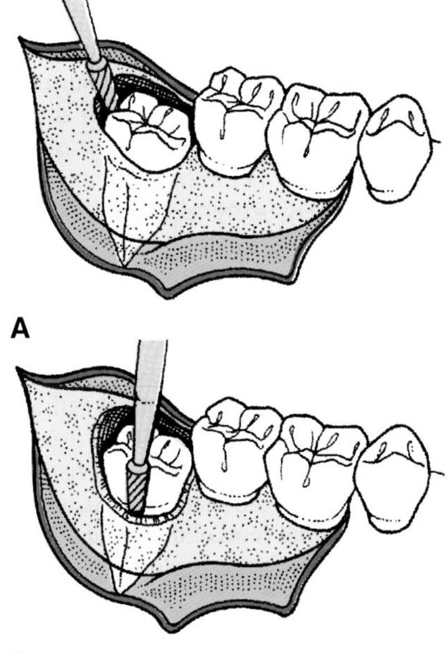

FIGURE 9-44 A, After soft tissue has been reflected, bone overlying occlusal surface of tooth is removed with a fissure bur. B, Bone on buccodistal aspect of impacted tooth is then removed with a bur.

with a periosteal elevator, rather than a bur. Additional bone must usually be removed on the mesial aspect of the tooth to allow an elevator an adequate purchase point to deliver the tooth.

Step 3: Sectioning the tooth. Once sufficient amounts of bone have been removed from around the impacted tooth, the surgeon should assess the need to section the tooth. Sectioning allows portions of the tooth to be removed separately with elevators through the opening provided by bone removal.

The direction in which the impacted tooth should be divided depends primarily on the angulation of the impacted tooth. Although minor modifications are necessary for teeth with divergent roots or for teeth that are more or less deeply impacted, the most important determinant is the angulation of the tooth.

Tooth sectioning is performed with a bur, and the tooth is sectioned three fourths of the way toward the lingual aspect. The bur should not be used to section the tooth completely through in the lingual direction because this is more likely to injure the lingual nerve. A straight elevator is inserted into the slot made by the bur and rotated to split the tooth.

The mesioangular mandibular impaction is usually the least difficult to remove of the four basic angulation types. After sufficient bone has been removed, the distal half of the crown is sectioned off at the buccal groove to just below the cervical line on the distal aspect. This portion is removed. The remainder of the tooth is removed with a No. 301 elevator placed at the mesial aspect of the cervical line. A mesioangular impaction can also be removed by preparing a purchase point in the tooth with the drill and using a Crane pick elevator to elevate the tooth from the socket (Fig. 9-45).

The next most difficult impaction to remove is the horizontal impaction. After sufficient bone has been removed down to the cervical line to expose the superior aspect of the distal root and the majority of the buccal surface of the crown, the tooth is sectioned by dividing the crown of the tooth from the roots at the cervical line. The crown of the tooth is removed, and the roots are displaced with a Cryer elevator into the space previously occupied by the crown. If the roots of an impacted third molar are divergent, they may require sectioning into two separate portions to be delivered individually (Fig. 9-46).

The vertical impaction is one of the two most difficult impactions to remove. The procedure of bone removal and sectioning is similar to the mesioangular impaction; that is, the occlusal buccal and distal bone is removed. The distal half of the crown is sectioned and removed, and the tooth is elevated by applying an elevator at the mesial aspect of the cervical line of the tooth. This is more difficult than a mesioangular removal because access around the mandibular second molar is difficult to obtain and requires the removal of substantially more bone on the buccal and distal sides (Fig. 9-47).

The most difficult tooth to remove is the distoangular impaction. After sufficient bone is removed from the buccoocclusal and the distal sides of the tooth, the crown is sectioned from the roots just above the cervical line. The entire crown is usually removed because it interferes with visibility and access to the root structure of the tooth. If the roots are fused, a Cryer or straight elevator can be used to elevate the tooth into the space previously occupied by the crown. If the roots are divergent, they are usually sectioned into two pieces and individually delivered. Extracting this impaction is

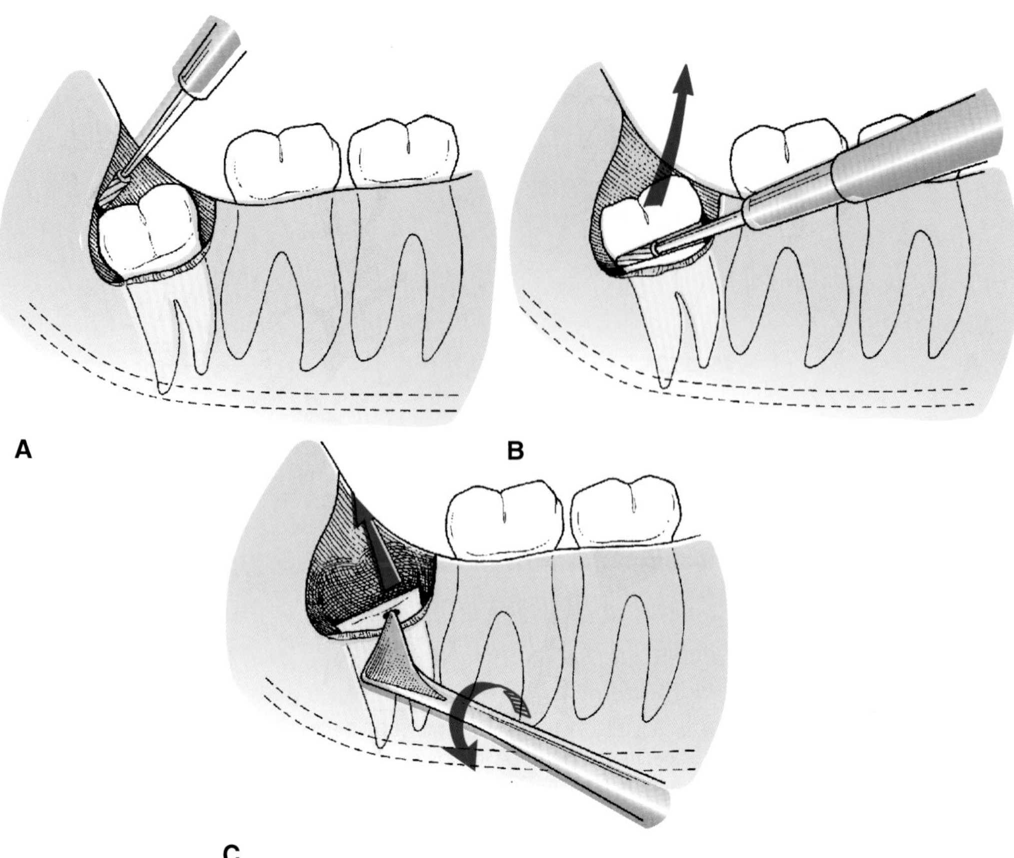

FIGURE 9-48 A, For distoangular impaction, occlusal, buccal, and distal bone is removed with bur. It is important to remember that more distal bone must be taken off than for vertical or mesioangular impaction. B, Crown of tooth is sectioned off with bur, and crown is delivered with straight elevator. C, Purchase point is put into remaining root portion of tooth, and roots are delivered by Cryer elevator with wheel-and-axle type of motion. If roots diverge, it may be necessary in some cases to split them into independent portions.

Step 5: Preparing for wound closure. A bone file is used to smooth any sharp, rough edges of bone particularly where an elevator was in bony contact. The surgeon should next direct attention to removing all particulate bone chips and debris from the wound. This is done with vigorous irrigation with sterile saline. Special care should be taken to irrigate thoroughly under the reflected soft tissue flap. A mosquito hemostat can be used to remove any remnants of the dental follicle if present. Once the follicle is grasped, it is lifted with a slow, steady pressure and will pull free from the surrounding hard and soft tissue. A final irrigation and a thorough inspection should be performed before the wound is closed.

The surgeon should check for adequate hemostasis. Bleeding can occur from a vessel in the flap, from the bone marrow that has been cut with a bur, or the inferior alveolar vessels. Specific bleeding points should be controlled if they exist. If brisk generalized ooze is seen after the sutures are placed, the surgeon should apply firm pressure with a small, moistened gauze pack. Postoperative bleeding to a certain degree occurs relatively frequently after third molar extraction but is usually self-limited if adequate hemostasis is achieved at the time of the operation.

At this point many surgeons apply an antibiotic such as tetracycline to the sockets of lower third molars to help prevent osteitis sicca from occurring.

The closure of the incision made for an impacted third molar is usually a primary closure. If the flap was well designed and not traumatized during the surgical procedure, it will fit into its original position. The initial suture should be placed through the attached tissue on the posterior aspect of the second molar. Additional sutures are placed posteriorly from that position and anteriorly through the papilla on the mesial side of the second molar. Usually two or three sutures are necessary to close an envelope incision. If a releasing incision was used, attention must be directed to closing that portion of the incision as well. If the flap for a maxillary third molar rests passively in place postoperatively, suturing may not be necessary.

PERIOPERATIVE PATIENT MANAGEMENT

The removal of impacted third molars is a surgical procedure that is usually associated with a great deal of patient anxiety. In addition, this surgical procedure can involve unpleasant noises and sensations. As a result, surgeons who routinely remove impacted third molars commonly recommend to their patients some type of profound anxiety control such as deep intravenous sedation or general anesthesia.

The choice of technique is based on the surgeon's preference. However, the goals are to achieve a level of patient consciousness that allows the surgeon to work efficiently and that limits the number of unpleasant memories for the patient.

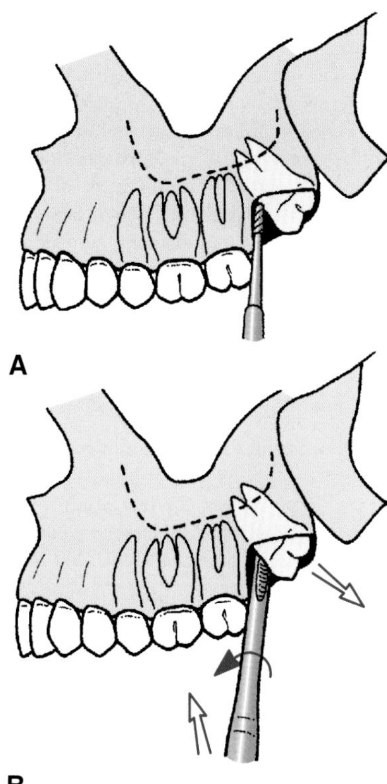

FIGURE 9-49 Delivery of impacted maxillary third molar. **A**, Once soft tissue has been reflected, small amount of buccal bone is removed with bur or the pointed end of a periosteal elevator. **B**, Tooth is then delivered by small straight elevator, with rotational and lever motion. Tooth is delivered in distobuccal and occlusal direction. Note that in most circumstances, bone removal using a bur is not required when removing impacted maxillary third molars.

In addition to the increased need for anxiety control, a variety of medications are used to control the sequelae of third molar extraction surgery. The use of long-acting local anesthetics should be considered in the mandible. These anesthetics provide the patient with a pain-free period of 4 to 8 hours during which prescriptions can be filled and analgesics taken. Analgesics are best begun at the point when the patient first begins to recognize the return of sensation. Some surgeons even have patients begin analgesics before any return of sensation. The surgeon should consider writing a prescription for a potent oral analgesic for every patient who undergoes surgical removal of an impacted third molar, and if the surgeon does separate consultation appointments, he or she should prescribe postoperative medications at that time so the patient and the patient's escort do not need to stop on the way home from the procedure. Enough doses should be prescribed to last for at least 3 or 4 days. Combinations of codeine, codeine congeners, or oxycodone with aspirin or acetaminophen are commonly used. Nonsteroidal antiinflammatory drugs such as ibuprofen may be of value for patients as well to use when the discomfort is less significant.

To minimize the swelling common after the surgical removal of impacted third molars, some surgeons give parenteral corticosteroids. Intravenous administration of a glucocorticoid steroid provides sufficient antiinflammatory activity to greatly limit edema. Although many different regimens and protocols for intravenous steroid administration exist, a relatively common one is the single administration of 8 mg dexamethasone before surgery. Dexamethasone is a long-acting steroid, and its efficacy in controlling third molar postsurgical edema is documented. This drug can then be continued in an oral dose of 0.75 to 1.25 mg twice a day for 2 to 3 days to continue edema control. Although steroids given in this manner have few side effects or contraindications, the general philosophy of weighing the risks and benefits of drug administration must be carefully followed before the decision is made to give any drugs routinely.

Some surgeons recommend the use of ice packs on the face to help prevent postoperative swelling, even though studies show that it is unlikely that the ice has much effect on preventing or limiting swelling. However, patients frequently report that the ice makes them feel more comfortable. Use of ice also provides patients the opportunity to participate in their postoperative care, which is important for many patients.

Another medication that is sometimes used is an antibiotic. If a patient has a preexisting pericoronitis or periapical abscess, it is common to prescribe antibiotics for a few days after surgery. However, if the patient is healthy and the clinician finds no systemic indication for antibiotics or a preexisting local infection, systemic antibiotics are usually not indicated. The use of a topical antibiotic such as tetracycline has been scientifically shown to greatly lower the incidence of osteitis sicca (dry socket) in mandibular molar extraction sites. One fourth of the contents of a 250-mg capsule is adequate to give the desired protection.

The normal postoperative experience of a patient after surgical removal of an impacted third molar is more involved than after a routine extraction. The patient can expect a modest amount of edema in the area of the surgery for 3 to 4 days, with the swelling completely dissipating by about 5 to 7 days. The amount of swelling depends on the degree of tissue trauma and variability among patients in their potential to swell.

A modest amount of discomfort usually follows the procedure, the degree of which depends on the amount of surgical trauma necessary to remove the teeth. This discomfort can be effectively controlled with potent oral analgesics. Patients usually require potent analgesics for 2 or 3 days routinely and intermittently (particularly at bedtime) for several more days. The patient may have some mild soreness in the region for up to 2 to 3 weeks after the surgery.

Patients who have had mandibular third molars surgically removed frequently have mild to moderate trismus. This inability to open the mouth interferes with the patient's normal oral hygiene and eating habits. Patients should be warned that they will be unable to open their mouths normally after surgery. The trismus gradually resolves, and the ability to open the mouth should return to normal by 7 to 10 days after surgery.

If pain, edema, and trismus have not greatly improved by 7 days after surgery, the surgeon should investigate why.

All of the sequelae of the surgical removal of impacted teeth are of less intensity in the young, healthy patient and of far greater intensity in the older, more debilitated patient. Even healthy adult patients between the ages of 35 to 40 years have a significantly more difficult time after the extraction of impacted third molars than do most healthy teenaged patients.

See Chapter 10 for a more detailed description of postoperative care.

REFERENCES

1. Venta I, Murtomaa H, Turtola L et al: Assessing the eruption of lower third molars on the basis of radiographic features, *Br J Oral Maxillofac Surg* 29:259-262, 1991.
2. Venta I, Murtomaa H, Turtola L et al: Clinical follow-up study of third molar eruption from ages 20 to 26 years, *Oral Surg Oral Med Oral Pathol* 72:150-153, 1991.
3. Bruce RA, Frederickson GC, Small GS: Age of patients and morbidity associated with mandibular third molar surgery, *J Am Dent Assoc* 101:240, 1980.
4. Marmary J, Brayer L, Tzokert A et al: Alveolar bone repair following extraction of impacted mandibular third molars, *Oral Surg Oral Med Oral Pathol* 61:324, 1986.
5. Meister F Jr, Nery EB, Angell DM et al: Periodontal assessment following surgical removal of mandibular third molars, *Gen Dent* 14:120-123, 1986.
6. Osborne WH, Snyder AJ, Tempel TR: Attachment levels and crevicular depths at the distal aspect of mandibular second molars following removal of adjacent third molars, *J Periodontol* 53:93, 1982.
7. Lysell L, Rohlin M: A study of indications used for removal of the mandibular third molar, *Int J Oral Maxillofac Surg* 17:161, 1988.
8. Nordenram A, Hultin M, Kjellman O et al: Indications for surgical removal of the mandibular third molar, *Swed Dent J* 11:23-29, 1987.
9. Leone SA, Edenfield MJ, Coehn ME: Correlation of acute pericoronitis and the position of the mandibular third molar, *Oral Surg Oral Med Oral Pathol* 62:245, 1986.
10. Stanley HR, Alattar M, Collett WK et al: Pathological sequelae of "neglected" impacted third molars, *J Oral Pathol* 17:113-117, 1988.
11. Richardson ME: The effect of mandibular first premolar extraction on third molar space, *Angle Orthod* 59:291-294, 1989.
12. Richardson ME: The role of the third molar in the cause of late lower arch crowding: a review, *Am J Orthod Dentofacial Orthop* 95:79, 1989.
13. Kugelberg CF: Periodontal healing two and four years after impacted lower third molar surgery, *Int J Oral Maxillofac Surg* 19:341, 1990.
14. Kugelberg CF, Ahlstrom U, Ericson S et al: The influence of anatomical, pathophysiological and other factors on periodontal healing after impacted lower third molar surgery, *J Clin Periodontol* 18:37-43, 1991.
15. Kugelberg CF, Ahlstrom U, Ericson S et al: Periodontal healing after impacted lower third molar surgery in adolescents and adults, *Int J Oral Maxillofac Surg* 20:18-24, 1991.

Bibliography

Bean LR, King DR: Pericoronitis: its nature and etiology, *J Am Dent Assoc* 83:1074, 1971.

Pell GJ, Gregory GT: Report on a ten-year study of a tooth division technique for the removal of impacted teeth, *Am J Orthod* 28:660, 1942.

Perciaccante VJ: Management of impacted teeth, *Oral Maxillofac Surg Clin North Am* 19:1-140, 2007.

Quee TA, Gosselin D, Millar EP et al: Surgical removal of the fully impacted mandibular third molar: the influence of flap design and alveolar bone height on the periodontal status of the second molar, *J Periodontol* 56:625-630, 1985.

von Wowern N, Nielsen HO: The fate of impacted lower third molars after the age of 20, *Int J Oral Maxillofac Surg* 18:277, 1989.

CHAPTER 10

Postoperative Patient Management

JAMES R. HUPP

CHAPTER OUTLINE

Many patients worry about having surgery more because of fears about what it will be like after the surgery than what will occur during the operation. This is particularly true if they trust the effectiveness of the planned method of anesthesia. There are several things the surgeon can do after surgery to diminish these patient concerns and lower the chances of postoperative problems. This chapter discusses those strategies.

Once the surgical procedure has been completed, patients and any accompanying family members should be given proper instructions on how to care for common postsurgical sequelae for the remainder of the day of surgery and a few days thereafter. Postoperative instructions should describe what the patient is likely to experience, explain why these phenomena occur, and tell the patient how to manage and control typical postoperative situations. The instructions must be given to the patient verbally and on a written sheet, and easily understood lay terms should be used. The instruction sheet should describe the typical problems and their management. Instructions should also include a telephone number at which the surgeon or covering doctor can be reached in an emergency.

If the patient is to receive intravenous sedation, the postoperative management instructions must be discussed before the sedation is given and must be repeated to the patient's escort before discharge from the office. In addition, a written set of postextraction instructions should be given to patients or their escorts. A typical postoperative instruction sheet is found in Appendix V.

CONTROL OF POSTOPERATIVE HEMORRHAGE

Once an extraction has been completed, the initial maneuver to control postoperative bleeding is the placement of a small gauze directly over the socket. Large packs that cover the occlusal surfaces of teeth adjacent to the extraction site do not apply pressure to the bleeding socket and so are ineffective (Fig. 10-1). The gauze may be moistened so that the oozing blood does not coagulate in the gauze and then dislodge the clot when the gauze is removed. The patient should be instructed to bite firmly on this gauze for at least 30 minutes and not to chew on the gauze. The patient should hold the gauze in place without opening or closing the mouth. Talking should be kept to a minimum for 2 to 3 hours.

Patients should be informed that it is normal for a fresh extraction site to ooze slightly for up to 24 hours after the extraction procedure. Patients should be warned that a small amount of blood and a large amount of saliva might appear to be a large amount of blood. If the bleeding is more than a slight ooze, the patient should be told how to reapply a small gauze directly over the area of the extraction. The patient should be instructed to hold this second gauze pack in place for as long as 1 hour to gain control of bleeding. Further control can be attained if necessary by having the patient bite on a tea bag for 30 minutes. The tannic acid in regular tea serves as a local vasoconstrictor.

Patients should be cautioned to avoid things that may aggravate the bleeding. Patients who smoke should be encouraged to avoid smoking for the first 12 hours or, more commonly, if they must smoke, to draw on the cigarette very lightly. Tobacco smoke and nicotine interfere with wound healing. The patient should also be told not to suck on a straw when drinking because this also creates negative pressure. The patient should not spit during the first 12 hours after surgery. The process of spitting involves negative pressure and mechanical agitation of the extraction site, which may trigger fresh bleeding. Patients who object to having blood in the mouth should be encouraged to bite firmly on a piece of gauze to control the hemorrhage and to swallow their saliva instead of spitting it out. Finally, no strenuous exercise should be performed for the first 12 to 24 hours after extraction because the increased blood pressure may result in greater bleeding.

Patients should be warned that there may be some oozing during the night and that they will probably have some blood stains on their pillows. This will prevent many frantic telephone calls to the surgeon in the middle of the night. Patients should also be instructed that if they are worried about their

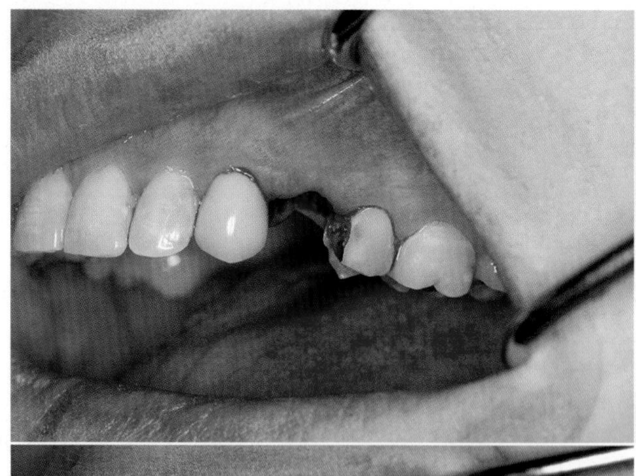

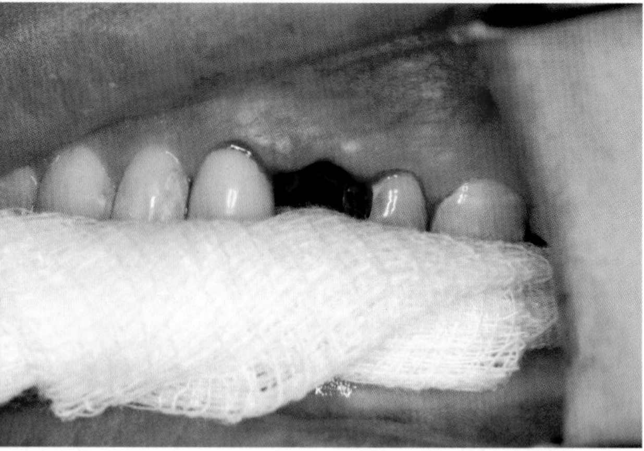

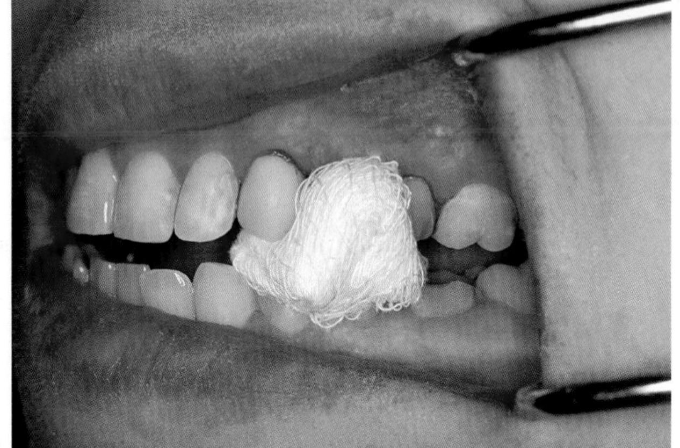

FIGURE 10-1 A, Fresh extraction site will bleed excessively unless a properly positioned gauze pack is placed, B, Small gauze pack is placed to fit only in area of extraction; this permits pressure to be applied directly to socket. C, Large or mispositioned gauze pack is not effective in controlling bleeding because the pressure of biting is not precisely directed onto the socket.

bleeding, they should call to get additional advice. Prolonged oozing, bright red bleeding, or large clots in the patient's mouth are indications for a return visit. The dentist should then examine the area closely and apply appropriate measures to control the hemorrhage (see Chapter 11).

CONTROL OF POSTOPERATIVE PAIN AND DISCOMFORT

All patients expect a certain amount of pain after a surgical procedure, so it is important for the dentist to discuss this issue carefully with each patient before discharge from the office. The surgeon must help the patient to have a realistic expectation of what type of pain may occur and must pay attention to the patient's concerns of how much pain is likely to occur.

Patients who tell the surgeon that they expect a great deal of pain after surgery should not be ignored and told to take an over-the-counter analgesic if it hurts; these patients are the ones most likely to experience pain postoperatively. It is important for the surgeon to assure patients, especially the latter group, that their postoperative discomfort can be effectively managed.

The pain a patient may experience after a surgical procedure, such as tooth extraction, is highly variable and depends a great deal on the patient's preoperative frame of mind. The surgeon who spends several minutes discussing these issues with the patient before surgery will be able to recommend the most appropriate medication.

All patients should be given advice concerning analgesics before they are discharged. Even when the surgeon believes that no prescription analgesics are necessary, the patient should be told to take ibuprofen or acetaminophen postoperatively to prevent initial discomfort when the effect of the local anesthetic disappears. Patients who are expected to have a higher level of pain should be given a prescription analgesic that will control the pain. The surgeon should also take care to advise the patient that the goal of analgesic medication is management of pain and not elimination of all soreness.

The surgeon must understand the three characteristics of the pain that occurs after tooth extraction. First, the pain is usually not severe and can be managed in most patients with mild analgesics. Second, the peak pain experience occurs about 12 hours after the extraction and diminishes rapidly after that. Finally, significant pain from extraction rarely persists longer than 2 days after surgery. With these factors in mind, patients can best be advised regarding the effective use of analgesics.

The first dose of analgesic medication should be taken before the effect of the local anesthetic subsides. If this is done, the patient is less likely to experience the intense, sharp pain after the loss of the local anesthesia. By preventing the sudden onset of surgical pain, the subsequent control of it is more predictably achieved with mild analgesics. Postoperative pain is much more difficult to overcome if administration of analgesic medication is delayed. If the patient waits to take the first dose of analgesic until the effects of the local anesthesia have disappeared, it may take up to 90 minutes for the analgesic to become effective. During this time, the patient is likely to become impatient and take additional medication that will increase the risk of nausea and vomiting.

The strength of the analgesic is also important. Potent analgesics are not required in most routine extraction situations;

instead, analgesics with a lower potency per dose are effective. The patient can then be told to take one, two, or three unit doses as necessary to control pain. By allowing the patient to assume an active role in determining the amount of medication to take, more precise control can be achieved.

Patients should be warned that taking too much of narcotic medications will result in drowsiness and an increased chance of gastric upset. In most situations, patients should take medication with some type of food to decrease its irritating effect on the stomach.

Ibuprofen has been demonstrated to be an effective medication to control the pain and discomfort of a tooth extraction. This drug works primarily peripherally, interfering with prostaglandin synthesis. Ibuprofen has the disadvantage of causing a decrease in platelet aggregation and bleeding time, but this does not appear to have a clinically important effect on postoperative bleeding. Acetaminophen does not interfere with platelet function, and it may be useful in certain situations where the patient has a platelet defect and is likely to bleed. If the surgeon prescribes a combination drug of acetaminophen and narcotic, it should be a combination that delivers 500 to 650 mg of acetaminophen per dose.

Drugs useful in situations with varying degrees of pain are listed in Table 10-1. Centrally acting opioid analgesics are also frequently used to control pain after tooth extraction. The most commonly used drugs are codeine and the codeine congeners oxycodone and hydrocodone. These narcotics are well absorbed from the gut and can produce drowsiness and gastrointestinal upset. Opioid analgesics are rarely used alone; instead, they are formulated with other analgesics, primarily aspirin or acetaminophen. When codeine is used, the amount of codeine is frequently designated by a numbering system. Compounds labeled No. 1 have 7.5 mg of codeine; No. 2, 15 mg; No. 3, 30 mg; and No. 4, 60 mg. When a combination of analgesic drugs is used, the dentist must keep in mind that it is necessary to provide 500 to 1000 mg of aspirin or acetaminophen every 4 hours to achieve maximal effectiveness from the nonnarcotic. Many of the compound drugs have only 300 mg of aspirin or acetaminophen added to the narcotic. An example of a rational approach would be to prescribe a compound containing 300 mg of acetaminophen and 15 mg of codeine (No. 2). The usual adult dose would be two tablets of this compound every 4 hours. This two-tablet (30 mg of codeine and 600 mg of acetaminophen) dose provides a nearly ideal analgesic. Should the patient require stronger analgesic action, three tablets can be taken with increased effectiveness of acetaminophen and codeine. Doses that supply 30 to 60 mg of codeine but only 300 mg of acetaminophen fail to take full advantage of the analgesic effect of acetaminophen (Table 10-2).

The Drug Enforcement Administration controls narcotic analgesics. To write prescriptions for these drugs, the dentist must have a Drug Enforcement Administration permit and number. The drugs are categorized into four basic schedules based on their liability for abuse. Several important differences exist between schedule II and schedule III drugs concerning writing prescriptions (see Appendix III).

It is important to emphasize that the most effective method of controlling pain is to build a close relationship between surgeon and patient. Specific time must be spent discussing the issue of postoperative discomfort, with concern clearly expressed by the surgeon. Prescriptions should be given with clear instructions about when to begin the medication and how to take it at each interval. If these procedures are followed, mild analgesics given for a short time (usually no longer than 2 to 3 days) may be all that is required.

Diet

Patients who have had extractions may avoid eating because of local pain or fear of pain when eating. Therefore, they should be given specific instructions regarding their postoperative diet. A high-calorie, high-volume liquid diet is best for the first 12 to 24 hours.

TABLE 10-1

Analgesics for Postextraction Pain

Oral Narcotic	Usual Dose
MILD PAIN SITUATIONS	
Ibuprofen	400-800 mg q4h
Acetaminophen	500-1000 mg q4h
MODERATE PAIN SITUATIONS	
Codeine	15-60 mg
Hydrocodone	5-10 mg
SEVERE PAIN SITUATIONS	
Oxycodone	2.5-10 mg

TABLE 10-2

Commonly Used Combination Analgesics

Brand Name	Amount (mg)	Amount (mg)
CODEINE-ACETAMINOPHEN	**CODEINE**	**ACETAMINOPHEN**
Tylenol		
No. 2	15.0	300
No. 3	30.0	300
No. 4	60.0	300
OXYCODONE-ASPIRIN	**OXYCODONE**	**ASPIRIN**
Percodan	5.0	325
Percodan-demi	2.5	325
OXYCODONE ACETAMINOPHEN	**OXYCODONE**	**ACETAMINOPHEN**
Percocet	2.5	325
	5.0	325
	7.5	500
	10.0	650
Tylox	5.0	500
HYDROCODONE-ASPIRIN	**HYDROCODONE**	**ASPIRIN**
Lortab ASA	5.0	500
HYDROCODONE-ACETAMINOPHEN	**HYDROCODONE**	**ACETAMINOPHEN**
Vicodin	5.0	500
Vicodin ES	7.5	750
Lorcet HD	5.0	500
Lorcet Plus	7.5	650
Lorcet 10/650	10.0	650
Lortab 2.5/500	2.5	500
Lortab 5/500	5.0	500
Lortab Elixir	2.5 mg/5 mL	170 mg/5 mL

The patient must have an adequate intake of fluids, usually at least 2 L, during the first 24 hours. The fluids can be juices, milk, water, or any other beverage that appeals to the patient.

Food in the first 12 hours should be soft and cool. Cool and cold foods help keep the local area comfortable. Ice cream and milkshakes, unlike solid foods, tend not to cause local trauma or initiate rebleeding episodes.

If the patient had multiple extractions in all areas of the mouth, a soft diet is recommended for several days after the surgical procedure. The patient should be advised to return to a normal diet as soon as possible.

Patients who are diabetic should be encouraged to return to their normal insulin and caloric intake as soon as possible. For such patients the surgeon may plan surgery on only one side of the mouth at each surgical sitting, thereby not overly interfering with normal dietary intake.

Oral Hygiene

Patients should be advised that keeping the teeth and mouth reasonably clean results in a more rapid healing of their surgical wounds. Postoperatively on the day of surgery patients may gently brush the teeth that are away from the area of surgery in the usual fashion. They should avoid brushing the teeth immediately adjacent to the extraction site to prevent a new bleeding episode, avoid disturbing sutures, and to avoid pain.

The next day, patients should begin gentle rinses with warm water. The water should be warm but not hot enough to burn the tissue. Most patients can resume preoperative oral hygienic methods by the third or fourth day after surgery. Dental floss should be used in the usual fashion on teeth anterior and posterior to the extraction sites as soon as the patient is sufficiently comfortable.

If oral hygiene is likely to be difficult after extractions in multiple areas of the mouth, mouth rinses with agents such as dilute hydrogen peroxide may be used. Rinsing 3 to 4 times a day for approximately 1 week after surgery may result in more rapid healing.

Edema

Many surgical procedures result in a certain amount of edema or swelling after surgery. Routine extraction of a single tooth will probably not result in swelling that the patient can see, whereas the extraction of multiple impacted teeth with reflection of soft tissue and removal of bone may result in moderately large amounts of swelling (Fig. 10-2). Swelling usually reaches its maximum 24 to 48 hours after the surgical procedure. Swelling begins to subside on the third or fourth day and is usually resolved by the end of the first week. Increased swelling after the third day may be an indication of infection rather than continued postsurgical edema.

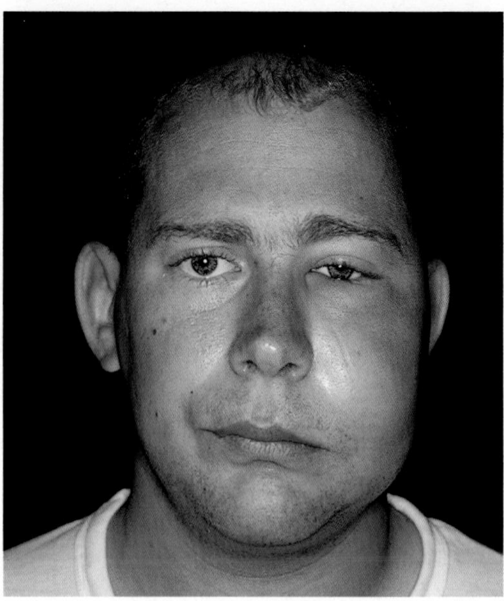

FIGURE 10-2 Extraction of impacted right maxillary and mandibular third molars was performed 2 days before this photograph was taken. Patient exhibits moderate amount of facial edema, which will resolve within 1 week of surgery.

Once the surgery is completed and the patient is ready to be discharged, some dentists use ice packs to help minimize the swelling and make the patient feel more comfortable; however, there is no evidence that the cooling actually controls this type of edema. Ice should not be placed directly on the skin, but rather a layer of dry cloth should be placed between the ice container and the tissue to prevent superficial tissue damage. An ice bag or small bag of frozen peas should be kept on the local area for 20 minutes and then left off for 20 minutes for 12 to 24 hours.

On the second postoperative day, neither ice nor heat should be applied to the face. On the third and subsequent postoperative days, application of heat may help to resolve the swelling more quickly. Heat sources such as hot water bottles and heating pads are recommended. Patients should be warned to avoid high-level heat for long periods to keep from injuring the skin.

Most important is that patients anticipate some amount of swelling. They should also be warned that the swelling may tend to wax and wane, occurring more in the morning and less in the evening because of postural variation. Patients should be informed that a moderate amount of swelling is a normal and healthy reaction of the tissue to the trauma of surgery. Patients should not be concerned or frightened by swelling, because it will resolve within a few days.

Prevention and Recognition of Infection

The principal way to prevent infection following routine extractions is for the surgeon to adhere carefully to the basic principles of surgery. These principles are to minimize tissue damage, remove sources of infection, and cleanse the wound. No other special measures must be taken with the average patient. However, some patients, especially those with depressed host-defense responses, may require antibiotics to prevent infection. Antibiotics in these patients should be administered before the surgical procedure is begun (see Chapter 15). Additional antibiotics after the surgery are usually not necessary for routine extraction in healthy patients.

Infections after routine extractions are unusual. The typical signs are development of a fever, increasing edema or worsening pain 3 to 4 days after surgery. Infected wounds looked inflamed, and some purulence is usually present.

Trismus

Extraction of teeth may result in trismus, or limitation in mouth opening. Trismus results from inflammation involving the muscles of mastication. The trismus may result from multiple injections of local anesthetic, especially if the injections have penetrated muscles. The muscle most likely to be involved is the

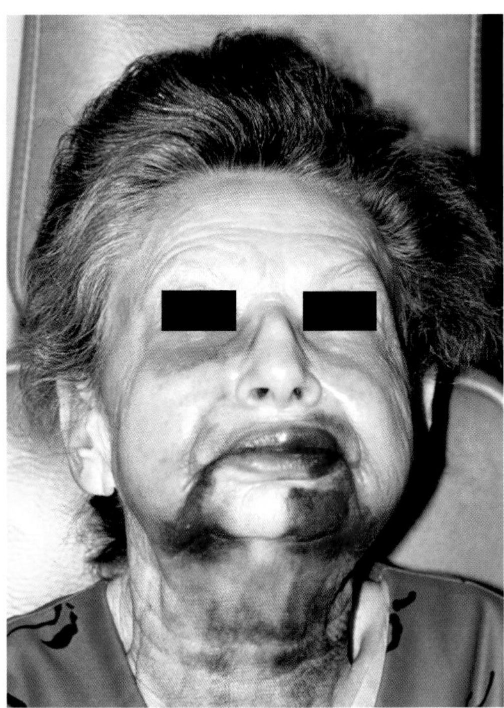

FIGURE 10-3 Moderate widespread ecchymosis of right side of face and neck is exhibited in an older patient after extraction of several mandibular teeth.

medial pterygoid muscle, which may be penetrated by the local anesthetic needle during the inferior alveolar nerve block.

Surgical extraction of impacted mandibular third molars usually results in some degree of trismus because the inflammatory response to the surgical procedure is sufficiently widespread to involve several muscles of mastication. Trismus is usually not severe and does not hamper the patient's activity. However, to prevent alarm, patients should be warned that this phenomenon might occur.

Ecchymosis

In some patients, blood oozes submucosally and subcutaneously, which appears as a bruise in the oral tissues and/or on the face (Fig. 10-3). Blood in the submucosal or subcutaneous tissues is known as *ecchymosis*. Ecchymosis is usually seen in older patients because of their decreased tissue tone, increased capillary fragility, and weaker intercellular attachment. Ecchymosis is not dangerous and does not increase pain or infection. Patients, however, should be warned that ecchymosis may occur, because if they awaken on the second postoperative day and see bruising in the cheek, submandibular area, or anterior neck, they may become apprehensive. This anxiety is easily prevented by postoperative instructions. Typically, the onset of ecchymosis is 2 to 4 days after surgery and usually resolves within 7 to 10 days.

POSTOPERATIVE FOLLOW-UP VISIT

All patients seen by novice surgeons should be given a return appointment so that the surgeon can check the patient's progress after the surgery and learn the appearance of a normally healing socket. In routine, uncomplicated procedures, a follow-up visit at 1 week is usually adequate. If sutures are to be removed, that can be done at a 1-week postoperative appointment.

Patients should be informed that if any question or problem arises, they should call the dentist and, if necessary, request an earlier follow-up visit. The most likely reasons for an earlier visit are prolonged bleeding, pain that is not responsive to the prescribed medication, and suspected infection.

If a patient who has had surgery begins to develop swelling with surface redness, fever, and/or pain on the third postoperative day or later, the patient can be assumed to have developed an infection until proved otherwise. The patient should be instructed to call for an appointment at the dentist's office immediately. The surgeon must then inspect the patient carefully to confirm or rule out the diagnosis of infection. If an infection is diagnosed, appropriate therapeutic measures should be taken (see Chapter 15).

Postsurgical pain that decreases at first but on the third or fourth day begins to increase, yet is not accompanied by swelling or other signs of infection, is probably a sign of "dry socket." This problem is usually confined to lower molar sockets. This annoying problem is simple to manage but may require that the patient return to the office several times (see Chapter 11).

OPERATIVE NOTE FOR THE RECORDS

The surgeon must enter into the records a note of what transpired during each visit. Some critical factors should be entered into the chart. The first is the date of the operation and a brief identification of the patient; then the surgeon states the diagnosis and reason for the extraction (e.g., nonrestorable caries or severe periodontal disease).

Comments regarding the patient's pertinent medical history, medications, and vital signs should be mentioned in the chart. This information should be noted in the chart before the surgery is performed to confirm that the dentist has reviewed these issues with the patient and that the patient's current status is satisfactory for the surgical procedure.

A brief mention should be made of the oral examination. During any routine long-term care of a patient, the dentist should examine the soft tissues of the face, mouth, and upper neck periodically. If this is done at the time of surgery, it should be noted in the chart.

The surgeon should enter into the chart the type and amount of anesthetic used. For example, if the drug were lidocaine with a vasoconstrictor, the dentist would write down the number of milligrams of lidocaine and of epinephrine.

The surgeon should then write a brief note concerning the procedure that was performed, which should include a description of surgery and any complications. A description of the patient's tolerance of the procedure can also be included.

A comment concerning the discharge instructions, including mention of the postoperative instruction that was given to the patient, is recorded.

The prescribed medications are listed, including the name of the drug, its dose, and the total number of tablets. Alternatively, a copy of the prescriptions can be added to the chart. Finally, the need for a return appointment is recorded in the chart if indicated (Box 10-1). (See Appendix II.)

BOX 10-1

Elements of an Operative Note

1. Date
2. Patient name and identification (may be on an adhesive label)
3. Diagnosis of problem to be managed surgically
4. Review of medical history, medications, and vital signs
5. Oral examination
6. Anesthesia (amount used)
7. Procedure (including description of surgery and complications)
8. Discharge instructions
9. Medications prescribed and their amounts (or attach copy of prescription)
10. Need for follow-up appointment
11. Signature (legible or printed underneath)

CHAPTER 11

Prevention and Management of Surgical Complications

JAMES R. HUPP

CHAPTER OUTLINE

This chapter discusses the most common complications occurring during or after oral surgical procedures. Some are minor, whereas others are more serious. These are surgical, not medical, complications; the latter are discussed in Chapter 3.

PREVENTION OF COMPLICATIONS

As is the case of medical complications, the best and easiest way to manage a surgical complication is to prevent it from happening. Prevention of surgical complications is best accomplished by a thorough preoperative assessment and comprehensive treatment plan and careful execution of the surgical procedure. Only when these are routinely performed can the surgeon expect to have few complications. One must realize that even with such planning and with excellent surgical technique, complications occasionally occur. In situations in which the dentist has planned carefully, the complication is often predictable and can be managed routinely. For example, when extracting a maxillary first premolar that has long, thin roots, it is far easier to remove the buccal root than the palatal root. Therefore the surgeon uses more force toward the buccal root than toward the palatal root. If a root does fracture, it is the buccal root rather than the palatal root, and the subsequent buccal root retrieval is more straightforward.

Dentists must perform surgery that is within their limitations of capabilities. They must therefore carefully evaluate their training and ability before deciding to perform a specific surgical task. Thus, for example, it is inappropriate for a dentist with limited experience in the management of impacted third molars to undertake the surgical extraction of an embedded tooth. The incidence of operative and post-operative complications is unacceptably high in this situation. Surgeons must be cautious of unwarranted optimism, which clouds their judgment and prevents them from delivering the best possible care to the patient. The dentist must keep in mind that referral to a specialist is an option that should always be exercised if the planned surgery is beyond the dentist's own skill level. In some situations, this is not only a moral obligation but also wise medicolegal risk management.

In planning a surgical procedure, the first step is always a thorough review of the patient's medical history. Several of the complications to be discussed in this chapter can be caused by inadequate attention to medical histories that would have revealed the presence of a factor increasing surgical risk.

One of the primary ways to prevent complications is by obtaining adequate images and carefully reviewing them (see Chapter 7). Radiographs must include the entire area of surgery, including the apices of the roots of the teeth to be extracted and the local and regional anatomic structures, such as adjacent parts of the maxillary sinus and the inferior alveolar canal. The surgeon must look for the presence of abnormal tooth root morphology or signs that the tooth may be ankylosed. After careful examination of the radiographs, the surgeon must occasionally alter the treatment plan to prevent or limit the magnitude of the complications that might be anticipated with a closed extraction. Instead, the surgeon should consider surgical approaches to removing teeth in such cases.

After an adequate medical history has been taken and the radiographs have been analyzed, the surgeon must do the preoperative planning. This is not simply a preparation of a detailed surgical plan and instrumentation but is also a plan for managing patient pain and anxiety and postoperative recovery (instructions and modifications of normal activity for the patient). Thorough preoperative instructions and explanations for the patient are essential in preventing or limiting the impact of the majority of complications that occur in the postoperative period. If the instructions are not carefully explained and the importance of compliance made clear, the patient is less likely to comply with them.

Finally, to keep complications at a minimum, the surgeon must always follow basic surgical principles. There should always be clear visualization and access to the operative field, which requires adequate light, adequate soft tissue retraction and reflection (including lips, cheeks, tongue, and soft tissue flaps), and adequate suction. The teeth to be removed must have an unimpeded pathway for removal. Occasionally, bone must be removed and teeth must be sectioned to achieve this goal. Controlled force is of paramount importance; this means "finesse," not "force." The surgeon must follow the principles of asepsis, atraumatic handling of tissues, hemostasis, and thorough débridement of the wound after the surgical procedure. Violation of these principles leads to an increased incidence and severity of surgical complications.

SOFT TISSUE INJURIES

Injuries to the soft tissue of the oral cavity are almost always the result of the surgeon's lack of adequate attention to the delicate nature of the mucosa, attempts to do surgery with inadequate access, or the use of excessive and uncontrolled force. The surgeon must continue to pay careful attention to the soft tissue while working on bone and tooth structures (Box 11-1).

Tear of a Mucosal Flap

The most common soft tissue injury during oral surgery is the tearing of the mucosal flap during surgical extraction of a tooth. This usually results from an initially inadequately sized envelope flap, which is then forcibly retracted beyond the ability of the tissue to stretch as the surgeon tries to gain needed surgical access (Fig. 11-1). This results in a tearing, usually at one end of the incision. Prevention of this complication is threefold: (1) create adequately sized flaps to prevent excess tension on the flap, (2) use controlled amounts of retraction force on the flap, and (3) create releasing incisions when indicated. If a tear does occur in the flap, the flap should be carefully repositioned once the surgery is complete. Or if the surgeon or assistant sees a flap beginning to tear, the hard tissue surgery can be stopped and the incision can be lengthened to gain better access before continuing the hard tissue surgery. In most patients, careful suturing of the tear results in adequate but somewhat delayed healing. If the tear is especially jagged, the surgeon may consider excising the edges of the torn flap to create a smooth flap margin before closure. This latter step should be performed with caution because excision of excessive amounts of tissue leads to closure of the wound under tension and probable wound dehiscence, or it might compromise the amount of attached gingiva adjacent to a tooth.

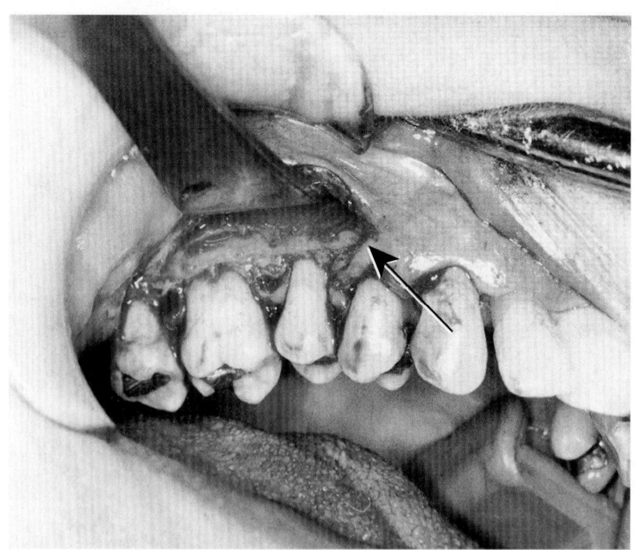

FIGURE 11-1 Periosteal elevator (Seldin elevator) is used to reflect mucoperiosteal flap. Elevator placed perpendicular to bone and held in place by pushing firmly against bone, not by pushing it apically against soft tissue (*arrow*).

BOX 11-1

Prevention of Soft Tissue Injuries

1. Pay strict attention to soft tissue injuries.
2. Develop adequate-sized flaps.
3. Use minimal force for retraction of soft tissue.

Puncture Wound

The second soft tissue injury that occurs with some frequency is inadvertent puncturing of the soft tissue. Instruments, such as a straight elevator or periosteal elevator, may slip from the surgical field and puncture or tear into adjacent soft tissue.

Once again, this injury is the result of using uncontrolled force and is best prevented by the use of controlled force, with special attention given to using finger rests or support from the opposite hand in anticipation of slippage. If the instrument slips from the tooth or bone, the fingers thus catch the hand before injury occurs (Fig. 11-2). When a puncture wound does occur, the treatment is primarily aimed at preventing infection and allowing healing to occur, usually by secondary intention. If the wound bleeds excessively, it should be controlled by direct pressure applied to the wound. Once hemostasis is achieved, the wound is usually left open unsutured so that if a small infection were to occur, there is an adequate pathway for drainage.

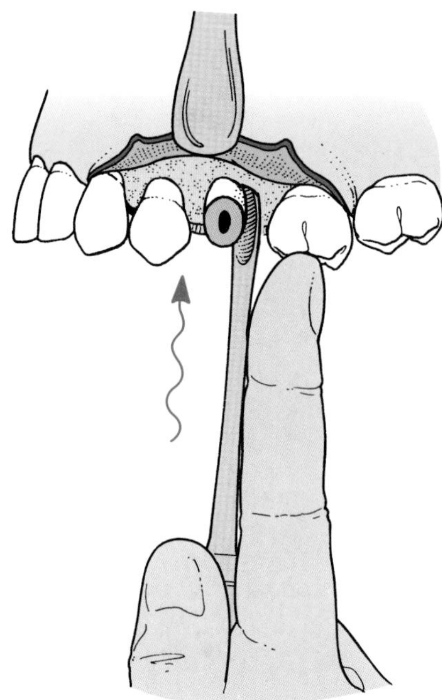

FIGURE 11-2 Small, straight elevator can be used as shoehorn to luxate broken root. When straight elevator is used in this position, hand must be securely supported on adjacent teeth to prevent inadvertent slippage of instrument from tooth and subsequent injury to adjacent tissue.

Stretch or Abrasion

Abrasions or burns of the lips, corners of the mouth, or flaps usually result from the rotating shank of the bur rubbing on the soft tissue or on a metal retractor in contact with soft tissue (Fig. 11-3). When the surgeon is focused on the cutting end of the bur, the assistant should be aware of the location of the shank of the bur in relation to the cheeks and lips. However, the surgeon should also remain aware of shaft location. If an area of oral mucosa is abraded or burned, little treatment is possible other than keeping the area clean with regular oral rinsing. Usually such wounds heal in 4 to 7 days (depending on the depth of damage) without scarring. If such an abrasion or burn does develop on the skin, the dentist should advise the patient to keep it covered with an antibiotic ointment. The patient must keep the ointment only on the abraded area and not spread onto intact skin because the ointment is likely to cause a rash. These abrasions usually take 5 to 10 days to heal. The patient should keep the area moist with the ointment during the entire healing period to prevent eschar formation and delayed healing, as well as to keep the area reasonably comfortable. Scarring or permanent discoloration of the affected skin may occur but is limited by proper wound care.

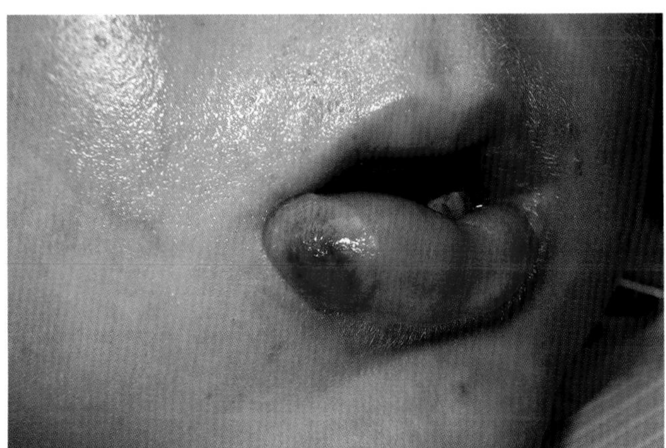

FIGURE 11-3 Abrasion of lower lip as a result of shank of burr rotating on soft tissue. Abrasion represents a combination of friction and heat damage. Wound should be kept covered with antibiotic ointment until an eschar forms, taking care to keep the ointment off uninjured skin as much as possible.
(Photo courtesy Dr. Myron Tucker.)

PROBLEMS WITH A TOOTH BEING EXTRACTED

Root Fracture

The most common problem associated with the tooth being extracted is fracture of its roots. Long, curved, divergent roots that lie in dense bone are the most likely to be fractured. The main methods of preventing fracture of roots is to perform surgery in the manner described in previous chapters or to use an open extraction technique and remove bone to decrease the amount of force necessary to remove the tooth (Box 11-2). Recovery of a fractured root with a surgical approach is discussed in Chapter 8.

Root Displacement

The tooth root that is most commonly displaced into unfavorable anatomic spaces is the maxillary molar root, when it is forced or lost into the maxillary sinus. If a fractured root of a maxillary molar is being removed with a straight elevator being used with excess apical pressure, the tooth root can be displaced into the maxillary sinus. If this occurs, the surgeon must make several assessments to determine the appropriate treatment. First, the surgeon must identify the size of the root lost into the sinus. It may be a root tip of several millimeters or an entire tooth root. The surgeon must next assess whether there has been any infection of the tooth or periapical tissues. If the tooth was not infected, management is more straightforward than if the tooth had been acutely infected. Finally, the surgeon must assess the preoperative condition of the maxillary sinus. For the patient who has a healthy maxillary sinus, it is easier to manage a displaced root than if the sinus is or has been chronically infected.

If the displaced tooth fragment is a small (2 or 3 mm) root tip and the tooth and sinus have no preexisting infection, the surgeon should make a brief attempt at removing the root. First, a radiograph of the fractured tooth root should be taken to document its position and size. Once that has been accomplished, the surgeon should irrigate through the small opening

BOX 11-2

Prevention of Root and Displacement Fracture

1. Always plan for root fracture.
2. Use surgical (i.e., open) extraction if high probability of fracture exists.
3. Do not use strong apical force on a broken root.

in the socket apex and then suction the irrigating solution from the sinus via the socket. This occasionally flushes the root apex from the sinus through the socket. The surgeon should check the suction solution and confirm radiographically that the root has been removed. If this technique is not successful, no additional surgical procedure should be performed through the socket, and the root tip should be left in the sinus. The small, noninfected root tip can be left in place because it is unlikely to cause any troublesome sequelae. Additional surgery in this situation causes more patient morbidity than leaving the root tip in the sinus. If the root tip is left in the sinus, measures should be taken similar to those taken when leaving any root tip in place. The patient must be informed of the decision and given proper follow-up instructions for regular monitoring of the root and the sinus.

The oroantral communication should be managed as discussed later, with a figure-of-eight suture over the socket, sinus precautions, antibiotics, and a nasal spray to lessen the chance of infection by keeping the ostium open. The most likely occurrence is that the root apex will fibrose onto the sinus membrane with no subsequent problems. If the tooth root is infected or the patient has chronic sinusitis, the patient should be referred to an oral and maxillofacial surgeon for removal of the root tip via a Caldwell-Luc approach.

If a large root fragment or the entire tooth is displaced into the maxillary sinus, it should be removed (Fig. 11-4). The usual method is a Caldwell-Luc approach into the maxillary sinus in the canine fossa region and then removal of the tooth. Oral and maxillofacial surgeons perform this procedure (see Chapter 19).

Impacted maxillary third molars are occasionally displaced into the maxillary sinus (from which they are removed via a Caldwell-Luc approach). But if displacement occurs, it is more commonly into the infratemporal space. During elevation of the tooth, the elevator may force the tooth posteriorly through the periosteum into the infratemporal fossa. The tooth is usually lateral to the lateral pterygoid plate and inferior to the lateral pterygoid muscle. If good access and light are available, the surgeon should make a single cautious effort to retrieve the tooth with a hemostat. However, the tooth is usually not visible, and blind probing results in further displacement. If the tooth is not retrieved after a single effort, the incision should be closed and the operation stopped. The patient should be informed that the tooth has been displaced and will be removed later. Antibiotics should be given to help decrease the possibility of an infection, and routine postoperative care should be provided. During the initial healing time, fibrosis occurs and stabilizes the tooth in a firm position. The tooth is removed later by an oral and maxillofacial surgeon after radiographic localization.

The lingual cortical bone over the roots of the molars becomes thinner as it progresses posteriorly. Mandibular third molars, for example, frequently have dehiscence in the overlying lingual bone and may be actually sitting in the submandibular space preoperatively. Fractured mandibular molar roots that are being removed with apical pressures may be displaced through the lingual cortical plate and into the submandibular space. Even small amounts of apical pressure can result in displacement of the root into that space. Prevention of displacement into the submandibular space is primarily achieved by avoiding all apical pressures when removing the mandibular roots.

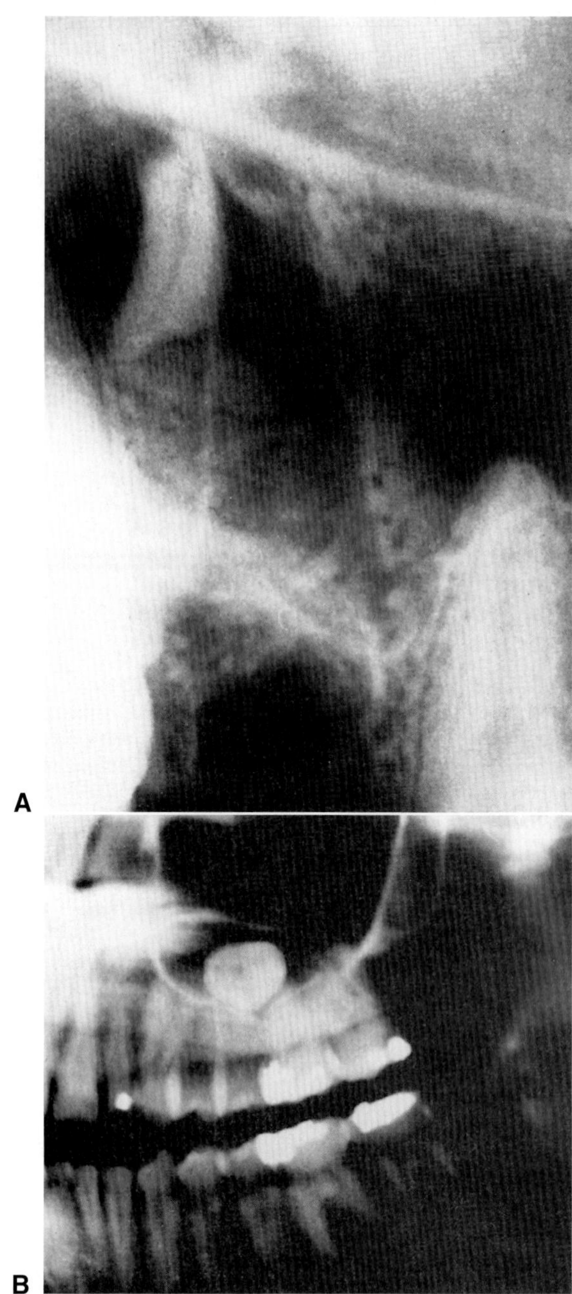

FIGURE 11-4 **A**, Large root fragment displaced into maxillary sinus. Fragment should be removed with Caldwell-Luc approach. **B**, Tooth in maxillary sinus is maxillary third molar that was displaced into sinus during elevation of tooth. This tooth must be removed from sinus, probably via a Caldwell-Luc approach.

Triangular-shaped elevators, such as the Cryer, are usually used to elevate broken tooth roots of mandibular molars. If the root disappears during the root removal, the dentist should make a single effort to remove it. The index finger of the left hand is inserted onto the lingual aspect of the floor of the mouth in an attempt to place pressure against the lingual aspect of the mandible and force the root back into the socket. If this works, the surgeon may be able to tease the root out of the socket with a root tip pick. If this effort is not successful on the initial attempt, the dentist should abandon the procedure and refer the patient to an oral and maxillofacial surgeon. The usual, definitive procedure for removing such a root tip is to reflect a soft tissue flap on the lingual aspect of the mandible and gently dissect the overlying mucoperiosteum until the root tip can be found. As with teeth that are displaced into the maxillary sinus, if the root fragment is small and was not infected preoperatively, the oral and maxillofacial surgeon may elect to leave the root in its position because surgical retrieval of the root may be an extensive procedure or risk serious injury to the lingual nerve.

Tooth Lost into the Pharynx

Occasionally, the crown of a tooth or an entire tooth might be lost into the pharynx. If this occurs, the patient should be turned toward the surgeon and placed into position with the mouth toward the floor as much as possible. The patient should be encouraged to cough and spit the tooth out onto the floor. The suction device can sometimes be used to help remove the tooth.

In spite of these efforts, the tooth may be swallowed or aspirated. If the patient has no coughing or respiratory distress, it is most likely that the tooth was swallowed and has traveled down the esophagus into the stomach. However, if the patient has a violent episode of coughing or shortness of breath, the tooth may have been aspirated through the vocal cords into the trachea and from there on to a main stem bronchus.

In either case the patient should be transported to an emergency room, and chest and abdominal radiographs should be taken to determine the specific location of the tooth. If the tooth has been aspirated, consultation should be requested regarding the possibility of removing the tooth with a bronchoscope. The urgent management of aspiration is to maintain the patient's airway and breathing. Supplemental oxygen may be appropriate if respiratory distress appears to be occurring.

If the tooth has been swallowed, it is highly probable that it will pass through the gastrointestinal tract within 2 to 4 days. Because teeth are not usually jagged or sharp, unimpeded passage occurs in almost all situations. However, it may be prudent to have the patient go to an emergency room and have a radiograph of the abdomen taken to confirm the presence of the tooth in the gastrointestinal tract instead of in the respiratory tract. Follow-up radiographs are probably not necessary because the usual fate of swallowed teeth is passage.

INJURIES TO ADJACENT TEETH

When the dentist extracts a tooth, the focus of attention is on that particular tooth and the application of forces to luxate and deliver it. When the surgeon's total attention is thus focused, likelihood of injury to the adjacent teeth increases. Injury is often due to use of a bur to remove bone or divide a tooth for removal. The surgeon should take care to avoid getting too close to adjacent teeth when surgically removing a tooth. This usually requires the surgeon to keep some of the focus on structures adjacent to the site of the surgery.

Fracture or Dislodgment of an Adjacent Restoration

The most common injury to adjacent teeth is the inadvertent fracture or dislodgment of a restoration or of a severely carious tooth while the surgeon is attempting to luxate the tooth to be removed with an elevator (Fig. 11-5). If a large restoration

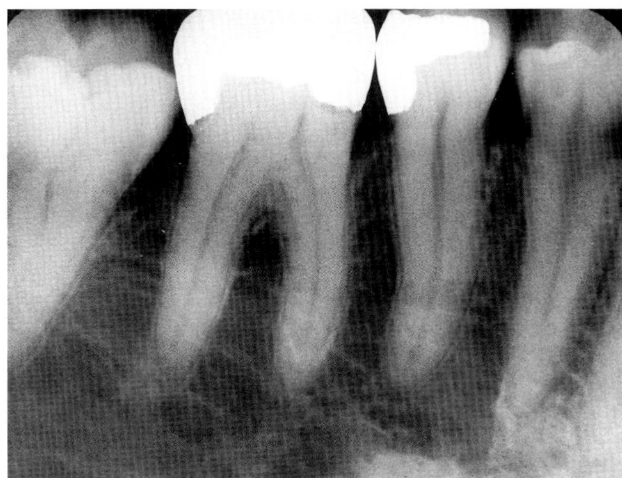

FIGURE 11-5 Mandibular first molar. If first molar is to be removed, surgeon must take care not to fracture amalgam in second premolar with elevators or forceps.

exists, the surgeon should warn the patient preoperatively about the possibility of fracturing it during the extraction. Prevention of such a fracture is primarily achieved by avoiding application of instrumentation and force on the restoration (Box 11-3). This means that the straight elevator should be used with great caution, inserting it entirely into the periodontal ligament space, or not used at all to luxate the tooth before extraction when the adjacent tooth has a large restoration. If a restoration is dislodged or fractured, the surgeon should make sure that the displaced restoration is removed from the mouth and does not fall into the empty tooth socket. Once the surgical procedure has been completed, the injured tooth should be treated by replacement of the displaced crown or placement of a temporary restoration. The patient should be informed if a fracture of a tooth or restoration has occurred and that a replacement restoration is needed (see Chapter 12).

Teeth in the opposite arch may also be injured as a result of uncontrolled forces. This usually occurs when buccolingual forces inadequately mobilize a tooth and/or excessive tractional forces are used. The tooth suddenly releases from the socket, and the forceps strikes the teeth of the opposite arch, chipping or fracturing a cusp. This is more likely to occur with extraction of lower teeth because these teeth may require more vertical tractional forces for their delivery, especially when using the No. 23 (cowhorn) forceps. Prevention of this type of injury can be accomplished by several methods. First and primarily, the surgeon should avoid the use of excessive tractional forces. The tooth should be adequately luxated with apical, buccolingual, and rotational forces to minimize the need for tractional forces.

BOX 11-3

Prevention of Injury to Adjacent Teeth

1. Recognize the potential to fracture a large restoration.
2. Warn patient preoperatively.
3. Use elevators judiciously.
4. Ask assistant to warn surgeon of pressure on adjacent teeth.

Even when this is done, however, occasionally a tooth releases unexpectedly. The surgeon or assistant should protect the teeth of the opposite arch by holding a finger or suction tip against them to absorb the blow should the forceps be released in that direction. If such an injury occurs, the tooth should be smoothed or restored as necessary to keep the patient comfortable until a permanent restoration can be constructed.

Luxation of an Adjacent Tooth

Inappropriate use of the extraction instruments may luxate an adjacent tooth. Luxation is prevented by judicious use of force with elevators and forceps. If the tooth to be extracted is crowded and has overlapping adjacent teeth, as is commonly seen in the mandibular incisor region, a thin, narrow forceps such as the No. 286 forceps may be useful for the extraction (Fig. 11-6). Forceps with broader beaks should be avoided because they will cause injury and luxation of adjacent teeth.

If an adjacent tooth is significantly luxated or partially avulsed, the treatment goal is to reposition the tooth into its appropriate position and stabilize it so that adequate healing occurs. This usually requires that the tooth simply be repositioned in the tooth socket and left alone. The occlusion should be checked to ensure that the tooth has not been displaced into a hypererupted and traumatic occlusion. Occasionally, the luxated tooth is mobile. If this is the case, the tooth should be stabilized with semirigid fixation to maintain the tooth in its position. A simple silk suture that crosses the occlusal table and is sutured to the adjacent gingiva is usually sufficient. Rigid fixation with circumdental wires and arch bars results in increased chances for external root resorption and ankylosis of the tooth and therefore should usually be avoided (see Chapter 23).

Extraction of the Wrong Tooth

A complication that every dentist believes can never happen—but happens surprisingly often—is extraction of the wrong tooth. This is usually the most common cause of malpractice lawsuits against dentists. Extraction of the wrong tooth should never occur if appropriate attention is given to the planning and execution of the surgical procedure.

This problem may be the result of inadequate attention to the preoperative assessment. If the tooth to be extracted is grossly carious, it is less likely that the wrong tooth will be removed. A common reason for removing the wrong tooth is that a dentist removes a tooth for another dentist. The use of differing tooth numbering systems or differences in the mounting of radiographs can easily lead the treating dentist to misunderstand the instructions from the referring dentist. Thus the wrong tooth is sometimes extracted when the dentist is asked to remove teeth for orthodontic purposes, especially from patients who are in mixed dentition stages and whose orthodontists have asked for unusual extractions. Careful preoperative planning, good communications with referring dentists, and clinical assessment of which tooth is to be removed before the elevator and forceps are applied are the main methods of preventing this complication (Box 11-4).

If the wrong tooth is extracted and the surgeon realizes this error immediately, the tooth should be replaced quickly into the tooth socket. If the extraction is for orthodontic purposes, the surgeon should contact the orthodontist immediately and discuss whether the tooth that was removed can substitute for the tooth that should have been removed. If the orthodontist believes the original tooth must be removed, the correct extraction should be deferred for 4 or 5 weeks until the fate of the replanted tooth can be assessed. If the wrongfully extracted

BOX 11-4

Prevention of Extraction of Wrong Teeth

1. Focus attention on procedure.
2. Check with patient and assistant to ensure that correct tooth is being removed.
3. Check, then recheck, images and records to confirm the correct tooth.

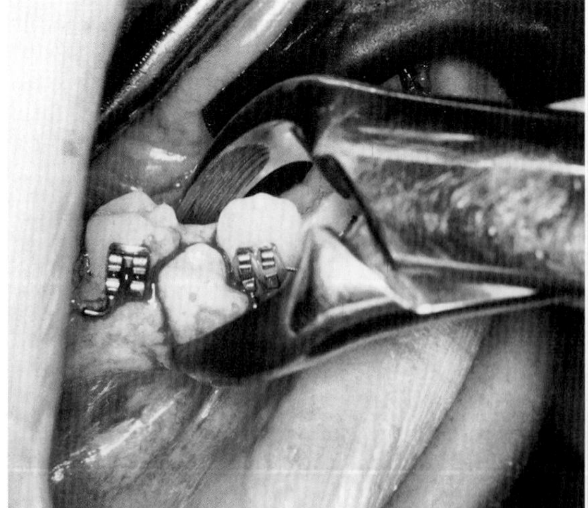

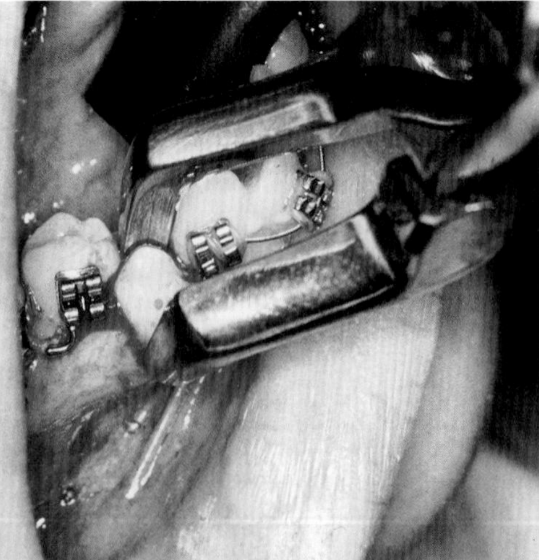

FIGURE 11-6 A, No. 151 forceps, which are too wide to grasp premolar to be extracted without luxating adjacent teeth. B, Maxillary root forceps, which can be adapted easily to tooth for extraction.

tooth has regained its attachment to the alveolar process, then the originally planned extraction may proceed. In addition, the surgeon should not extract the contralateral tooth until a definite alternative treatment plan is made.

If the surgeon does not recognize that the wrong tooth was extracted until the patient returns for a postoperative visit, little can be done to correct the problem. Replantation of the extracted tooth after it has dried cannot be successfully accomplished.

When the wrong tooth is extracted, it is important to inform the patient, the patient's parents (if the patient is a minor), and any other dentist involved with the patient's care, such as the orthodontist. In some situations the orthodontist may be able to adjust the treatment plan so that extraction of the wrong tooth necessitates only a minor adjustment. And if the case did not involve orthodontic care, a dental implant-supported restoration may totally restore the patient's dental status as it was before the inadvertent extraction.

INJURIES TO OSSEOUS STRUCTURES

Fracture of the Alveolar Process

The extraction of a tooth usually requires that the surrounding alveolar bone be expanded to allow an unimpeded pathway for tooth removal. However, in some situations the bone fractures and is removed with the tooth instead of expanding. The most likely cause of fracture of the alveolar process is the use of excessive force with forceps, which fractures large portions of cortical plate. If the surgeon realizes that excessive force is necessary to remove a tooth, a soft tissue flap should be elevated, and controlled amounts of bone should be removed so that the tooth can be easily delivered or in the case of multirooted teeth, sectioning of the tooth. If this principle is not adhered to and the surgeon continues to use excessive or uncontrolled force, fracture of the bone commonly occurs.

The most likely places for bony fracture are the buccal cortical plate over the maxillary canine, the buccal cortical plate over the maxillary molars (especially the first molar), the portions of the floor of the maxillary sinus associated with maxillary molars, the maxillary tuberosity, and the labial bone on mandibular incisors (Fig. 11-7). All of these bony injuries are caused by excessive force from the forceps.

The primary method of preventing these fractures is to perform a careful preoperative examination of the alveolar process, clinically and radiographically (Box 11-5). Surgeons should inspect the root form of the tooth to be removed and assess the proximity of the roots to the maxillary sinus (Fig. 11-8). Surgeons should also check the thickness of the buccal cortical plate overlying the tooth to be extracted (Fig. 11-9). If the roots diverge widely, if they lie close to the sinus, or if the patient has a heavy buccal cortical bone, surgeons must take special measures to prevent fracturing excessive portions of bone. Age is a factor to be considered because the bones of older patients are likely to be less elastic and therefore are more likely to fracture than to expand.

BOX 11-5

Prevention of Fracture of Alveolar Process

1. Conduct a thorough preoperative clinical and radiographic examination.
2. Do not use excessive force.
3. Use surgical (i.e., open) extraction technique to reduce force required.

The surgeon who preoperatively determines that a high probability exists for bone fracture should consider performing the extraction by the open surgical technique. Using this method the surgeon can remove a smaller, more controlled amount of bone, which results in more rapid healing and a more ideal ridge form for prosthetic reconstruction.

When the maxillary molar lies close to the maxillary sinus, surgical exposure of the tooth, with sectioning of the tooth roots into two or three portions prevents the removal of a portion of the maxillary sinus floor. This then prevents the formation of a chronic oroantral fistula, which requires secondary procedures to close.

In summary, prevention of fractures of large portions of the cortical plate depends on preoperative radiographic and clinical assessment, avoidance of the use of excessive amounts of uncontrolled force, and the early decision to perform an open extraction with removal of controlled amounts of bone and sectioning of multirooted teeth. During a forceps extraction, if the appropriate amount of tooth mobilization does not occur early, then the wise and prudent surgeon will alter the treatment plan to the surgical technique instead of pursuing the closed method.

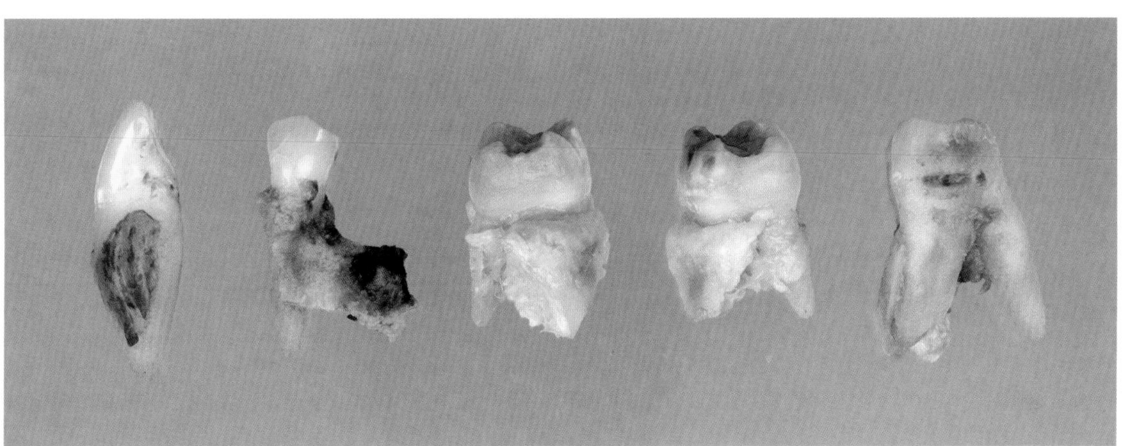

FIGURE 11-7 Forceps extraction of these teeth resulted in removal of bone and tooth instead of just tooth.

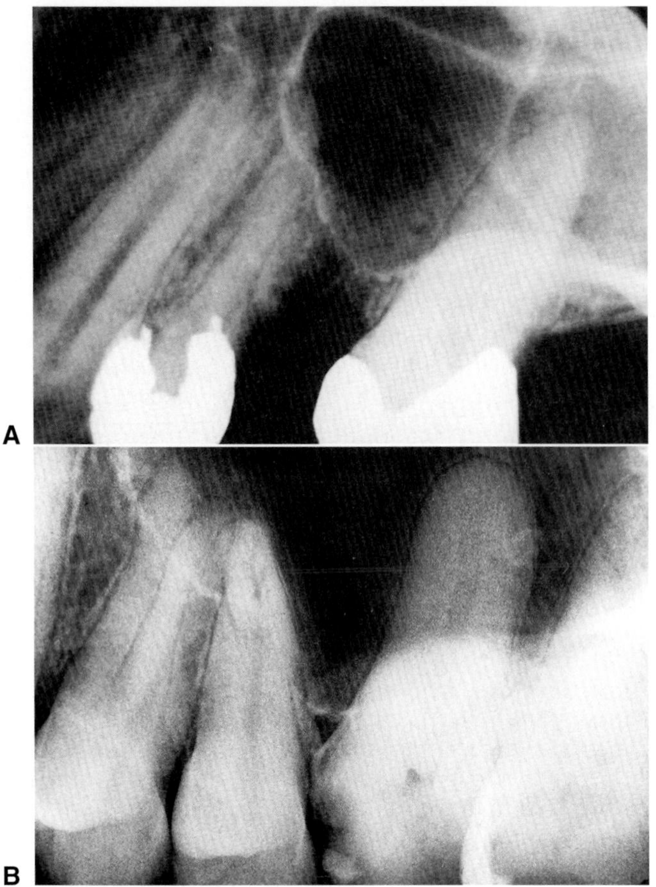

FIGURE 11-8 A, Floor of sinus associated with roots of teeth. If extraction is required, tooth should be removed surgically. B, Maxillary molar teeth immediately adjacent to sinus present increased danger of sinus exposure.

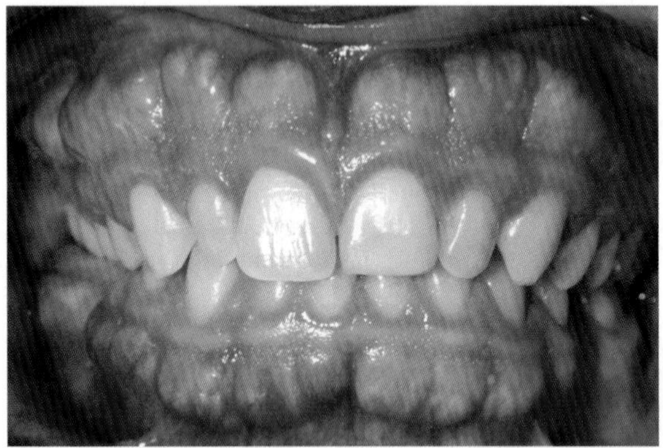

FIGURE 11-9 Patient with heavy buccal cortical plate who requires open extraction. (From Neville BW, Damm DD, Allen CM et al: *Oral and maxillofacial pathology*, ed 2, St Louis, 2002, Saunders.)

Management of fractures of the alveolar bone takes several different forms, depending on the type and severity of the fracture: If the bone has been completely removed from the tooth socket along with the tooth, it should *not* be replaced. The surgeon should simply make sure that the soft tissue has been repositioned as best as possible over the remaining bone to prevent delayed healing. The surgeon must also smooth any sharp edges that may have been caused by the fracture. If such sharp edges of bone exist, the surgeon should reflect a small amount of soft tissue and use a bone file to round off the sharp edges or rongeur to remove the sharpness.

The surgeon who has been supporting the alveolar process with the fingers during the extraction usually feels the fracture of the buccal cortical plate when it occurs. At this time the bone remains attached to the periosteum and usually heals if it can be separated from the tooth and left attached to the overlying soft tissue. The surgeon must carefully dissect the bone with its attached associated soft tissue away from the tooth. For this procedure the tooth must be stabilized with the forceps, and a small sharp instrument, such as a No. 9 periosteal elevator, should be used to elevate the buccal bone from the tooth root. One must realize that if the soft tissue flap is reflected from the bone, the blood supply to the overlying bone will be severed and the bone will then undergo necrosis. Once the bone and soft tissue have been elevated from the tooth, the tooth is removed and the bone and soft tissue flap are reapproximated and secured with sutures. When treated in this fashion, it is highly probable that the bone will heal in a more favorable ridge form for prosthetic reconstruction than if the bone had been removed along with the tooth. Therefore, it is worth the special effort to dissect the bone from the tooth.

Fracture of the Maxillary Tuberosity

Fracture of a large section of bone in the maxillary tuberosity area is a situation of special concern. The maxillary tuberosity is important for the construction of a stable retentive maxillary denture. If a large portion of this tuberosity is removed along with the maxillary tooth, denture stability is likely to be compromised. The maxillary tuberosity fractures most commonly result from extraction of an erupted maxillary third molar or from extraction of the second molar if it is the last tooth in the arch (Fig. 11-10).

If a tuberosity fracture occurs during an extraction, the treatment is similar to that just discussed for other bony fractures. The surgeon, using finger support for the alveolar process during the fracture (if the bone remains attached to the periosteum), should take measures to ensure the survival of

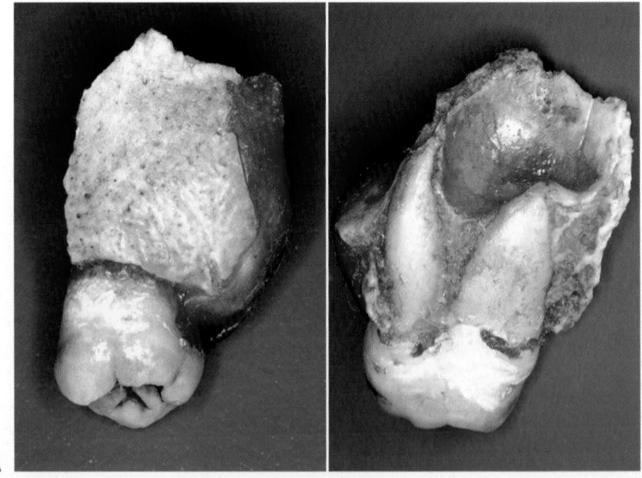

FIGURE 11-10 Tuberosity removed with maxillary second molar, which eliminates important prosthetic retention area and exposes maxillary sinus. A, Buccal view of bone removed with tooth. B, Superior view, looking onto sinus floor, which was removed with tooth. (Courtesy Dr. Edward Ellis III.)

that bony segment. If at all possible, the bony segment should be dissected away from the tooth, and the tooth should be removed in the usual fashion. The tuberosity is then stabilized with mucosal sutures as previously indicated.

However, if the tuberosity is excessively mobile and cannot be dissected from the tooth, the surgeon has several options. The first option is to splint the tooth being extracted to adjacent teeth and defer the extraction for 6 to 8 weeks, allowing time for the bone to heal. The tooth is then extracted with an open surgical technique. The second option is to section the crown of the tooth from the roots and allow the tuberosity and tooth root section to heal. After 6 to 8 weeks the surgeon can reenter the area and remove the tooth roots in the usual fashion. If the maxillary molar tooth was infected before surgery, these two techniques should be used with caution.

If the maxillary tuberosity is completely separated from the soft tissue, the usual steps are to smooth the sharp edges of the remaining bone and to reposition and suture the remaining soft tissue. The surgeon must carefully check for an oroantral communication and treat as necessary.

Fractures of the maxillary tuberosity should be viewed as a significant complication. The major therapeutic goal of management is to maintain the fractured bone in place and to provide the best possible environment for healing. This may be a situation that can best be handled by referral to an oral and maxillofacial surgeon.

INJURIES TO ADJACENT STRUCTURES

During the process of tooth extraction, it is possible to injure adjacent tissues. The prudent surgeon preoperatively evaluates all adjacent anatomic areas and designs a surgical procedure to lessen the chance of injury to these tissues.

Injury to Regional Nerves

The branches of the fifth cranial nerve, which provide innervation to the mucosa and skin, are the adjacent structures most likely to be injured during extraction. The most frequently involved specific branches are the mental nerve, the lingual nerve, the buccal nerve, and the nasopalatine nerve. The nasopalatine and buccal nerves are frequently sectioned during the creation of flaps for removal of impacted teeth. The area of sensory innervation of these two nerves is relatively small, and reinnervation of the affected area usually occurs rapidly. Therefore the nasopalatine and long buccal nerves can be surgically sectioned without long-lasting sequelae or much bother to the patient.

Surgical removal of mandibular premolar roots or impacted mandibular premolars and periapical surgery in the area of the mental nerve and mental foramen must be performed with great care. If the mental nerve is injured, the patient will have a paresthesia or anesthesia of the lip and chin. If the injury is the result of flap reflection or manipulation, normal sensation usually returns in a few days to a few weeks. If the mental nerve is sectioned at its exit from the mental foramen or torn along its course, it is likely that mental nerve function will not return, and the patient will have a permanent state of anesthesia. If surgery is to be performed in the area of the mental nerve or the mental foramen, it is imperative that surgeons have a keen awareness of the potential morbidity from injury to this nerve (Box 11-6). If surgeons have any question concerning their ability to perform the indicated surgical procedure, they should refer the patient to an oral and maxillofacial surgeon. If a three-corner flap is to be used in the area of the mental nerve, the vertical-releasing incision must be placed far enough anterior to avoid severing any portion of the mental nerve. Rarely is it advisable to make the vertical-releasing incision at the interdental papilla between the canine and second premolar.

BOX 11-6

Prevention of Nerve Injury

1. Be aware of nerve anatomy in the surgical area.
2. Avoid making incisions or affecting periosteum in the nerve area.

The lingual nerve is usually anatomically located directly against the lingual aspect of the mandible in the retromolar pad region. Occasionally, the path of the lingual nerve takes it into the retromolar pad area itself. The lingual nerve rarely regenerates if it is severely traumatized. Incisions made in the retromolar pad region of the mandible should be placed so as to avoid coming close to this nerve. Therefore, incisions made for surgical exposure of impacted third molars or of bony areas in the posterior molar region should be made well to the buccal aspect of the mandible. Similarly, if dissecting a flap involving the retromolar pad, care must be taken to avoid excessive dissection or stretching of the tissues on the lingual aspect of the retromolar pad. Prevention of injury to the lingual nerve is of paramount importance for avoiding this difficult complication.

Finally, the inferior alveolar nerve may be traumatized along the course of its intrabony canal. The most common place of injury is the area of the mandibular third molar. Removal of impacted third molars may bruise, crush, or sharply injure the nerve in its canal. This complication is common enough during the extraction of third molars that it is important routinely to inform patients preoperatively that it is a possibility. The surgeon must then take every precaution possible to avoid injuring the nerve during the extraction.

Injury to the Temporomandibular Joint

Another major structure that can be traumatized during an extraction procedure in the mandible is the temporomandibular joint. Removal of mandibular molar teeth frequently requires the application of a substantial amount of force. If the jaw is inadequately supported during the extraction to help counteract the forces, the patient may experience pain in this region. Controlled force and adequate support of the jaw prevents this. The use of a bite block on the contralateral side may provide an adequate balance of forces so that injury does not occur (Box 11-7). The surgeon or assistant should also support the jaw by holding the lower border of the mandible. If the patient complains of pain in the temporomandibular joint immediately after the extraction procedure, the surgeon should recommend the use of moist heat, rest for the jaw, a soft diet, and 600 to 800 mg of ibuprofen every 4 hours for several days. Patients who cannot tolerate nonsteroidal antiinflammatory drugs may take 500 to 1000 mg of acetaminophen.

BOX 11-7

Prevention of Injury to the Temporomandibular Joint

1. Support the mandible during extraction.
2. Do not open the mouth too widely.

OROANTRAL COMMUNICATIONS

Removal of maxillary molars occasionally results in communication between the oral cavity and the maxillary sinus. If the maxillary sinus is greatly pneumatized, if little or no bone exists between the roots of the teeth and the maxillary sinus, and if the roots of the tooth are widely divergent, it is common for a portion of the bony floor of the sinus to be removed with the tooth or a communication to be created even if no bone comes out with the tooth. If this problem occurs, appropriate measures are necessary to prevent a variety of sequelae. The two sequelae of most concern are postoperative maxillary sinusitis and formation of a chronic oroantral fistula. The probability that either of these two sequelae will occur is related to the size of the oroantral communication and the management of the exposure.

As with all complications, prevention is the easiest and most efficient method of managing the situation. Preoperative radiographs must be carefully evaluated for the tooth-sinus relationship whenever maxillary molars are to be extracted. If the sinus floor seems to be close to the tooth roots and the tooth roots are widely divergent, the surgeon should avoid a closed extraction and perform a surgical removal with sectioning of tooth roots (Fig. 11-8). Large amounts of force should be avoided in the removal of such maxillary molars (Box 11-8).

Diagnosis of the oroantral communication can be made in several ways: The first is to examine the tooth once it is removed. If a section of bone is adhered to the root ends of the tooth, the surgeon should assume that a communication between the sinus and mouth exists. If a small amount of bone or no bone adheres to the molars, a communication may exist anyway. Some advocate using the nose-blowing test to confirm the presence of a communication. This test involves pinching the nostrils together to occlude the patient's nose and asking the patient to blow gently through the nose while the surgeon observes the area of the tooth extraction. If a communication exists, there will be passage of air through the tooth socket and bubbling of blood in the socket area. However, if there is not a communication, forceful blowing like this may create a communication. Thus this test should be done only if it will alter treatment.

After the diagnosis of oroantral communication has been established or a strong suspicion exists, the surgeon should guess the approximate size of the communication because the treatment depends on the size of the opening. Probing a small opening may enlarge it, so if no bone came out with the tooth, the communication is likely to be 2 mm or less in diameter. However, if a sizable piece of bone comes out with the tooth, the size of the opening is measurable. If the communication is small (2 mm in diameter or less), no additional surgical treatment is necessary. The surgeon should take measures to ensure the formation of a high-quality blood clot in the socket and then advise the patient to take *sinus precautions* to prevent dislodgment of the blood clot.

BOX 11-8

Prevention of Oroantral Communications

1. Conduct a thorough preoperative radiographic examination.
2. Use surgical extraction early, and section roots.
3. Avoid excessive apical pressure.

Sinus precautions are aimed at preventing increases or decreases in the maxillary sinus air pressure that would dislodge the clot. Patients should be advised to avoid blowing the nose, violent sneezing, sucking on straws, and pipe or cigar smoking. Patients who smoke and who cannot stop (even temporarily) should be advised to smoke in small puffs, not in deep drags, to avoid pressure changes.

The surgeon must not probe through the socket into the sinus with a dental curette or a root tip pick. The bone of the sinus possibly may have been removed without perforation of the sinus lining. To probe the socket with an instrument might unnecessarily lacerate the membrane. Probing of the communication may also introduce foreign material, including bacteria, into the sinus and thereby further complicate the situation. Probing of the communication is therefore contraindicated.

If the opening between the mouth and sinus is of moderate size (2 to 6 mm), additional measures should be taken. To help ensure the maintenance of the blood clot in the area, a figure-of-eight suture should be placed over the tooth socket (Fig. 11-11). Some surgeons also place some clot-promoting substances such as a gelatin sponge (Gelfoam) into the socket before suturing. The patient should also be told to follow sinus precautions. Finally, the patient should be prescribed several medications to help lessen the possibility that maxillary sinusitis will occur. Antibiotics—usually amoxicillin, cephalexin, or clindamycin—should be prescribed for 5 days. In addition, a decongestant nasal spray should be prescribed to shrink the nasal mucosa to maintain ostium patency. As long as the ostium is patent and normal sinus drainage can occur, sinusitis and sinus infection are less likely. An oral decongestant is also sometimes recommended.

If the sinus opening is large (7 mm or larger), the surgeon should consider having the sinus communication repaired with a flap procedure. This usually requires that the patient be referred to an oral and maxillofacial surgeon because flap development and closure of a sinus opening are complex procedures that require special skills and experience.

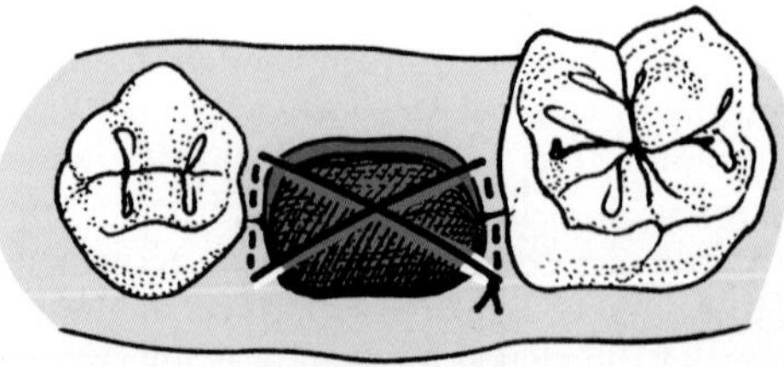

FIGURE 11-11 A figure-of-eight stitch is usually performed to help maintain piece of oxidized cellulose in tooth socket.

The most commonly used flap for small openings is a buccal flap. This technique mobilizes buccal soft tissue to cover the opening and provide for a primary closure. This technique should be performed as soon as possible, preferably on the same day in which the opening occurred. The same sinus precautions and medications are usually required (see Chapter 19).

The recommendations just described hold true for patients who have no preexisting sinus disease. If a communication does occur, it is important that the dentist inquire specifically about a history of sinusitis and sinus infections. If the patient has a history of chronic sinus disease, even small oroantral communications may heal poorly and may result in a chronic oroantral communication and eventual fistula. Therefore, creation of an oroantral communication in patients with chronic sinusitis is cause for referral to an oral and maxillofacial surgeon for definitive care (see Chapter 19).

The majority of oroantral communications treated in the methods just recommended heal uneventfully. Patients should be followed carefully for several weeks to ensure that healing has occurred. Even patients who return within a few days with a small communication usually heal spontaneously if no maxillary sinusitis exists. These patients should be followed closely and referred to an oral and maxillofacial surgeon if the communication persists for longer than 2 weeks. Closure of oroantral fistulae is important because air, water, food, and bacteria go from the oral cavity into the sinus, usually causing a chronic sinusitis. Additionally, if the patient is wearing a full maxillary denture, suction is not as strong; therefore retention of the denture is compromised.

POSTOPERATIVE BLEEDING

Extraction of teeth is a surgical procedure that presents a severe challenge to the hemostatic mechanism of the body. Several reasons exist for this challenge: First, the tissues of the mouth and jaws are highly vascular. Second, the extraction of a tooth leaves an open wound, with soft tissue and bone open, which allows additional oozing and bleeding. Third, it is almost impossible to apply dressing material with enough pressure and sealing to prevent additional bleeding during surgery. Fourth, patients tend to explore the area of surgery with their tongues and occasionally dislodge blood clots, which initiates secondary bleeding. The tongue may also cause secondary bleeding by creating small negative pressures that suction the blood clot from the socket. Finally, salivary enzymes may lyse the blood clot before it has organized and before the ingrowth of granulation tissue.

As with all complications, prevention of bleeding is the best way to manage this problem (Box 11-9). One of the prime factors in preventing bleeding is taking a thorough patient history regarding problems with coagulation. Several questions should be asked of the patient concerning any history of bleeding, particularly after injury or surgery, because affirmative answers to these questions should trigger special efforts to control bleeding (see Chapter 1).

BOX 11-9

Prevention of Postoperative Bleeding

1. Obtain a history of bleeding.
2. Use atraumatic surgical technique.
3. Obtain good hemostasis at surgery.
4. Provide excellent patient instructions.

The first question that patients should be asked is whether they have ever had a problem with bleeding in the past. The surgeon should inquire about bleeding after previous tooth extractions or other previous surgery or persistent bleeding after accidental lacerations. The surgeon must listen carefully to the patient's answers to these questions because the patient's idea of "persistent" may actually be normal. For example, it is normal for a socket to ooze small amounts of blood for the first 12 to 24 hours after extraction. However, if a patient relates a history of bleeding that persisted for more than a day or that required special attention from the surgeon, then his or her degree of suspicion should be substantially elevated.

The surgeon should inquire about any family history of bleeding. If anyone in the patient's family has or had a history of prolonged bleeding, further inquiry about its cause should be pursued. Most congenital bleeding disorders are familial, inherited characteristics. These congenital disorders vary from mild to profound, the latter requiring substantial efforts to control.

The patient should next be asked about any medications currently being taken that might interfere with coagulation. Drugs such as anticoagulants may cause prolonged bleeding after extraction. Patients receiving anticancer chemotherapy or aspirin, or who are alcoholics or have severe liver disease may also tend to bleed excessively.

The patient who has a known or suspected coagulopathy should be evaluated by laboratory testing before surgery is performed to determine the severity of the disorder. It is usually advisable to enlist the aid of a hematologist if the patient has a hereditary coagulation disorder.

The means to measure the status of therapeutic anticoagulation is the international normalized ratio (INR). This value takes into account the patient's prothrombin time and the standardized control. Normal anticoagulated status for most medical indications has an INR of 2.0 to 3.0. It is reasonable to perform extractions on patients who have an INR of 2.5 or less without reducing the anticoagulant dose. With special precautions, it is reasonably safe to do minor amounts of surgery in patients with an INR of up to 3.0, if special local hemostatic measures are taken. If the INR is higher than 3.0, the patient's physician should be contacted to determine whether the physician would lower the anticoagulant dosage to allow the INR to fall.

Primary control of bleeding during routine surgery depends on gaining control of all factors that may prolong bleeding. Surgery should be as atraumatic as possible, with clean incisions and gentle management of the soft tissue. Care should be taken not to crush the soft tissue because crushed tissue tends to ooze for longer periods. Sharp bony spicules should be smoothed or removed. All granulation tissue should be curetted from the periapical region of the socket and from around the necks of adjacent teeth and soft tissue flaps; however, this should be deferred when anatomic restrictions, such as the sinus or inferior alveolar canal, are present (Fig. 11-12). The wound should be carefully inspected for the presence of any specific bleeding arteries. If such arteries exist in the soft tissue, they

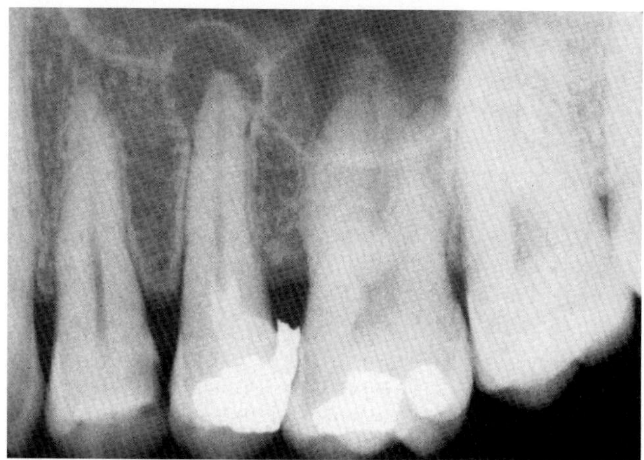

FIGURE 11-12 Granuloma of second premolar. Surgeon should not curette periapically around this second premolar to remove granuloma because risk for sinus perforation is high.

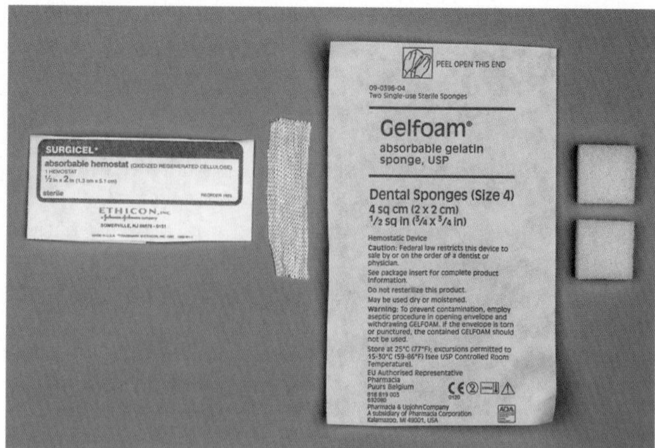

FIGURE 11-13 Examples of materials used to help control bleeding from an extraction socket. Surgical is oxidized regenerated cellulose and comes in a silky fabriclike form, whereas Gelfoam is absorbable gelatin that comes as latticework that is easily crushed with pressure. Both promote coagulation.

should be controlled with direct pressure or, if pressure fails, by clamping the artery with a hemostat and ligating it with a resorbable suture.

The surgeon should also check for bleeding from the bone. Occasionally, a small, isolated vessel bleeds from a bony foramen. If this occurs, the foramen can be crushed with the closed end of a hemostat, thereby occluding the bleeding vessel. Once these measures have been accomplished, the bleeding socket is covered with a damp gauze sponge that has been folded to fit directly into the area from which the tooth was extracted. The patient bites down firmly on this gauze for at least 30 minutes. The surgeon should not dismiss the patient from the office until hemostasis has been achieved. This requires that the surgeon check the patient's extraction socket about 30 minutes after the completion of surgery. The patient should open the mouth widely, the gauze should be removed, and the area should be inspected carefully for any persistent oozing. Initial control should have been achieved. New damp gauze is then folded and placed into position, and the patient is told to leave it in place for an additional 30 minutes.

If bleeding persists but careful inspection of the socket reveals that it is not of an arterial origin, the surgeon should take additional measures to achieve hemostasis. Several different materials can be placed in the socket to help gain hemostasis (Fig. 11-13). The most commonly used and the least expensive is the absorbable gelatin sponge (e.g., Gelfoam). This material is placed in the extraction socket and is held in place with a figure-of-eight suture placed over the socket. The absorbable gelatin sponge forms a scaffold for the formation of a blood clot, and the suture helps maintain the sponge in position during the coagulation process. A gauze pack is then placed over the top of the socket and is held with pressure.

A second material that can be used to control bleeding is oxidized regenerated cellulose (e.g., Surgicel). This material promotes coagulation better than the absorbable gelatin sponge because it can be packed into the socket under pressure. The gelatin sponge becomes friable when wet and cannot be packed into a bleeding socket. When the cellulose is packed into the socket, it almost always causes some delayed healing of the socket. Therefore packing the socket with cellulose is reserved for more persistent bleeding.

If the surgeon has special concerns about the ability of the patient's blood to clot, a liquid preparation of topical thrombin (prepared from human recombinant thrombin) can be saturated onto a gelatin sponge and inserted into the tooth socket. The thrombin bypasses steps in the coagulation cascade and helps to convert fibrinogen to fibrin enzymatically, which forms a clot. The sponge with the topical thrombin is secured in place with a figure-of-eight suture. A gauze pack is placed over the extraction site in the usual fashion.

A final material that can be used to help control a bleeding socket is collagen. Collagen promotes platelet aggregation and thereby helps accelerate blood coagulation. Collagen is currently available in several different forms. Microfibular collagen (e.g., Avitene) is available as a fibular material that is loose and fluffy but can be packed into a tooth socket and held in by suturing and gauze packs, as with the other materials. A more highly cross-linked collagen is supplied as a plug (e.g., Collaplug) or as a tape (e.g., Collatape). These materials are more readily packed into a socket (Fig. 11-14) and are easier to use, but they are also more expensive.

Even after primary hemostasis has been achieved, patients occasionally call the dentist with bleeding from the extraction site, referred to as secondary bleeding. The patient should be told to rinse the mouth gently with chilled water and then to place appropriate-sized, damp gauze over the area and bite firmly. The patient should sit quietly for 30 minutes, biting firmly on the gauze. If the bleeding persists, the patient should repeat the cold rinse and bite down on a damp tea bag. The tannin in the tea frequently helps stop the bleeding. If neither of these techniques is successful, the patient should return to the dentist.

The surgeon must have an orderly, planned regimen to control this secondary bleeding. Ideally, a trained dental assistant is present to help. The patient should be positioned in the dental chair, and all blood, saliva, and fluids should be suctioned from the mouth. Such patients frequently have large "liver clots" (clotted blood that resembles fresh liver) in their mouth that must be removed. The surgeon should visualize the bleeding site carefully with good light to determine the precise source of bleeding. If it is clearly seen to be a generalized oozing, the bleeding site is covered with a folded, damp gauze

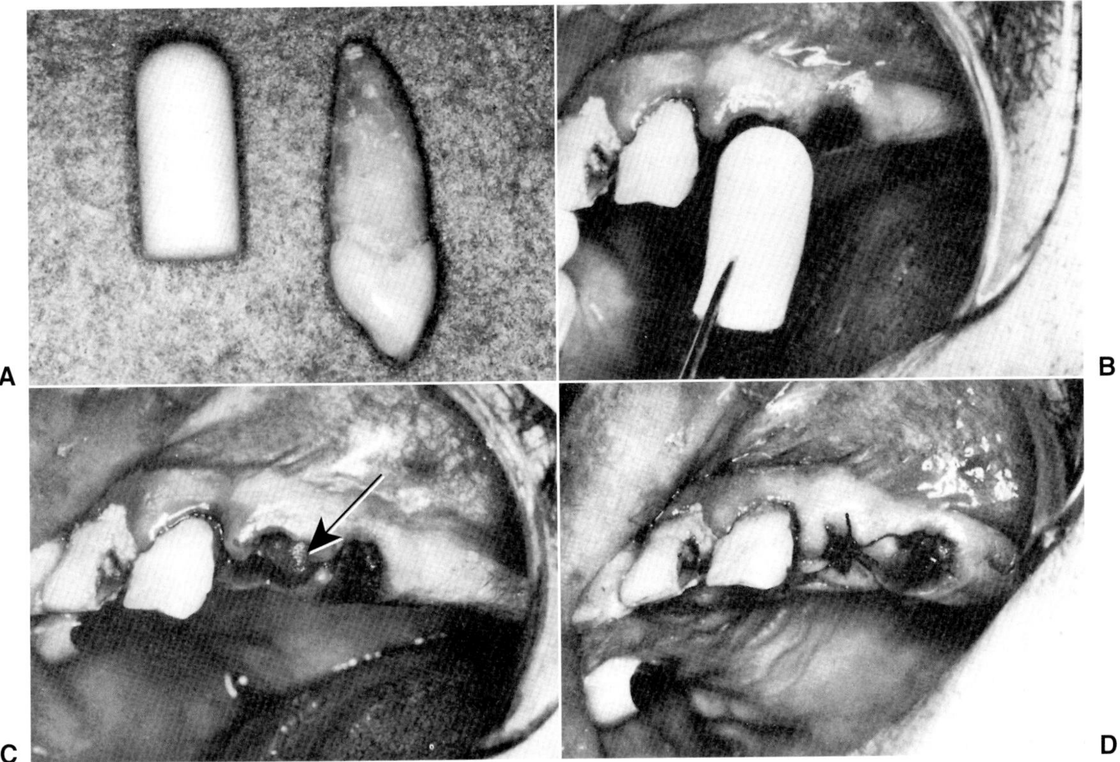

FIGURE 11-14 **A**, Collagen shaped into the form of a plug is similar in size to the root of a maxillary canine. **B** and **C**, The collagen plug is placed into the socket with cotton pliers (*arrow*). **D**, A figure-of-eight suture is placed over the socket to maintain the collagen in the socket.

sponge held in place with firm pressure by the surgeon's finger for at least 5 minutes.

This measure is sufficient to control most bleeding. The reason for the bleeding is usually some secondary trauma that is potentiated by the patient's continuing to suck on the area or to spit blood from the mouth instead of continuing to apply pressure with a gauze sponge.

If 5 minutes of this treatment does not control the bleeding, the surgeon must administer a local anesthetic so that the socket can be treated more aggressively. Block techniques are to be encouraged instead of local infiltration techniques. Infiltration with solutions containing epinephrine causes vasoconstriction and may control the bleeding temporarily. However, when the effects of the epinephrine dissipate, rebound hemorrhage with recurrent bothersome bleeding may occur.

Once regional local anesthesia has been achieved, the surgeon should gently curette out the tooth extraction socket and suction all areas of old blood clot. The specific area of bleeding should be identified as clearly as possible. As with primary bleeding, the soft tissue should be checked for diffuse oozing versus specific arterial bleeding. The bone tissue should be checked for small nutrient artery bleeding or general oozing. The same measures described for control of primary bleeding should be used. The surgeon must then decide whether a hemostatic agent should be inserted into the bony socket. The use of an absorbable gelatin sponge with topical thrombin held in position with a figure-of-eight stitch and reinforced with application of firm pressure from a small, damp gauze pack is standard for local control of secondary bleeding. This technique works well in almost every bleeding socket. In many situations an absorbable gelatin sponge and gauze pressure are adequate. The patient should be given specific instructions on how to apply the gauze packs directly to the bleeding site should additional bleeding occur. Before the patient with secondary bleeding is discharged from the office, the surgeon should monitor the patient for at least 30 minutes to ensure that adequate hemostasis has been achieved.

If hemostasis is not achieved by any of the local measures just discussed, the surgeon should consider performing additional laboratory screening tests to determine whether the patient has a profound hemostatic defect. The dentist usually requests a consultation from a hematologist, who orders the typical screening tests. Abnormal test results will prompt the hematologist to investigate the patient's hemostatic system further.

A final hemostatic complication relates to intraoperative and postoperative bleeding into the adjacent soft tissues. Blood that escapes into tissue spaces, especially subcutaneous tissue spaces, appears as bruising of the overlying soft tissue 2 to 5 days after the surgery. This bruising is termed *ecchymosis* (see Chapter 10).

DELAYED HEALING AND INFECTION

Infection

The most common cause of delayed wound healing is infection. Infections are a rare complication after routine dental extraction and are primarily seen after oral surgery that involves the reflection of soft tissue flaps and bone removal. Careful asepsis and thorough wound débridement after surgery can best prevent infection after surgical flap procedures. This means that the area of bone removal under the flap must be copiously irrigated with saline under pressure and that all visible foreign debris must be removed with a curette. Some patients are predisposed to postoperative wound infections and should be given antibiotics perioperatively for prophylaxis (see Chapter 15).

Wound Dehiscence

Another problem of delayed healing is wound dehiscence (separation of the wound edges; Box 11-10). If a soft tissue flap is replaced and sutured without an adequate bony foundation, the unsupported soft tissue flap often sags and separates along the line of incision. A second cause of dehiscence is suturing the wound under tension. This occurs when the surgeon must pull the edges of a wound together with sutures. The closure is under tension if the suture is the only force keeping the edges approximated. If the edges would spring apart if the suture were removed just after being placed, the wound closure is under tension. If the soft tissue flap is sutured under tension, the sutures cause ischemia of the flap margin with subsequent tissue necrosis, which allows the suture to pull through the flap margin and results in wound dehiscence. Therefore, sutures should always be placed in tissue without tension and tied loosely enough to prevent blanching of the tissue.

A common area of exposed bone after tooth extraction is the internal oblique ridge. After extraction of the first and second molar, during the initial healing, the lingual flap becomes stretched over the internal oblique (mylohyoid) ridge. Occasionally, the bone perforates through the thin mucosa, causing a sharp projection of bone in the area.

The two major treatment options are (1) to leave the projection alone or (2) to smooth it with bone file. If the area is left to heal untreated, the exposed bone will slough off in 2 to 4 weeks. If the irritation of the sharp bone is low, this is the preferred method. If a bone file is used, no flap should be elevated because this will result in an increased amount of exposed bone. The file is used only to smooth off the sharp projections of the bone. This procedure usually requires local anesthesia.

Dry Socket

Dry socket or alveolar osteitis is delayed healing but is not associated with an infection. This postoperative complication causes moderate to severe pain but is without the usual signs and symptoms of infection, such as fever, swelling, and erythema. The term *dry socket* describes the appearance of the tooth extraction socket when the pain begins. In the usual clinical course, pain develops on the third or fourth day after removal of the tooth. Almost all dry sockets occur after the removal of lower molars. On examination the tooth socket appears to be empty, with a partially or completely lost blood clot, and some bony surfaces of the socket are exposed. The exposed bone is sensitive and is the source of the pain. The dull, aching pain is moderate to severe, usually throbs, and frequently radiates to the patient's ear. The area of the socket has a bad odor, and the patient frequently complains of a foul taste.

The cause of alveolar osteitis is not absolutely clear, but it appears to result from high levels of fibrinolytic activity in and around the tooth extraction socket. This fibrinolytic activity results in lysis of the blood clot and subsequent exposure of the bone. The fibrinolytic activity may result from subclinical infections, inflammation of the marrow space of the bone, or other factors. The occurrence of a dry socket after a routine tooth extraction is rare (2% of extractions), but it is frequent after the removal of impacted mandibular third molars (20% of extractions in some series).

Prevention of the dry socket syndrome requires that the surgeon minimize trauma and bacterial contamination in the area of surgery. The surgeon should perform atraumatic surgery with clean incisions and soft tissue reflection. After the surgical procedure, the wound should be irrigated thoroughly with large quantities of saline delivered under pressure, such as from a plastic syringe. Small amounts of antibiotics (e.g., tetracycline) placed in the socket alone or on a gelatin sponge have been shown to help substantially to decrease the incidence of dry socket in mandibular third molars. The incidence of dry socket can also be decreased by preoperative and postoperative rinses with antimicrobial mouth rinses, such as chlorhexidine. Well-controlled studies indicate that the incidence of dry socket after impacted mandibular third molar surgery can be reduced by 50% or more with these measures.

The treatment of alveolar osteitis is dictated by the single therapeutic goal of relieving the patient's pain during the period of healing. If the patient receives no treatment, no sequela other than continued pain exists (treatment does not hasten healing).

Treatment is straightforward and consists of irrigation and insertion of a medicated dressing. First, the tooth socket is gently irrigated with sterile saline. The socket should not be curetted down to bare bone because this increases the amount of exposed bone and the pain. Usually the entire blood clot is not lysed, and the part that is intact should be retained. The socket is carefully suctioned of all excess saline, and a small strip of iodoform gauze soaked with the medication is inserted into the socket. The medication contains the following principal ingredients: eugenol, which obtunds the pain from the bone tissue; a topical anesthetic, such as benzocaine; and a carrying vehicle, such as balsam of Peru. The medication can be made by the surgeon's pharmacist or can be obtained as a commercial preparation from dental supply houses.

The medicated gauze is gently inserted into the socket, and the patient usually experiences profound relief from pain within 5 minutes. The dressing is changed every other day for the next 3 to 6 days, depending on the severity of the pain. The socket is gently irrigated with saline at each dressing change. Once the patient's pain decreases, the dressing should not be replaced, because it acts as a foreign body and further prolongs wound healing.

BOX 11-10

Prevention of Wound Dehiscence

1. Use aseptic technique.
2. Perform atraumatic surgery.
3. Close the incision over intact bone.
4. Suture without tension.

FRACTURES OF THE MANDIBLE

Fracture of the mandible during extraction is a rare complication; it is associated almost exclusively with the surgical removal of impacted third molars. A mandibular fracture is usually the result of the application of a force exceeding that needed to remove a tooth and often occurs during the forceful use of dental elevators. However, when lower third molars are deeply impacted, even small amounts of force may cause a fracture. Fractures may also occur during removal of impacted teeth from a severely atrophic mandible. Should such a fracture occur, it must be treated by the usual methods used for jaw fractures. The fracture must be adequately reduced and stabilized. Usually this means that the patient should be referred to an oral and maxillofacial surgeon for definitive care.

SUMMARY

Prevention of complications should be a major goal of the surgeon. Skillful management of complications when they do occur is the *sine qua non* of the wise and mature surgeon.

The surgeon who anticipates a high probability of an unusual specific complication should inform the patient and explain the anticipated management and sequelae. Notation of this should be made on the informed consent form that the patient signs.

CHAPTER 12

Medicolegal Considerations

VICTORIA J. STERLING AND MYRON R. TUCKER

CHAPTER OUTLINE

In recent years there has been an increase in the number of malpractice claims brought against dentists. This trend has had a profound impact on several aspects of dentistry. Some of the most common lawsuits are related to extraction of the wrong tooth, failure to diagnose a problem, and lack of proper informed consent. The stress associated with the increased possibility of litigation influences the entire office. Malpractice insurance premiums are high, contributing to increased patient costs. Dentists feel pressured into practicing "defensive dentistry," second-guessing sound clinical decisions based on concerns about potential litigation.

The influence of litigation on dentistry has resulted in an effort by the profession to reduce the risk of legal liability by more closely examining treatment decisions, improved documentation, and better dentist-patient relationships. Reviewing all aspects of dental practice to provide the best possible patient care and to reduce unnecessary legal liability is termed *risk management*.

Although no substitute exists for sound clinical practice, non–treatment issues prompt many lawsuits. These issues often include miscommunication and misunderstanding between the dentist and patient and poor record keeping, which in turn present opportunities for patient's lawyers to criticize. This chapter reviews concepts of liability, risk management, methods of risk reduction, and actions that should be taken if a malpractice suit is filed.

LEGAL CONCEPTS INFLUENCING LIABILITY

To understand the responsibility of the dentist in risk management, it is important to review several legal concepts pertaining to the practice of dentistry.

Malpractice is generally defined as professional negligence. Professional negligence occurs when treatment provided by the dentist fails to comply with the standard of care exercised by other dentists in similar situations. In other words, professional negligence occurs when professionals fail to have or exercise the degree of skill ordinarily possessed and demonstrated by members of their profession practicing under similar circumstances.

In most states the standard of care is defined as that which an ordinarily skilled, educated, and experienced dentist would do under similar circumstances. Many states adhere to a national standard for dental specialists. The dentist is considered to have practiced negligently when a patient convinces a judge or jury that the dentist failed to comply with this minimal level of care and that such failure caused a resulting injury.

In most malpractice cases the patient must prove all of the following four elements of a malpractice claim: (1) the existence of a duty, usually implied by the doctor-patient relationship; (2) a breach of the duty—in malpractice, a breach of the standard of care; (3) damages—in nonlegal terms, an injury; and (4) causation, a causal connection between the failure to meet the standard of care and the injury alleged. The initial burden of proving malpractice lies with the plaintiff (patient). The patient must prove by a preponderance of the evidence all four elements of the claim.

First, there must be a professional relationship between the dentist and patient before a legal duty or obligation is owed to exercise appropriate care. This relationship can be established if the dentist accepts the patient or otherwise begins treatment. Second, a breach or failure to provide treatment that satisfies the standard of care must be demonstrated. This standard of care does not obligate the dentist to provide the highest level of treatment exercised by the most skilled dentist or that which is taught in dental school. The standard of care is intended to be a common denominator defined by what average practitioners would ordinarily do under similar circumstances. Third, it must be shown that the failure to provide this standard of care was the cause of the patient's injury. Fourth, there must have been some form of damage demonstrated.

Dentists are not liable for inherent risks of treatment that occur in the absence of negligence. For example, a dentist is not liable if a patient experiences a numb lip after a properly performed third molar extraction. This is a recognized complication. A dentist can be legally liable for a numb lip if the patient proves it was caused by negligence (e.g., the numbness was caused by a careless incision, careless use of a bur, or other instrument).

Recently, many lawsuits include allegations of *unfair trade practices* or a *breach of contract*. Lately, this has become a popular mechanism of the plaintiff's attorneys to force dentists into settling questionable claims. This charge has traditionally been applied to business transactions and has not normally been used in disputes between patients and dentists. However, some courts have recently ruled that a patient and dentist may actually have a contractual agreement to produce a specific result and that failure to achieve this objective may result in a breach of contract. In many states an alleged promise or guarantee as to the result is not enforceable unless it is in writing. Overly aggressive marketing can lead to contractual liability.

Marketing pressures sometimes lead to written advertisements or promotions that can be interpreted as guaranteed results. Patients who have difficulty chewing after delivery of new dentures, if originally promised that they would be able to eat any type of food without difficulty, might consider such promises breach of contract. Dissatisfaction with esthetics or function is often linked to unreasonable expectations, sometimes fueled by ineffective communication or excessive salesmanship.

The *statute of limitations* generally provides a time limit for filing a malpractice suit against an individual or a corporation. This limit, however, varies widely from state to state. In some states the statute of limitations begins when an incident occurs. In other states the statute of limitations is extended for a short period after the alleged malpractice is discovered (or when a "reasonable" person would have discovered it).

Several other factors can extend the statute of limitations in many states. These factors include children under 18 or the age of majority, fraudulent concealment of negligent treatment by the dentist, or leaving a nontherapeutic foreign object in the body (e.g., broken bur or file). As mentioned before, the more recent development of trade practices and breach of contract claims can be traced, in part, to a longer statute of limitations period for contract actions and the common treble damages provisions of the deceptive trade practices acts.

RISK REDUCTION

The foundation for all dental practice should be sound clinical procedures. However, properly addressing other aspects of patient care and office policy may considerably reduce potential legal liability. These aspects include dentist-patient and staff-patient communication, patient information, informed consent, proper documentation, and appropriate management of complications. Additionally, clinicians should note that patients with reasonable expectations and a favorable relationship with their dentist are less likely to sue and more likely to tolerate complications.

Patient Information and Office Communication

A solid dentist-patient relationship is the key to any risk management program. Well-informed patients generally have a much better understanding of potential complications and more realistic expectations about treatment outcomes. This can be accomplished by providing patients with as much information as possible on proposed treatment, alternatives and risks, and benefits and limitations of each. If done properly, the informed consent process can improve rapport. Patients are given this information to help them better understand their care so that they can make informed decisions. The information should be communicated in a positive manner and not presented in a defensive way.

Patients value and expect a discussion with their dentist about their care. Brochures and other types of informational packages help provide patients with general and specific information about general dental and oral surgical care. Patients requiring oral surgical procedures will benefit from information on the nature of their problem, recommended treatment and alternatives, expectations, and possible complications. This information should have a well-organized format that is easily understood and is written in nonprofessional's language. Informed consent is discussed in detail in the following section.

When a dentist has a specific discussion with a patient or gives a patient an informational package, it should be documented in the patient's chart. Information about complications discussed earlier can be reviewed if they occur later. In general, patients with reasonable expectations create fewer problems (a theme repeated throughout this chapter).

INFORMED CONSENT

In addition to providing quality care, effective communication and good rapport should become a standard part of office management objectives. Dentists can be sued not only for negligent treatment but also for failing to inform patients properly about the diagnosis, the treatment to be rendered, the reasonable alternatives, and the reasonable benefits, risks, and complications of each. In some states, treatment without a proper informed consent is considered battery.

The concept of informed consent is that the patient has a right to consider known risks and complications inherent to treatment. This enables the patient to make a knowledgeable, voluntary decision whether to proceed with recommended treatment or elect another option. If a patient is properly advised of inherent risks and a complication occurs in the absence of negligence, the dentist is not legally liable. However, a dentist can be held liable when an inherent risk occurs after the dentist fails to obtain the patient's *informed consent*. The rationale for liability is that the patient was denied the opportunity to refuse treatment after being properly advised of risks associated with the treatment and reasonable options.

Current concepts of informed consent are based as much on providing the patient with the necessary information as on actually obtaining a consent or signature for a procedure. In addition to fulfilling the legal obligations, obtaining the proper informed consent from patients benefits the clinician in several ways. First, well-informed patients who understand the nature of the problem and have realistic expectations are less likely to sue. Second, a properly presented and documented informed consent often prevents frivolous claims based on misunderstanding or unrealistic expectations. Finally, obtaining an informed consent offers the dentist the opportunity to develop better rapport with the patient by demonstrating a greater personal interest in the patient's well-being.

The requirements of an informed consent vary from state to state. Initially, informed consent was to inform patients that bodily harm or death may result from a procedure. Informed consent did not require discussion of minor, unlikely complications that seldom occur and infrequently result in ill effects. However, some states have currently adopted the concept of "material risk," which requires dentists to discuss *all* aspects material to the patient's decision to undergo treatment, even if it is not customary in the profession to provide such information. A risk is material when a reasonable person is likely to attach significance to it in assessing whether to have the proposed therapy.

In most states, dentists have a duty to obtain the patient's consent; they cannot delegate the entire responsibility. Although staff can present the consent form, the dentist should review treatment recommendations, options, and the risks and benefits of each option; the dentist must also be available to answer questions. Although not required by the standard of care in many states, it is advisable to get the patient's written consent for invasive dental procedures. Parents or guardians must sign for minors. Legal guardians must sign for individuals with mental or similar incapacities. In certain regions of the country, it is helpful to have consent forms written in other languages or have multilingual staff members available to assist with the communications.

Informed consent consists of three phases: (1) discussion, (2) written consent, and (3) documentation in the patient's chart. When obtaining informed consent, the clinician should conduct a frank discussion and provide information about seven areas: (1) specific problem, (2) proposed treatment, (3) anticipated or common side effects, (4) possible complications and approximate frequency of occurrence, (5) anesthesia, (6) treatment alternatives, and (7) uncertainties about final outcome, including a statement that the treatment has no absolute guarantees.

This information must be presented so that the patient has no difficulty understanding it. A variety of video presentations, including Internet-based interactive education, are available describing dental and surgical procedures and the associated risks and benefits. These can be used as part of the informed consent process but should not replace direct discussions between the dentist and patient. At the conclusion of the presentation, the patient should be given an opportunity to ask any additional questions.

After these presentations or discussions, the patient should sign a written informed consent. The written consent should summarize in easily understandable terms the items presented. Some states presume that if the information is not on the form, it was not discussed. Whether the patient can read and speak English should also be documented; if the patient does not read or speak English, the presentation and written consent should be given in the patient's language. To ensure that the patient understands each specific paragraph of the consent form, the dentist should consider having the patient initial each paragraph on the form.

An example of an informed consent document appears in Appendix V. At the conclusion of the discussion, the patient, dentist, and at least one witness should sign the informed consent document. In the case of a minor, the patient and the parent or legal guardian should sign the informed consent. In some states, minors may sign the informed consent for their own treatment if they are married or pregnant. Before assuming this to be the case, the dentist should verify local regulations.

The third and final phase of the informed consent procedure is to document in the patient's chart that an informed consent was obtained after the dentist discussed treatment options, risks, and benefits. The dentist should record the fact that consent discussions took place and should also record other events, such as videos shown and brochures given. The written consent form should be included.

Three special situations exist in which an informed consent may deviate from these guidelines: First, a patient may specifically ask not to be informed of all aspects of the treatment and complications (this must be specifically documented in the chart).

Second, it may be harmful in some cases to provide all of the appropriate information to the patient. This is termed the *therapeutic privilege* for not obtaining a complete informed consent. Therapeutic privilege is controversial and would rarely apply to routine oral surgical and dental procedures. Third, a complete informed consent may not be necessary in an emergency, when the need to proceed with treatment is so urgent that unnecessary delays to obtain an informed consent may result in further harm to the patient. This also applies to management of complications during a surgical procedure.

It is assumed that if failure to manage a condition immediately would result in further patient harm, then treatment should proceed without a specific informed consent.

Patients have the right to know whether any risks are associated with their decision to reject certain forms of treatment. This *informed refusal* should be clearly documented in the chart, along with specific information informing the patient of the risks and consequences of refusing treatment. Patients who do not appear for needed treatment should be sent a letter warning of potential problems that may arise if they do not seek treatment. Copies of these letters should be kept in the patient's chart.

RECORDS AND DOCUMENTATION

Poor record keeping is one of the most common problems encountered in the defense of a malpractice suit. When the quality of patient care is questioned, the records supposedly reflect what was done and why. Poor records provide plaintiff attorneys with an opportunity to claim that patient care also must have been substandard. Even though a perfect record is neither possible nor required, records should reasonably reflect the diagnosis, treatment, consent, complications, and other key events.

Adequate documentation of the diagnosis and treatment is one of the most important aspects of patient care. A well-documented chart is the cornerstone of any risk management program. If dentists do not document fundamental clinical findings supporting the diagnosis and treatment, attorneys may question the need for treatment in the first place. Some argue that if an item is not charted, it did not happen. The following eleven items are helpful when recorded in the chart:

1. Chief complaint
2. Dental history
3. Medical history
4. Current medication
5. Allergies
6. Clinical and radiographic findings and interpretations
7. Recommended treatment and other alternatives
8. Informed consent
9. Therapy actually instituted
10. Recommended follow-up treatment
11. Referrals to other general dentists, specialists, or other medical practitioners

Ten frequently overlooked pieces of information should be recorded in the chart:

1. Prescriptions and refills dispensed to the patient
2. Messages or other discussions related specifically to patient care (including telephone calls)
3. Consultations obtained
4. Results of laboratory tests
5. Clinical observations of progress or outcome of treatment
6. Recommended adjunct follow-up care
7. Appointments made or recommended
8. Postoperative instructions and orders given
9. Warnings to the patient, including issues related to lack of compliance, failure to appear for appointments, failure to obtain or take medication, instructions to see other dentists or physicians, or instructions on participation in any activity that might jeopardize the patient's health
10. Missed appointments

Corrections should be made by drawing a single line through any information to be deleted. Correct information can be inserted above or added below, along with a contemporaneous date. The single-line deletion should be initialed and dated. No portion of the chart should be discarded, obliterated, erased, or altered in any fashion. In some states, it is a felony to alter records with the intent to deceive.

REFERRAL TO ANOTHER GENERAL DENTIST OR SPECIALIST

In many cases dentists may think that the recommended treatment is beyond their level of training or experience and may choose to refer a patient to another general dentist or specialist. A referral slip or letter should clearly indicate the basis for referral and what the specialist is being asked to do. The referral should be recorded in the chart. A written referral to a specialist may ask the specialist to provide a written report detailing the diagnosis and treatment plan.

A patient's refusal to pursue a referral should be clearly noted in the chart. If a patient refuses to seek treatment from a specialist, the dentist must decide whether the recommended treatment is within the dentist's own expertise. If not, the dentist should not provide this particular treatment, even if the patient insists. A patient's refusal to seek care from a specialist does not relieve the dentist of liability for injuries or complications resulting from care outside the dentist's level of training and expertise.

Dental specialists should carefully evaluate all referred patients. For example, extracting or treating the wrong tooth is a common allegation in court. When in doubt, the specialist should contact the referring dentist and discuss the case. Any change in the treatment plan provided by the specialist should be documented in the referring dentist's and specialist's charts. To avoid informed consent problems, the patient must approve any revised plan or recommendation.

COMPLICATIONS

Less-than-desirable results can occur despite the dentist's best efforts in diagnosis, treatment planning, and surgical technique. A poor result does not necessarily suggest that a practitioner is guilty of negligence or other wrongdoing. However, when complications occur, it is mandatory that the dentist immediately begin to address the problem in an appropriate fashion.

In most instances the dentist should advise the patient of the complication. Examples of such situations are loss of or failure to recover a root tip; breaking a dental instrument, such as an endodontic file, in a tooth; perforation of the maxillary sinus; damage to adjacent teeth; or inadvertent fracture of surrounding bone. In these instances the dentist should clearly outline proposed management of the problem, including specific instructions to the patient, further treatment that may be necessary, and referral to an oral and maxillofacial surgeon when appropriate.

It is advisable to consider and discuss alternative treatment options that may still produce reasonable results. For example, when teeth are extracted for orthodontic purposes, the first premolar may accidentally be extracted when the orthodontist preferred extraction of the second premolar. Before removing any other teeth or alarming the patient and parents, the dentist should call the orthodontist to discuss the effect on treatment outcome and available treatment modifications. The patient and parents should be notified that the wrong tooth was extracted but that the orthodontist indicated that the treatment can proceed without significantly compromising the result.

The lack of reasonable modifications of the original treatment plan is more challenging. The dentist may have to consider a more expensive plan, such as implants, and should also consider funding additional treatment.

Another common complication is altered sensation following third molar removal. The chart should reflect the existence and extent of the problem. It may be useful to use a diagram to document the area involved. The density and severity of the deficit should be noted after testing, if possible. The chart should reflect the progress of the condition each time the patient returns for follow-up. Ultimately, the patient may require a referral to an oral and maxillofacial surgeon with experience in diagnosing and treating nerve injuries. In most cases the referral should occur within 3 months after the injury if no significant improvement is seen. Excessive delays may limit the effectiveness of future treatment. Documentation of the patient's progress helps justify any decision to delay the referral.

PATIENT MANAGEMENT PROBLEMS

Noncompliant Patient

Dentists and staff should routinely chart lack of compliance, including missed appointments, cancellations, and failure to follow advice to take medications, seek consultations, wear appliances, or return for routine visits. Efforts to advise patients of risks associated with failing to follow instructions should also be recorded.

When the patient's health may be jeopardized by continued noncompliance, the clinician should consider writing a letter to the patient that identifies the potential harm and advises the patient that the office will not be responsible if these and other problems develop as a result of the patient's noncompliance. If the patient's care is eventually terminated, the accumulation of detailed chart entries documenting the noncompliance should justify why the dentist is unwilling to continue care.

Patient Abandonment

A legal duty is owed to the patient once a doctor-patient relationship is established. Generally, duty is established when a patient has been accepted by the office, the initial evaluation has been completed, and treatment has begun. The dentist is usually obligated to provide care until the treatment is completed. There may be instances, however, when it is impossible or unreasonable for a dentist to complete a treatment plan because of several problems. Such problems include the patient's failure to return for necessary appointments, follow explicit instructions, take medication, seek recommended consultations, or stop activities that may inhibit the treatment plan or otherwise jeopardize the dentist's ability to achieve acceptable results. This may include a total breakdown of communication and loss of rapport between the dentist and patient.

In these cases, it is usually necessary for the dentist to follow certain steps before discontinuing treatment to avoid being accused of patient abandonment. First, the chart must document the activities leading to the patient's termination. The patient should be adequately warned (if possible) that termination will result if the undesired activity does not stop. The patient should be warned of the potential harm that may result if such activity continues and the reason why the harm may occur. After being told why the office is no longer willing to provide treatment, the patient should be given a reasonable opportunity to find a new dentist (30 to 45 days is common). The office should continue treatment during this period if the patient is in need of emergency care or care is required to avoid harm to the patient's health or to treatment progress.

When it has been decided that the dentist-patient relationship cannot continue, the dentist must take the following steps to terminate the relationship.

A letter should be sent to the patient, indicating the intent to withdraw from the case and the unwillingness to provide further treatment. The letter should include five important pieces of information:

1. The reasons supporting the decision to discontinue treatment
2. If applicable, the potential harm caused by the patient (or parent's) undesired activity
3. Past warnings by the office that did not alter the patient's actions and continued to put the patient at risk (or jeopardized the dentist's ability to achieve an acceptable result)
4. A warning that the patient's treatment is not completed; therefore the patient should immediately seek another dentist or go to a hospital or teaching clinic in the area for immediate examination or consultation. (The clinician should include a warning that if the patient fails to follow this advice, the patient's dental health may continue to be jeopardized and any treatment progress may be lost or worse.)
5. An offer to continue treating the patient for a specified reasonable period and for emergencies until the patient locates another dentist

This letter should be sent by certified mail to ensure and document that the patient did in fact receive it. If other dentists are treating the patient, the clinician should consider advising them of this decision. The clinician should consult local counsel if any concerns of confidentiality or a particularly sensitive reason behind this decision exists.

The dentist must continue to remain available for treatment of emergency problems until the patient has had adequate time to seek treatment from another dentist. This must be communicated in the letter outlined previously.

The dentist must offer to forward copies of all pertinent records that affect patient care. Nothing must be done to inhibit efforts of subsequent treatment to complete patient care.

Patients who have tested positive for the human immunodeficiency virus or who have similar diseases cannot be terminated because of their disease, because this action may violate the Americans with Disabilities Act (ADA) and other federal or state laws. These patients cannot be refused treatment based on their disease. Patients who have tested positive for human immunodeficiency virus or who have acquired immunodeficiency syndrome are considered handicapped under these laws.[1] Legal counsel should be consulted if the clinician has another valid reason to terminate such a patient.

Exceptions do exist to these suggested guidelines. Dentists must evaluate each situation carefully. Occasions may occur when the dentist does not wish to lose contact with a patient or lose the ability to observe and follow a complication. Terminating treatment will often anger a patient, who may in turn seek legal advice if experiencing a complication. The office may elect to complete treatment in such cases.

If treatment continues, the chart should carefully reflect all warnings to the patient about potential harm and the increased chance that acceptable results may not be achieved.

In certain cases the patient may be asked to sign a revised consent form that includes three important points:

1. The patient realizes that he or she has been noncompliant or has otherwise not followed advice.
2. The previously mentioned activities jeopardized the patient's health or the dentist's ability to achieve acceptable results or have unreasonably increased the chances of complications.
3. The dentist will continue treatment but makes no assurances that the results will be acceptable. Complications may occur requiring additional care, and the patient (or the patient's legal guardian) will accept full responsibility if any of the foregoing events occur.

COMMON AREAS OF DENTAL LITIGATION

Litigation has involved all aspects of dental practice and nearly every specific type of treatment. A few types of dental treatment have a higher incidence of legal action.

Removal of the wrong tooth usually results from a communication breakdown between the general dentist and oral surgeon or the patient and dentist. When in doubt, the dentist must confirm the tooth to be extracted by radiograph, clinical examination, or discussion with the referring dentist. If opinions differ regarding the proposed treatment, the patient and the referring dentist should be notified and the outcome of any subsequent conversation documented. A short follow-up letter confirming the final decision may also be helpful in documenting this decision. If the wrong tooth is extracted, this should be handled in the manner described previously in this chapter.

Nerve injuries are often grounds for suits, with attorneys claiming that the nerve injuries resulted from extractions, implants, endodontic treatment, or other procedures. These allegations are usually coupled with allegations of insufficient informed consent.

Because nerve injuries are a known complication of mandibular extractions or mandibular implants posterior to the mental foramen, patient advocates claim that the patient had a right to accept these risks as part of treatment. If the dentist can visualize conditions that increase this risk, the patient should be advised and the condition documented. An example would be to note specifically the relationship of the inferior alveolar nerve to the third molar tooth to be extracted, when these appear to be in proximity.

Failure to diagnose can be related to several areas of dentistry: One of the most common problems is a lesion that is seen on examination but is not adequately documented and no treatment or follow-up is instituted. If the lesion causes further problems or a subsequent biopsy documents a long-standing pathologic condition or a malignancy, this may be viewed as negligence. This problem can be avoided by following up on any potentially abnormal finding. The clinician should chart an initial diagnosis or seek a consultation from a specialist. If the lesion has resolved by the next visit, the clinician should record that fact so that the issue is closed. If the patient is referred to another doctor, the referring clinician should follow up to document the patient's progress, including whether the patient's condition was successfully treated.

Failure to diagnose periodontal disease is often the area of criticism and legal action. A periodontal examination should be a part of routine dental evaluations and therefore becomes the primary responsibility of the general dentist. The status of the problem, suggestions for treatment, referrals, and progress or resolution of the problem must be clearly documented.

Implant complications or failure is another common area of litigation. As with any procedure, the patient should be informed of the associated reconstruction and long-term outcome of the complication. The need for careful long-term hygiene and follow-up should be explained. The potential detrimental effect of patient habits such as smoking should be explained and documented. Dentists placing implants should consider using a customized consent form, summarizing common complications, and stressing the importance of patient follow-up care and oral hygiene.

Failure to provide appropriate referral to another dentist or specialist can be a source of legal problems. Dentists usually determine the appropriate time to refer a patient to a specialist for initial care or management of a complication. Failure to refer patients for complicated treatment not routinely performed by the dentist or delayed referral for management of a complication frequently becomes the basis for litigation. Referrals to specialists can greatly reduce liability risks. Specialists are accustomed to treating more difficult cases and complications. Specialists with whom the dentist has a good relationship can also diffuse patient management problems by being objective and caring and by reassuring angry patients. The general dentist and specialist may discuss ways of relieving the expense of addressing a complication and completing treatment.

Temporomandibular joint disorders sometimes become more apparent after dental procedures requiring prolonged opening or manipulation, such as tooth extraction or endodontic treatment. Documentation of any preexisting condition in the pretreatment assessment is important. The risk of temporomandibular joint pain or other dysfunction as a result of a procedure should be included in the informed consent when indicated. If the patient is in dire need of care that may aggravate or cause a temporomandibular joint condition, a customized consent form should be drafted and signed. The form should clearly define the problem, giving the patient options and confirming the patient's authorization to proceed.

WHEN A PATIENT THREATENS TO SUE

Whenever a patient, the patient's attorney, or any other representative of the patient informs the dentist that a malpractice suit is being considered, several precautions should be taken.

First, all such threats should be documented and reported immediately to the malpractice insurance carrier. The dentist should follow the advice of the malpractice carrier, institutional risk management team, or the attorney assigned to the case. These individuals will usually respond to the threat. Because the first indication of a potential claim is usually a request for records, the office should comply with state law regarding what must be provided (usually copies of care and treatment records, not the originals).

Patients sometimes request the original chart and radiographs for a variety of reasons. The law in most states indicates that the dental office owns the records and has a legal obligation to maintain original records for a specified period. Patients are entitled to a legible copy, and dental offices are entitled to a reasonable reimbursement for the same. Patients do not own the records merely because they paid for care and treatment.

Second, the dentist and staff should not discuss the case with the patient (or representative of the patient) once a lawsuit is threatened or made. All requests for information or other contact should be forwarded to the insurance carrier or attorney representing the dentist. All arguments with the patient or representative should be avoided. The dentist must not admit liability or fault or agree to waive fees. Any such statement or admission made to the patient or patient's representative may be used against the dentist later as an "admission against the dentist's interest."

Third, it is *imperative* that no additions, deletions, or changes of any sort be made in the patient's dental record. Records must not be misplaced or destroyed. The clinician should seek legal advice before attempting to clarify an entry.

During the process of malpractice litigation, dentists may be called to give a deposition. This may be as the defendant in a case, as a subsequent treater, or as an expert witness. Although this is common for attorneys, the procedure is often unnerving and emotional for dentists, particularly when testifying in their own defense.

The following are six suggestions that should be considered when giving a deposition related to a malpractice case:

1. The clinician should be prepared and have complete knowledge of the records. All chart entries, test results, and any other relevant information should be reviewed. In complex cases, the clinician should consider reviewing textbook knowledge of the subject; however, an attorney should be consulted before anything other than the clinician's own record is reviewed.
2. The clinician should never answer a question unless the clinician completely understands it. The clinician should listen carefully to the question, provide a succinct answer to it, and stop talking after the answer is given. A lawsuit cannot be won at a deposition, but it can be lost.
3. The clinician should not speculate. If a review of the records, radiographs, or other information is necessary, the clinician should do so before answering a question, rather than guessing.
4. The clinician should be careful when agreeing that any particular expert author or text is "authoritative." Once such a statement is made, the clinician may be placed in a situation in which the clinician did something or disagreed with something the "expert" has written. In most states a clinician can be impeached by anything an author states, once the clinician agrees that the author is "authoritative."
5. The clinician should not argue unnecessarily with the other attorney. The clinician's temper should not be shown (this will only alert the clinician's adversary as to what will upset the clinician in front of a jury, who will expect the dentist to act professionally).
6. The advice of the clinician's lawyer should be followed. (Even if retained by the insurance company, the attorney is required to represent the clinician's interests, not that of the insurance company or anyone else.)

Most anxiety related to litigation comes from the fear of the unknown. Most dental practitioners have limited or no exposure to litigation. One must keep in mind that dentists prevail in most cases. Only about 10% of cases go to trial, and dentists win well more than 80% of these cases.

Unfortunately, a malpractice trial requires a tremendous investment of time, energy, and emotion, all of which detracts from patient care. Most dentists have no choice; they must defend themselves. Dentists who are prepared and who possess reasonable expectations of each step of the litigation process usually experience less anxiety.

MANAGED CARE ISSUES

The influence of managed health care has greatly changed many aspects of dentistry. This includes the doctor-patient relationship and the way decisions are made regarding which treatment alternatives are most appropriate. Dentists are often placed in the middle of a conflict between a desire to provide optimal treatment and the willingness of a health care plan to approve payment for appropriate or needed care.

Traditionally, the patient chooses whether to elect a compromised treatment plan or even no treatment. Under managed care, however, some patients are being forced to accept compromised treatment or no treatment, based on administrative decisions that may be driven more by cost containment pressures than sound dental judgment.

The American Dental Association Council on Ethics, Bylaws, and Judicial Affairs issued the following statement underscoring dentists' obligation to provide appropriate care:

> Dentists who enter into managed care agreements may be called upon to reconcile the demands placed on them to contain costs with the needs of their patients. Dentists must not allow these demands to interfere with the patient's right to select a treatment option based on informed consent. Nor should dentists allow anything to interfere with the free exercise of their professional judgment or their duty to make appropriate referrals if indicated. Dentists are reminded that contract obligations do not excuse them from their ethical duty to put the patient's welfare first.[2]

Dentists have a responsibility to advise patients that a "compromised" treatment plan has been approved by the managed care organization. The dentist should seek the patient's consent to provide such treatment after the pertinent risks, complications, and limitations have been reviewed, along with an explanation of more optimal treatment options. Dentists should advise in writing, both patients and third-party payers, of reasonably expected outcomes when the appropriate treatment is not available because of improper decisions by third-party providers.

The law has evolved in the area of managed care, and recent court decisions[3,4] create some additional responsibilities for the dentist in advocating for appropriate patient care. Ultimately, each dentist has a duty to treat the patient and not his or her insurance plan. This often entails challenging, in writing, the denial of payment by the plan administrators for the recommended course of treatment by appealing on behalf of the patient for medically appropriate dental care. A letter addressing this situation should include the following elements:

1. A statement that the patient has been under the dentist's care for a specific condition (diagnosis) and the dentist's recommended course of treatment
2. The clinical indications for the recommended treatment
3. The risks and complications involved in failing to undergo the recommended treatment
4. A statement that the dentist believes that the previous denial of authorization by plan administrators is inappropriate. It may be helpful to use key language from the court decision stating, "It is essential that cost limitation programs not be permitted to interfere with decisions based on medical/dental judgment."

Two other documents are needed to close the loop on the communications aspect of a managed care denial. First, a form for patients to sign that advises them of their diagnosis, recommended treatment, risks of not undergoing the treatment, an acknowledgment that alternative forms of treatment may create less desirable results than those of the recommended treatment, and an acknowledgment that they understand that they can pay for the recommended treatment from their own funds. A second letter should be sent to the patient who refuses recommended treatment that has been denied payment under the patient's insurance plan, asking the patient to reconsider the decision, expressing the dentist's concern for the consequences, and urging the patient to appeal the decision directly to the plan administrators.

TELEMEDICINE, ELECTRONIC RECORDS, AND THE INTERNET

Technologic developments have induced changes associated with medical and dental practices. The increasing popularity of computers and the Internet has given birth to new potential duties and liability concerns. Digital imaging, combined with the Internet capabilities for communication and even videoconferencing, has created situations in which patients may receive advice without the traditional doctor-patient interaction. The conversion to electronic rather than paper charts is a growing technology, with many potential applications for a modern dental practice.

The increasing use of electronic records has raised several issues about the validity of office notes, other written documents, and radiographs. As with any medical record it is important that records are not altered, in any way, after they are initially created and placed in a chart or digital file. Although alterations can be made on electronically generated documents, most software packages have tracking mechanisms in place that can detect whether documents, radiographs, or other images have been altered and when this occurred. If a change to an office note or other document is required, this should always be done as an addendum, entered into the record separately, rather than by changing the original document.

Because many offices are completely "paperless," many documents are signed electronically. Electronic signatures are as valid as the system in place to protect them from fraud, not unlike paper records where a signature can be forged. Most systems have some type of security measures imbedded within the software to protect the integrity of the system. As with many computer security issues this requires the use of user identification and passwords that protect access to the documents by unauthorized individuals. When generated, stored, and protected in the appropriate manner, electronic records are as valid as any other type of medical record.

The Internet access to health care information has changed the dynamics of traditional dentist-patient interaction. A dentist's legal duty to a patient is currently linked to the existence of a doctor-patient relationship. Determining whether this relationship exists, however, is no longer a simple task. The advent of Internet marketing, telemedicine, and other modes of providing information or advice through an electronic media, without the direct ability to examine, diagnose, and recommend treatment, has clouded the issue of whether a doctor-patient relationship (and a legal duty owed to a particular patient) exists. Courts make decisions that may provide some guidance related to these evolving issues, although disagreement by jurisdictions still exists. One court decision has determined that a physician who consults with a treating physician over the telephone owes no legal duty to the treating physician's patient when treatment options were relayed during a telephone call.[5] However, another court ruled that a doctor-patient relationship could be implied when an on-call physician is consulted by telephone by an emergency department physician who relied on the consulting physician's advice.[6]

Defining clear rules that can be relied upon by practicing dentists who provide direct or indirect advice over the telephone, Internet, or through websites will not be an easy task. Many questions remain unanswered. Do the laws of the state in which the patient lives or those in which the dentist practices actually control this issue? Is the dentist practicing dentistry in another state without a license? In general, courts have found that practitioners must be licensed in the state from which the patient initiates the consultation and that the laws of that jurisdiction control.

Is the advice offered by electronic means intended for general information and not intended to be relied upon by patients or the treating dentist for specific care? If so, then a prominent disclaimer should be posted and acknowledged before proceeding with the interaction. Will the electronic transfer of the information such as the patient's chart or billing information violate state or federal privacy laws? Under the Health Insurance Portability and Accountability Act (HIPAA) Security and Privacy regulations, duties are clearly defined as described later. Can the dentist protect the information from manipulation or misuse if sent electronically? Today, forensic computer science can track any attempts to change records, and therefore caveats about corrections to documentation apply in the same way they do for paper and film documentation.

Over the coming years, it will be important for practitioners to monitor trends in dental care as the Internet, information storage and transfer, and doctor-patient relationships are affected by advancing technology.

RULES AND REGULATIONS AFFECTING PRACTICE

HIPAA Privacy and Security

The Health Insurance Portability and Accountability Act of 1996[7] is also known as the Kennedy-Kasselbaum Act. In recent years, the public has grown increasingly concerned about disclosures of confidential health information by virtually all parts of the health care industry, including hospitals, pharmacies, managed care organizations, laboratories, and health care providers.

HIPAA was enacted to protect such information. Originally intended to codify an employee's right to continue to receive health insurance should he or she change jobs, quit, or be terminated, Congress used this legislation as a springboard to address several additional health care issues such as reduction of health care fraud and abuse, and security and confidentiality of electronic health information.

The privacy regulations apply to "covered entities," which include health plans, health care clearinghouses, and health care providers who transmit health information electronically. This also includes practices that employ third parties to process and transmit electronic claims on their behalf. The regulations require covered entities to protect "individually identifiable health information." It is important to state that practices are permitted by the privacy laws to make uses and disclosures of a patient's health information for purposes of *treatment, payment, and health care operations.* In other words, a consent form completed by the patient will allow the practice to use protected patient information in its regular business. Additional uses and disclosures of protected information require separate consent. Compliance with these regulations includes the following:

1. Each practice must maintain a confidentiality statement, known as a Notice of Privacy Practices, posted in a prominent place in the office and on the website of the practice, if applicable.

2. Each patient must sign a consent form that allows the release of his or her health information as necessary to conduct the business of the practice.
3. All staff must be educated about the privacy and confidentiality rules and regulations.

HIPAA security regulations cover protected health information and information that is maintained or transmitted in electronic form. The security regulations require that a covered entity protect the *confidentiality, integrity, and availability* of electronic protected health information that it creates, stores, maintains, or transmits. By "confidentiality," the regulations mean ensuring the privacy of the information; by "integrity," ensuring that the information is not improperly altered or destroyed; and by "availability," ensuring that the information is accessible and usable to authorized persons.

Title VI, Limited English Proficiency

Title VI of the Civil Rights Act of 1964[8] prohibits discrimination based on race, color, or national origin by any entity that receives federal financial assistance. Individuals with limited English proficiency (LEP) have also been determined to be protected under this law. Dentists who treat such patients are required to take necessary steps to ensure that LEP persons can meaningfully access programs and services. The key to meaningful access for LEP persons is effective communication. These requirements apply to practices that treat patients who receive financial assistance. Medicaid and Medicare patients are the most common patients assisted by the Department of Health and Human Services. There are varying levels of requirements based on the number of LEP persons served by a practice:

1. For practices in which the LEP language group consists of *fewer than 100* persons, all such persons must be provided with *written notice* in the primary language of the LEP language group of the right to receive competent oral translation of written materials.
2. For practices in which an eligible LEP language group constitutes *5% of the practice or 1000 persons,* whichever is less, the practice must provide translations for *vital documents* for patient interactions.
3. For practices in which an eligible LEP language group constitutes *10% of the practice or 3000 persons,* whichever is less, the practice must provide *translated written materials,* which includes vital documents for patient interactions in the primary language of the LEP language group.

If a practice falls under these boundaries, certain rules apply to serve LEP persons. To ensure compliance with these rules, a provider should develop and implement a comprehensive written language assistance program. This program should include the following:

- An assessment of the language needs of the patient population by identifying the non-English languages likely to be encountered, estimating the number of LEP persons eligible for services and their language needs, and identifying the resources needed to provide effective language assistance.
- The development of a policy on language access for providing oral language interpretation such as bilingual staff, staff interpreters, or outside interpreters, as well as translation of written materials (such as health history forms, consent forms, and privacy notices). The practice should post signs in regularly encountered languages about the available services and right to free language assistance services.
- Ensuring that the staff is trained in LEP policies and procedures and how to work effectively with in-person and telephone interpreters and inclusion of such training in orientation for new employees.

It is illegal for a practice to encourage language minority patients to provide their own interpreters as an alternative to maintaining bilingual employees or interpreters. Confidentiality issues aside, a patient might naturally be reluctant to disclose or discuss intimate details of personal and family life in front of a family member or complete stranger who has no formal training or obligation to observe confidentiality.

Americans with Disabilities Act

ADA,[9] enacted in 1990, is one of the nation's most comprehensive civil rights statutes. Many doctors have heard of the act but do not realize the significant implications the ADA can have on the provision of dental care for even the smallest health care practice.

The basic requirements of the law mandate that private practitioners accept patients with disabilities for treatment; provide "auxiliary aids" when necessary for effective communication with patients with disabilities; and make health care facilities physically accessible and usable by patients with disabilities if this is "readily achievable."

The ADA provisions apply to "places of public accommodation." "The professional office of a health care professional" is specifically included in this category. The law applies to health care offices irrespective of their size.

Under Title III of the ADA, a health care provider may not discriminate in providing services to individuals with disabilities. A dentist may not refuse to treat a patient nor refuse to accept a new patient because of the patient's disability. The ADA also imposes new obligations upon health care providers to provide "auxiliary aids and services" to enable a patient with a disability to benefit from the services of the office. The obligation can be as uncomplicated as the provision of additional assistance to a patient who has difficulty getting into an examination chair and as extensive as the provision of qualified interpreters for deaf patients.

In selecting an auxiliary aid, a doctor must take into account the specific abilities or limitations of the patient. For instance, the National Center for Law and Deafness points out a number of misconceptions regarding the abilities of deaf patients that may lead to ineffective communication. As an example, lip-reading is effective for only a few deaf patients. The vast majority of deaf adults rate themselves as having poor ability or complete inability to lip-read. The center also notes that the average deaf high school graduate reads and writes on a third-grade level; therefore the exchange of written communication may also not be effective for many deaf patients. Some patients may ask the doctor to provide an interpreter for them. Under the ADA laws, deaf patients have the right to ask for an interpreter. If asked, a dental office *must* provide an interpreter for the patient. If the office refuses to provide an interpreter, the office may be subject to a claim for discrimination. The cost of the interpreter must be borne by the office and may not be passed on to the patient.

In some situations, such as obtaining informed consent before surgery, it may be necessary to use a qualified interpreter. A qualified interpreter is defined by the ADA as someone "who is able to interpret effectively, accurately, and impartially, both receptively and expressively, using any necessary specialized vocabulary." Interpreters need not be specially accredited or affiliated with a particular group. In some instances, a family member or friend may be qualified to interpret. A good idea is to have the interpreter complete a Translator's Statement form before performing interpretation services.

Dentists and office staff members must be aware that there may be some instances when a family member may not be able to render the necessary interpretation because of emotional or personal involvement. Confidentiality considerations may also adversely affect the ability to interpret "effectively, accurately, and impartially." If there are concerns that a family member or friend may not be able to interpret for the reasons cited, it is best to obtain an impartial interpreter.

EMTALA

More formally known as the Emergency Medical Treatment and Active Labor Act, EMTALA[10] was enacted to prevent hospitals from refusing to treat patients who were unable to pay or from transferring such patients to other health care facilities before the emergency condition was identified and stabilized. EMTALA imposes four main duties on hospitals:

1. To provide a medical screening to any patient who presents to a hospital emergency department
2. To determine whether an emergency medical condition exists
3. To stabilize the condition so that transfer or discharge does not threaten a deterioration of the patient's condition
4. To transfer the patient to another facility if warranted but only if the benefits outweigh the risks of the transfer

The courts have been clear that EMTALA is intended only to prevent hospitals from purposefully withholding treatment from nonpaying patients in an emergency condition or dumping patients onto other health care providers or facilities. Dentists become involved with EMTALA issues when patients are referred to the practice by the hospital emergency room and the hospital administrators tell the practitioner that the dentist will be in violation of the antidumping statute, EMTALA, unless the dentist treats the nonpaying patient. This kind of threat is unfounded and should be challenged by asking for the statutory authority of the hospital in making such statements.

In two situations liability under EMTALA may extend to practitioners. First, if the dentist is on call with the hospital and the hospital sends a patient to the dentist's office (for the convenience of using an appropriately equipped facility), then the dentist most likely has an obligation to examine and stabilize the patient and make an appropriate referral to a facility that treats indigent patients. Second, if the dentist has agreed to be bound by EMTALA duties through a specific contract or under the by-laws of the hospital where he or she holds privileges, these regulations will apply.

SUMMARY

In addition to providing sound technical care, the dentist must address several other aspects of patient care to minimize unnecessary legal liability. The dentist should develop the best possible rapport with patients through improved communication and by providing any information that may enhance patient understanding of treatment. Adequate documentation of all aspects of patient care is also necessary. Clinicians face a constant struggle to document quality care and advice to the patient. The law only requires that such efforts be reasonable, not perfect.

This chapter is intended to provide suggestions to be considered by individual dentists. This chapter is not intended to establish, influence, or modify the standard of care. Medical and dental malpractice laws vary from state to state. When confronted with medicolegal issues, all health care providers should consult local counsel familiar with the laws and regulations that apply in their jurisdiction.

REFERENCES

1. *Americans with Disabilities Act of 1990,* 42 USC, § 12101.
2. ADA Counsel on Ethics, Bylaws, and Judicial Affairs: How to reconcile participation in managed care plans with their ethical obligations, *ADA News* Feb 6, 1995.
3. *Wickline v. State of California* (1986) 192 Cal.App.3d 1630 [239 Cal.Rptr. 810].
4. *Fox v. HealthNet of California,* No. 219692, 1993 WL 794305 (Riverside County Superior Court/Central Cal. Dec. 23, 1993).
5. *Hill v. Koksky,* 186 Mich. App. 300, 1993.
6. *Oja v. Kin,* 229 Mich. App. 184, 1998.
7. *Health Insurance Portability and Accountability Act,* 42 USC, § 1395 et. seq., 1996.
8. Title VI of the Civil Rights Act of 1964, 42 USC, § 2000d et. seq.
9. *Americans with Disabilities Act of 1990,* 42 USC, § 12101 et. seq.
10. *Emergency Medical Treatment and Active Labor Act,* 42 US Code 1395dd et. seq.

Bibliography

Golder D: Practicing dentistry in the age of telemedicine, *J Am Dent Assoc* 131:734-744, 2000.

Nora RL: Dental malpractice: its causes and cures, *Quintessence Int* 17:121, 1986.

OMS National Insurance Company, RRG: *The informed consent process,* Rosemont, Ill, 1994 (and subsequent editions), The Company.

Prednis P: De-fanging COBRA, *The Monitor,* 9(3): 1, 4, 8, 1998.

Sfikas PM: Teledentistry: legal and regulatory issues explored, *J Am Dent Assoc* 128:1716-1718, 1997.

Small RL: How to avoid being sued for malpractice, *J Mich Dent Assoc* 75:45, 1993.

PART III

Preprosthetic and Implant Surgery

Despite the improved ability of dentistry to maintain the dentition, many individuals continue to require replacement of some or all of their teeth. Surgical improvement of the denture-bearing area and surrounding tissue (preprosthetic surgery) offers an interesting and demanding challenge to the dental practice.

Many minor modifications of the alveolar ridge and vestibular areas can greatly improve denture stability and retention. In some cases, patients have severe bone changes or soft tissue abnormalities that require extensive surgical preparation before the prosthetic appliance can be properly constructed and worn. Procedures that improve prosthesis retention and stability are discussed and illustrated in Chapter 13.

One of the most exciting frontiers in dentistry is implantology. Proper bony and soft tissue reconstruction followed by placement of implants and subsequent prosthetic reconstruction can provide patients with a more natural and efficient substitute for their lost dentition. Depending on the circumstances, several types of implant systems may be used. Chapter 14 discusses the various types of implant systems currently in use and their advantages, disadvantages, and indications for use.

CHAPTER 13

Preprosthetic Surgery

MYRON R. TUCKER, BRIAN B. FARRELL, AND BART C. FARRELL

CHAPTER OUTLINE

After the loss of natural teeth, bony changes in the jaws begin to take place immediately. Because the alveolar bone no longer responds to stresses placed in this area by the teeth and periodontal ligament, bone begins to resorb. The specific pattern of resorption is unpredictable in a given patient because great variation exists among individuals. In many patients, this resorption process tends to stabilize after a period, whereas in others a continuation of the process eventually results in total loss of alveolar bone and underlying basal bone (Fig. 13-1). The results of this resorption are accelerated by wearing dentures and tend to affect the mandible more severely than the maxilla because of the decreased surface area and less favorable distribution of occlusal forces.[1]

OBJECTIVES OF PREPROSTHETIC SURGERY

Despite the enormous progress in the technology available to preserve the dentition, prosthetic restoration and rehabilitation of the masticatory system is still needed in patients who are edentulous or partially edentulous. General systemic and local factors are responsible for the variation in the amount and pattern of alveolar bone resorption.[2] Systemic factors include the presence of nutritional abnormalities and systemic bone disease, such as osteoporosis, endocrine dysfunction, or any other systemic condition that may affect bone metabolism. Local factors affecting alveolar ridge resorption include alveoloplasty techniques used at the time of tooth removal and localized trauma associated with loss of alveolar bone. Denture wearing also may contribute to alveolar ridge resorption because of improper ridge adaptation of the denture or inadequate distribution of occlusal forces. Variations in facial structure may contribute to resorption patterns in two ways: First, the actual volume of bone present in the alveolar ridges varies with facial form.[3] Second, individuals with low mandibular plane angles and more acute gonial angles are capable of generating higher bite force, thereby placing greater pressure on the alveolar ridge areas. The long-term result of combined general and local factors is the loss of the bony alveolar ridge,

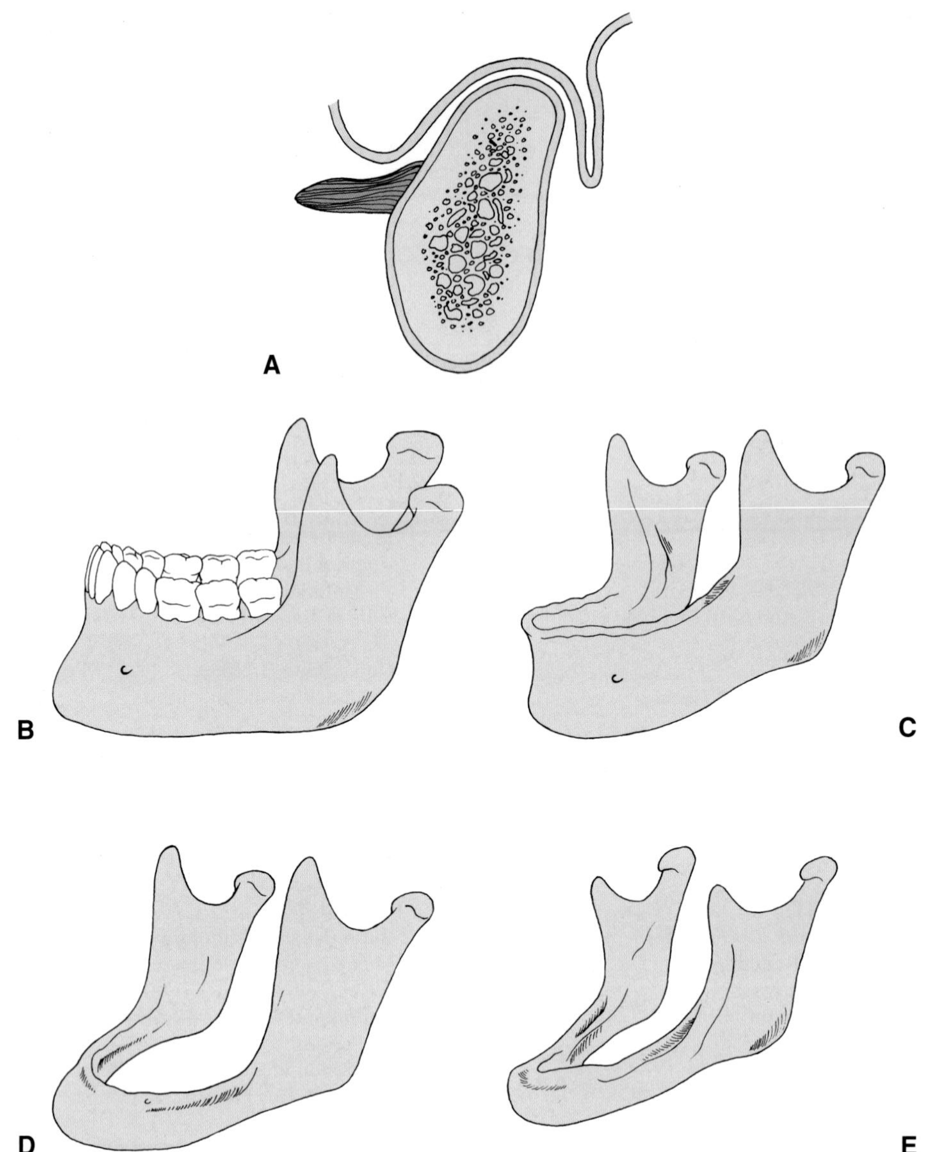

FIGURE 13-1 A, Ideal shape of alveolar process in denture-bearing area. B to E, Diagrammatic representation of progression of bone resorption in mandible after tooth extraction.

increased interarch space, increased influence of surrounding soft tissue, decreased stability and retention of the prosthesis, and increased discomfort from improper prosthesis adaptation. In the most severe cases of resorption a significant increase in the risk of spontaneous mandibular fracture exists.

The prosthetic replacement of lost or congenitally absent teeth frequently involves surgical preparation of the remaining oral tissues to support the best possible prosthetic replacement. Often oral structures, such as frenal attachments and exostoses, have no significance when teeth are present but become obstacles to proper prosthetic appliance construction after tooth loss. The challenge of prosthetic rehabilitation of the patient includes restoration of the best masticatory function possible, combined with restoration or improvement of dental and facial esthetics. Maximal preservation of hard and soft tissue during preprosthetic surgical preparation is also mandatory. The oral tissues are difficult to replace once they are lost.

The objective of preprosthetic surgery is to create proper supporting structures for subsequent placement of prosthetic appliances. The best denture support has the following 11 characteristics[4]:

1. No evidence of intraoral or extraoral pathologic conditions
2. Proper interarch jaw relationship in the anteroposterior, transverse, and vertical dimensions
3. Alveolar processes that are as large as possible and of the proper configuration (The ideal shape of the alveolar process is a broad U-shaped ridge, with the vertical components as parallel as possible [Fig. 13-1].)
4. No bony or soft tissue protuberances or undercuts
5. Adequate palatal vault form
6. Proper posterior tuberosity notching
7. Adequate attached keratinized mucosa in the primary denture-bearing area
8. Adequate vestibular depth for prosthesis extension
9. Added strength where mandibular fracture may occur

10. Protection of the neurovascular bundle
11. Adequate bony support and attached soft tissue covering to facilitate implant placement when necessary

PRINCIPLES OF PATIENT EVALUATION AND TREATMENT PLANNING

Before any surgical or prosthetic treatment, a thorough evaluation outlining the problems to be solved and a detailed treatment plan should be developed for each patient. It is imperative that no preparatory surgical procedure be undertaken without a clear understanding of the desired design of the final prosthesis.

Preprosthetic surgical treatment must begin with a thorough history and physical examination of the patient. An important aspect of the history is to obtain a clear idea of the patient's chief complaint and expectations of surgical and prosthetic treatment. Esthetic and functional goals of the patient must be assessed carefully and a determination made as to whether these expectations can be met. A thorough assessment of overall general health is especially important when considering more advanced preprosthetic surgical techniques because many of the approaches described require general anesthesia, donor site surgery to harvest autogenous graft material, and multiple surgical procedures. Specific attention should also be given to possible systemic diseases that may be responsible for the severe degree of bone resorption. Laboratory tests, such as serum levels of calcium, phosphate, parathyroid hormone, and alkaline phosphatase, may be useful in pinpointing potential metabolic problems that may affect bone resorption. Psychological factors and the adaptability of patients are important determinants of their ability to function adequately with full or partial dentures. Information on success or failure with previous prosthetic appliances may be helpful in determining the patient's attitude toward and adaptability to prosthetic treatment. The history should include important information such as the patient's risk status for surgery, with particular emphasis on systemic diseases that may affect bone or soft tissue healing.

An intraoral and extraoral examination of the patient should include an assessment of the existing occlusal relationships if any remain, the amount and contour of remaining bone, the quality of overlying soft tissue, the vestibular depth, location of muscle attachments, the jaw relationships, and the presence of soft tissue or bony pathologic condition.

Evaluation of Supporting Bony Tissue

Examination of the supporting bone should include visual inspection, palpation, radiographic examination, and in some cases evaluation of models. Abnormalities of the remaining bone can often be assessed during the visual inspection; however, because of bony resorption and location of muscle or soft tissue attachments, many bony abnormalities may be obscured. Palpation of all areas of the maxilla and mandible, including the primary denture-bearing area and vestibular area, is necessary.

Evaluation of the denture-bearing area of the maxilla includes an overall evaluation of the bony ridge form. No bony undercuts or gross bony protuberances that block the path of denture insertion should be allowed to remain in the area of the alveolar ridge, buccal vestibule, or palatal vault. Palatal tori that require modification should be noted. Adequate post-tuberosity notching must exist for posterior denture stability and peripheral seal.

The remaining mandibular ridge should be evaluated visually for overall ridge form and contour, gross ridge irregularities, tori, and buccal exostosis. In cases of moderate to severe resorption of alveolar bone, ridge contour cannot be adequately assessed by visual inspection alone. Muscular and mucosal attachments near the crest of the ridge may obscure underlying bony anatomy, particularly in the area of the posterior mandible, where a depression can frequently be palpated between the external oblique line and mylohyoid ridge areas. The location of the mental foramen and mental neurovascular bundle can be palpated in relation to the superior aspect of the mandible, and neurosensory disturbances can be noted.

Evaluation of the interarch relationship of the maxilla and the mandible is important and includes an examination of the anteroposterior and vertical relationships, as well as any possible skeletal asymmetries that may exist between the maxilla and mandible. In partially edentulous patients, the presence of supraerupted or malpositioned teeth should also be noted. The anteroposterior relationship must be evaluated with the patient in the proper vertical dimension. Overclosure of the mandible may result in a Class III skeletal relationship but may appear normal if evaluated with the mandible in the proper postural position. Lateral and posteroanterior cephalometric radiographs with the jaws in proper postural position may be helpful in confirming a skeletal discrepancy. Careful attention must be paid to the interarch distance, particularly in the posterior areas, where vertical excess of the tuberosity, either bony tissue or soft tissue, may impinge on space necessary for placement of a prosthesis that is properly constructed (Fig. 13-2).

Proper radiographs are an important part of the initial diagnosis and treatment plan. Panoramic radiographic techniques provide an excellent overview assessment of underlying bony structure and pathologic conditions.[5] Radiographs should disclose bony pathologic lesions, impacted teeth or portions of remaining roots, the bony pattern of the alveolar ridge, and pneumatization of the maxillary sinus (Fig. 13-3).

Cephalometric radiographs may also be helpful in evaluating the cross-sectional configuration of the anterior mandibular

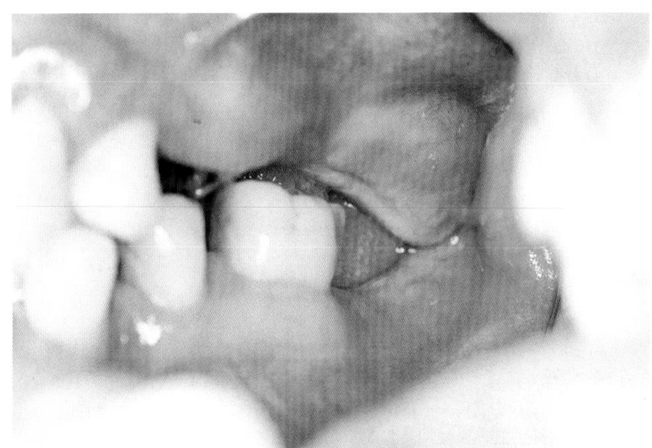

FIGURE 13-2 Examination of interarch relationships in proper vertical dimension often reveals lack of adequate space for prosthetic reconstruction. In this case, bony and fibrous tissue excess in tuberosity area must be reduced to provide adequate space for partial denture construction.

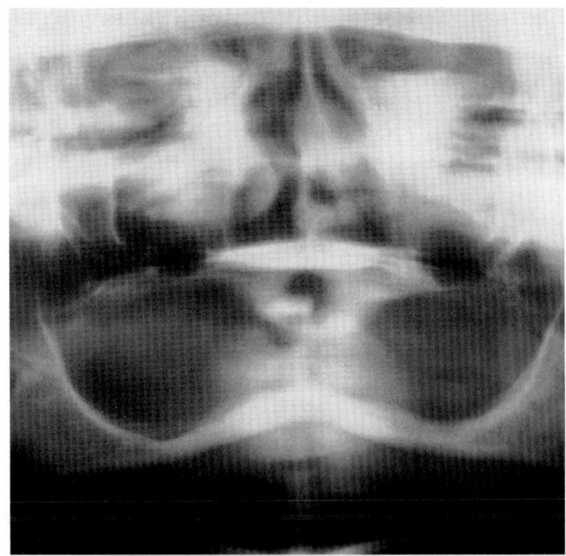

FIGURE 13-3 Radiograph demonstrating atrophic mandibular and maxillary alveolar ridges. Pneumatization of maxillary sinus is demonstrated.

ridge area and ridge relationships (Fig. 13-4). To evaluate the ridge relationship in the vertical and anteroposterior dimensions, it may be necessary to obtain the cephalometric radiograph in the appropriate vertical dimension. This often requires adjusting or reconstructing dentures to this position or making properly adjusted bite rims to be used for positioning at the time the radiograph is taken.

More sophisticated radiographic studies, such as computed tomography scans, may provide further information. Computed tomography scans are particularly helpful in evaluating the cross-sectional anatomy of the maxilla, including ridge form and sinus anatomy. The cross-sectional anatomy of the mandible can be evaluated more precisely, including the configuration of basal bone along with the alveolar ridge and the location of the inferior alveolar nerve.

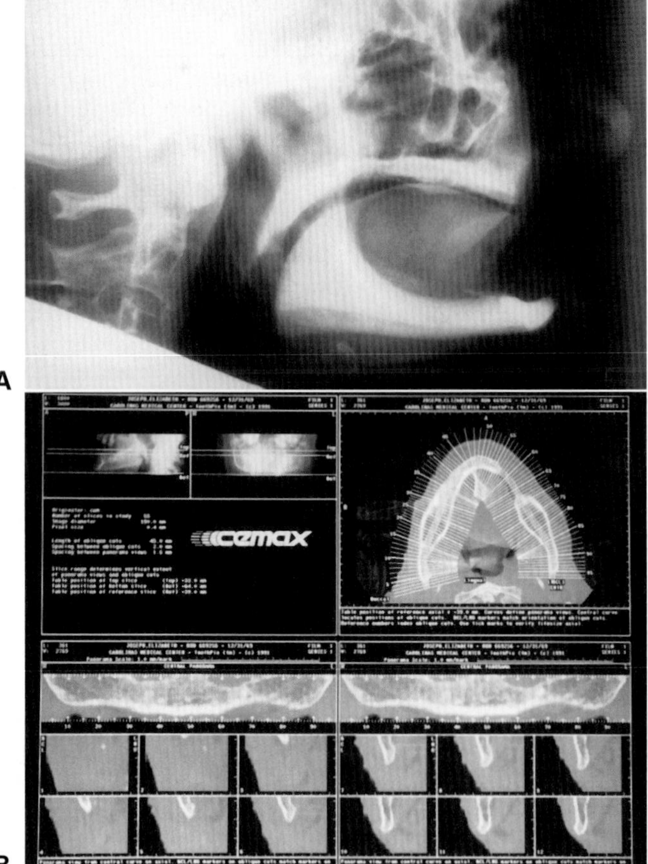

FIGURE 13-4 A, Cephalometric radiograph illustrating cross-sectional anatomy of the anterior mandible (patient is overclosed, giving the relative appearance of a Class III jaw relationship). B, Computed tomography showing detailed cross-sectional anatomy of mandible.

Evaluation of Supporting Soft Tissue

Assessment of the quality of tissue of the primary denture-bearing area overlying the alveolar ridge is of utmost importance. The amount of keratinized tissue firmly attached to the underlying bone in the denture-bearing area should be distinguished from poorly keratinized or freely movable tissue. Palpation discloses hypermobile fibrous tissue inadequate for a stable denture base (Fig. 13-5).

The vestibular areas should be free of inflammatory changes, such as scarred or ulcerated areas caused by denture pressure or hyperplastic tissue resulting from an ill-fitting denture. Tissue at the depth of the vestibule should be supple and without irregularities for maximal peripheral seal of the denture. Assessment of vestibular depth should include manual manipulation of the adjacent muscle attachments. By tensing the soft tissue adjacent to the area of the alveolar ridge, the dentist can note muscle or soft tissue attachments (including frena) that approximate the crest of the alveolar ridge and are often responsible for the loss of peripheral seal of the denture during speech and mastication.

The lingual aspect of the mandible should be inspected to determine the level of attachment of the mylohyoid muscle in relation to the crest of the mandibular ridge and the attachment of the genioglossus muscle in the anterior mandible. The linguovestibular depth should be evaluated with the tongue in several positions, because movement of the tongue accompanied by elevation of the mylohyoid and genioglossus muscles is a common cause of movement and displacement of the lower denture.

Treatment Planning

Before any surgical intervention, a treatment plan addressing the patient's identified oral problems should be formulated. The dentist responsible for prosthesis construction should assume responsibility for seeking surgical consultation when necessary. Long-term maintenance of the underlying bone and soft tissue, as well as of the prosthetic appliances, should be kept in mind at all times. When severe bony atrophy exists, treatment must be directed at correction of the bony deficiency and alteration of the associated soft tissue. When some degree of bony support remains despite alveolar atrophy, improvement of the denture-bearing area may be accomplished by directly

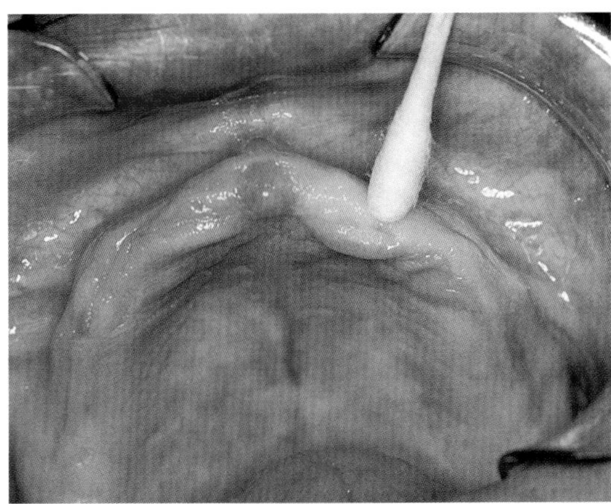

FIGURE 13-5 Palpation reveals hypermobile tissue that will not provide adequate base in denture-bearing area.

treating the bony deficiency or by compensating for it with soft tissue surgery. The most appropriate treatment plan should consider ridge height, width, and contour. Several other factors should also be considered: In an older patient in whom moderate bony resorption has taken place, soft tissue surgery alone may be sufficient for improved prosthesis function. In an extremely young patient who has undergone the same degree of atrophy, bony augmentation procedures may be indicated. The role of implants may alter the need for surgical modification of bone or soft tissue.

Hasty treatment planning, without consideration for long-term results, can often result in unnecessary loss of bone or soft tissue and improper functioning of the prosthetic appliance. For example, when there appears to be redundant or loose soft tissue over the alveolar ridge area, the most appropriate long-term treatment plan may involve grafting bone to improve the contour of the alveolar ridge or support endosteal implants. Maintenance of the redundant soft tissue may be necessary to improve the results of the grafting procedure. If this tissue were removed without any consideration of the possible long-term benefits of a grafting procedure, the opportunity for improved immediate function and the opportunity for long-term maintenance of bony tissue and soft tissue would be lost. If bony augmentation is indicated, maximum augmentation frequently depends on availability of adjacent soft tissue to provide tension-free coverage of the graft. Soft tissue surgery should be delayed until hard tissue grafting and appropriate healing have occurred. This is especially true for conservation of gingiva and keratinized soft tissues, which provide a better implant environment. Therefore, it is usually desirable to delay definitive soft tissue procedures until underlying bony problems have been adequately resolved. However, when extensive grafting or other, more complex treatment of bony abnormalities is not required, bony and soft tissue preparation sometimes can be completed simultaneously.

RECONTOURING OF ALVEOLAR RIDGES

Irregularities of the alveolar bone found at the time of tooth extraction or after a period of initial healing require recontouring before final prosthetic construction. This chapter focuses primarily on preparation of ridges for removable prostheses, but some emphasis is placed on the possibility of future implant placement and the obvious need to conserve as much bone and soft tissue as possible.

Simple Alveoloplasty Associated with Removal of Multiple Teeth

The simplest form of alveoloplasty consists of the compression of the lateral walls of the extraction socket after simple tooth removal. In many cases of single tooth extraction, digital compression of the extraction site adequately contours the underlying bone, provided no gross irregularities of bone contour are found in the area after extraction. When multiple irregularities exist, more extensive recontouring often is necessary. A conservative alveoloplasty in combination with multiple extractions is carried out after all of the teeth in the arch have been removed as described in Chapter 8. The specific areas requiring alveolar recontouring are obvious if this sequence is followed. Whether alveolar ridge recontouring is performed at the time of tooth extraction or after a period of healing, the technique is essentially the same. Bony areas requiring recontouring should be exposed using an envelope type of flap. A mucoperiosteal incision along the crest of the ridge, with adequate extension anteroposterior to the area to be exposed, and flap reflection allow adequate visualization and access to the alveolar ridge. Where adequate exposure is not possible, small vertical-releasing incisions may be necessary.

The primary objectives of mucoperiosteal flap reflection are to allow for adequate visualization and access to the bony structures that require recontouring and to protect soft tissue adjacent to this area during the procedure. Although releasing incisions often create more discomfort during the healing period, this technique is certainly preferred to the possibility of an unanticipated tear in the edges of a flap when inadequate exposure could not be achieved with an envelope flap. Regardless of flap design, the mucoperiosteum should be reflected only to the extent that adequate exposure to the area of bony irregularity can be achieved. Excessive flap reflection may result in devitalized areas of bone, which will resorb more rapidly after surgery, and a diminished soft tissue adaptation to the alveolar ridge area.

Depending on the degree of irregularity of the alveolar ridge area, recontouring can be accomplished with a rongeur, a bone file, or a bone bur in a handpiece, alone or in combination (Fig. 13-6). Copious saline irrigation should be used throughout the recontouring procedure to avoid overheating and bone necrosis. After recontouring, the flap should be reapproximated by digital pressure and the ridge palpated to ensure that all irregularities have been removed (Fig. 13-7). After copious irrigation to ensure removal of debris, the tissue margins can be reapproximated with interrupted or continuous sutures. Resorbable sutures are usually used to approximate tissue and add tensile strength across the wound margins. The resorbable material is broken down by salivary proteolytic enzymes or hydrolysis over several days to weeks, eliminating the need for removal.[6] If an extensive incision has been made, continuous suturing tends to be less annoying to the patient and provides for easier postoperative hygiene because of the elimination of knots and loose suture ends along the incision line. The initial soft tissue redundancy created with reduction of the bony irregularities often shrinks and readapts over the alveolus, allowing preservation of attached gingiva.

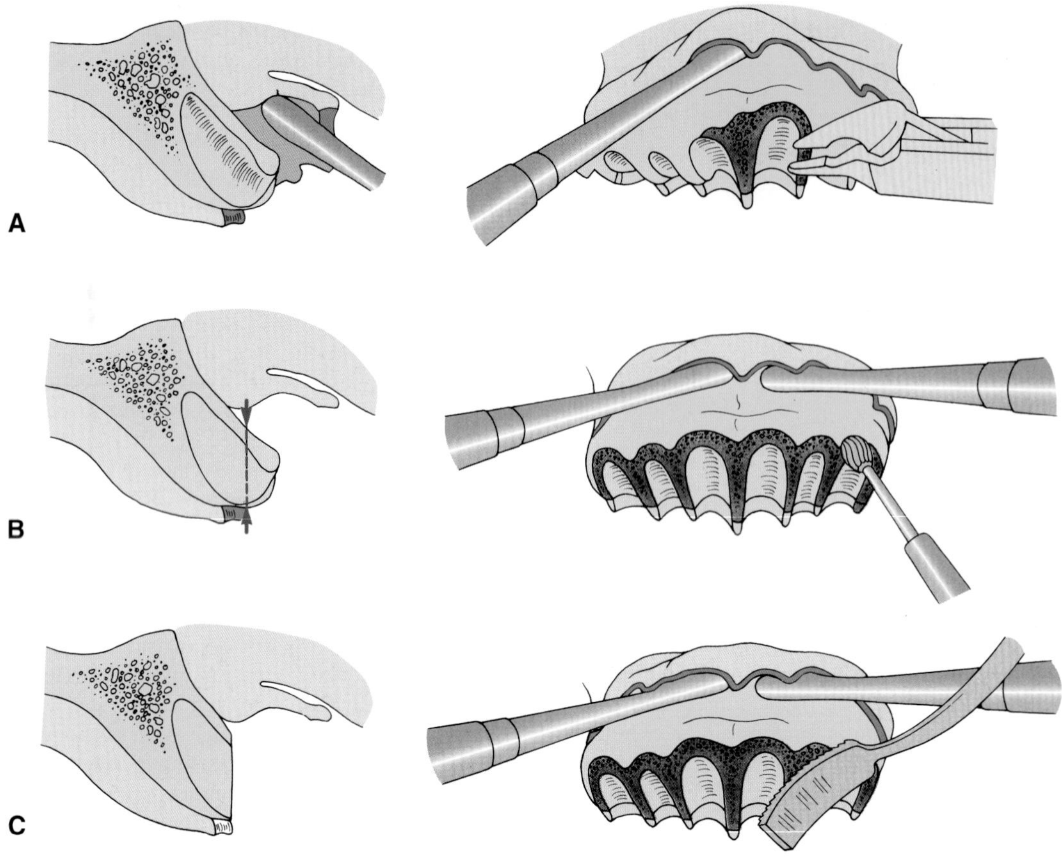

FIGURE 13-6 Simple alveoloplasty eliminates buccal irregularities and undercut areas by removing labiocortical bone. A, Elevation of mucoperiosteal flap, exposure of irregularities of alveolar ridge, and removal of gross irregularity with rongeur. B, Bone bur in rotating handpiece can also be used to remove bone and smooth labiocortical surface. C, Use of bone file to smooth irregularities and achieve final desired contour.

When a sharp knife-edge ridge exists in the mandible, the sharp superior portion of the alveolus can be removed in a manner similar to that described for simple alveoloplasty. After local anesthesia is obtained, a crestal incision is made, extending along the alveolar ridge, approximately 1 cm beyond either end of the area requiring recontouring (Fig. 13-8). After minimal reflection of the mucoperiosteum, a rongeur can be used to remove the major portion of the sharp area of the superior aspect of the mandible. A bone file is used to smooth the superior aspect of the mandible. After copious irrigation, this area is closed with continuous or interrupted sutures. Before removal of any bone, strong consideration should be given to reconstruction of proper ridge form using grafting procedures (discussed later in this chapter).

Intraseptal Alveoloplasty

An alternative to the removal of alveolar ridge irregularities by the simple alveoloplasty technique is the use of an intraseptal alveoloplasty, or Dean's technique, involving the removal of intraseptal bone and the repositioning of the labial cortical bone, rather than removal of excessive or irregular areas of the labial cortex.[7] This technique is best used in an area where the ridge is of relatively regular contour and adequate height but presents an undercut to the depth of the labial vestibule because of the configuration of the alveolar ridge. The technique can be accomplished at the time of tooth removal or in the early initial postoperative healing period.

After exposure of the crest of the alveolar ridge by reflection of the mucoperiosteum, a small rongeur can be used to remove the intraseptal portion of the alveolar bone (Fig. 13-9). After adequate bone removal has been accomplished, digital pressure should be sufficient to fracture the labiocortical plate of the alveolar ridge inward to approximate the palatal plate area more closely. Occasionally, small vertical cuts at either end of the labiocortical plate facilitate repositioning of the fractured segment. By using a bur or osteotome inserted through the distal extraction area, the labial cortex is scored without perforation of the labial mucosa. Digital pressure on the labial aspect of the ridge is necessary to determine when the bony cut is complete and to ensure that the mucosa is not damaged. After positioning of the labiocortical plate, any slight areas of bony irregularity can be contoured with a bone file and the alveolar mucosa can be reapproximated with interrupted or continuous suture techniques. A splint or an immediate denture lined with a soft lining material can then be inserted to maintain the bony position until initial healing has taken place.

This type of technique has several advantages: The labial prominence of the alveolar ridge can be reduced without significantly reducing the height of the ridge in this area. The periosteal attachment to the underlying bone can also be

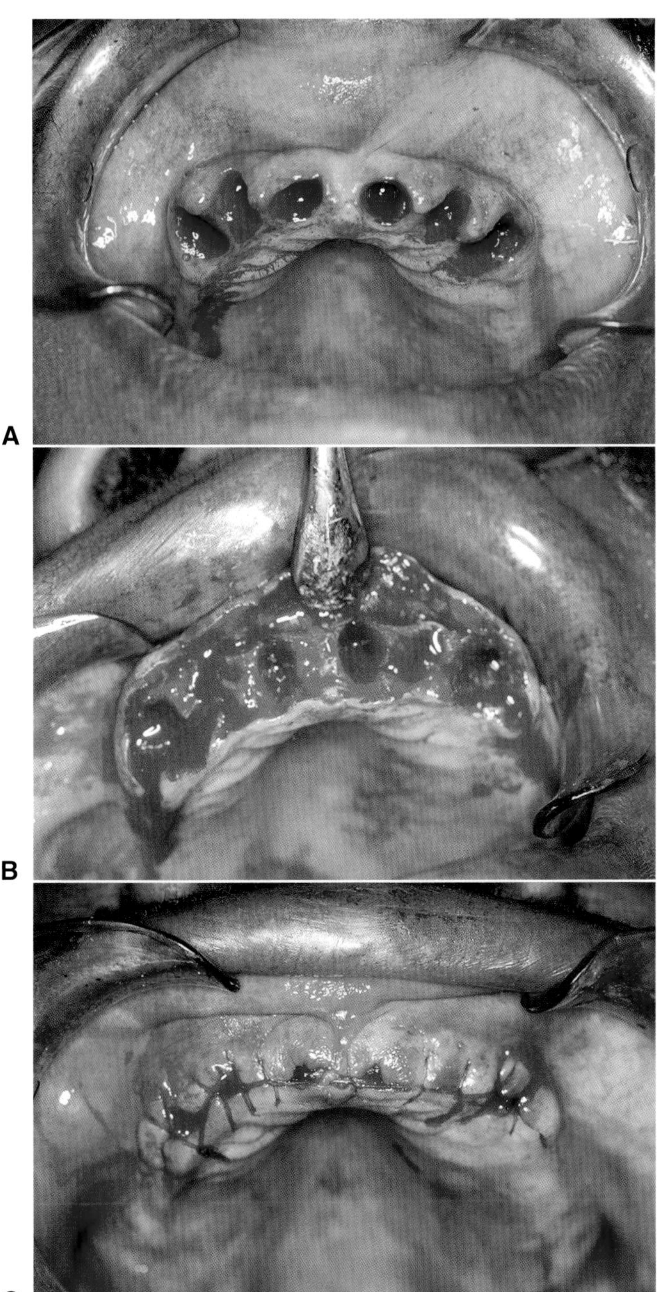

FIGURE 13-7 A, Clinical appearance of maxillary ridge after removal of teeth. B, Minimal flap reflection for recontouring. C, Proper alveolar ridge form free of irregularities and bony undercuts after recontouring.

maintained, thereby reducing postoperative bone resorption and remodeling. Finally, the muscle attachments to the area of the alveolar ridge can be left undisturbed in this type of procedure. Michael and Barsoum[8] reported the results of a study comparing the effects of postoperative bone resorption after three alveoloplasty techniques. In their study, nonsurgical extraction, labial alveoloplasty, and an intraseptal alveoloplasty technique were compared to evaluate postoperative bony resorption. The initial postoperative results were similar, but the best long-term maintenance of alveolar ridge height was achieved with nonsurgical extractions, and the intraseptal alveoloplasty technique resulted in less resorption than did removal of labiocortical bone for reduction of ridge irregularities.

The main disadvantage of this technique is the decrease in ridge thickness that obviously occurs with this procedure. If the ridge form remaining after this type of alveoloplasty is excessively thin, it may preclude placement of implants in the future. For this reason the intraseptal alveoloplasty should reduce the thickness of the ridge in an amount sufficient only to reduce or eliminate undercuts in areas where a plan to place endosteal implants does not exist. Methods for preservation of alveolar width with simultaneous grafting into the extraction site are addressed later in the chapter.

Maxillary Tuberosity Reduction (Hard Tissue)

Horizontal or vertical excess of the maxillary tuberosity area may be a result of excess bone, an increase in the thickness of soft tissue overlying the bone, or both. A preoperative radiograph or selective probing with a local anesthetic needle are often useful to determine the extent to which bone and soft tissue contribute to this excess and to locate the floor of the maxillary sinus. Recontouring of the maxillary tuberosity area may be necessary to remove bony ridge irregularities or to create adequate interarch space, which allows proper construction of prosthetic appliances in the posterior areas. Surgery can be accomplished using local anesthetic infiltration or posterosuperior alveolar and greater palatine blocks. Access to the tuberosity for bone removal is accomplished by making a crestal incision that extends up the posterior aspect of the tuberosity area. The most posterior aspect of this incision is often best made with a No. 12 scalpel blade. Reflection of a full-thickness mucoperiosteal flap is completed in the buccal and palatal directions to allow adequate access to the entire tuberosity area (Fig. 13-10). Bone can be removed using a side-cutting rongeur or rotary instruments, with care taken to avoid perforation of the floor of the maxillary sinus. If the maxillary sinus is inadvertently perforated, no specific treatment is required, provided that the sinus membrane has not been violated. After the appropriate amount of bone has been removed, the area should be smoothed with a bone file and copiously irrigated with saline. The mucoperiosteal flaps can then be readapted.

Excess, overlapping soft tissue resulting from the bone removal is excised in an elliptical fashion. A tension-free closure over this area is important, particularly if the floor of the sinus has been perforated. Sutures should remain in place for approximately 7 days. Initial denture impressions can be completed approximately 4 weeks after surgery.

In the event of a gross sinus perforation involving an opening in the sinus membrane, the use of postoperative antibiotics and sinus decongestants is recommended. Amoxicillin is usually the antibiotic of choice, unless contraindicated by allergy. Sinus decongestants, such as pseudoephedrine with or without an antihistamine, are adequate. The antibiotic and decongestant should be given for 7 to 10 days postoperatively. The patient is informed of the potential complications and cautioned against creating excessive sinus pressure, such as nose blowing or sucking with a straw for 10 to 14 days.

Buccal Exostosis and Excessive Undercuts

Excessive bony protuberances and resulting undercut areas are more common in the maxilla than the mandible. A local

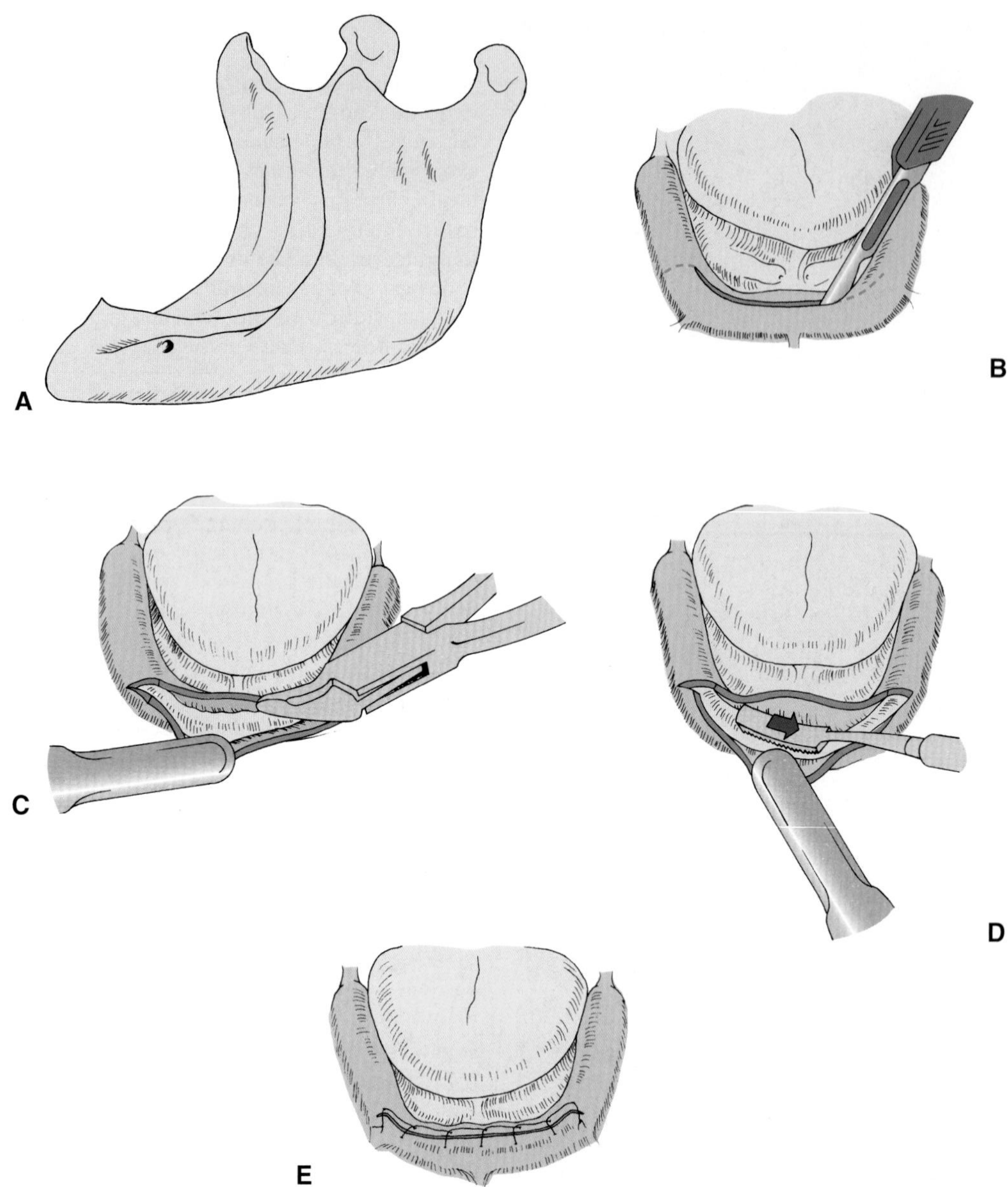

FIGURE 13-8 Recontouring of a knife-edge ridge. A, Lateral view of mandible, with resorption resulting in knife-edge alveolar ridge. B, Crestal incision extends 1 cm beyond each end of area to be recontoured (vertical-releasing incisions are occasionally necessary at posterior ends of initial incision). C, Rongeur used to eliminate bulk of sharp bony projection. D, Bone file used to eliminate any minor irregularities (bone bur and handpiece can also be used for this purpose). E, Continuous suture technique for mucosal closure.

anesthetic should be infiltrated around the area requiring bony reduction. For mandibular buccal exostosis, inferior alveolar blocks may also be required to anesthetize bony areas. A crestal incision extends 1.0 to 1.5 cm beyond each end of the area requiring contour, and a full-thickness mucoperiosteal flap is reflected to expose the areas of bony exostosis. If adequate exposure cannot be obtained, vertical-releasing incisions are necessary to provide access and prevent trauma to the soft tissue flap. If the areas of irregularity are small, recontouring with a bone file may be all that is required; larger areas may necessitate use of a rongeur or rotary instrument (Fig. 13-11). After completion of the bone recontouring, soft tissue is readapted, and visual inspection and palpation ensure that no irregularities or bony undercuts exist. Interrupted or continuous suturing techniques are used to close the soft tissue incision. Denture impressions can be completed 4 weeks postoperatively.

Although extremely large areas of bony exostosis generally require removal, small undercut areas are often best treated by being filled with autogenous or allogeneic bone material. Such a situation might occur in the anterior maxilla or mandible, where removal of the bony buccal protuberance results in a narrowed crest in the alveolar ridge area and a less desirable area of support for the denture, as well as an area that may resorb more rapidly.

Local anesthetic infiltration is generally sufficient when filling in buccal undercut areas. The undercut portion of the

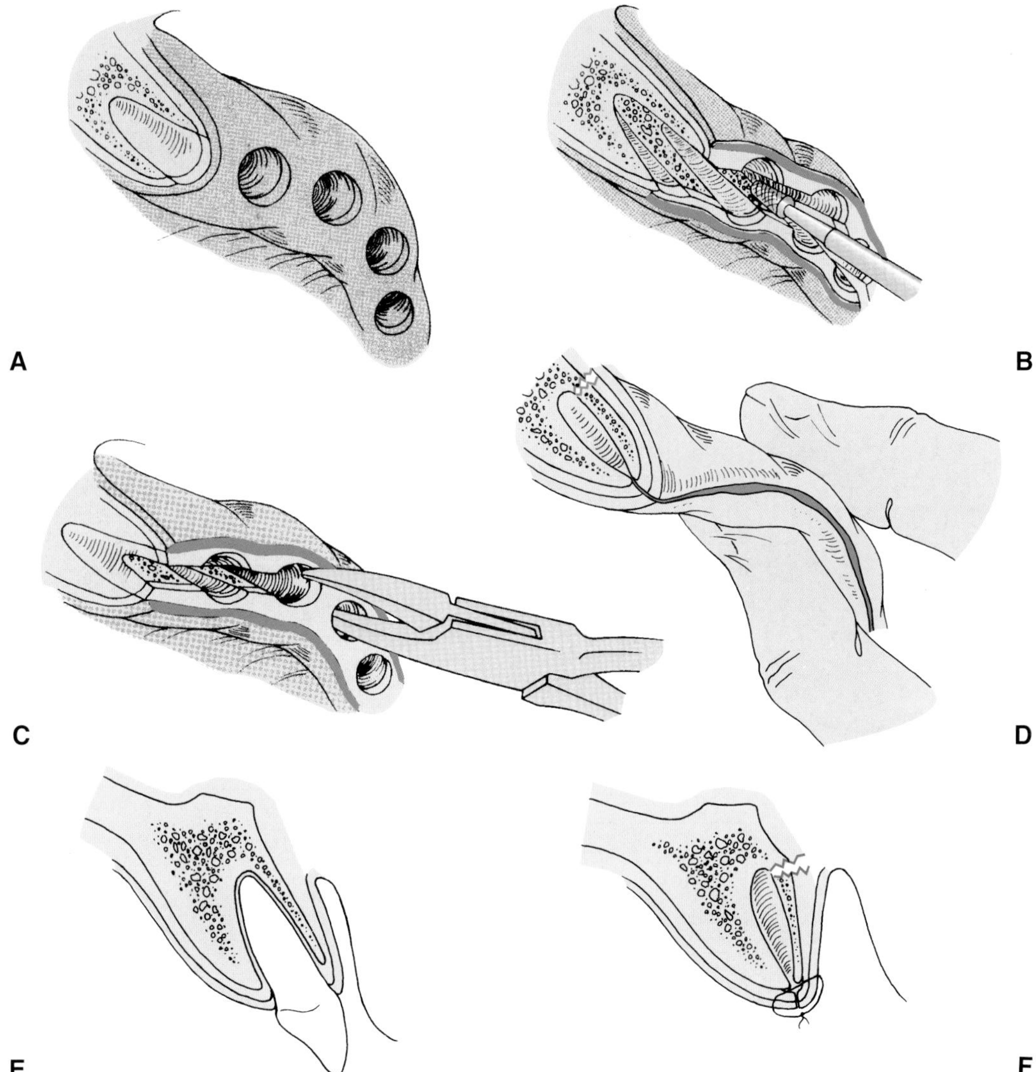

FIGURE 13-9 Intraseptal alveoloplasty. A, Oblique view of alveolar ridge, demonstrating slight facial undercut. B, Minimal elevation of mucoperiosteal flap, followed by removal of intraseptal bone using fissure bur and handpiece. C, Rongeur used to remove intraseptal bone. D, Digital pressure used to fracture labiocortex in palatal direction. E, Cross-sectional view of alveolar process. F, Cross-sectional view of alveolar process after tooth removal and intraseptal alveoloplasty. By fracturing labiocortex of alveolar process in palatal direction, labial undercut can be eliminated without reducing vertical height of alveolar ridge.

ridge is exposed with a crestal incision and standard dissection, or the undercut area can be accessed with a vertical incision made in the anterior maxillary or mandibular areas (Fig. 13-12). A small periosteal elevator is then used to create a subperiosteal tunnel extending the length of the area to be filled in with bone graft. Autogenous or allogeneic material can then be placed in the defect and covered with a resorbable membrane. Impressions for denture fabrication can be taken after tissue healing 3 to 4 weeks after surgery. A modification of this technique is also discussed in Chapter 14.

Lateral Palatal Exostosis

The lateral aspect of the palatal vault may be irregular because of the presence of lateral palatal exostosis. This presents problems in denture construction because of the undercut created by the exostosis and the narrowing of the palatal vault. Occasionally, these exostoses are large enough that the mucosa covering the area becomes ulcerated.

Local anesthetic in the area of the greater palatine foramen and infiltration in the area of the incision are necessary. A crestal incision is made from the posterior aspect of the tuberosity, extending slightly beyond the anterior area of the exostosis, which requires recontouring (Fig. 13-13). Reflection of the mucoperiosteum in the palatal direction should be accomplished with careful attention to the area of the palatine foramen to avoid damage to the blood vessels as they leave the foramen and extend forward. After adequate exposure, a rotary instrument or bone file can be used to remove the excess bony projection in this area. The area is irrigated with sterile saline and closed with continuous or interrupted sutures. No surgical splint or packing is generally required, and the apparent redundant soft tissues will adapt after this procedure.

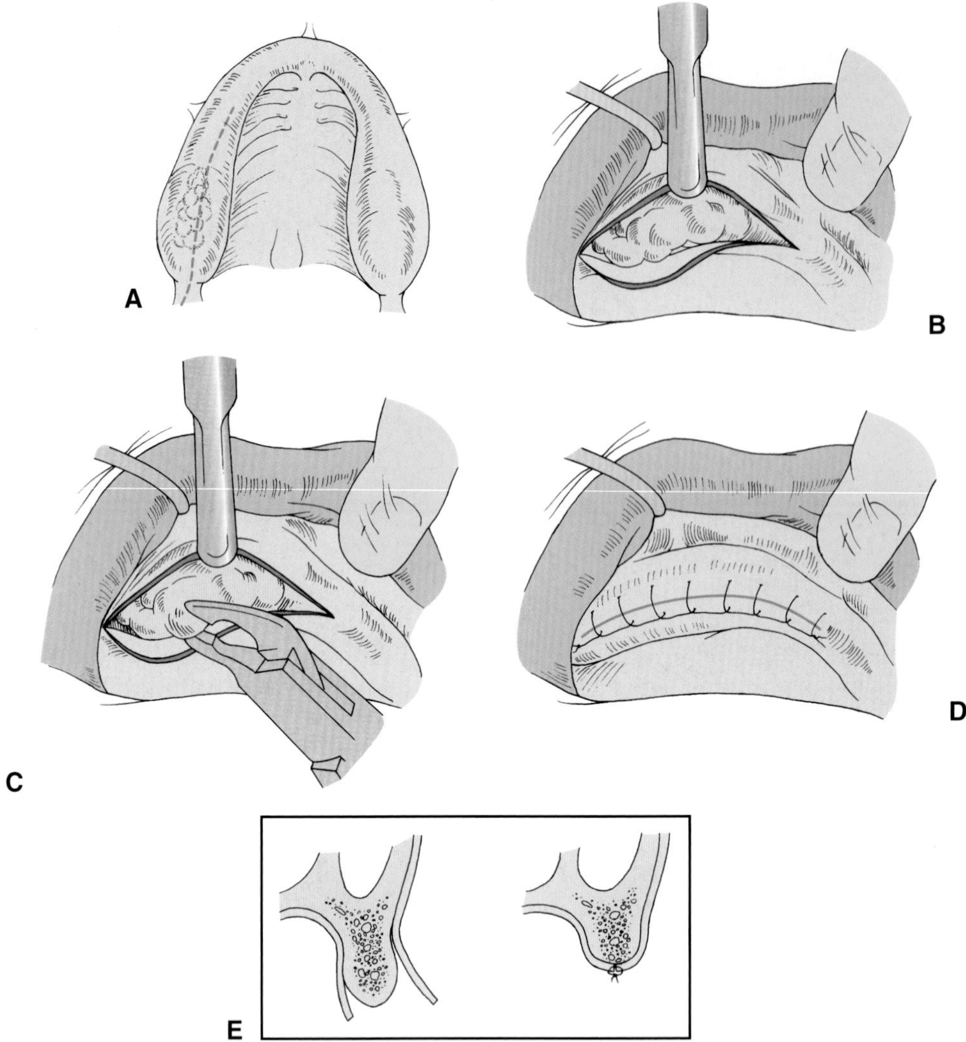

FIGURE 13-10 Bony tuberosity reduction. **A**, Incision extended along crest of alveolar ridge distally to superior extent of tuberosity area. **B**, Elevated mucoperiosteal flap provides adequate exposure to all areas of bony excess. **C**, Rongeur used to eliminate bony excess. **D**, Tissue reapproximated with continuous suture technique. **E**, Cross-sectional view of posterior tuberosity area, showing vertical reduction of bone and reapposition of mucoperiosteal flap. (In some cases, removal of large amounts of bone produces excessive soft tissue, which can be excised before closure to prevent overlapping.)

Mylohyoid Ridge Reduction

One of the more common areas interfering with proper denture construction in the mandible is the mylohyoid ridge area. In addition to the actual bony ridge, with its easily damaged thin covering of mucosa, the muscular attachment to this area often is responsible for dislodging the denture. When this ridge is extremely sharp, denture pressure may produce significant pain in this area. (Relocation of the mylohyoid muscle to improve this condition is discussed later in this chapter.) In cases of severe resorption, the external oblique line and the mylohyoid ridge area may actually form the most prominent areas of the posterior mandible, with the midportion of the mandibular ridge existing as a concave structure. In such cases, augmentation of the posterior aspect of the mandible, rather than removal of the mylohyoid ridge, may be beneficial. However, some cases can be improved by reduction of the mylohyoid ridge area.

Inferior alveolar, buccal, and lingual nerve blocks are required for mylohyoid ridge reduction. A linear incision is made over the crest of the ridge in the posterior aspect of the mandible. Extension of the incision too far to the lingual aspect should be avoided because this may cause potential trauma to the lingual nerve. A full-thickness mucoperiosteal flap is reflected, which exposes the mylohyoid ridge area and mylohyoid muscle attachments (Fig. 13-14). The mylohyoid muscle fibers are removed from the ridge by sharply incising the muscle attachment at the area of bony origin. When the muscle is released, the underlying fat is visible in the surgical field. After reflection of the muscle, a rotary instrument with careful soft tissue protection or bone file can be used to remove the sharp prominence of the mylohyoid ridge. Immediate replacement of the denture is desirable, because it may help facilitate a more inferior relocation of the muscular attachment; however, this is unpredictable and

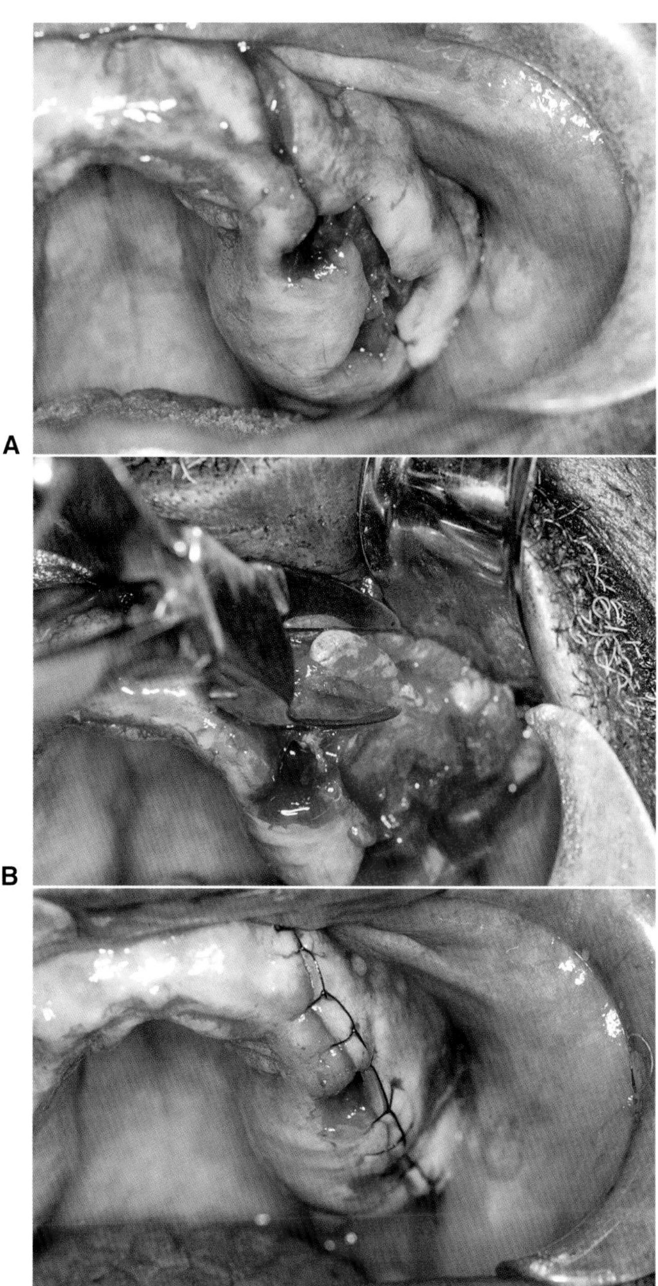

FIGURE 13-11 Removal of buccal exostosis. A, Gross irregularities of buccal aspect of alveolar ridge. After tooth removal, incision is completed over crest of alveolar ridge. (Vertical-releasing incision in cuspid area is demonstrated.) B, Exposure and removal of buccal exostosis with rongeur. C, Soft tissue closure using continuous suture technique.

may actually be best managed by a procedure to lower the floor of the mouth.

Genial Tubercle Reduction

As the mandible begins to undergo resorption, the area of the attachment of the genioglossus muscle in the anterior portion of the mandible may become increasingly prominent. In some cases the tubercle may actually function as a shelf against which the denture can be constructed, but it usually requires reduction to construct the prosthesis properly. Before a decision to remove this prominence is made, consideration should be given to possible augmentation of the anterior portion of the mandible rather than reduction of the genial tubercle. If augmentation is the preferred treatment, the tubercle should be left to add support to the graft in this area. Local anesthetic infiltration and bilateral lingual nerve blocks should provide adequate anesthesia. A crestal incision is made from each premolar area to the midline of the mandible. A full-thickness mucoperiosteal flap is dissected lingually to expose the genial tubercle. The genioglossus muscle attachment can be removed by a sharp incision.

Smoothing with a bur or a rongeur followed by a bone file removes the genial tubercle. The genioglossus muscle is left to reattach in a random fashion. As with the mylohyoid muscle and mylohyoid ridge reduction, a procedure to lower the floor of the mouth may also benefit the anterior mandible.

TORI REMOVAL

Maxillary Tori

Maxillary tori consist of bony exostosis formation in the area of the palate. The origin of maxillary tori is unclear. Tori are found in 20% of the female population, approximately twice the prevalence in males.[9] Tori may have multiple shapes and configurations, ranging from a single smooth elevation to a multiloculated pedunculated bony mass. Tori present few problems when the maxillary dentition is present and only occasionally interfere with speech or become ulcerated from frequent trauma to the palate. However, when the loss of teeth necessitates full or partial denture construction, tori often interfere with proper design and function of the prosthesis. Nearly all large maxillary tori should be removed before full or partial denture construction. Smaller tori may often be left because they do not interfere with prosthetic construction or function. Even small tori necessitate removal when they are irregular, extremely undercut, or in the area where a posterior palatal seal would be expected.

Bilateral greater palatine and incisive blocks and local infiltration provide the necessary anesthesia for tori removal. A linear incision in the midline of the torus with oblique vertical-releasing incisions at one or both ends is generally necessary (Fig. 13-15). Because the mucosa over this area is extremely thin, care must be taken in reflecting the tissue from the underlying bone, a particularly difficult task when the tori are multiloculated. A full palatal flap can sometimes be used for exposure of the tori. An incision is made along the crest of the ridge when the patient is edentulous or a palatal sulcular incision is used when teeth are present. Tissue reflection with this type of incision is often difficult if the tori have large undercuts where the bony exostosis is fused with the palate. When tori with a small pedunculated base are present, an osteotome and mallet may be used to remove the bony mass. For larger tori, it is usually best to section the tori into multiple fragments with a bur in a rotary handpiece. Careful attention must be paid to the depth of the cuts to avoid perforation of the floor of the nose. After sectioning, individual portions of the tori can be removed with a mallet and osteotome or a rongeur; then the area can be smoothed with a large bone bur. The entire bony projection does not necessarily require removal, but a smooth regular area without undercuts should be created, without

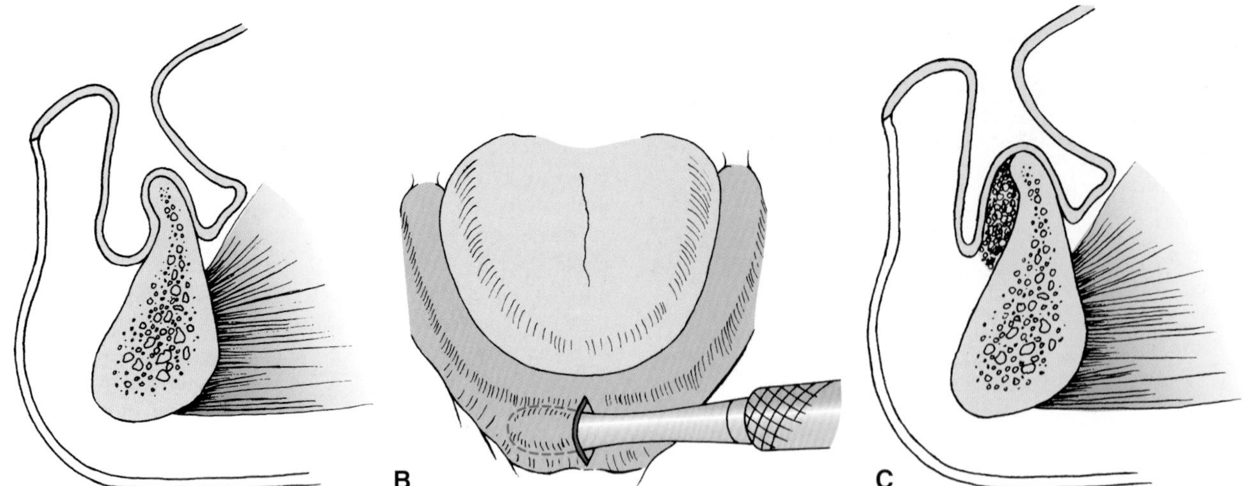

FIGURE 13-12 Removal of mandibular buccal undercut. A, Cross-sectional view of anterior portion of mandible, which, if corrected by removal of labiocortical home, would result in knife-edge ridge. B, Vertical incision is made and subperiosteal tunnel developed in depth of undercut area. C, Cross-sectional view after filling defect with graft material. The material is contained within the boundaries of the subperiosteal tunnel.

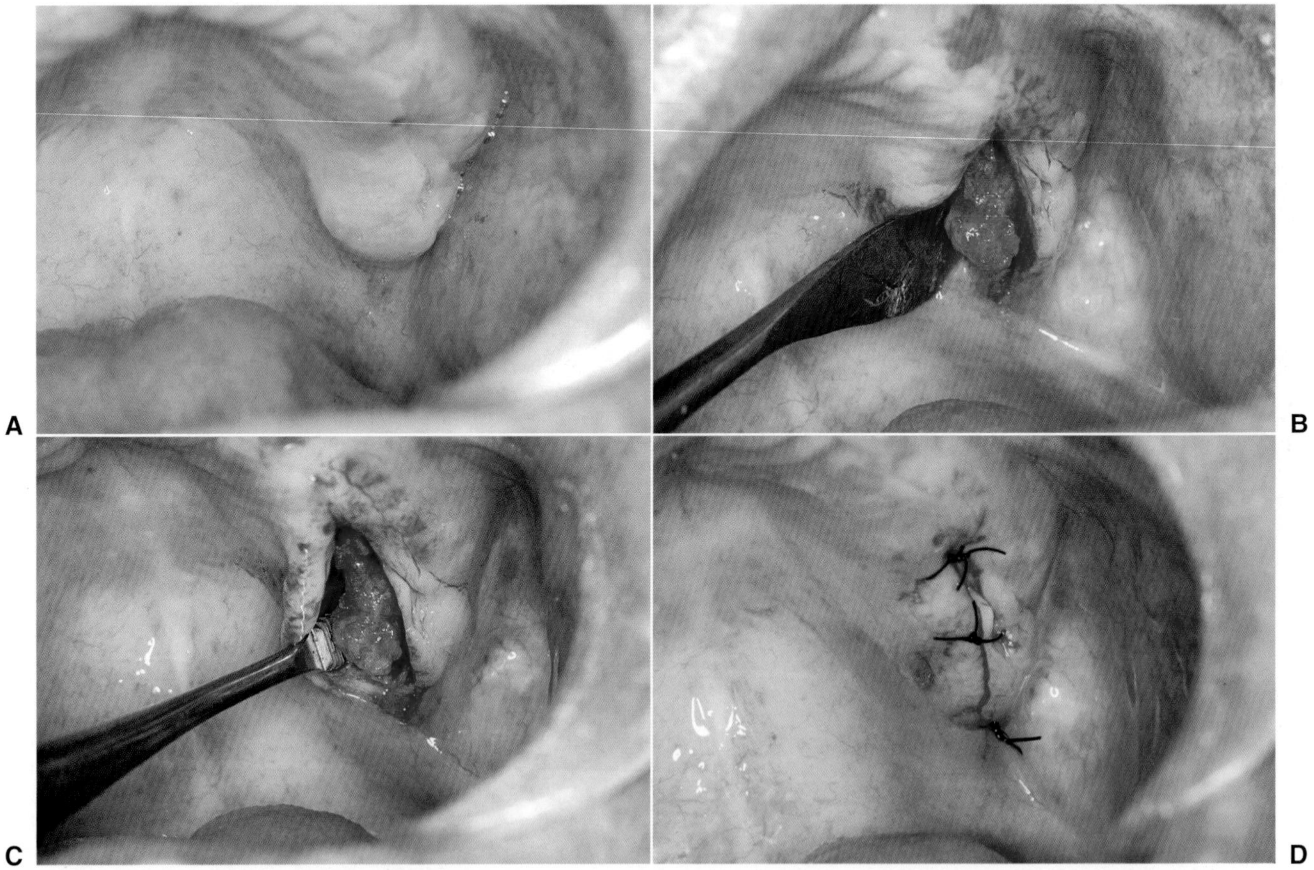

FIGURE 13-13 Removal of palatal bony exostosis. A, Small palatal exostosis that interferes with proper denture construction in this area. B, Crestal incision and mucoperiosteal flap reflection to expose palatal exostosis. C, Use of bone file to remove bony excess. D, Soft tissue closure.

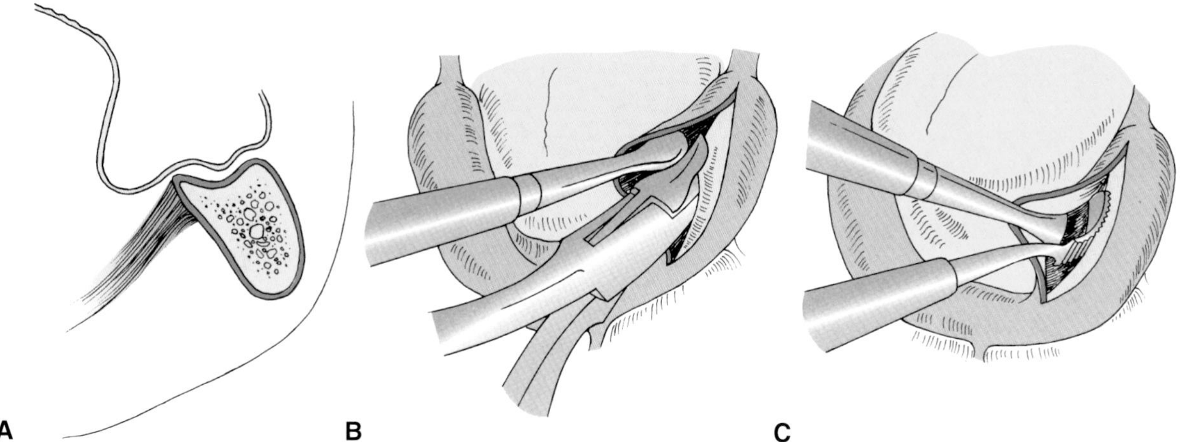

FIGURE 13-14 Mylohyoid ridge reduction. A, Cross-sectional view of posterior aspect of mandible, showing concave contour of the superior aspect of ridge from resorption. Mylohyoid ridge and external oblique lines form highest portions of ridge. (This can generally best be treated by alloplastic augmentation of mandible but in rare cases may also require mylohyoid ridge reduction.) B, Crestal incision and exposure of lingual aspect of mandible for removal of sharp bone in mylohyoid ridge area. Rongeur or bur in rotating handpiece can be used to remove bone. C, Bone file used to complete recontouring of mylohyoid ridge.

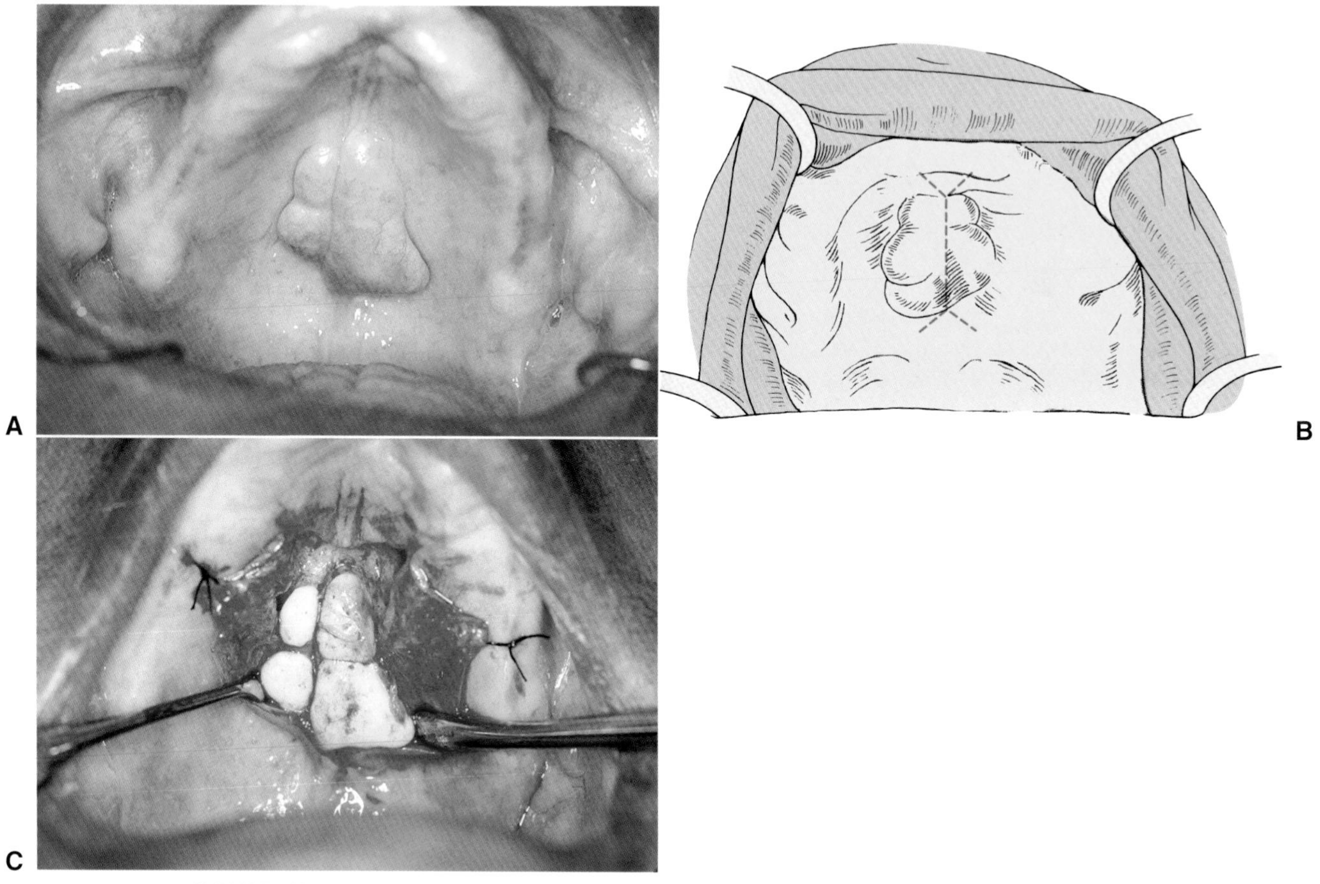

A

B

C

FIGURE 13-15 Removal of palatal torus. A, Typical appearance of maxillary torus. B, Midline incision with anteroposterior oblique releasing incisions. C, Mucoperiosteal flaps retracted with silk sutures to improve access to all areas of torus.

Continued

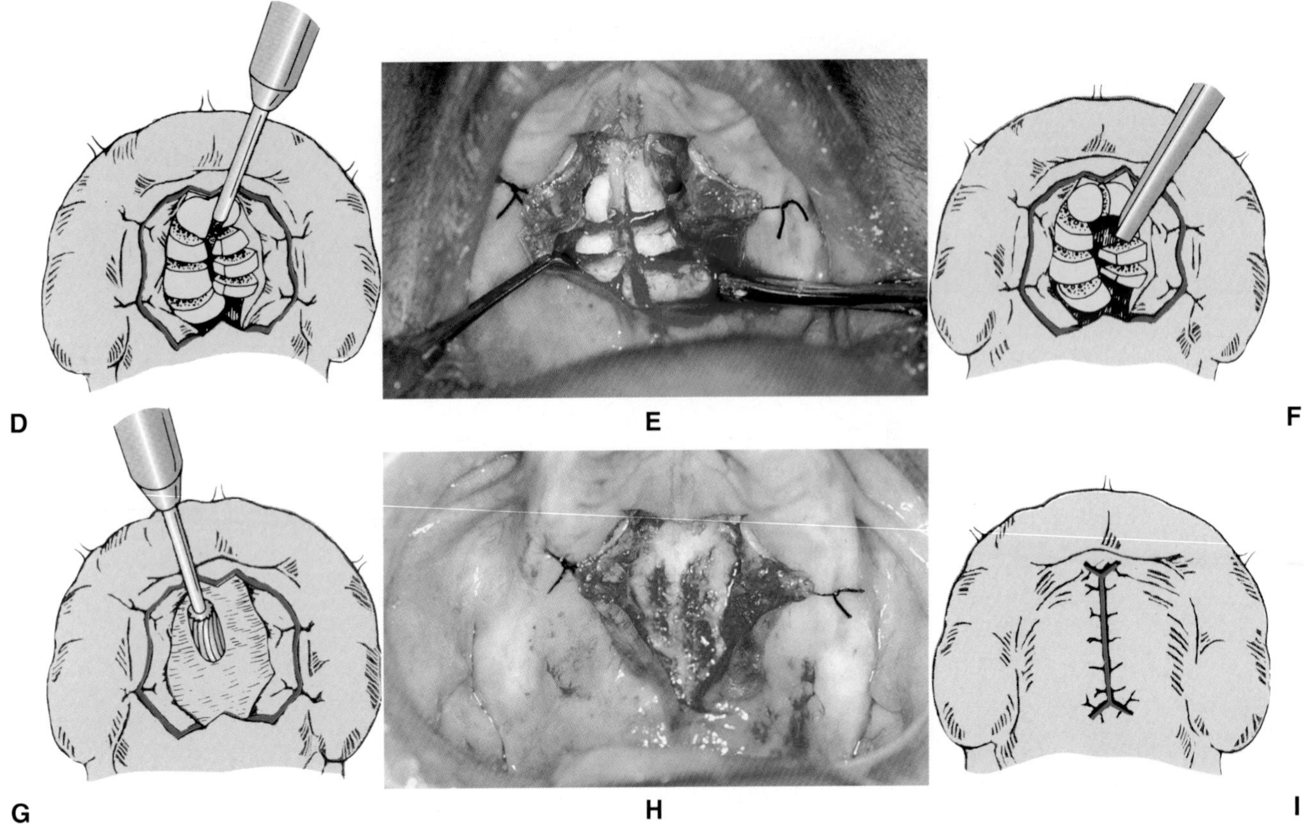

FIGURE 13-15, cont'd Removal of palatal torus. **D** and **E**, Sectioning of torus using fissure bur. **F**, Small osteotome used to remove sections of torus. **G** and **H**, Large bone bur used to produce the final desired contour. **I**, Soft tissue closure.

extension into the area where a posterior palatal seal would be placed. Tissue is readapted by finger pressure and is inspected to determine the amount of excess mucosa that may require removal. Retention of enough tissue to allow a tension-free closure over the entire area of exposed bone is important. The mucosa is reapproximated and sutured; an interrupted suture technique is often required because the thin mucosa may not retain sutures well. To prevent hematoma formation, some form of pressure dressing must be placed over the area of the palatal vault. A temporary denture or prefabricated splint with a soft liner placed in the center of the palate to prevent pressure necrosis can also be used to support the thin mucosa and prevent hematoma formation.

The major complications of maxillary tori removal include postoperative hematoma formation, fracture or perforation of the floor of the nose, and necrosis of the flap. Local care, including vigorous irrigation, good hygiene, and support with soft tissue conditioners in the splint or denture, usually provides adequate treatment.

Mandibular Tori

Mandibular tori are bony protuberances on the lingual aspect of the mandible that usually occur in the premolar area. The origins of this bony exostosis are uncertain, and the growths may slowly increase in size. Occasionally, extremely large tori interfere with normal speech or tongue function during eating, but these tori rarely require removal when teeth are present. After the removal of lower teeth and before the construction of partial or complete dentures, it may be necessary to remove mandibular tori to facilitate denture construction.

Bilateral lingual and inferior alveolar injections provide adequate anesthesia for tori removal. A crest of the ridge incision should be made, extending 1 to 1.5 cm beyond each end of the tori to be reduced. When bilateral tori are to be removed simultaneously, it is best to leave a small band of tissue attached at the midline between the anterior extent of the two incisions. Leaving this tissue attached helps eliminate potential hematoma formation in the anterior floor of the mouth and maintains as much of the lingual vestibule as possible in the anterior mandibular area. As with maxillary tori, the mucosa over the lingual tori is generally very thin and should be reflected carefully to expose the entire area of bone to be recontoured (Fig. 13-16).

When the torus has a small pedunculated base, a mallet and osteotome may be used to cleave the tori from the medial aspect of the mandible. The line of cleavage can be directed by creating a small trough with a bur and a handpiece before using an osteotome. It is important to ensure that the direction of the initial bur trough (or the osteotome if it is used alone) is parallel with the medial aspect of the mandible to avoid an unfavorable fracture of the lingual or inferior cortex. The bur can also be used to deepen the trough so that a small instrument can be levered against the mandible to fracture the lingual tori to allow its removal. A bone bur or file can then be used to smooth the lingual cortex. The tissue should be readapted and palpated to evaluate contour and elimination of undercuts.

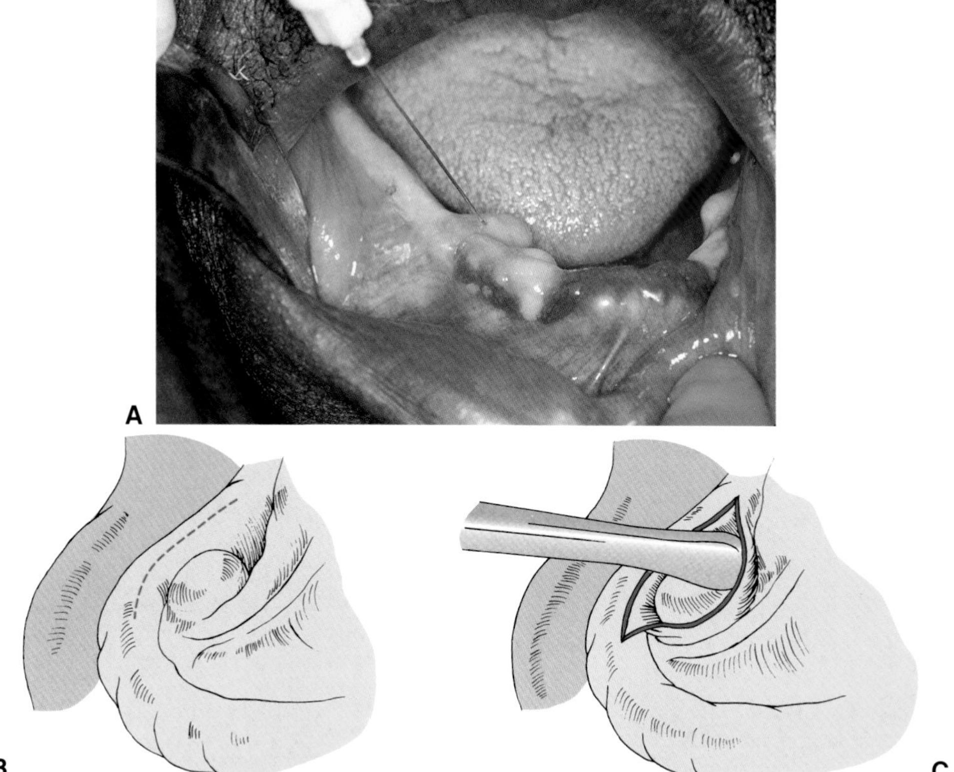

FIGURE 13-16 Removal of mandibular tori. A, After block, local anesthetic is administered; ballooning of thin mucoperiosteum over area of tori can be accomplished by placing bevel of local anesthetic needle against torus and injecting local anesthetic subperiosteally. (This greatly facilitates reflection of mucoperiosteal flap.) B, Outline of crestal incision. C, Exposure of torus.

Continued

An interrupted or continuous suture technique is used to close the incisions. Gauze packs placed in the floor of the mouth and retained for several hours are generally helpful in reducing postoperative edema and hematoma formation. In the event of wound dehiscence or exposed bone in the area of a mucosal perforation, treatment with local care, including frequent vigorous saline irrigation, is usually sufficient.

SOFT TISSUE ABNORMALITIES

Abnormalities of the soft tissue in the denture-bearing and peripheral tissue areas include excessive fibrous or hypermobile tissue; inflammatory lesions, such as inflammatory fibrous hyperplasia of the vestibule and inflammatory papillary hyperplasia of the palate; and abnormal muscular and frenal attachments. With the exception of pathologic and inflammatory lesions, many of the other conditions do not present problems when the patient has a full dentition. However, when loss of teeth necessitates prosthetic reconstruction, alteration of the soft tissue is often necessary. Immediately after tooth removal, muscular and frenal attachments initially do not present problems but may eventually interfere with proper denture construction as bony resorption takes place.

Long-term treatment planning before any soft tissue surgery is mandatory. Soft tissue that initially appears to be flabby and excessive may be useful if future ridge augmentation or grafting procedures are necessary. Oral mucosa is difficult to replace once it is removed. The only exception to this usefulness of excess tissue is when pathologic soft tissue lesions require removal.

Maxillary Tuberosity Reduction (Soft Tissue)

The primary objective of soft tissue maxillary tuberosity reduction is to provide adequate interarch space for proper denture construction in the posterior area and a firm mucosal base of consistent thickness over the alveolar ridge denture-bearing area. Maxillary tuberosity reduction may require the removal of soft tissue and bone to achieve the desired result. The amount of soft tissue available for reduction can often be determined by evaluating a presurgical panoramic radiograph. If a radiograph is not of the quality necessary to determine soft tissue thickness, this depth can be measured with a sharp probe after local anesthesia is obtained at the time of surgery.

Local anesthetic infiltration in the posterior maxillary area is sufficient for a tuberosity reduction. An initial elliptical incision is made over the tuberosity in the area requiring reduction, and this section of tissue is removed (Fig. 13-17). After tissue removal, the medial and lateral margins of the excision must be thinned to remove excess soft tissue, which allows further soft tissue reduction and provides a tension-free soft tissue closure. This can be accomplished by digital pressure on the mucosal surface of the adjacent tissue while sharply excising tissue tangential to the mucosal surface (Fig. 13-18). After the flaps are thinned, digital pressure can be used to approximate

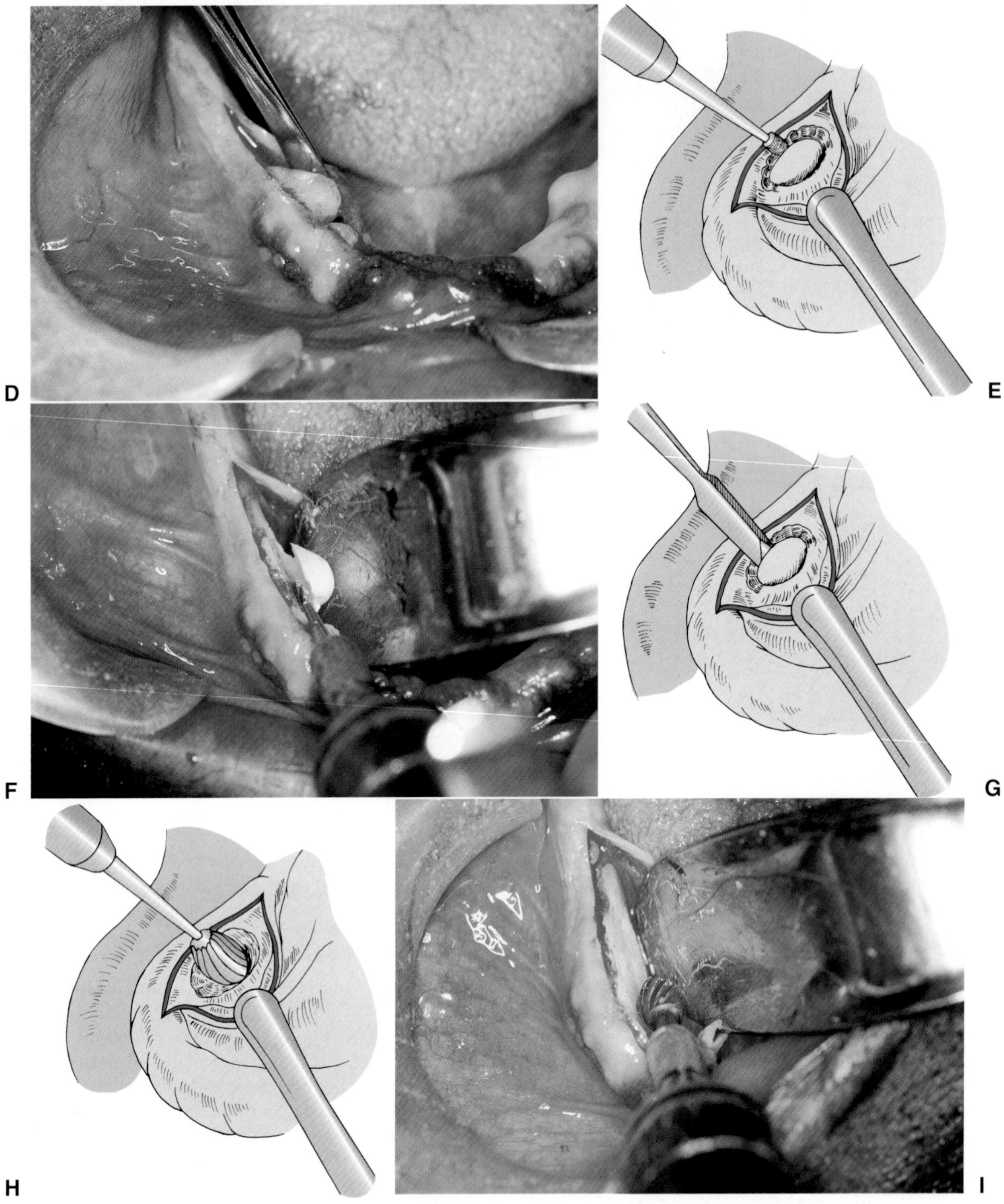

FIGURE 13-16, cont'd Removal of mandibular tori. **D**, Exposure of torus. **E** and **F**, Fissure bur and handpiece used to create small trough between mandibular ridge and torus. **G**, Use of small osteotome to complete removal of torus from the mandible. **H** to **J**, Use of bone bur and bone file to eliminate minor irregularities.

the tissue to evaluate the vertical reduction that has been accomplished. If adequate tissue has been removed, the area is sutured with interrupted or continuous suturing techniques. If too much tissue has been removed, no attempt should be made to close the wound primarily. A tension-free approximation of the tissue to bone should be accomplished, which allows the open wound area to heal by secondary intention.

Mandibular Retromolar Pad Reduction

The need for removal of mandibular retromolar hypertrophic tissue is rare. It is important to determine that the patient is not posturing the mandible forward or vertically overclosed during clinical evaluation and with treatment records and mounted casts. Local anesthetic infiltration in the area requiring excision is sufficient. An elliptical incision is made to

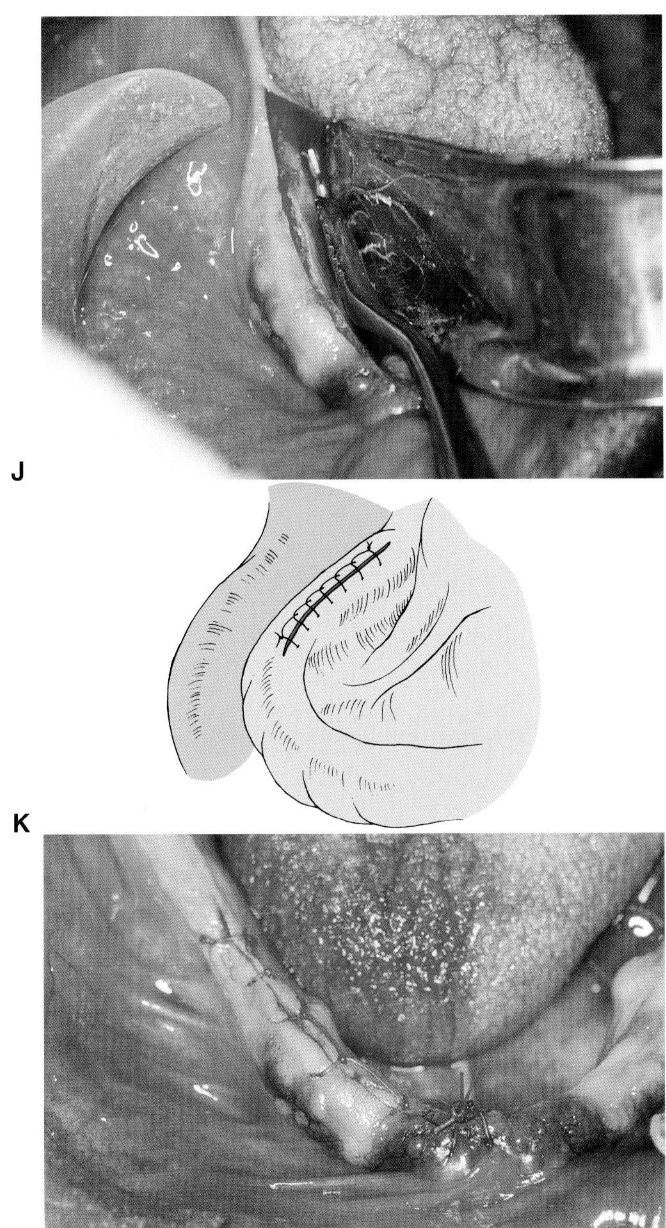

FIGURE 13-16, cont'd Removal of mandibular tori. **J**, Use of bone bur and bone file to eliminate minor irregularities. **K** and **L**, Tissue closure.

excise the greatest area of tissue thickness in the posterior mandibular area. Slight thinning of the adjacent areas is carried out with the majority of the tissue reduction on the labial aspect. Excess removal of tissue in the submucosal area of the lingual flap may result in damage to the lingual nerve and artery. The tissue is approximated with continuous or interrupted sutures. Another option for tissue removal in this area is with the use of a laser. Laser-assisted recontouring of the retromolar area allows reduction of the tissue excess without incisions and limits the postoperative healing period.[10] The most common laser used in oral surgery is the carbon dioxide laser.[11] Tissue ablation allows for controlled removal of tissue in layers based on intensity and depth of penetration.[12]

Lateral Palatal Soft Tissue Excess

Soft tissue excess on the lateral aspect of the palatal vault often interferes with proper construction of the denture. As with bony abnormalities of this area, soft tissue hypertrophy often narrows the palatal vault and creates slight undercuts, which interfere with denture construction and insertion.

One technique suggested for removal of lateral palatal soft tissue involves submucosal resection of the excess tissue in a manner similar to the previously described soft tissue tuberosity reduction. However, the amount and extension of soft tissue removal under the mucosa is much more extensive and creates the risk of damage to the greater palatine vessels, with possible hemorrhaging or sloughing of the lateral palatal soft tissue area.

The preferred technique requires superficial excision of the soft tissue excess. Local anesthetic infiltrated in the greater palatine area and anterior to the soft tissue mass is sufficient. With a sharp scalpel blade in the tangential fashion, the superficial layers of mucosa and underlying fibrous tissue can be removed to the extent necessary to eliminate undercuts in soft tissue bulk (Fig. 13-19). After removal of this tissue, a surgical splint lined with a tissue conditioner can be inserted for 5 to 7 days to aid in healing.

Unsupported Hypermobile Tissue

Excessive hypermobile tissue without inflammation on the alveolar ridge is generally the result of resorption of the underlying bone, ill-fitting dentures, or both. Before the excision of this tissue, a determination must be made of whether the underlying bone should be augmented with a graft. If a bony deficiency is the primary cause of soft tissue excess, then augmentation of the underlying bone is the treatment of choice. If adequate alveolar height remains after reduction of the hypermobile soft tissue, then excision may be indicated.

A local anesthetic is injected adjacent to the area requiring tissue excision. Removal of hypermobile tissue in the alveolar ridge area consists of two parallel full-thickness incisions on the buccal and lingual aspects of the tissue to be excised (Fig. 13-20). A periosteal elevator is used to remove the excess soft tissue from the underlying bone. A tangential excision of small amounts of tissue in the adjacent areas may be necessary to allow for adequate soft tissue adaptation during closure. These additional excisions should be kept to a minimum whenever possible to avoid removing too much soft tissue and to prevent detachment of periosteum from underlying bone. Continuous or interrupted sutures are used to approximate the remaining tissue. Denture impressions can usually be taken 3 to 4 weeks after surgery. One possible complication of this type of procedure is the obliteration of the buccal vestibule as a result of tissue undermining necessary to obtain tissue closure.

Hypermobile tissue in the crestal area of the mandibular alveolar ridge frequently consists of a small cordlike band of tissue. If no underlying sharp bony projection is present, this tissue can best be removed by a supraperiosteal soft tissue excision. Local anesthetic is injected adjacent to the area requiring tissue removal. The cordlike band of fibrous connective tissue can be elevated by using pickups and scissors, and the scissors can be used to excise the fibrous tissue at the attachment to the alveolar ridge (Fig. 13-21). Generally, no suturing is necessary for this technique, and a denture with a soft liner can be reinserted immediately.

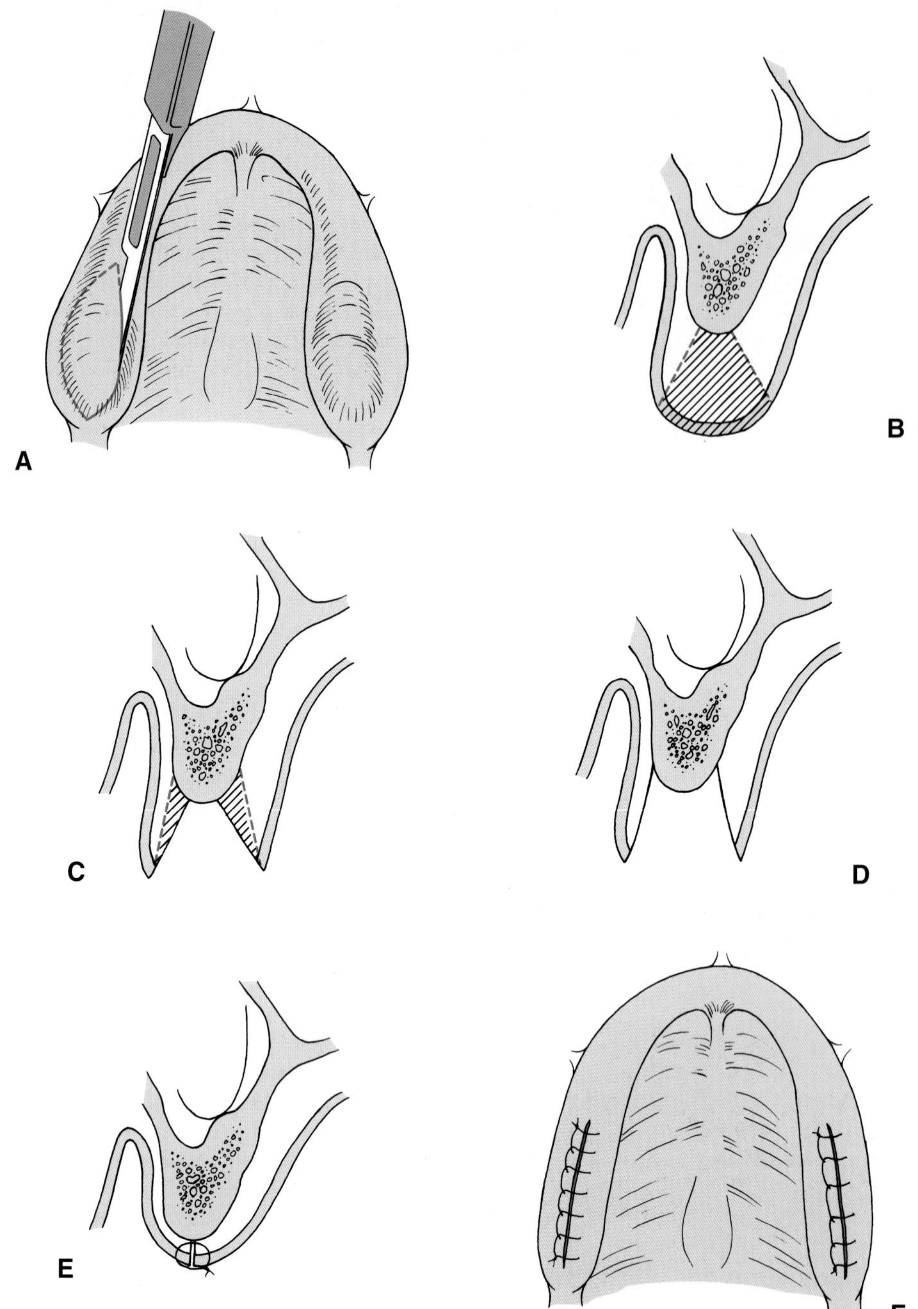

FIGURE 13-17 Maxillary soft tissue tuberosity reduction. **A**, Elliptical incision around soft tissue to be excised in tuberosity area. **B**, Soft tissue area excised with initial incision. **C**, Undermining of buccal and palatal flaps to provide adequate soft tissue contour and tension-free closure. **D**, View of final tissue removal. **E**, and **F**, Soft tissue closure.

Inflammatory Fibrous Hyperplasia

Inflammatory fibrous hyperplasia, also called *epulis fissurata* or *denture fibrosis*, is a generalized hyperplastic enlargement of mucosa and fibrous tissue in the alveolar ridge and vestibular area, which most often results from ill-fitting dentures. In the early stages of fibrous hyperplasia, when fibrosis is minimal, nonsurgical treatment with a denture in combination with a soft liner is frequently sufficient for reduction or elimination of this tissue. When the condition has been present for some time, significant fibrosis exists within the hyperplastic tissue. This tissue does not respond to nonsurgical treatment (Fig. 13-22); excision of the hyperplastic tissue is the treatment of choice.

Three techniques can be used for successful treatment of inflammatory fibrous hyperplasia. Local anesthetic infiltration in the area of the redundant tissue is sufficient for anesthesia. When the area to be excised is minimally enlarged, electrosurgical or laser techniques provide good results for tissue excision. If the tissue mass is extensive, large areas of excision using electrosurgical techniques may result in excessive vestibular scarring. Simple excision and reapproximation of

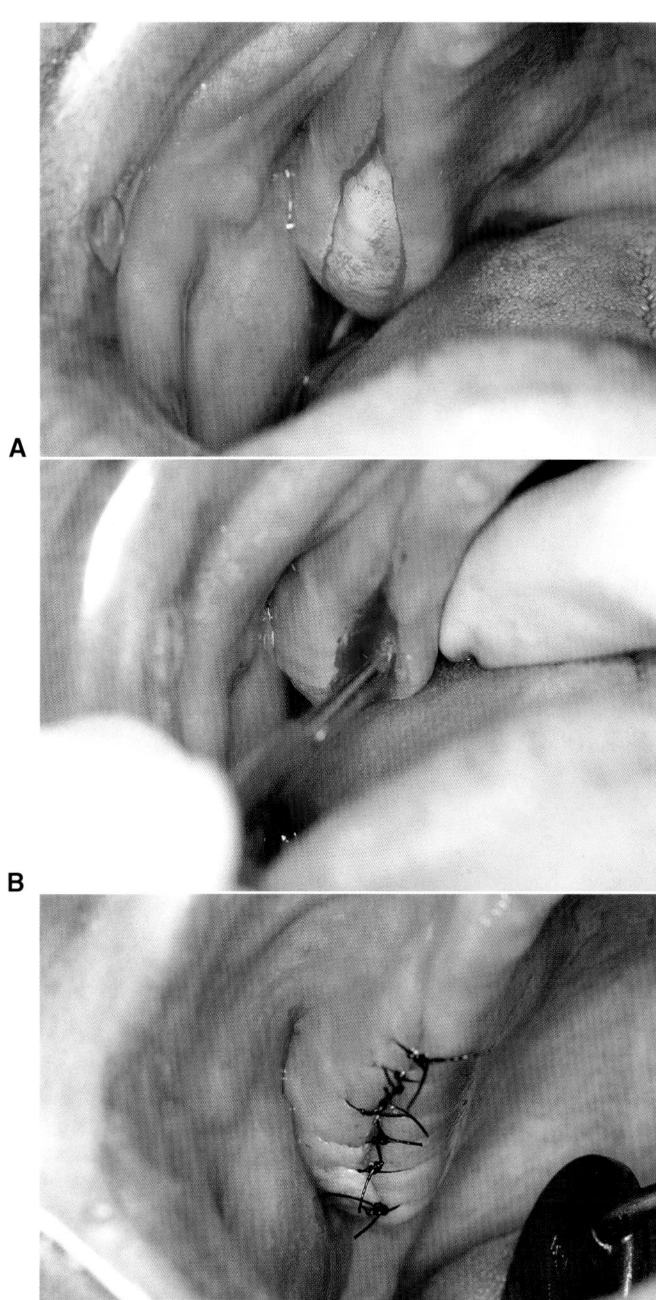

FIGURE 13-18 Maxillary soft tissue tuberosity reduction. A, Elliptical incision. B, Thinning of mucosal flaps by removal of underlying soft tissue. Digital pressure used to stabilize the tissue flaps during submucosal excision. C, Tension-free readaptation of flaps.

the remaining tissue is preferred. The redundant areas of tissue are grasped with tissue pickups, a sharp incision is made at the base of the excessive fibrous tissue down to the periosteum, and the hyperplastic tissue is removed (Fig. 13-23). The adjacent tissue is gently undermined and reapproximated using interrupted or continuous sutures.

When areas of gross tissue redundancy are found, excision frequently results in total elimination of the vestibule. In such cases, excision of the epulides, with peripheral mucosal repositioning and secondary epithelialization, is preferable.

In this procedure the hyperplastic soft tissue is excised superficial to the periosteum from the alveolar ridge area. A clean supraperiosteal bed is created over the alveolar ridge area, and the unaffected margin of the tissue excision is sutured to the most superior aspect of the vestibular periosteum with an interrupted suture technique. A surgical splint or denture lined with soft tissue conditioner is inserted and worn continuously for the first 5 to 7 days, with removal only for oral saline rinses. Secondary epithelialization usually takes place, and denture impressions can be made within 4 weeks. Laser excision of large epulis allows complete removal without excessive scarring or bleeding. A soft relined denture can provide for additional postoperative comfort from a procedure that initially creates minimal pain but with pain that peaks several days later.

The hyperplastic tissue usually represents only the result of an inflammatory process; however, other pathologic conditions may exist. It is therefore imperative that representative tissue samples *always* be submitted for pathologic examination after removal.

Labial Frenectomy

Labial frenal attachments consist of thin bands of fibrous tissue covered with mucosa, extending from the lip and cheek to the alveolar periosteum. The level of frenal attachments may vary from the height of the vestibule to the crest of the alveolar ridge and even to the incisal papilla area in the anterior maxilla. With the exception of the midline labial frenum in association with a diastema, frenal attachments generally do not present problems when the dentition is intact. However, the construction of a denture may be complicated when it is necessary to accommodate a frenal attachment. Movement of the soft tissue adjacent to the frenum may create discomfort and ulceration and may interfere with the peripheral seal and dislodge the denture.

Multiple surgical techniques are effective in removal of frenal attachments: (1) the simple excision technique, (2) the Z-plasty technique, (3) localized vestibuloplasty with secondary epithelialization, and (4) the laser-assisted frenectomy. The simple excision and Z-plasty are effective when the mucosal and fibrous tissue band is relatively narrow. A localized vestibuloplasty with secondary epithelialization is often preferred when the frenal attachment has a wide base. Laser-assisted techniques are versatile in creating local excision and ablation of excessive mucosal tissue and fibrous tissue attachments, allowing secondary epithelialization.

Local anesthetic infiltration is often sufficient for surgical treatment of frenal attachments. Care must be taken to avoid excessive anesthetic infiltration directly in the frenum area because it may obscure the anatomy that must be visualized at the time of excision. In all cases, it is helpful to have the surgical assistant elevate and evert the lip during this procedure. For the simple excision technique, a narrow elliptical incision around the frenal area down to the periosteum is completed (Fig. 13-24). The fibrous frenum is then sharply dissected from the underlying periosteum and soft tissue, and the margins of the wound are gently undermined and reapproximated. Placement of the first suture should be at the maximal depth of the vestibule and should include both edges of mucosa and underlying periosteum at the height of the vestibule beneath the anterior nasal spine. This technique reduces hematoma formation and allows for

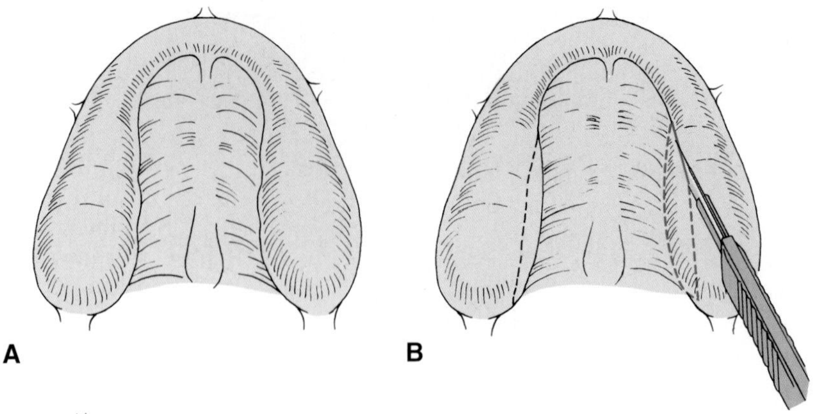

FIGURE 13-19 Removal of lateral palatal soft tissue. A, View of excessive palatal tissue creating narrow palatal vault and undercut areas. B, Tangential excision of excess soft tissue.

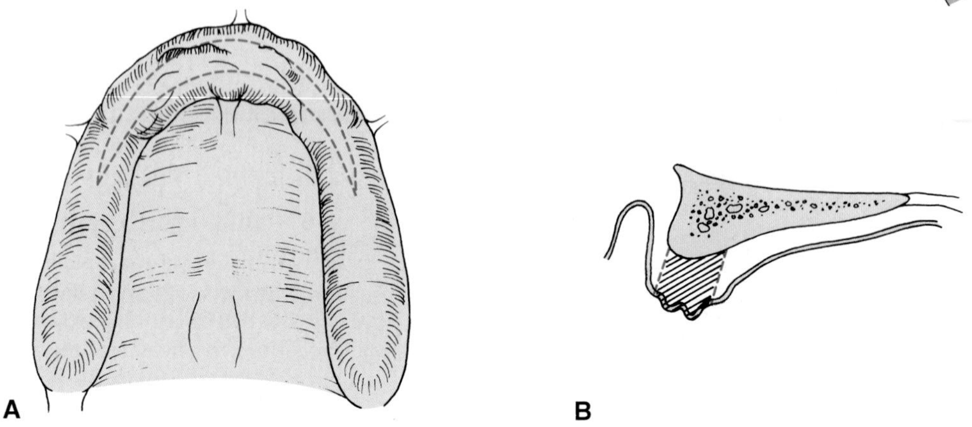

FIGURE 13-20 Removal of hypermobile unsupported tissue. A, Outline of incisions for removal of crestal area of hypermobile tissue. B, Cross-sectional area demonstrating amount of tissue to be excised. (This type of tissue excision should be considered only if adequate ridge height will remain after removal of tissue. If excision of this tissue will result in inadequate ridge height and obliteration of vestibular depth, some type of augmentation procedure should be considered.)

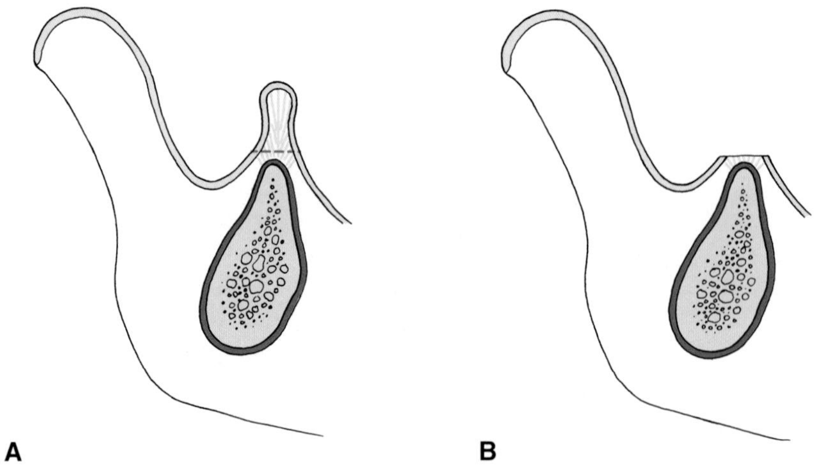

FIGURE 13-21 Supraperiosteal removal of hypermobile tissue on mandibular alveolar ridge. A, Hypermobile tissue on superior aspect of ridge. B, Pickups and scissors are used to excise the cordlike mobile fibrous tissue without perforating periosteum.

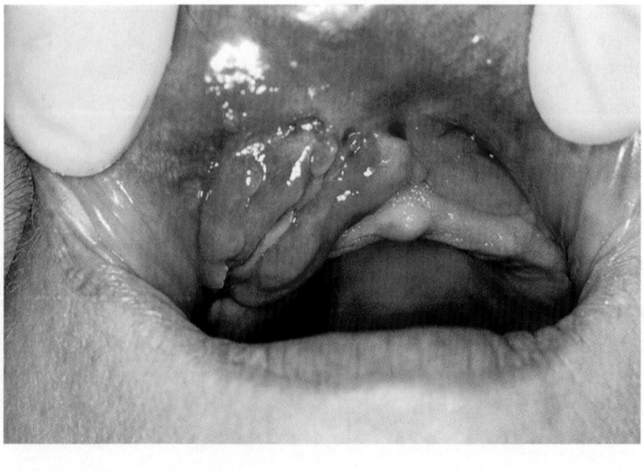

FIGURE 13-22 Inflammatory fibrous hyperplasia of vestibule.

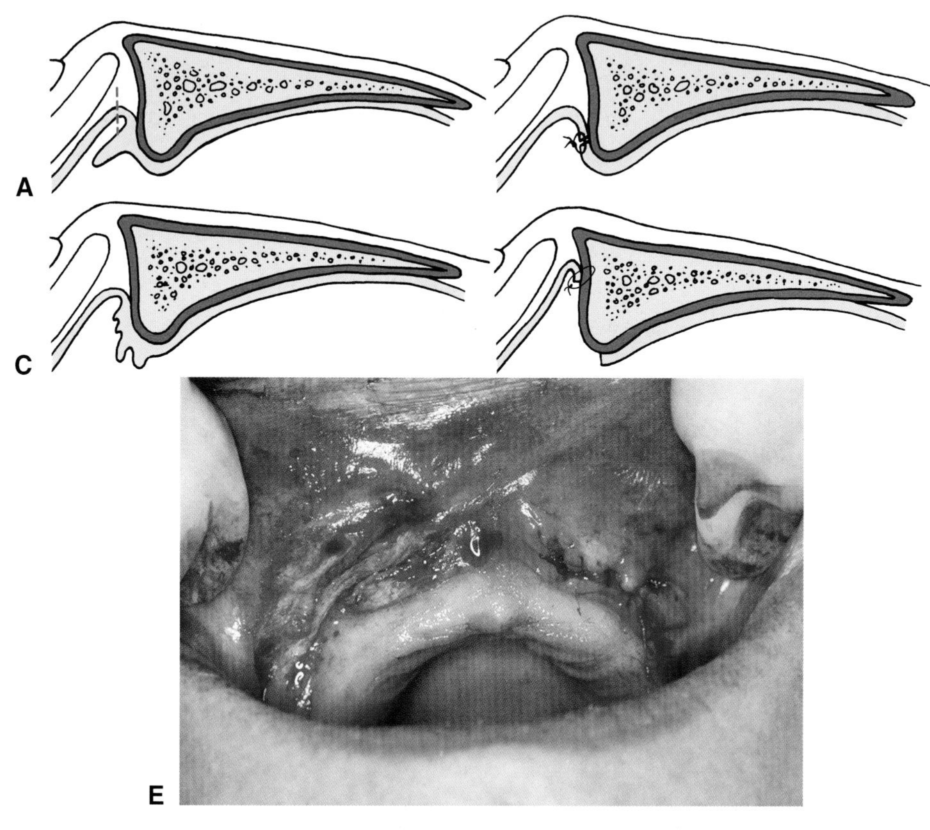

FIGURE 13-23 A, Small, well-localized area of fibrous hyperplasia. This area can be removed with simple excision. B, Closure of wound margins. C, Large area of inflammatory fibrous hyperplasia. Removal and primary closure would result in elimination of labial vestibule. D, After supraperiosteal removal of excess tissue, mucosal edge is sutured to periosteum at depth of vestibule. E, Postoperative view of Figure 13-22. The smaller well-localized area on patient's left has been removed and closed primarily. The larger area of excessive tissue on right has been removed and wound margin sutured to periosteum at depth of vestibule, which leaves exposed periosteum.

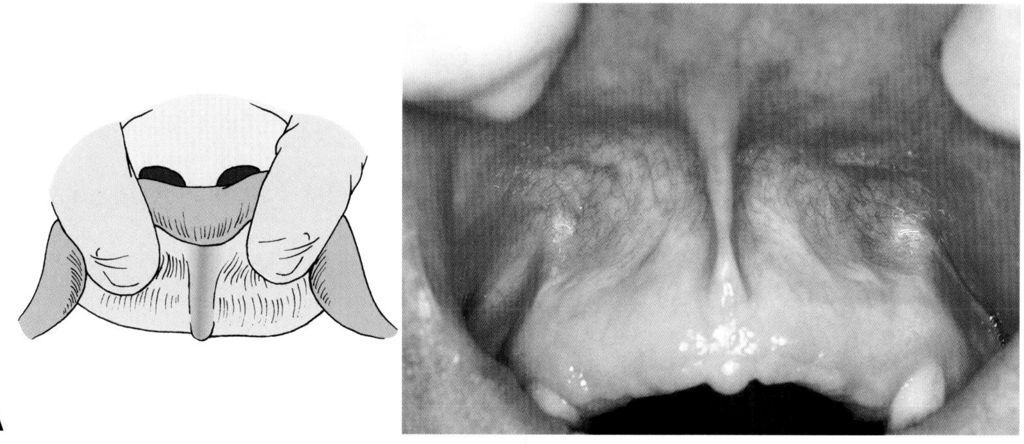

FIGURE 13-24 Simple excision of maxillary labial frenum. A and B, Eversion and exposure of frenal attachment area.

Continued

adaptation of the tissue to the maximal height of the vestibule. The remainder of the incision should then be closed with interrupted sutures. Occasionally, it is not possible to approximate the portion of the excision closest to the alveolar ridge crest; this will undergo secondary epithelialization without difficulty.

In the Z-plasty technique, an excision of the fibrous connective tissue is done similar to that in the simple excision procedure. After excision of the fibrous tissue, two oblique incisions are made in a Z fashion, one at each end of the previous area of excision (Fig. 13-25). The two pointed flaps are then gently undermined and rotated to close the initial vertical incision horizontally. The two small oblique extensions also require closure. This technique may decrease the amount of vestibular ablation sometimes seen after linear excision of a frenum.

A third technique for elimination of the frenum involves a localized vestibuloplasty with secondary epithelialization. This procedure is especially advantageous when the base of the frenal attachment is extremely wide, as in many mandibular anterior frenal attachments. Local anesthetic is infiltrated primarily in the supraperiosteal areas along the margins of the frenal attachments. An incision is made through mucosal tissue and underlying submucosal tissue, without perforating the

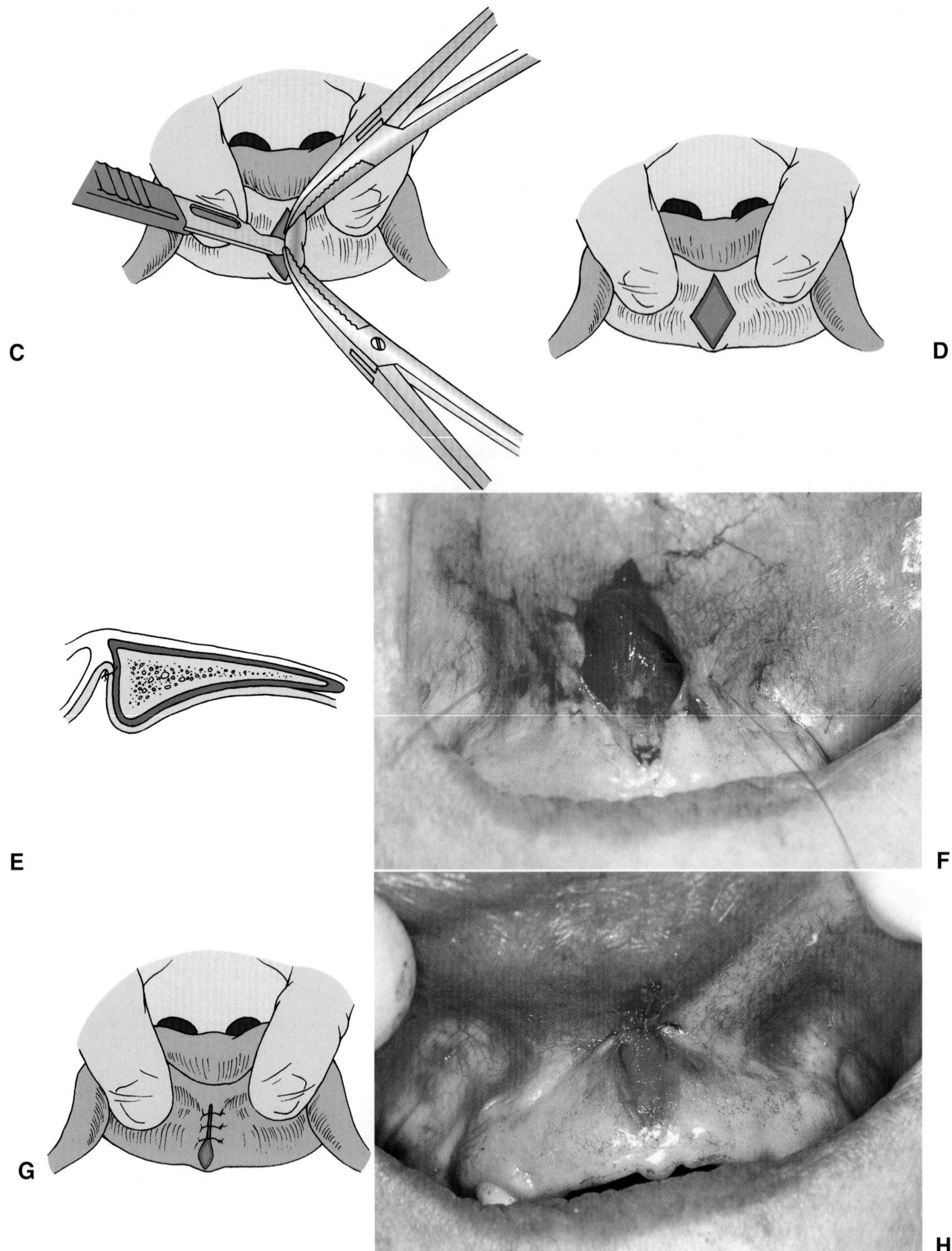

FIGURE 13-24, cont'd Simple excision of maxillary labial frenum. C and D, Excision along lateral margins of frenum. Tissue is removed, exposing underlying periosteum. E and F, Placement of suture through mucosal margins and periosteum, which closes mucosal margin and sutures mucosa to periosteum at depth of vestibule. G and H, Wound closure. Removal of tissue in areas adjacent to attached mucosa sometimes prevents complete primary closure at most inferior aspect of wound margin.

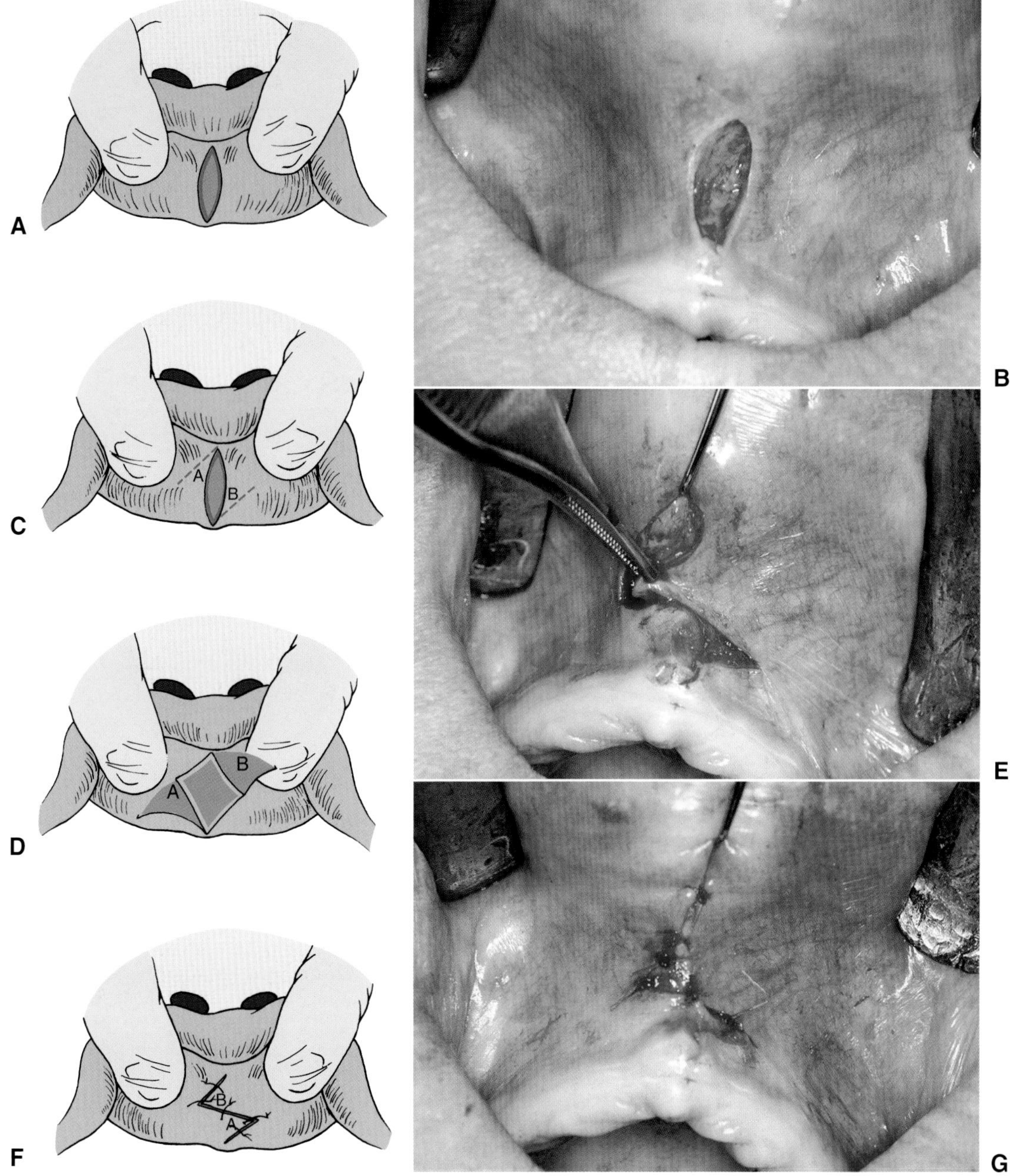

FIGURE 13-25 Z-plasty technique for elimination of labial frenum. A and B, Small elliptical excision of mucosa and underlying loose connective tissue. C to E, Flaps are undermined and rotated to desired position. F and G, Closure with interrupted sutures.

periosteum. A supraperiosteal dissection is completed by undermining the mucosal and submucosal tissue with scissors or by digital pressure on a sponge placed against the periosteum. After a clean periosteal layer is identified, the edge of the mucosal flap is sutured to the periosteum at the maximal depth of the vestibule and the exposed periosteum is allowed to heal by secondary epithelialization (Fig. 13-26). A surgical splint or denture containing soft tissue liner is often useful in the initial healing period. This technique is also useful in localized broad-based muscle attachments, such as those frequently seen in the lateral maxillary areas.

The excision of frenum attachments can also be accomplished through a laser. The tendinous frenum attachment is ablated with the laser and often does not require suture reapproximation of the tissue because reepithelialization occurs from the wound margins (Fig. 13-27). Frenectomies completed with the laser often respond well with fewer postoperative complaints of swelling and pain.

Lingual Frenectomy

An abnormal lingual frenal attachment usually consists of mucosa, dense fibrous connective tissue, and occasionally, superior fibers of the genioglossus muscle. This attachment binds the tip of the tongue to the posterior surface of the mandibular alveolar ridge. Even when no prosthesis is required, such attachments can affect speech. After loss of teeth, this

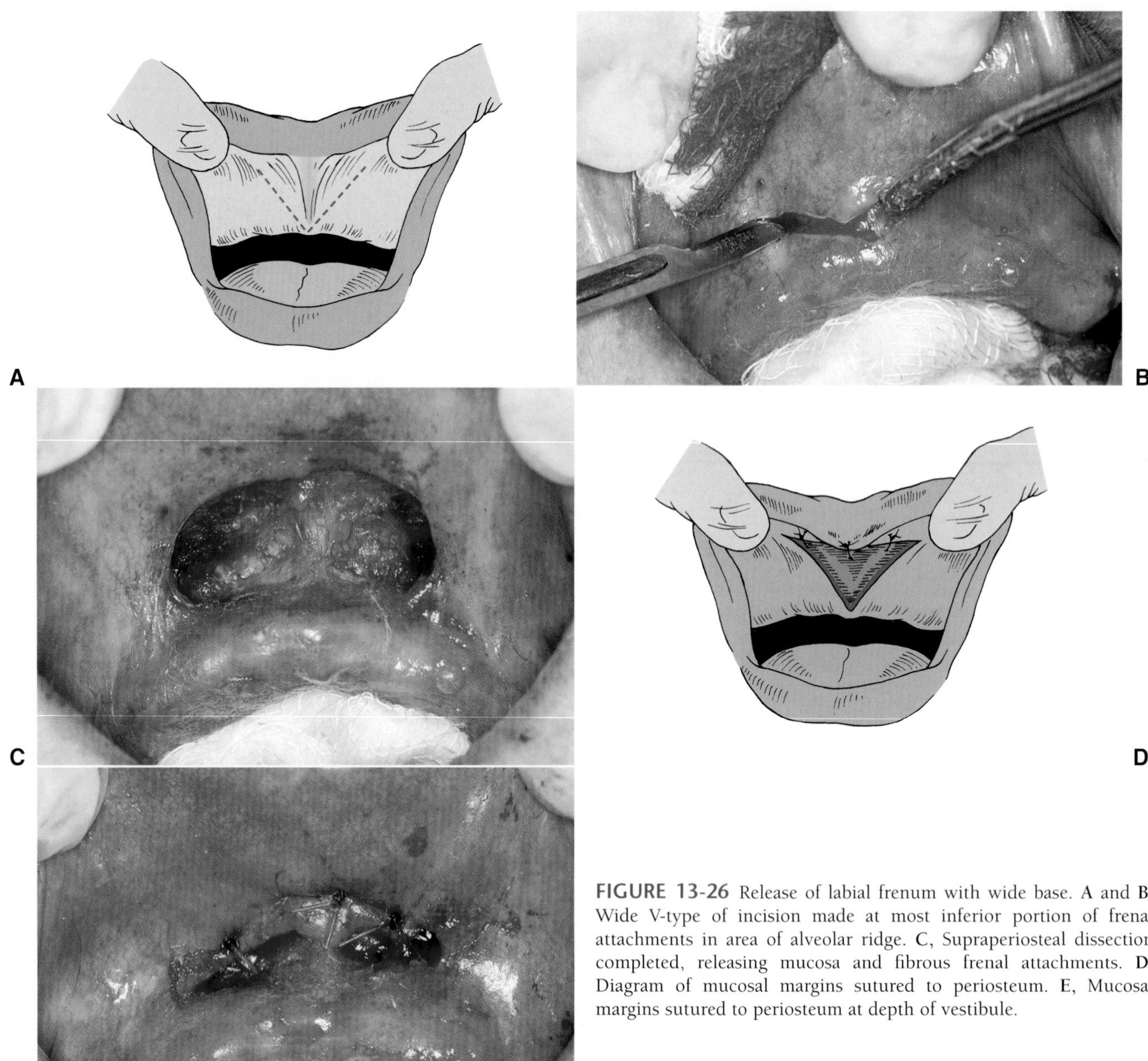

FIGURE 13-26 Release of labial frenum with wide base. A and B, Wide V-type of incision made at most inferior portion of frenal attachments in area of alveolar ridge. C, Supraperiosteal dissection completed, releasing mucosa and fibrous frenal attachments. D, Diagram of mucosal margins sutured to periosteum. E, Mucosal margins sutured to periosteum at depth of vestibule.

frenal attachment interferes with denture stability, because each time the tongue is moved, the frenal attachment is tensed and the denture is dislodged.

Bilateral lingual blocks and local infiltration in the anterior area provide adequate anesthesia for a lingual frenectomy. The tip of the tongue is best controlled with a traction suture. Surgical release of the lingual frenum requires incising the attachment of the fibrous connective tissue at the base of the tongue in a transverse fashion, followed by closure in a linear direction, which completely releases the anterior portion of the tongue (Fig. 13-28). A hemostat can be placed across the frenal attachment at the base of the tongue for approximately 3 minutes, which provides vasoconstriction and a nearly bloodless field during the surgical procedure. After removal of the hemostat, an incision is created through the area previously closed within the hemostat. The tongue is retracted superiorly, and the margins of the wound are carefully undermined and closed parallel to the midline of the tongue. Careful attention must be given to blood vessels at the inferior aspect of the tongue and floor of the mouth and to the submandibular duct openings. Trauma to these vital structures during the incision or closure may result in postoperative hemostatic concerns and obstruction of salivary flow.

Occasionally, a lingual frenum release must also be accompanied by a small soft tissue–releasing procedure performed between the opening of the submandibular duct and the lingual aspect of the mandible. If access is available, this can be done in a fashion similar to the release above the sub-

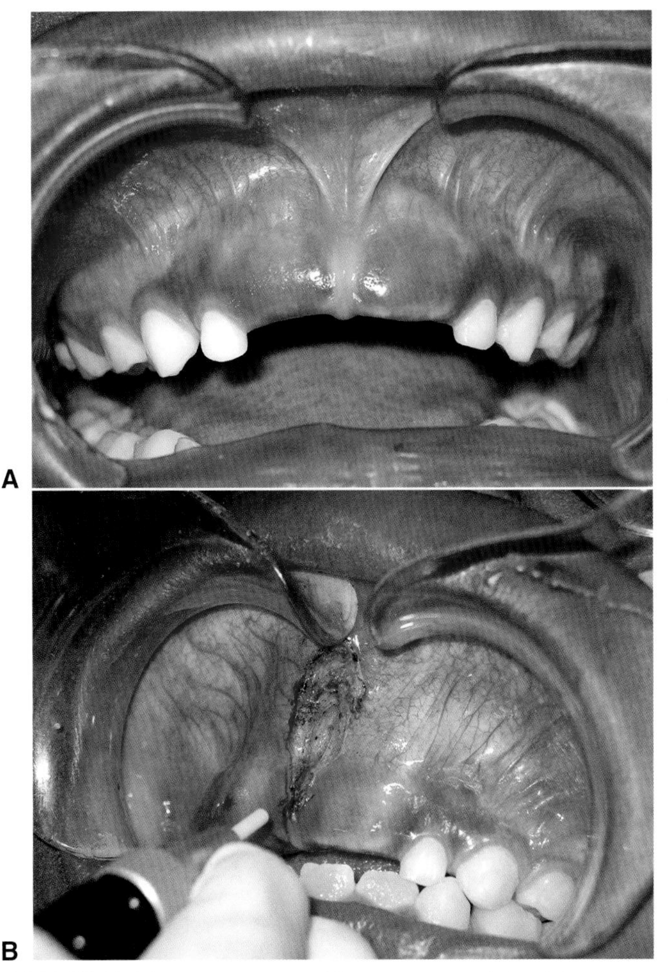

FIGURE 13-27 Laser excision of frenum. A, Broad-based frenum in anterior maxilla. B, Supraperiosteal ablation of mucosal and dense fibrous frenal attachments. Healing occurs by secondary epithelialization.

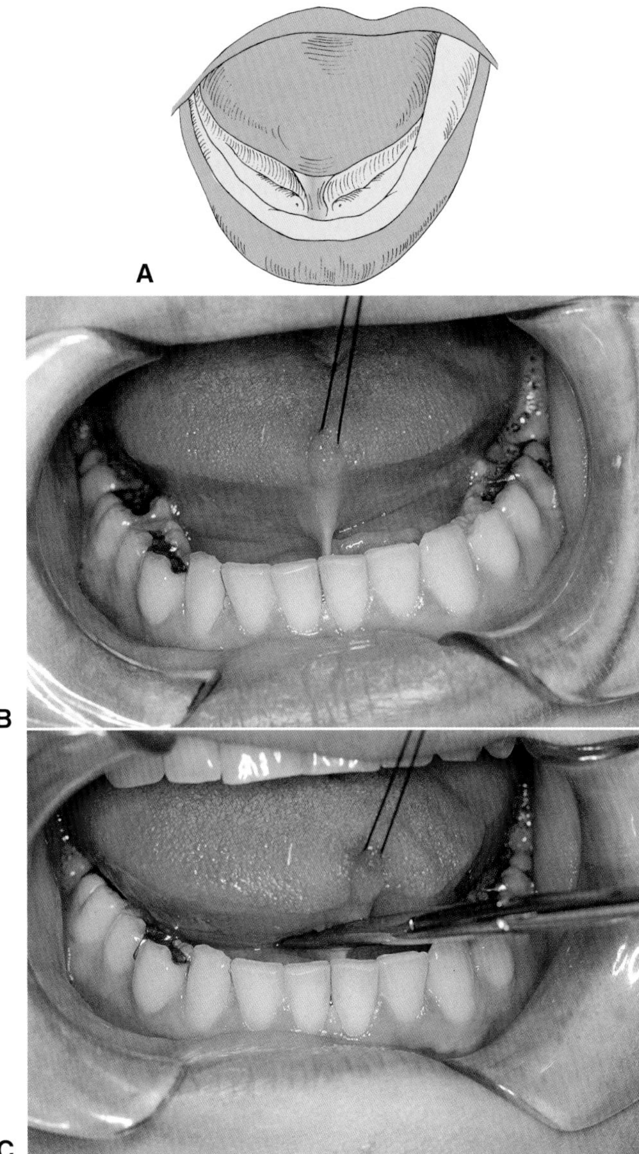

FIGURE 13-28 Lingual frenum release. A, Frenal attachment connecting tip of tongue to lingual aspect of mandible. In edentulous patients, movement of tongue will dislodge denture. B, Traction suture placed in tip of tongue. C, Hemostat used to compress frenum area for 2 to 3 minutes allows improved hemostasis.

Continued

mandibular ducts. However, if only a short tissue band exists in this area, a localized supraperiosteal dissection removing the fibrous attachment from the lingual aspect of the alveolar ridge is sufficient.

IMMEDIATE DENTURES

The decision may be made to insert dentures at the time of tooth removal and bony recontouring. Hartwell[13] cites several advantages of an immediate denture technique. The insertion of a denture after extraction offers immediate psychological and esthetic benefits to patients, whereas alternatively they may be edentulous for some time. The immediate insertion of a denture after surgery also functions to splint the surgical site, which results in the reduction of postoperative bleeding and edema and improved tissue adaptation to the alveolar ridge. Another advantage is that the vertical dimension can be most easily reproduced with an immediate denture technique. Disadvantages include the need for frequent alteration of the denture postoperatively and the construction of a new denture after initial healing has taken place.

Anterior and posterior teeth can be extracted and dentures inserted in a single stage, although this requires meticulous planning and construction of the prosthesis. Surgical treatment for immediate denture insertion can also be accomplished in stages, with extraction of the posterior dentition in the maxilla and the mandible done before anterior extraction. This allows for initial healing of the posterior areas and facilitates improved adaptation of the denture over the alveolus and tuberosity. Before extraction of the remaining anterior teeth, new records are taken and models are mounted on a semiadjustable articulator. The models allow for fabrication of dentures maintaining proper vertical height and esthetics. The cast of the alveolar ridge area is then carefully recontoured in anticipation of the extraction of the remaining anterior teeth and recontouring of the bony alveolus (Fig. 13-29). A clear acrylic

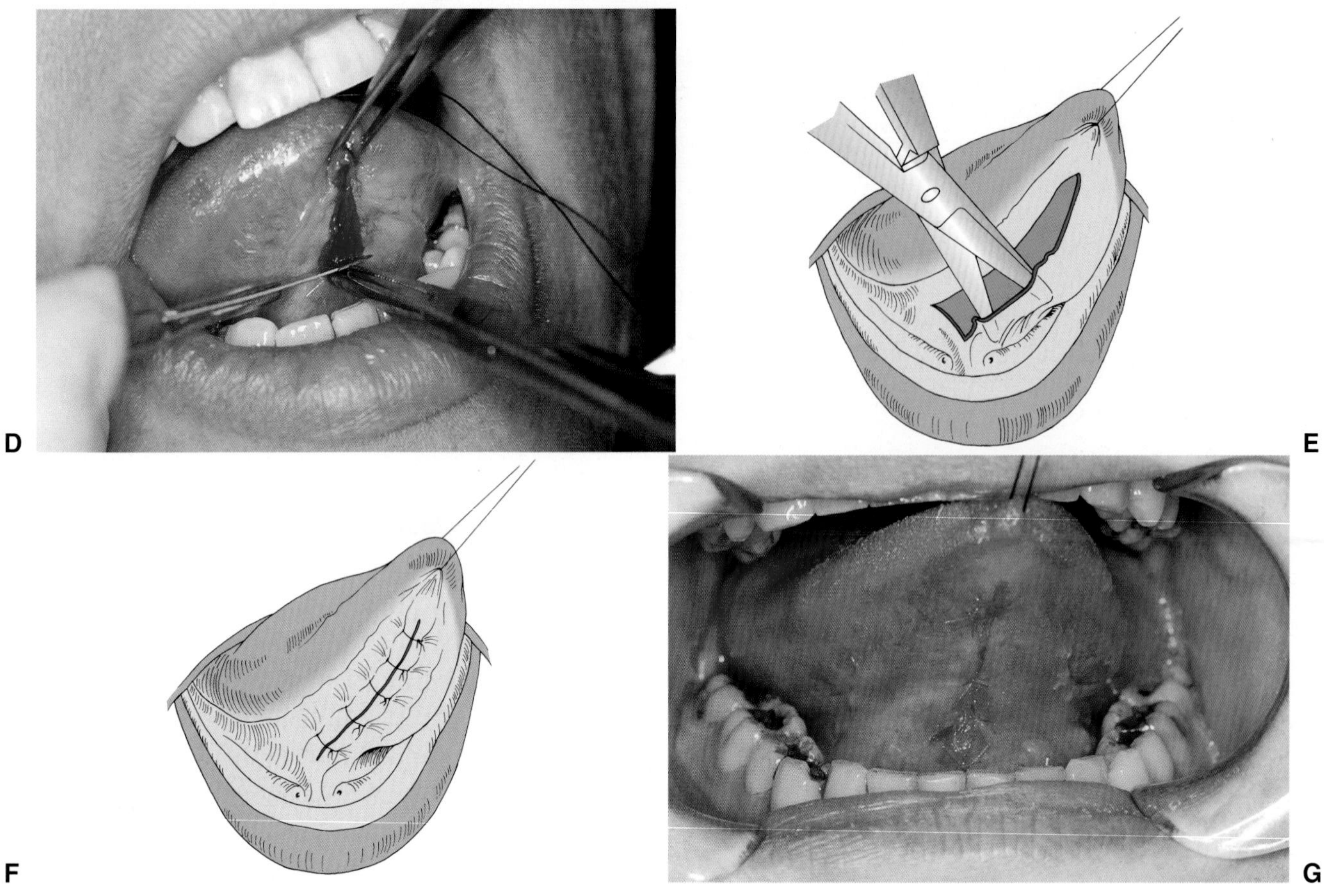

FIGURE 13-28, cont'd Lingual frenum release. **D**, Incision made at superior portion of frenal attachment through the serrations created by the hemostat to inferior surface of tongue. **E**, Lateral borders of wound margin are undermined. **F** and **G**, Soft tissue closure.

splint is fabricated from the recontoured presurgical casts to replicate the desired alveolar ridge form. The dentures are also constructed on these casts.

Immediate denture surgery involves the most conservative technique possible in removal of the remaining teeth. Simple minimal recontouring or an intraseptal alveoloplasty, preserving as much vertical height and cortical bone as possible, is generally indicated (Fig. 13-30). After the bony recontouring and elimination of gross irregularities is completed, the tissue is approximated with digital pressure, and the clear acrylic surgical guide is inserted. Any areas of tissue blanching or gross irregularities are then reduced until the clear surgical guide is adapted to the alveolar ridge in all areas. Incisions are closed with continuous or interrupted sutures. The immediate denture with a soft liner is inserted. Care should be taken not to extrude any reline material into the fresh wound. The occlusal relationships are checked and adjusted as necessary. The patient is instructed to wear the denture continuously for 24 hours and to return the next day for a postoperative check. Bupivacaine or another similar long-acting local anesthetic injected at the conclusion of the surgical procedure greatly improves comfort in the first 24-hour postoperative period. At that time the denture is gently removed, and the underlying mucosa and alveolar ridge areas are inspected for any areas of excessive pressure. The denture is cleaned and reinserted, and the patient is instructed to wear the denture for 5 to 7 days and to remove it only for oral saline rinses.

ALVEOLAR RIDGE PRESERVATION

The majority of this chapter is devoted to management of the dentoalveolar area following extraction and subsequent bony and soft tissue changes. An important aspect of preprosthetic surgery can actually be accomplished at the time of tooth extraction by attempting to maintain and regain as much bone in the extraction area as possible. If a tooth is deemed nonrestorable and planned for extraction, simultaneous preservation of the socket using a variety of bone materials can aid in the maintenance of alveolar height and width.[14] The adjunctive measures maintain ridge form as the alloplastic materials are slowly resorbed through bony remodeling. Several allogeneic and xenogeneic bone materials have been used to maintain the bony architecture, limiting the morbidity of harvesting autogenous bone from an adjacent intraoral site.[15] These anorganic materials are derived from a bovine source (xenograft) or processed cadaveric bone.[16,17]

Atraumatic extraction with maintenance of the buccal and lingual cortical walls is essential to preservation of alveolar bone.[18] The site is curetted and irrigated after removal of the tooth in entirety. The graft material is placed into the extrac-

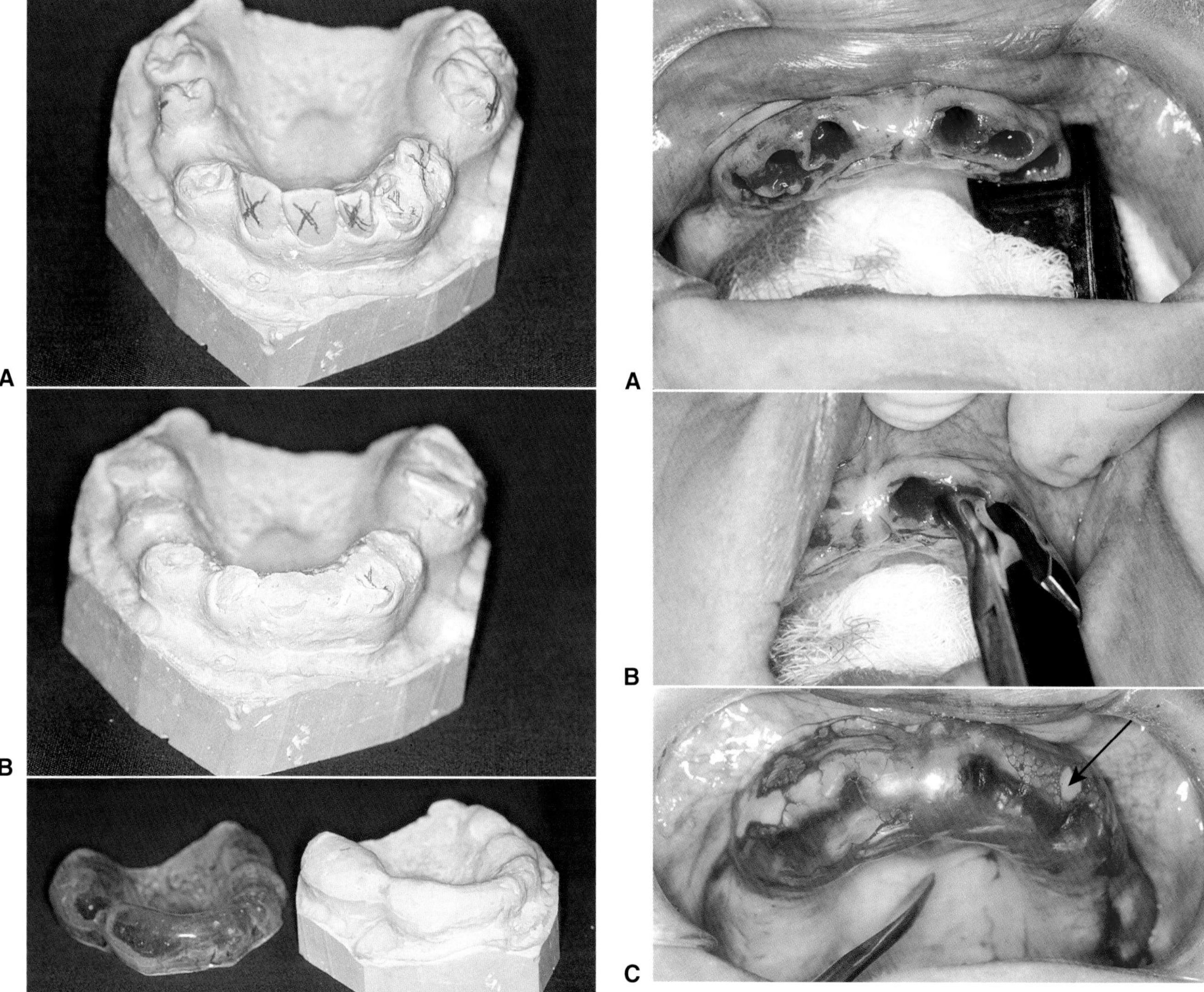

FIGURE 13-29 Construction of clear acrylic surgical guide for immediate denture surgery. **A**, Presurgical cast. **B**, Cast after removal of teeth exhibiting bony irregularity. **C**, Recontoured maxillary cast and surgical guide.

FIGURE 13-30 **A**, Appearance of maxillary alveolar ridge after removal of teeth. **B**, Intraseptal removal of bone with rongeur. **C**, Clear acrylic surgical guide in place. Any areas that interfere with seating of template or cause blanching of tissue from excess bone or underlying soft tissue should be removed (*arrow*).

tion site and compressed to the level of the alveolar crest (Fig. 13-31). The extraction site usually is not closed primarily. In most cases the graft material is covered with some type of collagen material that is held in place with resorbable sutures. The use of a resorbable membrane requires limited soft tissue reflection of the adjacent margins to place the membrane under the attached gingiva. Mucosal reepithelialization occurs over the grafted site within a few weeks.

Implant placement in a site preserved with grafted bone material usually proceeds in 2 to 6 months.

OVERDENTURE SURGERY

Alveolar bone is maintained primarily in response to stresses transferred to the bone through the teeth and periodontal ligament during mastication. By maintaining teeth wherever possible, resorption of bone under a prosthetic appliance may be minimized. An overdenture technique attempts to maintain teeth in the alveolus by transferring force directly to the bone and improving masticatory function with prosthetic restoration. The presence of teeth may also improve proprioception during function, and special retentive attachments can be incorporated into the retained teeth to improve denture retention and stability. Overdentures should be considered wherever several teeth exist with adequate bone support and when good periodontal health can be maintained and the teeth can be properly restored. Bilateral canines are generally best suited for this type of treatment. Because this technique also requires endodontic and prosthetic treatment of retained teeth, financial considerations must also be taken into account.

A complete discussion of periodontal considerations is not within the scope of this chapter; however, it is important to evaluate any potentially retained teeth before preparing the patient for an overdenture. Adequate clinical and radiographic

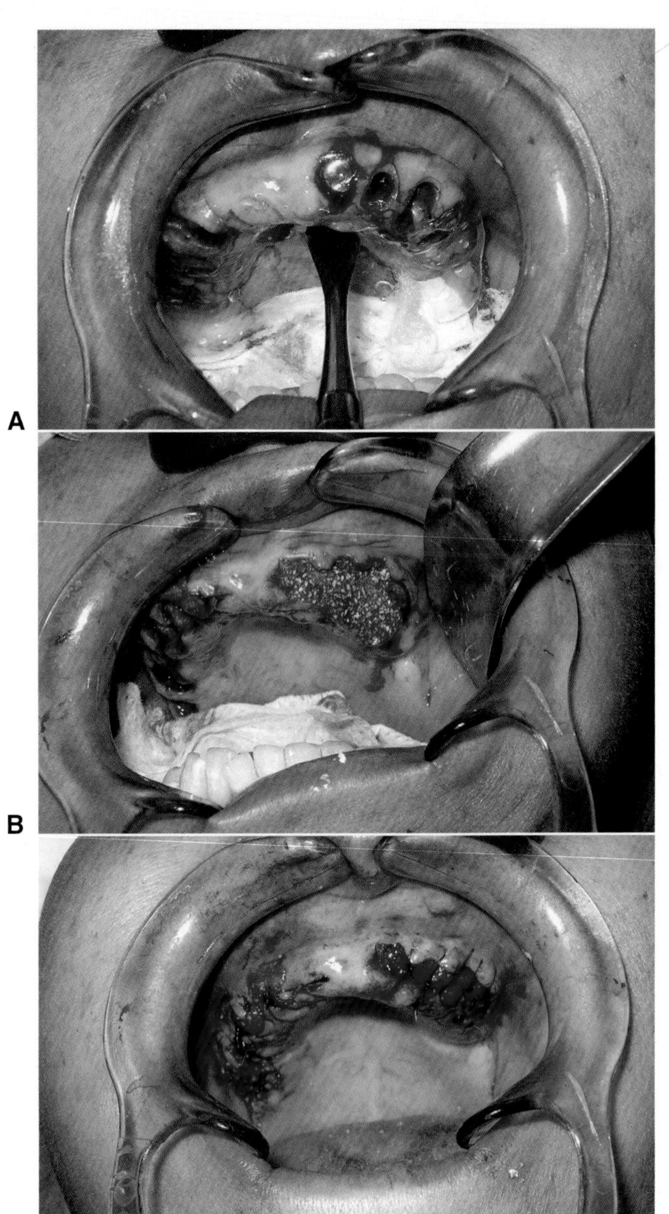

FIGURE 13-31 Alveolar ridge preservation. A, Extraction of teeth maintaining alveolar height. B, Allogeneic material is placed in extraction site to height of alveolar crest. C, Resorbable membrane placed over graft and stabilized with bolster stitches to allow secondary intention over crest.

evaluation of these teeth should be completed, including a clinical examination, evaluation of pocket depth around the teeth, and evaluation of the attached gingiva.

MANDIBULAR AUGMENTATION

Augmentation grafting adds strength to an extremely deficient mandible and improves the height and contour of the available bone for implant placement on denture-bearing areas. Sources of graft material include autogenous or allogeneic bone and alloplastic materials. Historically, autogenous bone has been the most biologically acceptable material used in mandibular augmentation. Disadvantages of the use of autogenous bone include the need for donor site surgery and the possibility of resorption after grafting. The use of allogeneic bone eliminates the need for a second surgical site and has been shown to be useful in augmenting small areas of deficiency in the mandible.[19] The increased popularity of implants has renewed enthusiasm for use of autogenous bone grafts alone or in combination with other biologic materials for bony augmentation.

Superior Border Augmentation

Superior border augmentation with a bone graft is often indicated when severe resorption of the mandible results in inadequate height and contour and potential risk of fracture or when the treatment plan calls for placement of implants in areas of insufficient bone height or width. Neurosensory disturbances from inferior alveolar nerve dehiscence at the location of the mental foramen at the superior aspect of the mandible also can be corrected with this technique.

The use of autogenous corticocancellous blocks of iliac crest bone was described by Thoma and Holland[20] in 1951 for superior border augmentation. However, as much as 70% resorption of iliac crest bone can occur with this technique.[21] This large amount of resorption may be the result of movement of the bone graft segments that were initially wired to the mandible, allowing slight movement combined with the external rather than internal loads placed on the graft after healing. The cortical nature of the iliac crest allows rigid fixation to secure the graft to the mandible via multiple screws, minimizing graft mobility (Fig. 13-32). In some cases, implants can be placed at the same time the bone graft augmentation is completed.

Augmentation of the Mandible with Alternative Biologic Materials

Autogenous bone remains the gold standard for reconstruction in the maxillofacial region. The donor site morbidity associated with harvesting autogenous bone from a second surgical site continues to be the primary disadvantage. The problems associated with bone grafting, including donor site morbidity, resorption, and the potential need for hospitalization have been responsible in part for the search for alternative materials

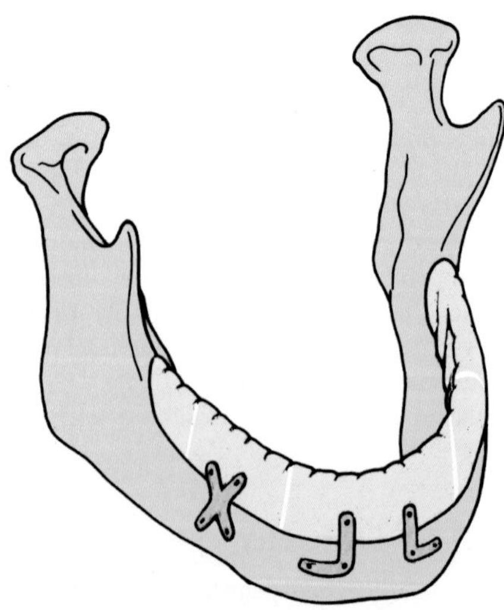

FIGURE 13-32 Superior border grafting of atrophic mandible. Corticocancellous iliac crest contoured to adapt to configuration of mandible; stabilized with rigid fixation screws.

that would function as an adequate graft material. The continued research into the physiology, chemistry, and genetics of bone has greatly enhanced bone reconstruction. The formation of new bone (osteogenesis) requires osteoinduction and osteoconduction. Bone formation through the recruitment of progenitor cells is osteoinduction. Osteoconduction facilitates bone growth by providing a framework for bone deposition.

Allogeneic bone grafts procured from cadavers are processed to provide sterility and decrease the potential for immune response. The processing destroys the osteoinductive nature of the graft; however, the graft provides a scaffold allowing bone ingrowth (osteoconduction).[16] Bony incorporation followed by remodeling and resorption occurs during the healing phase.[17] Granular forms of allogeneic graft material provide increased surface area and improved adaptation within the graft and are the most commonly used form for augmenting alveolar ridge contour defects. The advantages of allogeneic bone grafting include the avoidance of an additional donor site and unlimited availability and that most patients can undergo this type of procedure in an outpatient setting. Xenografts from a processed bovine source have minimal immune response based on the absence of antigenic protein. These grafts facilitate osteoconduction rather than osteoinduction. The anorganic graft has a slow rate of resorption with nonincorporated remnants of the original graft identified in several studies.[22]

Continued advancements have led to the identification of a series of proteins involved in regulating bone physiology. Bone morphogenetic proteins (BMP) are growth factors that have been isolated and applied to reconstruction of the maxillofacial skeleton.[16] Recombinant BMP has been isolated and has now been produced and packaged for use in grafting procedures. The BMP is usually combined with osteoconductive allogeneic materials to expand the graft and help place, shape, and contain the graft material. BMP with a collagen matrix carrier can be used for sinus lifting and reconstruction of non–load-bearing bony defects. The recombinant materials have been positioned around implants placed immediately into extraction sites aiding in osteointegration. Further research is ongoing on the applications of BMP to the maxillofacial region; however, the benefit of avoiding the morbidity of a second surgical site for graft harvesting and the ability to induce native bone offers tremendous promise.

Guided Bone Regeneration (Osteopromotion)

In guided bone regeneration, a membrane (nonresorbable or resorbable) is used to cover an area where bone graft healing or bone regeneration is desired. The concept of guided regeneration, or osteopromotion, is based on the ability to exclude undesirable cell types, such as epithelial cells or fibroblasts, from the area where bone healing is taking place.

In 1982, Nyman et al.[23] described a technique to improve periodontal ligament regeneration using a membrane barrier to exclude undesirable cells from the area where periodontal ligament healing or regeneration was required. Dahlin et al.[24] showed that bone growth around implants could be facilitated using a similar technique. By placing a membrane covering over a bone graft, faster-growing fibroblasts and epithelial cells can be walled off, allowing bone to grow in a relatively protected environment without epithelial ingrowth.

Many types of materials have been used as a membrane to cover graft sites, including resorbable and nonresorbable barriers. Expanded polytetrafluoroethylene or Gortex is the most popular nonresorbable membrane. This material must be removed after adequate bone healing occurs. Resorbable membranes were developed to avoid the need for a second surgical intervention for removal. The resorbable membranes, synthetic polymers such as polylactin, and collagen have been used with increased frequency. The resorbable sheets are degraded via hydrolysis over the course of several weeks in a process similar to that seen with suture material.[25] These materials and the concept of guided tissue regeneration are discussed fully in Chapter 14.

MAXILLARY AUGMENTATION

Severe resorption of the maxillary alveolar ridge presents a significant challenge to prosthetic reconstruction of the dentition. When moderate to severe maxillary resorption does occur, the larger denture-bearing area of the maxilla may allow prosthetic rehabilitation without bony augmentation. In certain cases a severe increase in interarch space, loss of palatal vault, interference from the zygomatic buttress area, and absence of posterior tuberosity notching may prevent construction of proper dentures, and augmentation must be considered.

Onlay Bone Grafting

Bone grafting of the edentulous atrophic maxilla with an autogenous rib was first described by Terry et al.[26] Maxillary onlay bone grafting is indicated primarily when severe resorption of the maxillary alveolus is seen that results in the absence of a clinical alveolar ridge and loss of adequate palatal vault form.[27]

Maxillary onlay grafting currently is usually accomplished using corticocancellous blocks of iliac crest bone. The blocks can be secured to the maxilla with small screws, eliminating mobility and decreasing resorption (Fig. 13-33). Cancellous bone is then packed around the grafts to improve contour. Implants can be placed at the time of grafting in some cases, but placement is often delayed to allow initial healing of the grafted bone.

Interpositional Bone Grafts

Maxillary interpositional bone grafting maintains the blood supply to the repositioned portion of the maxilla and generally results in more predictability with less extensive resorption postoperatively. Interpositional bone grafting in the maxilla is indicated in the bone-deficient maxilla, where the palatal vault is found to be adequately formed but ridge height is insufficient (particularly in the zygomatic buttress and posterior tuberosity areas and when excessive interarch space exists).[28] Anteroposterior and transverse discrepancies between the maxilla and mandible can also be corrected by interpositional bone-grafting techniques (Fig. 13-34).

Interpositional grafting techniques provide stable and predictable results by changing the maxillary position in the vertical, anteroposterior, and transverse directions and may eliminate the need for secondary soft tissue procedures. Disadvantages of this type of procedure include the need to harvest bone from an iliac crest donor site and possible secondary soft tissue surgery.

Sinus Lift

Rehabilitation of the maxilla using implants is frequently problematic because of the extension of the maxillary sinus

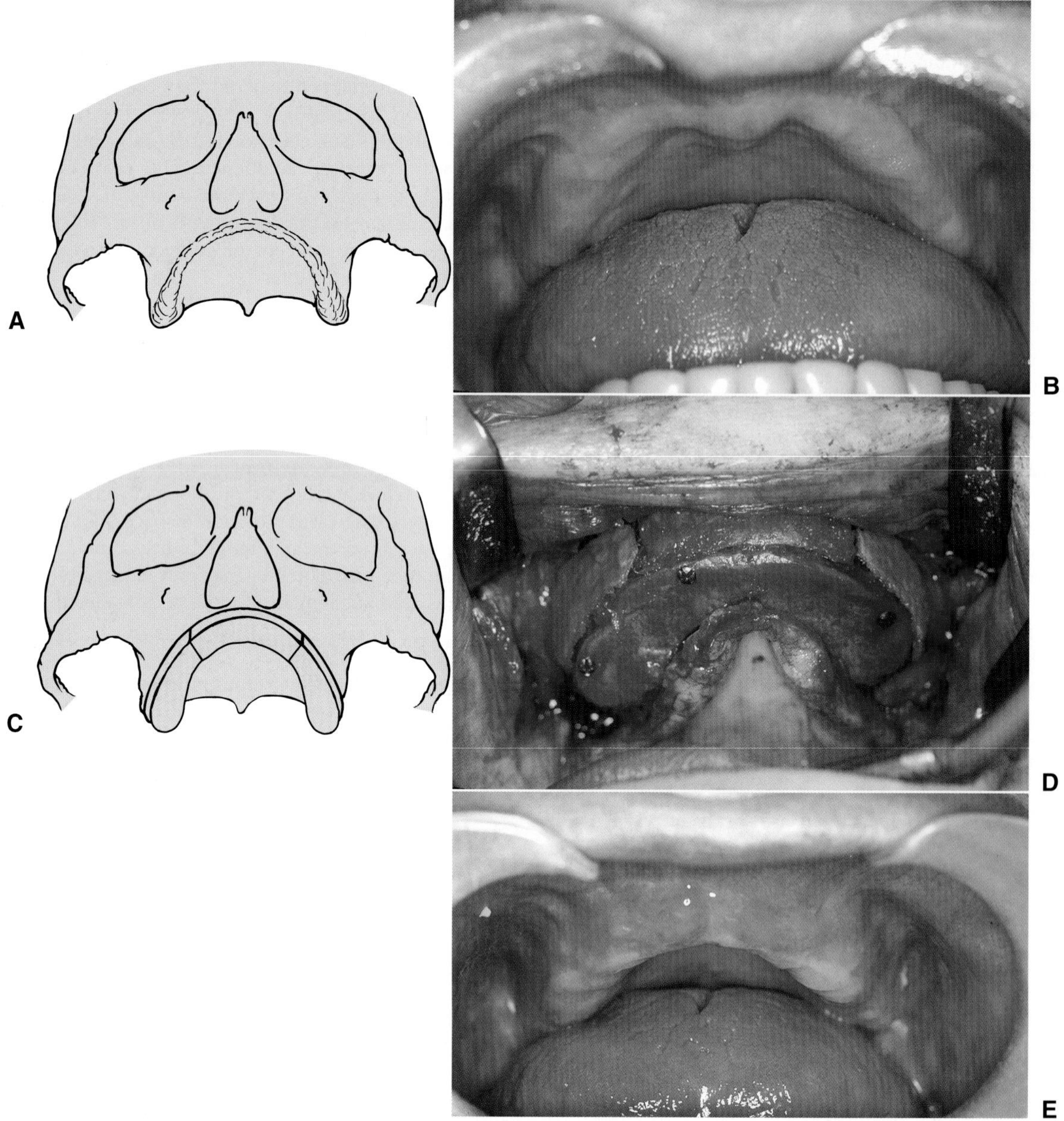

FIGURE 13-33 Iliac crest onlay bone reconstruction of maxilla. A, Diagram of atrophic maxilla. B, Clinical photograph illustrating inadequate alveolar ridge for reconstruction. C, Three segments of bone are secured in place. D, Stabilization of the onlay grafting with rigid fixation. Small defects are filled with cancellous bone. E, Postoperative result demonstrating improved alveolar ridge height and contour.

into the alveolar ridge area. In many cases the actual size and configuration of the maxilla are satisfactory in terms of height and width of the alveolar ridge area. However, extension of the maxillary sinuses into the alveolar ridge may prevent placement of implants in the posterior maxillary area because of insufficient bony support. A sinus lift procedure is a bony augmentation procedure that places graft material inside the sinus and augments the bony support in the alveolar ridge area.

In this technique an opening is made in the lateral aspect of the maxillary wall, and the sinus lining is carefully elevated from the bony floor of the sinus (Fig. 13-35). Allogeneic, autogenous, xenogeneic bone, BMP, or a combination of these materials can be used as a graft source.[16,29] The current method of choice usually incorporates some autogenous bone material in the sinus graft. After elevation of the sinus membrane the graft material is placed in the inferior portion of the sinus, below the sinus membrane. Perforation of the sinus membrane can occur during exposure of the maxillary sinus floor. Perforations are usually covered with redundancy of the elevated membrane and a resorbable membrane material. These measures allow placement of the graft material with protection from a direct sinus communication.[30] The graft is allowed to heal for 3 to 6 months, after which the first stage of implant placement can begin in the usual fashion described in Chapter 14. This procedure can be performed as outpatient surgery and does not affect postoperative denture wearing.

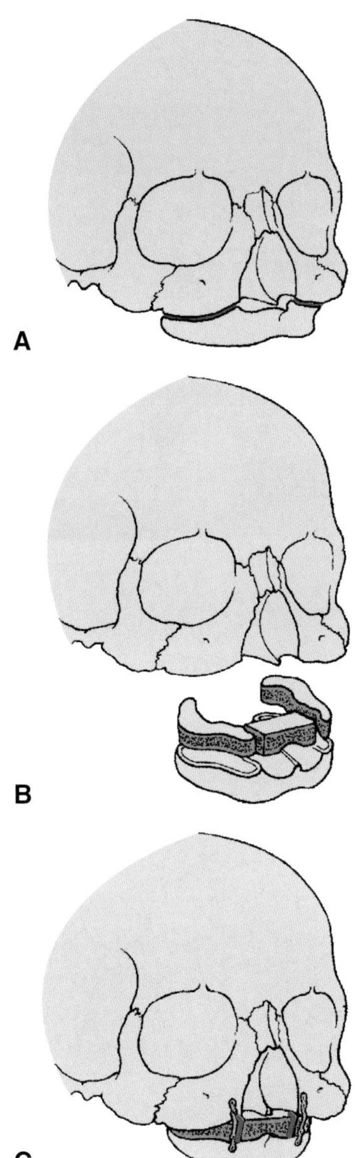

FIGURE 13-34 Interpositional (Le Fort I) augmentation of maxilla. **A**, Diagrammatic representation of atrophic maxillary alveolar ridge. **B**, Augmentation is completed by down-fracturing maxilla and placing interpositional graft using autogenous iliac crest. **C**, The maxilla is stabilized using rigid fixation plates.

ALVEOLAR RIDGE DISTRACTION

Trauma, congenital defects, and resection of bony pathologic conditions often create a bone defect inadequate for immediate reconstruction with implants. Considerable soft tissue defects including loss of attached gingiva or mucosa frequently accompany the bony discrepancy. Distraction osteogenesis has been applied to correct alveolar deficiencies.[31-33] Distraction osteogenesis involves cutting an osteotomy in the alveolar ridge (Fig. 13-36). An appliance is then screwed directly into the bone segments. After an initial latency period of 5 to 7 days, the appliance is gradually activated to separate the bony segments at approximately 1 mm per day. The gradual tension placed on the distracting bony interface produces continuous bone formation. Additionally, the adjacent tissue including mucosa and attached gingiva expands and adapts to this gradual tension. Because the adaptation and tissue genesis involves a variety of tissue types in addition to bone, this concept should also include the term *distraction histiogenesis*. The distracted segment and newly generated bone (termed *regenerate*) is allowed to heal for 3 to 4 months. The distraction appliance is then removed, and implants are usually placed at the time of distractor removal. Horizontal distraction of the alveolus to increase width followed by implant placement has also been completed successfully.[34]

SOFT TISSUE SURGERY FOR RIDGE EXTENSION OF THE MANDIBLE

As alveolar ridge resorption takes place, the attachment of mucosa and muscles near the denture-bearing area exerts a greater influence on the retention and stability of dentures. In addition, the amount and quality of fixed tissue over the denture-bearing area may be decreased. Soft tissue surgery performed to improve denture stability may be carried out alone or may be done after bony augmentation. In either case the primary goals of soft tissue preprosthetic surgery are to provide an enlarged area of fixed tissue in the primary denture-bearing or implant area and to improve extension in the area of the denture flanges by removing the dislodging effects of muscle attachments in the denture-bearing or vestibular areas.

Transpositional Flap Vestibuloplasty (Lip Switch)

A lingually based flap vestibuloplasty was first described by Kazanjian.[35] In this procedure a mucosal flap pedicled from the alveolar ridge is elevated from the underlying tissue and sutured to the depth of the vestibule (Fig. 13-37). The inner portion of the lip is allowed to heal by secondary epithelialization. This procedure has been modified, and the use of a technique transposing a lingually based mucosal flap and a labially based periosteal flap (transpositional flap) has become popular.[36]

When adequate mandibular height exists, this procedure increases the anterior vestibular area, which improves denture retention and stability. The primary indications for the procedure include adequate anterior mandibular height (at least 15 mm), inadequate facial vestibular depth from mucosal and muscular attachments in the anterior mandible, and the presence of an adequate vestibular depth on the lingual aspect of the mandible.

These techniques provide adequate results in many cases and generally do not require hospitalization, donor site surgery, or prolonged periods without a denture. Disadvantages of these techniques include unpredictability of the amount of relapse of the vestibular depth, scarring in the depth of the vestibule, and problems with adaptation of the peripheral flange area of the denture to the depth of the vestibule.[37,38]

Vestibule and Floor-of-Mouth Extension Procedures

In addition to the attachment of labial muscles and soft tissues to the denture-bearing area, the mylohyoid and genioglossus muscles in the floor of the mouth present similar problems on the lingual aspect of the mandible. Trauner[39] described detaching the mylohyoid muscles from the mylohyoid ridge area and

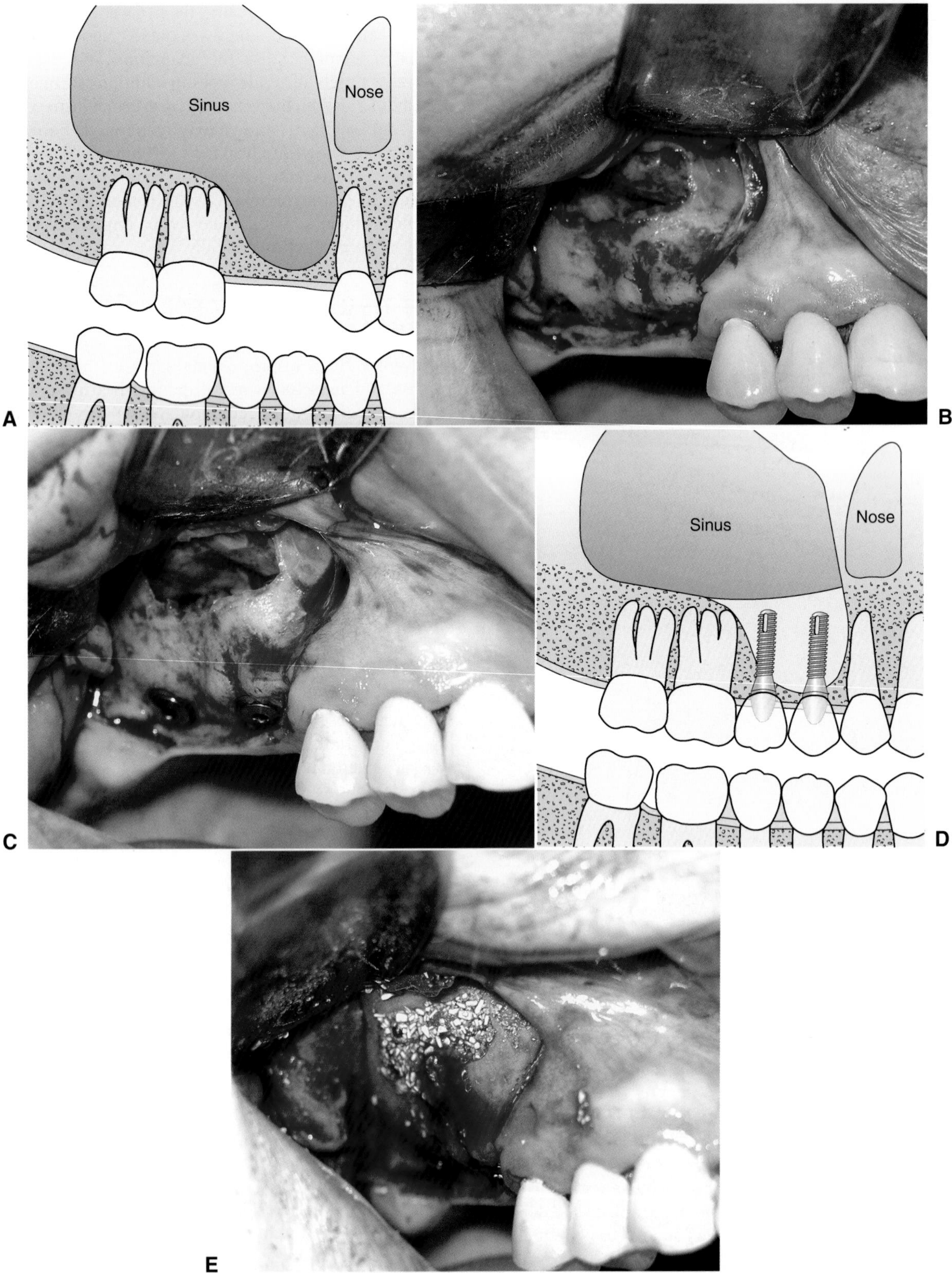

FIGURE 13-35 Sinus lift procedure. A, Diagram illustrating pneumatization of the maxillary sinus into the alveolar ridge with inadequate bone support for reconstruction. B, Bone window provides access; sinus membrane is elevated. C, Implants are placed, protruding into the sinus. D, Diagram depicting elevation of the sinus membrane, implant placement, and grafting of area around implants below sinus membrane. E, Graft (a combination of autogenous bone and allograft material) in place.

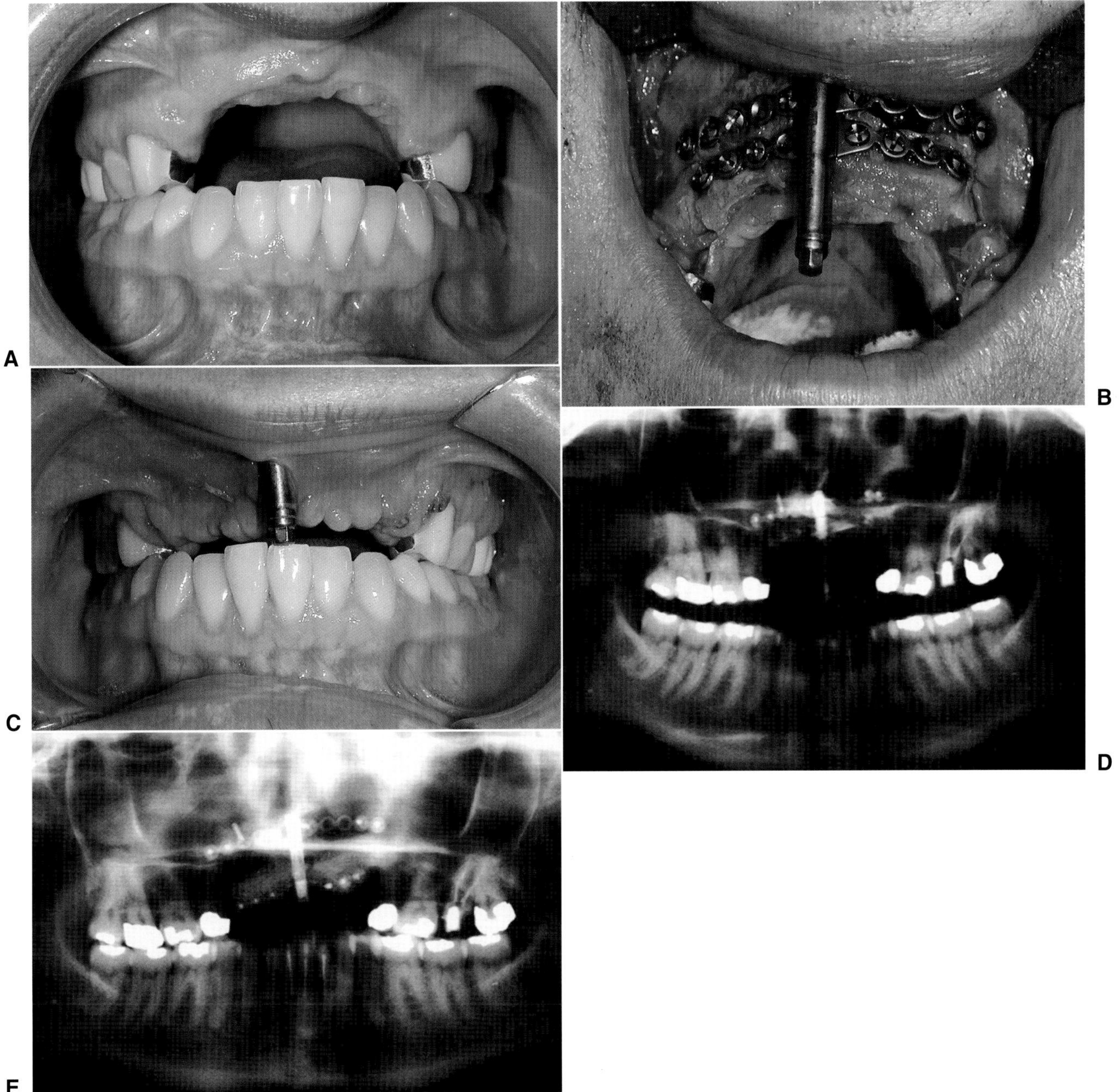

FIGURE 13-36 Alveolar distraction osteogenesis A, Pronounced vertical alveolar deficiency of the anterior maxilla. B, Positioning of distractor on alveolus. C, Improved alveolar positioning is evident with distraction of the segment at 2 weeks. D, Preoperative radiograph illustrating vertical alveolar deficiency. E, Postdistraction radiograph indicating improved alveolar height.

repositioning them inferiorly, effectively deepening the floor of the mouth area and relieving the influence of the mylohyoid muscle on the denture. MacIntosh and Obwegeser[40] later described the effective use of a labial extension procedure combined with Trauner's procedure to provide maximal vestibular extension to the buccal and lingual aspects of the mandible. The technique for extension of the labial vestibule is a modification of a labially pedicled supraperiosteal flap described by Clark.[41] After the two vestibular extension techniques, a skin graft can be used to cover the area of denuded periosteum (Fig.13-38). The combination procedure effectively eliminates the dislodging forces of the mucosa and muscle attachments and provides a broad base of fixed keratinized tissue on the primary denture-bearing area (Fig.13-39). Soft tissue grafting with the buccal vestibuloplasty and floor-of-mouth procedure is indicated when adequate alveolar ridge for a denture-bearing area is lost but at least 15 mm of mandibular bone height remains. The remaining bone must have adequate contour so that the form of the alveolar ridge exposed after the procedure is adequate for denture construction. Endosteal

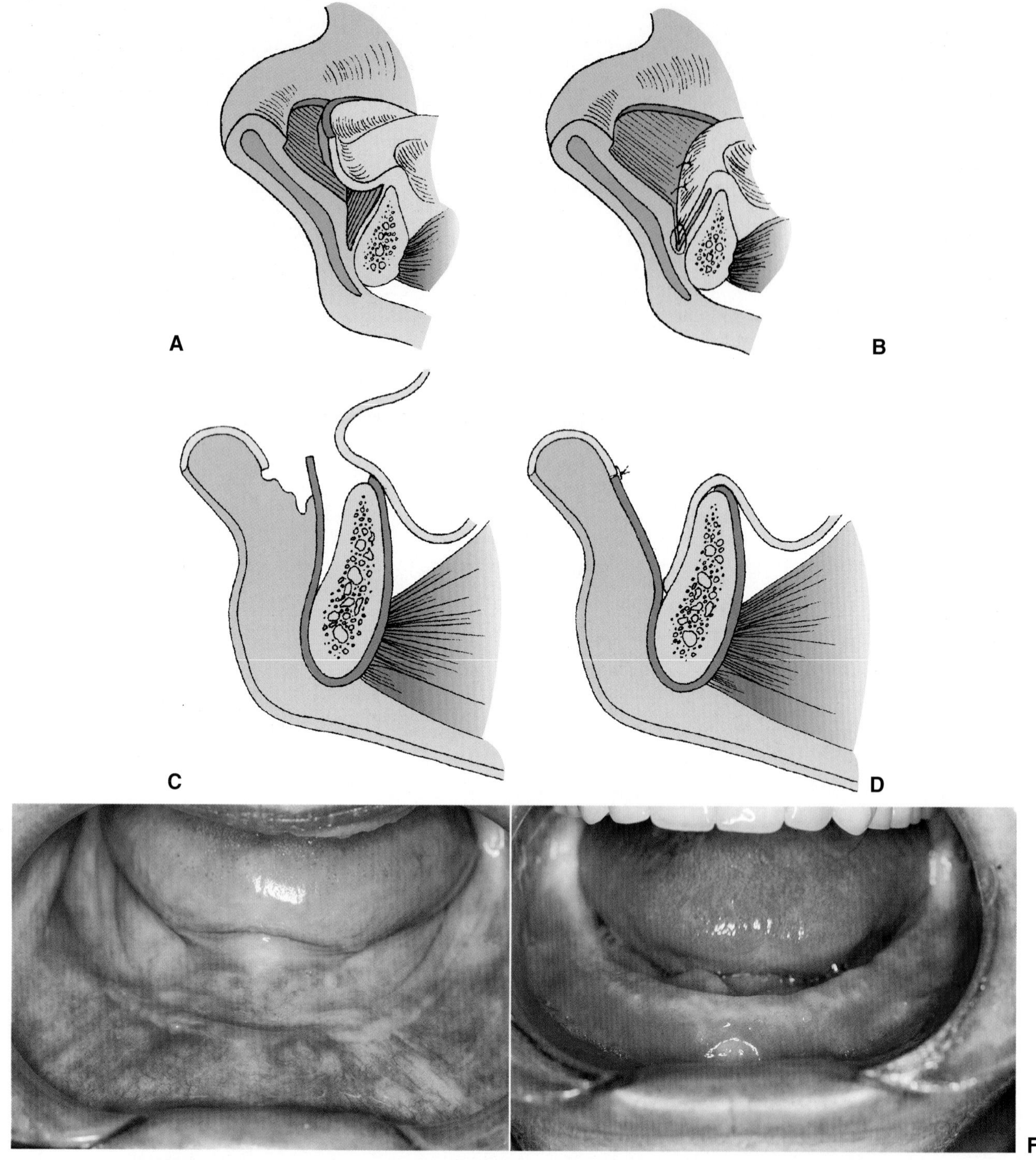

FIGURE 13-37 Transpositional flap vestibuloplasty (i.e., lip switch). A, Incision is made in labial mucosa, and thin mucosal flap is dissected from underlying tissue. Supraperiosteal dissection is also performed on anterior aspect of the mandible. B, Flap of labial mucosa is sutured to depth of vestibule. Exposed labial tissue heals by secondary intention. C, Modification of technique by incising periosteum at crest of alveolar ridge and suturing free periosteal edge to denuded area of labial mucosa. D, Mucosal flap is then sutured over denuded bone to periosteal junction at depth of vestibule. E, Preoperative photograph. F, Six-month postoperative result.

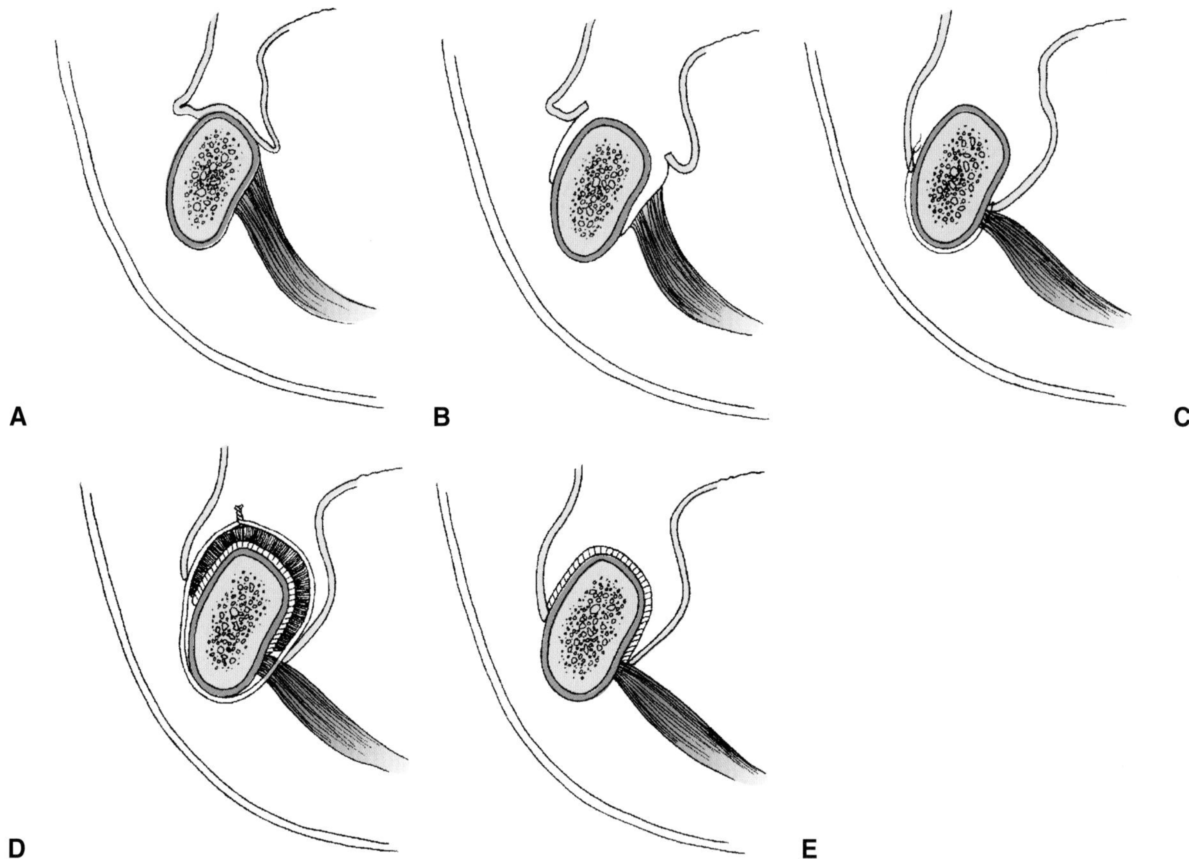

FIGURE 13-38 Labial vestibuloplasty, floor-of-mouth lowering procedure, and skin grafting (i.e., Obwegeser's technique). A, Preoperative muscle and soft tissue attachments near crest of remaining mandible. B, A crestal incision is made. Buccal and lingual flaps are created by a supraperiosteal dissection. C, Sutures are passed under the inferior border of the mandible tethering the labial and lingual flaps near the inferior border of the mandible. D, Graft held over the supraperiosteal dissection with a stent stabilized with circummandibular wires. E, Postoperative view of newly created vestibular depth and floor-of-mouth area.

implants are generally a much more suitable treatment, and therefore vestibuloplasty with grafting is not commonly performed. If gross bony irregularities exist, such as large concavities in the superior aspect of the posterior mandible, they should be corrected through grafting or minor alveoloplasty procedures before the soft tissue procedure.

The technique has the advantage of early covering of the exposed periosteal bed, which improves patient comfort and allows earlier denture construction. In addition, the long-term results of vestibular extension are predictable. The need for hospitalization and donor site surgery combined with the moderate swelling and discomfort experienced by the patient postoperatively are the primary disadvantages. Patients rarely complain about the appearance or function of skin in the oral cavity. If the skin graft is too thick at the time of harvesting, hair follicles may not totally degenerate, and hair growth may occasionally be seen in isolated areas of the graft.

Tissue other than skin has been used effectively for grafting over the alveolar ridge. Palatal tissue offers the potential advantages of providing a firm, resilient tissue, with minimal contraction of the grafted area.[42] Although palatal tissue is relatively easy to obtain at the time of surgery, the limited amount of tissue and the discomfort associated with donor site harvesting are the primary drawbacks. In areas where only a small localized graft is required, palatal tissue is usually adequate.

Full-thickness buccal mucosa harvested from the inner aspect of the cheek provides advantages similar to those of palatal tissue. However, the need for specialized mucotomes to harvest buccal mucosa and extensive buccal mucosa scarring after harvesting of a full-thickness graft are disadvantages. This mucosa does not become keratinized, is generally mobile, and often results in an inadequate denture-bearing surface.

SOFT TISSUE SURGERY FOR MAXILLARY RIDGE EXTENSION

Maxillary alveolar bone resorption frequently results in mucosal and muscle attachments that interfere with denture construction, stability, and retention. Because of the large denture-bearing area of the maxilla, adequate denture construction and stability can often be achieved after extensive bone loss. However, excess soft tissue may accompany bony resorption, or soft tissue may require modification as an adjunct to previous augmentation surgery. Several techniques provide additional fixed mucosa and vestibular depth in the maxillary denture-bearing area.

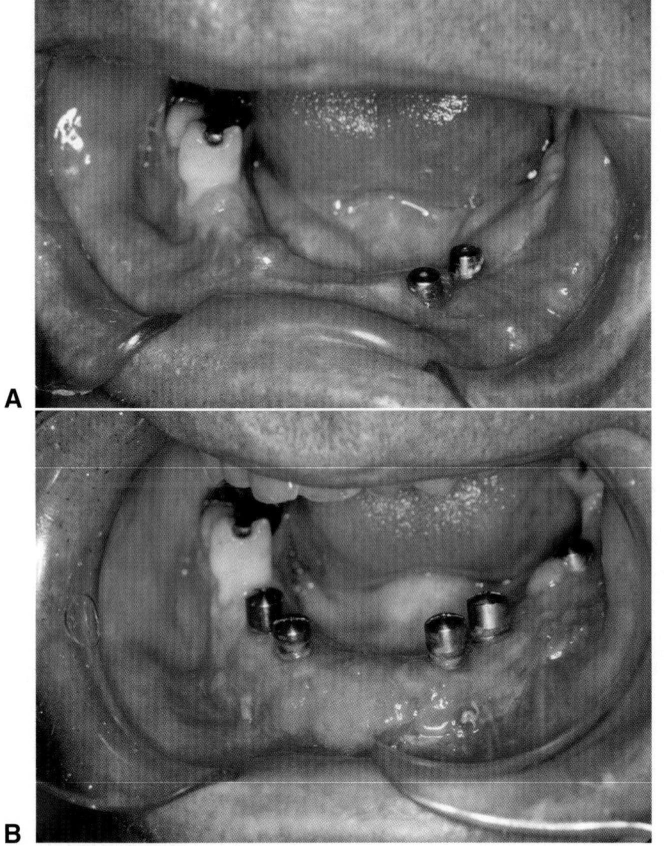

FIGURE 13-39 Vestibuloplasty, floor of the mouth lowering, and palatal soft tissue grafting. A, Preoperative photograph showing lack of facial and lingual vestibular depth and absent keratinized tissue adjacent to implant abutments. B, Improved vestibular depth with sound attached tissue over the alveolar ridge.

Submucosal Vestibuloplasty

The submucosal vestibuloplasty as described by Obwegeser[43] may be the procedure of choice for correction of soft tissue attachment on or near the crest of the alveolar ridge of the maxilla. This technique is particularly useful when maxillary alveolar ridge resorption has occurred but the residual bony maxilla is adequate for proper denture support. In this technique, underlying submucosal tissue is excised or repositioned to allow direct apposition of the labiovestibular mucosa to the periosteum of the remaining maxilla.

To provide adequate vestibular depth without producing an abnormal appearance of the upper lip, adequate mucosal length must be available in this area. A simple test to determine whether adequate labiovestibular mucosa is present is performed by placing a dental mouth mirror under the upper lip and elevating the superior aspect of the vestibule to the desired postoperative depth (Fig. 13-40). If no inversion or shortening of the lip occurs, then adequate mucosa is present to perform a proper submucosal vestibuloplasty.

The submucosal vestibuloplasty can generally be performed with local anesthetic and intravenous sedation in an outpatient setting. A midline incision is made in the anterior maxilla, and the mucosa is undermined and separated from the underlying submucosal tissue. A supraperiosteal tunnel is then developed by dissecting the muscular and submucosal attachments from the periosteum. The intermediate layer of tissue created by the two tunneling dissections is incised at its attachment area near the crest of the alveolar ridge. This submucosal and muscular tissue can be repositioned superiorly or excised. After closure of the midline incision, a preexisting denture or prefabricated splint is modified to extend into the vestibular areas and is secured with palatal screws for 7 to 10 days to hold the mucosa over the ridge in close apposition to the periosteum. When healing takes place, usually within 3 weeks, the mucosa is closely adapted to the anterior and lateral walls of the maxilla at the required depth of the vestibule.

These techniques provide a predictable increase in vestibular depth and attachment of mucosa over the denture-bearing area. A properly relined denture can often be worn immediately after the surgery or after removal of the splint, and impressions for final denture relining or construction can be completed 2 to 3 weeks after surgery.

Maxillary Vestibuloplasty with Tissue Grafting

When insufficient labiovestibular mucosa exists and lip shortening would result from a submucosal vestibuloplasty technique, other vestibular extension techniques must be used. In such cases a modification of Clark's vestibuloplasty technique using mucosa pedicled from the upper lip and sutured at the depth of the maxillary vestibule after a supraperiosteal dissection can be used.[44] The denuded periosteum over the alveolar ridge heals by secondary epithelialization. Moderate discomfort can occur in the postoperative period, and a longer healing time is required (6 to 8 weeks) before denture construction. Maintenance of the maxillary vestibular depth is unpredictable. The use of a labially pedicled mucosal flap combined with tissue grafting over the exposed periosteum of the maxilla provides the added benefits of more rapid healing over the area of previously exposed periosteum and more predictable long-term maintenance of vestibular depth (Fig. 13-41).

CORRECTION OF ABNORMAL RIDGE RELATIONSHIPS

Approximately 5% of the population has a severe skeletal discrepancy between their upper and lower jaws that results in a severe malocclusion. When the teeth are lost, an abnormal ridge relationship can result that complicates construction of prosthetic appliances. When a preexisting Class III ridge relationship exists, loss of teeth and the pattern of bony resorption increase the severity of the Class III skeletal problem. In patients with partially missing dentition, the absence of opposing occlusal forces may allow the supraeruption of teeth, which may complicate subsequent prosthetic restoration.

The assessment of ridge relationships is an important, often overlooked aspect of the evaluation of patients for prosthetic treatment. In partially edentulous patients the evaluation should include an examination of the direction of the occlusal plane and a determination of interarch distances that may be affected by supraerupted teeth or segments. In totally edentulous patients the interarch space and the anteroposterior and transverse relationships of the maxilla and mandible must be evaluated with the patient's jaw at the proper occlusal vertical dimension. This determination in the diagnostic phase may require the

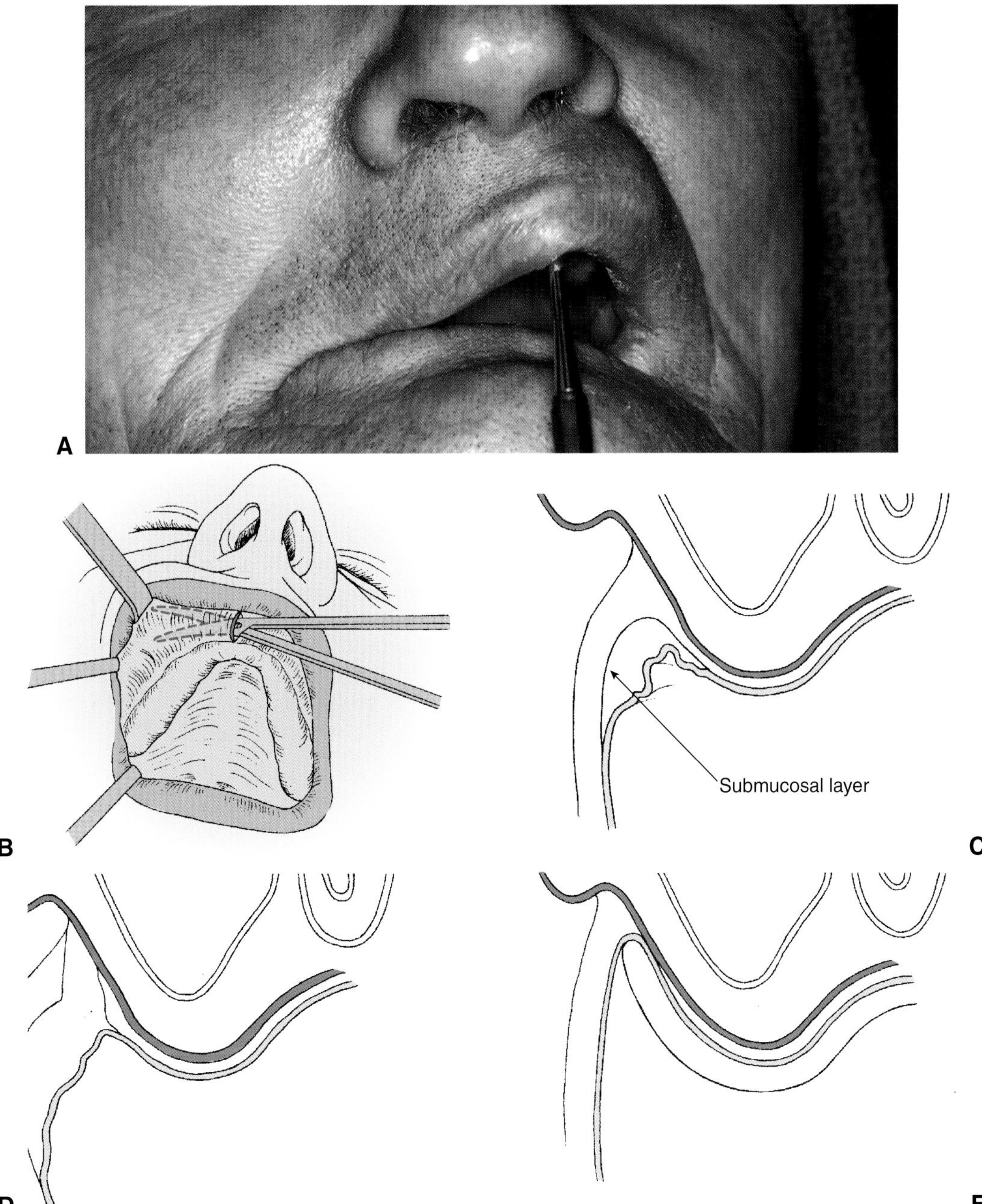

FIGURE 13-40 Submucosal vestibuloplasty. A, Mouth mirror placed in maxillary vestibule under upper lip and elevated against anterior wall of maxilla to desired postoperative vestibular depth. If no abnormal lip shortening occurs, then adequate mucosa exists to perform submucosal vestibuloplasty. B, Anterior vertical incision is used to create submucosal and then supraperiosteal tunnel along lateral aspects of maxilla. C, Cross-sectional view showing submucosal tissue layer. D, Excision of submucosal soft tissue layer. E, Splint in place holding mucosa against periosteum at depth of vestibule until healing occurs.

Continued

construction of bite rims with proper lip support. Lateral cephalometric radiographs are also necessary in this evaluation to confirm the clinical impression.

Segmental Alveolar Surgery in the Partially Edentulous Patient

Supraeruption of teeth and bony segments into an opposing edentulous area may decrease interarch space and preclude the construction of an adequate fixed or removable prosthetic appliance in this area. The loss of teeth in one arch may increase the difficulty of obtaining a functional and esthetic prosthetic appliance with prosthetic teeth located properly over the underlying ridge. Several alternatives exist to restore the dentition in these patients, including extraction of teeth in the malpositioned segment or repositioning of these teeth with segmental surgery.

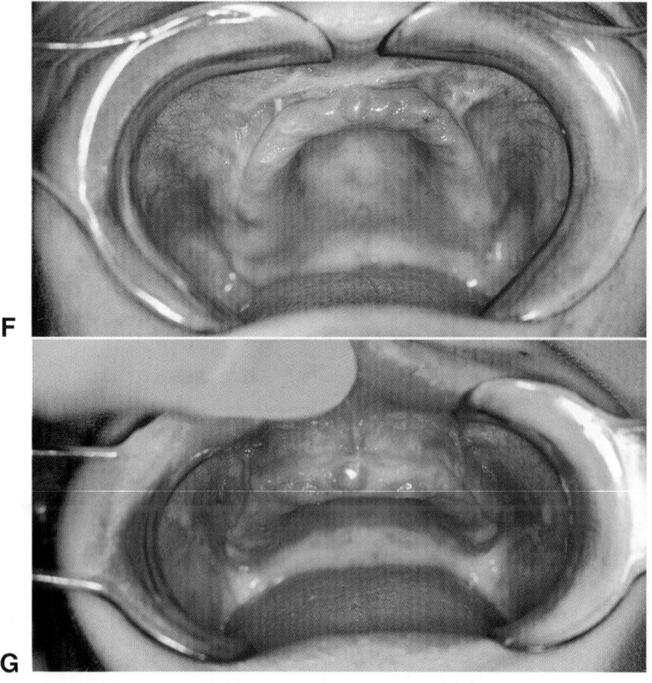

FIGURE 13-40, cont'd Submucosal vestibuloplasty. F, Preoperative photograph. G, Postoperative result.

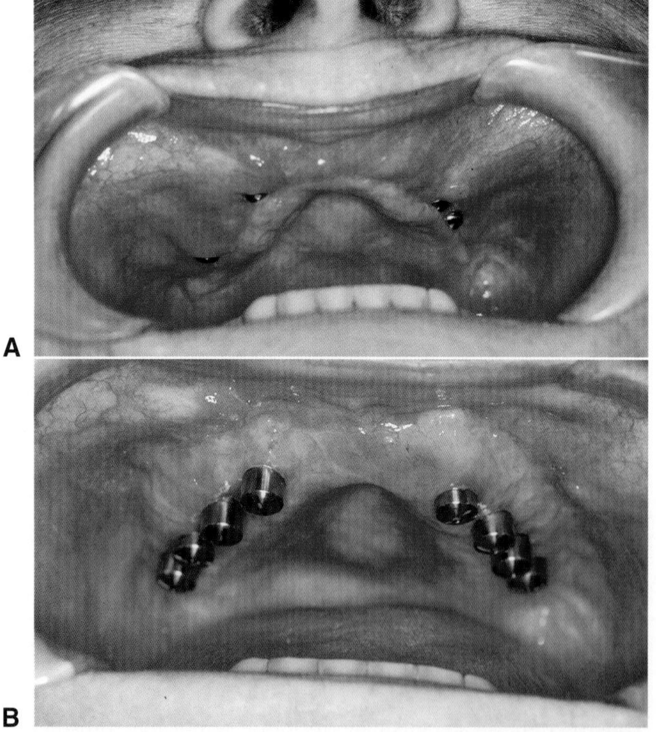

FIGURE 13-41 Improved soft tissue contours for implant reconstruction. A, Lack of facial vestibule and deficient keratinized tissue overlying maxillary alveolus. B, One-month postoperative result illustrating improved soft tissue contours for implant supported restoration.

Preoperative considerations should include facial esthetic quality, an intraoral occlusal examination, panoramic and cephalometric radiographs, and models properly mounted on an articulator. If segmental surgery is to be considered, the models can be cut and teeth repositioned in their desired location. The dentist responsible for final prosthetic restoration of the patient must make the final determination of the placement of the segments on the articulated models. Presurgical orthodontic preparation may be necessary to align teeth properly and allow proper segmental positioning. After model surgery, a splint is fabricated to locate placement of segments precisely at the time of surgery and to provide stability during the postoperative healing period. When possible, the splint should be stabilized by contacting other teeth rather than resting on soft tissue. Palatal and lingual flanges on the splint should be avoided because pressure from the splint may interfere with blood supply important for the viability of the bone and teeth that were repositioned with segmental surgery. In some cases, construction of the splint must include contact on the alveolar ridge tissue of the opposing arch to maintain the interridge distance. The patient's deformity and the surgeon's preference and experience dictate the specific surgical procedure performed. Segmental procedures for correction of abnormalities in the maxilla and the mandible are described in Chapter 25 and in other textbooks (Fig. 13-42).[45] A final fixed and removable prosthetic rehabilitation follows the surgical procedure and an adequate postoperative healing period.

Correction of Skeletal Abnormalities in the Totally Edentulous Patient

After the appropriate clinical and radiographic evaluation, casts should be mounted on an articulator for determination of the ideal ridge relationship. The dentist responsible for prosthetic construction should be responsible for determining the final desired position of the maxilla and mandible after surgery. In the case of the totally edentulous patient in whom the maxilla, mandible, or both are to be repositioned, the esthetic facial result must also be considered with the functional result of ridge repositioning. Casts with simulated surgical changes, cephalometric prediction tracings, and experienced clinical judgment are required to determine the desired postoperative jaw position (Chapter 25). Once the desired postoperative skeletal position has been determined, splints are made to allow positioning of the jaws into their proper relationship at the time of surgery. Rigid fixation techniques following repositioning of the maxilla or mandible are reviewed in Chapter 25 and are useful in stabilizing bone segments at the time of surgery and in eliminating a prolonged period of jaw immobilization.

Denture construction can begin within 3 months after surgical repositioning of the maxilla and mandible. The combination of orthognathic surgery and prosthetic rehabilitation of the patient provides satisfactory functional and esthetic results in many patients with skeletal abnormalities who would otherwise present significant problems in prosthetic reconstruction.

SUMMARY

The success of preprosthetic surgical preparation depends on careful evaluation and treatment planning. In general, bony abnormalities should be managed first. Associated soft tissue correction is often delayed until bone augmentation and

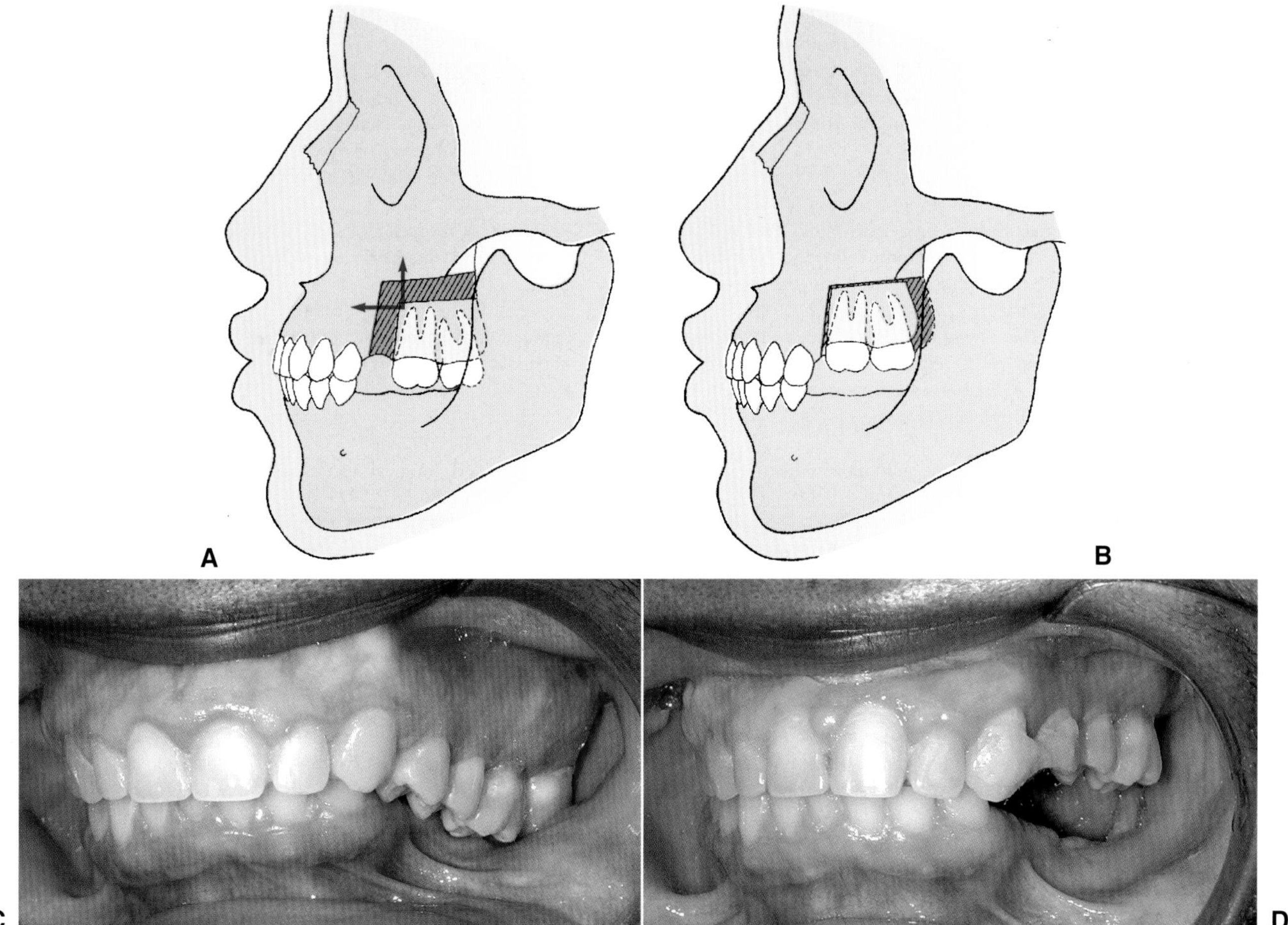

FIGURE 13-42 Segmental osteotomies. A and B, Posterior maxillary osteotomy for superior and anterior repositioning of posterior segment of maxilla. This improves interarch space for implant placement or construction of a removable partial denture. C, Clinical appearance of supraerupted maxillary teeth. D, Postoperative view demonstrating superior repositioning of isolated segment to improve interarch distance.

contouring is complete. Simultaneous bony augmentation is attempted when bony augmentation is aimed at improving contour rather than creating significant augmentation in alveolar height or width. Final prosthesis design and goals of long-term function, esthetic quality, and tissue maintenance must be considered during all phases of treatment.

REFERENCES

1. Tallgren A: The continuing reduction of residual alveolar ridges in complete denture wearers: mixed longitudinal study covering 25 years, *J Prosthet Dent* 27:120-132, 1972.
2. Bays RA: The pathophysiology and anatomy of edentulous bone loss. In Fonseca R, Davis W, editors: *Reconstructive preprosthetic oral and maxillofacial surgery,* Philadelphia, 1985, WB Saunders.
3. Mercier P, Lafontant R: Residual alveolar ridge atrophy: classification and influence of facial morphology, *J Prosthet Dent* 41:90-100, 1979.
4. Starshak TJ: Oral anatomy and physiology. In Starshak TJ, Sanders B, editors: *Preprosthetic oral and maxillofacial surgery,* St Louis, 1980, Mosby.
5. Crandell CE, Trueblood SN: Roentgenographic findings in edentulous areas, *Oral Surg Oral Med Oral Pathol* 13:1343, 1960.
6. Jenkins WS, Brandt MT, Dembo JB: Suturing principles in dentoalveolar surgery, *Oral and Maxillofacial Surgery Clinics of North America* 14:213-229, 2002.
7. Dean OT: Surgery for the denture patient, *J Am Dent Assoc* 23:2124, 1936.
8. Michael CG, Barsoum WM: Comparing ridge resorption with various surgical techniques in immediate dentures, *J Prosthet Dent* 35: 142-155, 1976.
9. Kalas S, Halperin V, Jefferis K et al: The occurrence of torus palatinus and torus mandibularis in 2478 dental patients, *Oral Surg Oral Med Oral Pathol* 6:1134, 1953.
10. Strauss RA: Laser management of discrete lesions. In Catone G, Alling C, editors: *Laser applications in oral and maxillofacial surgery,* Philadelphia, 1997, WB Saunders.
11. Atkinson T: Fundamentals of the carbon dioxide laser. In Catone G, Alling C, editors: *Laser applications in oral and maxillofacial surgery,* Philadelphia, 1997, WB Saunders.
12. Pick RM: Use of the laser for treatment of gingival diseases, *Oral and Maxillofacial Surgery Clinics of North America* 9:1-19, 1997.
13. Hartwell CM Jr: *Syllabus of complete dentures,* Philadelphia, 1968, Lea & Febiger.
14. Bartee BK: Extraction site reconstruction for alveolar ridge preservation. 1. Rationale and materials selection, *J Oral Implantol* 27(4): 187-193, 2001.

15. Feuille F, Knapp CI, Brunsvold MA et al: Clinical and histological evaluation of bone replacement grafts in the treatment of localized alveolar ridge defects. I. Mineralized freeze dried bone allograft, *Int J Periodontics Restorative Dent* 23:29-35, 2003.
16. Hosney M: Recent concepts in bone grafting and banking, *J Craniomandibular Pract* 5:170-182, 1987.
17. Alexopoulou M, Semergidis T, Serti M: Allogenic bone grafting of small and medium defects of the jaws. Congress of the European Association for Cranio-maxillofacial Surgery, Helsinki, Finland, 1998.
18. Sclar AG: Preserving alveolar ridge anatomy following tooth removal in conjunction with immediate implant placement: the Bio-col technique, *Atlas Oral Maxillofac Surg Clin North Am* 7(2):39-59, 1999.
19. Terry BC: Subperiosteal onlay grafts. In Stoelinga PJW, editor: *Proceedings consensus conference: Eighth International Conference on Oral Surgery,* Chicago, 1984, Quintessence International.
20. Thoma KH, Holland DJ: Atrophy of the mandible, *Oral Surg Oral Med Oral Pathol* 4:1477, 1951.
21. Curtis T, Ware W: Autogenous bone graft procedures for atrophic edentulous mandibles, *J Prosthet Dent* 38:366-379, 1977.
22. Taylor JC, Cuff SE, Leger JP et al: In vitro osteoclast resorption of bone substitute biomaterials used for implant site augmentation: a pilot study, *Int J Oral Maxillofac Implants* 17:321-330, 2002.
23. Nyman S, Lindhe J, Karring T et al: New attachment following surgical treatment of human periodontal disease, *J Clin Periodontol* 9:290-296, 1982.
24. Dahlin C, Sennerby L, Lekholm U et al: Generation of new bone around titanium implants using a membrane technique: an experimental study in rabbits, *Int J Oral Maxillofac Implants* 4:19-25, 1989.
25. Camargo PM, LekovicV, Karring T: Alveolar bone preservation following tooth extraction: a perspective of clinical trials utilizing osseous grafting and guided bone regeneration, *Oral and Maxillofacial Surgery Clinics of North America* 16(1):9-18, 2004.
26. Terry BC, Albright JE, Baker RD: Alveolar ridge augmentation in the edentulous maxilla with use of autogenous ribs, *J Oral Surg* 32:429-434, 1974.
27. Baker RD, Connole PW: Preprosthetic augmentation grafting: autogenous bone, *J Oral Surg* 35:541-551, 1977.
28. Bell WH, Buche WA, Kennedy JW 3rd et al: Surgical correction of the atrophic alveolar ridge: a preliminary report on a new concept of treatment, *Oral Surg Oral Med Oral Pathol* 43:485-498, 1977.
29. Boyne PJ, Lilly LC, Marx RE et al: De novo bone induction by recombinant human bone morphogenetic protein-2 (rhBMP-2) in maxillary sinus floor augmentation, *J Oral Maxillofac Surg* 63:1693-1707, 2005.
30. Proussaefs P, Lozada J, Kim J et al: Repair of the perforated sinus membrane with a resorbable collagen membrane: a human study, *Int J Oral Maxillofac Implants* 10(3):413-420, 2004.
31. Block MS, Chang A, Crawford C: Mandibular alveolar ridge augmentation in the dog using distraction osteogenesis, *J Oral Maxillofac Surg* 54(3):309-314, 1996.
32. Rachmiel A, Srouji S, Peled M: Alveolar ridge augmentation by distraction osteogenesis, *Int J Oral Maxillofac Surg* 30(6):510-517, 2001.
33. Jensen OT, Cockrell R, Kuhlke L et al: Anterior maxillary alveolar distraction osteogenesis: a prospective 5-year clinical study, *Int J Oral Maxillofac Implants* 17(1):52-68, 2002.
34. Laster Z, Rachmiel A, Jensen OT: Alveolar width distraction osteogenesis for early implant placement, *J Oral Maxillofac Surg* 63(12):1724-1730, 2005.
35. Kazanjian VH: Surgical operations as related to satisfactory dentures, *Dental Cosmos* 66:387, 1924.
36. Keithley JL, Gamble JW: The lip switch: a modification of Kazanjian's labial vestibuloplasty, *J Oral Surg* 36:701, 1978.
37. Hillerup S: Preprosthetic vestibular sulcus extension by the operation of Edlan and Mejchar. I. A 2-year follow-up study, *Int J Oral Surg* 8:333, 1979.
38. Hillerup S: Profile changes of bone and soft tissue following vestibular sulcus extension by the operation of Edlan and Mejchar. II. A 2-year follow-up study, *Int J Oral Surg* 8:340-346, 1979.
39. Trauner R: Alveoloplasty with ridge extensions on the lingual side of the lower jaw to solve the problem of a lower dental prosthesis, *Oral Surg Oral Med Oral Pathol* 5:340, 1952.
40. MacIntosh RB, Obwegeser HL: Preprosthetic surgery: a scheme for its effective employment, *J Oral Surg* 25:397-413, 1967.
41. Clark HB Jr: Deepening of the labial sulcus by mucosa flap advancement: report of a case, *J Oral Surg* 11:165, 1953.
42. Hall HD, O'Steen AN: Free grafts of palatal mucosa in mandibular vestibuloplasty, *J Oral Surg* 28:565-574, 1970.
43. Obwegeser H: Die Submukose Vestibulumplastik, *Dtsch Zahnarztl Z* 14:629, 1959.
44. Obwegeser HL: Surgical preparation of the maxilla for prosthesis, *J Oral Surg* 22:127, 1964.
45. Bell WH, Proffit WR, White RP Jr: *Surgical correction of dentofacial deformities,* Philadelphia, 1980, WB Saunders.

CHAPTER 14

Contemporary Implant Dentistry

PETER E. LARSEN AND EDWIN A. MCGLUMPHY

CHAPTER OUTLINE

The dental professional must use considerable clinical skill to help patients cope with the effects of partial or complete edentulism. Dental problems that were historically the most difficult can be solved today with the assistance of dental implants. Completely edentulous patients now enjoy the security and function of fixed restorations (Fig. 14-1). Patients missing a posterior abutment, who would ordinarily require a distal extension removable partial denture, may now enjoy the benefits of a fixed restoration with dental implants (Fig. 14-2). Trauma victims who are missing teeth and bone can be successfully rehabilitated with fixed restorations (Fig. 14-3).

Even the patient missing only a single tooth can receive a restoration more analogous to the missing natural tooth (Fig. 14-4). Likewise, a patient with adequate alveolar bone can receive a complete fixed implant rehabilitation (Fig. 14-5). These examples illustrate advantageous and predictable alternatives to edentulism that are becoming the standard of care within the dental community.

The dental profession has not always had a positive opinion of dental implants. Implants had their beginnings around the middle of the twentieth century. Early types of dental implants came into relatively common use during the 1960s because of patient demand, although little or no scientifically sound research had been done to characterize implant success rates.

In a May 1982 conference held in Toronto, the North American dental profession was introduced to a body of scientific literature on Swedish research into the bone-to-implant interface—a concept called *osseointegration.* This new concept is based on atraumatic implant placement and delayed implant loading. These factors contribute to a remarkably higher degree of implant predictably than was previously possible. The Swedish research team led by P.I. Branemark

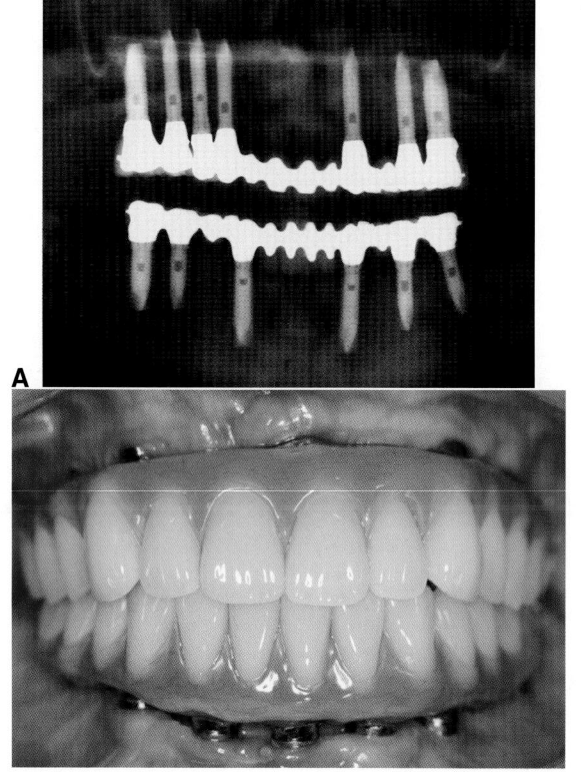

FIGURE 14-1 A, Radiograph showing fixed restorations supported by seven implants in the maxilla and six in the mandible. B, Metal-resin restorations are the treatment of choice for edentulous patients with moderate bone resorption. (Rosenstiel SF, Land MF, Fujimoto J: *Contemporary fixed prosthodontics,* ed 4, St Louis, 2006, Mosby.)

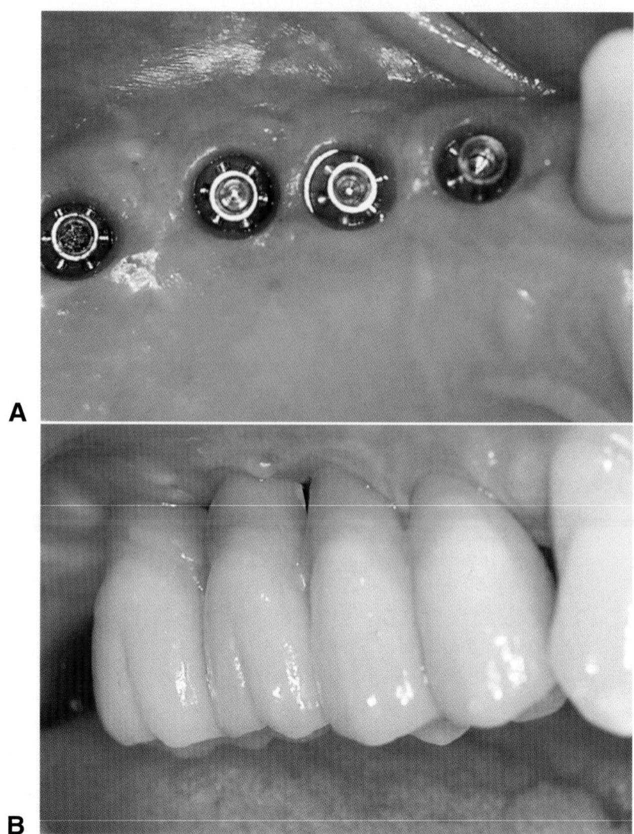

FIGURE 14-2 Implant-supported fixed prosthesis. Four dental implants (A) supporting a fixed dental prosthesis (B). (Rosenstiel SF, Land MF, Fujimoto J: *Contemporary fixed prosthodontics,* ed 4, St Louis, 2006, Mosby.)

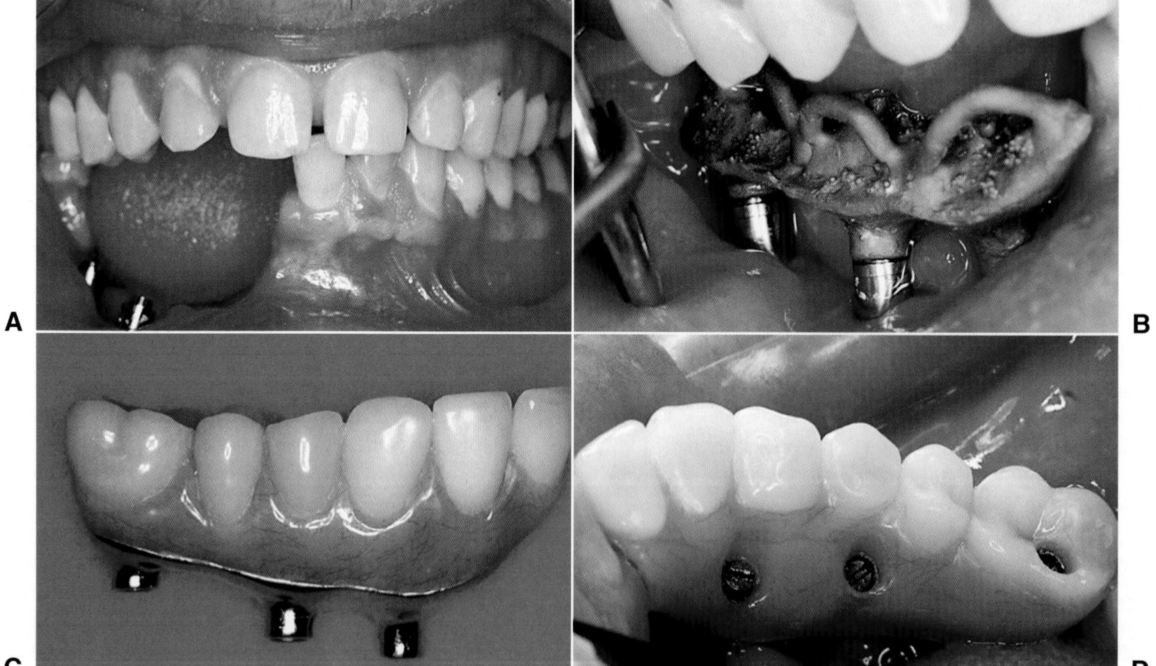

FIGURE 14-3 A, Large mandibular defect created by a shotgun wound. B, Metal substructure of a metal-resin prosthesis tied onto three implants in this defect. C, Denture resin can more effectively recreate the soft tissue color and contours in the completed restoration than dental porcelain. D, Metal-resin restorations over the defect. (Rosenstiel SF, Land MF, Fujimoto J: *Contemporary fixed prosthodontics,* ed 4, St Louis, 2006, Mosby.)

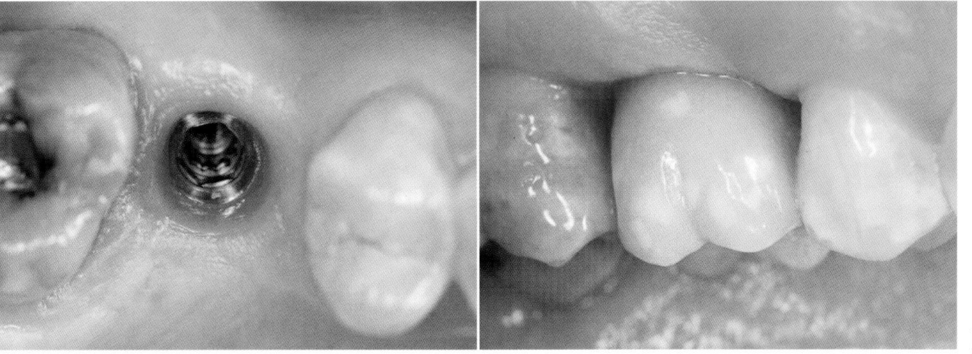

FIGURE 14-4 A, Single-tooth implant with an internal antirotational feature. B, Implant crown replacing a single missing tooth (cement retained). (Rosenstiel SF, Land MF, Fujimoto J: *Contemporary fixed prosthodontics,* ed 4, St Louis, 2006, Mosby.)

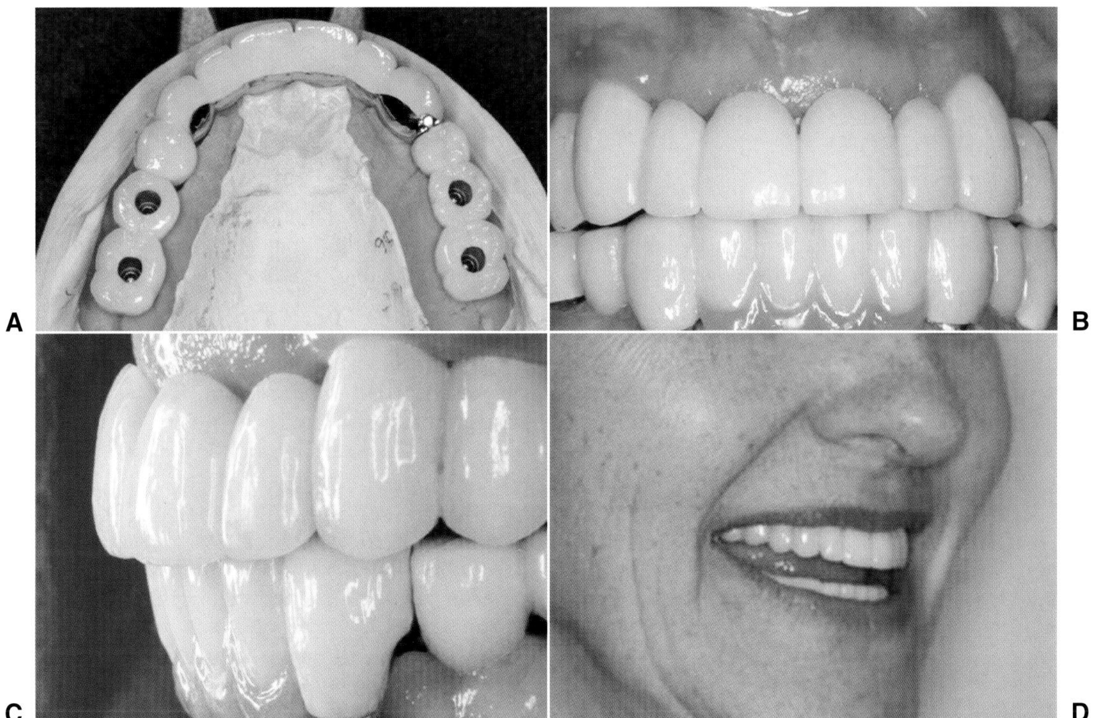

FIGURE 14-5 A to D, A metal-ceramic implant restoration may be indicated if adequate bone and soft tissue contours are available. (Rosenstiel SF, Land MF, Fujimoto J: *Contemporary fixed prosthodontics,* ed 4, St Louis, 2006, Mosby.)

reported high success in the mandible for more than 15 years. The knowledge gained from the experience of the Swedish team was used in the development of other systems currently available on the market. Today the American Dental Association has also approved many other systems.

In 1988 a National Institutes of Health consensus conference was held in Washington, D.C. This conference evaluated the long-term effectiveness of dental implants and established indications and contraindications for the various types of dental implants. Stringent criteria for success were proposed and have gained general acceptance (Box 14-1). By these criteria, success rates of 85% at the end of a 5-year observation period and 80% at the end of a 10-year period are minimal levels for success.

BOX 14-1

Generally Accepted Implant Success Criteria

1. The individual unattached implant is immobile when tested clinically.
2. No evidence of periimplant radiolucency is present, as assessed on an undistorted radiograph.
3. The mean vertical bone loss is less than 0.2 mm annually after the first year of service.
4. No persistent pain, discomfort, or infection is attributable to the implant.
5. The implant design does not preclude placement of a crown or prosthesis with an appearance that is satisfactory to the patient and the dentist.

From Smith D, Zarb GA: Criteria for success for osseointegrated endosseous implants, *J Prosthet Dent* 62:567, 1989.

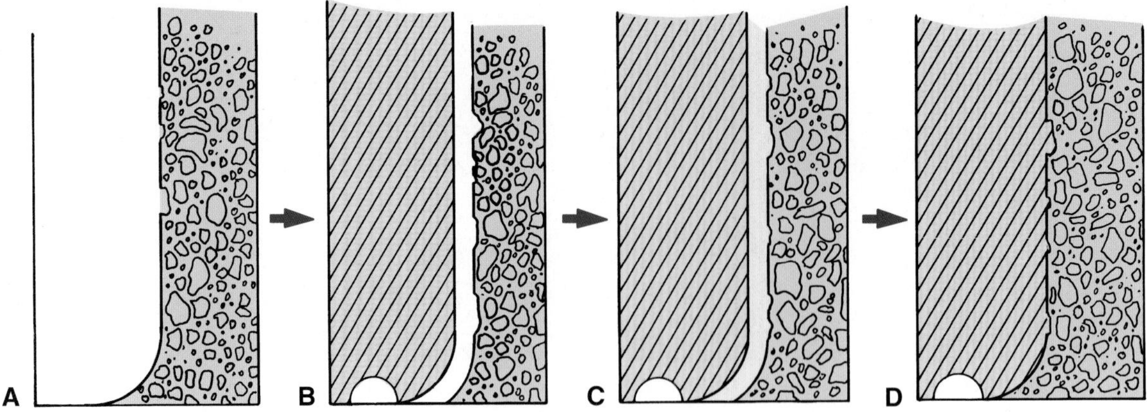

FIGURE 14-6 **A**, Implant site prepared in bone using irrigation to keep temperatures below 47° C to prevent cell damage and death in area. **B**, Precisely machined implant placed in site. Gap between implant and bone should be much less than 1 mm. **C**, If gap between implant and bone is small enough, embryonic bone will rapidly bridge gap. **D**, If implant is left undisturbed during healing phase, embryonic bone on the implant surface will mature to lamellar load-bearing bone.

BIOLOGIC CONSIDERATIONS FOR OSSEOINTEGRATION

The recent success of dental implants relates directly to the discovery of methods to maximize the amount of bone and implant contact. Osseointegration is a histologic definition meaning "a direct connection between living bone and load-bearing endosseous implant at the light microscopic level." Four main factors are required to achieve a successful osseo-integrated bone-to-implant interface: (1) a biocompatible material, (2) an implant precisely adapted to the prepared bony site, (3) atraumatic surgery to minimize tissue damage, and (4) an immobile, undisturbed healing phase. A biocompatible material is necessary to promote healing without a foreign-body rejection reaction by the host tissue. If biocompatible materials are not used, the body attempts to isolate the foreign-body implant material by surrounding it with granulation and then connective tissue. It has been demonstrated that titanium and certain calcium-phosphate ceramics are biologically inert.

The size of the gap between the implant and the bone immediately after implant placement is critical to achieving osseointegration. The gap size can be controlled primarily by the preparation of a precise cylindrically shaped surgical bed into which the implant is placed. Precision instrumentation and a technically sound surgical procedure help minimize the distance between the implant and host bone.

Atraumatic surgery is required to allow minimal mechanical and thermal injury to occur. Sharp, high-quality burs that are run at low speed by high-torque drills are essential to precise atraumatic implant site preparation. Copious irrigation by internal or external methods must keep the bone temperatures to levels below 56° C, which is the level beyond which irreversible bone damage occurs. It has been shown that bone tissue damage occurs when the bone temperature reaches 47° C for more than 1 minute. If the temperature rises, alkaline phosphatase within the bone is denatured, this prevents alkaline calcium synthesis. If the gap between the implant and the bone can be minimized and surgery is atraumatic, embryonic bone will be laid down rapidly between the implant and the bone and will then mature into the lamellar load-bearing bone (Fig. 14-6).

Implant immobility during the healing phase is affected by the precision of site preparation, bone quality, and quantity in the vertical and buccal-lingual dimensions. Areas of the jaws that have a high percentage of cortical bone, such as the anterior mandible, are more likely to anchor the implant successfully. Areas of the jaws with a high percentage of cancellous bone make initial stability of the implant more difficult to achieve. If the superior and inferior cortical plates can be engaged by the implant, this also is advantageous for initial implant stability (Fig. 14-7). This is frequently possible in the anterior mandible and the maxilla; however, the inferior alveolar canal prevents this from occurring in the posterior mandible. Regardless of the anatomy in the area of implant placement, it is crucial to obtain primary stabilization for successful osseointegration. Once the implant is placed, a healing cover is inserted and the mucosa is sutured over the implant. In some cases the implant is not covered and a short healing screw protrudes through the gingival. In all cases the implant is protected from occlusal forces.

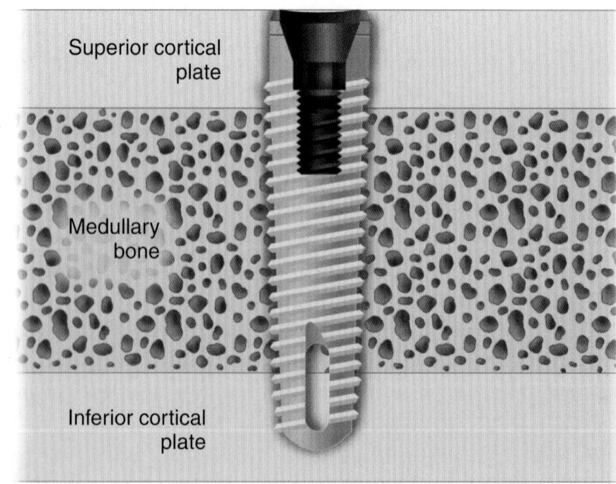

FIGURE 14-7 Whenever possible, implants should engage two cortical plates of bone. (Rosenstiel SF, Land MF, Fujimoto J: *Contemporary fixed prosthodontics,* ed 4, St Louis, 2006, Mosby.)

Once the initial stability of the implant has been achieved, it must be maintained throughout the healing phase. Should the patient desire to continue to wear the removable prosthesis during the healing period, it is important that a soft liner be placed in the removable denture to further decrease load transfer to the implant. The bone in the mandible is generally denser than the bone in the maxilla with a higher ratio of cortical to cancellous bone. Because the maxilla is primarily cancellous bone and the cortical bone is much thinner than in the mandible, osseointegration requires a longer healing period.

The achievement of successful osseointegration is first assessed at the second-stage surgery when the implant is uncovered, the healing cover is removed, and a prosthetic abutment is inserted. Once the abutment is attached to the implant body, the surgeon should carefully check for any signs of clinically detectable mobility. An immobile implant at this stage usually indicates successful osseointegration. Detectable mobility at this stage indicates that fibrous connective tissue has encapsulated the implant, in which case the implant should be removed at that time. The failed site is allowed to heal, and another implant can be placed at a later time. Once a successful osseointegrated bone-to-implant interface has been achieved, masticatory function at least equal that of natural dentition is generally possible.

The major mechanisms for the destruction of osseointegration are similar to those of natural teeth. Disease activity in the periimplant soft tissue environment and biomechanical overload of the individual implant are the two factors most commonly associated with the potential breakdown of osseointegration.

Soft Tissue–to–Implant Interface

The successful dental implant should have an unbroken, perimucosal seal between the soft tissue and the implant abutment surface. To maintain the integrity of this seal, the patient must maintain a high level of oral hygiene specific to dental implants. Clinicians, dental hygienists, and patients must understand and appreciate the necessity for a comprehensive implant maintenance program, including regularly scheduled recall visits. In the natural dentition the junctional epithelium provides a seal at the base of the gingival sulcus against the penetration of chemical and bacterial substances. It has been demonstrated that epithelial cells attach to the surface of titanium in much the same manner in which the epithelial cells attach to the surface of the natural tooth, that is, through a basal lamina and by the formation of hemidesmosomes. The connection differs from that occurring with natural teeth at the connective tissue attachment level. In the natural dentition, Sharpey's fibers extend from the bundle bone of the lamina dura and insert into the cementum of the tooth root surface. Because no cementum or fiber insertion is found on the surface of an endosseous implant, the epithelial surface attachment is all-important. If this seal is lost, the periodontal pocket can extend directly to the osseous structures. Therefore, if the seal breaks down or is not present, the area of the bone-implant interface is subject to periimplant gingival disease.

Although the abutment–to–junctional epithelium attachment is not mechanically strong, it is adequate to resist bacterial invasion with the assistance of adequate home care. When implants are stable and they have a highly polished titanium collar transversing the tissue, gingival and periimplant health is relatively easy to maintain. The lack of a definitive gingival connective tissue attachment appears to be less of a problem in osseointegrated implants than it was in implants with fibrous connective tissue attachments. Because osseointegrated implants have a different relationship between the implant and bone, there appears to be different mechanisms working against inflammation caused by bacteria and their by-products. The pathogenicity of the bacteria seems to be particularly diminished in the completely edentulous patient restored with dental implants. Inflammation around the natural dentition in the partially edentulous patient may contribute to a slightly higher incidence of periimplant disease in these patients.

Biomechanical Factors Affecting Long-Term Implant Success

Bone resorption around dental implants can be caused by premature loading or repeated overloading. Vertical or angular bone loss is usually characteristic of bone resorption caused by occlusal trauma. When pressure from traumatic occlusion is concentrated, bone resorption occurs by osteoclastic activity. In the natural dentition, bone redeposition would typically occur once the severe stress concentration is reduced or eliminated. However, in the osseointegrated implant system, after bone resorbs, it usually does not reform. Because dental implants can resist forces directed primarily in the long axis of the implant more effectively than they can resist lateral forces, lateral forces on implants should be minimized. Lateral forces in the posterior part of the mouth have higher impact and are more destructive than lateral forces in the anterior part of the mouth. When lateral forces cannot be completely eliminated from the implant prosthesis, efforts should be made to distribute the lateral forces equally over as many teeth and implants as possible.

Divergent implant placement (varying the angle of placement of adjacent implants) can also improve the vectors through which force is transferred to the bone-to-implant interface. Such force could potentially exceed the threshold for bone resorption. Inadequate implant distribution, which leads to excessive cantilevers, can also potentially overload the system (Fig. 14-8).

Connecting a single osseointegrated implant to one natural tooth with a fixed partial denture may effectively create an excessive cantilever situation, as well. Because of the relative

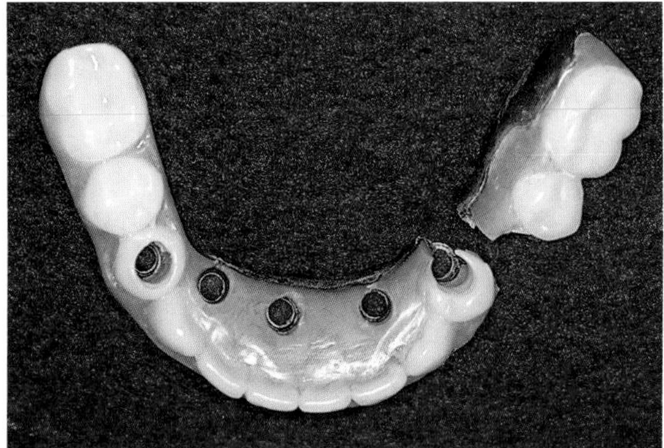

FIGURE 14-8 Cantilever fracture of a metal-resin prosthesis. (Rosenstiel SF, Land MF, Fujimoto J: *Contemporary fixed prosthodontics*, ed 4, St Louis, 2006, Mosby.)

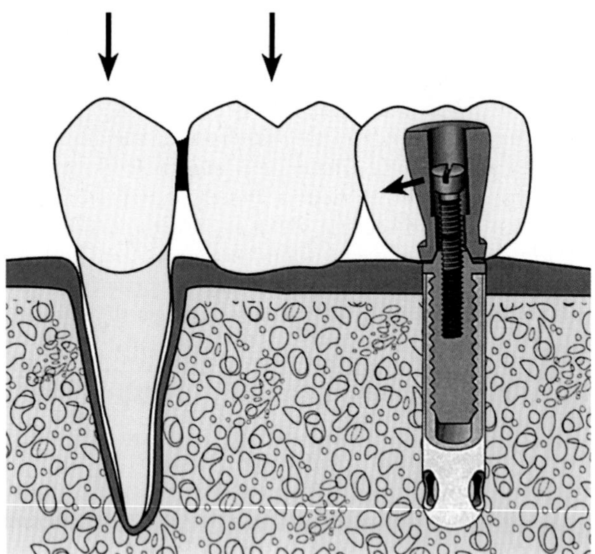

FIGURE 14-9 When a single implant is attached to a natural tooth, biting forces on the natural tooth and pontic cause stress to be concentrated at the superior portion of the implant. (Rosenstiel SF, Land MF, Fujimoto J: *Contemporary fixed prosthodontics*, ed 4, St Louis, 2006, Mosby.)

BOX 14-2

Potential Problems with Tooth- and Implant-Supported Fixed Partial Dentures

1. Breakdown of osseointegration
2. Cement failure on natural abutments
3. Screw or abutment loosening
4. Failure of implant prosthetic component

immobility of the osseointegrated implant compared with the functional mobility of a natural tooth when loads are applied to the bridge, the tooth can move within the limits of its periodontal ligament. This can create stresses at the neck of the implant up to 2 times the applied load on the prosthesis (Fig. 14-9). Potential problems with this type of restoration are described in Box 14-2. Therefore, freestanding implant restorations not attached to any natural teeth should be planned whenever possible.

Additionally, pathogenic forces can be placed on implants by nonpassively fitting frameworks. If screws are tightened to close gaps between the abutment and the nonpassive framework, compressive force is placed on the interfacial bone. Excessive force of this nature can lead to implant failure (Fig. 14-10).

PREOPERATIVE MEDICAL EVALUATION OF IMPLANT PATIENT

As with any surgery, the implant patient must be assessed preoperatively to evaluate the patient's ability to tolerate the proposed procedure. The predictable risks and the expected benefits should be weighed for each patient because surgical placement of dental implants may be associated with certain risks.

Of concern are the immediate surgical and anesthetic risks associated with implant placement. Because implant placement is a relatively atraumatic procedure, little immediate surgical risk exists. Absolute contraindications to implant placement based on immediate surgical and anesthetic risks are limited primarily to patients who are acutely ill, those with uncontrolled metabolic disease, and pregnant patients. These contraindications are applicable to virtually all elective surgical procedures. These conditions are also generally limited in duration; once the illness resolves, the pregnancy is over, or the metabolic disorder is controlled, the patient may become a good implant candidate. Relative contraindications may also exist. Many implant patients are elderly and have preexisting chronic systemic medical conditions such as diabetes mellitus that may effect long-term success of implant treatment. Although the presence of a chronic medical condition is rarely a contraindication to surgical placement of implants, each patient must be evaluated for anesthesia and surgery in light of the preexisting disease process, as discussed in Chapter 1.

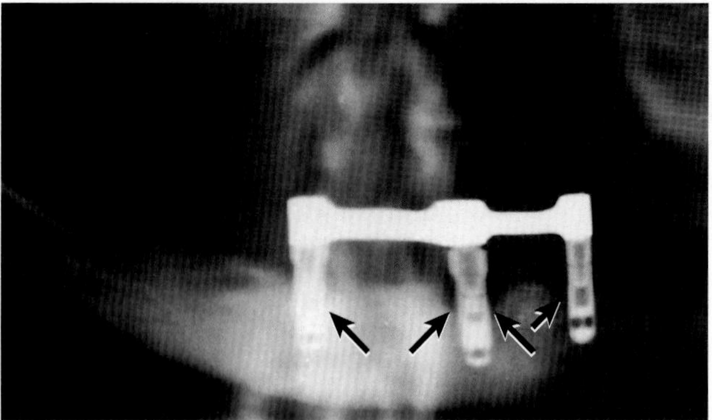

FIGURE 14-10 Stress produced by nonpassive framework can cause bone resorption at implant interface (arrows denote bone loss).

Local and systemic conditions that threaten long-term retention of the implants must be evaluated. Implants may be contraindicated in patients with abnormal bone metabolism, poor oral hygiene, and previous radiation to the implant site or who are smokers. Smoking has been conclusively linked with increased implant failure. Although smoking is not an absolute contraindication, patients who smoke should be counseled on cessation and informed of the increased risk of failure.

Although osteoporosis is prevalent in the geriatric female population, these patients show no documented decrease in the success of implants. Bisphosphonate medications are often used orally for control of osteoporosis. These medications may also be used via an intravenous route as adjunctive therapy for certain malignancies. Although the impact of oral therapy on implant bone healing has not been established, it is clear that previous intravenous bisphosphonate therapy is an absolute contraindication to implant surgery. These patients have high risk of refractory bone necrosis when even minor surgery is performed (see Chapter 18). Other metabolic bone disorders, including osteopetrosis, fibrous dysplasia, chronic diffuse sclerosing osteomyelitis, and florid osseous dysplasia, may contraindicate implant placement.

Most patients who present for implant placement became edentulous from caries and periodontal disease resulting from poor oral hygiene. Suspicion that inadequate hygiene is likely to continue is a relative contraindication to implant placement. Patients must be motivated and educated in oral hygienic techniques as part of their preparation for implants. Some patients

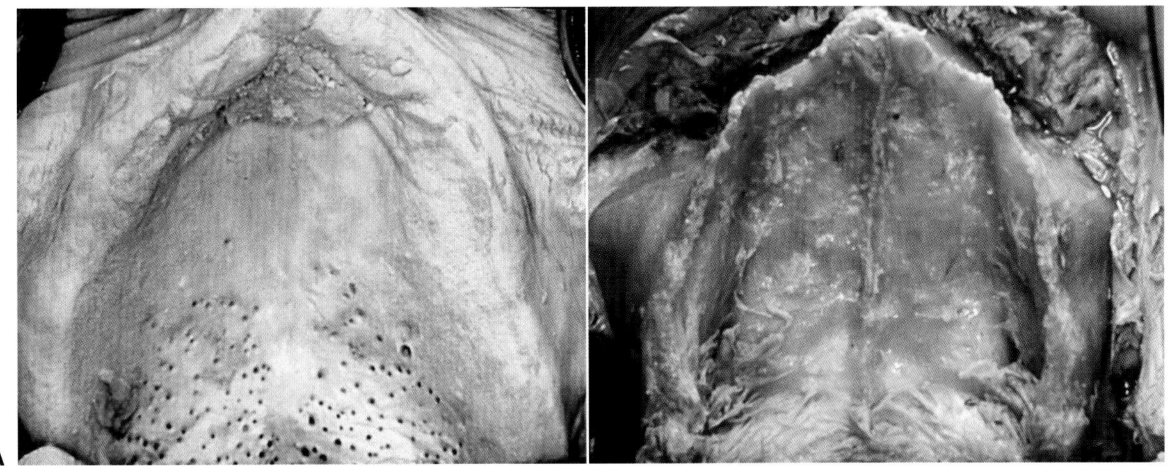

FIGURE 14-11 A, Cadaver specimen of edentulous maxilla that appears to have adequately wide ridge. B, Same specimen with soft tissue removed. Very thin and knife edge ridge is present, which was not evident from clinical examination.

may not be able to improve their hygiene, such as those suffering from paralysis of the arms, debilitating arthritis, cerebral palsy, and severe mental retardation. Implants are contraindicated in these patients, unless caregivers will provide adequate hygiene. A summary of contraindications to implant placement is presented in Box 14-3.

SURGICAL PHASE: TREATMENT PLANNING

Clinical and radiographic evaluation of the planned implant site is essential to treatment planning, to determine whether adequate bone exists and to evaluate the proximity of anatomic structures that may interfere with implant placement.

Evaluation of Implant Site

Evaluation of the planned site begins with a thorough clinical examination. Visual inspection and palpation allow the detection of movable redundant tissue, narrow bony ridges, and sharp underlying ridges and undercuts that may limit implant placement. Clinical inspection alone may not be adequate if the thick overlying soft tissue is dense, immobile, fibrous tissue (Fig. 14-11).

Radiographic evaluation is also necessary, with the best initial film being a panoramic radiograph. Because variations in magnification may occur (Fig. 14-12), a small radiopaque reference object of known size placed at the area of the proposed implant placement allows correction for any magnification. A ball bearing placed in wax on a denture base plate or within polyvinyl siloxane putty adapted to the ridge works well (Fig. 14-13). The known size of the metallic ball bearing can be compared to the size seen on the radiograph, and the degree of magnification can be determined precisely.

Bone width is not revealed on panoramic films but can be evaluated in the anterior maxilla and mandible with a lateral cephalometric film. Width of the posterior mandible and maxilla are primarily determined by clinical examination. Specialized computed tomography scans are useful to determine the location of the inferior alveolar canal and maxillary sinus and to evaluate ridge form (Fig. 14-14). Once only available in limited settings, cone-beam computed tomography has become more commonly available in many dental offices. Such equipment may become the standard of care in the future. For the present time, these imaging devices should be viewed as

BOX 14-3

Contraindications to Implant Placement

- Acute illness
- Terminal illness
- Pregnancy
- Uncontrolled metabolic disease
- Tumoricidal radiation including the implant site*
- History of intravenous bisphosphonate therapy
- Unrealistic expectations
- Improper motivation
- Lack of operator experience
- Unable to restore prosthodontically

*Perioperative hyperbaric therapy may allow implant placement.

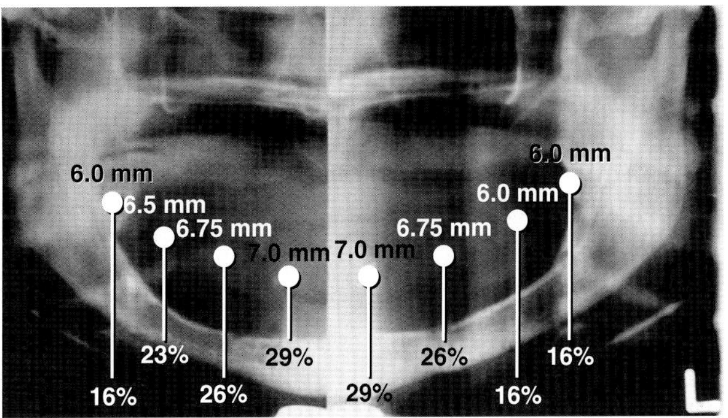

FIGURE 14-12 Panoramic radiograph with standard-sized steel ball bearings placed along ridge. Magnification varies from site to site.

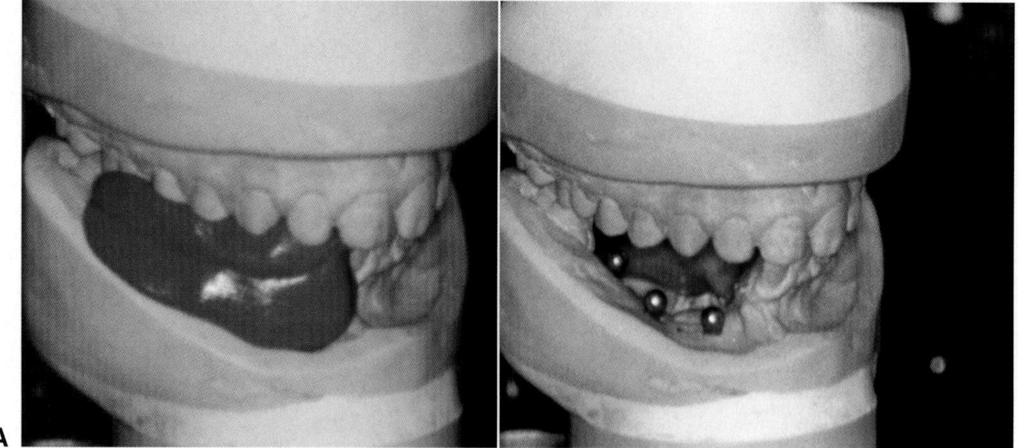

FIGURE 14-13 A, Steel ball bearings of known diameter are placed on cast at points at which implants are to be placed. B, Polyvinyl siloxane impression material is placed over bearings. This can be carried to mouth and used to produce a radiograph with ball bearings as a standard to calculate effect of magnification.

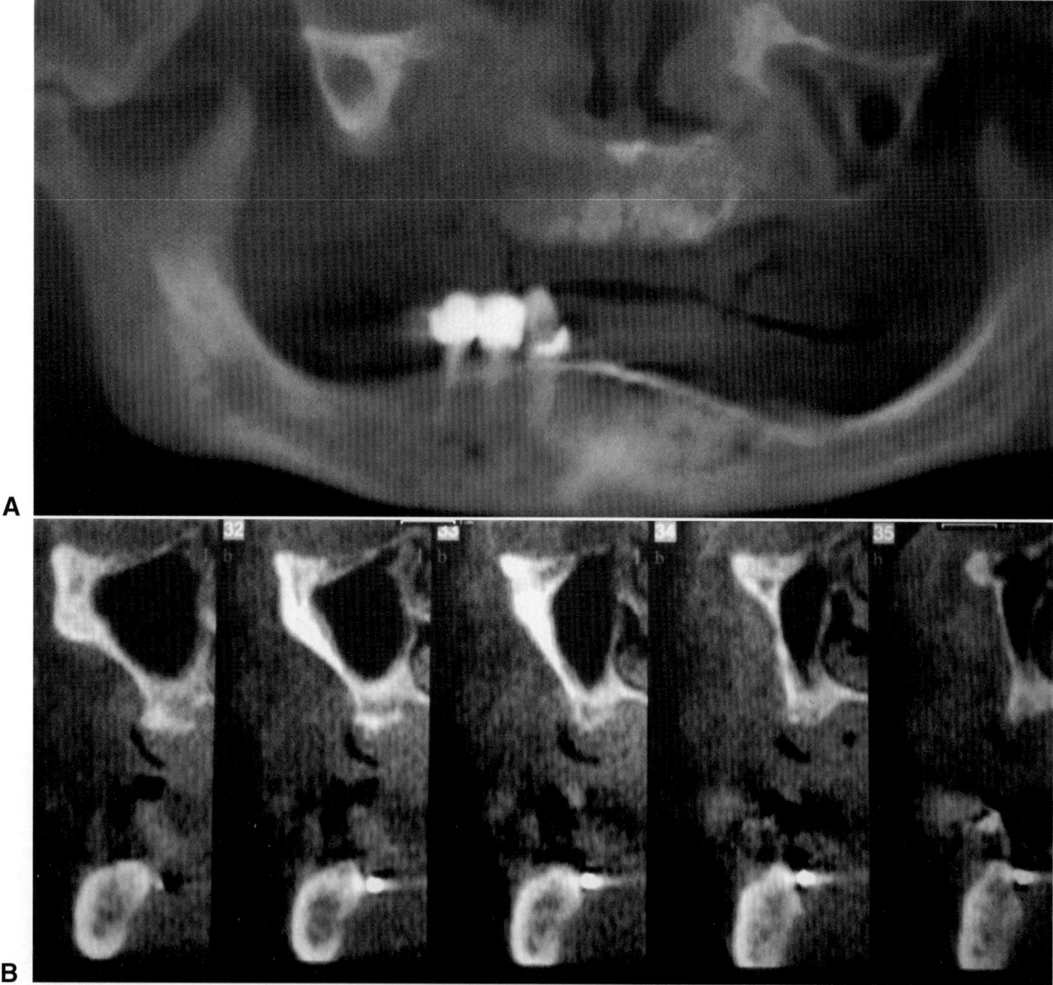

FIGURE 14-14 A, Panoramic film shows possible pneumatization of the maxillary sinus. Determination of the quantity of bone available for implant placement is difficult. B, Reformatted computed tomographic scan allows direct visualization of bone morphology in several areas of the maxilla.

adjunctive tools because their routine use is not required and has not been demonstrated to improve outcome or decrease morbidity.

Bone Height, Width, and Anatomic Limitations

Bone quality and quantity are important considerations. In general, more cortical bone and denser cancellous bone (i.e., anterior mandible) is associated with higher implant success compared with thinner cortical bone and loose cancellous marrow (i.e., posterior maxilla). Bone quality has been classified as types I to IV (Fig. 14-15). In type I to III bone, implant success, regardless of length, is predictably high. However, in type IV bone, short implants (<10 mm) have significantly higher failure rates.

To maximize the chance for success, there must be adequate bone width to allow 1 mm of bone on the lingual aspect and 1 mm on the facial aspect of the implant. There should also be adequate space between the implants. The minimal distance between implants varies slightly among implant systems but is generally accepted as 3 mm. This minimal space is necessary to ensure bone viability between the implants and to allow adequate oral hygiene once the restorative dentistry is complete.

Specific limitations as a result of anatomic variations between different areas of the jaws must also be considered. Implant length, diameter, proximity to adjacent structures, and time required to achieve integration varies in areas within the jaws. The anterior maxilla, posterior maxilla, anterior mandible, and posterior mandible each require special consideration when placing implants. Some common guidelines for implant placement are summarized in Table 14-1.

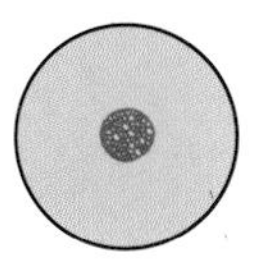

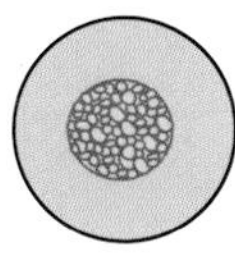

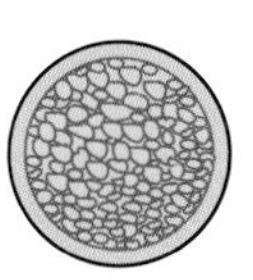

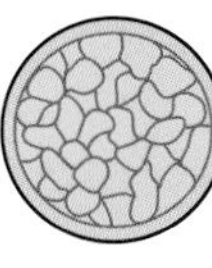

FIGURE 14-15 Bone types based on quantity of cortical bone and density of cancellous marrow. (Misch CE: *Contemporary implant dentistry*, ed 3, St Louis, 2008, Mosby.)

TABLE 14-1

Anatomic Limitations to Implant Placement

Structure	Minimum Required Distance Between Implant and Indicated Structure
Buccal plate	1 mm
Lingual plate	1 mm
Maxillary sinus	1 mm
Nasal cavity	1 mm
Incisive canal	Avoid midline maxilla
Interimplant distance	3 mm between outer edge of implants
Inferior alveolar canal	2 mm from superior aspect of bony canal
Mental nerve	5 mm from anterior of bony foramen
Inferior border	1 mm
Adjacent natural tooth	1 mm

After tooth loss, resorption of the ridge follows a pattern that results in crestal bone thinning and changes in angulation of the residual ridge, which is most often a problem in the anterior mandible and maxilla. The altered anatomy of the residual ridge may lead to intraoperative problems of achieving ideal implant angulation or lack of adequate bone along the labial aspect of the implant. This is a particular problem in the esthetic zone. Techniques for intraoperative management of these problems are discussed later, but the potential for such problems must be anticipated in the preoperative phase to allow adequate management.

The anterior maxilla must be evaluated for proximity of the nasal cavity. A minimum of 1 mm of bone should be left between the apical end of the implant and the nasal cavity. The incisive foramen may be located near the residual ridge as a result of resorption of anterior maxillary bone. This is especially true in patients in whom the edentulous maxilla has been allowed to function against natural mandibular anterior dentition. Anterior maxillary implants should be located slightly off midline on either side of the incisive foramen.

Implant placement in the posterior maxilla poses two specific concerns: First, as previously discussed, the *quality* of the bone in the maxilla, particularly the posterior maxilla, is poorer than mandibular bone. Larger marrow spaces and thinner, less dense cortical bone affect treatment planning because increased time must be allowed for integration of implants. Generally, a minimum of 6 months is necessary for adequate integration of implants placed in the maxilla (Table 14-2).

The second concern is that the maxillary sinus is in proximity to the edentulous ridge in the posterior maxilla. Frequently, as a result of resorption of bone and increased pneumatization of the sinus, only a few millimeters of bone are found between the ridge and the sinus (Fig. 14-16). In treat-

TABLE 14-2

Traditional Minimum Integration Times

Region of Implant Placement	Minimum Integration Time
Anterior mandible	3 months
Posterior mandible	4 months
Anterior maxilla	6 months
Posterior maxilla	6 months
Into bone graft	6 to 9 months

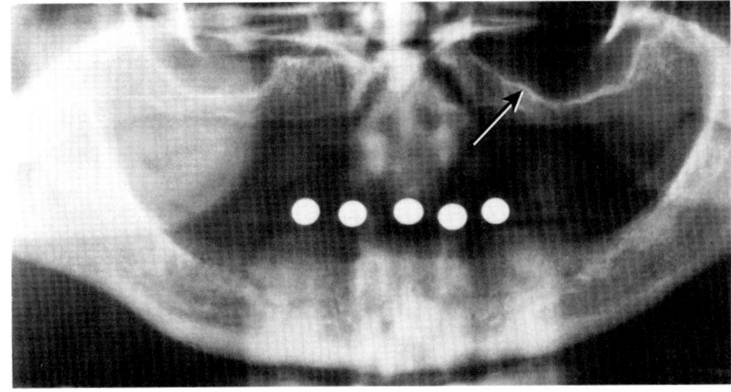

FIGURE 14-16 Radiograph illustrates how pneumatization of maxillary sinus and crestal bone loss together produce residual ridge that is not capable of supporting implant (*arrow*).

ment planning of implants in the posterior maxilla, the surgeon should plan to leave 1 mm of bone between the floor of the sinus and the implant. This allows the implant to be anchored apically into the cortical bone of the sinus floor. Adequate bone height for implant stability can usually be found in the area between the nasal cavity and maxillary sinus. If inadequate bone exists for implant placement and support, bony augmentation through the sinus may be performed as discussed in the section on advanced surgical techniques.

The posterior mandible poses some limitations on implant placement. The inferior alveolar nerve traverses the mandibular body in this region. Treatment planning of implant length must allow for a 2-mm margin from the apical end of the implant to the superior aspect of the inferior alveolar canal (Fig. 14-17), which is an inviolable guideline to avoid damaging the inferior alveolar nerve and causing numbness of the lower lip. If inadequate length is present for even the shortest available implant, then nerve repositioning, grafting, or a conventional non–implant-borne prosthesis can be considered. These procedures are discussed further in the section on advanced surgical techniques.

Implants placed in the posterior mandible are usually shorter, do not engage cortical bone inferiorly, and must support increased biomechanical occlusal force once loaded. As a result, slightly increased time for integration may be beneficial. Additionally, if short implants (8 to 10 mm) are used, it is advisable to "overengineer" and to place more implants than usual to withstand the occlusal load.

The width of the residual ridge must also be carefully evaluated in the posterior mandible. Attachment of the mylohyoid muscle may maintain bony width along the superior aspect of the ridge, although a deep lingual depression forms immediately below (Fig. 14-18). This area should be palpated at the time of evaluation and visualized at surgery.

The anterior mandible is usually the most straightforward area for treatment planning with respect to anatomic limitations. The mandible is usually wide enough and tall enough to provide adequate bone for implant placement. The bone quality is usually excellent, which makes this the area of the jaw that requires the least time for integration to occur. In the premolar area, care must be taken to ensure that the implant is placed anterior to the mental foramen. The inferior alveolar nerve usually courses anterior to the mental foramen before turning posteriorly and superiorly to exit the mental foramen. Because the nerve may be as much as 3 mm anterior to the foramen, the most posterior extent of the implant should be a minimum of 5 mm anterior to the mental foramen (Fig. 14-19).

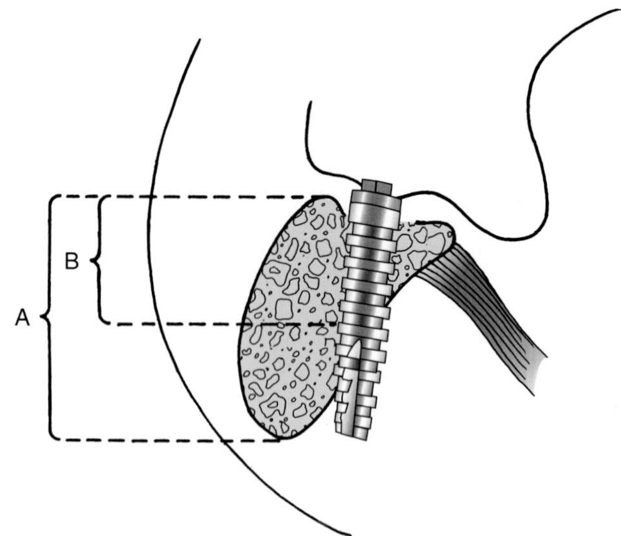

FIGURE 14-18 Mylohyoid muscle will maintain bone along its attachment on medial of mandibular body. Frequently, a significant depression is found just below this. If implant position and angulation do not compensate, lingual perforation may result. Apparent bone height on radiograph (*A*) and actual height in desired area (*B*) are demonstrated.

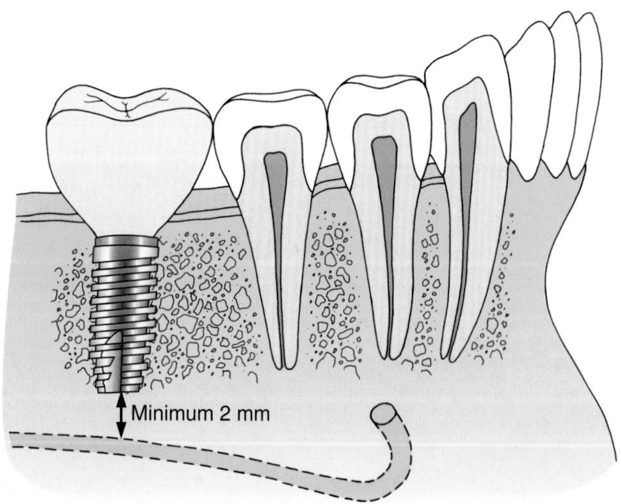

FIGURE 14-17 Implants should be placed a minimum of 2 mm from inferior alveolar canal.

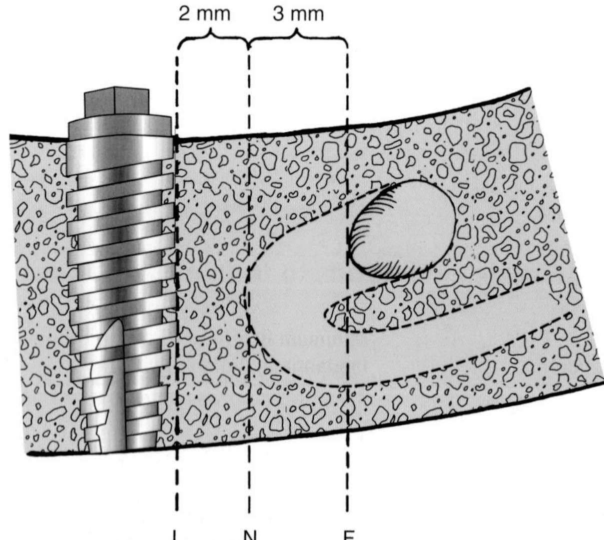

FIGURE 14-19 Most anterior extent of bony mental foramen (*F*) is frequently located posterior to most anterior extent of mental nerve before its exit from bone (*N*). Most posterior aspect of implant (*I*) should be placed a minimum of 2 mm from nerve. This means that implant must be placed 5 mm anterior to most anterior aspect of bony mental foramen.

Informed Consent

Once adequate information is obtained to allow formulation of a treatment plan, informed consent is obtained before surgery. This step is best accomplished using a team approach involving the surgeon and the restorative dentist. The combined surgical and restorative plan and feasible nonimplant alternatives are presented to the patient so that he or she can make an informed decision whether to proceed with treatment.

Models of various implant-supported prostheses can be used to demonstrate the proposed treatment. The patient should be informed about the timing of surgery, the possible necessity of two surgical procedures, and the expected time between the initial surgery and the delivery of the finished prosthesis. The patient should also be informed of the need to leave existing dentures out and the length of time this must be done. The patient should be informed about potential short- and long-term risks, such as nerve injury, infection, and implant failure. Finally, a clear understanding of the expected cost of the proposed treatment should be reached. After this information is discussed, the patient should sign a written informed consent document.

Surgical Guide Template

The coordination of the surgical and prosthetic procedures through proper treatment planning is one of the most critical factors in obtaining an ideal esthetic and functional result for the implant restoration. The surgical guide template is a critical factor for implants placed in an esthetic area because even slight variations of angulation can have large effects on the appearance of the final restoration. The construction of the surgical guide template is nearly indispensable for those patients for whom it is necessary to optimize implant placement to ensure correct emergence profiles in the anterior esthetic zone. The four objectives of using a surgical template for the partially edentulous patient are as follows: (1) delineate embrasure, (2) locate implant within tooth contour, (3) align implants with long axis of completed restoration, and (4) identify level of cementoenamel junction or tooth emergence from the soft tissue. The template most useful in the anterior esthetic zone is a clear resin template, which allows a surgeon ease of access to the bone and uninterrupted visual confirmation of frontal and sagittal angulations (Fig. 14-20). Although the underlying bone may dictate some minor variation, the surgeon must stay as close as possible to the template during implant placement (Fig. 14-21). The ultimate result should allow the surgeon to place the implant optimally in bone while maintaining the angulation that will provide the least compromise of the final restoration.

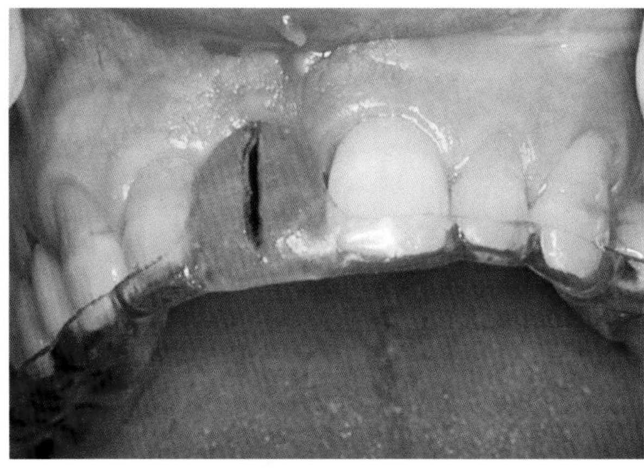

FIGURE 14-20 Anterior surgical guide. Thickness should equal that of porcelain on final restoration. Distance from facial of tooth to be restored and lingual extent of template should be approximately 2 mm. The embrasures, tooth form, position, angulation, and cementoenamel junction are clearly identifiable.

In posterior edentulous areas, a similar template is fabricated with directional holes drilled through the template. This surgical template provides the surgeon with a guide to locate the implant placement accurately and direct the long-access inclination of the implant (Fig. 14-22).

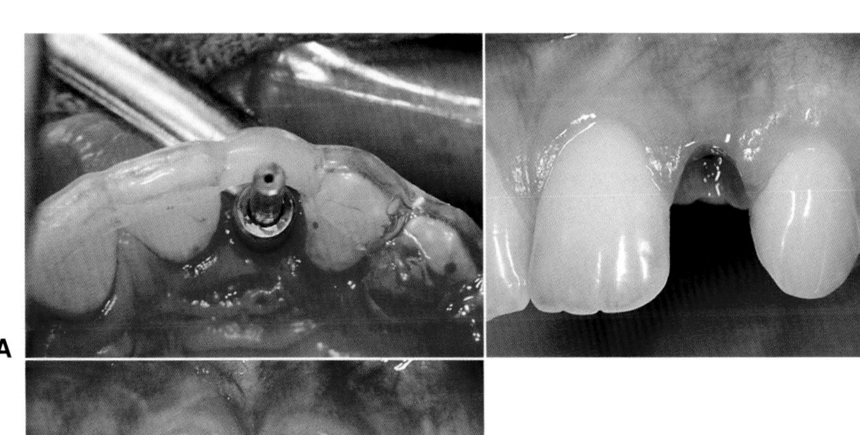

FIGURE 14-21 A, Surgical guide in place with paralleling pin identifying the position of the implant, which is well within the contours of the planned restoration. B, Resulting implant position, angulation, and depth produces natural contours that (C) result in ideal form of the final restoration.

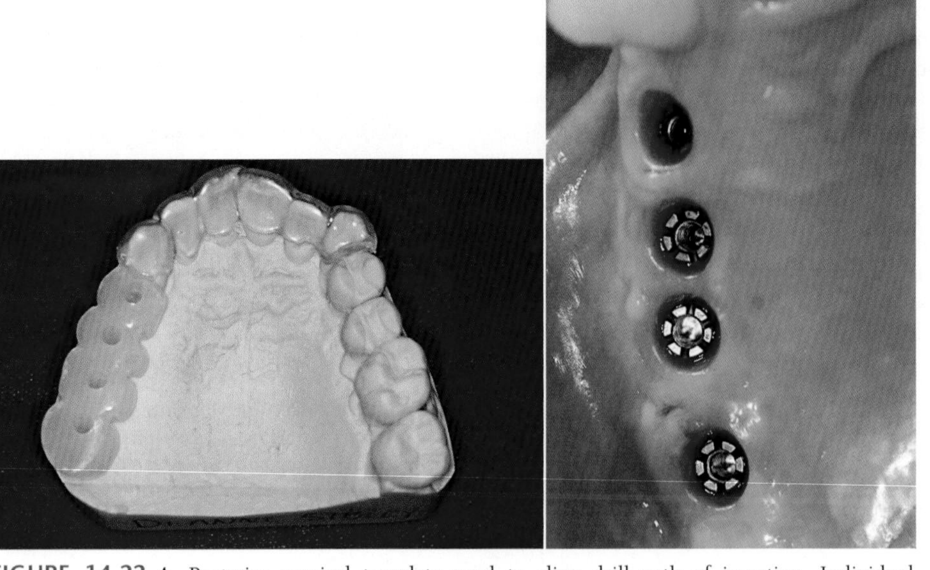

FIGURE 14-22 A, Posterior surgical template used to align drill path of insertion. Individual embrasure spaces are delineated by template. B, Resulting position of implants.

The surgical template for the completely edentulous mandible should allow the surgeon maximal flexibility to select the implant position in the resorbed bone but yet provide guidance as to the angulation requirements of the restorative dentist. A template with a labial flange that simulates the labial surface of the anticipated position of the denture teeth but that is cut out on the lingual aspect satisfies these two requirements (Fig. 14-23). The surgeon places the implants within the arch form, as close to the surgical template as possible, to prevent the placement of the implants too far lingually or labially.

BASIC SURGICAL TECHNIQUE

Before Implant Placement

Successful implant placement relies on adequate bone quantity and quality. The availability of bone at the implant site is based on many variables. Some of the variables controlled by the dentist include use of atraumatic extraction techniques, preservation of the bony socket, selection of an interim prosthesis, and timing of implant placement.

Atraumatic Extraction

An intact socket is critical to achieve full bony regeneration. A "four-walled" defect produced by an intact socket will regenerate bone with minimal loss of width and contour. Lone standing teeth and teeth with prominent labial roots pose a risk to the labial plate. Atraumatic extraction with a periotome preserves the contour and integrity of this bone.

Socket Preservation

After extraction, some marginal resorption of bone takes place and the residual ridge may thin. This bone loss can compromise ideal implant placement. To encourage consistent healing and lessen the time between extraction and implant placement, reconstruction of the socket may be considered. A number of alloplastic and allogeneic grafts or xenografts are

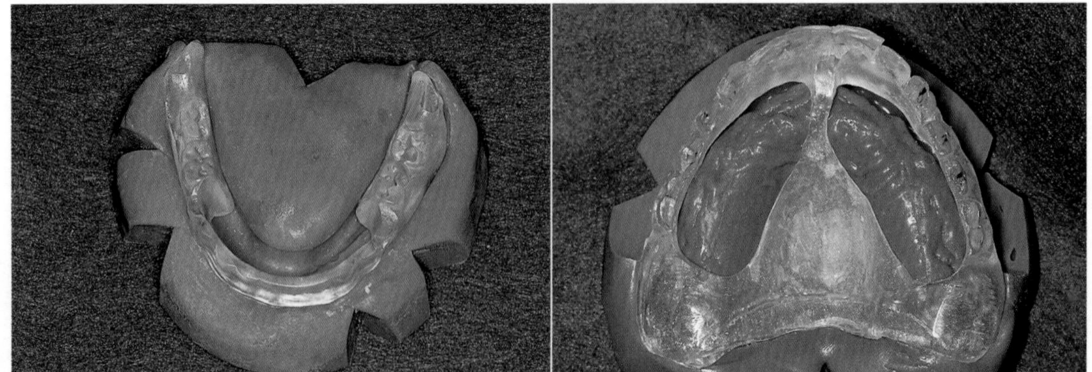

FIGURE 14-23 A and B, Edentulous surgical templates should delineate arch form and facial tooth location. Access for the surgeon and maximal flexibility to select the implant position in the resorbed bone while guiding angulation is achieved. A template with a labial flange that simulates the labial surface of the anticipated position of the denture teeth but that is cut out on the lingual aspect satisfies these two requirements.

available. Alternatively, the implant itself may be placed into the residual socket. If there is adequate stability, this may aid in preservation of the bony contour. Indications for this are discussed later in this chapter. Even if the extraction site meets the requirements for immediate implant placement, it may be desirable to delay implant placement. If the socket is reconstructed with a graft, as little as 2 months is an adequate waiting period before implant placement. During this time the overlying soft tissue heals, and primary closure is easier at the time of implant placement.

This time is generally long enough to allow remodeling of the socket and, in the case of multirooted teeth, some filling of the socket with bone. In this situation, implants are placed using the same technique described for routine implant placement. The bone in the area of surgery is softer but generally allows preparation of the implant recipient site with little modification. No increase in integration time is generally necessary in this situation.

Interim Prosthesis Design

The interim prosthesis should be designed to aid in contouring the residual soft tissue. It is important that the tissue-borne provisional prosthesis not produce excess pressure on the underlying soft tissue and bone, particularly on the interdental papilla. An ovate style pontic with open embrasures to allow room for the normal papilla anatomy is preferable to a ridge lap design (Fig. 14-24).

Timing of Implant Placement

Excessive delay between extraction and implant placement may result in bone loss. Although a period of 2 to 6 months following extraction can aid in improved bone quality, longer delay may result in bone resorption. Implant placement produces functional stresses in the bone that helps maintain contour and bulk. In the absence of a natural tooth or an implant, bone will resorb. Excessive resorption may necessitate grafting procedures before an implant can be placed. Patients undergoing extraction should be educated about this window of opportunity.

Implant Placement

Patient Preparation

Implant surgery can be performed in an ambulatory setting with local anesthesia. Such surgery requires more time than other surgical procedures, so the use of conscious sedation is often beneficial. Although implant placement is less traumatic than tooth extraction, the patient has the expectation that it will be more so. Preoperative patient education and conscious sedation help to lessen anxiety.

Preoperative antibiotic prophylaxis is usually recommended. An oral dose of 2 g penicillin V 1 hour preoperatively or an intravenous dose of 1 million units penicillin G immediately preoperatively are effective. Alternative medications include 600 mg clindamycin orally or intravenously. No postoperative antibiotic administration is necessary.

Profound local anesthesia is required for precise implant placement. In the atrophic anterior mandible, block anesthesia, as well as infiltration anesthesia, is sometimes required to achieve this goal.

Adequate aseptic technique minimizes the risk for postoperative infection. The patient can rinse with 15 mL 0.12% chlorhexidine gluconate (Peridex) for 30 seconds immediately before the start of surgery. This significantly reduces the oral microbial count and maintains a reduced level for 1 hour or more. The surgeon and assistants should follow sound aseptic techniques using masks, sterile gloves, and sterile instrumentation. A complete sterile surgical gown is not required.

Proper implant placement is a technically demanding procedure requiring precision. Therefore, adequate visualization is critical. Carefully directed lighting and adequate retraction are necessary.

Soft Tissue Incision

Several types of incisions can be used to gain access to the residual ridge for implant placement. The incision should be designed to allow convenient retraction of the soft tissue for unimpeded implant placement. The incision should preserve or increase the quantity of attached tissue and preserve local soft tissue esthetics. Access can be gained through open or closed techniques. The closed technique uses a tissue punch to gain access only to the crestal bone. The closed technique relies on the surgeon's ability to determine bone morphology without direct visualization and works best with wide, uniform ridges.

An open approach is more predictable but also more invasive. When the quantity of attached tissue is adequate and

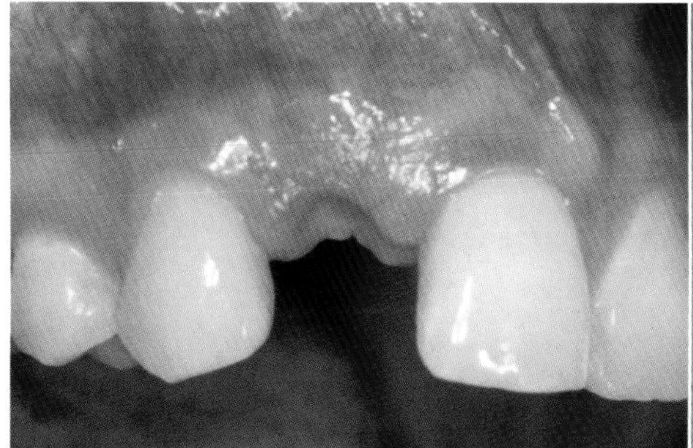
A

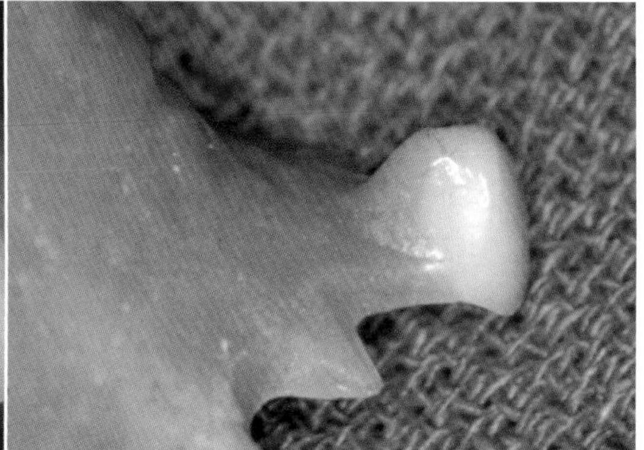
B

FIGURE 14-24 A, The interim prosthesis should be designed to aid in contouring the residual soft tissue. B, An ovate-style pontic with open embrasures to allow room for the papilla is preferable to a ridge lap design.

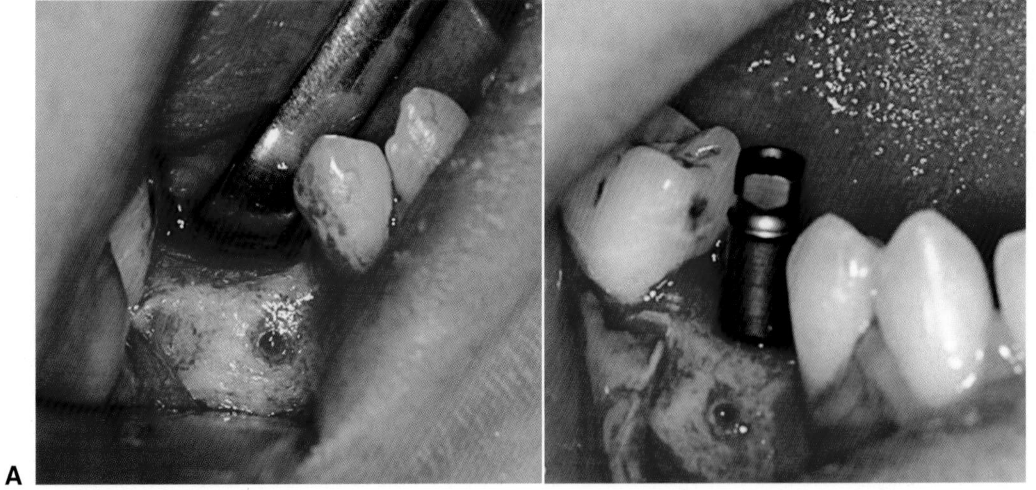

FIGURE 14-25 A, A simple crestal incision allows good access to the ridge when adequate bone contour and soft tissue health is present. B, Implant position is easily visualized with this access.

the underlying bone is expected to be of adequate width, a simple crestal incision is the incision of choice (Fig. 14-25). Closure of the incision must be done carefully, because the implants lie directly beneath the incision. This approach works well in the mandible and posterior maxilla. An incision placed slightly palatal may be a better choice in the anterior maxilla, especially when esthetics is of concern, because it preserves facial contour and soft tissue bulk. In the esthetic zone, an incision that preserves the adjacent papilla may be helpful.

Preparation of the Implant Site

After the bone is exposed, the surgical guide template is positioned and a preliminary assessment of the implant site is made. The residual ridge may have areas of unevenness or sharp ridges that are best reduced with a rongeur or a bur before drilling for implant placement. Fibrous tissue should also be removed so that it will not be incorporated into the implant site.

Placement procedures for all implant systems require atraumatic preparation of the recipient site. A low-speed (1500 to 2000 rpm), high-torque handpiece and copious irrigation are necessary to prevent excess thermal injury to the bone. Irrigation may be externally applied or internally directed through the drills. Recommendations of the specific implant manufacturer should be followed because they relate to the type of irrigation and the allowable speed of the drilling equipment.

The implant site is located using the surgical guide template, which may also assist in directing the angulation of the implant. All implant systems have an initial small-diameter drill that is used to mark the implant site. With the initial drill the center of the implant recipient site is marked and the initial pilot hole is prepared (Fig. 14-26). The implant recipient site preparation continues by drilling with a series of gradually larger burs.

A paralleling pin is placed in the initial preparation to check alignment and angulation (Fig. 14-27).

Once the initial preparation for the implant is determined to be appropriate, it is sequentially enlarged to a dimension that precisely conforms to the dimensions of the implant. Care must be taken to maintain the angulation and depth established by the initial drill. Tapered implants may require separate drills for each depth. Failure to follow implant manufacuturer protocols correctly regarding drilling sequence may result in implants that are placed too deep or too shallow or that have inadequate stability or excessive insertion forces leading to bone necrosis.

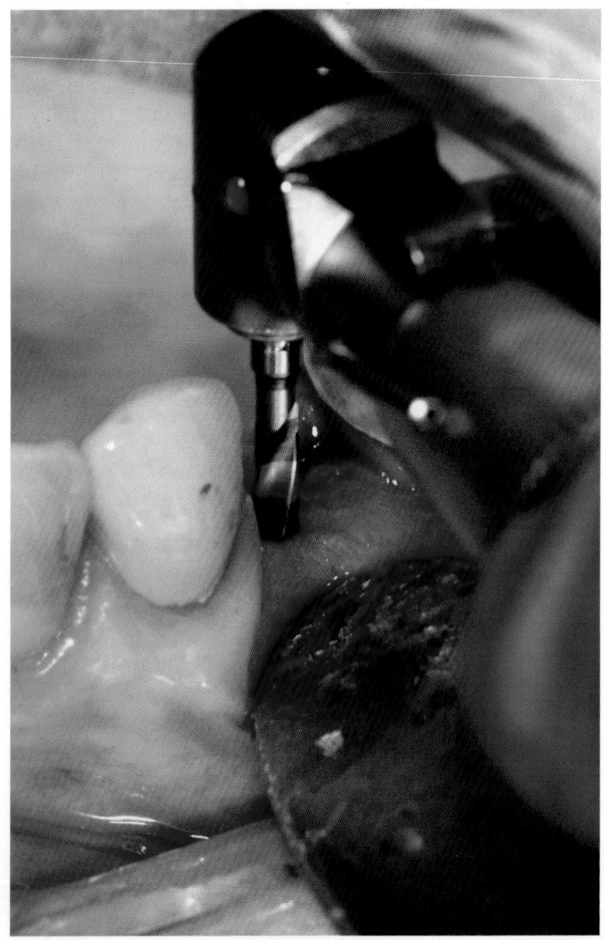

FIGURE 14-26 Initial position, angulation, and depth is established with the first twist drill in the sequence.

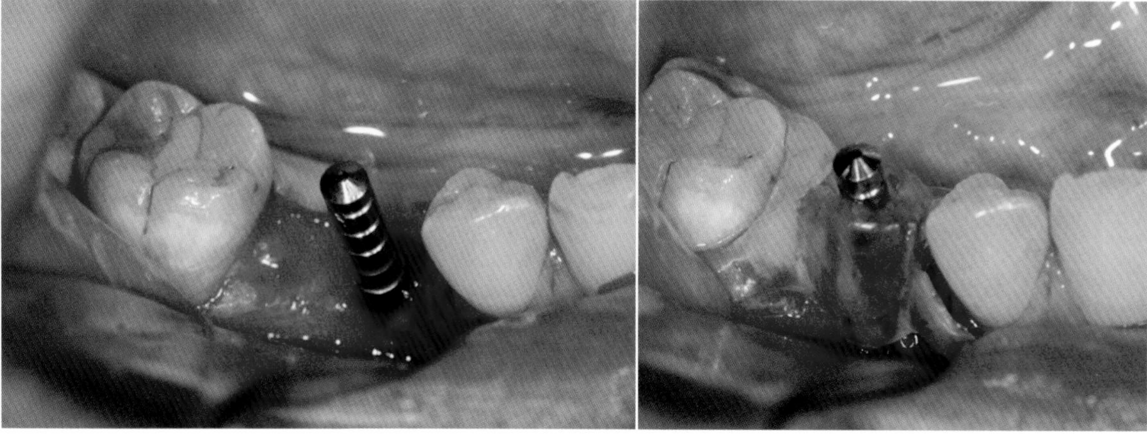

FIGURE 14-27 A, Initial osteotomy has been prepared, and paralleling pin is placed to evaluate position and angulation. B, The surgical guide can be placed over the paralleling pin for confirmation.

Implant Placement

After the desired depth and diameter of the recipient site is accomplished, the implant is placed. For titanium implants, an uncontaminated surface oxide layer is necessary to obtain osseointegration. Contamination by touching the implant with instruments made of a dissimilar metal or by contact with cloth, soft tissue, or even surgical gloves may affect the degree of osseointegration. Hydroxyapatite-coated implants are also sensitive to contamination. Hydroxyapatite is porous and easily absorbs liquids or oils and becomes contaminated with fibers from cloth drapes or powder from surgical gloves.

Although some implants are pressed into place, most are threaded and must be screwed into place. Implants can be screwed in place by a handpiece at very low speeds (e.g., 15 rpm) or by hand (Fig. 14-28). Final tightening in most cases is done by hand with a ratchet. Modern threaded implants are self-tapping. However, in very dense bone, the recipient site may need to be tapped to produce threads within the bone, thereby avoiding excess torque and heat during implant placement. Excess torque can damage the anti-rotational features of the implant, may crush the bone leading to necrosis, or may even induce fractures.

After all implants are placed, the wound is closed. A tension-free closure is important to prevent wound dehiscence.

In some cases the surgeon may plan to leave the implant exposed following placement. In these cases a longer healing post is added to the implant and the soft tissue is contoured around the post that extends from the top of the implant through the soft tissue into the oral cavity. This technique eliminates the need for a second-stage uncovering of the implant and may produce a more mature gingival contour. This technique increases requirements for oral hygiene care of the exposed implant because of the increased risk of trauma and mobility and should be reserved for implants with good primary stability at the time of placement.

Postoperative Care

A radiograph should be taken postoperatively to evaluate the position of the implant in relation to adjacent structures, such as the sinus and inferior alveolar canal, and relative to other implants.

Patients should be provided analgesics. Mild- to moderate-strength analgesics are usually sufficient. Rarely are potent oral analgesics required. Patients can also be instructed to use 0.12% chlorhexidine gluconate (Peridex) rinses for 2 weeks after surgery to help keep bacterial populations at a minimum during healing. The patient is evaluated weekly until soft tissue wound healing is complete (approximately 2 to 3 weeks). If the patient wears a tissue-borne denture over the area of

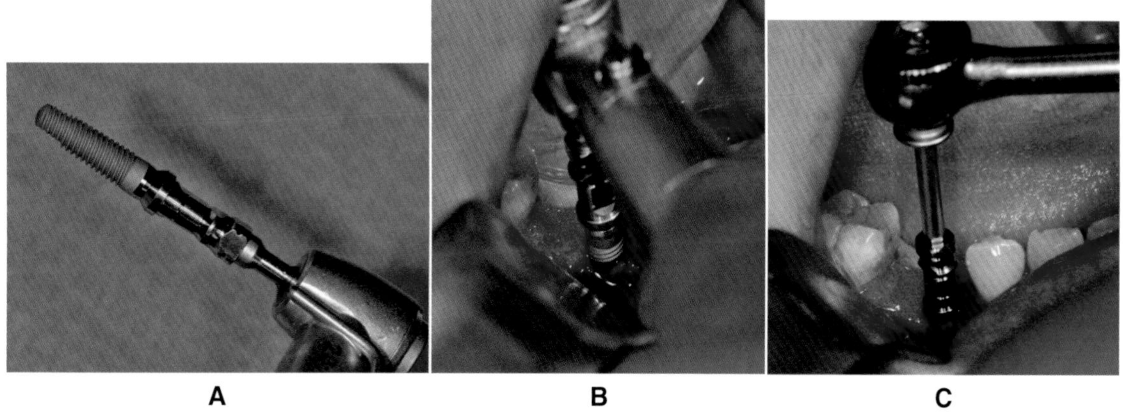

FIGURE 14-28 A, Most implants are threaded and must be screwed into place. B, This can be done by handpiece at very low speeds (e.g., 15 rpm) or by hand. C, Final tightening is done with a ratchet.

implant placement, the denture can be relined with a soft liner after 1 week and may be worn. Interim partial dentures or orthodontic retainers with an attached pontic may be worn immediately but must be contoured to avoid soft tissue loading over the implant site.

Uncovering

The length of time necessary to achieve integration varies from site to site and may require modification based on the particular situation. Successful loading with shorter integration times has been reported when various protocols are followed, and immediate loading in controlled settings has reported success (Table 14-2 gives conventionally accepted times for integration based on historical experience, which should serve as a reference point). Although shorter times may be possible, longer times may be required if the bone quality at surgery was poor or if there was a question regarding the adequacy of bone-to-implant interface at the time of placement.

In a single-stage system the implant remains exposed after surgery and throughout the healing phase. After appropriate integration time, restoration can proceed. In a two-stage system the implant must be uncovered before restoration. The goals of surgical uncovering are to attach the abutment accurately to the implant, preserve attached tissue, and recontour and thin tissue or add form and thickness to existing tissue. This may be accomplished by one of the following general techniques: the tissue punch, crestal incision, flap repositioning, or soft tissue grafting. Each has its own advantages and indications (Box 14-4).

The simplest method of implant uncovering is the tissue punch (Fig. 14-29). This method of uncovering is easy to perform, only minimally disturbs the tissue surrounding the implant, and produces minimal patient discomfort. To use this technique, the implant must be located with certainty below the tissue. Use of the punch is contraindicated if inadequate attached tissue will remain after the punch is used. The punch also has the slight disadvantage of not allowing visualization of the bone. If a graft was placed or if there was some question regarding the relationship between the marginal bone and the implant, this technique would not allow assessment at the time of uncovering, and nonresorbable guided tissue regeneration membranes could not be removed. This technique also makes visualization of the abutment–to–implant body interface difficult. The operator must rely on tactile sense to determine whether the abutment is completely seated on the implant body.

If the implants cannot be palpated or the clinician needs to visualize the marginal bone, a crestal incision over the implant is indicated. If sufficient attached tissue is found, a punch or scissors can be used to contour the edge of the flap to conform to the implant before wound closure. This technique also heals rapidly because primary closure exists. This technique also requires adequate attached tissue.

If attached tissue surrounding the implant is limited or inadequate, an apically repositioned flap is the uncovering method of choice. A crestal incision developed in a supraperiosteal plane is performed to develop a split-thickness flap. The flap is then sutured over the facial surface at a more apical level. Healing occurs by secondary intention. This technique requires the longest healing time and is more painful. The technique preserves and increases the amount of attached soft tissue but does not improve tissue thickness.

BOX 14-4

Indications for Various Uncovering Techniques

TISSUE PUNCH

Requirements

Adequate attached tissue
Implant can be palpated

Advantages

Least traumatic
Periosteum not reflected—less bone resorption
Early impressions are possible

Disadvantages

Sacrifice of attached tissue
Unable to visualize bone
Unable to visualize implant and superstructure interface

CRESTAL INCISION

Requirement

Adequate attached tissue

Advantages

Does not require implants to be palpable
Easy access
Minimal trauma
Able to visualize bone
Able to visualize implant and superstructure interface

Disadvantage

Periosteum reflected—may lead to bone loss

APICALLY REPOSITIONED FLAP

Advantage

Improves vestibular depth and attached tissue

Disadvantages

Longer healing time
Bone loss as a result of reflection of periosteum
Technically more difficult

In some situations the bulk of soft tissue is not adequate to produce proper contour around the implant. This is especially a problem in the anterior maxilla where, despite adequate osseous contour and proper implant placement, a localized depression at the facial margin of the crown is found that will compromise esthetics. In this situation a pedicled or free connective tissue graft is an effective way to restore soft tissue form around the implant (Fig. 14-30). These procedures allow minor changes in the tissue height around the implant crown but cannot substitute for adequate osseous form that must always be maintained (or reestablished first).

In situations in which the overlying tissue is thick, it may be necessary to recontour tissue. A carbon dioxide laser or electrocautery is effective. Laser or bipolar cautery poses less risk of damage to the implant or bone than conventional monopolar cautery.

After the implant is exposed, the implant abutment is placed. Two approaches can be used to do this: One approach is to place the abutment that the restorative dentist will use in the restoration. This is effective in the mandible and posterior maxilla where esthetics is of less concern. The other technique is to place a temporary healing abutment that will remain until the tissue heals and will then be discarded and replaced by the final prosthesis. This may be a factory or custom-made

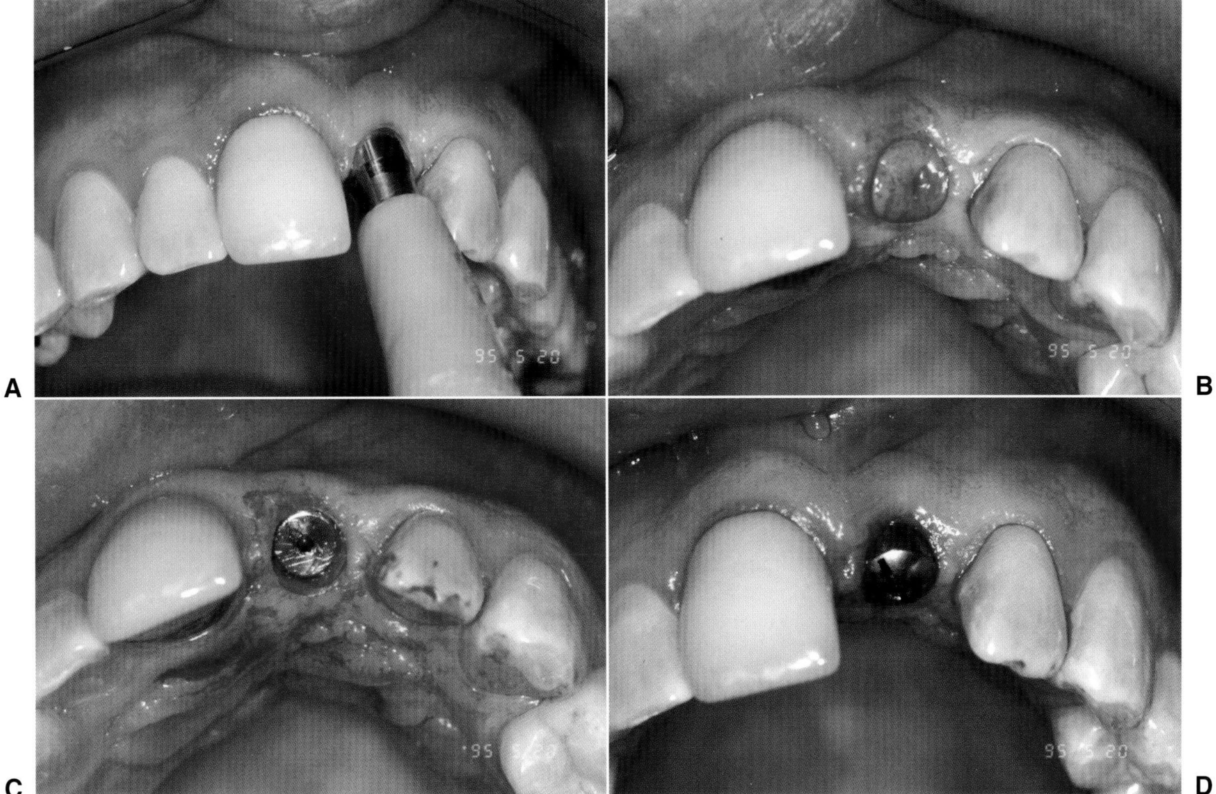

FIGURE 14-29 A to D, The simplest method of implant uncovering is the tissue punch. This method of uncovering is easy to perform, only minimally disturbs the tissue surrounding the implant, and produces minimal patient discomfort. To use this technique, the implant must be located with certainty below the tissue.

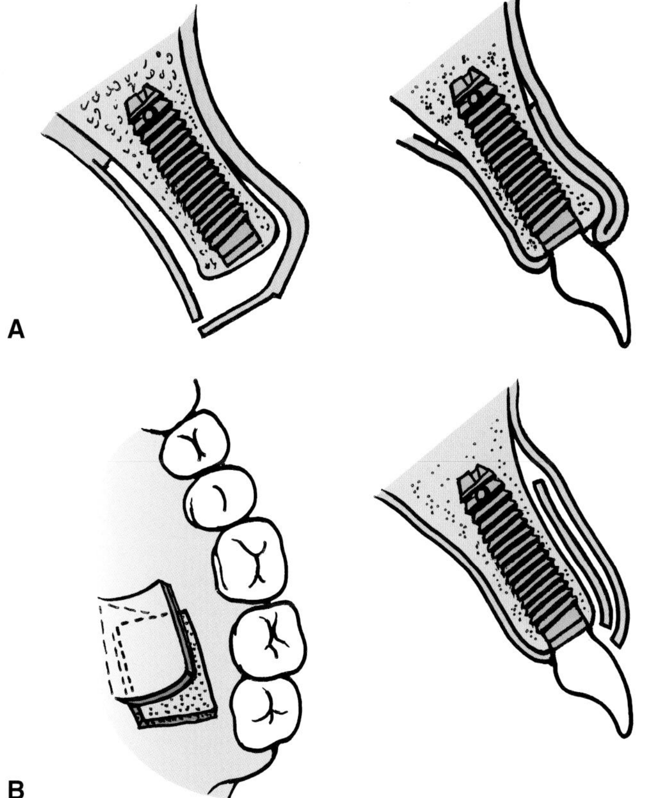

FIGURE 14-30 A, Pedicled connective tissue graft from the palate can be used to augment the labial soft tissue contour. B, Free connective tissue graft can also be used to provide the same outcome.

abutment. A custom abutment helps contour soft tissue for better esthetic results. Custom abutments are made from an index of implant position recorded at the time of placement.

When the abutment is placed, it is important that it be completely seated on the implant body without gaps or intervening soft or hard tissue. In systems that have antirotational facets built into the implant, these must be aligned to allow complete seating of the abutment. The abutment-to-implant interface should be evaluated radiographically immediately after uncovering. If a gap is present, the abutment must be repositioned.

COMPLICATIONS

Potential complications of implant placement include improper angulation or positioning of the implants; perforation of the inferior border, the maxillary sinus, or the inferior alveolar canal; dehiscence of the buccocortical or linguocortical plate; mandibular fracture; and soft tissue wound dehiscence.

Variation in the position or angulation of the implant results when the anatomy found at surgery requires implant placement different from that planned preoperatively. This should be avoided by grafting bone and/or soft tissue to allow implant placement in the desired location and angle. In the event that ideal angulation has not been achieved, a variety of prosthodontic attachments are available to salvage implants that have nonideal angulation.

Sinus perforation occurring during drilling for implant placement is unlikely to cause serious sequelae. Shorter implant length than planned may be necessary to prevent the implant from extending too far into the sinus. Usually the resistance provided by the cortical bone of the maxillary sinus floor is encountered before a perforation results and can serve as an indicator that maximum depth has been reached. If perforation does occur and the implant is placed only a short distance into the maxillary sinus, a problem is not likely. Similar guidelines exist for perforation of the inferior border of the mandible. The apical portion of the implant should be within the cortical bone of the inferior border.

Perforation of the inferior alveolar canal is a serious problem. Local infiltration over the bone crest rather than inferior alveolar nerve block may facilitate identification of this at surgery because the patient will be adequately anesthetized for implant placement but feel a sharp pain if the canal is perforated. Perforation of the canal may also be accompanied by sudden increased bleeding. If this occurs, an implant shorter than planned should be used. If the implant appears to extend into the inferior alveolar canal on the postoperative radiographs, the implant should be removed immediately and a shorter implant should be placed. If no indication of perforation exists and no radiographic evidence of violation of the canal is noted, patients may still have postoperative neurosensory alteration. This may be from traction on the mental nerve, from direct injury during implant placement, or from extraosseous hematoma or soft tissue swelling. These patients should be followed closely. Deficits of this nature generally resolve with time but may require surgical intervention if they persist and are bothersome to the patient.

Perforation of the buccocortical or linguocortical plates may occur when resorption has resulted in a thin ridge along the planned implant site. A simple solution is to countersink the implant until the depth of the implant recipient site is adequate for the length of the implant. This may leave excess bone height on the lingual, mesial, and distal surfaces. At the time of uncovering there may be bone growth over the implant that requires removal. If the sharp crest is generalized and several implants are to be placed, the entire crest can be reduced down to a suitable width. If a dehiscence does occur, it should be evaluated and a decision should be made regarding treatment. A small, 1- to 2-mm bony dehiscence on the buccal aspect of an implant generally requires no additional treatment. Larger defects, particularly if the implant is short, may compromise stability. If this results, the defect can be grafted with bone or a bone substitute (Fig. 14-31). This technique is more fully discussed in the section on advanced surgical techniques.

An unusual complication of implant placement in the mandible is mandibular fracture. Fracture is most likely when the mandible is extremely atrophic, when preexisting metabolic disease (e.g., osteoporosis) is seen, or when the patient has a history of postoperative trauma. Failure to tap threaded implants in very dense mandibular bone may also be associated with fracture. Management may require routine fracture management with rigid internal fixation and bone grafting to increase the bone mass of the mandible.

Soft tissue wound dehiscence may occur, allowing part of the implant to become exposed. If this occurs, no attempt should be made to resuture the wound because the only result will be increased wound dehiscence. Chlorhexidine rinses can be used until soft tissue healing has occurred. If the tissue is healthy but the implant remains exposed, a soft toothbrush dipped in chlorhexidine should be used to keep the implant clean throughout the integration period. This generally does not result in increased implant failure because single-stage implants are purposely left exposed throughout osseointegration and have comparable success as two-stage systems.

CLINICAL IMPLANT COMPONENTS

Osseointegrated implants are generally designed to support screw- and cement-retained implant restorations. Contemporary implant systems offer many advantages over conventional dental restorations and original systems (Box 14-5).

BOX 14-5

Advantages of Osseous Integrated Implants

SURGICAL

Documented success rate
In-office procedure
Adaptable to multiple intraoral locations
Precise implant site preparation
Reversibility in the event of implant failure

PROSTHETIC

Multiple restorative options
Versatility of second-stage components
- Angle correction
- Esthetics
- Crown contours
- Screw- or cement-retained options

Retrievability in the event of prosthodontic failure

From Rosenstiel SF, Land MF, Fujimoto J: *Contemporary fixed prosthodontics*, ed 4, St Louis, 2006, Mosby.

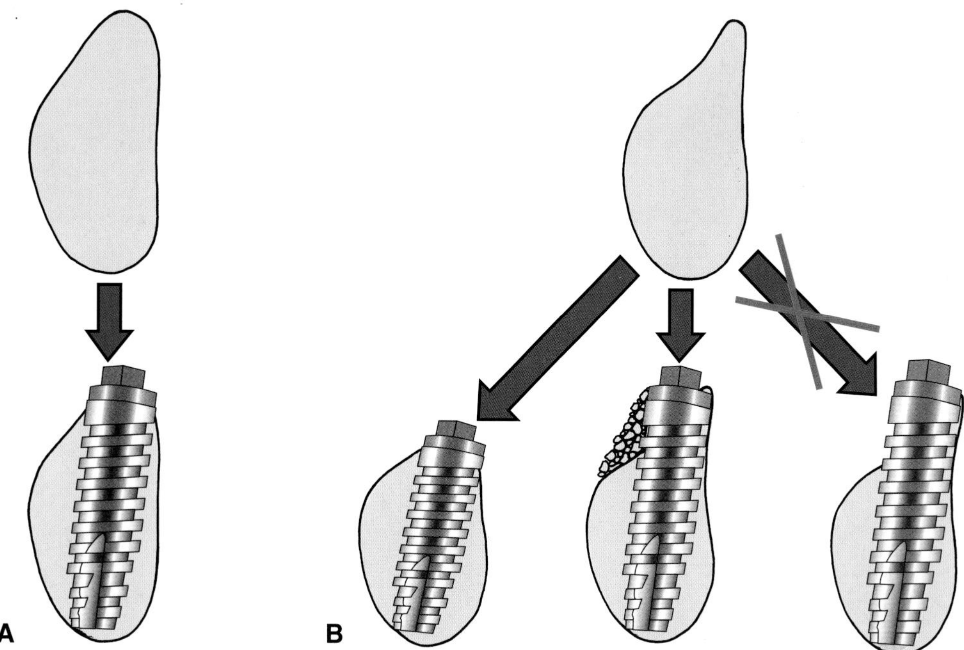

FIGURE 14-31 In an ideal situation (A), adequate bone on buccolingual areas for implant placement exists. This may not occur when there has been resorption of buccal bone (B). Acceptable ways to handle this include removal of sharp crest to level of adequate width for implant or placement of bone graft over buccal dehiscence that results.

Implant restorations require the use of several component parts that heretofore had not been routinely described in conventional dental education. For the inexperienced implant clinician, the sheer number of parts within one system often creates an overwhelming obstacle to getting involved in implant dentistry. This section describes in generic terms the component parts typically necessary to restore a screw-retained, osseointegrated implant. It should be noted that the components might differ slightly in design and materials among implant systems.

Implant Body

The dental implant body, often referred to as the fixture, is the component placed within the bone during first-stage surgery. The implant body may be a threaded or nonthreaded root form and is ordinarily made of titanium or titanium alloy of varying surface roughness, with or without a hydroxyapatite coating (Fig. 14-32). Although some controversy exists regarding the optimum shape and surface coating for an implant in different parts of the mouth, the significant factors for success are precise placement, atraumatic surgery, unloaded healing, and passive restoration. All contemporary dental implants have an internally threaded portion that can accept second-stage screw placements. These implants also may incorporate an antirotational feature within the design of the fixture body. If it is incorporated, the antirotational feature may be internal or external. Implant bodies can also be classified as *one-stage* or *two-stage*. One-stage implants project through the soft tissue immediately after stage I surgery. Two-stage implants are typically covered with soft tissue at the time of surgery. When a tall *healing screw* or cap is placed on a two-stage implant to project it through the tissue at the time of placement, this is referred to as "using a two-stage implant with a one-stage protocol."

Healing Screw

During the healing phase after first-stage surgery, a screw is normally placed in the superior aspect of the fixture. The screw is usually low in profile to facilitate the suturing of soft tissue in the two-stage implant or to minimize loading in the one-stage implant (Fig. 14-33). At second-stage surgery, the screw is removed and replaced by subsequent components. In some

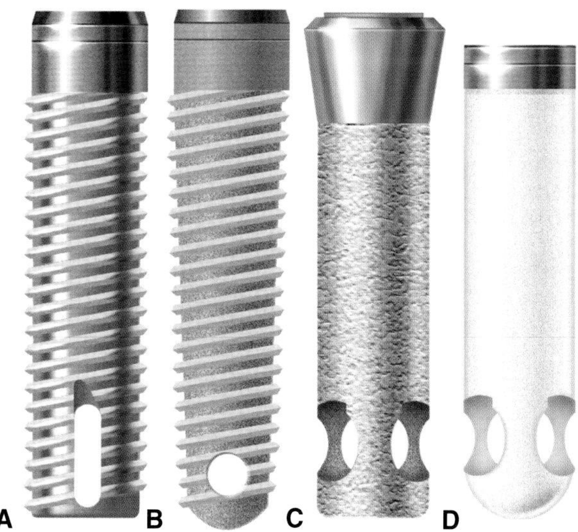

FIGURE 14-32 Four main categories of osseous integrated implants. A, Titanium screw. B, Hydroxyapatite-coated screw. C, Titanium plasma-sprayed cylinder. D, Hydroxyapatite-coated cylinder. (Rosenstiel SF, Land MF, Fujimoto J: *Contemporary fixed prosthodontics*, ed 4, St Louis, 2006, Mosby.)

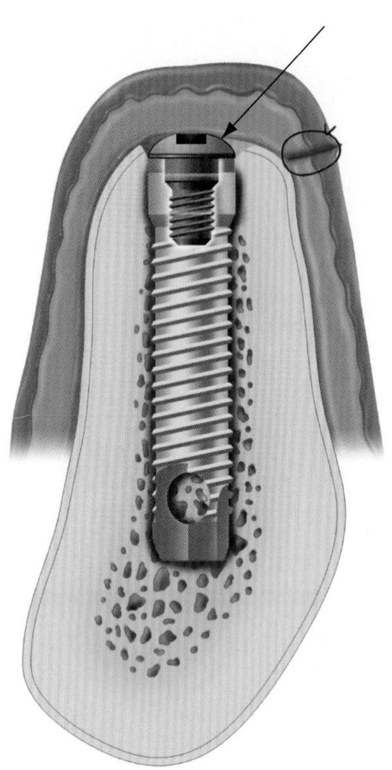

FIGURE 14-33 Healing screw (*arrow*) in place during the initial implant healing phase. Soft tissue is sutured over the implant. A removable prosthesis can be worn over this area during healing. (Rosenstiel SF, Land MF, Fujimoto J: *Contemporary fixed prosthodontics,* ed 4, St Louis, 2006, Mosby.)

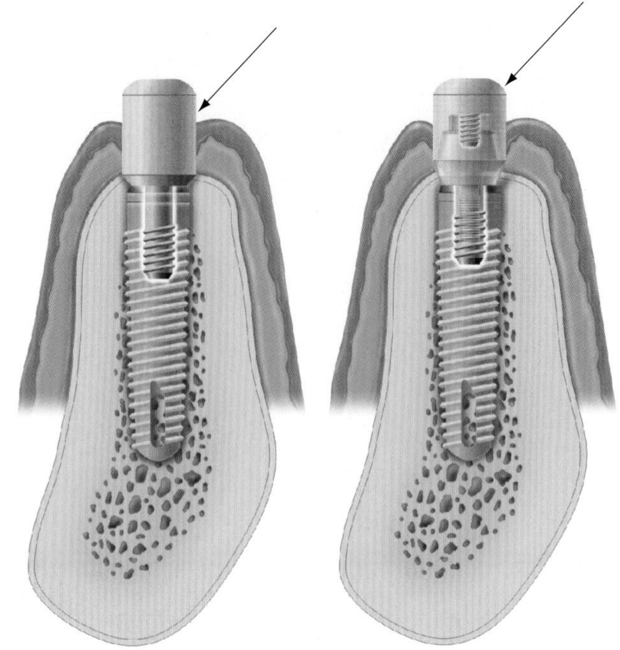

FIGURE 14-34 Components that allow for soft tissue healing after second-stage surgery. **A**, This interim abutment screws into the implant. **B**, The healing cap screws into the abutment. (Rosenstiel SF, Land MF, Fujimoto J: *Contemporary fixed prosthodontics,* ed 4, St Louis, 2006, Mosby.)

systems the screw is made slightly larger than the diameter of the implant, which facilitates abutment placement by ensuring that bone does not grow over the edge of the implant. The implant surgeon should always be sure that the healing screw is completely seated after stage I surgery to prevent bone from growing between the screw and the implant. If this occurs, removing the bone may damage the superior surface of the implant and affect the fit of subsequent components.

Interim Abutment

Interim abutments are dome-shaped screws placed after second-stage surgery and before insertion of the prosthesis. The abutments range in length from 2 to 10 mm and project through the soft tissue into the oral cavity. The abutments may screw directly into the fixture or, in some systems, onto the abutment immediately after second-stage surgery. Those abutments that screw onto the abutment are commonly referred to as *healing caps* (Fig. 14-34). Both components are made of titanium or titanium alloy. In areas where esthetics is paramount, healing after second-stage surgery should be sufficiently complete around an interim abutment to stabilize the gingival margin before final prosthesis construction. At this time, abutments of appropriate length are selected to ensure that the metal-porcelain interface of the restoration will be located subgingivally. In areas where tissue esthetics is not crucial, adequate healing for impressions usually takes 2 weeks after second-stage uncovering. In esthetic zones, 3 to 5 weeks may be required before abutment selection.

Abutment

Abutments are the component of the implant system that screw directly into the implant. Abutments eventually support the prosthesis in screw-retained restorations, inasmuch as they accept the retaining screw of the prosthesis. For cement-retained restorations, abutments may be shaped like a conventional crown preparation. Abutments take many forms (Fig. 14-35). The walls of abutments are usually smooth, polished, and straight-sided titanium or titanium alloy. The lengths range from 1 to 10 mm. In nonesthetic areas, 1 to 2 mm of titanium should be allowed to penetrate the soft tissue to maximize the patient's ability to clean the prosthesis (Fig. 14-36). In esthetic areas an abutment can be selected to allow porcelain to be carried subgingivally for optimum esthetics (Fig. 14-37). In implant systems that incorporate an antirotational feature, the abutment must have two components that move independently of each other: One engages the antirotational feature, and the other secures the abutment within the fixture (Fig. 14-38). With angled abutments a similar technique is used to correct divergently placed implants (Fig. 14-39). Some systems have included tapered or wide-base abutments, which allow teeth with larger cross-sectional diameters to be restored with more physiologic contours. The nonsegmented implant crown (UCLA) bypasses the abutment portion by means of a sleeve waxed directly to the implant. Use of nonsegmented implant crowns may be necessary when soft tissue thickness is less than 2 mm. Abutments made entirely of ceramic onto which all-ceramic crowns can be cemented are gaining popularity for the anterior part of the mouth. The ceramic components are usually made of sintered alumina, zirconia, or a combination of the two (Fig. 14-40).

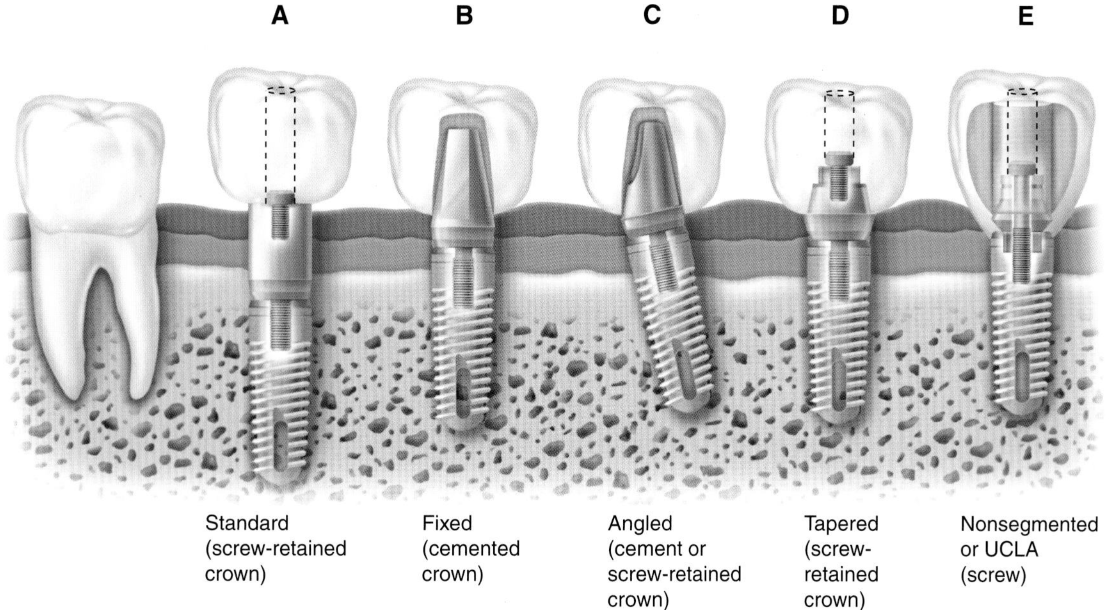

FIGURE 14-35 Types of abutments (*left to right*). **A**, Standard. Length can be selected to make the margin subgingival or supragingival. **B**, Fixed. This abutment is much like a conventional post and core. It is screwed into the implants, has a prepared finish line, and receives a cemented restoration. **C**, Angled. This type is available when implant angles must be corrected for esthetic or biomechanical reasons. **D**, Tapered. This type can be used to make the transition to restoration more gradual in larger teeth. **E**, Nonsegmented, or direct. This type is used in areas of limited interarch distance or areas where an esthetic outcome is important. The restoration can be built directly on the implant, so there is no intervening abutment. This direct restoration technique as been called the UCLA abutment. (Rosenstiel SF, Land MF, Fujimoto J: *Contemporary fixed prosthodontics,* ed 4, St Louis, 2006, Mosby.)

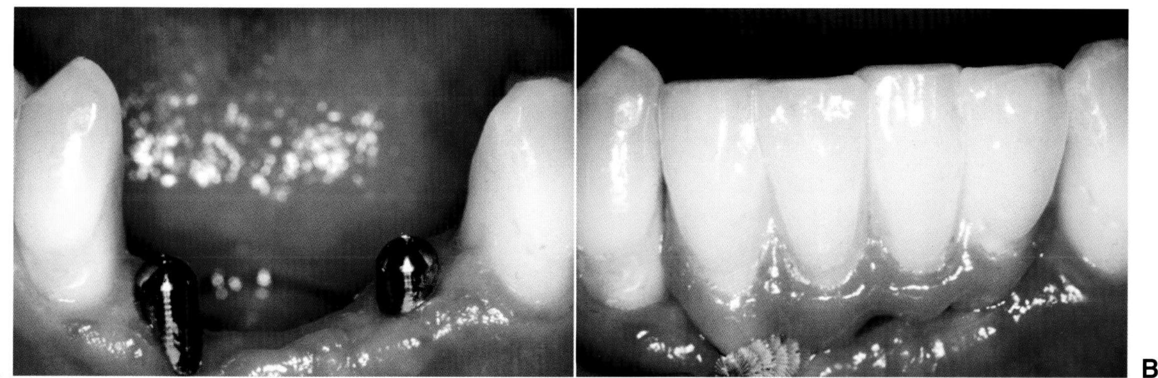

FIGURE 14-36 **A**, Interim abutments projecting through the soft tissue. **B**, Implant restorations supported by standard abutments that allow easy access for oral hygiene. (Rosenstiel SF, Land MF, Fujimoto J: *Contemporary fixed prosthodontics,* ed 4, St Louis, 2006, Mosby.)

The choice of abutment size depends on the vertical distance between the fixture base and opposing dentition, the existing sulcular depth, and the esthetic requirements in the area being restored. For acceptable appearance, an anterior maxillary crown may require 2 to 3 mm of subgingival porcelain at the facial gingival margin to create the proper emergence profile and appearance, whereas fixtures in the posterior maxilla or mandible may have margin termination at or below the gingival crest.

Impression Coping

Impression copings facilitate transfer of the intraoral location of the implant or abutment to a similar position on the laboratory cast. Impression copings may screw into the implant or onto the abutment and are customarily subdivided into fixture types or abutment types (Fig. 14-41).

Both types can be further subdivided into transfer (indirect) and pickup (direct) types. With the transfer impression coping

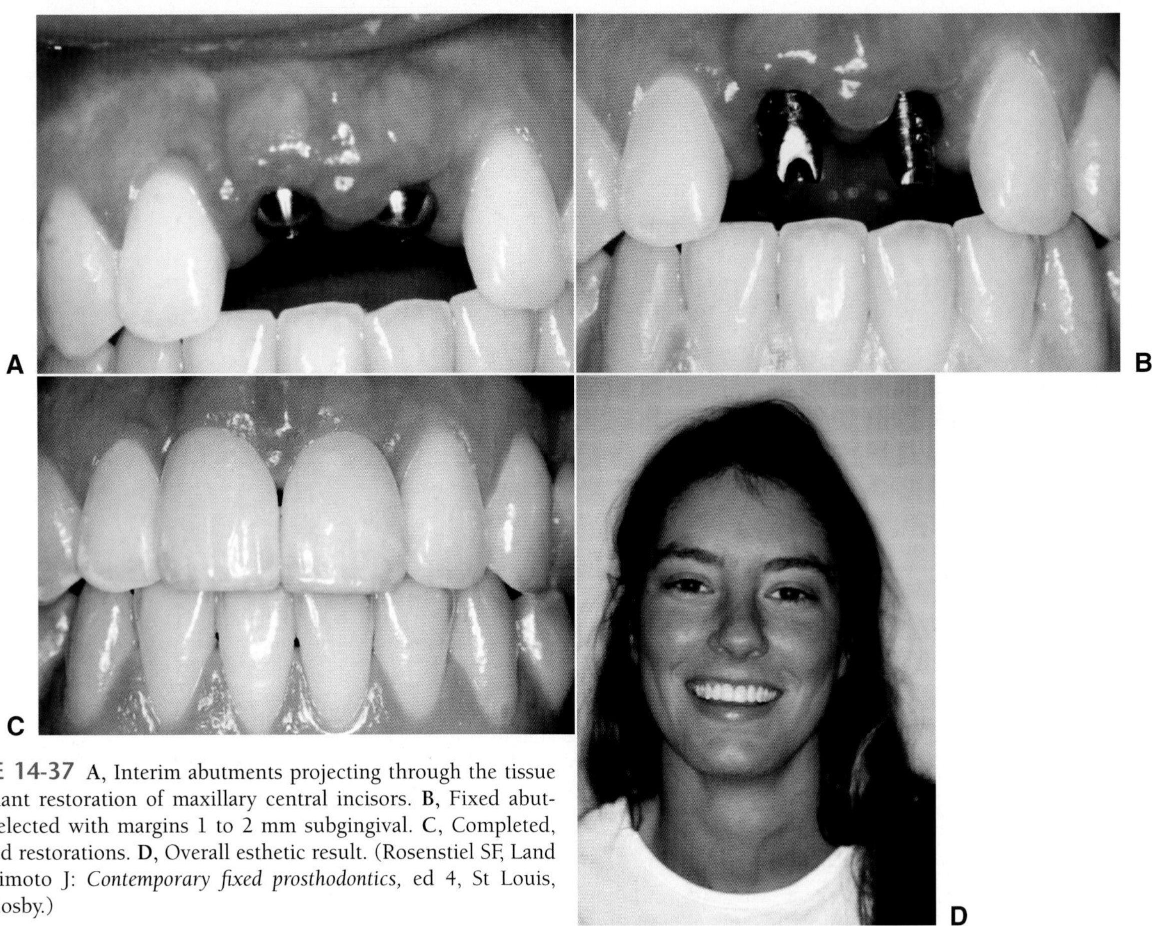

FIGURE 14-37 A, Interim abutments projecting through the tissue for implant restoration of maxillary central incisors. B, Fixed abutments selected with margins 1 to 2 mm subgingival. C, Completed, cemented restorations. D, Overall esthetic result. (Rosenstiel SF, Land MF, Fujimoto J: *Contemporary fixed prosthodontics,* ed 4, St Louis, 2006, Mosby.)

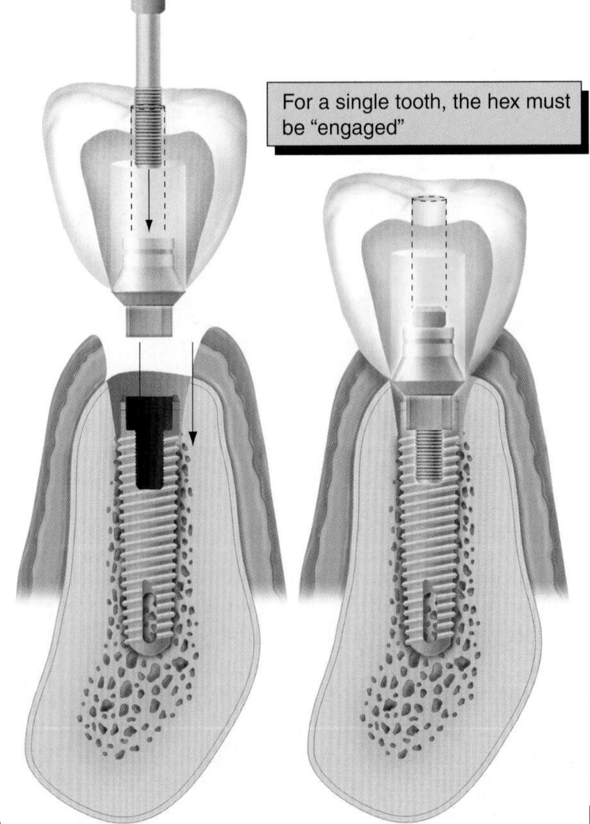

FIGURE 14-38 A and B, When an antirotational feature is to be engaged by the abutment, one component of the abutment (the sleeve) must fit the hexagon, whereas the other (the screw) independently tightens the components together. (Rosenstiel SF, Land MF, Fujimoto J: *Contemporary fixed prosthodontics,* ed 4, St Louis, 2006, Mosby.)

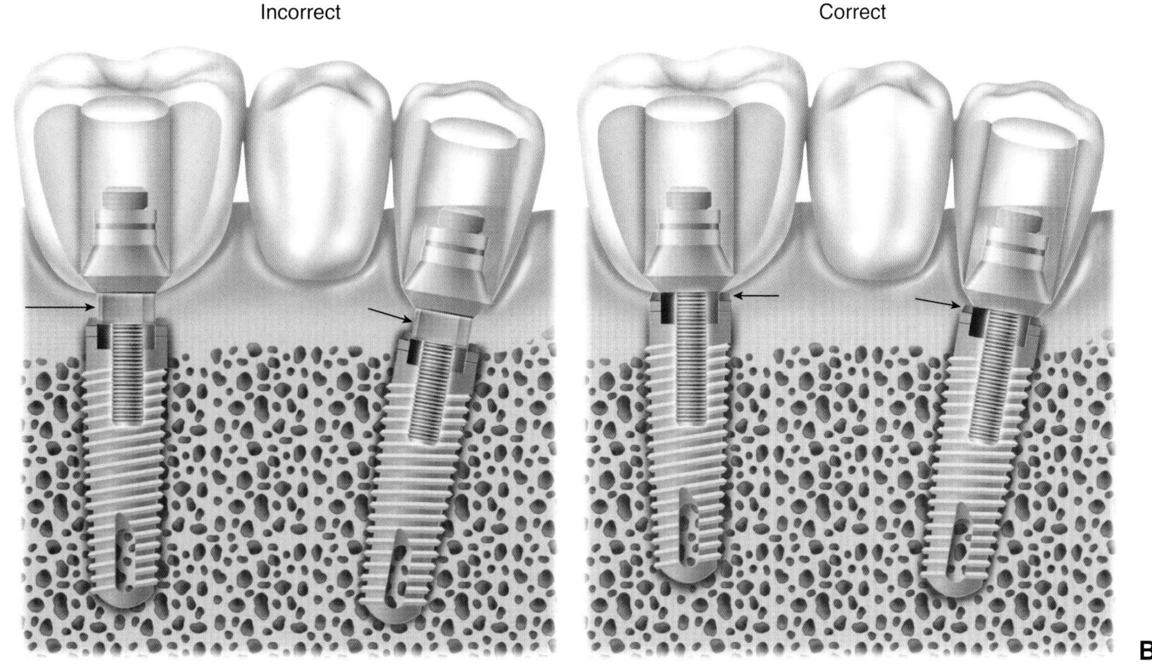

FIGURE 14-39 For a multiple unit restoration, the hexes *(arrows)* usually cannot be "engaged" (**A**) because of lack of parallelism of the implants. So nonengaging direct abutments *(arrows)* must be used (**B**). (Rosenstiel SF, Land MF, Fujimoto J: *Contemporary fixed prosthodontics,* ed 4, St Louis, 2006, Mosby.)

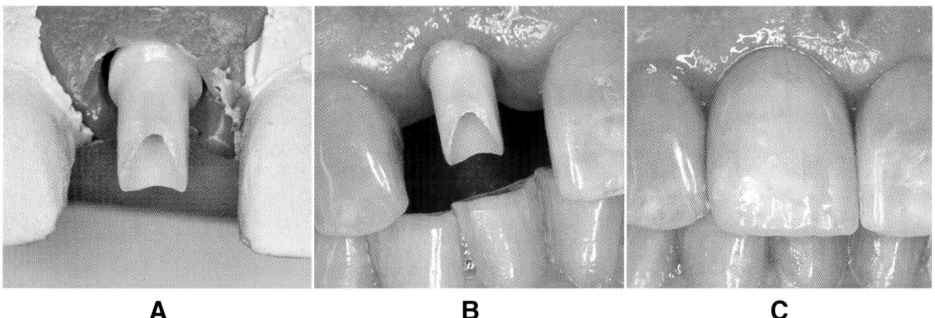

FIGURE 14-40 **A**, Zirconia abutment seated on the cast and ready for fabrication of all-ceramic restoration. **B**, Zirconia abutment seated in the mouth. **C**, All-ceramic restoration.

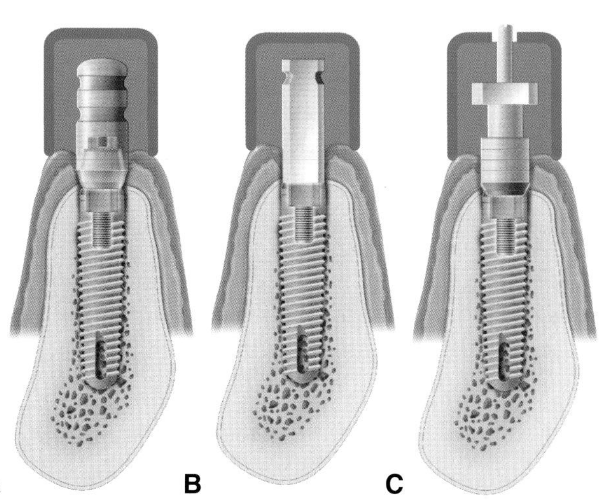

FIGURE 14-41 Types of impression copings. **A**, A one-piece coping (screws onto abutment) is used if the abutment does not need to be changed on the laboratory cast. **B**, A two-piece coping (transfer/closed tray) is attached directly to the fixture if the abutment does need to be changed on the cast (it should have a flat side if angle correction is necessary). **C**, A two-piece coping (pickup/open tray), used to orient the antirotational feature or to make impressions of very divergent implants. (Rosenstiel SF, Land MF, Fujimoto J: *Contemporary fixed prosthodontics,* ed 4, St Louis, 2006, Mosby.)

in place, an impression is made intraorally, after radiographs are taken to confirm that the implant components are properly assembled. This requirement is especially important when an antirotational feature is involved. Heavier body impression materials (e.g., polyvinyl siloxane and polyether) are usually recommended, although any conventional impression material can be used. When the impression is removed from the mouth, the impression coping remains in place on the implant abutment or on the fixture. The coping is then removed from the mouth and joined to the *implant analog* before being transferred to the impression in the proper orientation. Before an implant impression is taken, a radiograph should be made to ensure that the components are properly assembled. This is especially important when an antirotational feature is involved.

Implant Analog

Implant analogs are made to represent exactly the top of the implant fixture or the abutment in the laboratory cast. Therefore, analogs can be classified as fixture analogs and abutment analogs (Fig. 14-42). Both types of analog screw directly into the impression coping after it has been removed from the mouth, and the joined components are returned to the impression before pouring. The final impression should be poured in dental stone or die stone. The gingival tissues can be reproduced by injecting an elastomer (e.g., Permadyne, 3M, St. Paul, Minnesota) to represent soft tissue around the implant analog before pouring. This facilitates removal of the impression coping from the stone cast and the placement of subsequent abutments without breaking the stone and losing the reference point of the soft tissue (Fig. 14-43).

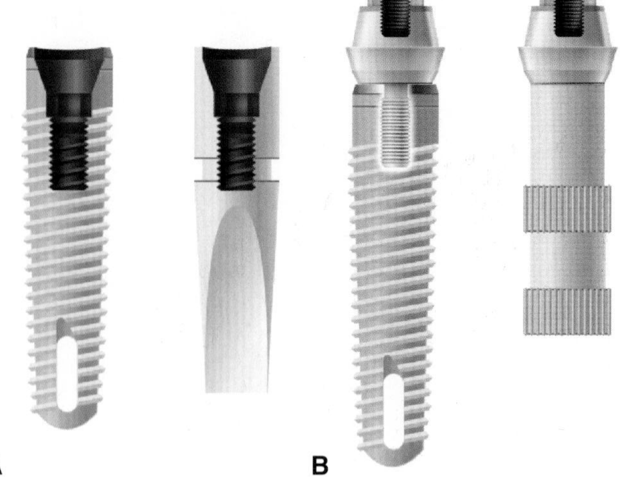

FIGURE 14-42 Implant analogs. These represent implants or abutments. **A**, Analog that duplicates the top of the implant. **B**, Analog that duplicates the top of the abutment. (Rosenstiel SF, Land MF, Fujimoto J: *Contemporary fixed prosthodontics*, ed 4, St Louis, 2006, Mosby.)

Abutment analogs are generally attached to an implant impression coping. Implant body impression copings are normally attached to implant body analogs. The advantage of using the implant body analog is that the abutments can be

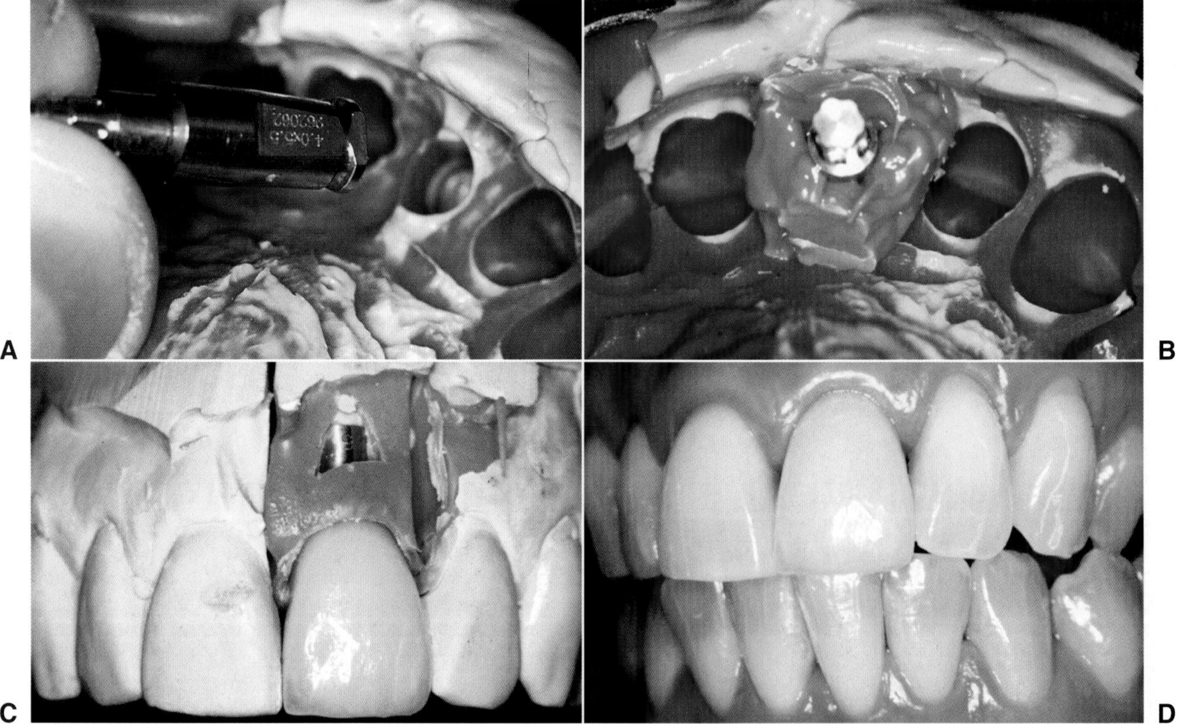

FIGURE 14-43 **A** and **B**, Polyether impression material injected around an implant analog before the impression is poured. The gingival material should not cover any retention features of the analog. **C**, The impression material reproduces the patient's soft tissue contours adjacent to the implant. The impression coping may be removed and other components inserted without losing the associated anatomic landmarks. **D**, Completed restorations. (Rosenstiel SF, Land MF, Fujimoto J: *Contemporary fixed prosthodontics*, ed 4, St Louis, 2006, Mosby; courtesy Dr. C. Pechous.)

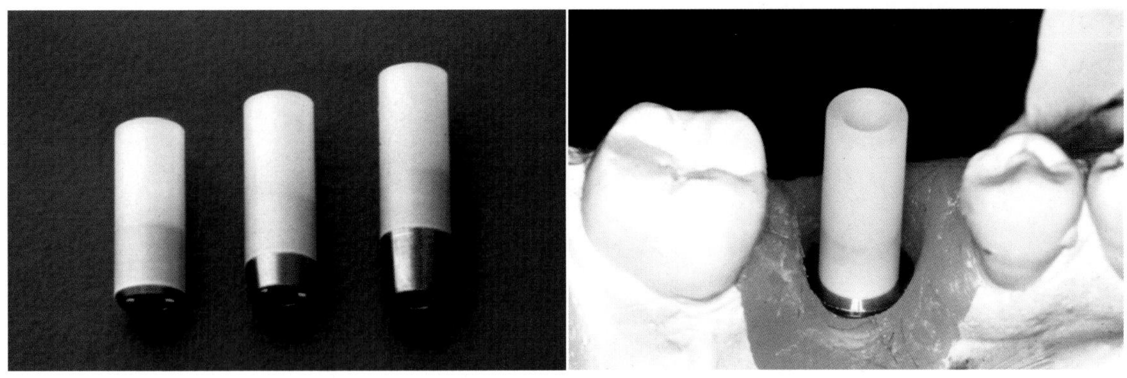

FIGURE 14-44 A, Waxing sleeves with gold alloy base and plastic extension. B, On the laboratory cast the technician can wax to the plastic extension. The wax and plastic are burned out, and the new alloy is "cast to" the original alloy base. (Rosenstiel SF, Land MF, Fujimoto J: *Contemporary fixed prosthodontics,* ed 4, St Louis, 2006, Mosby.)

changed in the laboratory. Also, if a flat-sided impression coping has been used to orient the threads or the hexagon of the implant body analog properly, the decision to correct for less than optimal implant angulation can be deferred until the laboratory stage. If the clinician is confident that the appropriate abutment has been selected, using the abutment impression coping and abutment analog can simplify the procedure. If a supragingival abutment margin has been selected, a soft tissue cast is not necessary.

Waxing Sleeve

Waxing sleeves are attached to the abutment by the relating screw on the laboratory model. The sleeves eventually become part of the prosthesis. In nonsegmented implant crowns, the sleeves are attached directly to the implant body analog in the cast. Commonly referred to as *UCLA abutments,* the sleeves may be plastic patterns that are burned out and cast as part of the restoration framework, precious metal that is incorporated in the framework when it is cast to the precious alloy cylinder, or a combination of each. Use of a metal waxing sleeve ensures that two machined surfaces are always in contact. The cast surface of the plastic waxing sleeve may be retooled before it is returned to the fixture. Waxing sleeves are available in several vertical dimensions. Tall ones can be shortened to conform to the requirements of the occlusal plane. Today, most waxing sleeves are a combination of gold alloy and plastic (Fig. 14-44). This combination allows the advantage of plastic at the waxing surface and precise metal-to-metal tolerances at the implant level.

Prosthesis-Retaining Screw

Prosthesis-retaining screws penetrate the fixed restoration and secure it to the abutment (Fig. 14-45). The screws are tightened with a screwdriver and attach nonsegmented crowns to the body of the implant. The screws generally are made of titanium, titanium alloy, or gold alloy and may be long (which allows them to penetrate the total length of the implant crown) or short (which requires countersinking them into the occlusal surface of the restoration). Screws that are countersunk must be covered by an initial layer of resilient material (e.g., gutta-percha, cotton, or silicone). A subsequent seal of composite resin is placed over the resilient plug.

IMPLANT PROSTHETIC OPTIONS

Completely Edentulous Patients

At least three prosthetic implant options exist for the completely edentulous patient. The options include (1) the implant- and tissue-supported overdenture, (2) the all implant-supported overdenture, and (3) the complete implant-supported fixed prosthesis.

Implant- and Tissue-Supported Overdenture

Completely edentulous patients have the most difficulty with the mandibular denture. Long-time denture wearers with a progressively worsening lower denture fit may derive great benefit from an implant- and tissue-supported overdenture. For this type of prosthesis, most commonly two implants are placed in the mandibular symphysis area between the mental foramina. These implants are used to retain and support the lower denture (Fig. 14-46).

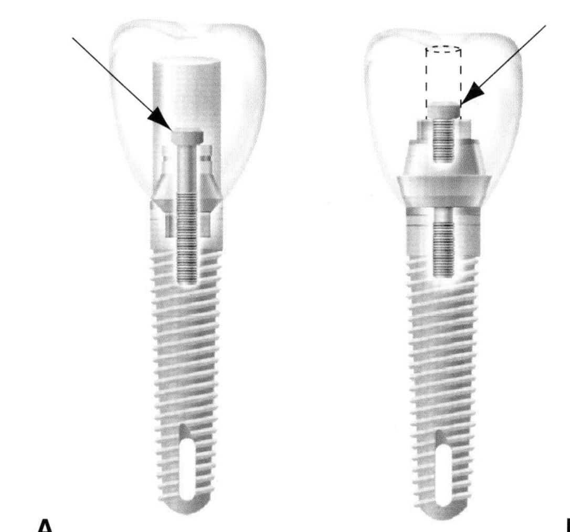

FIGURE 14-45 Two types of prosthesis-retaining screws. A, Nonsegmented crown retained to implant. B, Crown retained on abutment. (Rosenstiel SF, Land MF, Fujimoto J: *Contemporary fixed prosthodontics,* ed 4, St Louis, 2006, Mosby.)

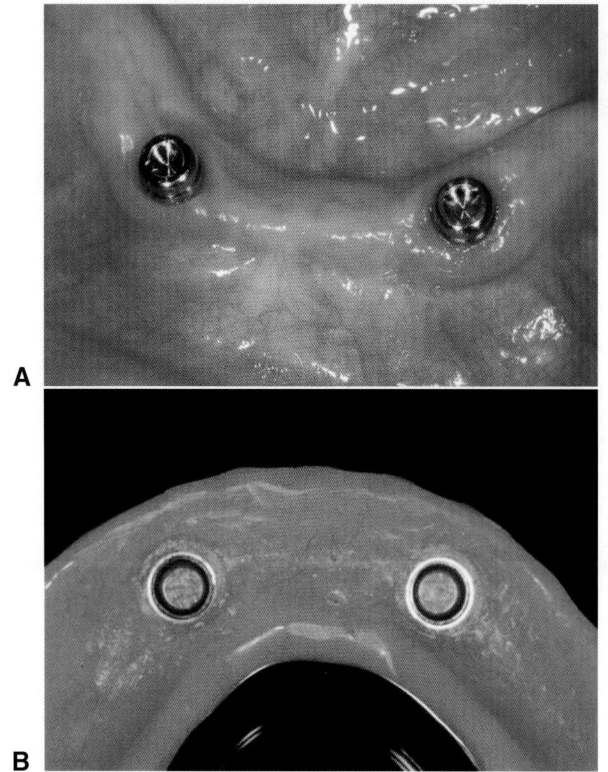

FIGURE 14-46 A and B, Implant- and tissue-supported overdenture retained by individual attachments.

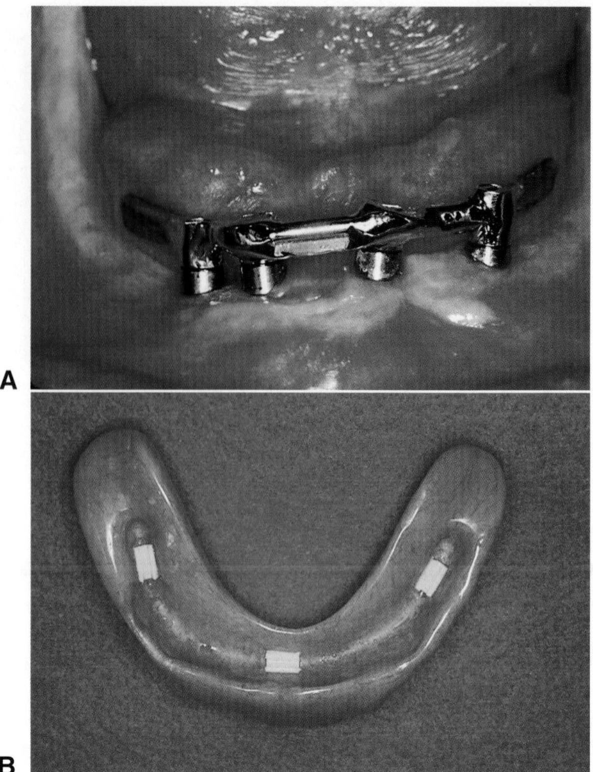

FIGURE 14-47 A, More extensive bar design with distal cantilevers joining four mandibular implants. B, Three Hader clips in an all implant-supported overdenture.

Implant- and tissue-supported overdentures require a precise prosthetic technique. It is important that the retentive devices engage at the same time the posterior extensions contact the tissue and at the same time the teeth meet in occlusion. Although this option is not the answer for all patients, it provides an economical alternative for the patient who only needs additional retention and stability for a lower denture.

All Implant-Supported Overdenture

For those patients requiring more retention and stability for an upper and lower denture, the all implant-supported overdenture may be the answer. For implants to support the entire load, it is recommended that a minimum of four implants be placed in the lower jaw and six implants in the upper jaw. These implants are connected by a more extensive bar design using multiple clips for retention (Fig. 14-47).

This type of prosthesis can provide the advantages of minimal tissue pressure, optimal access for hygiene, and optimal esthetics because the denture covers all metalwork. In the maxilla, this prosthesis can also have the additional advantages that the palate can be removed from the denture and that all air holes can be covered, which provides the patient with a better phonetic result. The disadvantage to this prosthesis is that it is still a removable prosthesis and must be removed for cleaning and maintenance, which does not satisfy that patient who seeks implant treatment for the psychological benefits of having a permanently retained restoration. A further disadvantage is that clip mechanisms wear over time and must be replaced.

Fixed Porcelain-Metal and Resin-Metal Restorations

For those completely edentulous patients who require nonremovable restorations the two options are (1) a fixed porcelain-fused-to-metal prosthesis (Figs. 14-5 and 14-48) or (2) a resin-metal fixed prosthesis (Fig. 14-49). The resin-metal prosthesis is a cast framework with resin denture material and teeth processed to the framework. Both of these options require a minimum of five implants in the mandible and six implants in the maxilla. One major determining factor for selecting the appropriate option is the amount of bone loss. Complete-mouth fixed rehabilitation can only be made esthetically pleasing if minimal bone loss has occurred. This

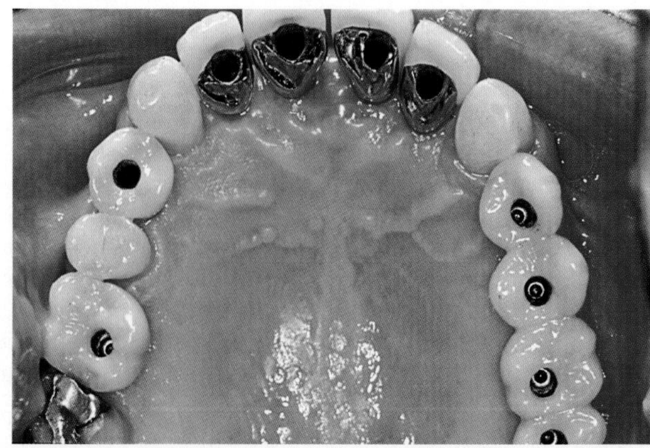

FIGURE 14-48 Occlusal view of a porcelain-fused-to-metal implant-supported rehabilitation.

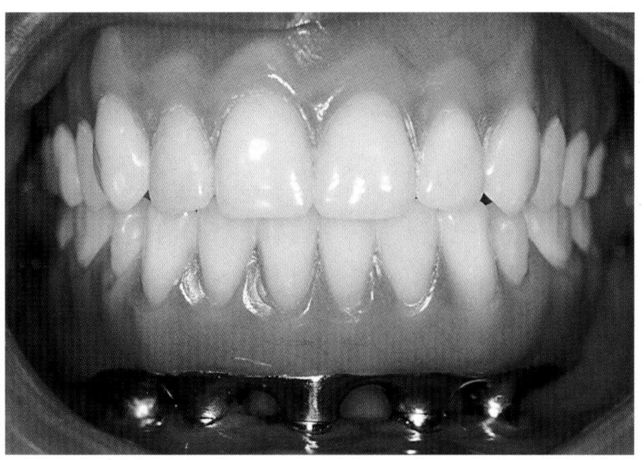

FIGURE 14-49 Facial view of mandibular metal-resin (hybrid) prosthesis. This prosthesis consists of precious metal substructure with acrylic resin and denture teeth processed to it.

type of restoration is best suited for those patients who have recently lost their natural dentition.

For patients who have moderate bone loss, the prosthesis must replace bone and soft tissue, as well as teeth. In this case, the resin-metal prosthesis can best mimic soft tissue replacement. The advantage to the completely fixed restoration (the resin or porcelain prosthesis) is that it is completely retained by the patient at all times. Patients derive the maximal psychological benefit by having a restoration that is most like their natural teeth. Movement within the system is minimized, so the component parts tend to wear out less quickly.

Potential disadvantages for the complete-mouth fixed rehabilitation is that implants must be precisely placed, especially in the maxillary anterior esthetic zone, to achieve the ideal esthetic result. The relative benefit to each restorative option can be described to the edentulous patient (Box 14-6).

Partially Edentulous Patients

Major advantages from implant support can be derived in the partially edentulous patient. The two main indications for implant restorations in this patient are (1) the free-end distal extension when no terminal abutment is available and (2) a long edentulous span. In both of these situations the conventional dental treatment plan would include a removable partial denture. In the short edentulous span (including single-tooth restorations), the implant option is becoming a more popular choice. This selection is often made because natural abutments do not have to be prepared and improved access for hygiene can be realized. If the implants are 10 mm long or less, definite consideration should be given to adding a third implant to support a three-unit fixed partial denture.

Free-End Distal Extension

The implant dentist has two options in treating the patient missing terminal posterior abutments: (1) a single implant placed distal to the most posterior natural abutment and (2) a fixed prosthesis made to connect the implant and a natural tooth abutment. This situation is associated with a higher incidence of implant failure because of forces placed on the implant (Fig. 14-49). Alternatively, two or more implants can be placed posterior to the most distal natural tooth, and an implant restoration can be fabricated (Fig. 14-50).

Single-Tooth Implant Restorations

The use of single implants in restoring missing teeth is an attractive option for the patient and the dentist. This procedure requires careful implant placement and precise control of all prosthetic components. Single-tooth restorations supported by implants may be indicated in four situations: (1) patients with otherwise intact dentition, (2) dentition with spaces that would be more complicated to treat with conventional fixed prosthodontics, (3) distally missing teeth when cantilevers or removable partial dentures are not indicated, and (4) patient desire for treatment that will most closely mimic the missing natural tooth.

The five requirements for single-tooth crown are as follows: (1) esthetics, especially when a visible metal collar from the abutment is unacceptable; (2) antirotation to avoid prosthetic component loosening and allow accurate transfer of angle corrections; (3) simplicity, to minimize the number of components used; (4) accessibility, so the patient can maintain optimal oral hygiene; and (5) variability, so the clinician can easily control the height, diameter, and angulation of the implant restoration. Many systems have been developed to comply with the demands of single-tooth replacement. Very small teeth may be best restored with cemented crowns. Larger teeth (i.e., molars, premolars/canines, and central incisors) may be more easily restored with screw retention (Fig. 14-51).

Implant survival depends on proper and timely home care and maintenance. The dentist must ensure that the patient receives thorough instruction in maintenance techniques. The goal of implant maintenance is to eradicate microbial populations. Recall visits should be scheduled at least every 3 months for the first year. The sulcular area should be débrided of calculus by using plastic or wooden scalers. A rubber cup with low abrasive polishing paste or tin oxide may be used to polish implant abutments. Implant mobility should be evaluated, and bleeding upon probing should be documented. Framework fit and occlusion should also be checked at recall appointments. These biomechanical factors are as important as oral hygiene for the long-term success of the dental implant.

Failing Implant

Implant failure occurs at three distinct times: (1) at the time of (or shortly after) stage II surgery, (2) approximately 18 months after stage II surgery, and (3) more than 18 months after stage II surgery.

A few implants fail to integrate. This failure often is identified at the time of (or shortly after) stage II surgery. Failure in this period may be related to a variety of factors.

BOX 14-6

Patient Benefit Scale

0	No teeth
2	Dentures
4	Implant and tissue overdenture
6	All implant-supported overdenture
8	Fixed implant restoration
20	Natural teeth

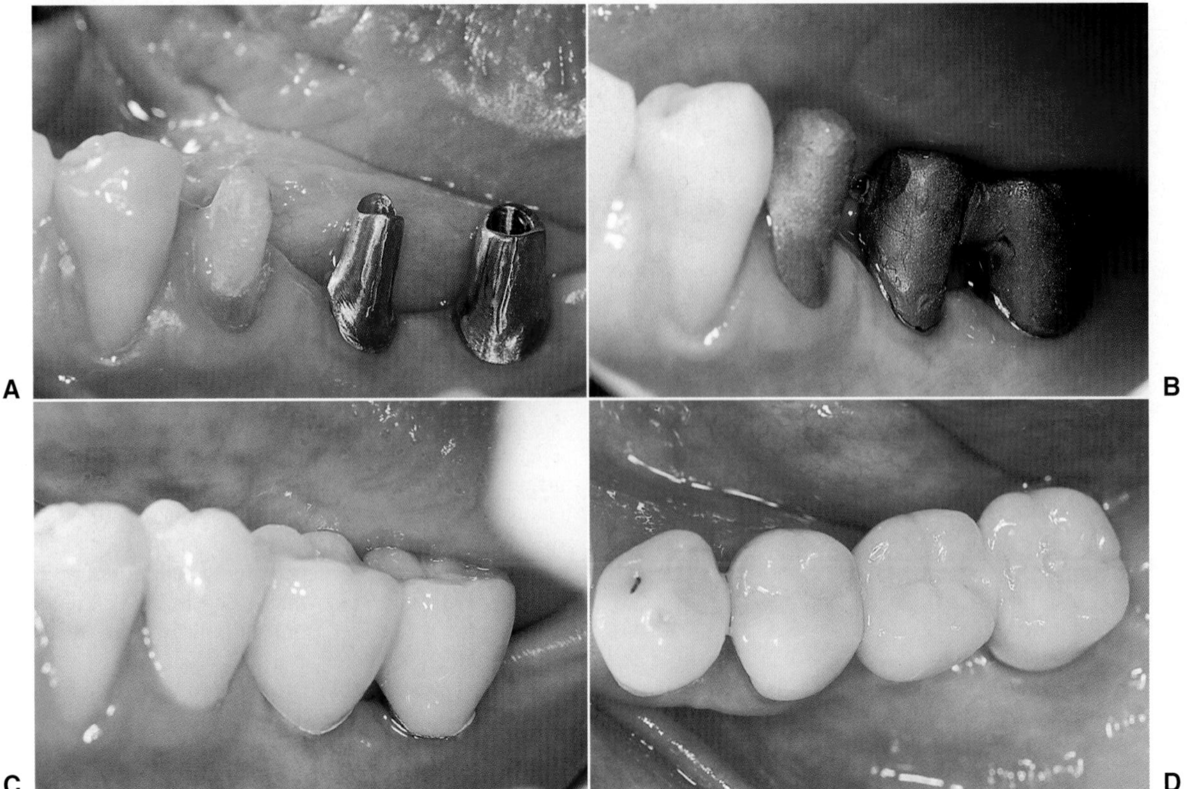

FIGURE 14-50 A, Two implants placed distal to the mandibular premolar. B to D, The completed restoration is not connected to the crown on the natural tooth. (Rosenstiel SF, Land MF, Fujimoto J: *Contemporary fixed prosthodontics,* ed 4, St Louis, 2006, Mosby; courtesy Dr. R.B. Miller.)

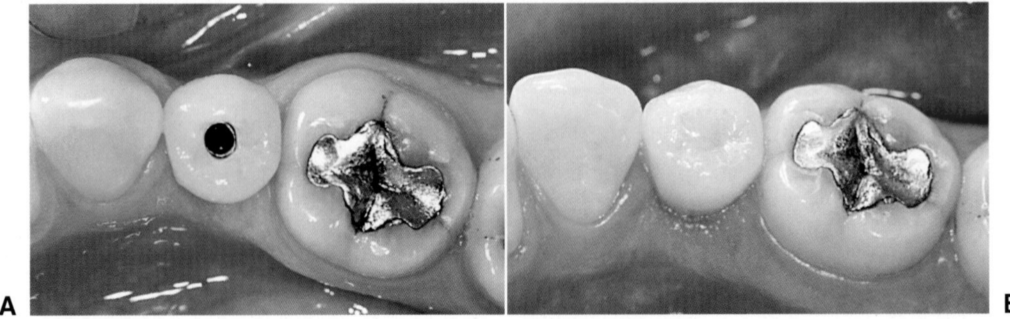

FIGURE 14-51 A, Occlusal view of a single-tooth implant crown replacing a fractured mandibular premolar. B, Implant crown with screw access restored. (Rosenstiel SF, Land MF, Fujimoto J: *Contemporary fixed prosthodontics,* ed 4, St Louis, 2006, Mosby.)

Overheating of the bone during placement or failure to achieve a precise implant fit with primary stability may lead to failure of integration. Postoperative infection, excessive pressure on the integrating implant (with movement of the implant), or wound-healing problems may also jeopardize implant integration.

After loading with a prosthesis, bone loss occurs for approximately 18 months, after which time a steady state will be achieved. During this 18-month period, additional implant failure may occur. Failure in this period is often associated with excessive biomechanical forces on the implant or compromised periimplant soft tissue health resulting from lack of attached tissue, poor hygiene, or both. Smoking is also associated with increased failure in this period and later periods. Late failure (i.e., more than 18 months after placement of the prosthesis) may also occur. This is rare, and frequently the cause is not identifiable. In general, these implants are identified as "ailing" during routine recall. Progressive bone loss in spite of rigorous hygiene measures is often seen. A combined prosthodontic and surgical intervention can often restore health to these ailing implants.

Once periimplant bone loss has been identified, efforts should initially be focused on optimizing hygiene. This may even require removal of the prosthesis to facilitate access. If bone loss is severe or progressive, surgical intervention is necessary. The implant must be exposed surgically and all soft tissue adjacent to the implant surface removed. The surface of the implant is then cleaned with hydrogen peroxide, after

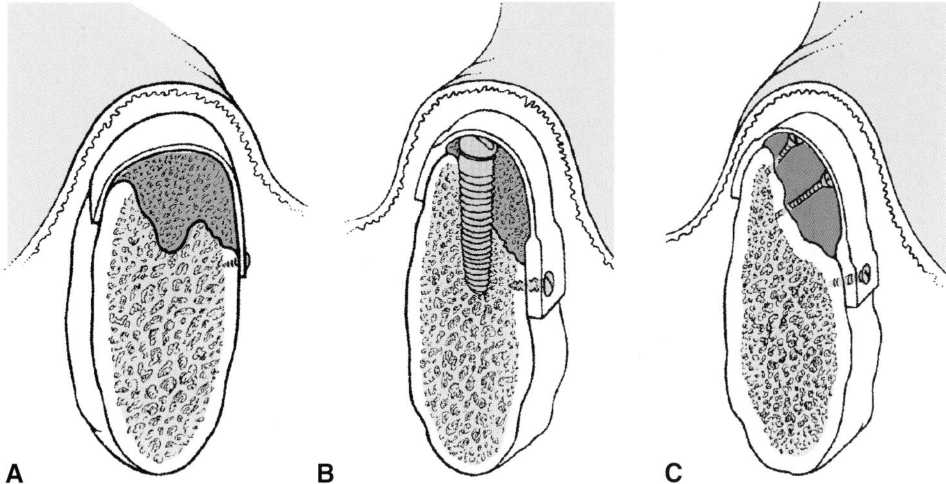

FIGURE 14-52 Various applications of guided bone regeneration. A, Membrane and "filler material" such as allogeneic bone is used to augment the ridge. B, Same as in A except that an implant is placed simultaneously. C, The membrane is supported by screws that preserve the space beneath the graft to allow bone fill.

which citric acid is used. Tetracycline powder can be placed along the implant surface and into the bony defect, and the defect can be reconstructed with a graft. Healing for a minimum of 4 months is allowed, after which the implant is uncovered and the prosthesis is replaced.

ADVANCED SURGICAL TECHNIQUES

Guided Bone Regeneration

Guided bone regeneration is a process that allows bone growth while retarding the ingrowth of fibrous connective tissue and epithelium. Most bone defects will regenerate with new bone if the invasion of connective tissue from adjacent soft tissue can be prevented. Guided bone regeneration uses a barrier that is placed over the bone defect and prevents fibrous tissue ingrowth while the bone underlying the barrier has time to grow and fill the defect (Fig. 14-52). This technique is particularly useful in the treatment of buccal dehiscence, where labiobuccal augmentation of bone is required. Guided bone regeneration can be performed simultaneously with implant placement or before stage I. A variety of materials may serve as barriers to fibrous tissue ingrowth. Ideal characteristics of a membrane are outlined in Box 14-7. Expanded polytetrafluoroethylene (Gore-Tex) is the most extensively tested material. Resorbable materials are also now available, eliminating the necessity of removal.

BOX 14-7

Characteristics of an Ideal Membrane

- Effective
- Ease of handling
- Inexpensive
- Resorbable
- Tolerates exposure

Block Bone Grafting

Guided bone regeneration is most often used for lateral ridge augmentation. Some authors have described vertical augmentation, but it is less predictable.

Corticocancellous bone grafts are an alternative to guided bone regeneration techniques. Bone can be harvested from the genial region, mandibular ramus, or iliac crest and used to augment lateral or vertical height of the atrophic ridge (Fig. 14-53). The defect is approached and prepared for grafting by perforating the cortical bone and creating a site to receive the graft. The corticocancellous block is harvested and trimmed to fit into the defect. Stabilization of the graft and primary closure is paramount. After 4 to 6 months of healing, the implant surgery can be accomplished (Fig. 14-54).

Alveolar Distraction

All grafting techniques are compromised when inadequate soft tissue is present. This is particularly problematic in the

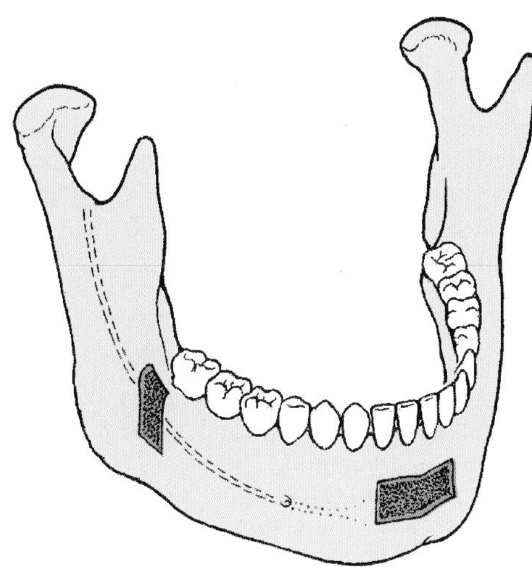

FIGURE 14-53 Graft sites from the genial region or from the buccal shelf.

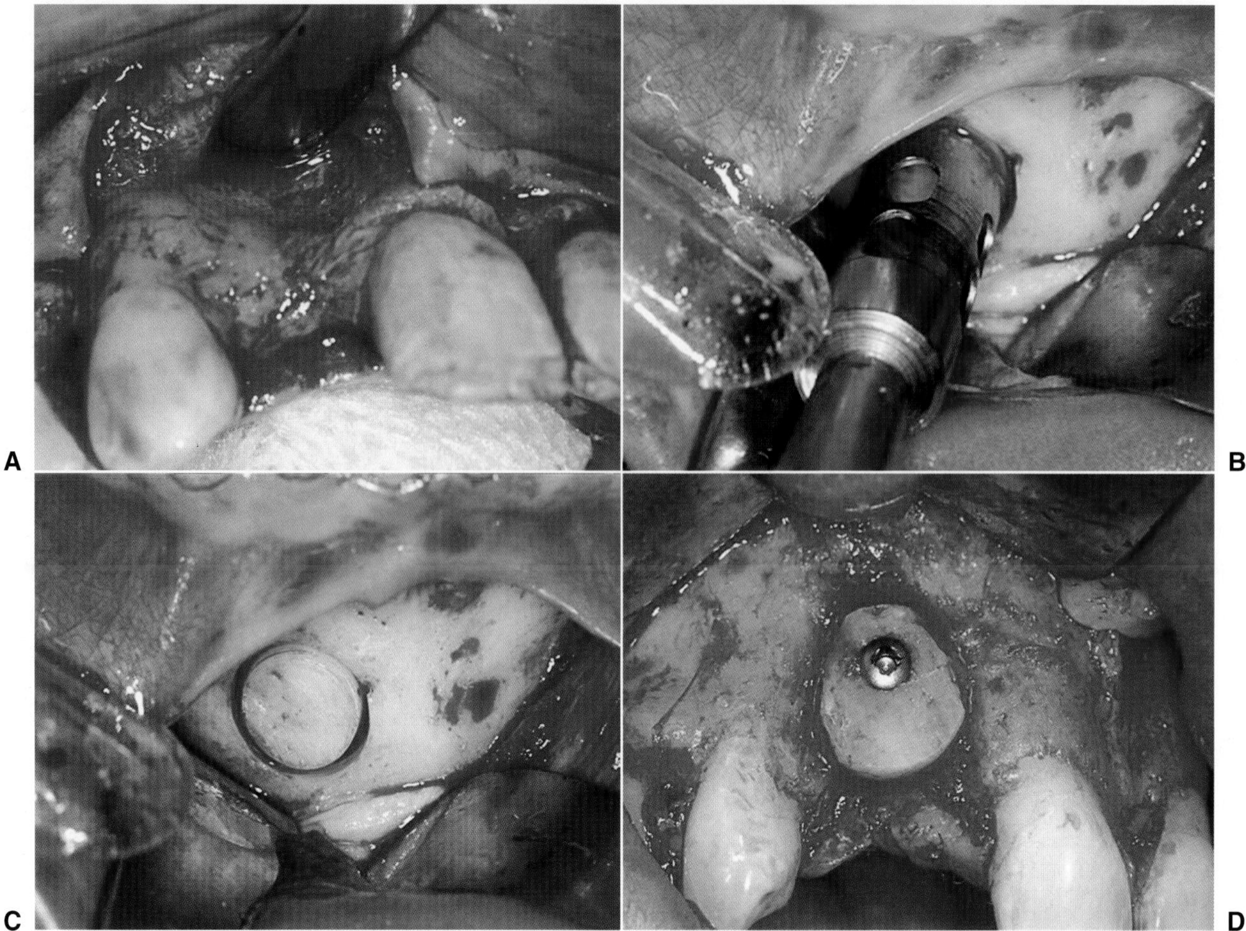

FIGURE 14-54 A, A bony defect is suspected in the anterior maxilla caused by congenitally missing lateral incisor. B, View of the defect after the bone is exposed. C, Harvest of a cortical cancellous bone graft from the genial region with a trephine. D, The graft is placed and stabilized with a screw.

anterior maxilla when vertical hard and soft tissue defects exist after trauma or treatment of a pathologic condition. Tightly bound tissue in this area makes primary closure difficult. Distraction osteogenesis techniques take advantage of the development of bone that results when an osteotomized segment of bone is slowly moved, allowing new bone formation within the gap. This technique was initially used to lengthen long bones, but the principles have been applied to the jaws and to alveolar bone (also refer to Chapters 13 and 25). The technique has the disadvantage of increased cost associated with the distraction device and esthetic compromise during the distraction phase. However, it is a predictable way to gain large vertical increases of soft and hard tissue, especially in difficult areas such as the anterior maxilla (Fig. 14-55).

Transantral Grafting (Sinus Lift)

After tooth loss, alveolar resorption occurs. In the posterior maxilla, crestal bone resorption is also accompanied by sinus pneumatization. In situations in which inadequate bone exists to place implants of appropriate length, sinus floor augmentation can be performed. This can be done indirectly through the implant osteotomy site or directly by an approach through the lateral wall of the maxillary sinus.

When only a few millimeters of augmentation is needed in conjunction with simultaneous implant placement, indirect sinus lift is effective. This procedure relies on the lack of density found in maxillary cancellous bone. The initial drill is used to locate the angulation and position of the planned implant. The depth is drilled just short of the sinus floor. Osteotomes are then used to enlarge the site progressively. The osteotome is cupped on the end and compresses the walls of the osteotomy site; it also scrapes bone from the sides of the wall, pushing it ahead. The bone of the sinus floor is pushed upward, elevating the sinus membrane and depositing the bone from the lateral wall of the osteotomy into the sinus below the membrane (Fig. 14-56). If needed, additional graft material can be introduced through the implant site.

Undetected perforation may occur with this technique. This procedure is only possible when a few millimeters of bone are needed for an implant that has adequate primary stability in native bone.

If several implants are to be placed or more than 4 to 5 mm of augmentation is needed, a direct approach is required. A window is created in the lateral wall of the sinus, the sinus membrane is elevated, and the floor is grafted to increase vertical bone height (Fig. 14-57). Implants may be placed simultaneously with the grafting procedure if adequate native bone is present for primary implant stability. This is usually defined as 4 mm or more of bone. If less than 4 mm of bone is available, the procedure should be staged with initial grafting

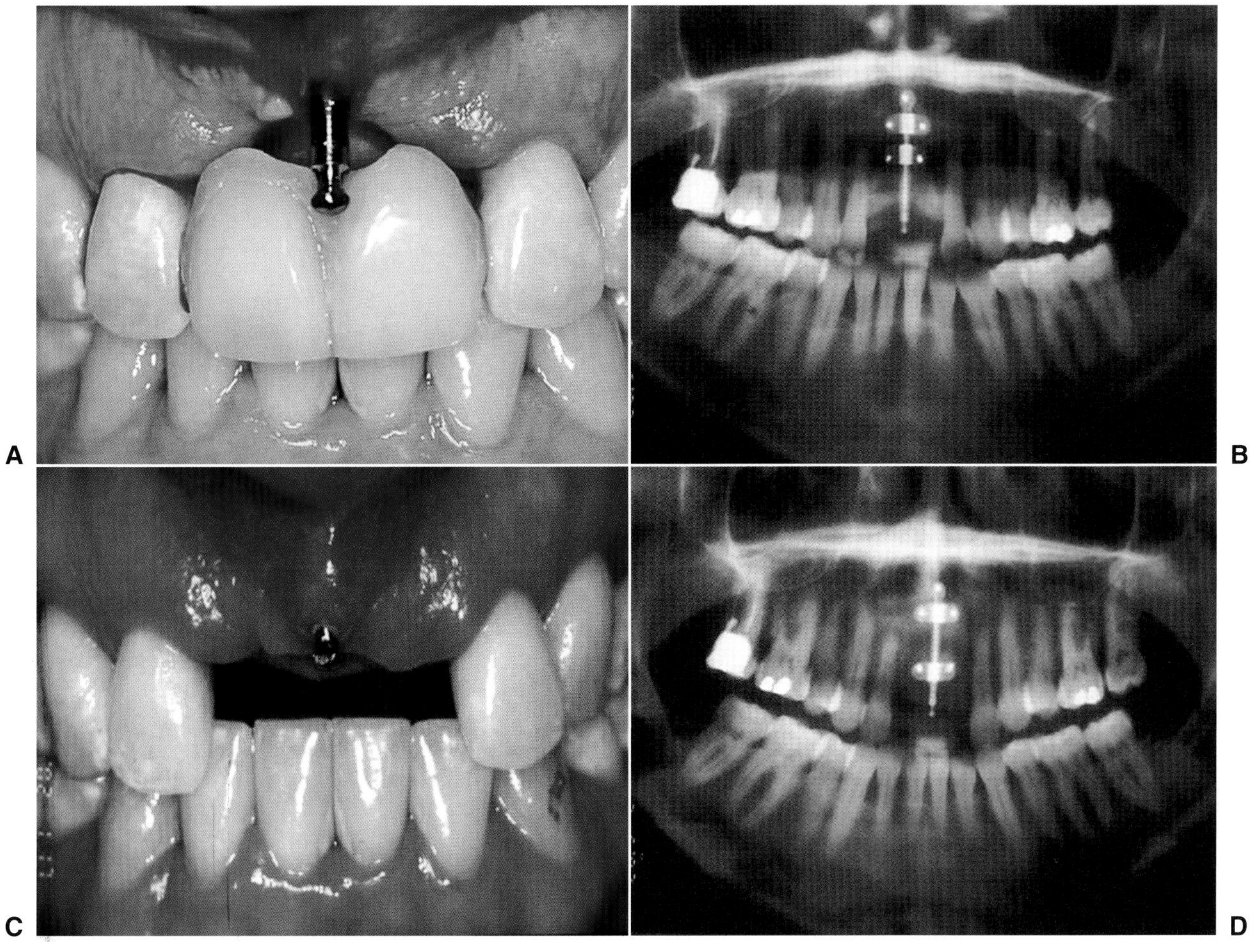

FIGURE 14-55 A, A large anterior maxillary defect is the result of trauma. A distraction device is in place. B, Radiograph of distraction device in place. C, Clinical presentation after distraction. Note increase bone height. D, Radiograph showing expanded distractor and increased bone height.

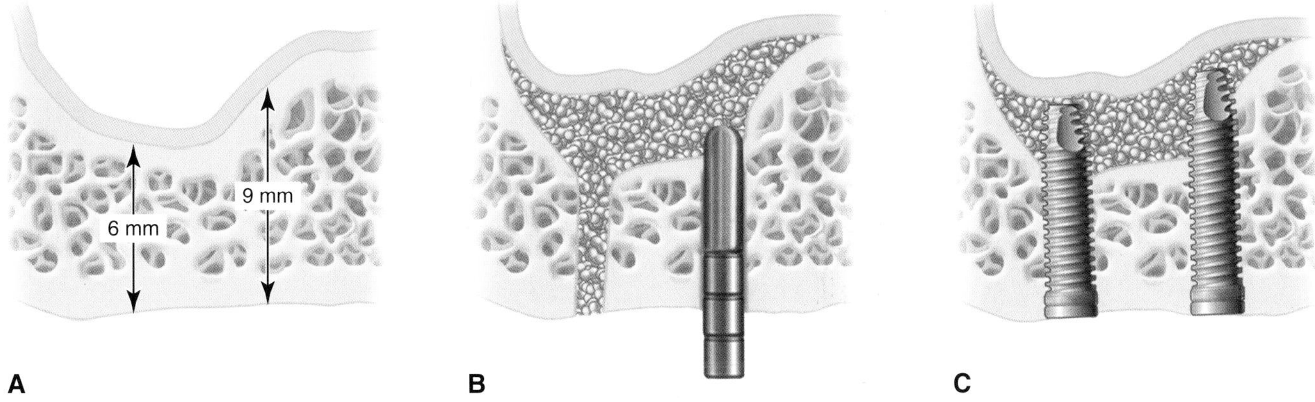

FIGURE 14-56 Indirect sinus elevation procedure. A, Pneumatized sinus with adequate bone for primary stability. B, After drilling pilot holes, osteotomes are used to enlarge the osteotomy while placing graft material. C, The pressure created by the graft material as it is inserted into the osteotomy expands the intact sinus membrane and elevates the floor of the sinus, allowing implant placement.

alone, after which the graft is consolidated and the implant is placed. Transantral grafting (i.e., sinus lift) procedures can be performed in an outpatient setting using autogenous bone, allogeneic bone, or bone substitutes. Success is similar for all these materials. Autogenous bone requires less time than allogeneic or xenogeneic bone to consolidate (4 to 6 months versus 7 to 12 months).

The available bone to support the implant can be significantly improved with these techniques. Patients who smoke have a significant increased failure rate, and some authors

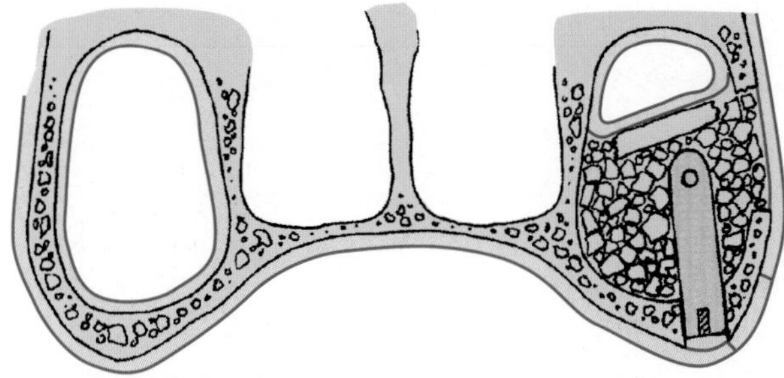

FIGURE 14-57 Direct sinus lift procedure.

suggest that smoking is a contraindication to sinus lift. In addition, a much higher incidence of infection after this procedure is found than with other implant surgery. Antibiotic prophylaxis is paramount. Patients must also refrain from wearing a prosthesis over the surgical area for a minimum of 1 week.

SPECIAL SITUATIONS

Postextraction Placement of Implants

When implant placement is planned before extraction of the tooth, consideration should be given to the most desirable time for implant placement. The implant may be placed immediately (i.e., at the time of extraction), early (i.e., 2 months after extraction), or late (i.e., more than 6 months after extraction). Each of these times has its indications, advantages, and disadvantages.

Immediate placement allows the overall shortest healing time and combines the tooth extraction with the surgical implant placement. Immediate placement can be considered if the tooth to be removed is not infected and can be removed without the loss of alveolar bone. Once the tooth is removed, the implant is placed at least 4 mm apical to the apex of the tooth (Fig. 14-58). The implant should be countersunk slightly below the height of the crestal bone to allow for resorption of the bone resulting from extraction.

The gap between the implant and the residual tooth socket must be evaluated and managed according to its size. If the gap is less than 1 mm, no treatment modification is needed. If the gap is greater than 1 mm, grafting with a particulate material may be necessary.

After implant placement, every effort should be made to achieve a primary soft tissue closure. If this is not possible, a resorbable collagen pellet may be placed over the implant and held in place with a figure-of-eight suture. The surgeon may consider extending the time allowed for integration before loading.

Anterior Maxilla Esthetic Zone

In the esthetic zone of the anterior maxilla, successful integration alone is not adequate. The implant must have proper position, angulation, and depth for esthetic restoration. These parameters are prosthodontically determined and communicated to the surgeon by the surgical stent. The stent must show the ideal position; labial thickness of porcelain and metal; and location of the cementoenamel junction of the final prosthesis. If inadequate bone is present to place the implant with proper position and angulation, grafting is necessary. Esthetic concerns and compromised bone often present in the situation of congenitally missing teeth. Failure of tooth formation is associated with severe hypoplasia of the alveolar bone. Grafting using guided bone regeneration techniques or corticocancellous blocks must be considered (see Fig. 14-54). Implant depth is also important to allow proper emergence profile. Excessive depth leads to increased pocket depth, and

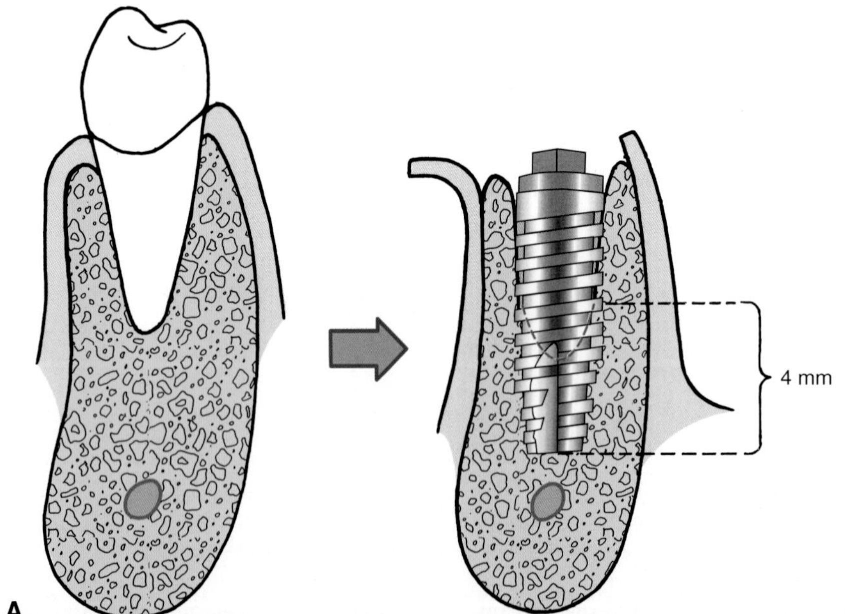

FIGURE 14-58 Implants placed in fresh extraction sockets must have 4 mm of precise fit along apical aspect of implant. Implants should be countersunk slightly below the crest of bone, and any gap between sides of extraction socket and implant should be less than 1 mm. If the gap is greater than 1 mm, grafting with a scientifically validated particulate graft material of the surgeon's choice should be considered.

too shallow placement can result in a poorly contoured crown or metal showing at the gingival margin. As a general rule, the top of the implant should be placed 3 mm below the planned position of the cementoenamel junction of the final restoration.

Atrophic Anterior Mandible

In the atrophic mandible (i.e., less than 8 mm of vertical height), the shortest implant may be longer than the available bone. Implants may be placed by purposefully perforating the inferior cortex. This may decrease the crown-to-root ratio or increase the risk of fracture. Recent studies have shown that after restoration of the atrophic mandible with an entirely implant-supported prosthesis, bone height and density increase, presumably as a result of the functional stresses that result from the prosthesis.

Therefore an effective approach in the atrophic mandible is to place five implants, leaving 2 to 3 mm above the height of the residual bone. An entirely implant-supported hybrid prosthesis is then fabricated. Alternatively, the transmandibular implant has also been shown to be effective in the atrophic mandible, with similar remodeling and formation of new bone. Either of these techniques may be considered in the atrophic mandible where 6 mm or more of bone height is found. If the bone height is less than 6 mm, augmentation of the bony height in this area with autogenous grafts may be necessary. Autogenous grafts onlayed onto the residual ridge undergo resorption if conventional dentures are placed but are generally maintained well if an implant-borne prosthesis is placed.

Atrophic Posterior Mandible

As discussed before, the posterior mandible poses unique problems. Presence of the inferior alveolar nerve limits implant length. This, coupled with increased occlusal load, is one reason for the higher implant failure rate in this region. Overengineering with placement of more implants can improve the prognosis. When less than 8 mm of vertical height overlying the inferior alveolar nerve is found, implant success will be severely compromised. Bone may be grafted to increase height as previously described.

However, if supereruption of the posterior maxillary dentition exists, a graft of adequate thickness to improve implant stability may result in inadequate interarch space for the prosthesis. In this case the inferior alveolar nerve may be repositioned to allow use of the entire height of the mandibular body (Fig. 14-59). This procedure carries the risk of permanent anesthesia or painful dysesthesia. The magnitude of this complication requires that a surgeon experienced with nerve surgery and postoperative assessment of neurosensory function perform this operation. The advantage is that with repositioning of the nerve, a longer implant can be placed, with stabilization in the superior and inferior cortical bone.

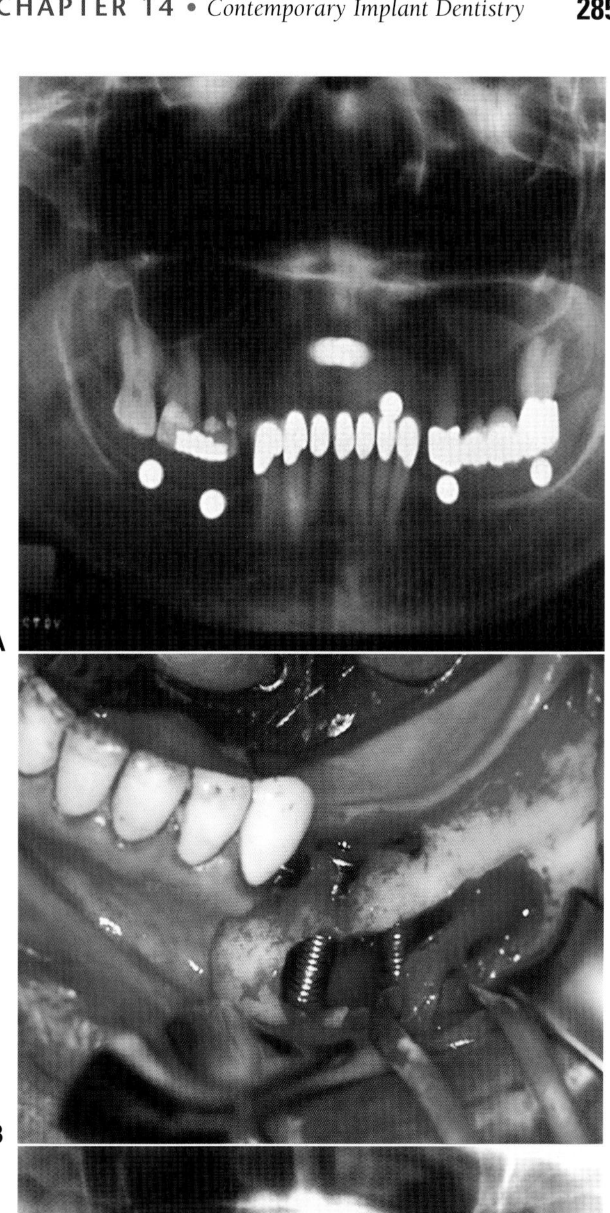

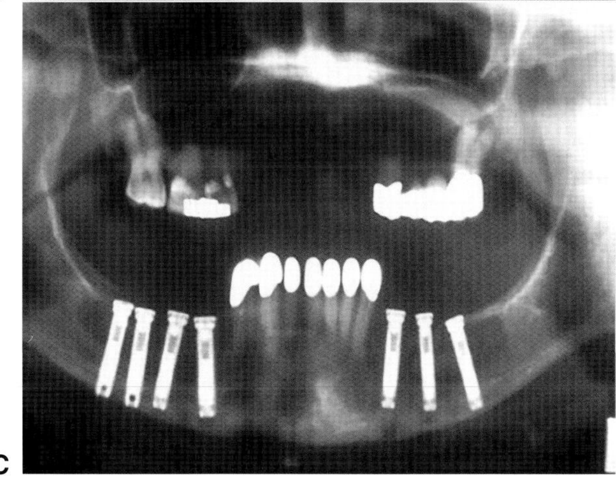

FIGURE 14-59 A, Panoramic radiograph reveals supereruption of the posterior maxillary dentition with loss of interarch space. Inadequate room for implants above the inferior alveolar nerve and no room for a graft is found. B, The inferior alveolar nerve is positioned buccally to allow implants to be placed. C, Postoperative panoramic radiograph shows implants of adequate length extending to the inferior border.

Atrophic Maxilla

Initial implant restorative approaches for the fully edentulous maxilla concentrated on implant placement in the anterior region, similar to the edentulous mandible. However, the resulting prosthesis was often unsatisfactory. If adequate space was allowed for proper hygiene, phonetics and esthetics were severely compromised. If the prosthesis was developed in such a way as to eliminate these problems, hygiene became virtually impossible. The cantilever effect of this type of prosthesis on implants placed within the compromised bone of the maxilla also resulted in increased failures. If implants are placed bilaterally in the posterior maxilla, a prosthesis with ideal esthetics, phonetics, and hygiene access can be created. However, the bone overlying the sinus is frequently inadequate to place the implant and to allow suitable bony support. In these situations the sinus floor may be grafted to increase the quantity of bone for implant placement.

Some patients are unwilling to wait the time required for sinus lift consolidation or are unwilling to undergo grafting. A relatively new technique that places very long implants into the body of the zygoma (Zygomaticus system), along with short anterior implants, is an effective way to support a maxillary overdenture without need for sinus lift surgery (Fig. 14-60).

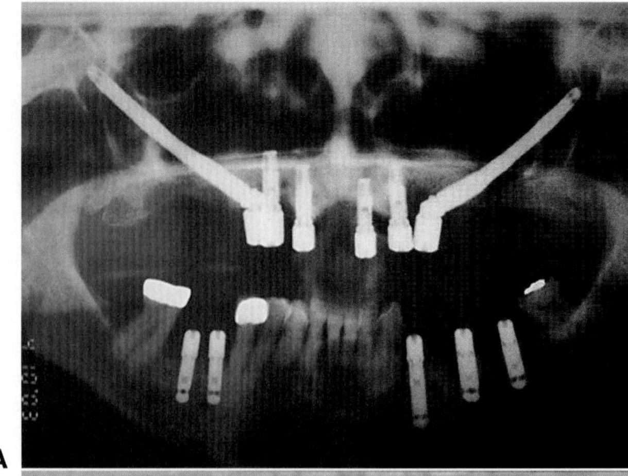

A

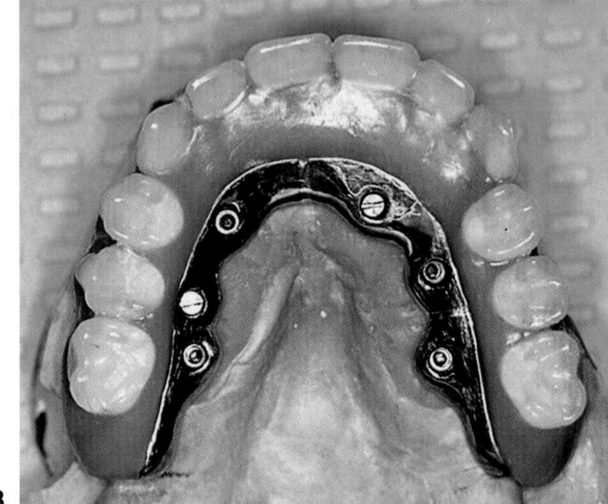

B

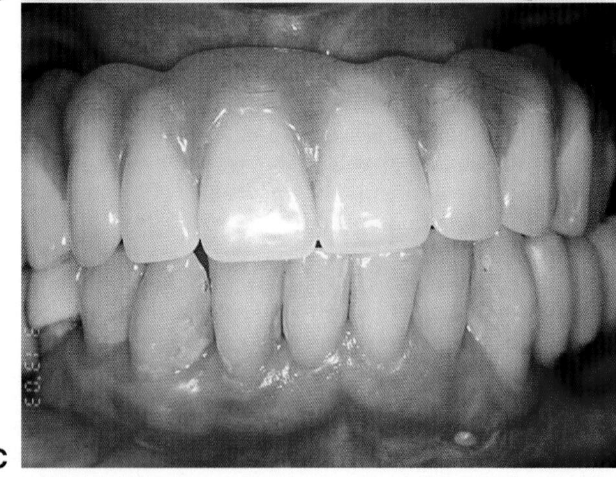

C

FIGURE 14-60 A, As an alternative to grafting the sinus floor, the Zygomaticus implant is placed along with four conventional implants in the anterior maxilla. B and C, An implant-supported maxillary denture is fabricated without the need for sinus lift.

Implants in Growing Patients

Children may have edentulous spaces resulting from congenital absence of teeth or loss of teeth from trauma, infection, or neoplasia. The ability to restore the lost function without damage to adjacent virgin teeth that would occur from conventional restorative methods is appealing. Evidence suggests that implants can be successfully placed into growing patients. In the fully edentulous patient, an implant-supported prosthesis can be fabricated as soon as the patient is old enough to cooperate with hygiene requirements. This is usually defined as age 7. In patients who have lost a portion of the jaw from tumor resection or trauma, an implant-supported prosthesis can likewise be used as early as age 7. However, when the edentulous area in question is associated with unerupted natural teeth, no implants should be placed until eruption of the natural dentition and alveolar growth are complete (i.e., at approximately 16 years of age). Implants placed before this time behave in similar fashion to an ankylosed tooth, with progressive submersion of the implant as a result of eruption of adjacent teeth and alveolar bone growth.

Implants in Irradiated Bone

Cancer patients frequently suffer from surgery- and irradiation-associated soft and hard tissue defects that significantly compromise conventional prosthodontic rehabilitation. An implant-supported prosthesis could improve function and esthetics; however, concern regarding the compromised wound healing that results after tumoricidal irradiation to the jaws has contraindicated even minor surgery and implant placement in these patients. It now appears that it may be possible to place implants in this group of patients (see Chapter 18). Careful soft tissue handling and perioperative hyperbaric oxygen treatments have been used for patients receiving implants in irradiated tissue, with results comparable to that found in nonirradiated patients. Little is known about the long-term results in these patients, and potential for increased failure and serious sequelae (e.g., osteoradionecrosis) still exists. As a result, an experienced implant surgeon should manage implant placement in this group of patients.

Early Loading

Since staged implant systems were first introduced, there have been efforts to define the minimum time required for osseointegration. Generally accepted integration times are based on experience and tradition with little experimental data. Research continues to attempt to define ideal minimum integration times. Factors that are likely important in determining what these minimum times should be include bone quality, implant material, and surface and prosthesis configuration. Some studies have shown that early loading (i.e., 6 weeks) is successful, even in typically difficult areas such as the posterior mandible.

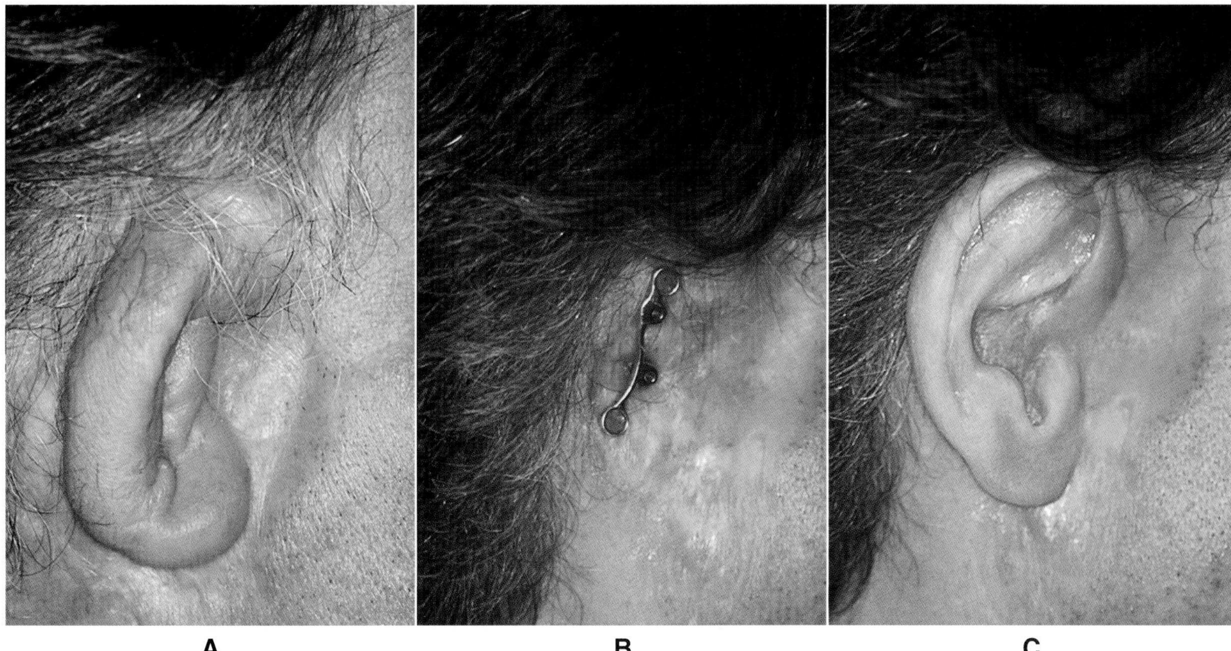

FIGURE 14-61 A, Congenitally absent ear with unsatisfactory autogenous reconstruction. B, Endosseous implants placed into temporal bone with framework. C, Implant-supported prosthetic ear.

Clearly, there are more variables to consider in these cases, and not all patients or restorative situations are amenable. The most extreme variation on the theme of early loading is immediate loading. There are emerging data to suggest that immediate loading of implants in controlled situations can be successful as well. Initial primary stability, good bone, controlled occlusal forces, and patient compliance are factors that must be considered.

Extraoral Implants

Recognizing the success of implants for oral applications, maxillofacial prosthodontists and surgeons have expanded use of titanium fixtures to extraoral application. Extraoral implants are now used to anchor prosthetic ears, eyes, and noses for patients with defects resulting from congenital conditions, trauma, or pathologic conditions (Fig. 14-61).

Bibliography

Adell R: Long-term treatment results. In Branemark PI, Zarb G, Albrektson I, editors: *Tissue-integrated prostheses,* Chicago, 1985, Quintessence.

Adell R, Lekholm U, Rockler B et al: A 15-year study of osseointegrated implants in the treatment of the edentulous jaw, *Int J Oral Surg* 10:387, 1981.

Bain CA, May PK: The association between the failure of dental implants and cigarette smoking, *Int J Oral Maxillofac Implants* 8:609, 1993.

Dahlin C, Sennerby L, Lekholm U et al: Generation of new bone around titanium implants using a membrane technique: an experimental study in rabbits, *Int J Oral Maxillofac Implants* 4:19, 1989.

Eriksson AR, Albrektsson T: Temperature threshold levels for heat-induced bone tissue injury: a vital microscopic study in the rabbit, *J Prosthet Dent* 50:101, 1983.

Granström G, Bergström K, Tjellström A et al: A detailed analysis of titanium implants lost in irradiated tissue, *Int J Oral Maxillofac Implants* 9:653, 1994.

Jensen OT, Shulman LB, Block MS et al: Report of the Sinus Consensus Conference of 1996, *Int J Oral Maxillofac Implants* 13:11-41, 1998.

Lazzara RJ: Immediate implant placement into extraction sites: surgical and restorative advantages, *Int J Periodontics Restorative Dent* 9:333, 1989.

McKinney RV, Steflik DE, Roth DL: The biologic response to single crystal sapphire endosteal implant: SEM observations, *J Prosthet Dent* 51:372, 1984.

Perrott, DH, Shama AB, Vargerik K: Endosseous implants for pediatric patients, *Oral Maxillofac Clin N Am* 6:79, 1994.

Peterson LJ, McGlumphy EA, Larsen PE et al: Comparison of mandibular bone response to implant overdentures versus implant-supported hybrid, *J Dent Res* 75:333, 1996.

Peterson LJ, Larsen PE, McGlumphy EA et al: Long-term antibiotic prophylaxis is not necessary for placement of dental implants, *J Oral Maxillofac Surg* 54(suppl 3):76, 1996.

Quirynen M, Alsaadi G, Pauwels M et al: Microbiological and clinical outcomes and patient satisfaction for two treatment options in the edentulous lower jaw after 10 years of function, *Clin Oral Implants Res* 16:277-287, 2005.

Rosen PS, Summers R, Mellado JR et al: PA. The bone-added osteotome sinus floor elevation technique: multicenter retrospective report of consecutively treated patients, *Int J Oral Maxillofac Implants* 14:853-858, 1999.

Sammartino G, Marenzi G, di Lauro AE et al: Aesthetics in oral implantology: biological, clinical, surgical, and prosthetic aspects, *Implant Dent* 16:54-65, 2007.

Sclar AG: Strategies for management of single-tooth extraction sites in aesthetic implant therapy, *J Oral Maxillofac Surg* 62(9 suppl 2):90-105, 2004.

Smith D, Zarb GA: Criteria for success for osseointegrated endosseous implants, *J Prosthet Dent* 62:567, 1989.

Stanford CM: Application of oral implants to the general dental practice, *J Am Dent Assoc* 36:1092-100, 2005.

Tarnow DP, Magner AW, Fletcher P: The effect of the distance from the contact point to the crest of gone on the presence or absence of the interproximal dental papilla, *J Periodontol* 63:995-996, 1992.

U.S. Department of Health and Human Services: Dental implants, NIH Consensus Development Conference Statement, 7:108.

Veksler AE, Kayrouz GA, Newman MG: Chlorhexidine reduces salivary bacteria during scaling and root planing, *J Dent Res* 69:240, 1990.

Woo SB, Hellstein JW, Kalmar JR: Systematic review: bisphosphonates and osteonecrosis of the jaws, *Ann Intern Med* 2006:144:753-761.

PART IV

Infections

Odontogenic infections are generally caused by bacteria that have a propensity to cause abscess formation. In addition, the roots of the teeth provide a pathway for infecting bacteria to enter the deep tissues of the periodontium and periapical regions. Therefore odontogenic infections cause deeply seated abscesses, and they almost always require some form of surgical therapy, ranging from endodontic therapy and gingival curettage to extraction, and incision and drainage of the deep fascial spaces of the head and neck. Antibiotic therapy is an adjunctive treatment to the required surgery. Prophylactic antibiotic therapy may prevent distant infections resulting from bacteremias caused by oral surgical procedures, and such therapy may also prevent some postoperative wound infections.

This section presents the principles of infection management and prevention in dental patients.

Chapter 15 describes the basic management techniques, including surgery and antibiotic administration, for the treatment of odontogenic infections. This chapter also discusses the principles of antibiotic prophylaxis for the prevention of wound infection and distant metastatic infection, such as infectious endocarditis.

Chapter 16 presents an overview of complex odontogenic infections that involve the deep fascial spaces and may require hospitalization of the patient for treatment. Osteomyelitis and other unusual infections are also discussed.

Chapter 17 presents the indications, rationale, and technical aspects of surgical endodontics. Although periapical surgery is occasionally necessary for successful endodontic management, it is necessary for the clinician to be wise in deciding when to choose this treatment modality. Therefore the discussion of the indications and contraindications for endodontic surgery is extensive, and the technical aspects of surgical endodontics are profusely illustrated.

Chapter 18 presents information about patients at risk for infection and other problems that are caused by patient host defense compromise as the result of radiotherapy or cancer chemotherapy. These patients are susceptible to a variety of problems, and the prevention and management of these problems are discussed.

Chapter 19 describes maxillary sinus problems that arise from odontogenic infections and other problems. Although general practitioners rarely see patients with these problems, they may have to provide diagnoses before referring these patients to the appropriate professional for definitive care.

Finally, Chapter 20 discusses salivary gland diseases, primarily the obstructive and infectious types. The major diagnostic and therapeutic modalities used in managing these problems are discussed.

CHAPTER 15

Principles of Management and Prevention of Odontogenic Infections

THOMAS R. FLYNN

CHAPTER OUTLINE

One of the most difficult problems to manage in dentistry is an odontogenic infection. Odontogenic infections arise from the teeth and have a characteristic flora. Caries, periodontal disease, and pulpitis are the initiating infections that can spread beyond the teeth to the alveolar process and the deeper tissues of the face, oral cavity, head, and neck. These infections may range from low-grade, well-localized infections that require only minimal treatment to severe, life-threatening deep fascial space infections. Although the overwhelming majority of odontogenic infections are readily managed by minor surgical procedures and supportive medical therapy that includes antibiotic administration, the practitioner must constantly bear in mind that these infections occasionally become severe and life-threatening in a short time.

This chapter is divided into several sections. The first section discusses the typical microbiologic organisms involved in odontogenic infections. Appropriate therapy of odontogenic infections depends on a clear understanding of the causative bacteria. The second section discusses the natural history of odontogenic infections. When infections occur, they may erode through bone and into the overlying soft tissue. Knowledge of the usual pathway of infection from the teeth and surrounding tissues through the bone and into the overlying soft tissue planes is essential when planning appropriate therapy. The third section of this chapter deals with the principles of management of odontogenic infections. A series of principles are discussed, with consideration of the microbiology and typical pathway of infection. The chapter concludes with a section on prophylaxis against infection. The prophylaxis of wound infection and of metastatic infection is discussed.

MICROBIOLOGY OF ODONTOGENIC INFECTIONS

The bacteria that cause infection are most commonly part of the indigenous bacteria that normally live on or in the host. Odontogenic infections are no exception because the bacteria that cause odontogenic infections are part of the normal oral flora: those that comprise the bacteria of plaque, those found on the mucosal surfaces, and those found in the gingival sulcus. These bacteria are primarily aerobic gram-positive cocci, anaerobic gram-positive cocci, and anaerobic gram-negative rods. These bacteria cause a variety of common diseases, such as dental caries, gingivitis, and periodontitis. When these bacteria gain access to deeper underlying tissues, as through a necrotic dental pulp or through a deep periodontal pocket, they cause odontogenic infections. As the infection progresses more deeply, different members of the infecting flora can find better growth conditions and begin to outnumber the previously dominant species.

Many carefully performed microbiologic studies of odontogenic infections have demonstrated the microbiologic composition of these infections. Several important factors must be noted. First, almost all odontogenic infections are caused by multiple bacteria. The polymicrobial nature of these infections makes it important that the clinician understand the variety of bacteria that are likely to cause the infection. In most odontogenic infections, the laboratory can identify an average of five species of bacteria. For as many as eight different species to be identified in a given infection is not unusual. On rare occasions a single species may be isolated. New molecular methods, which identify the infecting species by their genetic makeup, have allowed scientists to identify greater numbers and a whole new range of species not previously associated with these infections, including unculturable pathogens.

A second important factor is the oxygen tolerance of the bacteria causing odontogenic infections. Because the mouth flora is a combination of aerobic and anaerobic bacteria, it is not surprising to find that most odontogenic infections have anaerobic and aerobic bacteria. Infections caused by aerobic bacteria alone account for 6% of all odontogenic infections. Anaerobic bacteria alone are found in 44% of odontogenic infections. Infections caused by mixed anaerobic and aerobic bacteria compose 50% of all odontogenic infections (Table 15-1).

The predominant aerobic bacteria in odontogenic infections (found in about 65% of cases) are the *Streptococcus milleri* group, which consists of three members of the *S. viridans* group of bacteria: *S. anginosus, S. intermedius,* and *S. constellatus.* These facultative organisms, which can grow in the presence and the absence of oxygen, may initiate the process of spreading into the deeper tissues (Table 15-2). Miscellaneous bacteria contribute 5% or less of the aerobic species found in these infections. Rarely found bacteria include staphylococci, group D *Streptococcus* organisms, other streptococci, *Neisseria* spp., *Corynebacterium* spp., and *Haemophilus* spp.

The anaerobic bacteria found in odontogenic infections include an even greater variety of species (Table 15-2). Two main groups, however, predominate. The anaerobic gram-positive cocci are found in about 65% of cases. These cocci are anaerobic *Streptococcus* and *Peptostreptococcus*. Oral gram-negative anaerobic rods are cultured in about three quarters of the infections. The *Prevotella* and *Porphyromonas* spp. are found in about 75% of these, and *Fusobacterium* organisms are present in more than 50%.

Of the anaerobic bacteria, several gram-positive cocci (i.e., anaerobic *Streptococcus* and *Peptostreptococcus* spp.) and gram-negative rods (i.e., *Prevotella* and *Fusobacterium* spp.) play a more important pathogenic role. The anaerobic gram-negative cocci and the anaerobic gram-positive rods appear to have little or no role in the cause of odontogenic infections; instead, they appear to be opportunistic organisms.

The method by which mixed aerobic and anaerobic bacteria cause infections is known with some certainty. After initial inoculation into the deeper tissues, the facultative *S. milleri* group organisms can synthesize hyaluronidase, which allows the infecting organisms to spread through connective tissues, initiating a cellulitis type of infection. Metabolic by-products from the streptococci then create a favorable environment for the growth of anaerobes: the release of essential nutrients, lowered pH in the tissues, and consumption of local oxygen supplies. The anaerobic bacteria are then able to grow, and as the local oxidation-reduction potential is lowered further, the anaerobic bacteria predominate and cause liquefaction necrosis of tissues by their synthesis of collagenases. As collagen is broken down and invading white blood cells necrose and lyse, microabscesses form and may coalesce into a clinically recognizable abscess. In the abscess stage, the anaerobic bacteria predominate and may eventually become the only organisms found in culture. Early infections appearing initially as a cellulitis may be characterized as aerobic streptococcal infections, and late, chronic abscesses may be characterized as anaerobic infections.

Clinically, this progression of the infecting flora from aerobic to anaerobic seems to correlate with the type of swelling that can be found in the infected region. Thus, odontogenic infections seem to pass through four stages. In the first 3 days of

TABLE 15-1

Role of Anaerobic Bacteria in Odontogenic Infections

	Percentage
Anaerobic only	50
Mixed anaerobic and aerobic	44
Aerobic only	6

Brook I, Frazier EH, Gher ME: Aerobic and anaerobic microbiology of periapical abscess, *Oral Microbiol Immunol* 6:123-125, 1991.

TABLE 15-2

Major Pathogens in Odontogenic Infections

	Percent of Cases	
Microorganism	Sakamoto et al.* (1998)	Heimdahl et al.† (1985)
Streptococcus milleri group	65	31
Peptostreptococcus species	65	31
Other anaerobic streptococci	9	38
Prevotella species (e.g., *P. oralis* and *P. buccae*)	74	35
Porphyromonas species (e.g., *P. gingivalis*)	17	—
Fusobacterium species	52	45

*Sakamoto H, Kato H, Sato T, Sasaki J: Semiquantitative bacteriology of closed odontogenic abscesses, *Bull Tokyo Dent Coll* 39:103-107, 1998.
†Heimdahl A, Von Konow L, Satoh T et al: Clinical appearance of orofacial infections of odontogenic origin in relation to microbiological findings, *J Clin Microbiol* 22:299, 1985.

TABLE 15-3

Comparison of Edema, Cellulitis, and Abscess

Characteristic	Edema (Inoculation)	Cellulitis	Abscess
Duration	0-3 days	1-5 days	4-10 days
Pain, borders	Mild, diffuse	Diffuse	Localized
Size	Variable	Large	Smaller
Color	Normal	Red	Shiny center
Consistency	Jellylike	Boardlike	Soft center
Progression	Increasing	Increasing	Decreasing
Pus	Absent	Absent	Present
Bacteria	Aerobic	Mixed	Anaerobic
Seriousness	Low	Greater	Less

symptoms, a soft, mildly tender, doughy swelling represents the *inoculation stage,* in which the invading streptococci are just beginning to colonize the host. After 3 to 5 days, the swelling becomes hard, red, and acutely tender as the infecting mixed flora stimulates the intense inflammatory response of the *cellulitis stage*. At 5 to 7 days after the onset of swelling, the anaerobes begin to predominate, causing a liquefied abscess in the center of the swollen area. This is the *abscess stage*. Finally, when the abscess drains spontaneously through skin or mucosa or it is surgically drained, the *resolution stage* begins as the immune system destroys the infecting bacteria and the processes of healing and repair ensue. The clinical and microbiologic characteristics of edema, cellulitis, and abscess are summarized and compared in Table 15-3.

NATURAL HISTORY OF PROGRESSION OF ODONTOGENIC INFECTIONS

Odontogenic infections have two major origins: (1) periapical, as a result of pulpal necrosis and subsequent bacterial invasion into the periapical tissue, and (2) periodontal, as a result of a deep periodontal pocket that allows inoculation of bacteria into the underlying soft tissues. Of these two, the periapical origin is the most common in odontogenic infections.

Necrosis of the dental pulp as a result of deep caries allows a pathway for bacteria to enter the periapical tissues. Once this tissue has become inoculated with bacteria and an active infection is established, the infection spreads equally in all directions but preferentially along the lines of least resistance. The infection spreads through the cancellous bone until it encounters a cortical plate. If this cortical plate is thin, the infection erodes through the bone and enters the surrounding soft tissues. Treatment of the necrotic pulp by standard endodontic therapy or extraction of the tooth should resolve the infection. Antibiotics alone may arrest, but do not cure, the infection because the infection is likely to recur when antibiotic therapy has ended without treatment of the underlying dental cause. Thus the primary treatment of pulpal infections is endodontic therapy or tooth extraction, as opposed to antibiotics.

When the infection erodes through the cortical plate of the alveolar process, it spreads into predictable anatomic locations. The location of the infection arising from a specific tooth is determined by the following two major factors: (1) the thickness of the bone overlying the apex of the tooth and (2) the relationship of the site of perforation of bone to muscle attachments of the maxilla and mandible.

Figure 15-1 demonstrates how infections perforate through bone into the overlying soft tissue. In Figure 15-1, *A,* the labial

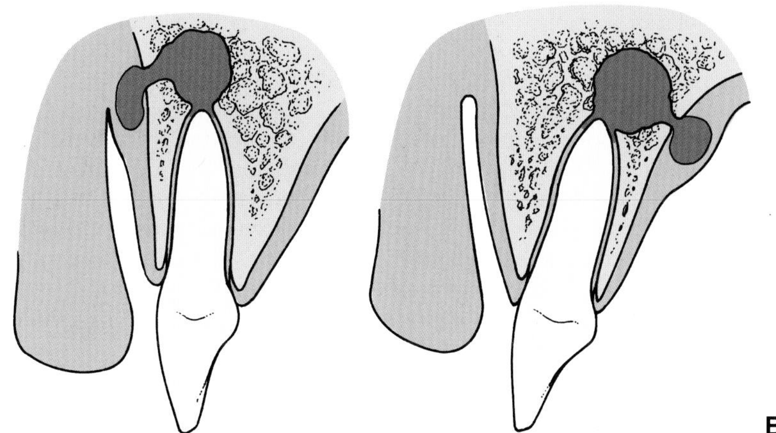

FIGURE 15-1 When infection erodes through bone, it will enter soft tissue through thinnest bone. A, Tooth apex is near thin labial bone, so infection erodes labially. B, Right apex is near palatal aspect, so palatal bone will be perforated.

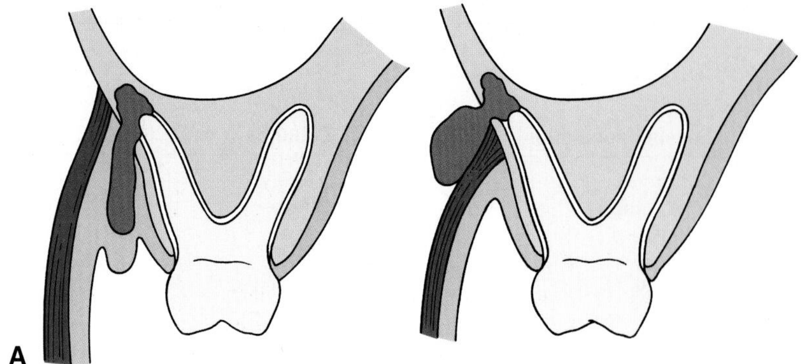

FIGURE 15-2 Relationship of point of bone perforation to muscle attachment determines fascial space involved. A, When tooth apex is lower than muscle attachment, vestibular abscess results. B, If apex is higher than muscle attachment, the adjacent fascial space is involved.

bone overlying the apex of the tooth is thin compared with the bone on the palatal aspect of the tooth. Therefore, as the infectious process spreads, it goes into the labial soft tissues. In Figure 15-1, *B*, the tooth is severely proclined, which results in thicker labial bone and a relatively thinner palatal bone. In this situation, as the infection spreads through the bone into the soft tissue, the infection is seen as a palatal abscess.

Once the infection has eroded through the bone, the precise location of the soft tissue infection is determined by the position of the perforation relative to the muscle attachments. In Figure 15-2, *A*, the infection has eroded through to the facial aspect of the tooth and inferior to the attachment of the buccinator muscle, which results in an infection that appears as a vestibular abscess. In Figure 15-2, *B*, the infection has eroded through the bone superior to the attachment of the buccinator muscle and is expressed as an infection of the buccal space because the buccinator muscle separates the buccal and vestibular spaces.

Infections from most maxillary teeth erode through the facial cortical plate. These infections also erode through the bone below the attachment of the muscles that attach to the maxilla, which means that most maxillary dental abscesses appear initially as vestibular abscesses. Occasionally, a palatal abscess arises from the apex of a severely inclined lateral incisor or the palatal root of a maxillary first molar or premolar (Fig. 15-3). More commonly, the maxillary molars cause infections that erode through the bone superior to the insertion of the buccinator muscle, which results in a buccal space infection. Likewise, on occasion a long maxillary canine root allows infection to erode through the bone superior to the insertion of the levator anguli oris muscle and causes an infraorbital (canine) space infection.

In the mandible, infections of the incisors, canines, and premolars usually erode through the facial cortical plate superior to the attachment of the muscles of the lower lip, resulting in vestibular abscesses. Mandibular molar teeth infections erode through the lingual cortical bone more frequently than with the anterior teeth. First molar infections may drain buccally or lingually. Infections of the second molar can perforate buccally or lingually (but usually lingually), and third molar infections almost always erode through the lingual cortical plate. The mylohyoid muscle determines whether infections that drain lingually go superior to that muscle into the sublingual space or below it into the submandibular space.

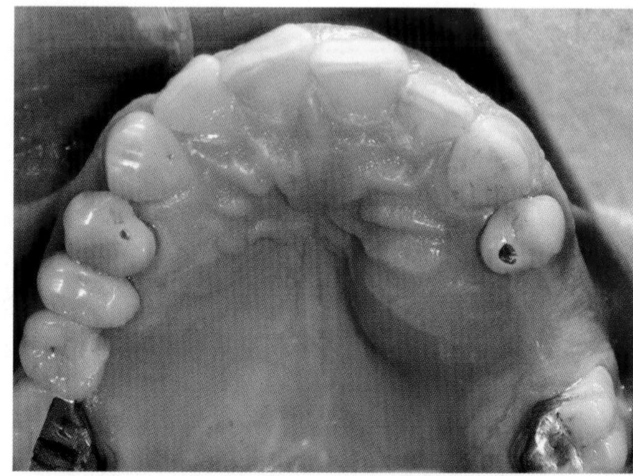

FIGURE 15-3 Palatal abscess arising from the palatal root of a maxillary first premolar.

The most common odontogenic deep fascial space infection is a vestibular space abscess (Fig. 15-4). Occasionally, patients do not seek treatment for these infections, and the process ruptures spontaneously and drains, resulting in resolution or chronicity of the infection. The infection recurs if the site of spontaneous drainage closes. Sometimes the abscess establishes a chronic sinus tract that drains to the oral cavity or to the skin (Fig. 15-5). As long as the sinus tract continues to drain, the patient experiences no pain. Antibiotic administration usually stops the drainage of infected material temporarily, but when the antibiotic course is over, the drainage recurs. Definitive treatment of a chronic sinus tract requires treatment of the original causative problem, which is usually a necrotic pulp. In such a case the necessary surgery is endodontic therapy or extraction of the infected tooth.

PRINCIPLES OF THERAPY OF ODONTOGENIC INFECTIONS

This section discusses the management of the odontogenic infection. A series of principles are discussed that are useful in treating patients who come to the dentist with infections related to the teeth and gingiva. The clinician must keep in mind the

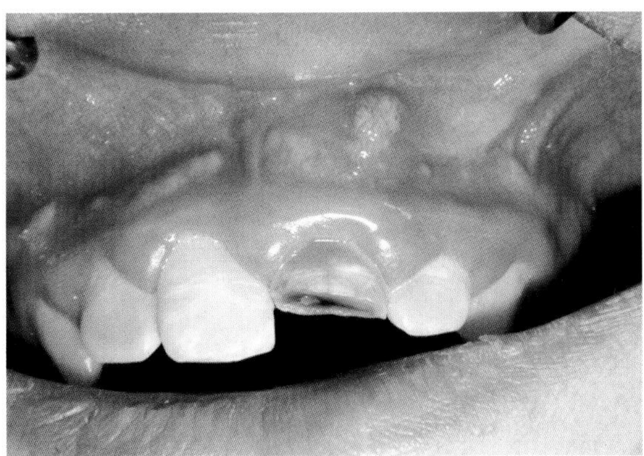

FIGURE 15-4 Vestibular abscess arising from maxillary incisor. Overlying mucosa is thin because pus is near surface. (From Flynn TR: Anatomy of oral and maxillofacial infections. In Topazian RG, Goldberg MH, Hupp JR, editors: *Oral and maxillofacial infections,* ed 4, Philadelphia, 2002, WB Saunders.)

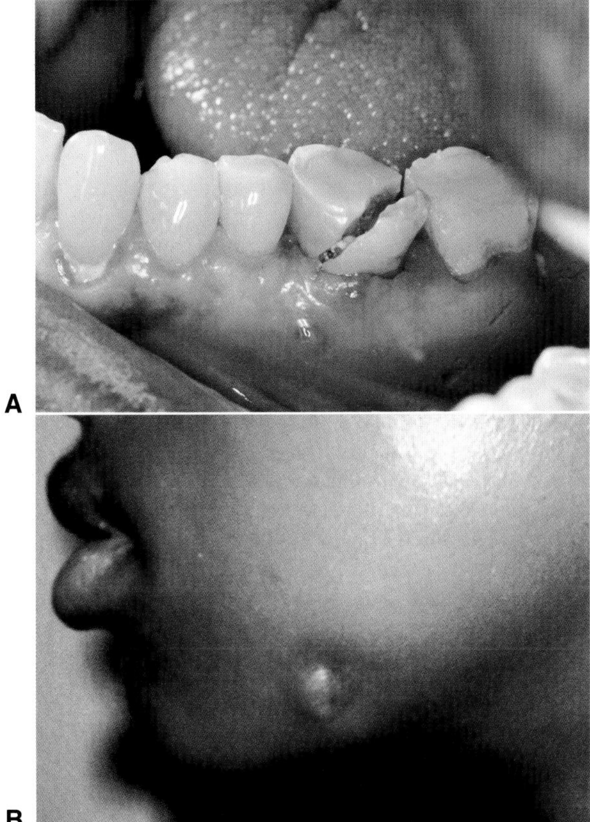

FIGURE 15-5 Chronic drainage sinus tracts that result from low-grade infections may drain intraorally (A) or extraorally (B). (A courtesy Sasha B. Ross, DMD. B from Flynn TR, Topazian RG: Infections of the oral cavity. In Waite D, editor: *Textbook of practical oral and maxillofacial surgery,* Philadelphia, 1987, Lea & Febiger.)

information in the preceding two sections of this chapter to understand these principles. By following these principles in stepwise fashion, the clinician may not always achieve the expected result, but he or she will certainly have met the standard of care. The first three principles are perhaps the most important in determining the outcome, yet they can be accomplished by the experienced practitioner within the first few minutes of the initial patient encounter.

Principle 1: Determine Severity of Infection

Most odontogenic infections are mild and require only minor surgical therapy. When the patient comes for treatment, the initial goal is to assess the severity of the infection. This determination is based on a complete history of the current infectious illness and a physical examination.

Complete History

The history of the patient's infection follows the same general guidelines as any history. The initial purpose is to find out the patient's chief complaint. Typical chief complaints of patients with infections are "I have a toothache," "My jaw is swollen," or "I have a gum boil in my mouth." The complaint should be recorded in the patient's own words.

The next step in taking of the history is determining how long the infection has been present. First, the dentist should inquire as to time of *onset* of the infection. How long ago did the patient first have symptoms of pain, swelling, or drainage, which indicated the beginning of the infection? The *course* of the infection is then discussed. Have the symptoms of the infection been constant, have they waxed and waned, or has the patient steadily grown worse since the symptoms were first noted? Finally, the practitioner should determine the *rapidity* of progress of the infection. Has the infection process progressed rapidly over a few hours, or has it gradually increased in severity over several days to a week?

The next step is eliciting the patient's symptoms. Infections are actually a severe inflammatory response, and the cardinal signs of inflammation are clinically easy to discern. These signs and symptoms are the Latin terms *dolor* (pain), *tumor* (swelling), *calor* (warmth), *rubor* (erythema, redness), and *functio laesa* (loss of function).

The most common complaint is pain. The patient should be asked where the pain actually started and how the pain has spread since it was first noted. The second sign is *tumor* (swelling). Swelling is a physical finding that is sometimes subtle and not obvious to the practitioner, although it is obvious to the patient. It is important that the dentist ask the patient to describe any area of swelling. The third characteristic of infection is calor (warmth). The patient should be asked whether the area has felt warm to the touch. Redness of the overlying area is the next characteristic to be evaluated. The patient should be asked if there has been or currently is any change in color, especially redness, over the area of the infection. Functio laesa should then be checked. When inquiring about this characteristic, the dentist should ask about trismus (difficulty in opening the mouth widely) and difficulty in chewing, swallowing (dysphagia), or breathing (dyspnea).

Finally, the dentist should ask how the patient feels in general. Patients who feel fatigued, feverish, weak, and sick are said to have *malaise.* Malaise usually indicates a generalized reaction to a moderate to severe infection (Fig. 15-6).

In the next step the dentist inquires about treatment. The dentist should ask about previous professional treatment and self-treatment. Many patients doctor themselves with leftover antibiotics, hot soaks, and a variety of other home or herbal remedies. Occasionally, a dentist sees a patient who received treatment in an emergency room 2 or 3 days earlier and was

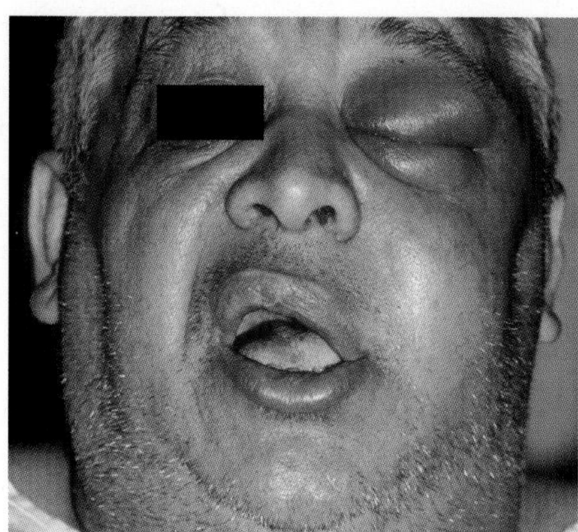

FIGURE 15-6 Patient with severe infection and elevated temperature, pulse rate, and respiratory rate. The patient feels sick and tired; he has a "toxic appearance." (From Flynn TR: *Atlas Oral Maxillofac Surg Clin North Am* 8:79, 2000.)

referred to a dentist by the emergency room physician. The patient may have neglected to follow that advice until the infection became severe. Sometimes, the patient did not take the prescribed antibiotic because he or she could not afford to purchase it.

The patient's complete medical history should be obtained in the usual manner by interview or by self-administered questionnaire with verbal follow-up of any positive findings.

Physical Examination

The first step in the physical examination is to obtain the patient's vital signs, including temperature, blood pressure, pulse rate, and respiratory rate. The need for evaluation of temperature is obvious. Patients who have systemic involvement of infection have elevated temperatures. Patients with severe infections have temperatures elevated to 101° F or higher (greater than 38.3° C).

The patient's pulse rate increases as the patient's temperature increases. Pulse rates of up to 100 beats/min are not uncommon in patients with infections. If pulse rates increase to greater than 100 beats/min, the patient may have a severe infection and should be treated more aggressively.

The vital sign that varies the least with infection is the patient's blood pressure. Only if the patient has significant pain and anxiety will there be an elevation in systolic blood pressure. However, severe septic shock results in hypotension.

Finally, the patient's respiratory rate should be closely observed. One of the major considerations in odontogenic infections is the potential for partial or complete upper airway obstruction as a result of extension of the infection into the deep fascial spaces of the neck. As respirations are monitored, the dentist should carefully check to ensure that the upper airway is clear and that breathing is without difficulty. The normal respiratory rate is 14 to 16 breaths per minute. Patients with mild to moderate infections may have elevated respiratory rates greater than 18 breaths/min.

Patients who have normal vital signs with only a mild temperature elevation usually have a mild infection that can be readily treated. Patients who have abnormal vital signs with elevation of temperature, pulse rate, and respiratory rate are more likely to have serious infection and require more intensive therapy and evaluation by an oral and maxillofacial surgeon.

Once vital signs have been taken, attention should be turned to physical examination of the patient. The initial portion of the physical examination should be inspection of the patient's general appearance. Patients who have more than a minor, localized infection have an appearance of fatigue, feverishness, and malaise. This is a "toxic appearance" (Fig. 15-6).

The patient's head and neck should be carefully examined for the cardinal signs of infection, and the patient should be inspected for any evidence of swelling and overlying erythema. The patient should be asked to open the mouth widely, swallow, and take deep breaths so that the dentist can check for trismus, dysphagia, or dyspnea. These are ominous signs of a severe infection, and the patient should be referred immediately to an oral and maxillofacial surgeon or emergency room. A recent study of severe odontogenic infections requiring hospitalization found trismus (maximum interincisal opening less than 20 mm) in 73% of cases, dysphagia in 78%, and dyspnea in 14%.

Areas of swelling must be examined by palpation. The dentist should gently touch the area of swelling to check for tenderness, amount of local warmth or heat, and the consistency of the swelling. The consistency of the swelling may vary from very soft and almost normal through a firmer, fleshy swelling (described as having a *doughy feeling*) to an even firmer or hard swelling (described as feeling *indurated*). An indurated swelling has similar firmness to a tightened muscle. Another characteristic consistency is *fluctuant*. Fluctuance is the feeling of a fluid-filled balloon. Fluctuant swelling almost always indicates an accumulation of pus in the center of an indurated area.

The dentist then performs an intraoral examination to try to find the specific cause of the infection. There may be severely carious teeth, an obvious periodontal abscess, severe periodontal disease, combinations of caries and periodontal disease, or an infected fracture of a tooth or the entire jaw. The dentist should look and feel for areas of gingival swelling and fluctuance and for localized vestibular swellings or draining sinus tracts.

The next step is to perform a radiographic examination. This usually consists of the indicated periapical radiographs. Occasionally, however, extraoral radiographs, such as a panoramic radiograph, may be necessary because of limited mouth opening or other extenuating circumstances.

After the physical examination, the practitioner should begin to have a sense of the stage of the presenting infection. Very soft, mildly tender, edematous swellings indicate the *inoculation* stage, whereas an indurated swelling indicates the *cellulitis* stage (Fig. 15-7), and central fluctuance indicates an *abscess* (Fig. 15-8). Soft tissue infections in the inoculation stage may be cured by removal of the odontogenic cause with or without supportive antibiotics, and infections in the cellulitis or abscess stages require removal of the dental cause of infection plus incision and drainage and antibiotics.

Distinctions between the inoculation, cellulitis, and abscess stages are typically in duration, pain, size, peripheral definition, and consistency on palpation, presence of purulence, infecting bacteria, and potential danger (Table 15-3). The duration of cellulitis is usually thought to be acute and is the most severe presentation of the infection. An abscess, however, is a sign of increasing host resistance to the infection. Cellulitis is usually described as more painful than an abscess, which may be the result of its acute onset and distention of tissues.

Edema, the hallmark of the inoculation stage, is typically diffuse and jellylike, with minimal tenderness to palpation.

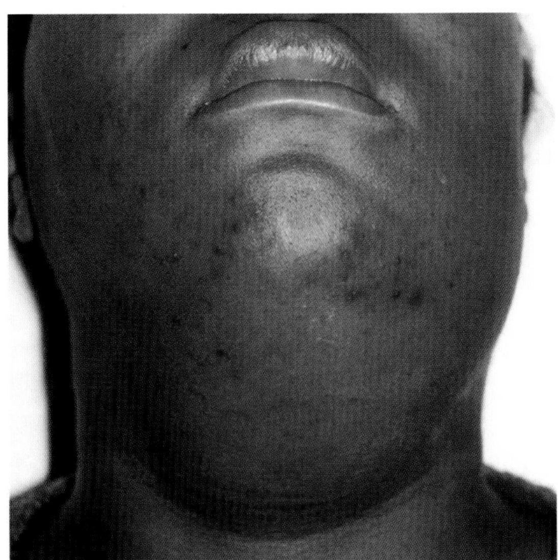

FIGURE 15-7 Cellulitis involving the submental and submandibular region. The cellulitis is indurated on palpation, and the patient is sick. (From Flynn TR: *Atlas Oral Maxillofac Surg Clin North Am* 8:79, 2000.)

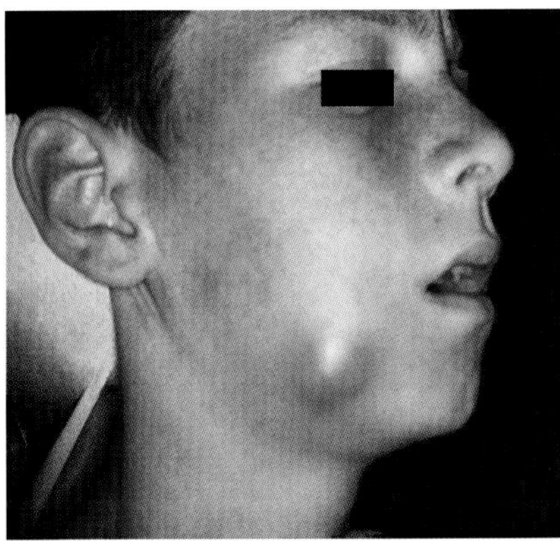

FIGURE 15-8 Well-localized abscess with fluctuance in the center and induration at its periphery. (Courtesy Richard G. Topazian, DDS.)

The size of a cellulitis is typically larger and more widespread than that of an abscess or edema. The periphery of a cellulitis is usually indistinct, with a diffuse border that makes it difficult to determine where the swelling begins or ends. The abscess usually has distinct and well-defined borders. Consistency to palpation is one of the primary distinctions among the stages of infection. When palpated, edema can be very soft or doughy; a severe cellulitis is almost always described as indurated or even as being "boardlike." The severity of the cellulitis increases as its firmness to palpation increases. On palpation, an abscess feels fluctuant because it is a pus-filled cavity in the tissue. Thus an infection may appear innocuous in its early stages and extremely dangerous in its more advanced, indurated, rapidly spreading stages. A localized abscess is typically less dangerous, because it is more chronic and less aggressive.

The presence of pus usually indicates that the body has locally walled off the infection and that the local host resistance mechanisms are bringing the infection under control. In many clinical situations, the distinction between severe cellulitis and abscess may be difficult to make, especially if an abscess lies deeply within the soft tissue. In some patients an indurated cellulitis may have areas of abscess formation within it (see Chapter 16).

Severe infections occupying multiple deep fascial spaces may be in an early stage in one anatomic space, and in a more severe, rapidly progressive stage in another fascial space. A severe, deeply invading infection may pass through ever deeper anatomic spaces in a predictable fashion like a fire in a house, where there may be smoke in one room, intense heat in another room, and open flames near the source of the fire. The goal of therapy in such infections is to abort the spread of the infection in all involved anatomic spaces. These infections are discussed in detail in Chapter 16.

In summary, edema represents the earliest, inoculation stage of infection that is most easily treated. A cellulitis is an acute, painful infection with more swelling and diffuse borders. Cellulitis has a hard consistency on palpation and contains no pus. Cellulitis may be a rapidly spreading process in serious infections. An acute abscess is a more mature infection with more localized pain, less swelling, and well-circumscribed borders. The abscess is fluctuant on palpation because it is a pus-filled tissue cavity. A chronic abscess is usually slow growing and less serious than a cellulitis, especially if it has drained spontaneously to the external environment.

Principle 2: Evaluate State of Patient's Host Defense Mechanisms

Part of the evaluation of the patient's medical history is designed to estimate the patient's ability to defend against infection. Several disease states and several types of drug use may compromise this ability. Compromised patients are more likely to have infections, and these infections often become serious more rapidly. Therefore, to manage their infections more effectively, it is important to be able to discern those patients who may have compromised host defenses.

Medical Conditions That Compromise Host Defenses

Delineation of those medical conditions that may result in decreased host defenses is important. These compromises allow more bacteria to enter the tissues or to be more active, or they prevent the humoral or cellular defenses from exerting their full effect. Several specific conditions may compromise patients' defenses (Box 15-1).

Uncontrolled metabolic diseases—such as uncontrolled diabetes, end-stage renal disease with uremia, and severe alcoholism with malnutrition—result in decreased function of leukocytes, including decreased chemotaxis, phagocytosis, and bacterial killing. Of these metabolic diseases, poorly controlled type 1 (insulin-dependent) and type 2 (non–insulin-dependent) diabetes are the most common immunocompromising diseases, and worsening control of hyperglycemia correlates directly with lowered resistance to all types of infections.

The second major group of immunocompromising diseases is those that interfere with host defense mechanisms, such as leukemias, lymphomas, and many types of cancer. These diseases result in decreased white cell function and decreased antibody synthesis and production.

Human immunodeficiency virus (HIV) infection attacks the T lymphocytes, affecting resistance to viruses and other intra-

BOX 15-1

Compromised Host Defenses

UNCONTROLLED METABOLIC DISEASES
- Poorly controlled diabetes
- Alcoholism
- Malnutrition
- End-stage renal disease

IMMUNE SYSTEM–SUPPRESSING DISEASES
- Human immunodeficiency virus/acquired immunodeficiency syndrome
- Lymphomas and leukemias
- Other malignancies
- Congenital and acquired immunologic diseases

IMMUNOSUPPRESSIVE THERAPIES
- Cancer chemotherapy
- Corticosteroids
- Organ transplantation

cellular pathogens. Fortunately, odontogenic infections are caused largely by extracellular pathogens (bacteria). Therefore, HIV-seropositive individuals are able to combat odontogenic infections fairly well until acquired immunodeficiency syndrome has progressed into advanced stages, when the B lymphocytes are also severely impaired. Nonetheless, care for the HIV-seropositive patient with an odontogenic infection is usually more intensive than for the otherwise normal patient.

Pharmaceuticals That Compromise Host Defenses

Patients taking certain drugs are also immunologically compromised. Cancer chemotherapeutic agents can decrease circulating white cell counts to low levels, commonly less than 1000 cells/mL. When this occurs, patients are unable to defend themselves effectively against bacterial invasion. Patients receiving immunosuppressive therapy, usually for organ transplantation or autoimmune diseases, are compromised. The common drugs in these categories are cyclosporin, corticosteroids, and azathioprine (Imuran). These drugs decrease T and B lymphocyte function and immunoglobulin production. Thus, patients taking these medications are more likely to have severe infections. The immunosuppressive effects of some cancer chemotherapeutic agents can last for up to a year after the completion of therapy.

In summary, when evaluating a patient whose chief complaint may be an infection, the patient's medical history should be carefully reviewed for the presence of diabetes, severe renal disease, alcoholism with malnutrition, leukemias and lymphomas, cancer chemotherapy, and immunosuppressive therapy of any kind. When the patient's history includes any of these, the patient with an infection must be treated much more vigorously because the infection may spread more rapidly. Referral to an oral-maxillofacial surgeon for early and aggressive surgery to remove the cause and initiate more intensive parenteral antibiotic therapy must be considered.

Additionally, when a patient with a history of one of these problems is seen for routine oral surgical procedures, it may be necessary to provide the patient with prophylactic antibiotic therapy to decrease the risk of postoperative wound infection. Use of the guidelines and regimens for prevention of endocarditis published by the American Heart Association and American Dental Association is a practical way to manage this problem.

Principle 3: Determine Whether Patient Should Be Treated by General Dentist or Oral and Maxillofacial Surgeon

Most odontogenic infections seen by the dentist can be managed with the expectation of rapid resolution. Odontogenic infections, when treated with minor surgical procedures and antibiotics, if indicated, almost always respond rapidly. However, some odontogenic infections are potentially life-threatening and require aggressive medical and surgical management. In these special situations, early recognition of the potential severity is essential, and these patients should be referred to an oral-maxillofacial surgeon for definitive management. As the specialist with the best training and experience in the management of severe odontogenic infections, the oral and maxillofacial surgeon can optimize the outcomes and minimize the complications of these infections. For some patients, hospitalization is required, whereas others can be managed as outpatients.

When a patient with an odontogenic infection comes for treatment, the dentist must have a set of criteria by which to judge the seriousness of the infection (Box 15-2). If some or all of these criteria are met, immediate referral must be considered.

Three main criteria indicate immediate referral to a hospital emergency room because of an impending threat to the airway. The first is a history of a *rapidly progressing infection*. This means that the infection began 1 or 2 days before the interview and is growing rapidly worse, with increasing swelling, pain, and other associated signs and symptoms. This type of odontogenic infection may cause swelling in deep fascial spaces of the neck, which can compress and deviate the airway. The second criterion is *difficulty in breathing* (dyspnea). Patients who have severe swelling of the soft tissue of the upper airway as the result of infection may have difficulty maintaining a patent airway. In these situations the patient often will not lie down, has muffled or distorted speech, and is obviously distressed with breathing difficulties. This patient should be referred directly to an emergency room because immediate surgical attention may be necessary to maintain an intact airway. The third urgent criterion is *difficulty in swallowing* (dysphagia). Patients with acutely progressive deep fascial space infections may also have difficulty swallowing their saliva.

BOX 15-2

Criteria for Referral to an Oral and Maxillofacial Surgeon

- Difficulty breathing
- Difficulty swallowing
- Dehydration
- Moderate to severe trismus (interincisal opening less than 20 mm)
- Swelling extending beyond the alveolar process
- Elevated temperature (greater than 101° F)
- Severe malaise and toxic appearance
- Compromised host defenses
- Need for general anesthesia
- Failed prior treatment

This is an ominous sign because the inability to control one's secretions frequently indicates a narrowing of the oropharynx and potential for acute airway obstruction. This patient should also be transported to the hospital emergency room because surgical intervention or intubation may be required for airway maintenance. Definitive treatment of the infection can follow once the airway is secure.

Several other criteria should indicate referral to an oral and maxillofacial surgeon. Patients who have involvement of extraoral fascial spaces, such as buccal space infections or submandibular space infections, may require extraoral surgical incision and drainage (I&D), as well as hospitalization. Next, although infection frequently causes an elevated temperature, a temperature higher than 101° F indicates a greater likelihood of severe infection, and this patient should be referred. Another important sign is trismus, which is the inability to open the mouth widely. In odontogenic infections, trismus results from the involvement of the muscles of mastication in the inflammatory process. Mild trismus can be defined as a maximum interincisal opening between 20 and 30 mm; moderate trismus is between 10 and 20 mm; and severe trismus is an interincisal opening of less than 10 mm.

Moderate or severe trismus may be an indication of the spread of the infection into the masticator space (surrounding the muscles of mastication) or worse, the lateral pharyngeal and/or retropharyngeal spaces surrounding the pharynx and trachea. In this situation, referral to a specialist is necessary for evaluation of upper airway patency. In addition, systemic involvement of an odontogenic infection is an indication for referral. Patients with systemic involvement have a typical toxic facial appearance: glazed eyes, open mouth, and a dehydrated, sick appearance. When this is seen, the patient is usually fatigued, has a substantial amount of pain, has an elevated temperature, and is dehydrated. Finally, if the patient has compromised host defenses, hospitalization is likely to be required. An oral and maxillofacial surgeon is qualified to admit the patient expeditiously to the hospital for definitive care.

In summary, within the first few minutes of the initial patient encounter, the aforementioned three principles allow the dentist to assess the severity of the infection, evaluate host defenses, and decide expeditiously on the best setting for the patient's care. In doubtful situations, it is always best to err on the side of caution and refer the patient for a higher level of care. Appropriate decision making at this stage can prevent serious morbidity and the occasional mortality that still occurs because of odontogenic infections.

Principle 4: Treat Infection Surgically

The primary principle of management of odontogenic infections is to perform surgical drainage and to remove the cause of the infection. Surgical treatment may range from something as simple as an endodontic access opening and extirpation of the necrotic tooth pulp to treatment as complex as the wide incision of soft tissue in the submandibular and neck regions for a severe infection or even open drainage of the mediastinum.

The primary goal in surgical management of infection is to remove the cause of the infection, which is most commonly a necrotic pulp or deep periodontal pocket. A secondary goal is to provide drainage of accumulated pus and necrotic debris.

When a patient has a typical odontogenic infection, the most likely appearance is a carious tooth with a periapical radiolucency and a small vestibular abscess. With this presentation, the dentist has the following surgical options: endodontic treatment or extraction, with or without I&D. If the tooth is not to be extracted, it should be opened and its pulp removed, which results in elimination of the cause and limited drainage through the apical foramen of the tooth. If the tooth cannot be salvaged or is not restorable, it should be extracted as soon as possible.

Extraction provides removal of the cause of the infection and drainage of the accumulated periapical pus and debris. In addition to the endodontic procedure or extraction of the tooth, an I&D procedure may be required for an infection that has spread beyond the periapical region. Incision of the abscess or cellulitis allows removal of the accumulated pus and bacteria from the underlying tissue. Evacuation of the abscess cavity dramatically decreases the load of bacteria and necrotic debris. Evacuation also reduces the hydrostatic pressure in the region by decompressing the tissues, which improves the local blood supply and increases the delivery of host defenses to the infected area. I&D of a cellulitis serves to abort the spread of the infection into deeper anatomic spaces. The I&D procedure includes the insertion of a drain to prevent premature closure of the mucosal incision, which could allow the abscess cavity to reform. It is important to remember that the surgical goal is to achieve adequate drainage. If endodontic opening of the tooth does not provide adequate drainage of the abscess, it is essential to perform an I&D.

The technique for I&D of a vestibular abscess or cellulitis is straightforward (Fig. 15-9). The preferred site for intraoral incision is directly over the site of maximum swelling and inflammation. However, it is important to avoid incising across a frenum or the path of the mental nerve in the lower premolar region. When I&D procedures are performed extraorally, a more complex set of criteria must be met when selecting a site for the incision. Once the area of incision has been selected, a method of pain control must be used. Regional nerve block anesthesia is preferred when it can be achieved by injecting in an area away from the site of the incision. Alternatively, infiltration of local anesthetic solution into and around the area to be drained can be performed. Once the local anesthetic needle has been used in an infected site, however, it should not be reused in an uninfected area.

Before the actual incision of the abscess is performed, one must consider obtaining a specimen for culture and sensitivity (C&S) testing. If the decision is made to perform a culture, culture is carried out as the initial portion of the surgery (Box 15-3). After the site of surgery has been anesthetized, the surface mucosa is disinfected with a solution such as povidone-iodine (Betadine) and dried with sterile gauze. A large-gauge needle,

BOX 15-3

Indications for Culture and Antibiotic Sensitivity Testing

- Infection spreading beyond the alveolar process
- Rapidly progressive infection
- Previous, multiple antibiotic therapy
- Nonresponsive infection (after more than 48 hours)
- Recurrent infection
- Compromised host defenses

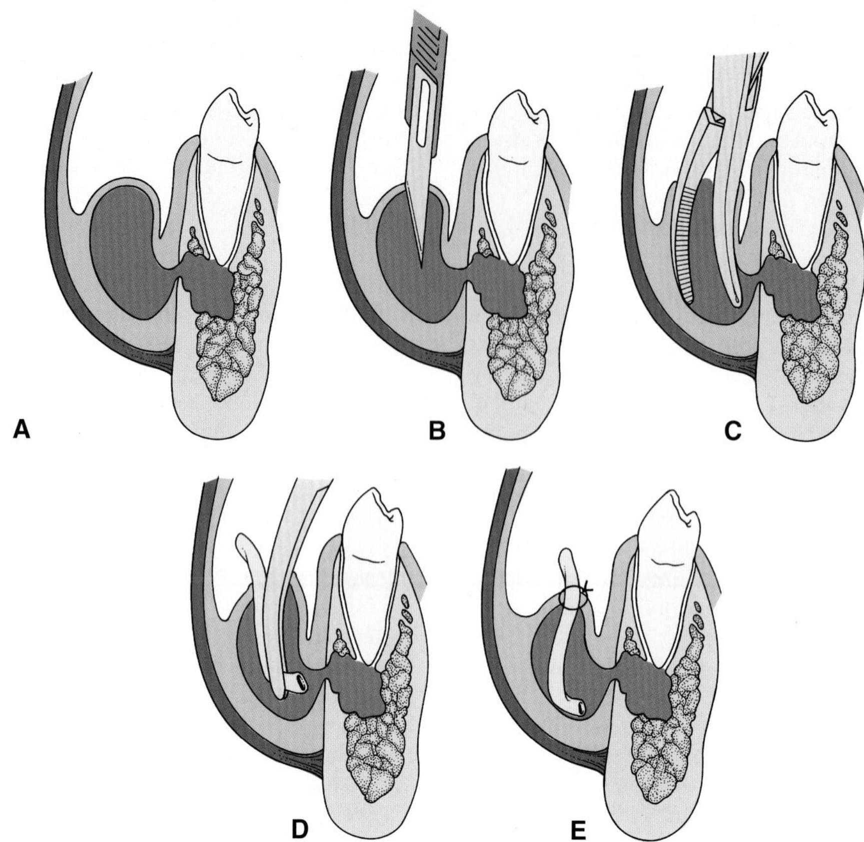

FIGURE 15-9 A, Periapical infection of lower premolar extends through buccal plate and creates sizable vestibular abscess. B, Abscess is incised with No. 11 blade. C, Beaks of hemostat are inserted through incision and opened so that beaks spread to break up any loculations of pus that may exist in abscessed tissue. D, Small drain is inserted to depths of abscess cavity with hemostat. E, Drain is sutured into place with single black silk suture.

usually 18 gauge, is used for specimen collection. A small syringe, usually 3 mL, is adequate. The needle is then inserted into the abscess or cellulitis, and 1 or 2 mL of pus or tissue fluid is aspirated. The specimen may contain only tissue fluid and blood instead of pus, yet it still most often provides sufficient bacteria for an accurate culture. The specimen is then inoculated directly into aerobic and anaerobic culturettes, which are sterile tubes containing a swab and bacterial transport medium. Culturettes and specimen bottles that are appropriate for aerobes and anaerobes are also available. All culturettes and specimen bottles have a limited shelf-life, so the expiration date should be checked before use. Care must be taken to keep the anaerobic culture tube upright while open to prevent the escape of the carbon dioxide that is needed to maintain the tube's anaerobic environment. As discussed before, anaerobic bacteria are almost always present in odontogenic infections, and therefore care must be taken to provide the laboratory the best opportunity to find them. The surgeon should request a Gram stain, aerobic and anaerobic cultures, and antibiotic sensitivity testing in writing.

Once the culture specimen is obtained, an incision is made with a scalpel blade just through the mucosa and submucosa into the abscess cavity (Fig. 15-9). The incision should be short, usually no more than 1 cm in length. Once the incision is completed, a closed curved hemostat is inserted through the incision into the abscess cavity. The hemostat is then opened in several directions to break up any small loculations or cavities of pus that have not been opened by the initial incision. Any pus or tissue fluid that drains out during this time should be aspirated into the suction and should not be allowed to drain into the patient's mouth. If, however, an adequate specimen has not been obtained by aspiration, aerobic and anaerobic culturette swabs may be carefully introduced into the wound without contaminating them on the surface mucosa. Adequate specimens can be obtained in this manner even if obvious pus is not present in the wound.

Once all areas of the abscess cavity have been opened and all pus has been removed, a small drain is inserted to maintain the opening. The most commonly used drain for intraoral abscesses is a $^{1}/_{4}$-inch sterile Penrose drain. A frequently used substitute is a small strip of sterilized rubber dam or surgical glove material. A piece of drain of adequate length to reach the depth of the abscess cavity is prepared and inserted into the cavity using a hemostat. The drain is then sutured to one edge of the incision with a nonresorbable suture. The suture should be placed in viable tissue to prevent loss of the drain because it might tear through friable, nonvital tissue.

The drain should remain in place until all the drainage has stopped, usually 2 to 5 days. Removal is done by simply cutting the suture and slipping the drain from the wound.

Inoculation stage infections that initially appear as edema with soft, doughy, diffuse, mildly tender swelling do not typically

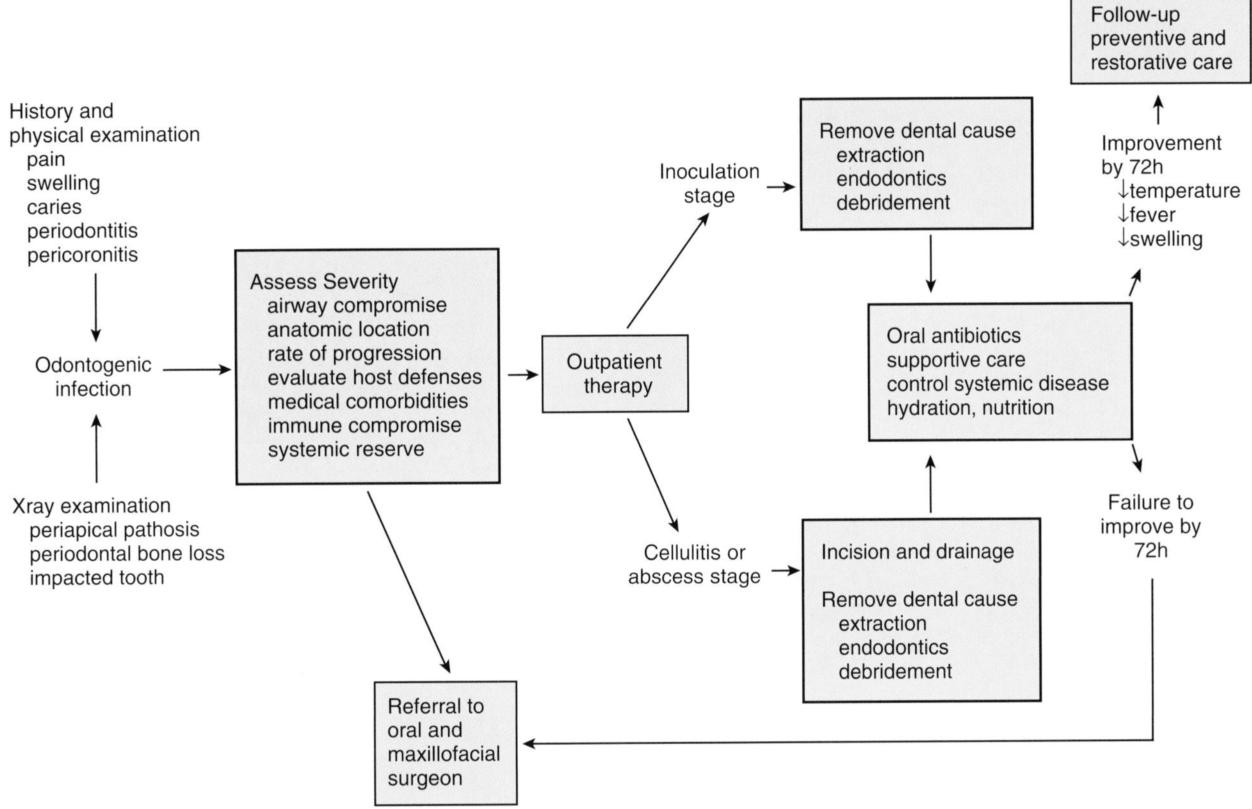

FIGURE 15-10 Management algorithm for odontogenic infections. (Adapted from Flynn TR: Deep fascial space infections. In Laskin DM, Abubaker AO, editors. *Decision making in oral and maxillofacial surgery,* Chicago, 2007, Quintessence.)

require I&D. Surgical management of infections of this type is limited to removal of the necrotic pulp or removal of the involved tooth. Adjunctive antibiotic therapy may be used, according to the following indications.

It is critical to keep in mind that the *primary* method for treating odontogenic infections is to perform surgery to remove the source of the infection and drain anatomic spaces affected by indurated cellulitis or abscess. Whenever an abscess or cellulitis is diagnosed, the surgeon must drain it. Failure to do so will result in worsening of the infection and failure of the infection to resolve, even if antibiotics are given. Even if the tooth cannot be opened or extracted, an I&D should be done.

Some clinicians believe that I&D of a cellulitis may allow the infection to spread into deeper tissues by opening them up to infecting bacteria. The experience of others has shown that establishing drainage for a cellulitis serves to abort the spread of infection. In a prospective study of 37 patients hospitalized for severe odontogenic infection, approximately 25% of the cases had drainage in the cellulitis stage.* On multivariate analysis the stage of infection had no significant effect on complications or the length of hospital stay.

The algorithm presented in Figure 15-10 is a decision pathway for the management of uncomplicated odontogenic infections, which follows the principles described in this chapter. After deciding to treat the patient in the outpatient setting, the dentist should determine whether the infection is in the inoculation (edema) stage or if it has progressed to a cellulitis or abscess. In the inoculation stage the dental cause of the infection should be treated surgically. An antibiotic may also hasten resolution of the infection at this stage. If the infection has progressed to cellulitis or abscess, then an I&D and the appropriate dental therapy should be performed. Sometimes, a separate I&D is not necessary if the abscess cavity drains completely through an extraction socket. Antibiotic therapy should be used when complete abscess drainage cannot be achieved by extraction alone.

The criteria for referral to an oral and maxillofacial surgeon are listed in Box 15-2. In summary, when there is potential or actual airway compromise, infection spreading beyond the alveolar process, medical or immune system compromise, or signs of systemic involvement, immediate referral to an oral and maxillofacial surgeon or, in life-threatening cases, referral to a hospital emergency room is indicated.

Principle 5: Support Patient Medically

A patient's systemic resistance to infection is perhaps the most important determinant of a good outcome. Host systemic resistance must be considered in three areas: immune system compromise, control of systemic diseases, and physiologic reserves.

Diseases that compromise the immune system are listed in Box 15-1. Odontogenic infections that occur in patients with

*Flynn TR, Shanti RM, Levy M et al: Severe odontogenic infections, part one: prospective report, *J Oral Maxillofac Surg* 64:1093-1103, 2006.

immune system compromise should be treated by a specialist. Often, hospitalization and medical consultation are required. The treatment team selects therapies designed to enhance the immune response, combat the infection medically with bactericidal antibiotics, and optimize surgical management of the infection.

Many systemic diseases also reduce the ability of the patient to resist infection and to undergo treatment. In diabetes, for example, the control of blood sugar is directly correlated with resistance to infection. Host response to a significant infection increases the blood sugar levels and therefore the insulin requirements of a diabetic person. Moreover, cardiovascular diseases decrease the ability of the host to respond to the stress of infection and surgery. Therefore, optimizing control of hypertension, cardiac dysrhythmias, and atherosclerotic heart disease is an essential part of the comprehensive management of odontogenic infections. Medications may also affect the treatment of odontogenic infections. For example, the patient receiving anticoagulant therapy with warfarin (Coumadin) may need reversal of the anticoagulation before surgery can be safely performed. Patients with systemic conditions, especially of the immune, cardiovascular, respiratory, hematologic, and metabolic systems, often need sophisticated medical support from a team of specialists.

Even patients without medically compromising diseases may have reduced or altered physiologic reserves to draw upon as they combat an odontogenic infection. Children, for example, are particularly susceptible to dehydration and high fevers. Elderly patients, however, have a reduced ability to mount a fever, and yet they are susceptible to dehydration. Fever increases daily fluid requirements in the adult by about 800 mL per degree Fahrenheit per day, and daily caloric requirements by 3% to 5% per degree per day. However, temperatures up to 103° F may be beneficial in combating infections. Therefore, judicious control of highly elevated fever along with active hydration and nutritional support are important components of the management of odontogenic infections.

Because of pain and/or difficulty swallowing, patients frequently have not had adequate fluid intake, nutritional intake, or rest. During the immediate posttreatment period, patients should be encouraged to drink sufficient water or juice to require them to need to urinate regularly and to take high-calorie nutritional supplements. Patients should also be prescribed adequate analgesics for relief of pain so that they can rest. Patients should be given careful postoperative instructions and should be able to manage their self-care. The clinician is responsible to make sure patients are provided careful instructions about these important issues.

Principle 6: Choose and Prescribe Appropriate Antibiotic

Choosing the appropriate antibiotic for treating an odontogenic infection must be done carefully. When all factors are weighed, the clinician may decide that no antibiotic is necessary at all, whereas in other situations, broad-spectrum or even combination antibiotic therapy may be indicated. A variety of factors must be considered when choosing an antibiotic from the nearly 70 antibiotics currently available. Antibiotics must be viewed as a double-edged sword. Although appropriate use may result in dramatic resolution and cure of patients with infections, misuse of antibiotics provides little benefit to offset the associated risks and expense of antibiotic administration. Recent studies have shown that even the administration of oral penicillin promotes the growth of penicillin-resistant organisms in the oropharyngeal flora of the patient, the patient's family, and even the patient's co-workers or classmates. Therefore the following guidelines are recommended for consideration when choosing a specific antibiotic.

Determine the Need for Antibiotic Administration

A common misconception is that all infections, by definition, require antibiotic administration. This is not necessarily the case. In some situations, antibiotics are not useful and may be contraindicated. In making this determination, three factors must be considered: The first factor is the seriousness of the infection when the patient comes to the dentist. If the infection has caused swelling, has progressed rapidly, or is a diffuse cellulitis, the evidence supports the use of antibiotics in addition to surgical therapy. The second factor is whether adequate surgical treatment can be achieved. In many situations, extraction of the offending tooth may result in rapid resolution of the infection. Contrary to widely held opinion, extraction of a tooth in the presence of infection does not promote the spread of infection. Several studies have shown that removal of a tooth in the presence of infection hastens its resolution and minimizes the complications of the infection, such as time out of work, hospitalization, and the need for extraoral I&D. Therefore, prompt removal of the offending tooth (teeth) in the presence of infection is to be encouraged; a prior period of antibiotic therapy is not necessary. However, when the appropriate surgery cannot be immediately performed, antibiotics may be useful to retard the progression of infection. The third consideration is the state of the patient's host defenses. A young, healthy patient may be able to mobilize host defenses and may not need antibiotic therapy for resolution of a minor infection. However, patients who have any type of decreased host resistance, such as those with severe metabolic disease or those receiving cancer chemotherapy, may require vigorous antibiotic therapy even for minor infections.

When these three factors are balanced, several definite indications for antibiotic use in dentistry become clear (Box 15-4). The first and most common indication is the presence of an acute-onset infection with diffuse swelling and moderate to severe pain. This infection is usually in the cellulitis stage; and with appropriate antibiotic therapy, I&D, and treatment of the offending tooth, rapid resolution is expected. The second indication is almost any type of infection in a patient who is medically compromised. Such patients who have infections of any severity should be considered candidates for antibiotic administration. The third indication for antibiotic therapy is

BOX 15-4

Indications for Therapeutic Use of Antibiotics

- Swelling extending beyond the alveolar process
- Cellulitis
- Trismus
- Lymphadenopathy
- Temperature higher than 101° F
- Severe pericoronitis
- Osteomyelitis

BOX 15-5

Situations in Which Use of Antibiotics Is Not Necessary

- Patient demand
- Toothache
- Periapical abscess
- Dry socket
- Multiple dental extractions in a noncompromised patient
- Mild pericoronitis (inflammation of the operculum only)
- Drained alveolar abscess

the presence of an infection that has progressed to involvement of the deep fascial spaces. In these situations, the infection is aggressive enough to have spread beyond the alveolar process of the jaws, indicating that the host defenses are inadequate to contain the infection. The fourth indication is severe pericoronitis, with temperatures higher than 100° F, trismus, and swelling of the lateral aspect of the face, which occurs most commonly around impacted mandibular third molars. Finally, the patient who has osteomyelitis requires antibiotic therapy in addition to surgery to achieve resolution of the infection.

Based on the same three criteria, antibiotic therapy is not indicated and is even contraindicated in other situations (Box 15-5). The first is a minor, chronic, well-localized abscess for which extraction of the offending tooth results in complete evacuation of a periapical abscess, assuming that the patient's host defenses are intact and that the patient has no other compromising conditions. An example of this is the patient without symptoms who may require the extraction of teeth with chronic periapical abscesses, a draining parulis, or severe periodontitis. A second, albeit similar, contraindication is a well-localized dentoalveolar abscess, with little or no facial swelling. In these situations, endodontic therapy can be performed or the tooth can be extracted along with I&D of the swelling on the alveolar process, which will result in rapid resolution in most patients. Third is a localized alveolar osteitis, or dry socket. Treatment of the dry socket is primarily palliative, and dry socket is not treated as an infection. Although bacterial pathogens may play a role in dry socket, the clinical problem of dry socket (alveolar osteitis) is self-limiting and appears to be due to premature fibrinolysis (loss of the blood clot). Fourth, patients who have mild pericoronitis with minor gingival edema and mild pain do not require antibiotics for resolution of their infection. Irrigation with hydrogen peroxide or chlorhexidine, plus extraction of the partially erupted tooth will result in resolution. Antibiotics should not prescribed simply because a patient demands them for a routine toothache or for dental extractions in a patient without immune system compromise.

In summary, antibiotics should be used when clear evidence exists of bacterial invasion into deeper tissues that is greater than the host defenses can overcome. Patients who have an impaired ability to defend themselves against infection and patients who have infections that are not immediately amenable to surgical treatment should be considered for antibiotic therapy. Antibiotics should not be used when no evidence of bacterial invasion of deeper tissues is found. Antibiotics do not hasten wound healing and do not provide any benefit for nonbacterial (e.g., viral) conditions. Patients who have inflammatory pulpitis have severe pain, but the pain results from the local inflammatory reaction within the pulp, not from bacterial infection spreading into deeper tissues. These patients should not routinely be given antibiotic therapy.

Use Empirical Therapy Routinely

Odontogenic infections are caused by a highly predictable group of bacteria. Additionally, the antibiotic sensitivity of these organisms is well known and consistent. As a result, the use of C&S testing is not necessary for routine odontogenic infections. The bacteria that cause odontogenic infections are overwhelmingly the facultative oral streptococci, anaerobic streptococci including peptostreptococci, and *Prevotella* and *Fusobacterium* species. Other species of bacteria may also be cultured from these infections, but they appear to be opportunistic rather than causative bacteria. Fortunately, the antibiotic susceptibility of the causative bacteria is fairly predictable. The orally administered antibiotics that are effective against odontogenic infections include penicillin, amoxicillin, clindamycin, azithromycin, metronidazole, and moxifloxacin (Box 15-6).

These antibiotics are effective against aerobic and facultative streptococci (except metronidazole) and oral anaerobes. Metronidazole is effective only against obligate anaerobic bacteria, yet the effectiveness of this antibiotic class in odontogenic infections has been shown in a prospective study. Several important variations can be found among these antibiotics. (See Appendix VI for detailed description of the various antibiotics.)

Because the microbiology and antibiotic sensitivity of the oral pathogens is well known, it is a reasonable therapeutic maneuver to use one of these antibiotics empirically; that is, to give the antibiotic with the assumption that an appropriate drug is being given. The drug of choice is usually penicillin. Alternative drugs for use in the penicillin-allergic patient are clindamycin and azithromycin. Metronidazole is useful only against anaerobic bacteria and should be reserved for a situation in which only anaerobic bacteria are suspected (or in combination with an antibiotic that has antiaerobic activity, such as penicillin).

Clearly, patients frequently fail to take the medication in the way in which it was prescribed. In fact, Socrates in 400 BC cautioned physicians to be aware that patients will lie about taking the medications prescribed.

Reliable data exist from many studies that demonstrate that patient compliance decreases with increasing number of pills per day. When it is necessary to take the prescription 1 time daily, patient compliance is approximately 80%. However, when it is necessary to take the pill 2 times daily, compliance decreases to 69%, and drops even further to 35% for 4 times daily. Therefore, if the clinician has a reasonable choice, anti-

BOX 15-6

Effective Orally Administered Antibiotics Useful for Odontogenic Infections

- Penicillin
- Amoxicillin
- Clindamycin
- Azithromycin
- Metronidazole
- Moxifloxacin

biotics should be prescribed that can be given the fewest times daily to improve patient compliance.

For example, amoxicillin and clindamycin are usually given 3 times daily instead of 4 times daily (as is penicillin). Azithromycin is given twice a day, instead of 4 times daily (as is erythromycin). Moxifloxacin is given once daily. Thus when other important factors, such as antibacterial effectiveness, side effects, drug interactions, and cost are reasonably equal, a drug that can be given less frequently is preferable. As is discussed subsequently, however, there are significant differences among these antibiotics in their side effects, drug interactions, and cost.

Routine C&S testing is not cost-effective for the routine odontogenic infection. However, in some cases the dentist should seriously consider sending a specimen for C&S testing (Box 15-3). The first is the rapid onset of severe infection and its rapid spread. Delay in bacterial identification may have disastrous consequences in this situation. The second case is postoperative infection. If a patient had no signs of infection when the original surgery was done but returns 3 or 4 days later with an infection, the possibility of nonindigenous bacteria causing the infection is increased. Precise identification of the causative bacteria early on may facilitate the timely administration of the appropriate antibiotic and thus the resolution of the infection. The third case is an infection that is not resolving. In these situations the clinician should make every effort to obtain a specimen of pus or tissue fluid for C&S testing. The fourth case is a recurrent infection. When the initial infectious problem has resolved and there has been an infection-free period of 2 days to 2 weeks but a second infection occurs, the probability is high that the infection is caused by bacteria that are resistant to the previously used antibiotic. The fifth case is the patient who has compromised host defenses. Patients with immune system compromise have a propensity to harbor unusual pathogens that can be identified by C&S testing.

In the foreseeable future, conventional C&S testing may be replaced by molecular methods that are currently used in research. Bacteria can be identified even after their demise by their genetic material, using the polymerase chain reaction to amplify tiny amounts of bacterial DNA and RNA. Single-stranded nucleic acids from the unknown sample can be hybridized to single-stranded genes from known species, resulting in a positive identification of the infecting bacteria. These methods have identified the involvement of a large number of unculturable pathogens in odontogenic infections the presence of which was only suspected in the past. In the future, these methods may be able to detect antibiotic-resistance genes directly as well, resulting in prompt diagnosis of the infecting species and their antibiotic sensitivity patterns.

Use the Narrowest-Spectrum Antibiotic

When an antibiotic is administered to a patient, most susceptible bacteria are killed. If the antibiotic is a narrow-spectrum antibiotic, it kills bacteria of a narrow range. For example, penicillin will kill streptococci and oral anaerobic bacteria but will have little effect on the staphylococci of the skin and almost no effect on gastrointestinal tract bacteria. As a result, penicillin has little or no effect on the gastrointestinal tract and does not expose a multitude of other bacteria to the opportunity to develop resistance. By contrast, drugs such as amoxicillin-clavulanate (Augmentin) are broad-spectrum antibiotics, inhibiting not only the streptococci and oral anaerobes but also a variety of staphylococci and enteric gram-negative rods. Thus when this antibiotic is given, it has an effect on skin and gastrointestinal bacteria that may result in problems caused by alterations of host flora and overgrowth of resistant bacteria. In addition, broad-spectrum antibiotics provide a multitude of bacteria with the opportunity to develop resistance, which can be communicated by our patients to their families, co-workers, and entire communities.

The American Dental Association's (ADA's) Council on Scientific Affairs has issued guidelines, based on a review of the available scientific literature, which recommends that dentists use only narrow-spectrum antibiotics for simple infections. Narrow-spectrum and broad-spectrum antibiotics are listed in Box 15-7. Broad-spectrum antibiotics may be used for complex infections, which are not defined in the ADA advisory statement. Nonetheless, a simple odontogenic infection can be defined as one involving only the alveolar process or the oral vestibule, in its first course of treatment, and in an immunocompetent individual. A complex infection may be defined as one that has spread beyond the alveolar process and oral vestibule, with prior treatment failures, or in an immunocompromised patient. The characteristics of simple and complex odontogenic infections are differentiated in Box 15-8.

In summary, antibiotics that have narrow-spectrum activity against the causative organisms are just as effective as antibiotics that have broad-spectrum activity, without the

BOX 15-7

Narrow- and Broad-Spectrum Antibiotics

NARROW-SPECTRUM ANTIBIOTICS USEFUL FOR SIMPLE ODONTOGENIC INFECTIONS

- Penicillin
- Clindamycin
- Metronidazole

BROAD-SPECTRUM ANTIBIOTICS USEFUL FOR COMPLEX ODONTOGENIC INFECTIONS

- Amoxicillin
- Amoxicillin with clavulanic acid (for sinus infections)
- Azithromycin
- Tetracycline
- Moxifloxacin

BOX 15-8

Simple Versus Complex Odontogenic Infections

SIMPLE ODONTOGENIC INFECTIONS

- Swelling limited to the alveolar process and vestibular space
- First attempt at treatment
- Nonimmunocompromised patient

COMPLEX ODONTOGENIC INFECTIONS

- Swelling extending beyond the vestibular space
- Failed prior treatment
- Immunocompromised patient

problems of upsetting normal host microflora populations and increasing the chance of bacterial resistance.

Use the Antibiotic with the Lowest Incidence of Toxicity and Side Effects

Most antibiotics have a variety of toxicities and side effects that limit their usefulness. These range from mild to so severe that the antibiotic cannot be used in clinical practice. The older antibiotics usually used for odontogenic infections have a surprisingly low incidence of toxicity-related problems. The newer antibiotics, however, can have significant toxicities and drug interactions. Therefore, it is becoming increasingly important for the clinician to understand the toxicities, side effects, and drug interactions of the drugs he or she may prescribe.

Allergy is the major side effect of penicillin. Approximately 2% or 3% of the total population is allergic to penicillin. Patients who have allergic reactions to penicillin, as exhibited by hives, itching, or wheezing, should not be given penicillin again. Penicillin does not have other major side effects or toxicities in the normal dose range used by dentists.

Likewise, azithromycin and clindamycin have a low incidence of toxicity and side effects. Clindamycin may cause a severe diarrhea, called *pseudomembranous colitis*. Several other drugs, such as ampicillin and the oral cephalosporins, also cause this problem. However, with clindamycin and other antibiotics, this problem is usually confined to severely ill and debilitated patients and is rare in other patients. The elimination of much of the anaerobic gut flora allows the overgrowth of an antibiotic-resistant bacterium, *Clostridium difficile*. This bacterium produces toxins that injure the gut wall, which results in colitis. Patients who take clindamycin, amoxicillin, or cephalosporins should be warned of the possibility of profuse watery diarrhea and should be told to contact their prescribing dentist if it occurs.

Among the new members of the macrolide (erythromycin) family, azithromycin has the best combination of effectiveness, low toxicity, and infrequent drug interactions. Erythromycin is no longer considered effective against the oral pathogens, and it shares with clarithromycin a propensity to cause drug interactions involving the liver microsomal enzyme system.

Moxifloxacin is a new member of the fluoroquinolone class of antibiotics that has much better effectiveness against the oral pathogens than older members of this class. However, it has significant toxicities, including muscle weakness and mental clouding, and serious, potentially fatal drug interactions with many of the commonly used cardiovascular drugs. Moxifloxacin is also contraindicated in children and pregnant females. As a new antibiotic, moxifloxacin is expensive. Moxifloxacin should be reserved for use by specialists treating severe, recalcitrant infections for which no other effective drug is available.

The oral cephalosporins, such as cephalexin and cefadroxil, have lost much of their effectiveness in odontogenic infections. These antibiotics are no longer commonly used for odontogenic infections, even though they are associated with only mild toxicity problems. As with penicillin, the cephalosporins may cause allergic reactions. Cephalosporins should be given cautiously to patients with penicillin allergies because these patients may also be allergic to the cephalosporins. Patients who have experienced an anaphylactic type of reaction to penicillin should *not* be given a cephalosporin because of increased chance for that life-threatening event to recur.

The tetracyclines, like the cephalosporins, are no longer considered useful for odontogenic infections, except when they are used topically in very high local concentrations, such as when they are inserted into periodontal pockets. They have minor toxicities for most patients (i.e., the commonly encountered gastrointestinal problems of nausea, abdominal cramping, and diarrhea). Some patients may have a photosensitivity while they are taking this drug systemically and should be warned to stay out of the sun. Finally, tetracyclines may produce tooth discoloration if given to patients who are pregnant or who are in the tooth development stages of their lives (under 12 years of age). This discoloration is the result of chelation of the tetracycline to calcium, which results in incorporation of the tetracycline into developing teeth.

Metronidazole has mild toxicities, the most prominent being the typical gastrointestinal disturbances discussed previously. The drug may also produce a disulfiram effect; that is, the patient taking metronidazole who also drinks ethanol may experience sudden, violent abdominal cramping and vomiting.

Use a Bactericidal Antibiotic, If Possible

Antibiotics may kill bacteria (i.e., bactericidal antibiotics) or interfere with their reproduction (i.e., bacteriostatic antibiotics). Bactericidal antibiotics usually interfere with cell wall production in newly forming, growing bacteria. The resultant defective cell wall is not able to withstand the osmotic pressure differential between the cytoplasm and the environment, and the bacteria virtually explode. The antibiotic actually kills the bacteria, whereas the white blood cells, complement, and antibodies of the host play a less important role in fighting the bacteria.

Bacteriostatic antibiotics interfere with bacterial reproduction and growth. This slowing of bacterial reproduction allows the host defenses to move into the area of infection, phagocytize the existing bacteria, and kill them. Bacteriostatic antibiotics require reasonably intact host defenses. This type of antibiotic should be avoided in patients who have compromised host defense systems.

For patients with compromised host defenses, bactericidal antibiotics should be the drug of choice. For example, the bactericidal antibiotic penicillin would be preferred over the bacteriostatic antibiotic azithromycin in a patient who is receiving cancer chemotherapy.

Be Aware of the Cost of Antibiotics

Antibiotics vary widely in their cost to patients. Newer drugs tend to be more expensive, whereas older drugs, which are made by a variety of companies, tend to be less expensive. Drugs prescribed generically also tend to be less expensive than their brand-name counterparts. Generic prescriptions for newer drugs are not available. When other factors are equal, the clinician should prescribe the less expensive antibiotic. Table 15-4 provides a cost comparison among commonly used antibiotics.

Summary

Antibiotics should be used to assist the dentist in treating patients with infections that are spreading beyond the alveolar processes of the jaws and to prevent endocarditis or infection of prosthetic-implanted devices arising from bacteremia induced by dental manipulations. Surgical treatment of the infection remains the primary method of treatment in most patients; antibiotic therapy plays an adjunctive role. Anti-

TABLE 15-4

Cost Comparison of Orally Administered Antibiotics

Antibiotic	Usual Dose	Usual Interval	Wholesale Cost, 2006*	1-Week Retail Cost, 2006†	Penicillin V Cost Ratio
PENICILLINS					
Penicillin V	500 mg	6 hours	$ 0.39	$ 12.19	1.00
Amoxicillin	500 mg	8 hours	$ 0.13	$ 13.99	1.15
Augmentin‡	500 mg	8 hours	$ 2.87	$ 71.59	5.87
Augmentin XR	2000 mg	12 hours	$ 5.84	$ 113.99	9.35
Dicloxacillin	500 mg	6 hours	$ 0.20	$ 24.99	2.05
CEPHALOSPORINS (GENERATION)					
Cephalexin (first)	500 mg	6 hours	$ 0.44	$ 23.59	1.94
Cefadroxil (first)	500 mg	12 hours	$ 2.48	$ 49.49	4.06
Cefuroxime (second)	500 mg	8 hours	$10.95	$ 84.99	6.97
Ceclor CD 500 (second)	500 mg	12 hours	$ 3.50	$ 83.59	6.86
Cefaclor ER (generic)‡	500 mg	12 hours	$ 3.79	$ 31.69	2.60
Cefdinir (third)	600 mg	24 hours	$ 9.50	$ 93.99	7.71
ERYTHROMYCINS					
Clarithromycin (Biaxin XL)	500 mg	24 hours	$ 9.86	$ 59.99	4.92
Azithromycin (Zithromax)	250 mg	12 hours	$ 7.53	$ 96.59	7.92
Dirithromycin (Dynabac)	500 mg	24 hours	$ 9.50	$ 75.59	6.20
ANTIANAEROBIC					
Clindamycin (generic)‡	150 mg	6 hours	$ 1.12	$ 31.79	2.61
Clindamycin (generic)‡	300 mg	6 hours	$ 2.24	$ 59.99	4.92
Metronidazole	500 mg	6 hours	$ 0.21	$ 32.59	2.67
OTHER					
Vancomycin	125 mg	6 hours	$ 9.15	$ 487.99	40.03
Ciprofloxacin	500 mg	12 hours	$ 5.80	$ 33.09	2.71
Moxifloxacin (Avelox)	400 mg	24 hours	$10.00	$ 98.99	8.12
Doxycycline	100 mg	12 hours	$ 0.08	$ 11.99	0.98
Linezolid (Zyvox)	600 mg	12 hours	$65.00	$1145.99	94.01

Usual doses and intervals are for moderate infections and are not to be considered prescriptive.
Penicillin cost ratio = Retail cost of antibiotic for 1 week/Retail cost of penicillin V for 1 week.
*Source: Gilbert DN, Moellering RC Jr, Eliopoulos GM, Sande MA: *The Sanford guide to antimicrobial therapy 2006,* ed 36, Sperryville, Va, 2006, Antimicrobial Therapy. Prices are wholesale cost per dose, generic when available.
†Retail cost/1 Week = Retail price charged for a 1-week prescription at a large pharmacy chain in the Boston region. Courtesy Gabriela Hoffens, CPHT.
‡Pharmacy cost per pill from *Mosby's drug consult 2006,* St Louis, 2006, Mosby.

biotics are especially important in patients who have infections that are spreading beyond the alveolar process and in patients who have compromise of their host defense mechanisms. When antibiotic therapy is to be used a simple odontogenic infection, empiric antibiotic therapy with a narrow-spectrum antibiotic is recommended because the microbiology of odontogenic infections is well known and usually consistent from patient to patient. The antibiotic of choice for odontogenic infections is still penicillin. Penicillin has been shown to be as effective as other antibiotics in several prospective studies. Penicillin is bactericidal; has a narrow spectrum that includes streptococci and the oral anaerobes, which are responsible for odontogenic infections; has low toxicity; and is inexpensive.

Although about 25% of *Prevotella* strains are resistant to penicillin, when used in conjunction with adequate surgery, penicillin almost always results in cure. Amoxicillin and amoxicillin/clavulanate (Augmentin) are broad-spectrum penicillins that should be reserved for complex infections. Amoxicillin may be used for prophylaxis of endocarditis and late prosthetic joint infections as per the formal guidelines of the ADA in conjunction with the American Heart Association and the American Academy of Orthopaedic Surgeons. An alternative drug is azithromycin, which is a useful medication for patients who are allergic to penicillin. Clindamycin is also a useful alternative for patients with penicillin allergy or in special situations in which resistant anaerobic bacteria are suspected. Metronidazole may be useful, especially when anaerobic bacteria are suspected. It may be used in combination with another antibiotic that kills the facultative and aerobic oral pathogens. Moxifloxacin, because of the need to limit the development of resistance and due to its toxicities and drug interactions, should be restricted to use by specialists in the treatment of severe infections.

Principle 7: Administer Antibiotic Properly

Once the decision is made to prescribe an antibiotic to the patient, the drug should be administered in the proper dose and at the proper dose interval. The manufacturer usually recommends the proper dosage and administration. Provision of plasma levels that are sufficiently high to kill the bacteria that are sensitive to the antibiotic but are not so high as to cause toxicity is adequate. The peak plasma level of the drug should usually be at least 4 or 5 times the minimal inhibitory concentration for the bacteria involved in the infection.

Clearly, some patients stop taking their antibiotics after acute symptoms have subsided and rarely take their drugs as prescribed after 4 or 5 days. Therefore the antibiotic that would have the highest compliance would be the drug that could be given once a day for 4 or 5 days. One study has shown that for odontogenic infections a 4-day course of penicillin, combined with the appropriate surgery, was as effective as a 7-day course of the antibiotic.

Additional administration of antibiotics may be necessary in some infections that have not resolved rapidly at the clinical follow-up examination. The clinician must make it clear to the patient that the entire prescription must be taken. If for some reason the patient is advised to stop taking the antibiotic early, all remaining pills or capsules should be discarded. Keeping small amounts of unused antibiotics in medicine cabinets for the anticipated sore throat next winter should be strongly discouraged. Casual self-administration of antibiotics is not useful and may be hazardous to the health of the individual and the community.

Principle 8: Evaluate Patient Frequently

Once the patient has been treated by surgery and antibiotic therapy has been prescribed, the patient should be followed carefully to monitor response to treatment and complications. In most situations the patient should be asked to return to the dentist 2 days after the original therapy. Typically, the patient is much improved. If therapy is successful, swelling and pain decreases dramatically. The dentist should check the I&D site to determine whether the drain should be removed at this time. Other parameters, such as temperature, trismus, swelling, and the patient's subjective feelings of improvement, should also be evaluated.

If there is not an adequate response to treatment, the patient should be examined carefully for clues to the reason for failure (Box 15-9). The most common cause of treatment failure is inadequate surgery. A tooth may have to be reevaluated for extraction, or an extension of the infection into an area not detected at the first treatment may have to be incised and drained. It may be necessary to admit such a patient to the hospital for purposes of airway security, further surgery, and intravenous antibiotic therapy.

A second reason for failure is depressed host defense mechanisms. A review of the patient's medical history should be performed, and more careful probing questions should be asked. In addition to immunocompromising diseases, conditions that diminish physiologic reserves, such as dehydration, malnutrition, and pain, should also be considered and corrected if necessary.

A third reason for treatment failure is the presence of a foreign body. Although this is unlikely in an odontogenic infection, the dentist may consider taking a careful history and a periapical radiograph of the area to help ensure that a radiopaque foreign body is not present. Dental implants are increasingly common foreign bodies, and the ability of bacteria to find shelter from the immune system in their surface gaps and irregularities can perpetuate the infection until the implant is successfully débrided or removed.

Finally, there may be problems with the antibiotic that was given to the patient. The dentist first ascertains whether the patient has been compliant. The patient must have the prescription filled and must take the antibiotic according to directions. Many patients fail to follow the orders of their dentists as carefully as they should. Sometimes, a patient may not have the prescription filled because he or she cannot afford it. The dentist should use the most cost-effective antibiotic available and can frankly ask whether a particular prescription is affordable to the patient. Another problem to consider is whether the antibiotic reached the infected area. The penetration of antibiotics into abscess cavities is poor. Failure of the antibiotic to reach the area may be related to inadequate surgery or drainage, inadequate blood supply to the local area, or a dose that is too low to be effective against the bacteria. Another antibiotic-related problem is an incorrect bacterial diagnosis. If a culture was not performed at the initial surgical treatment or if no surgical treatment was done at the initial therapy, the dentist should obtain a specimen for C&S testing. Finally, it is possible that the wrong antibiotic was prescribed for the infection, which may be because of an inaccurate bacterial diagnosis or the increasing antibiotic resistance of oral bacteria. For example, 25% to 35% of *Prevotella* organisms are resistant to penicillin but rarely cause persistent infection if penicillin is given and adequate surgery is done. However, if the patient has a persistent, low-grade infection that does not resolve despite adequate surgery, prescribing an antianaerobic antibiotic such as clindamycin is appropriate.

The clinician must also examine the patient to look specifically for toxicity reactions and untoward side effects. Patients may report complaints such as nausea and abdominal cramping but may fail to associate watery diarrhea with the drug administration. Specific questioning about the expected toxicities is important to their early recognition.

The dentist should also be aware of the possibility of secondary or superinfections. The most common secondary infection encountered by dentists is oral or vaginal candidiasis. This is the result of an overgrowth of *Candida* organisms because the normal oral flora has been altered by the antibiotic therapy. Other secondary infections may arise as normal host flora is altered, but they are not seen with any degree of frequency in the management of odontogenic infections.

BOX 15-9

Reasons for Treatment Failure

- Inadequate surgery
- Depressed host defenses
- Foreign body
- Antibiotic problems:
  - Patient noncompliance
  - Drug not reaching site
  - Drug dose too low
  - Wrong bacterial diagnosis
  - Wrong antibiotic

Finally, the dentist should follow the patient carefully once the infection has resolved to check for recurrent infection. Recurrence would be seen in a patient who had incomplete therapy for the infection. A variety of reasons may account for this. For example, the patient may have stopped taking the antibiotic too early. The drain may have been removed too early and the drainage site sealed too early, which reestablished the infectious process. If infection does recur, surgical intervention and reinstitution of antibiotic therapy should be considered.

PRINCIPLES OF PREVENTION OF INFECTION

The use of antibiotics to treat an established infection is a well-accepted and well-defined technique. These drugs provide major assistance for the patient in overcoming an established infection. The use of antibiotics for prevention (i.e., prophylaxis) of infection is less widely accepted. The final section of this chapter discusses the use of antibiotics for prophylaxis of two distinct types of infection. The use of antibiotics to prevent wound infection after surgery is presented first, followed by a discussion of antibiotic use to prevent metastatic infection.

PRINCIPLES OF PROPHYLAXIS OF WOUND INFECTION

The use of antibiotics for prophylaxis of postoperative wound infections may be effective and desirable in certain situations. On the other hand, there is little scientific evidence that demonstrates the effectiveness of prophylactic antibiotics in dentistry and oral and maxillofacial surgery. If, however, prophylactic antibiotics are effective in preventing postoperative wound infections and blood-borne infections of distant sites, they would have three distinct advantages. First, prophylactic antibiotics may reduce the incidence of postoperative infection and thereby reduce postoperative morbidity. When a patient becomes infected after surgery, wound healing and recovery are substantially delayed. Second, appropriate and effective antibiotic prophylaxis may reduce the cost of health care. By decreasing the incidence of postoperative infection, the patient can be saved the additional expense of returning to the dentist, buying additional antibiotics, and missing additional days of work. Third, appropriate use of prophylactic antibiotics requires a shorter-term administration than therapeutic use, thereby possibly decreasing the total amount of antibiotics used by the population. On the other hand, when they are used inappropriately, prophylactic antibiotics are actually associated with an increased risk of postoperative infection, typically by a bacterium resistant to the prophylactic antibiotic.

The use of prophylactic antibiotics also has several disadvantages: First, they may alter host flora. The body is populated with a variety of bacteria that have a symbiotic relationship with the host. When antibiotics are administered, some of these bacteria are eliminated, allowing the overgrowth of antibiotic-resistant and perhaps more pathogenic bacteria that may then cause infection. Second, several studies have shown that antibiotic administration in one patient allows antibiotic-resistant organisms to spread to the patient's family and community. Third, the antibiotic may provide no benefit, which means that in certain situations the risk of infection is so low that the antibiotic provides no additional decrease in the incidence of infection. Fourth, the use of prophylactic antibiotics may encourage lax surgical and aseptic technique on the part of the dentist. The attitude of, "Oh well, the patient is on antibiotics," is an unacceptable excuse when the principles of atraumatic tissue handling and surgical asepsis are violated. Fifth, the cost of the antibiotic must be considered. Although for a single event for a single patient the cost may be small, the cost for many surgeries for many patients can be enormous. Finally, the toxicity of the drug to the patient must be also kept in mind. All drugs have the potential to cause injury to the patient. Although most antibiotics used by dentists have low toxicity, the possibility of toxicity is always present. The principles of prophylactic antibiotic use are summarized in Box 15-10.

BOX 15-10

Principles of Prophylactic Antibiotic Use

- Risk of infection must be significant
- Correct narrow-spectrum antibiotic must be chosen
- Antibiotic level must be high
- Antibiotic must be in the target tissue before surgery
- Use the shortest effective antibiotic exposure

Principle 1: Procedure Should Have Significant Risk of Infection

For prophylactically administered antibiotics to reduce the incidence of infection, the surgical procedure must have a high enough incidence of infection to be reduced with antibiotic therapy. Clean surgery done with strict adherence to basic surgical principles usually has an incidence of infection of about 3%. Infection rates of 10% or more are usually considered unacceptable, and the prophylactic use of antibiotics must be strongly considered for such infection-prone procedures. For the dentist doing routine office surgery, this means that most office procedures performed on healthy patients do not require prophylactically administered antibiotics. The incidence of infection after tooth extraction, frenectomy, biopsy, minor alveoloplasty, and torus reduction is extremely low; therefore, antibiotics would provide no benefit. This is true even in the presence of periapical infection, severe periodontitis, and multiple extractions.

However, several surgical factors may influence the dentist to strongly consider the use of antibiotic prophylaxis (Box 15-11): The first and most obvious factor that may lead to infection is a bacterial inoculum of sufficient size. The usual surgical procedure performed in the mouth rarely involves sufficient

BOX 15-11

Factors Related to Postoperative Infection

- Size of bacterial inoculum
- Duration of surgery
- Presence of foreign body, implant, or dead space
- State of host resistance

bacterial inoculation to cause infection, unless an acute infection with cellulitis or abscess is already present. The second factor is surgical procedures that require prolonged surgery. In hospital surgeries, the incidence of postoperative infection increases significantly with operations lasting longer than 4 hours. A third factor that may suggest the use of antibiotics is the insertion or presence of a foreign body, most commonly a dental implant. Most data seem to suggest that the use of antibiotics may decrease the incidence of infection when foreign bodies, such as dental implants, are inserted into the jaws.

The final and most important factor for most dentists in determining which patients should receive prophylactically administered antibiotics is whether the patient has depressed host defenses. Patients who have a compromised ability to defend themselves against infection should receive antibiotics prophylactically because they are likely to have a higher incidence of more severe infection. All patients receiving cancer chemotherapy or immunosuppressives should receive antibiotics prophylactically, even when minor surgical procedures are performed. Patients receiving immunosuppressives for organ transplant will be taking these drugs for the remainder of their lives and should be given preventive antibiotics accordingly. Patients receiving cancer chemotherapy will receive cytotoxic drugs for 1 year or less but should be given antibiotics prophylactically for at least a 1-year period after the cessation of their chemotherapy. This is also wise for those receiving radiation therapy to the jaw. End-stage renal disease, including patients receiving kidney dialysis, is an immunocompromising disease that requires antibiotic prophylaxis for oral surgical procedures. The most common immunocompromising disease, however, is diabetes mellitus. The incidence of postoperative infection in diabetic persons is directly correlated with elevations of blood sugar. The oral surgical management of diabetic persons based on their blood glucose is summarized in Table 15-5. The glycosylated hemoglobin test, or hemoglobin A_{1c}, is a good measure of the level of diabetes control over the previous 3 to 4 months. Before complex reconstructive oral surgery, such as the placement of dental implants, the dentist is wise to ensure that acceptable intermediate-term control of blood sugar has been achieved, as measured by a hemoglobin A_{1c} of 8% or less. The American Diabetes Association recommends a therapeutic target hemoglobin A_{1c} level of 7%. Withholding dental implant therapy and working with the patient's physician can help motivate the patient to achieve good long-term control of diabetes. Although prophylactically administered antibiotics are helpful in diabetic patients, perioperative control of blood sugar levels is paramount.

TABLE 15-5

Dental Treatment for Diabetics Based on Fingerstick Blood Glucose Testing

Finger Stick Blood Glucose (mg/dL%)	Dental Treatment
Less than 85	Administer glucose; postpone elective treatment
85-200	Stress reduction; consider antibiotic prophylaxis for extraction
200-300	Stress reduction; antibiotic prophylaxis; referral to primary care physician
300-400	Avoid elective treatment; referral to primary care physician or emergency room at nearby hospital
Greater than 400	Avoid elective treatment; send to emergency room at nearby hospital

Principle 2: Choose Correct Antibiotic

The choice of antibiotic for prophylaxis against infections after surgery of the oral cavity should be based on the following criteria: First, the antibiotic should be *effective* against the organisms most likely to cause infection in the oral cavity. As previously discussed, the facultative streptococci are usually the originally invading organism in oral infection. Second, the antibiotic chosen should be a *narrow-spectrum* antibiotic.

By using a narrow-spectrum antibiotic, the disadvantage of altering host flora is minimized. Third, the antibiotic should be the *least toxic* antibiotic available for the patient. Finally, the drug selected should be a *bactericidal* antibiotic. Because many of the routine prophylactic uses of antibiotics in the dental office are for patients with compromised host defenses, it is important that the antibiotic effectively kill the bacteria.

Taking into account these four criteria, the antibiotic of choice for prophylaxis before oral surgery is penicillin or amoxicillin. These two antibiotics are effective against the causative organism (i.e., *Streptococcus*), are narrow-spectrum, have low toxicity, and are bactericidal. For patients allergic to penicillin, the best choice is clindamycin. Clindamycin is fairly effective against oral streptococci and is narrow-spectrum, but it is bacteriostatic. The third choice for oral administration for prophylaxis is azithromycin. Azithromycin is reasonably effective against the usual organisms and is narrow-spectrum, but it is also bacteriostatic.

Principle 3: Antibiotic Plasma Level Must Be High

When antibiotics are used prophylactically, the antibiotic level in the plasma must be higher than when antibiotics are used therapeutically. The peak plasma levels should be high to ensure diffusion of the antibiotic into all of the fluid and tissue spaces where the surgery is going to be performed. The usual recommendation for prophylaxis is that the drug be given in a dose at least 2 *times* the usual therapeutic dose. Use of the same prophylactic doses recommended by the American Heart Association for prophylaxis of infective endocarditis is reasonable. For penicillin or amoxicillin, this is 2 g; for clindamycin, 600 mg; and for azithromycin, 500 mg.

Principle 4: Time Antibiotic Administration Correctly

For the antibiotic to be maximally effective in preventing postoperative infection, the antibiotic must be given 2 hours or less *before* the surgery begins. The time of dosing before surgery varies by the route used, allowing for absorption of the antibiotic into the tissues at the time of wounding. For the oral route, this is usually 1 hour; with the intravenous route, a much shorter preoperative dosing interval is possible. This principle has been clearly established in many animal and human clinical trials. Antibiotic administration that occurs after surgery is greatly decreased in its efficacy or has no effect at all on preventing infection; there is evidence to indicate that prophylactically administered antibiotics given 2 hours or more after surgery may *increase* the risk of wound infection.

If the surgery is prolonged and an additional antibiotic dose is required, intraoperative dose intervals should be shorter (i.e., one half the usual therapeutic dose interval). Therefore, penicillin and clindamycin should be given every 3 hours. This ensures that the peak plasma levels will stay adequately high and avoids periods of inadequate antibiotic levels in the tissue fluids.

Principle 5: Use Shortest Antibiotic Exposure That Is Effective

For the antibiotic prophylaxis to be effective, the antibiotic must be given before the surgery begins, and adequate plasma levels must be maintained during the surgical procedure. Once the surgical procedure is completed, continued antibiotic administration produces little if any benefit. If the procedure is a short operation, a single preoperative dose of antibiotics is adequate. A plethora of animal and human clinical data demonstrates that the prophylactic use of antibiotics is necessary only for the time of surgery; after closure of the wounds and formation of the blood clots, migration of bacteria into the wound and underlying tissues occurs at such a low level that additional antibiotics are not necessary.

Summary

The use of antibiotics for prophylaxis of postoperative wound infection may be effective. It may reduce patient pain, morbidity, cost, and total antibiotic use. Appropriate antibiotic prophylaxis does little to alter host flora. Most dental procedures on healthy patients do not require antibiotic prophylaxis. A few select patients who are to undergo long surgical procedures or the insertion of foreign bodies, such as dental implants, should be considered for prophylaxis. Patients who have compromised host defenses because of poorly controlled metabolic diseases or certain diseases that interfere with host defenses or who are taking drugs that suppress the immune system should also be given prophylactic antibiotics. The drug of choice is a narrow-spectrum antibiotic that is effective against causative organisms, is nontoxic, and is bactericidal. Penicillin fits these criteria the best.

When the antibiotic is given, it should be taken before the surgery begins, at a normal dose twice that of therapeutically administered antibiotics. If the surgery is prolonged, interim doses at half the normal dose interval should be used. High plasma levels should be maintained during the surgical procedure, but no additional antibiotics are necessary after surgery.

PRINCIPLES OF PROPHYLAXIS AGAINST METASTATIC INFECTION

Metastatic infection is defined as infection that occurs at a location physically separate from the portal of entry of the bacteria. The classic and most widely understood example of this phenomenon is bacterial endocarditis, which may arise from bacteria that are introduced into the circulation as a result of tooth extraction. The incidence of metastatic infection can be reduced if antibiotic administration is used to eliminate the bacteria before they can establish an infection at the remote site.

BOX 15-12

Factors Necessary for Metastatic Infection

- Distant susceptible site
- Hematogenous bacterial seeding
- Impaired local defenses

For metastatic infection to occur, several conditions must be met (Box 15-12). The first and most important is that there must be a susceptible location in which an infection can be established. An example of this is the deformed heart valve with its altered endothelial surface onto which an irregularly surfaced vegetation has formed.

Bacterial seeding of the susceptible area must also take place. This seeding occurs as the result of a bacteremia in which bacteria from the mouth are carried to the susceptible site. Most likely, a quantitative factor is involved in this seeding process because the body experiences multiple episodes of small bacteremias as a result of normal daily activities, such as chewing and tooth brushing. Turbulent blood flow across a deformed heart valve can traumatize the endothelial lining of the valve, which can then precipitate the deposition of platelets and fibrin, resulting in nonbacterial thrombotic endocarditis (NBTE). Subsequently, bacterial proteins called adhesins recognize the fibrin and platelet matrix of NBTE. Some staphylococci and oral streptococci, especially *Streptococcus sanguis, Streptococcus mitis,* and *Streptococcus oralis,* have these adhesins, which explains their association with infective endocarditis.

Also necessary for the establishment of metastatic infection is some impairment of the local host defenses. Once bacteria have attached to NBTE, they are protected from white blood cell phagocytosis by a thin coating of fibrin and an extracellular matrix synthesized by the bacteria, resulting in biofilm. More than 90% of the bacteria existing within a mature cardiac vegetation are in a metabolically inactive state, which also renders them less susceptible to bactericidal antibiotics. Bacteria inhabiting such a biofilm coating on foreign bodies, such as prosthetic joint or dental implants, are not easily phagocytized by white blood cells or killed by antibiotics, as in endocarditis.

Prophylaxis Against Infectious Endocarditis

Historically, the rationale for antibiotic prophylaxis of infectious endocarditis (IE) after dental procedures has been based on the following facts: bacteremia has been shown to cause IE; *viridans*-group streptococci are part of the normal oral flora and have been commonly found in IE; dental procedures can cause bacteremias because of *Streptococcus viridans;* a large number of case reports associate dental procedures with subsequent IE; *S. viridans* is generally susceptible to the antiobiotics recommended for prophylaxis of IE; antibiotic prophylaxis prevents experimental endocarditis in animals because of *S. viridans;* and the risk of significant adverse reaction to the antibiotic is low in an individual patient, and the morbidity and mortality of IE are high. When this occurs, the patient must be treated in the hospital with high doses of intravenous (IV) antibiotics for prolonged periods. Often, the damaged native heart valve must be surgically replaced with a prosthetic valve. Although initial recovery from bacterial endocarditis approaches 100%, recurrent episodes reduce the 5-year survival rate of patients with this disease to approximately 60%.

Recent evidence puts into question the likelihood, however, that prophylactic antibiotics prevent IE in human beings. Antibiotics do no consistently prevent bacteremias after dental procedures. Bacteremias after chewing, toothbrushing, and other daily activities occur far more frequently than after dental procedures. Endocarditis has been shown to occur despite appropriate antibiotic prophylaxis for dental procedures. Only a small proportion of IE cases are from dental procedures, and very few cases of IE would be prevented by antibiotic prophylaxis for dental procedures, even it if were 100% effective.

The American Heart Association has had formal recommendations for the prevention of IE after dental treatments since 1960. The latest formal recommendations appeared in May 2007. Dentists must stay abreast of revised recommendations as they are published by the American Heart Association and the American Dental Association. These new guidelines take into account that a very small number of cases of IE are caused by dental procedures and can be prevented by antibiotic prophylaxis. New emphasis has been correctly placed on the establishment and maintenance of optimum oral health in patients with increased risk for IE.

The new guidelines indicate prophylaxis only for the patients at highest risk of endocarditis, including those with previous endocarditis, prosthetic heart valves, cyanotic congenital heart defects that have not been repaired or have remaining partial defects after repair, and heart transplant patients with valvulopathy. This will significantly decrease the number of dental patients for whom prophylaxis is indicated. A list of the conditions that pose the highest risk of endocarditis can be found in Box 15-13.

Recent evidence also indicates that the magnitude of bacteremia caused by a given dental procedure is not necessarily correlated with the incidence of IE. Therefore the new guidelines have simplified the description of dental procedures for which antibiotic prophylaxis should be used to the following description: "All dental procedures that involve manipulation of gingival tissue or the periapical region of teeth or perforation of the oral mucosa" (Box 15-14). Prophylaxis is not required for routine local anesthetic injections through noninfected tissue, dental radiographs, placement of removable prosthodontic or orthodontic appliances, adjustment of orthodontic appliances, placement of orthodontic brackets, shedding of deciduous teeth, and bleeding from trauma to the lips or oral mucosa (Box 15-15).

Bacterial endocarditis prophylaxis is achieved for most routine conditions with the administration of 2 g of amoxicillin orally ½ to 1 hour before the procedure (Table 15-6). Amoxicillin is the drug of choice because it is better absorbed from the gastrointestinal tract and provides higher and more sustained plasma levels. Amoxicillin is an effective killer of viridans-

BOX 15-13

Cardiac Conditions Associated with the Highest Risk of Adverse Outcome from Endocarditis for Which Prophylaxis with Dental Procedures Is Recommended

- Prosthetic cardiac valve
- Previous infective endocarditis
- Congenital heart disease (CHD)*
  - Unrepaired cyanotic CHD, including palliative shunts and conduits
  - Completely repaired congenital heart defect with prosthetic material or device, whether placed by surgery or by catheter intervention, during the first 6 months after the procedure†
  - Repaired CHD with residual defects at the site or adjacent to the site of a prosthetic patch or prosthetic device (which inhibit endothelialization)
- Cardiac transplantation recipients who have cardiac valculopathy

*Except for the conditions listed above, antibiotic prophylaxis is no longer recommended for any other form of CHD.
†Prophylaxis is recommended because endothelialization of prosthetic material occurs within 6 months after the procedure.

TABLE 15-6

Antibiotic Regimens for Prophylaxis of Bacterial Endocarditis

Situation	Agent	Regimen	30–60 Min Before Procedure
		Adults	Children*
Oral	Amoxicillin	2 g	50 mg/kg
Parenteral	Ampicillin	2 g IM or IV	50 mg/kg IM or IV
	Cefazolin/ceftriaxone†	1 g IM or IV	50 mg/kg IM or IV
PCN allergy, oral	Cephalexin†	2 g	50 mg/kg
	Clindamycin	600 mg	20 mg/kg
	Azithromycin/clarithromycin	500 mg	15 mg/kg
PCN, allergy, parenteral	Cefazolin/ceftriaxone†	1 g IM or IV	50 mg/kg IM or IV
	Clindamycin	600 mg IM or IV	20 mg/kg IM or IV

*Total children's dose should not exceed adult dose.
†Cephalosporins should not be used in patients with immediate-type hypersensitivity reaction to penicillins. Other first- or second-generation oral cephalosporins may be substituted in equivalent adult or pediatric doses.
IM, Intramuscularly; *IV,* intravenously.

BOX 15-14

Dental Procedures for Which Endocarditis Prophylaxis Is Recommended for Patients in Box 15-13

All dental procedures that involve manipulation of gingival tissue or the periapical region of teeth or perforation of the oral mucosa.*

The following procedures and events do not need prophylaxis: routine anesthetic injections through noninfected tissues, taking dental radiographs, placement of removable prosthodontic or orthodontic appliances, adjustment of orthodontic appliances, placement of orthodontic brackets, shedding of deciduous teeth, and bleeding from trauma to the lips or oral mucosa.

BOX 15-15

Dental Procedures in Which Prophylaxis Is *Not* Recommended

- Restorative dentistry
- Routine local anesthetic injection
- Intracanal endodontic therapy and placement of rubber dams
- Suture removal
- Placement of removable appliances
- Making of impressions
- Taking of oral radiographs
- Fluoride treatments
- Orthodontic appliance adjustment
- Shedding of primary teeth

group streptococci, which include the organisms that most commonly causes IE after dental procedures.

For patients who are allergic to penicillin, two alternative drugs have been recommended. The first recommended drug is clindamycin, with a dose of 600 mg orally 1 hour before the surgery. If the patient's allergy to penicillin is mild and not of an anaphylactic type, a first-generation cephalosporin, such as cephalexin, may be prescribed. Although erythromycin is no longer recommended, the newer macrolide antibiotics, azithromycin or clarithromycin, are acceptable alternative drugs. If the patient is unable to take oral medication, parenteral administration can be used.

For the pediatric patient, the dose of the drugs that are given must be reduced. The recommendations include clear guidelines for proper pediatric dosing (see Table 15-6).

Some patients at risk for bacterial endocarditis may be taking daily doses of penicillin to prevent recurrence of rheumatic fever or may already be taking an antibiotic for other reasons. In these patients, the streptococci may be relatively resistant to penicillin. The recommendation for this situation is that the dentist should use clindamycin, azithromycin, or clarithromycin for endocarditis prophylaxis. The cephalosporins should be avoided because of possible cross-resistance with the penicillins. If possible, the procedure should be postponed until 10 or more days after the antibiotic is completed, thus allowing a more normal oral flora to be reestablished.

If a particular patient requires a series of dental treatments that requires antibiotic prophylaxis, a period of 10 or more days between appointments is appropriate. The reason for the interval is that the administration of antibiotics for several days or more continuously may promote colonization of the patient by bacteria that are resistant to the antibiotic being given, thus making prophylaxis more likely to fail. The 10-or-more day antibiotic-free period may allow antibiotic-sensitive organisms to repopulate the oral flora. On the other hand, it has been shown that baseline antibiotic resistance levels are not reestablished for several months after a course of antibiotics. For this reason, the number of dental visits should also be minimized, consistent with the patient's tolerance level.

Occasionally, unexpected bleeding may occur during dental treatment in a patient who is at risk for endocarditis, or a patient may not inform the dentist of the indication for antibiotic prophylaxis before the beginning of the procedure. In this situation, appropriate antibiotic prophylaxis should be administered as soon as possible but definitely within 2 hours after the procedure. Prophylaxis given longer than 4 hours after the bacteremia has limited prophylactic benefit.

Patients at risk for IE should have a comprehensive prophylaxis program that includes excellent oral hygiene with excellent periodic professional care. Special care should be taken for the establishment of an effective preventive program, and all incipient dental and periodontal disease should be treated. If surgery is required, the mouth can be rinsed preoperatively with an antibacterial agent, such as chlorhexidine. Preoperative oral antiseptic rinses have been shown to reduce the magnitude of bacteremias (the number of bacteria entering the bloodstream), although they are not a substitute for antibiotic prophylaxis.

Finally, it is important for the dentist to understand that even when appropriate measures are taken to prevent bacterial endocarditis, it may still occur. Patients should be informed of this and advised to return to the dentist or to their primary care physician if any of the signs and symptoms of bacterial endocarditis, especially fever and malaise, occur.

Prosthetic valve endocarditis occurs when the tissue around the cardiac valve implant becomes infected. Such infections are caused by the same bacteria that cause typical native valve endocarditis. Prosthetic valve endocarditis is a much more serious illness than native valve endocarditis because the loosening of the heart valve may result in death. The 1-year survival rate for patients who have prosthetic valve endocarditis is about 50%. The American Heart Association currently states that the standard oral regimens are adequate for most patients with prosthetic heart valves.

Prophylaxis in Patients with Other Cardiovascular Conditions

Several other cardiovascular conditions require the clinician to consider the administration of prophylactic antibiotics for the prevention of metastatic infection. In *coronary artery bypass grafting* (CABG), the coronary arteries are reconstructed with vascular grafts. Because CABG does not predispose patients to metastatic infection, these patients should not be given prophylactic antibiotics before a dental procedure is performed.

Patients with a transvenous pacemaker have a battery pack implanted in their chests, with a thin wire that runs through the superior vena cava into the right side of the heart. These patients usually do not require prophylactic antibiotics when dental procedures are performed. Similarly, coronary artery angioplasty with or without stent placement is not an indi-

TABLE 15-7

Antibiotic Regimens for Prophylaxis of Total Joint Replacement Infection

Regimen	Drug	Dose
Standard oral prophylaxis	Amoxicillin, cephalexin, or cephradine	2 g orally 1 hour before procedure
Penicillin-allergic oral prophylaxis	Clindamycin	600 mg orally 1 hour before procedure
Parenteral prophylaxis	Cefazolin *or* ampicillin	1 g IV 1 hour before procedure 2 g IV 1 hour before procedure
Penicillin-allergic parenteral prophylaxis	Clindamycin	600 mg IV 1 hour before procedure

IV, Intravenous

cation for endocarditis prophylaxis. However, consultation with the patient's cardiologist may be used to confirm that this is the best management.

Patients receiving renal dialysis frequently have an arteriovenous shunt surgically constructed in their forearms to provide the dialysis team ready access to the bloodstream. Metastatic infection may occur in these shunts after bacteremia. Therefore the dentist should contact the patient's nephrologist or renal dialysis team to discuss the best management.

Patients who have hydrocephaly may have decompression with ventriculoatrial shunts. Because these shunts may induce valvular dysfunction, antibiotic prophylaxis may be required. Consultation with the patient's neurosurgeon should be considered.

Patients who have had severe atherosclerotic vascular disease and have had alloplastic vascular grafts placed to replace portions of their arteries do not appear to be at risk for metastatic infection from dental procedures. Therefore the American Heart Association does not recommend antibiotic prophylaxis for nonvalvular cardiovascular devices, including coronary artery stents and vena caval filters. The exception to this rule is for incision and drainage of abscesses at other sites, including the oral cavity.

Prophylaxis Against Total Joint Replacement Infection

Patients who have undergone total replacement of a joint with a prosthetic joint may be at risk for hematogenous spread of bacteria and subsequent infection. These late prosthetic joint infections result in severe morbidity because the implant is usually lost when infections occur. There has been great concern that the bacteremia caused by tooth extraction may result in such infections. However, the recent literature suggests that bacteremias from oral procedures are not likely to cause prosthetic joint infections. It appears that the bacteremia after oral surgery is of a transient nature and does not expose the implant and periimplant tissues to bacteria long enough to cause infection.

Instead it appears that the hematogenous spread of prosthetic joint infections is caused by chronic infections elsewhere in the body that result in chronic septicemias. These infections are typically urogenital, gastrointestinal, pulmonary, or skin infections, but established odontogenic infections may also cause a septicemia of sufficient magnitude to cause a total joint infection. Patients with orthopedic pins, plates, and screws do not need antibiotic prophylaxis.

In July of 2003 the American Dental Association (ADA) and the American Academy of Orthopaedic Surgeons (AAOS) issued a revised joint recommendation concerning the management of patients with prosthetic total joints. The recommendations of the ADA and AAOS recognize that most patients with a prosthetic joint are not at risk for joint infection after a dental surgical procedure. Instead the guidelines identify the high-risk patients who are potentially susceptible to such infections (Box 15-16). Likewise, it identifies those procedures that are most likely to cause joint infections and therefore require prophylaxis (Box 15-17). The joint statement recommends specific antibiotic regimens to help prevent infection in the susceptible patient who is undergoing one of the procedures that require prophylaxis (Table 15-7). Ultimately however, the revised guidelines make the following statement: "Practitioners must exercise their own clinical judgment in determining whether or not antibiotic prophylaxis is appropriate."

BOX 15-16

Conditions Placing Patients at Risk for Prosthetic Joint Infection

- Prosthetic joint placed within 2 years
- Rheumatoid arthritis
- Systemic lupus erythematosus
- Insulin-dependent diabetes
- Previous prosthetic joint infection
- Congenital or acquired immunosuppressive diseases
- Malnourishment
- Hemophilia

BOX 15-17

Procedures That Indicate Prophylaxis for Prosthetic Joint Infection

- Dental extractions
- Periodontal procedures, including scaling and root planing
- Dental implant placement and reimplantation of avulsed teeth
- Periapical endodontic procedures
- Initial placement of orthodontic bands but not brackets
- Intraligamentary local anesthetic injections
- Dental prophylaxis when bleeding is expected
- Subgingival placement of antibiotic fibers or strips

BOX 15-18

Indication for Parenteral Regimen

- Patient having general anesthetic and allowed nothing by mouth
- Unable to take oral medications
- High-risk patients, such as those with history of previous bacterial endocarditis

When the dentist decides to provide antibiotic prophylaxis of prosthetic joint infection, the recommended antibiotics are a first-generation cephalosporin and amoxicillin. For patients who are allergic to penicillin, clindamycin is recommended. As with bacterial endocarditis prophylaxis, only a single preoperative dose is recommended, with no follow-up doses. If patients are unable to take oral medication, a parenteral regimen is also suggested (Box 15-18).

If a patient who has a total joint replacement needs treatment of an infection, aggressive therapy for the infection is necessary to prevent seeding of the bacteria into the prosthesis, causing odontogenic infection of the prosthetic joint. This aggressive treatment should include extraction, I&D, and the use of high-dose bactericidal antibiotics, possibly given IV. The clinician should strongly consider performing C&S testing because if a prosthetic joint infection does occur, it would be useful to know which bacteria are likely the causative organisms along with their antibiotic sensitivity.

When there is disagreement between the dentist, the patient, or the patient's physician over the need for antibiotic prophylaxis, clear communication between all parties is required to clarify all relevant facts and scientific data and to arrive at a consensus. Ultimately, the dentist is responsible for his or her own treatment decisions and should not render care that he or she thinks is not in the best interest of the patient.

Bibliography

ADA Council on Scientific Affairs: Combating antibiotic resistance, *JADA* 135:484-487, 2004.

American Dental Association, American Academy of Orthopaedic Surgeons: Antibiotic prophylaxis dental patients with total joint replacements, *J Am Dent Assoc* 134:895-899, 2003.

Brook I, Frazier EH, Gher ME: Aerobic and anaerobic microbiology of periapical abscess, *Oral Microbiol Immunol* 6:123-125, 1991.

Chow AW, Roser SM, Brady FA: Orofacial odontogenic infections, *Ann Intern Med* 88:392, 1978.

Conover MA, Kaban LB, Mulliken JB: Antibiotic prophylaxis for major maxillocraniofacial surgery, *J Oral Maxillofac Surg* 43:865, 1985.

Conover MA, Kaban LB, Mulliken JB: Antibiotic prophylaxis for major maxillofacial surgery: one-day vs five-day therapy, *Otolaryngology* 95: 554, 1986.

Dajani AS, Taubert KA, Wilson W et al: Prevention of bacterial endocarditis: recommendations by the American Heart Association, *JAMA* 277:1794-1801, 1997.

Doern GV, Ferraro MJ, Brueggemann AB, Ruoff KL: Emergence of high rates of antimicrobial resistance among viridans group streptococci in the United States, *Antimicrob Agents Chemother* 40:891-894, 1996.

Fazakerley MW, McGowan P, Hardy P, Martin MV: A comparative study of cephradine, amoxycillin and phenoxymethylpenicillin in the treatment of acute dentoalveolar infection, *Br Dent J* 174:359-363, 1993 (see comments).

Field EA, Martin MV: Prophylactic antibiotics for patients with artificial joints undergoing oral and dental surgery: necessary or not? *Br J Oral Maxillofac Surg* 29:341-346, 1991.

Flynn TR, Halpern LR: Antibiotic selection in head and neck infections, *Oral Maxillofac Surg Clin North Am* 15:17-38, 2003.

Flynn TR, Shanti RM, Hayes C: Severe odontogenic infections, part two: prospective outcomes study, *J Oral Maxillofac Surg* 64:1104-1113, 2006.

Flynn TR, Shanti RM, Levy M et al: Severe odontogenic infections, part one: prospective report, *J Oral Maxillofac Surg* 64:1093-1103, 2006.

Fouad AF, Rivera EM, Walton RE: Penicillin as a supplement in resolving the localized acute apical abscess, *Oral Surg Oral Med Oral Pathol Oral Radiol Endod* 81:590-595, 1996.

Gilmore WC, Jacobus NV, Gorbach SL et al: A prospective double-blind evaluation of penicillin versus clindamycin in the treatment of odontogenic infections, *J Oral Maxillofac Surg* 46:1065-1070, 1988.

Heimdahl A, Nord CE: Treatment of orofacial infections of odontogenic origin, *Scand J Infect Dis* 46(suppl):101, 1985.

Heimdahl A, Von Konow L, Satoh T et al: Clinical appearance of orofacial infections of odontogenic origin in relation to microbiological findings, *J Clin Microbiol* 22:299, 1985.

Jacobson JJ, Schweitzer SO, Kowalski CJ: Chemoprophylaxis of prosthetic joint patients during dental treatment: a decision-utility analysis, *Oral Surg Oral Med Oral Pathol* 72:167, 1991.

Kaye D: Prophylaxis for infective endocarditis: an update, *Ann Intern Med* 104:419, 1986.

Kim Y, Flynn TR, Donoff RB et al: The gene: the polymerase chain reaction and its clinical application, *J Oral Maxillofac Surg* 60:808-815, 2002.

Kuriyama T, Absi EG, Williams DW, Lewis MA: An outcome audit of the treatment of acute dentoalveolar infection: impact of penicillin resistance, *Br Dent J* 198:759-763, 2005.

Kuriyama T, Karasawa T, Nakagawa K et al: Antimicrobial susceptibility of major pathogens of orofacial odontogenic infections to 11 beta-lactam antibiotics, *Oral Microbiol Immunol* 17(5):285-289, 2002.

Kuriyama T, Nakagawa K, Karasawa T et al: Past administration of beta-lactam antibiotics and increase in the emergence of beta-lactamase-producing bacteria in patients with orofacial odontogenic infections, *Oral Surg Oral Med Oral Pathol Oral Radiol Endod* 89:186-192, 2000.

Laskin DM: Anatomic considerations in diagnosis and treatment of odontogenic infections, *J Am Dent Assoc* 69:308, 1964.

Lewis MA, Carmichael F, MacFarlane TW, Milligan SG: A randomised trial of co-amoxiclav (Augmentin) versus penicillin V in the treatment of acute dentoalveolar abscess, *Br Dent J* 175:169-174, 1993.

Lewis MAO, MacFarlane TW, McGowan DA: Quantitative bacteriology of acute dento-alveolar abscesses, *J Med Microbiol* 2:101, 1986.

Lewis MAO, Parkhurst CL, Douglas CW et al: Prevalence of penicillin-resistant bacteria in acute suppurative oral infection, *J Antimicrob Chemother* 35:785-791, 1995.

Martin C, Karabouta I: Infection after orthognathic surgery, with and without preventative antibiotics, *Int J Oral Surg* 13:490, 1984.

Nager C, Murphy AA: Antibiotics and oral contraceptive pills, *Semin Reprod Endocrinol* 7:220, 1989.

Pallasch TJ: Antibiotic prophylaxis: problems in paradise, *Dent Clin North Am* 47:665-679, 2003.

Paterson SA, Curzon MEJ: The effect of amoxicillin versus penicillin V in the treatment of acutely abscessed primary teeth, *Br Dent J* 174:443, 1993.

Peterson LJ: Antibiotic prophylaxis against wound infections in oral and maxillofacial surgery, *J Oral Maxillofac Surg* 48:617, 1990.

Peterson LJ: Microbiology of head and neck infections, *Atlas Oral Maxillofac Surg Clin North Am* 3:247, 1991.

Peterson LJ: Contemporary management of deep infections of the neck, J Oral Maxillofac Surg 51:226,1993.

Polk HC Jr, Simpson CJ, Simmons BP, Alexander JW: Guidelines for prevention of surgical wound infection, *Arch Surg* 118:1213-1217, 1983.

Sakamoto H, Kato H, Sato T, Sasaki J: Semiquantitative bacteriology of closed odontogenic abscesses, *Bull Tokyo Dent Coll* 39:103-107, 1998.

Sclar DA, Tartaglione TA, Fine MJ: Overview of issues related to medical compliance with implications for outpatient management of infectious disease, *Infect Agents Dis* 3:266, 1994.

Takai S, Kuriyama T, Yanagisawa et al: Incidence and bacteriology of bacteremia associated with various oral and maxillofacial surgical procedures, *Oral Surg Oral Med Oral Pathol Oral Radiol Endod* 99:292-298, 2005.

Wilson W, Taubert KA, Gewitz M, et al: Prevention of infective endocarditis: guidelines from the American Heart Association: a guideline from the American Heart Association Rheumatic Fever, Endocarditis, and Kawasaki Disease Committee, Council on Cardiovascular Disease in the Young, and the Council on Clinical Cardiology, Council on Cardiovascular Surgery and Anesthesia, and the Quality of Care and Outcomes Research Interdisciplinary Working Group, *Circulation* 2007, doi:10.1161/CIRCULATIONAHA. 106.183095. Published online before print April 19, 2007. http://circ.ahajournals.org./cgi/content/abstract/CIRCULATIONAHA. 106.183095v1. Accessed May 19, 2007.

CHAPTER 16

Complex Odontogenic Infections

THOMAS R. FLYNN

CHAPTER OUTLINE

Odontogenic infections are usually mild and readily treated with the appropriate surgical procedure with or without supplemental antibiotic therapy. Infections that spread beyond the teeth into the oral vestibule are usually managed by intraoral incision and drainage (I&D) procedures, plus dental extraction, root canal therapy, or gingival curettage, as appropriate. The principles of management of routine odontogenic infections are discussed in Chapter 15. Some odontogenic infections are serious and require management by oral and maxillofacial surgeons, who have extensive training and experience in this area. Even after the advent of antibiotics and improved dental health, serious odontogenic infections still sometimes result in death. These deaths occur when the infection reaches areas distant from the alveolar process. The purpose of this chapter is to present an overview of deep fascial space infections of the head and neck originating in the teeth, as well as several less common but important infections of the oral cavity.

DEEP FASCIAL SPACE INFECTIONS

The pathways of odontogenic infection extending from the teeth through bone and into surrounding soft tissues are discussed in Chapter 15. As a general rule, infection erodes through the thinnest bone and causes infection in the adjacent tissue. Whether this becomes a vestibular or a deeper fascial space abscess is determined primarily by the relationship of the attachment of the nearby muscles to the point at which the infection perforates the bony cortical plate. Most odontogenic infections penetrate the facial cortical plate of bone to become vestibular abscesses. On occasion, infections erode into other deep fascial spaces directly (Fig. 16-1). Fascial spaces are fascia-lined tissue compartments filled with loose, areolar connective tissue that can become inflamed when invaded by microorganisms. The resulting process of inflammation passes through stages that are seen clinically as edema (inoculation), cellulitis, and abscess. In healthy persons, the deep fascial spaces are only potential spaces that do not exist. The loose areolar tissue within these spaces serves to cushion the muscles, vessels, nerves, glands, and other structures that it surrounds and to allow relative movement between these structures. During an infection, this cushioning and lubricating tissue has the potential to become greatly edematous in response to the exudation of tissue fluid and then to become indurated as polymorphonuclear leukocytes, lymphocytes, and macrophages migrate from the vascular space into the infected interstitial spaces. Ultimately, liquefactive necrosis of white blood cells and this connective tissue leads to abscess formation, and spontaneous or surgical drainage typically leads to resolution. This is the pathophysiology of the stages of infection that clinicians see as edema, when the bacteria are inoculating the tissues of a particular anatomic space; cellulitis, when an intense inflammatory response causes all of the classic signs of inflammation; and abscess, when small areas of liquefactive necrosis coalesce centrally to form pus within the tissues.

Based on the relationship between the point at which the infection erodes through the alveolar bone and the surrounding muscle attachments, infections arising from any maxillary or mandibular tooth can cause vestibular, buccal, or subcutaneous space infections. Infections passing beyond the alveolar process on the deep (toward the oral cavity) side of the nearby muscle of facial expression invade the vestibular space, and those that enter the soft tissues on the superficial (toward the skin) side of those muscles enter the buccal or the subcutaneous space. Infections arising from the maxillary teeth also tend to spread into the infraorbital, palatal, orbital, and infratemporal spaces, and the maxillary sinus (Box 16-1). Mandibular dental infections also tend to spread into the submandibular, sublingual, submental, and masticator spaces. Infections can extend beyond these primary spaces into the deeper fascial spaces of the neck, such as the lateral pharyngeal, retropharyngeal, carotid, and pretracheal spaces. From there, such infections can spread into the danger space and the mediastinum. In addition, infections can rise superiorly through

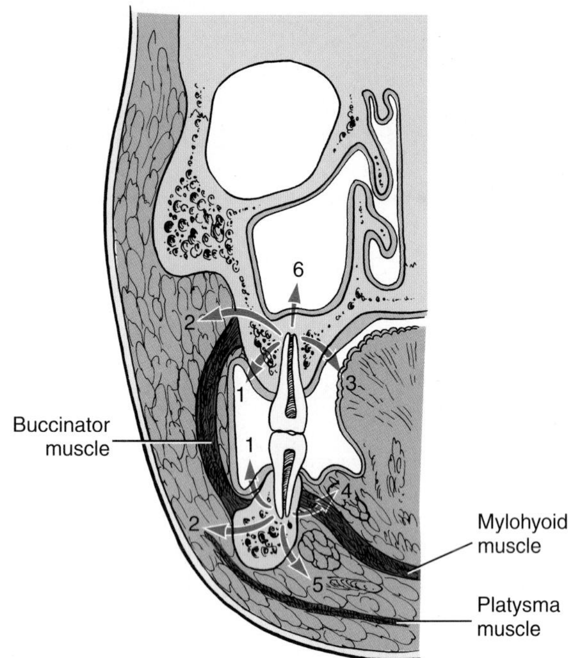

FIGURE 16-1 As infection erodes through bone, it can express itself in a variety of places depending on thickness of overlying bone and relationship of muscle attachments to site of perforation. This illustration notes six possible locations: vestibular abscess (*1*), buccal space (*2*), palatal abscess (*3*), sublingual space (*4*), submandibular space (*5*), and maxillary sinus (*6*). (From Cummings CW, Fredrickson JM, Harker LA, et al, editors: *Otolaryngology: head and neck surgery,* ed 3, vol 3, St Louis, 1998, Mosby.)

BOX 16-1

Anatomic Spaces Involved in Odontogenic Infections

DEEP FASCIAL SPACE INFECTIONS ASSOCIATED WITH ANY TOOTH
- Vestibular
- Buccal
- Subcutaneous

DEEP FASCIAL SPACE INFECTIONS ASSOCIATED WITH MAXILLARY TEETH
- Infraorbital
- Buccal
- Infratemporal
- Maxillary and other paranasal sinuses
- Cavernous sinus thrombosis

DEEP FASCIAL SPACE INFECTIONS ASSOCIATED WITH MANDIBULAR TEETH
- Space of the body of the mandible
- Perimandibular spaces
- Submandibular
- Sublingual
- Submental
- Masticator space
- Submasseteric
- Pterygomandibular
- Superficial temporal
- Deep temporal

DEEP FASCIAL SPACES OF THE NECK
- Lateral pharyngeal
- Retropharyngeal
- Pretracheal
- Danger space
- Prevertebral

the sinuses or vascular structures to invade the brain or the intracranial dural sinuses, such as the cavernous sinus.

Infections of the deep fascial spaces can be classified as having low, moderate, or high severity according to their likelihood of threatening the airway or other vital structures. Low-severity infections are not likely to threaten the airway or vital structures. Moderate-severity infections hinder access to the airway by causing trismus or elevation of the tongue, which can make endotracheal intubation difficult. High-severity infections can directly compress or deviate the airway or damage vital organs, such as the brain, heart, or lungs. Determining the exact anatomic location of infection is a key step in determining its severity. A classification of the deep fascial spaces according to their severity is listed in Box 16-2. Examples of low-, moderate-, and high-severity infections are shown in Figures 16-2 to 16-4. Table 16-1 lists the anatomic borders of the more commonly infected deep fascial spaces of the head and neck.

Infections Arising from Any Tooth

As discussed in Chapter 15 and previously in this chapter, maxillary or mandibular teeth can cause infections of the buccal, vestibular, or subcutaneous spaces. The buccal space is actually a portion of the subcutaneous space, which extends from head to toe. Thus a long-standing buccal space abscess tends to drain spontaneously through the skin at its inferior extent near the inferior border of the mandible. Table 16-2 lists the likely causative teeth, contents, neighboring spaces into which infection may spread, and surgical approaches for drainage of the more commonly infected deep fascial spaces of the head and neck.

Infections Arising from the Maxillary Teeth

Because the apices of the upper lateral incisors and the palatal roots of upper premolars and molars are closest to the palatal cortical plate, infection arising from these teeth can erode through the bone without perforating the periosteum. The potential subperiosteal space in the palate is the palatal space.

The infraorbital space is a thin potential space between the levator anguli oris and the levator labii superioris muscles. The infraorbital space becomes involved primarily as the result of infections from the maxillary canine tooth or by extension of infections from the buccal space. The canine root is often sufficiently long to allow erosion to occur through the alveolar bone superior to the origin of the levator anguli oris and below the origin of the levator labii superioris muscle. When this space is infected, swelling of the anterior face obliterates the nasolabial fold (Fig. 16-5). Spontaneous drainage of infections of this space commonly occurs near the medial or the lateral canthus of the eye because the path of least resistance is to either side of the levator labii superioris muscle, which attaches along the center of the inferior orbital rim.

The buccal space is bounded by the overlying skin of the face on the lateral aspect and the buccinator muscle on the medial aspect (Fig. 16-6). This space may become infected from extensions of infection from maxillary teeth through the

BOX 16-2

Relative Severity of Deep Fascial Space Infections

LOW SEVERITY—LITTLE THREAT TO THE AIRWAY OR VITAL STRUCTURES
- Vestibular
- Buccal
- Subperiosteal
- Space of the body of the mandible
- Infraorbital

MODERATE SEVERITY—HINDERED ACCESS TO THE AIRWAY
- Perimandibular spaces
- Submandibular
- Sublingual
- Submental
- Masticator space
- Submasseteric
- Pterygomandibular
- Superficial temporal
- Deep temporal (includes infratemporal)

HIGH SEVERITY—DIRECT THREAT TO THE AIRWAY OR VITAL STRUCTURES
- Deep neck spaces
- Lateral pharyngeal
- Retropharyngeal
- Pretracheal
- Danger space
- Mediastinum
- Intracranial infections
- Cavernous sinus thrombosis
- Brain abscess

bone superior to the attachment of the buccinator on the alveolar process of the maxilla. The posterior maxillary teeth, most commonly the molars, cause most buccal space infections.

Involvement of the buccal space usually results in swelling below the zygomatic arch and above the inferior border of the mandible. Infections may follow the extensions of the buccal fat pad into the superficial temporal space, the infratemporal space, the infraorbital space, and the periorbital space, as illustrated in Figure 16-7. Because the fascial layers that pass over the zygomatic arch are tightly bound down to the bone, swelling above and below the zygomatic arch can cause the relatively dimpled appearance over the left zygomatic arch in Figure 16-7. The zygomatic arch and the inferior border of the mandible remain palpable in buccal space infections.

The infratemporal space lies posterior to the maxilla. The space is bounded medially by the lateral pterygoid plate of the sphenoid bone and superiorly by the base of the skull. Laterally and superiorly, the infratemporal space is continuous with the deep temporal space (Fig. 16-8). Essentially, the infratemporal space is the bottom portion of the deep temporal space. The space contains branches of the internal maxillary artery and the pterygoid venous plexus. Importantly, emissary veins from the pterygoid plexus pass through foramina in the base of the skull to connect with the intracranial dural sinuses. Because the veins of the face and the orbit do not have valves, blood-borne infections may pass superiorly or inferiorly along their course. The infratemporal space is the origin of the posterior route by which infections may spread into the cavernous sinus (Fig. 16-9). The infratemporal space is rarely infected, but when it is, the cause is usually an infection of the maxillary third molar.

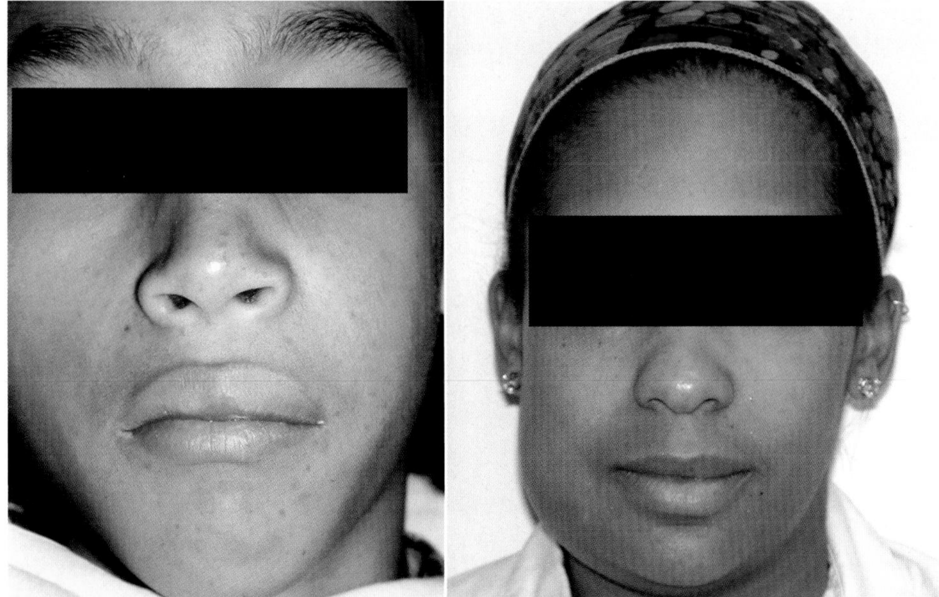

FIGURE 16-2 Low-severity infections that are not likely to threaten the airway or vital structures. A, Vestibular space abscess under the upper lip. B, Cellulitis of the space of the body of the mandible. (A from Flynn TR: Anatomy of oral and maxillofacial infections. In Topazian RG, Goldberg MH, Hupp JR, editors: *Oral and maxillofacial infections,* ed 4, Philadelphia, 2002, WB Saunders.)

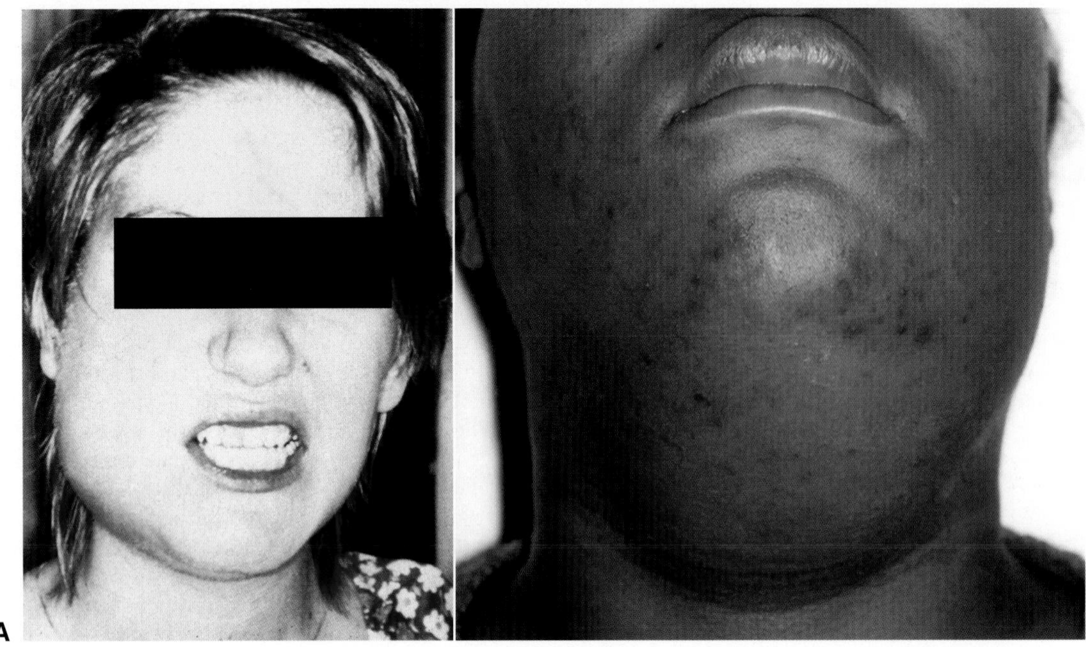

FIGURE 16-3 Moderate-severity infections that hinder access to the airway. **A**, Submasseteric space abscess that is causing severe trismus. **B**, Cellulitis of the submandibular and submental spaces. (A from Goldberg MH: Odontogenic infections and deep fascial space infections of odontogenic origin. In Topazian RG, Goldberg MH, Hupp JR, editors: *Oral and maxillofacial infections,* ed 4, Philadelphia, 2002, WB Saunders; **B** from Flynn TR: Surgical management of orofacial infections. *Atlas Oral Maxillofac Surg Clin North Am* 8:77-100, March 2000.)

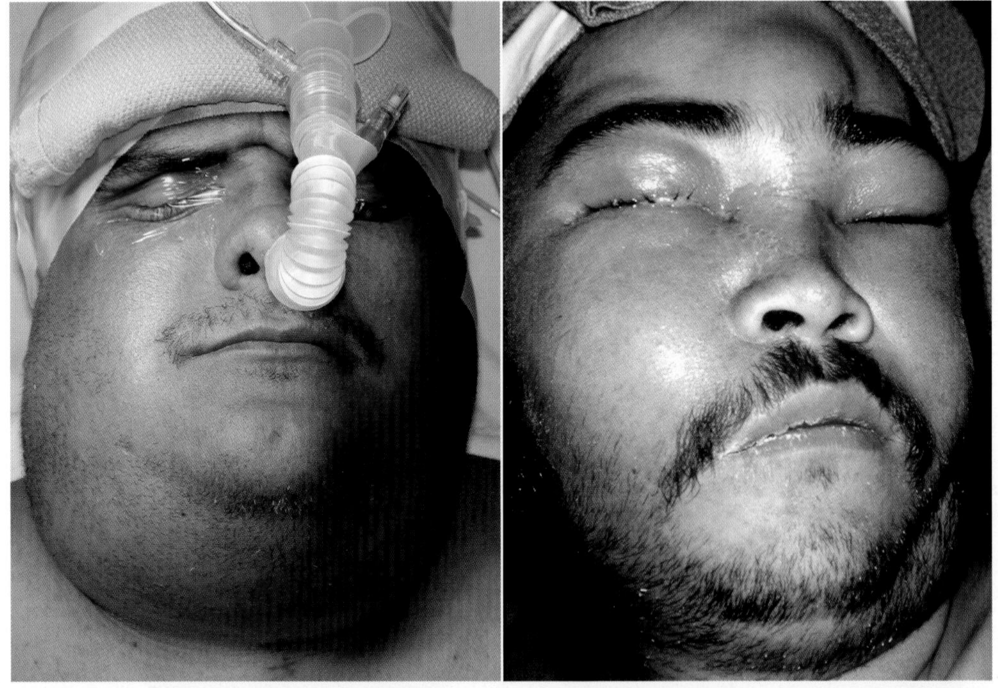

FIGURE 16-4 High-severity infections that are likely to obstruct the airway or threaten vital structures. **A**, Lateral pharyngeal space abscess. **B**, Cavernous sinus thrombosis. (From Flynn TR, Topazian RG: Infections of the oral cavity. In Waite D, editor: *Textbook of practical oral and maxillofacial surgery,* Philadelphia, 1987, Lea & Febiger.)

TABLE 16-1

Borders of the Deep Fascial Spaces of the Head and Neck

	Borders					
Space	**Anterior**	**Posterior**	**Superior**	**Inferior**	**Superficial or Medial***	**Deep or Lateral†**
Buccal	Corner of mouth	Masseter m. Pterygomandibular space	Maxilla Infraorbital space	Mandible	Subcutaneous tissue and skin	Buccinator m.
Infraorbital	Nasal cartilages	Buccal space	Quadratus labii superioris muscle	Oral mucosa	Quadratus labii superioris m	Levator anguli oris muscle Maxilla
Submandibular	Anterior belly digastric muscle	Posterior belly digastric muscle Stylohyoid muscle Stylopharyngeus m	Inferior and medial surfaces of mandible	Digastric tendon	Platysma muscle Investing fascia	Mylohyoid m. Hyoglossus muscle Superior constrictor muscles
Submental	Inferior border of mandible	Hyoid bone	Mylohyoid muscle	Investing fascia	Investing fascia	Anterior bellies of digastric muscles†
Sublingual	Lingual surface of mandible	Submandibular space	Oral mucosa	Mylohyoid m.	Muscles of tongue*	Lingual surface of mandible†
Pterygomandibular	Buccal space	Parotid gland	Lateral pterygoid m	Inferior border of mandible	Medial pterygoid muscle*	Ascending ramus of mandible†
Submasseteric	Buccal space	Parotid gland	Zygomatic arch	Inferior border of mandible	Ascending ramus of mandible*	Masseter muscle†
Lateral pharyngeal	Superior and middle pharyngeal constrictor muscles	Carotid sheath and scalene fascia	Skull base	Hyoid bone	Pharyngeal constrictors and retropharyngeal space*	Medial pterygoid muscle†
Retropharyngeal	Superior and middle pharyngeal constrictor muscles	Alar fascia	Skull base	Fusion of alar and prevertebral fasciae at C6-T4		Carotid sheath and lateral pharyngeal space†
Pretracheal	Sternothyroid-thyrohyoid fascia	Retropharyngeal space	Thyroid cartilage	Superior mediastinum	Sternothyroid-thyrohyoid fascia	Visceral fascia over trachea and thyroid gland

From Flynn TR: Anatomy of oral and maxillofacial infections. In Topazian RG, Goldberg MH, Hupp JR, editors: *Oral and maxillofacial infections,* ed 4, Philadelphia, 2002, WB Saunders.
*Medial border.
†Lateral border.

Periapical or periodontal infections of maxillary posterior teeth may erode superiorly through the floor of the maxillary sinus. Approximately 20% of cases of maxillary sinusitis are odontogenic. Odontogenic maxillary sinus infections may also spread superiorly through the ethmoid sinus or the orbital floor to cause secondary periorbital or orbital infections. Periorbital or orbital infection rarely occurs as the result of odontogenic infection, but when either does occur, the presentation is typical: redness and swelling of the eyelids and involvement of the vascular and neural components of the orbit. This is a serious infection and requires aggressive medical and surgical intervention from an oral and maxillofacial surgeon and other specialists. Figure 16-10 shows the clinical and radiographic appearance of a case of odontogenic infection extending from the maxillary sinus through the ethmoid sinus into the orbit.

When maxillary odontogenic infections erode into the infraorbital vein in the infraorbital space or the inferior ophthalmic vein via the sinuses, they can follow the common ophthalmic vein through the superior orbital fissure and extend directly into the cavernous sinus. This is the anterior route to the cavernous sinus. Intravascular inflammation caused by the invading bacteria stimulates the clotting pathways, resulting in a septic cavernous sinus thrombosis. Cavernous sinus thrombosis is an unusual occurrence that is rarely the result of an infected tooth.

TABLE 16-2

Relations of the Deep Fascial Spaces of the Head and Neck

Space	Likely Causes	Contents	Neighboring Spaces	Approach for Incision and Drainage
Buccal	Upper premolars Upper molars Lower premolars	Parotid duct Anterior facial artery and vein Transverse facial artery and vein Buccal fat pad	Infraorbital Pterygomandibular Infratemporal	Intraoral (small) Extraoral (large)
Infraorbital	Upper canine	Angular artery and vein Infraorbital nerve	Buccal	Intraoral
Submandibular	Lower molars	Submandibular gland Facial artery and vein Lymph nodes	Sublingual Submental Lateral pharyngeal Buccal	Extraoral
Submental	Lower anterior teeth Fracture of symphysis	Anterior jugular vein Lymph nodes	Submandibular (on either side)	Extraoral
Sublingual	Lower premolars Lower molars Direct trauma	Sublingual glands Wharton's ducts Lingual nerve Sublingual artery and vein	Submandibular Lateral Pharyngeal Visceral (trachea and esophagus)	Intraoral Intraoral-extraoral
Pterygomandibular	Lower third molars Fracture of angle of mandible	Mandibular division of trigeminal nerve Inferior alveolar artery and vein	Buccal Lateral pharyngeal Submasseteric Deep temporal Parotid Peritonsillar	Intraoral Intraoral-extraoral
Submasseteric	Lower third molars Fracture of angle of mandible	Masseteric artery and vein	Buccal Pterygomandibular Superficial temporal Parotid	Intraoral Intraoral-extraoral
Infratemporal and deep temporal	Upper molars	Pterygoid plexus Interior maxillary artery and vein Mandibular division of trigeminal nerve Skull base foramina	Buccal Superficial temporal Inferior petrosal sinus	Intraoral Extraoral Intraoral-extraoral
Superficial temporal	Upper molars Lower molars	Temporal fat pad Temporal branch of facial nerve	Buccal Deep temporal	Intraoral Extraoral Intraoral-extraoral
Lateral pharyngeal	Lower third molars Tonsils Infection in neighboring spaces	Carotid artery Internal jugular vein Vagus nerve Cervical sympathetic chain	Pterygomandibular Submandibular Sublingual Peritonsillar Retropharyngeal	Intraoral Intraoral-extraoral

From Flynn TR: Anatomy of oral and maxillofacial infections. In Topazian RG, Goldberg MH, Hupp JR, editors: *Oral and maxillofacial infections,* ed 4, Philadelphia, 2002, WB Saunders (with permission).

Like orbital cellulitis, cavernous sinus thrombosis is a serious, life-threatening infection that requires aggressive medical and surgical care. Cavernous sinus thrombosis has a high mortality even today. Figure 16-11 illustrates the rapid extension of a case of orbital cellulitis into cavernous sinus thrombosis; fortunately, the most vulnerable structure in the cavernous sinus, the abducens (sixth cranial) nerve, was spared.

Infections Arising from the Mandibular Teeth

Although many infections arising from the mandibular teeth erode into the vestibular space, they may also spread into other deep fascial spaces. Initially, such mandibular infections tend to enter the space of the body of the mandible, the submandibular, sublingual, submental, or masticator spaces. From

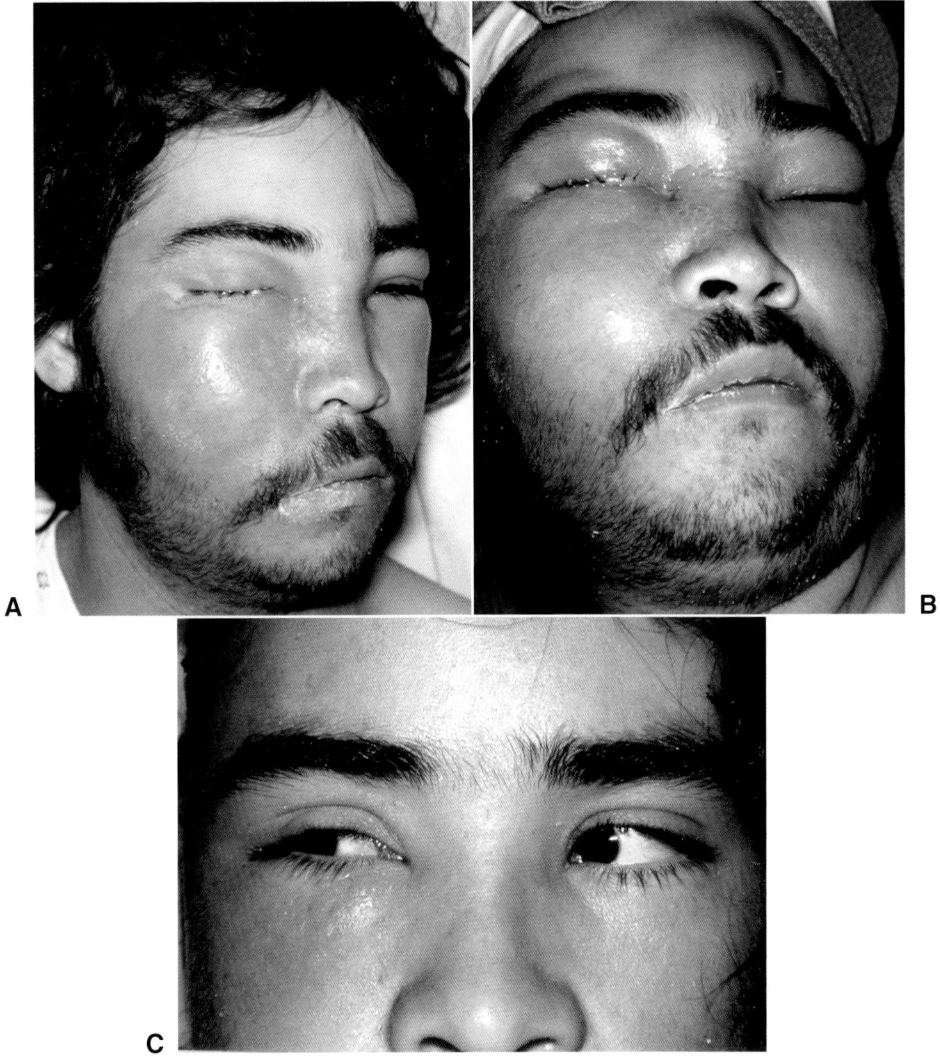

FIGURE 16-11 Cavernous sinus thrombosis. **A**, Infraorbital and buccal space abscess with extension into the periorbital and orbital spaces. **B**, The same patient, 4 hours later, with continued spread of the infection to the superficial and deep temporal spaces, cavernous sinus, and the opposite orbit. **C**, The same patient, 2 weeks later. On voluntary gaze toward the affected right side, both eyes turn toward the right, demonstrating that the right abducens nerve was not injured. (**A** and **B** from Flynn TR, Topazian RG: Infections of the oral cavity. In Waite D, editor: *Textbook of practical oral and maxillofacial surgery,* Philadelphia, 1987, Lea & Febiger.)

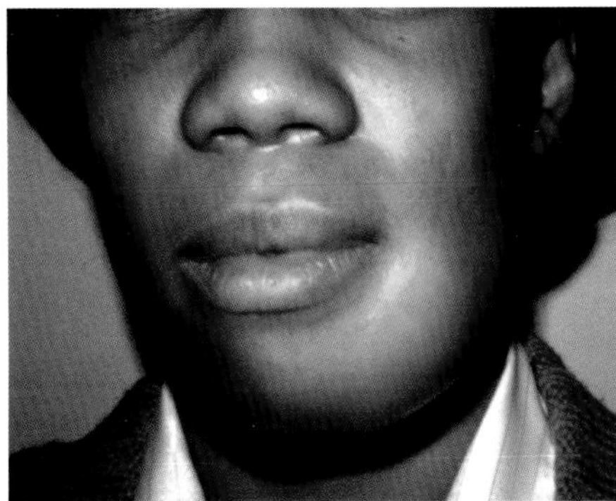

FIGURE 16-12 Space of the body of the mandible infection. It appears as if the mandible itself is enlarged by the subperiosteal collection of fluid. (From Flynn TR: The swollen face. *Emerg Med Clin North Am* 15:481-519, Aug 2000.)

infection is submandibular or sublingual is the attachment of the mylohyoid muscle on the mylohyoid ridge of the medial aspect of the mandible (Fig. 16-13). If the infection erodes through the medial aspect of the mandible above this line, the infection will be in the sublingual space. This is most commonly seen with premolars and the first molar. If the infection erodes through the medial aspect of the mandible inferior to the mylohyoid line, the submandibular space will be involved. The mandibular third molar is the tooth that most commonly involves the submandibular space primarily. The second molar may involve the sublingual or submandibular space, depending on the length of the individual roots.

The sublingual space lies between the oral mucosa of the floor of the mouth and the mylohyoid muscle (Fig. 16-14, *A*). The posterior border of the sublingual space is open, and therefore it freely communicates with the submandibular space.

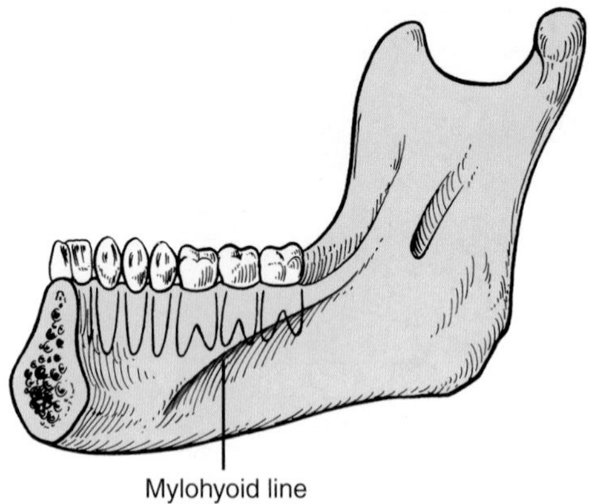

FIGURE 16-13 Mylohyoid line is area of attachment of mylohyoid muscle. Linguocortical plate perforation by infection from premolars and first molar causes sublingual space infection, whereas infection from third molar involves submandibular space. (From Cummings CW, Fredrickson JM, Harker LA et al, editors: *Otolaryngology: head and neck surgery,* vol 3, St Louis, 1998, Mosby.)

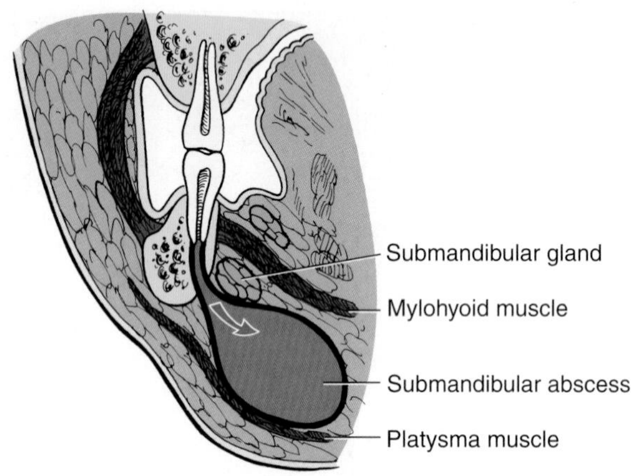

FIGURE 16-15 The submandibular space lies between the mylohyoid muscle and anterior layer of the deep cervical fascia, just deep to the platysma muscle, and includes the lingual and inferior surfaces of the mandible below the mylohyoid muscle attachment. (From Cummings CW, Fredrickson JM, Harker LA et al, editors: *Otolaryngology: head and neck surgery,* vol 3, St Louis, 1998, Mosby.)

Clinically, little or no extraoral swelling is produced by an infection of the sublingual space, but much intraoral swelling is seen in the floor of the mouth on the infected side. The infection usually becomes bilateral, and the tongue becomes elevated (Fig. 16-14, *B*).

The submandibular space lies between the mylohyoid muscle and the overlying superficial layer of the deep cervical fascia (Fig. 16-15). The posterior extent of the submandibular space communicates with the deep fascial spaces of the neck. Infection of the submandibular space causes swelling that can look like an inverted triangle, with the base at the inferior border of the mandible, the sides determined by the anterior and posterior bellies of the digastric muscle, and the apex at the hyoid bone (Fig. 16-16).

The submental space lies between the anterior bellies of the right and left digastric muscles and between the mylohyoid muscle and the overlying fascia (Fig. 16-17). Isolated submental space infections are rare, caused by infections of the mandibular incisors. More commonly, submental space involvement is the result of the spread of a submandibular space infection, which can easily pass around the anterior belly of the digastric muscle to enter the submental space. Such an aggressive infection can then easily pass from the submental space to the contralateral submandibular space to involve all three spaces.

When the perimandibular spaces (submandibular, sublingual, and submental) are bilaterally involved in an infection, it is known as *Ludwig's angina.* This infection is a rapidly spreading cellulitis that can obstruct the airway and commonly spreads posteriorly to the deep fascial spaces of the neck.

Severe swelling is almost always seen, with elevation and displacement of the tongue, and a tense, hard, bilateral induration of the submandibular region superior to the hyoid bone. The

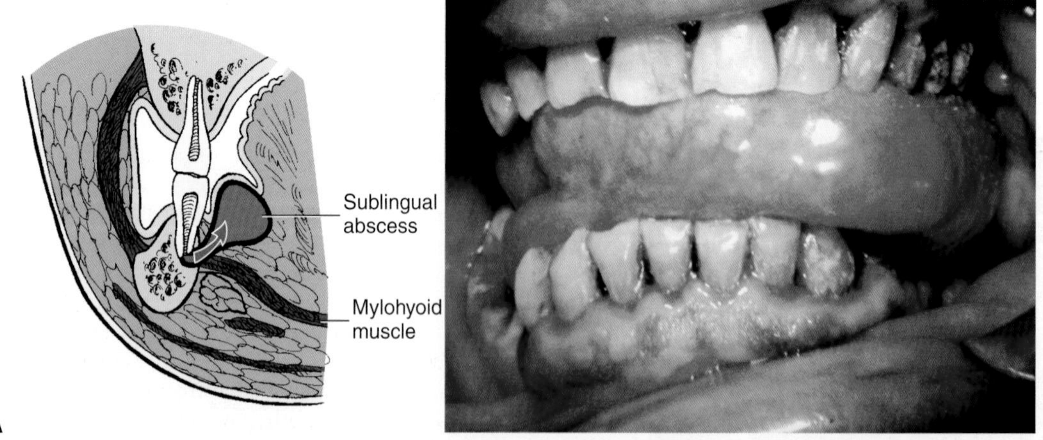

FIGURE 16-14 A, The sublingual space lies between the oral mucosa and the mylohyoid muscle. The space is primarily involved by infection from mandibular premolars and first molar. B, Severe sublingual space abscess that has elevated the tongue into the palate such that only the ventral surface of the tongue and floor of the mouth are visible. (From Flynn TR, Topazian RG: Infections of the oral cavity. In Waite D, editor: *Textbook of practical oral and maxillofacial surgery,* Philadelphia, 1987, Lea & Febiger.)

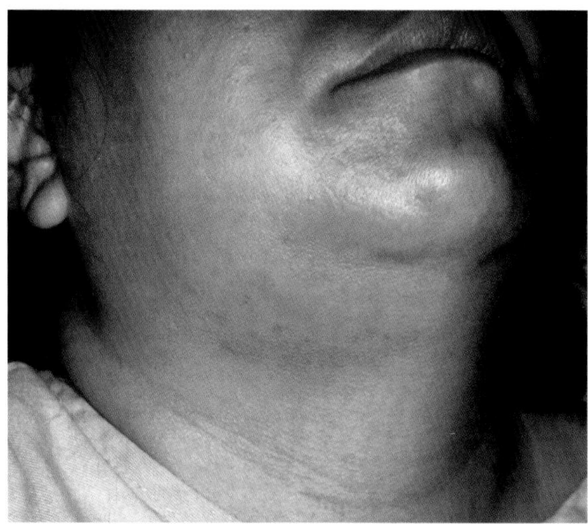

FIGURE 16-16 Typical submandibular space infection demarcated by both bellies of the digastric muscle, the inferior border of the mandible, and the hyoid bone. (From Flynn TR: The swollen face. *Emerg Med Clin North Am* 15:481-519, Aug 2000.)

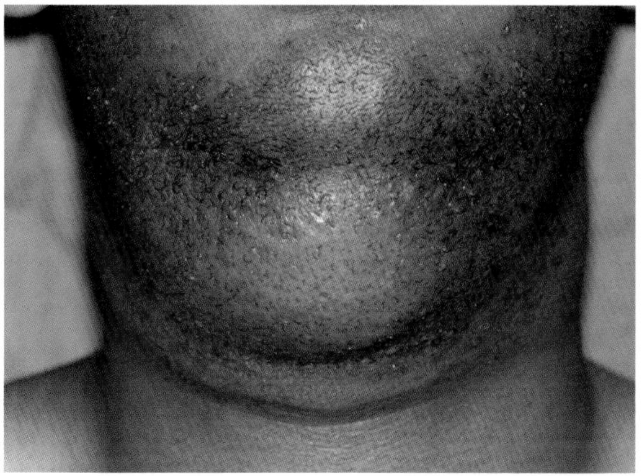

FIGURE 16-17 Submental space infection appears as discrete swelling in central area of submandibular region.

patient usually has trismus, drooling of saliva, and difficulty with swallowing and sometimes breathing. The patient often experiences severe anxiety concerning the inability to swallow and maintain an airway. This infection may progress with alarming speed and thus may produce upper airway obstruction that often leads to death. The most common cause of Ludwig's angina is an odontogenic infection. In the 1940s, before penicillin was available, Williams[4] and Williams and Guralnick[5] were able to reduce the mortality of Ludwig's angina from 54% to 10% by instituting a protocol of initially securing the airway and then performing early and aggressive I&D procedures. Their landmark studies established the principles of airway security and prompt, aggressive surgery and demonstrated that antibiotic therapy plays only a supportive role in the management of severe odontogenic infections.

The submandibular and sublingual spaces join together at the posterior edge of the mylohyoid muscle. At the posterior edge of this junction is the buccopharyngeal gap, where the styloglossus and stylohyoid muscles pass between the superior and middle pharyngeal constrictor muscles on their way to the tongue and the hyoid bone, respectively. Submandibular or sublingual space infections can pass through the buccopharyngeal gap to enter the lateral pharyngeal space, which is one of the deep fascial spaces of the neck. In addition, submandibular space infections can pass around the posterior belly of the digastric muscle to enter the lateral pharyngeal space directly. These are the pathways by which submandibular and sublingual space infections can spread into the deep fascial spaces of the neck and beyond.

In most of the reported case series of severe odontogenic infections, the submandibular space is the most frequently involved. In a recent series of severe odontogenic infections requiring hospitalization, however, the submandibular space was involved in 54% of cases, and the masticator space was involved in 78% of cases. The pterygomandibular portion of the masticator space was involved in 60% of cases. The mandibular third molar is the most commonly associated tooth, and it frequently causes infections of the pterygomandibular portion of the masticator space.[6,7]

The masticator space is formed by the splitting of the anterior layer of the deep cervical fascia, also called the superficial or the investing layer of the deep cervical fascia, to surround the muscles of mastication. This fascia separates at the inferior border of the mandible to pass laterally over the masseter muscle and medially over the medial surface of the medial pterygoid muscle. Medially, this fascia terminates at its attachment to the pterygoid plates and sphenoid bone. Laterally, this fascia, locally called the parotideomasseteric fascia, rises over the masseter muscle and fuses with the periosteum over the zygomatic arch. Above the zygomatic arch, this fascia, locally called the temporalis fascia, rises over the lateral surface of the temporalis muscle, and terminates at the insertion of the temporalis muscle on the cranium. This fascial envelope, and the surfaces of the skull that form its medial border, is the masticator space. Within this space, there are four compartments that are referred to as separate spaces. They are the submasseteric space, between the masseter muscle and the lateral surface of the ascending ramus of the mandible; the pterygomandibular space, between the medial pterygoid muscle and the medial surface of the ascending ramus; the superficial temporal space, between the temporalis fascia and the temporalis muscle; and the deep temporal space, between the temporalis muscle and the skull. The zygomatic arch separates the submasseteric and superficial temporal spaces, and the lateral pterygoid muscle separates the pterygomandibular and the deep temporal spaces. The infratemporal space is actually the inferior portion of the deep temporal space, between the lateral pterygoid muscle and the infratemporal crest of the sphenoid bone. These four compartments of the masticator space clinically behave like separate spaces because in most cases only one compartment of the masticator space becomes infected. However, particularly severe or long-standing masticator space infections can involve all four compartments, as illustrated in Figure 16-18.

The submasseteric space is involved by infection most commonly as the result of spread from the buccal space or from soft tissue infection around the mandibular third molar (pericoronitis). Occasionally, an infected mandibular angle fracture causes a submasseteric space infection. When the submasseteric space is involved, the masseter muscle also becomes inflamed and swollen, as seen clinically and radiographically in Figure 16-19. Because of the involvement of the masseter muscle, the patient also has moderate to severe trismus caused by inflammation of the masseter muscle.

The pterygomandibular space is the site into which local anesthetic solution is injected when an inferior alveolar nerve block is performed. Infections of this space spread primarily from the mandibular third molar. When the pterygomandibular space alone is involved, little or no facial swelling is observed; however, the patient almost always has significant trismus. Therefore, trismus without swelling is a valuable diagnostic

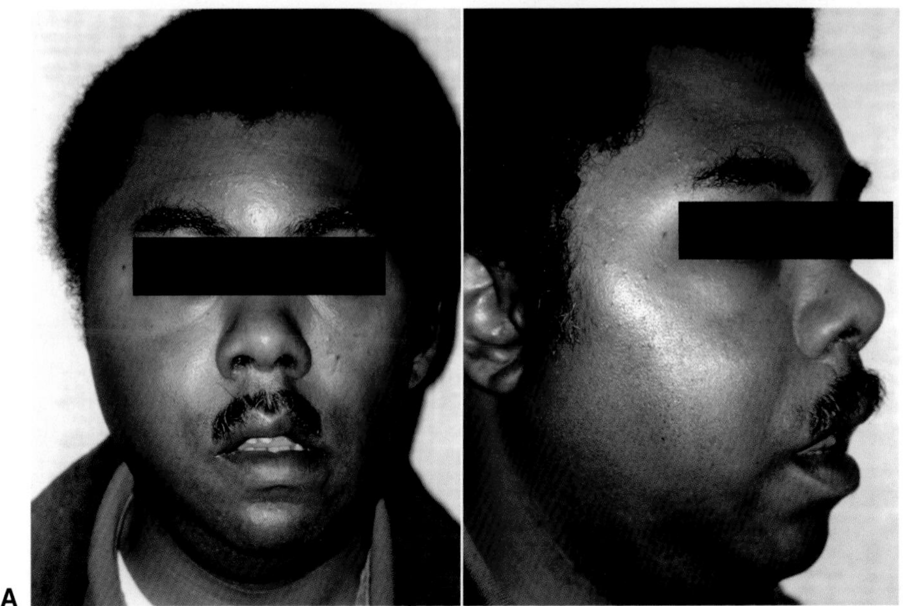

FIGURE 16-18 Masticator space infection, with all compartments involved. **A**, Frontal view demonstrating the swelling anterior to and obscuring the ear and in the temporal region. **B**, Oblique view demonstrating the dimpling of the swelling over the zygomatic arch, with temporal and submasseteric swelling above and below. (**A** from Flynn TR: *Emerg Med Clin North Am* 15:499, Aug 2000.)

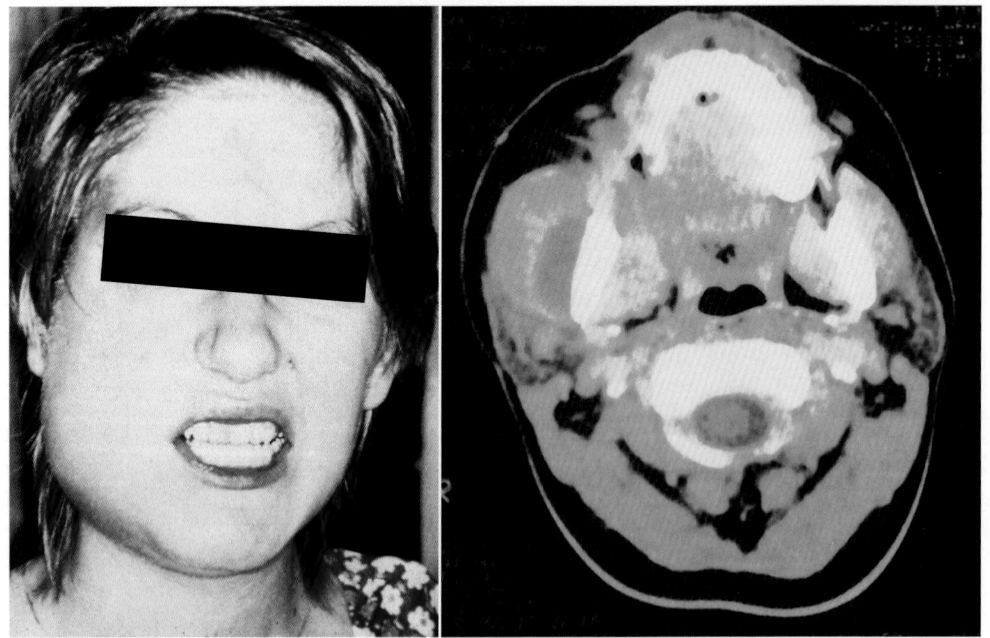

FIGURE 16-19 Submasseteric space abscess. **A**, Severe trismus. **B**, Computed tomography image of a submasseteric space abscess that illustrates the fluid between the edematous masseter muscle and the ascending ramus of the mandible. (**A** from Goldberg MH: Odontogenic infections and deep fascial space infections of odontogenic origin. In Topazian RG, Goldberg MH, Hupp JR, editors: *Oral and maxillofacial infections,* ed 4, Philadelphia, 2002, WB Saunders; **B** from Flynn TR: Anatomy of oral and maxillofacial infections. In Topazian RG, Goldberg MH, Hupp JR, editors: *Oral and maxillofacial infections,* ed 4, Philadelphia, 2002, WB Saunders.)

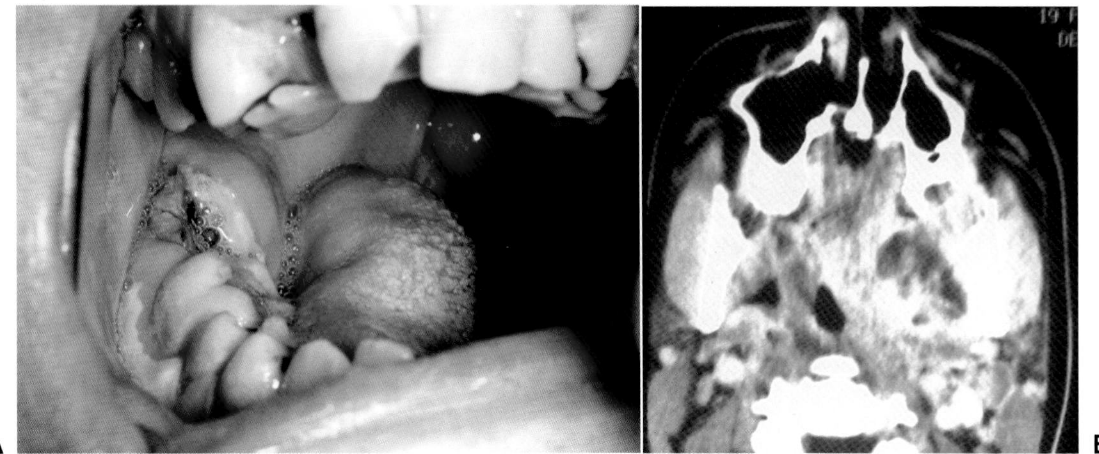

FIGURE 16-20 A, Pterygomandibular space abscess due to a carious lower third molar, with swelling of the anterior tonsillar pillar and deviation of the uvula to the opposite side. B, Computed tomography scan of a pterygomandibular space abscess due to a lower third molar. Note the fluid collection between the distended medial pterygoid muscle and the ascending ramus of the mandible, as well as the displacement and compression of the airway. (A from Flynn TR, Topazian RG: Infections of the oral cavity. In Waite D, editor: *Textbook of practical oral and maxillofacial surgery,* Philadelphia, 1987, Lea & Febiger; B from Flynn TR: The swollen face. *Emerg Med Clin North Am* 15:481-519, Aug 2000.)

clue for pterygomandibular space infection. On physical examination, with a good light and a tongue depressor, the clinician can see swelling and erythema of the anterior tonsillar pillar on the affected side and deviation of the uvula to the opposite side. On computed tomography examination, fluid collection may be detected between the medial pterygoid muscle and the mandible; the airway is often compressed and deviated by the swelling, as shown in Figure 16-20. Occasionally, this clinical picture is caused by needle tract infection from a mandibular block.

The superficial and deep temporal spaces rarely become infected and usually only in severe infections. When these spaces are involved, the swelling that occurs is evident in the temporal region, superior to the zygomatic arch and posterior to the lateral orbital rim. The tight attachment of the anterior layer of the deep cervical fascia to the zygomatic arch prevents swelling there, so that when either of the temporal spaces plus the submasseteric space are infected, an hourglass shape can be detected in the frontal view, as shown in Figures 16-7 and 16-18.

Deep Cervical Fascial Space Infections

Extension of odontogenic infections beyond the spaces described before is an uncommon occurrence. However, when it does happen, involvement of the deep cervical spaces may have serious life-threatening sequelae. Infection of the deep fascial spaces of the neck can compress, deviate, or completely obstruct the airway, invade vital structures such as the major vessels, and allow extension of the infection into the mediastinum and the vital structures it contains.

Infection extending posteriorly from the pterygomandibular, submandibular, or sublingual spaces first encounters the lateral pharyngeal space. This space extends from the base of the skull at the sphenoid bone to the hyoid bone inferiorly. The space is medial to the medial pterygoid muscle and lateral to the superior pharyngeal constrictor muscle (Fig. 16-21). The space is bounded anteriorly by the pterygomandibular raphe and extends posteromedially to the retropharyngeal space. The styloid process and associated muscles and fascia divide the lateral pharyngeal space into an anterior compartment, which contains primarily loose connective tissue, and a posterior compartment, which contains the carotid sheath and cranial nerves IX (glossopharyngeal), X (vagus), and XII (hypoglossal).

The clinical findings of lateral pharyngeal space infection include trismus as the result of inflammation of the medial pterygoid muscle; lateral swelling of the neck, especially between the angle of the mandible and the sternocleidomastoid muscle; and swelling of the lateral pharyngeal wall, toward the midline. Patients who have lateral pharyngeal space infections have difficulty swallowing and usually have a high temperature and become very sick. Figure 16-22 illustrates the clinical and computed tomography radiographic appearance of patients with lateral pharyngeal space infection.

Patients who have infection of the lateral pharyngeal space have several serious potential problems. When the lateral pharyngeal space is involved, the odontogenic infection is severe and may be progressing at a rapid rate. Another possible problem is the direct effect of the infection on the contents of the space, especially those of the posterior compartment. These problems include thrombosis of the internal jugular vein, erosion of the carotid artery or its branches, and interference with cranial nerves IX, X, and XII. A third serious complication arises if the infection progresses from the lateral pharyngeal space to the retropharyngeal space or beyond.

The retropharyngeal space lies behind the soft tissue of the posterior aspect of the pharynx. The retropharyngeal space is bounded anteriorly by the pharyngeal constrictor muscles and the retropharyngeal fascia and posteriorly by the alar fascia (see Fig. 16-21).

The retropharyngeal space begins at the base of the skull and ends inferiorly at a variable point between the sixth cervical (C6) and fourth thoracic (T4) vertebrae, where the alar fascia fuses anteriorly with the retropharyngeal fascia (Fig. 16-23). The retropharyngeal space contains only loose connective tissue and lymph nodes, so it provides little barrier

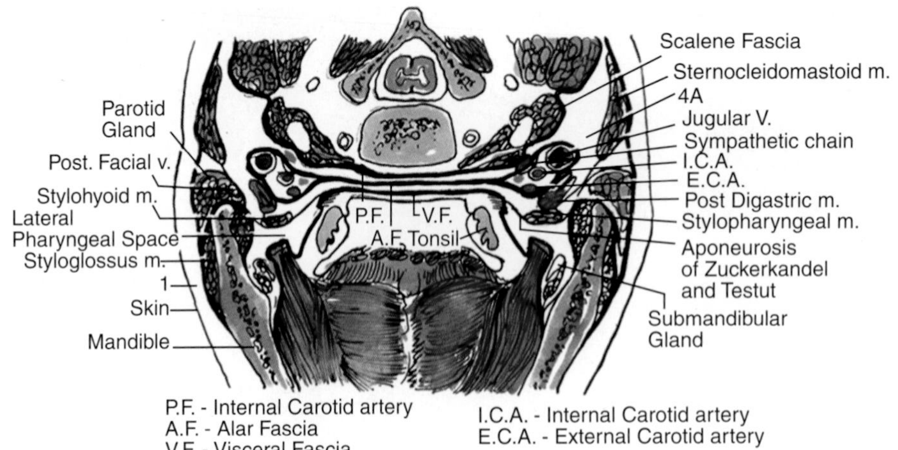

FIGURE 16-21 The lateral pharyngeal space is located between medial pterygoid muscle laterally and superior pharyngeal constrictor medially. The retropharyngeal and danger spaces lie between the pharyngeal constrictor muscles and the prevertebral fascia. The retropharyngeal space lies between the superior constrictor muscle and the alar fascia. The danger space lies between the alar layer and the prevertebral fascia.(From Flynn TR: Anatomy and surgery of deep fascial space infections. In Kelly JJ, editor: *Oral and maxillofacial surgery knowledge update 1994*, Rosemont, IL, 1994, American Association of Oral and Maxillofacial Surgeons.)

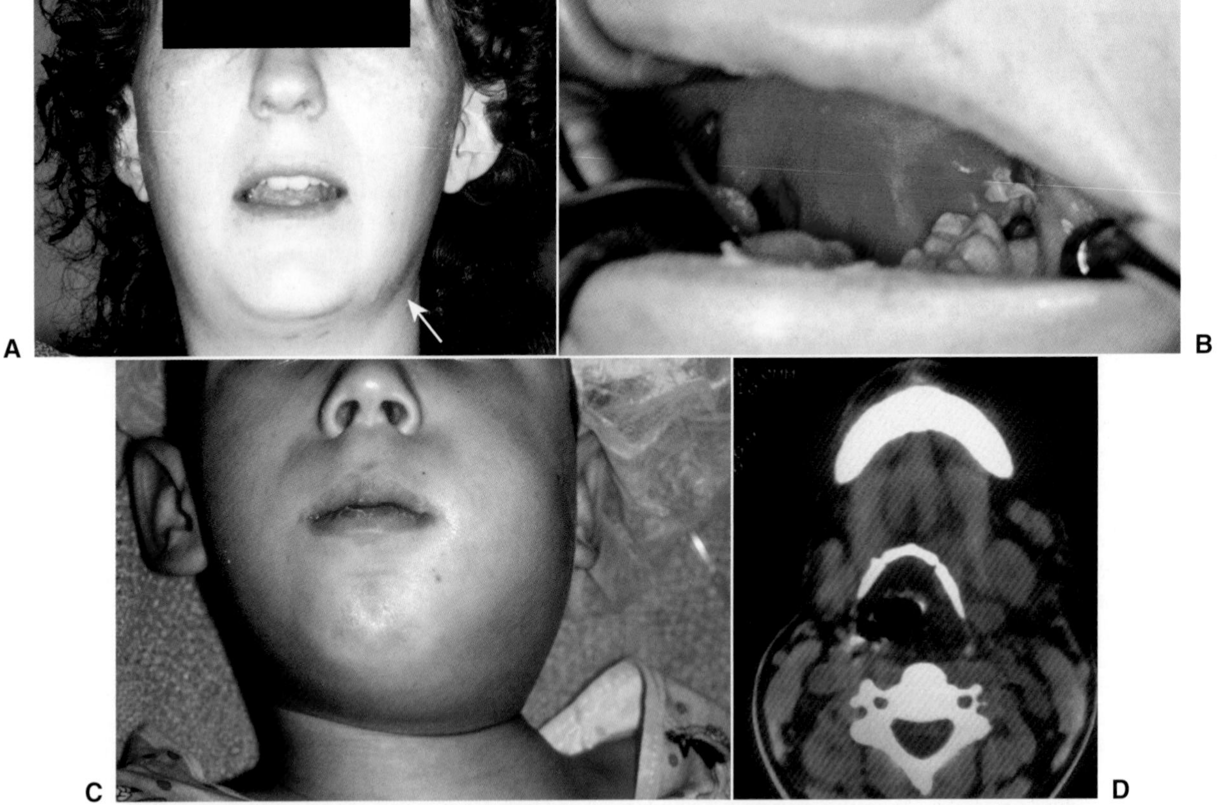

FIGURE 16-22 Lateral pharyngeal space abscess. **A**, Left lateral pharyngeal space abscess with extraoral swelling (*arrow*) and trismus. **B**, Intraoral view of the same patient, illustrating swelling of the anterior tonsillar pillar and blunting of the palatouvular fold. **C**, A boy with a left lateral pharyngeal space abscess who is deviating his head toward the right shoulder in order to place the upper airway over his deviated trachea. **D**, Computed tomography at the level of the hyoid bone, showing a lateral pharyngeal space infection that is deviating the airway to the opposite side. (From Flynn TR: Anatomy of oral and maxillofacial infections. In Topazian RG, Goldberg MH, Hupp JR, editors: *Oral and maxillofacial infections*, ed 4, Philadelphia, 2002, WB Saunders.)

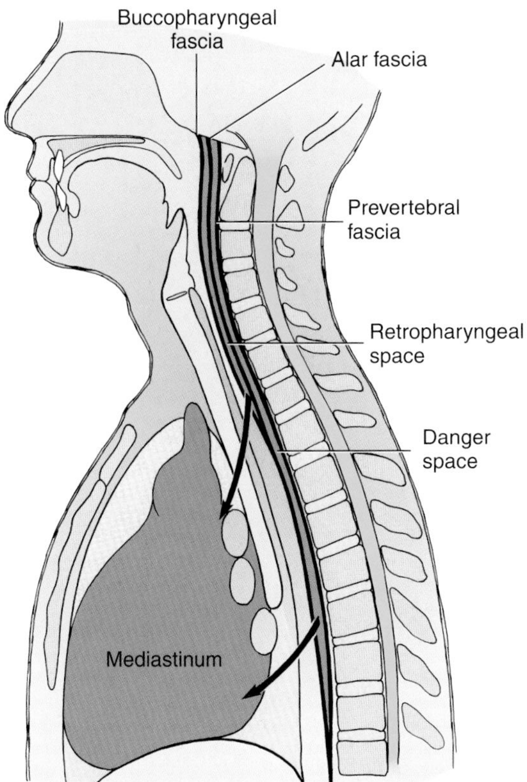

FIGURE 16-23 The retropharyngeal and the alar fascia fuse at a variable level between the C6 and T4 vertebrae, which forms a pouch at the inferior extent of the retropharyngeal space. If infection passes through the alar fascia to the danger space, the posterosuperior mediastinum will most likely soon become involved. The inferior boundary of the danger space is the diaphragm, which puts the entire mediastinum at risk.

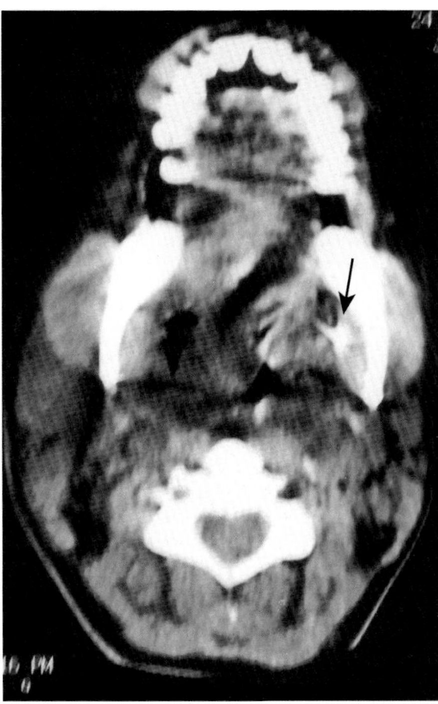

FIGURE 16-24 Postoperative computed tomography scan of a patient with a previously placed drain (*arrow*) in the left pterygomandibular space. The infection has now spread through the left lateral pharyngeal space and the retropharyngeal space to the right lateral pharyngeal space, thus encircling, compressing, and deviating the airway. (From Flynn TR: Surgical management of orofacial infections. *Atlas Oral Maxillofac Surg Clin North Am* 8:77-100, March 2000.)

to the spread of infection from one lateral pharyngeal space to the other to encircle the airway, as illustrated in Figure 16-24. Moreover, when the retropharyngeal space becomes involved, the major concern is that the infection can rupture the alar fascia posteriorly to enter the danger space (Fig. 16-25).

The danger space lies between the alar fascia anteriorly and the prevertebral fascia posteriorly. The danger space extends from the base of the skull to the diaphragm, and it is continuous with the posterior mediastinum (Fig. 16-23). The prevertebral space is rarely involved in odontogenic infections because the prevertebral fascia fuses with the periosteum of the vertebral bodies. Prevertebral space infections are usually caused by osteomyelitis of the vertebrae.

The mediastinum is the space between the lungs, and it contains the heart, the phrenic and vagus nerves, the trachea and the main stem bronchi, the esophagus, and the great vessels, including the aorta and the inferior and superior vena cava. A patient with mediastinitis can have an overwhelming infection that compresses the heart and lungs; interferes with the neurologic control of heart rate and respiration; ruptures into the lung, trachea, or esophagus; and even spreads into the abdominal cavity. The mortality of mediastinitis is high, even with modern methods of care, such as open thoracic surgical drainage and close follow-up with serial computed tomography scans.

Management of Fascial Space Infections

Management of infections, mild or severe, always has five general goals: (1) medical support of the patient, with special attention to protection of the airway and correcting host defense compromises where they exist; (2) surgical removal of the source of infection as early as possible; (3) surgical drainage of the infection, with proper placement of drains; (4) administration of correct antibiotics in appropriate doses; and (5) frequent reevaluation of the patient's progress toward resolution. Although the intensity of treatment is greater in complex odontogenic infections, the principles of surgical and medical management of fascial space infections are the same as those for less serious infections; these principles are described in detail in Chapter 15 and are summarized in Box 16-3. Conscientious application of these

BOX 16-3

Principles of Management of Odontogenic Infections

- Determine severity
- Evaluate host defenses
- Determine the setting of care
- Treat surgically
- Support medically
- Choose and prescribe appropriate antibiotic(s)
- Administer antibiotic appropriately
- Reevaluate frequently

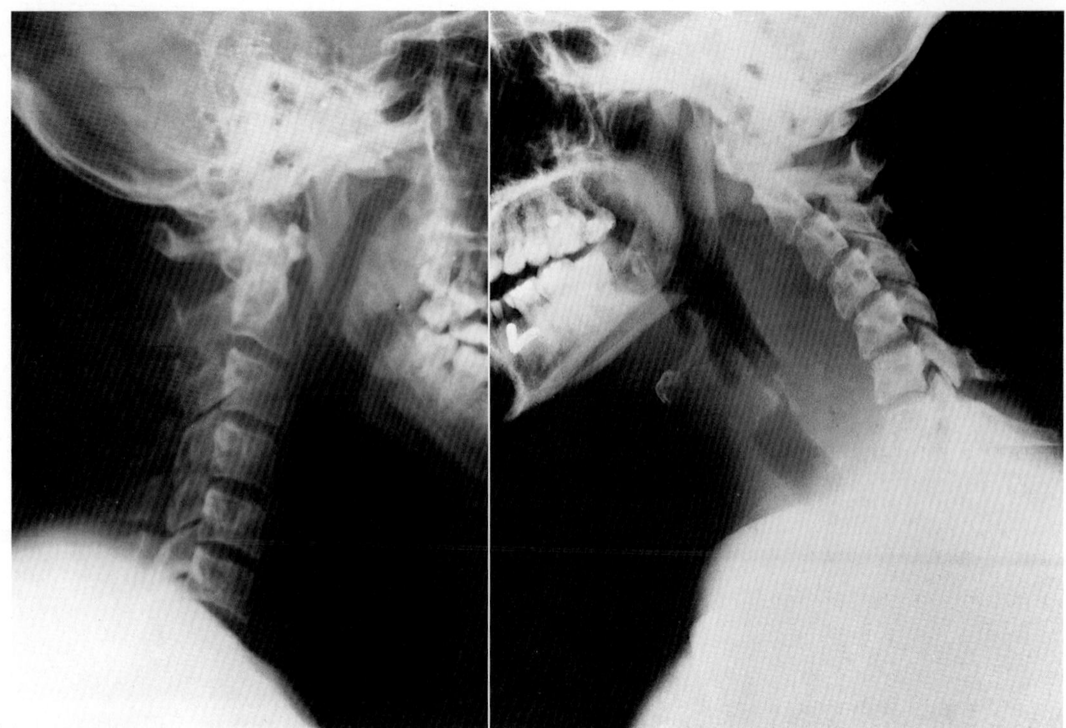

FIGURE 16-25 A, The normal retropharyngeal soft tissue shadow is narrow (6 mm or less) at C2 and 20 mm or less at C6 on plain x-ray films. B, When the retropharyngeal space is infected, the soft tissue becomes substantially thicker, and the width of the oropharyngeal air shadow decreases. (From Cummings CW, Fredrickson JM, Harker LA et al, editors: *Otolaryngology: head and neck surgery,* vol 3, St Louis, 1998, Mosby.)

principles cannot guarantee an ideal result in any given case, but it should ensure that the standard of care has been met.

The patient's airway must be continually monitored, and endotracheal intubation or tracheotomy should be performed if warranted. Airway security is the prime concern in the management of severe odontogenic infections. Medical management of the patient with a serious infection must include a thorough assessment and support of host defense mechanisms, including analgesics, fluid requirements, and nutrition. High-dose bactericidal antibiotics are usually necessary and are almost always administered intravenously.

Several large studies, performed as early as the 1950s, have shown that extraction of teeth in the presence of infection hastens the resolution of the infection and reduces the morbidity of the infection by measures such as decreased time out of work, shortened or avoided hospitalization, and reduced need for extraoral I&D. Occasionally, tooth extraction has been blamed for subsequent severe infections requiring hospitalization. In actuality, the infection that necessitated the tooth extraction had most likely become severe enough to warrant hospital care and more aggressive surgery.

Surgical management of fascial space infections almost always requires a generous incision and aggressive exploration of the involved fascial spaces with a hemostat. One or more drains are usually required to provide adequate drainage and decompression of the infected area. Because the I&D must be extensive, it is usually done in an operating room, with the patient under general anesthesia. The locations of various I&D sites are depicted in Figure 16-26. Ample clinical experience and experimental evidence indicate that, even if no abscess

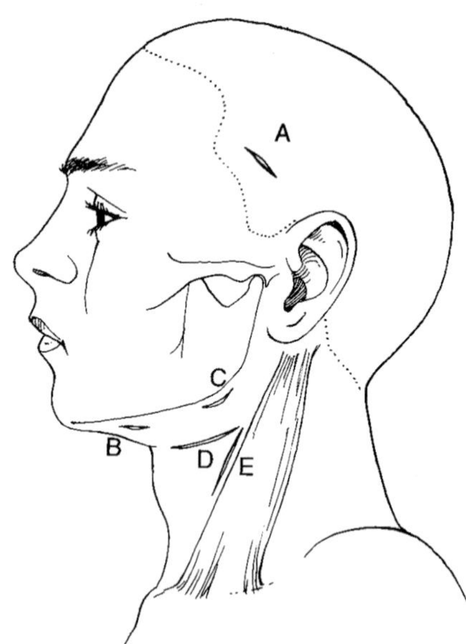

FIGURE 16-26 Placement of incisions for extraoral drainage of deep space infections. *A,* Superficial or deep temporal. *B,* Submental or submandibular. *C,* Submandibular, submasseteric, or submandibular. This incision may also be used with incision B for through-and-through drainage of the submental space or with incision A for through-and-through drainage of the temporal spaces. *D,* Lateral pharyngeal or the superior portion of the retropharyngeal space. *E,* Retropharyngeal space or carotid sheath. This incision may also be combined with incision D. (From Flynn TR: Surgical management of orofacial infections. *Atlas Oral Maxillofac Surg Clin North Am* 8:77-100, March 2000.)

formation can be detected by palpation, needle aspiration, radiographic examination, or open surgical drainage, an infection in the cellulitis stage will resolve more rapidly if incised and drained. The surgeon must not wait for unequivocal evidence of pus formation. In the preantibiotic era, surgical treatment was the only method of therapy for infections, and early and aggressive surgical therapy was frequently curative for these severe infections. One must remember that aggressive surgical exploration is still the primary method of therapy for serious odontogenic infections of the head and neck.

OSTEOMYELITIS

The term *osteomyelitis* literally means inflammation of the bone marrow. Clinically, osteomyelitis implies an infection of the bone. Osteomyelitis usually begins in the medullary cavity, involving the cancellous bone; then it extends and spreads to the cortical bone and eventually to the periosteum. Invasion of bacteria into the cancellous bone causes soft tissue inflammation and edema within the closed bony marrow spaces. As with the dental pulp, soft tissue edema that is enclosed by unyielding calcified tissue results in increased tissue hydrostatic pressure that rises above the blood pressure of the feeding arterial vessels. The resulting severe compromise of the blood supply then causes soft tissue necrosis. The failure of microcirculation in the cancellous bone is a critical factor in the establishment of osteomyelitis because the involved area becomes ischemic and the cellular component of the bone becomes necrotic. Bacteria can then proliferate because normal bloodborne defenses do not reach the tissue, and the osteomyelitis spreads until it is arrested by medical and surgical therapy.

Although the maxilla can also become involved in osteomyelitis, it does so rarely compared with the mandible. The primary reason for this is that the blood supply to the maxilla is much richer and is derived from several arteries, which form a complex network of feeder vessels. Because the mandible tends to draw its primary blood supply from the inferior alveolar artery and because the dense overlying cortical bone of the mandible limits penetration of periosteal blood vessels, the mandibular cancellous bone is more likely to become ischemic and therefore infected.

In spite of the many opportunities that bacteria have to enter into the cancellous bone via dental infections, osteomyelitis of the mandible rarely occurs if the host defenses are reasonably intact. The major predisposing factors for osteomyelitis of the jaws are preceding odontogenic infections and fractures of the mandible (Fig. 16-27). Even these two events rarely cause infections of the bone unless the host defenses are suppressed by problems such as diabetes, alcoholism, intravenous drug abuse, malnutrition, and myeloproliferative diseases, such as the leukemias, sickle cell disease, or chemotherapy-treated cancer.

Recent carefully performed investigations on the microbiology of osteomyelitis of the mandible have adequately demonstrated that the primary bacteria of concern are similar to those causing odontogenic infections, that is, streptococci, anaerobic cocci such as *Peptostreptococcus* spp., and anaerobic gram-negative rods such as those of the genera *Fusobacterium* and *Prevotella*. Traditional investigation of the microbiology of osteomyelitis of the jaws has used culture specimens from surface drainage of pus (contaminated with *Staphylococcus* organisms) and not anaerobic culture techniques (and thereby have not grown anaerobes). Thus, osteomyelitis of the mandible differs substantially from osteomyelitis of other bones in which staphylococci are the predominant bacteria.

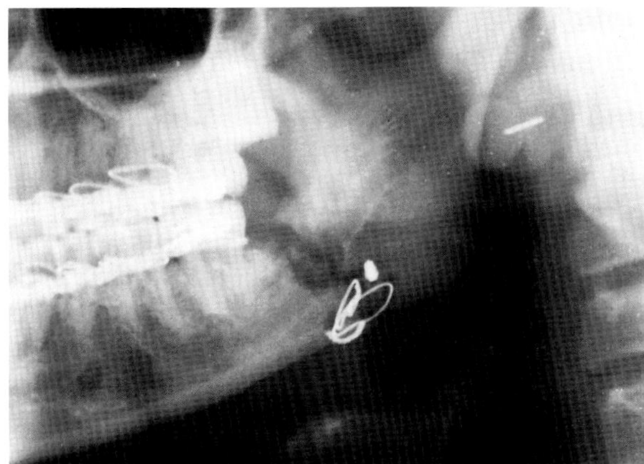

FIGURE 16-27 Osteomyelitis occurred in the area of a fracture of the mandible of a patient who was poorly nourished and abused ethanol. The sequestrum is surrounded by the radiolucency.

Acute suppurative osteomyelitis shows little or no radiographic change because at least 10 to 12 days are required for lost bone to be detectable radiographically. Chronic osteomyelitis usually demonstrates bony destruction in the area of infection. The appearance is one of increased radiolucency, which may be uniform in its pattern or patchy, with a moth-eaten appearance. Areas of radiopacity also may occur within the radiolucency. These radiopaque areas represent islands of bone that have not been resorbed and are known as *sequestra*. In long-standing chronic osteomyelitis, there may actually be an area of increased radiodensity surrounding the area of radiolucency called an involucrum. This is the result of a reaction in which bone production increases as a result of the inflammatory reaction.

Treatment of osteomyelitis is medical and surgical. Because patients with osteomyelitis may have depressed host defense mechanisms, the clinician must take these compromises into account during the treatment and seek medical consultation when necessary.

Acute osteomyelitis of the jaws is primarily managed by the administration of appropriate antibiotics. The precipitating event, condition, or both must also be carefully managed. If the event is a fracture of the mandible, careful attention must be given to its treatment. The antibiotics of choice include clindamycin, the penicillins, and the fluoroquinolones because of their effectiveness against the flora of odontogenic infections and their good to excellent bone penetration. If the patient has a serious acute osteomyelitis, hospitalization may be required for intravenous administration of antibiotics, which can then be followed by home intravenous therapy via a peripherally inserted central catheter or oral therapy, especially with the fluoroquinolones, which are very well absorbed orally. Surgical treatment of acute or chronic suppurative osteomyelitis consists primarily of removing obviously nonvital teeth in the area of the infection, any wires or bone plates that may have been used to stabilize a fracture in the area, or any obviously loose pieces of bone. Bone specimens are sent for aerobic and anaerobic culture and sensitivity testing and histopathologic examination. In addition, corticotomy (removal or perforation of the bony cortex) and excision of necrotic bone (until actively bleeding bone tissue is encountered) may be necessary. For acute osteomyelitis that results from jaw fracture, the surgeon must stabilize the mobile segments of the mandible, usually by open reduction and rigid internal fixation. Immobility of the fracture segments aids in the resolution of osteomyelitis.

Chronic osteomyelitis requires not only aggressive antibiotic therapy but also aggressive surgical therapy. Because of the severe compromise in the blood supply to the area of osteomyelitis, the patient is usually admitted to the hospital and given high-dose intravenous antibiotics to control the infection. The surgeon should obtain culture material at the time of surgery so that the selection of an antibiotic can be based on the specific microbiology of the infection.

Therapy for acute and chronic osteomyelitis, most authorities agree, should ensure that antibiotics are continued for a much longer time than is usual for odontogenic infections. For mild acute osteomyelitis that has responded well, antibiotics should be continued for at least 6 weeks after resolution of symptoms. For severe chronic osteomyelitis that has been difficult to control, antibiotic administration may continue for up to 6 months. This is especially true in actinomycotic osteomyelitis, which has a propensity to recur after long, symptom-free intervals.

Osteomyelitis of the mandible is a severe infection that may result in loss of a large portion of the mandible. Therefore a clinician who has the training and experience to handle the problem expeditiously should manage this infection. In addition, it is likely that medical consultation will be required to help correct any underlying compromise of host defenses.

ACTINOMYCOSIS

Actinomycosis is a relatively uncommon infection of the hard and soft tissues of the head and neck. Actinomycosis is usually caused by *Actinomyces israelii* but may also be caused by *A. naeslundii* or *A. viscosus*. *Actinomyces* is an endogenous bacterium of the oral cavity that was once thought to be an anaerobic fungus. However, it has now been clearly established that the actinomycetes are anaerobic bacteria.

Actinomycosis is a relatively uncommon disease because the bacteria have a low degree of virulence. For the infection to become established, the bacteria must be inoculated into an area of injury or locally increased susceptibility, such as areas of recent tooth extraction, severely carious teeth, bone fracture, or minor oral trauma. The infection is primarily one of soft tissue and progresses by direct extension into adjacent tissues and bone.

Unlike other infections, actinomycosis does not follow usual anatomic planes but rather burrows through them and becomes a lobular "pseudotumor." If the infection erodes through a cutaneous surface, which is common with orofacial actinomycosis, multiple sinus tracts typically develop. Once drainage is established, the patient has minimal pain, although the sinus tracts continue to drain spontaneously until the infection is brought under control (Fig. 16-28).

A definitive diagnosis depends on laboratory identification. *Actinomyces* is an anaerobic bacterium and therefore must be incubated in an anaerobic environment, usually on brain-heart agar or blood agar, for 4 to 6 days. In up to 50% of all actinomycotic infections, the organism is not grown. However, the clinical presentation of the patient with actinomycosis is characteristic. The diagnosis is often made on histopathologic examination of a pus specimen because of the presence of typical colonies of actinomyces that look like sulfur granules within the exudate. The patient has an atypical infection of the jaws that responds well to antibiotic therapy initially; however, after the antibiotic is stopped, the infection often recurs. The patient with this disease has frequently had multiple episodes of recurrent infection in the same area.

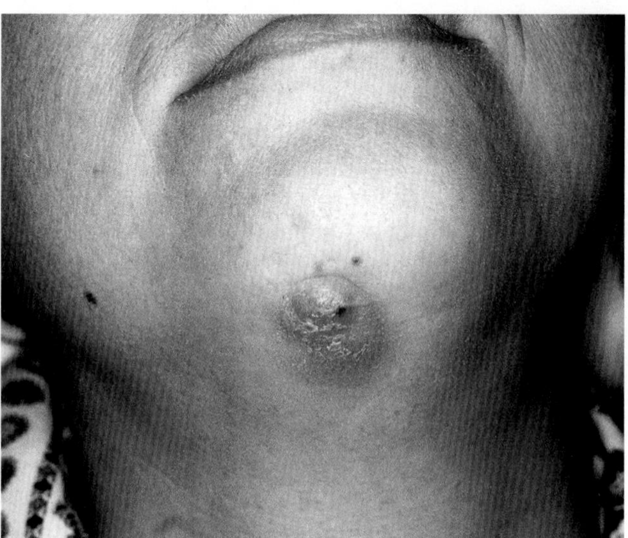

FIGURE 16-28 This actinomycosis had multiple recurrences. The patient experienced a small amount of swelling with multiple small sinus tracts.

Therapy of actinomycosis includes surgical I&D and excision of all sinus tracts. This portion of the treatment is important to ensure that adequate amounts of antibiotic are actually delivered to the infected area.

The antibiotic of choice for actinomycosis in the non-allergic patient is one of the intravenous penicillins initially, followed by long-term oral therapy. The reason for the prolonged administration of the antibiotic is to prevent the recurrence of the infection.

The alternative antibiotics include doxycycline or clindamycin. An advantage of doxycycline is that it can be administered orally once per day for long-term therapy.

In summary, actinomycosis is an indolent infection that tends to erode through tissues rather than to follow the typical fascial planes and spaces. Actinomycosis is difficult to eradicate using short-term antibiotic regimens. Therefore, I&D of any accumulation of pus and excision of chronic sinus tracts and necrotic bone and foreign bodies must be accomplished. Finally, high-dose antibiotic administration is recommended for initial control of the infection, with long-term antibiotic therapy to prevent recurrence of actinomycosis.

CANDIDIASIS

The organism *Candida albicans* is a naturally occurring yeast in the oral cavity. *Candida* rarely causes disease unless the patient's health becomes compromised. The two most common causes of compromise are administration of antibiotics, especially penicillin, for prolonged periods and immune system compromise, such as acquired immunodeficiency syndrome (AIDS) or chemotherapy for leukemias and other forms of cancer. In these situations, *Candida* organisms overgrow in the oral cavity

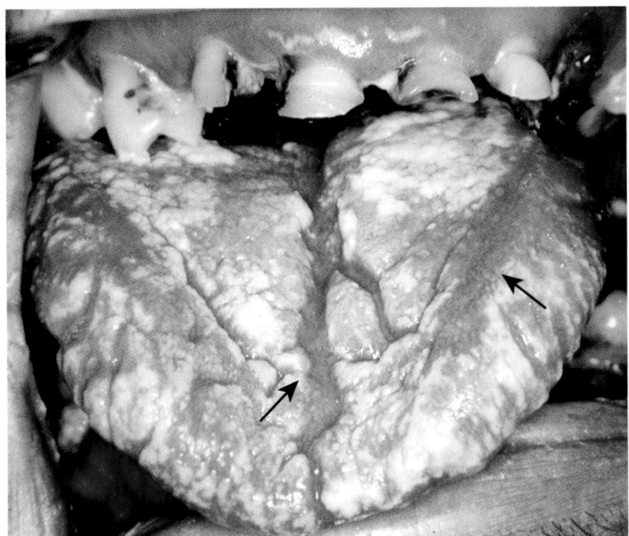

FIGURE 16-29 Candidiasis of the tongue. The white patches are the pseudomembranous type, and the eroded, glossy areas (*arrows*) are the erythematous type. (From Flynn TR, Piecuch JF, Topazian RG: Orofacial infections. In McMillan JA, DeAngelis CD, Feigin RD, Warshaw JB, editors: *Oski's pediatrics: principles and practice,* ed 4, Philadelphia, 2006, Lippincott Williams & Wilkins.)

and cause a superficial infection. Three forms of oral candidiasis have been described: pseudomembranous, which usually appears intraorally as distinct white patches that can be easily rubbed off with gauze to expose an underlying red, raw surface; erythematous, which appears simply as a raw surface, or as loss of the filiform papillae of the tongue; and angular cheilitis, which appears as white or ulcerated patches in the corners of the mouth. The pseudomembranous and erythematous types are visible in Figure 16-29. *Candida* spp. can be diagnosed by culture and by their typical appearance on Gram stain.

Angular cheilitis can be caused by *Candida* organisms. Most patients who have this problem are edentulous and have decreased vertical dimension between the upper and lower jaws, resulting in chronic wetness at the corner of the mouth and subsequent yeast growth.

Topical antifungal agents can usually deliver effective therapy for oral candidiasis. The two most commonly used drugs for this purpose are nystatin and clotrimazole. Both drugs are prepared as lozenges and are delivered by sucking on the lozenge until it is totally dissolved. Nystatin is preferred for initial therapy because of low toxicity and cost.

Clotrimazole, a newer antifungal, has a very low risk of toxicity and better taste but higher cost. The usual course of either preparation is one lozenge allowed to dissolve in the mouth 4 or 5 times per day for 2 weeks. Patients usually experience rapid resolution of the signs and symptoms of candidiasis but must be informed that there will be a recurrence of the infection unless they continue the therapy for the entire 14 days. If the patient has a denture, it should also be treated to eliminate yeast because it can serve as a reservoir of yeast organisms. Treatment of the denture involves removal of a thin layer of acrylic from the internal surface of the denture and antiseptic soaks overnight for the entire time of active treatment and periodically thereafter.

Systemically administered new antifungals, such as fluconazole, ketoconazole, and itraconazole, are used to treat oropharyngeal candidiasis in immunocompromised individuals, such as in AIDS. These antifungal drugs are effective, especially against some of the highly resistant strains of *Candida albicans* and other species such as *C. glabrata* that are seen more frequently in immunocompromised individuals. Because of their expense and occasionally life-threatening drug interactions, these newer, highly potent antifungals are generally reserved for immunocompromised individuals and use by specialists.

One must remember that candidiasis occurs most commonly in medically compromised patients. Patients without histories of recent antibiotic therapy, poorly controlled diabetes, AIDS, cancer chemotherapy, or other types of immunocompromise should be suspected of having an underlying systemic immunocompromising disease. Therefore, referral for evaluation and control of underlying medical conditions is important in the management of a patient with oral candidiasis that cannot be controlled by local means.

REFERENCES

1. Grodinsky M: Retropharyngeal and lateral pharyngeal abscesses, *Ann Surg* 110:177, 1939.
2. Grodinsky M: Ludwig's angina: an anatomical and clinical study with review of the literature, *Surgery* 5:678, 1939.
3. Grodinsky M, Holyoke EA: The fasciae and fascial spaces of the head, neck, and adjacent regions, *Am J Anat* 63:367, 1938.
4. Williams AC: Ludwig's angina, *Surg Gynecol Obstet* 70:140, 1940.
5. Williams AC, Guralnick WC: The diagnosis and treatment of Ludwig's angina: a report of twenty cases, *N Engl J Med* 1943;228:443.
6. Flynn TR, Shanti RM, Hayes C: Severe odontogenic infections, part two: prospective outcomes study, *J Oral Maxillofac Surg* 64:1104-1113, 2006.
7. Flynn TR, Shanti RM, Levy M et al: Severe odontogenic infections, part one: prospective report, *J Oral Maxillofac Surg* 64:1093-1103, 2006.

Bibliography

Balcerak RJ, Sisto JM, Bosack RC: Cervicofacial necrotizing fasciitis: report of three cases and literature review, *J Oral Maxillofac Surg* 46:450, 1988.

Bennett JD, Flynn TR: Anesthetic considerations in orofacial infections. In Topazian RG, Goldberg MH, Hupp JR, editors: *Oral and maxillofacial infections,* ed 4, Philadelphia, 2002, WB Saunders.

Carey JW, Dodson TB: Hospital course of HIV-positive patients with odontogenic infections, *Oral Surg Oral Med Oral Pathol Oral Radiol Endod* 91(1):23-27, 2001.

Flynn TR: Anatomy of oral and maxillofacial infections. In Topazian RG, Goldberg MH, Hupp JR, editors: *Oral and maxillofacial infections,* ed 4, Philadelphia, 2002, WB Saunders.

Flynn TR: Deep fascial space infections. In Laskin DM, Abubakar AO, editors: *Decision making in oral and maxillofacial surgery,* Chicago, 2007, Quintessence.

Flynn TR: Odontogenic infections, *Oral Maxillofac Surg Clin North Am* 3:311-329, 1991.

Flynn TR: Principles of management of odontogenic infections. In Miloro M, editor: *Peterson's principles of oral and maxillofacial surgery,* ed 2, Hamilton, Ontario, 2005, BC Decker.

Flynn TR: Surgical management of orofacial infections: *Atlas Oral Maxillofac Surg Clin North Am* 8:77-100, March 2000.

Flynn TR: The swollen face, *Emerg Med Clin North Am* 15:481-519, Aug 2000.

Flynn TR: The timing of incision and drainage. In Piecuch JF, editor: *Oral and maxillofacial surgery knowledge update 2002,* Rosemont, Ill, 2002, American Association of Oral and Maxillofacial Surgeons.

Flynn TR: Use of antibiotics. In Laskin DM, Abubaker AO, editors: *Decision making in oral and maxillofacial surgery,* Chicago, 2007, Quintessence.

Flynn TR, Halpern LR: Antibiotic selection in head and neck infections, *Oral and Maxillofacial Surgery Clinics of North America,* 15:17-38, Feb 2003.

Freeman RK, Vallieres E, Verrier ED et al: Descending necrotizing mediastinitis: an analysis of the effects of serial surgical debridement on patient mortality, *J Thorac Cardiovasc Surg* 119(2):260-267, 2000.

Gidley PW, Ghorayeb BY, Stiernberg CM: Contemporary management of deep neck space infections, *Otolaryngol Head Neck Surg* 116:16-22, 1997.

Hall HD, Gunter JW, Jamison HC et al: Effect of time of extraction on resolution of odontogenic cellulitis, *J Am Dent Assoc* 77:626, 1968.

Haug RH, Picard U, Indresano AT: Diagnosis and treatment of the retropharyngeal abscess in adults, *Br J Oral Maxillofac Surg* 28:34-38, 1990.

Heimdahl A, VonKonow L, Satoh T et al: Clinical appearance of orofacial infections of odontogenic origin in relation to microbiological findings, *J Clin Microbiol* 22:299, 1985.

Hought RT, Fitzgerald BE, Latta JE et al: Ludwig's angina: report of two cases and review of the literature from 1945 to January 1979, *J Oral Surg* 38:849, 1980.

Kim Y, Flynn TR, Donoff RB et al: The gene: the polymerase chain reaction and its clinical application, *J Oral Maxillofac Surg* 60:808-815, 2002.

Krogh HW: Extraction of teeth in the presence of acute infections, *J Oral Surg* 9:136, 1951.

Langford FPJ, Moon RE, Stolp BW et al: Treatment of cervical necrotizing fasciitis with hyperbaric oxygen therapy, *Otolaryngol Head Neck Surg* 112:274-278, 1995.

LeBlanc DJ, Flynn TR, Simos C et al: Antibiotics and the treatment of infectious diseases. In Lamont RJ, Burne RA, Lantz MS et al: editors: *Oral microbiology and immunology,* Washington, DC, 2006, ASM Press.

Marra S, Hotaling AJ: Deep neck infections, *Am J Otol* 17:287-298, 1996.

Martis CS, Karakasis DT: Extractions in the presence of acute infections, *J Dent Res* 54:59, 1975.

Marx RE: Chronic osteomyelitis of the jaws, *Oral and Maxillofacial Surgery Clinics of North America,* 3:367, 1991.

Miller EJ Jr, Dodson TB: The risk of serious odontogenic infections in HIV-positive patients: a pilot study, *Oral Surg Oral Med Oral Pathol Oral Radiol Endod* 86:406-409, 1998.

Miller WD, Furst IM, Sandor GKB et al: A prospective blinded comparison of clinical examination and computed tomography in deep neck infections, *Laryngoscope* 109:1873-1879, 1999.

O'Ryan F, Diloreto D, Barber HD et al: Orbital infections: clinical and radiographic diagnosis and surgical treatment, *J Oral Maxillofac Surg* 46:991, 1988.

Peterson LJ: Principles of surgical and antimicrobial infection management. In Topazian RG, Goldberg MH, Hupp JR, editors: *Oral and maxillofacial infections,* ed 4, Philadelphia, 2002, WB Saunders.

Scully C, McCarthy G: Management of oral health in persons with HIV infection, *Oral Surg Oral Med Oral Pathol Oral Radiol Endod* 73:215, 1992.

Telford G: Postoperative fever. In Condon RE, Nyhus LM, editors: *Manual of surgical therapeutics,* ed 6, Boston, 1985, Little, Brown.

Umeda M, Minamikawa T, Komatsubara H et al: Necrotizing fasciitis caused by dental infection: a retrospective analysis of 9 cases and a review of the literature, *Oral Surg Oral Med Oral Pathol Oral Radiol Endod* 95:283-290, 2003.

CHAPTER 17

Principles of Endodontic Surgery

STUART E. LIEBLICH

CHAPTER OUTLINE

Endodontic surgery is the management or prevention of periradicular pathosis by a surgical approach. In general, this includes abscess drainage, periapical surgery, corrective surgery, intentional replantation, and root removal (Box 17-1).

Conventional endodontic treatment is generally a successful procedure; however, in 10% to 15% of cases the symptoms can persist or spontaneously recur. Findings such as a draining fistula, pain on mastication, or the incidental noting of a radiolucency increasing in size indicate problems with the initial endodontic procedure. Many endodontic failures occur a year or more following the initial root canal treatment, often complicating a situation because a definitive restoration may have already been placed. This creates a higher "value" for the tooth because it now may be supporting a fixed partial denture.

Surgery has traditionally been an important part of endodontic treatment. However, until recently there was little research on indications and contraindications, techniques, success and failure (i.e., long-term prognosis), wound healing, and materials and devices to augment procedures. Because of this lack of information, referral for surgery—such as the routine correcting of failed endodontic treatment, removing of large lesions believed to be cysts, or performing of single-visit root canal treatment—may have been inappropriate. A decision on whether to approach the case surgically or to consider orthograde (through the coronal portion of the tooth) endodontic retreatment is dictated by various clinical and anatomic situations. Other treatment options, such as extraction of the tooth with placement of an implant, may be preferred and actually may be associated with a higher long-term success

BOX 17-1

Factors Associated with Success and Failures in Periapical Surgery

SUCCESS

Preoperative Factors

Dense orthograde fill

Healthy periodontal status
- No dehiscence
- Adequate crown/root ratio

Radiolucent defect isolated to apical one third of the tooth

Tooth treated
- Maxillary incisor
- Mesiobuccal root of maxillary molars

Postoperative Factors

Radiographic evidence of bone fill following surgery

Resolution of pain and symptoms

Absence of sinus tract

Decrease in tooth mobility

FAILURE

Preoperative Factors

Clinical or radiographic evidence of fracture

Poor or lack of orthograde filling

Marginal leakage of crown or post

Poor preoperative periodontal condition

Radiographic evidence of post perforation

Tooth treated
- Mandibular incisor

Postoperative Factors

Lack of bone repair following surgery

Lack of resolution of pain

Fistula does not resolve or returns

From Thomas P, Lieblich SE: Office-based surgery. In Ward-Booth P, Schendel S, Hausamen J-E, editors: *Maxillofacial surgery,* ed 2, London, 2007, Churchill Livingston.

rate. A recent consensus conference, however, concluded that endodontic therapy and implant procedures are considered to be equally successful. Additional procedures on the tooth, whether orthograde retreatment or periapical surgery, may reduce the long-term success rate of the tooth because each treatment is associated with additional tooth structure removal. When surgery is indicated, under the correct clinical situations it can maintain the tooth and its overlying restoration. Figure 17-1 is an algorithm to help guide the clinical decision as to whether endodontic surgery is indicated.

The purpose of this chapter is to present the indications and contraindications for endodontic surgery, the diagnosis and treatment planning, and the basics of endodontic surgical techniques. Most of the procedures presented should be performed by specialists, or on occasion, by specially trained experienced generalists. Surgical approaches are often in proximity to anatomic structures such as the maxillary sinus (Box 17-2) and inferior alveolar nerve, and expertise in working around these structures is mandatory. Nonetheless, the general dentist must be skilled in diagnosis and treatment planning and must be able to recognize which procedures are indicated in particular situations. When a patient is to be referred to a specialist for treatment, the general dentist must have knowledge sufficient to describe the surgical procedure to the patient. In addition, the generalist should assist in the follow-up care and long-term assessment of treatment outcomes. The final determination of success, such as when a definitive final restoration should be placed, is often the responsibility of the referring dentist.

BOX 17-2

Categories of Endodontic Surgery

- Abscess drainage
- Periapical surgery
- Hemisection/root amputation
- Intentional replantation
- Corrective surgery

The procedures discussed in this chapter are drainage of an abscess, apical (i.e., periradicular) surgery, and corrective surgery.

DRAINAGE OF AN ABSCESS

Drainage releases purulent or hemorrhagic transudates and exudates from a focus of liquefaction necrosis (i.e., abscess). Draining the abscess relieves pain, increases circulation, and removes a potent irritant. The abscess may be confined to bone or may have eroded through bone and periosteum to invade soft tissue. Managing these intraoral or extraoral swellings by incision for drainage is reviewed in Chapters 15 and 16. Draining the infection does not eliminate the cause of the infection, and definitive treatment of the tooth is still needed.

An abscess in bone resulting from an infected tooth may be drained by two methods: One method is by opening into the offending tooth coronally to obtain drainage through the pulp chamber and canal. The other approach to manage an abscess in bone is a formal incision and drainage with or without the placement of a drain. An incision and drainage is indicated if the spread of the infection is rapid, there is evidence of space involvement, or if opening the tooth coronally does not yield obvious purulence. An incision and drainage permits the dentist to obtain the pus for culture and sensitivity testing when indicated. Most community-acquired endodontic infections do not require culture and sensitivity testing unless the patient is medically compromised, has failed to respond to an empirical course of antibiotics, or the infection was acquired in a hospital setting, predisposing to resistant forms of bacteria.

PERIAPICAL SURGERY

Periapical (i.e., periradicular) surgery includes a series of procedures performed to eliminate the symptoms. Periapical surgery includes the following:

1. Appropriate exposure of the root and apical region
2. Exploration of the root surface for fractures or other pathologic conditions
3. Curettage of the apical tissues
4. Resection of the root apex
5. Retrograde preparation with the ultrasonic tips
6. Placement of the retrograde filling material
7. Appropriate flap closure to permit healing and minimize gingival recession

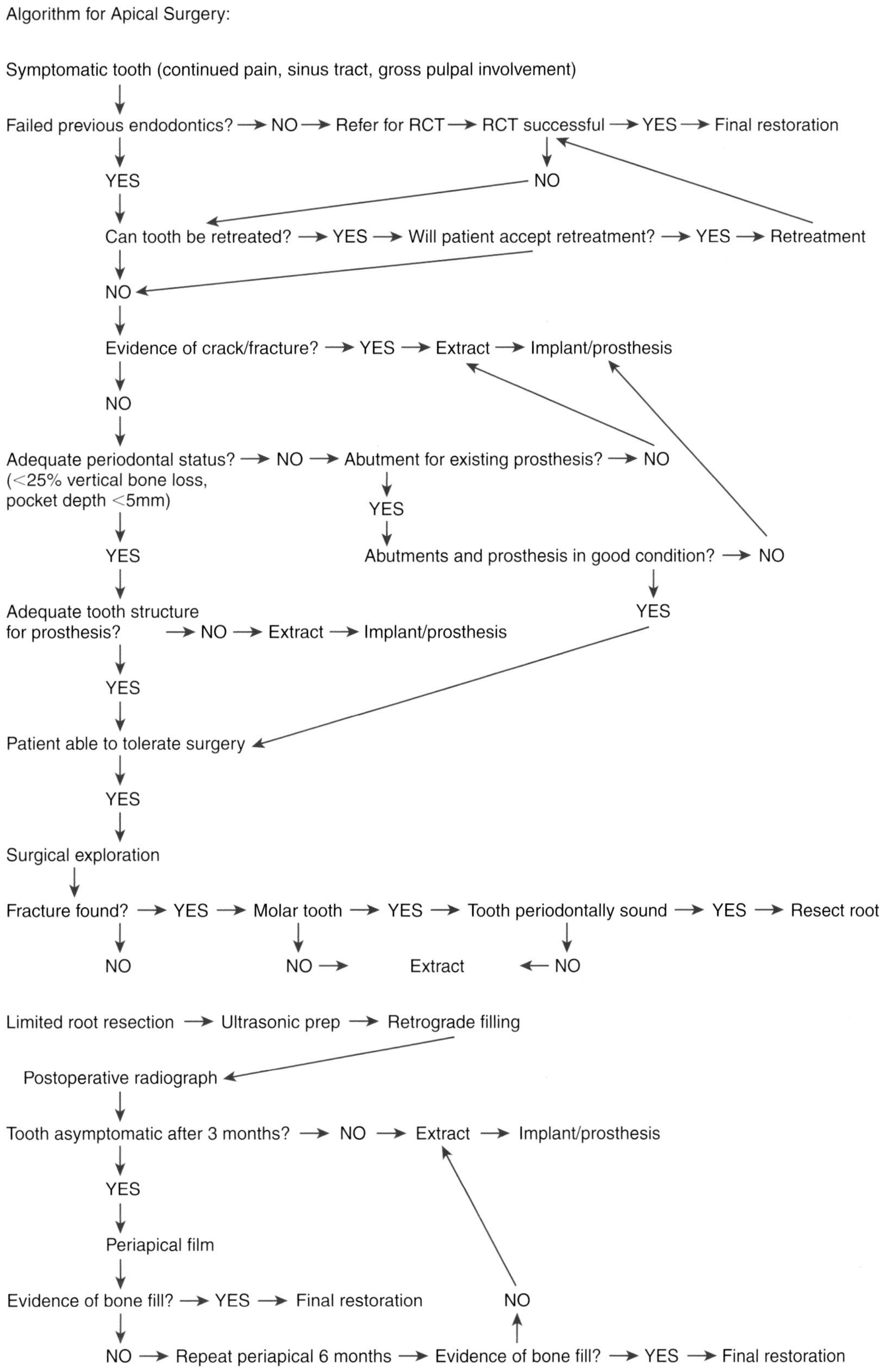

Algorithm for Apical Surgery:

Symptomatic tooth (continued pain, sinus tract, gross pulpal involvement)
↓
Failed previous endodontics? → NO → Refer for RCT → RCT successful → YES → Final restoration
↓ (RCT successful) ↓ NO → Can tooth be retreated?
YES
↓
Can tooth be retreated? → YES → Will patient accept retreatment? → YES → Retreatment → RCT successful
↓ (Will patient accept retreatment? NO → NO)
NO
↓
Evidence of crack/fracture? → YES → Extract → Implant/prosthesis
↓
NO
↓
Adequate periodontal status? → NO → Abutment for existing prosthesis? → NO → Extract
(<25% vertical bone loss,
pocket depth <5mm)
↓ (Abutment for existing prosthesis?) ↓ YES → Abutments and prosthesis in good condition? → NO → Implant/prosthesis
YES
↓ (Abutments and prosthesis in good condition?) ↓ YES → Patient able to tolerate surgery
Adequate tooth structure
for prosthesis? → NO → Extract → Implant/prosthesis
↓
YES
↓
Patient able to tolerate surgery
↓
YES
↓
Surgical exploration
↓
Fracture found? → YES → Molar tooth → YES → Tooth periodontally sound → YES → Resect root
↓ NO
Molar tooth ↓ NO → Extract
Tooth periodontally sound ↓ NO → Extract

Limited root resection → Ultrasonic prep → Retrograde filling
↓
Postoperative radiograph
↓
Tooth asymptomatic after 3 months? → NO → Extract → Implant/prosthesis
↓
YES
↓
Periapical film
↓
Evidence of bone fill? → YES → Final restoration
↓
NO → Repeat periapical 6 months → Evidence of bone fill? → YES → Final restoration
(Evidence of bone fill?) ↑ NO → Extract

FIGURE 17-1 Algorithm for apical surgery.

Indications

Following the completion of endodontics, symptoms associated with the tooth may lead to the recommendation for periapical surgery. Most commonly, patients have a chronic fistula and drainage. Other signs can include pain and the sudden onset of a vestibular space infection. Incidental findings of an increasing size of a radiolucent area found on routine radiographs may also lead to the decision to treat the periapical region surgically.

The success of apical surgery varies considerably, depending on the reason for and nature of the procedure. With failed root canal treatment, often retreatment is not possible or a better result cannot be achieved by a coronal approach. If the cause of the failure cannot be identified, surgical exploration may be necessary (Fig. 17-2). On occasion, an unusual entity in the periapical region requires surgical removal and biopsy for identification (Fig. 17-3). Those indications for periapical surgery are discussed in the following sections (Box 17-3).

It is important to tell the patient preoperatively that endodontic surgery is exploratory. The precise surgical procedure is dictated by the clinical findings once the site is exposed and explored. For example, a fracture of a root may be noted, and the decision whether to resect the root or extract the tooth will need to be made intraoperatively. If the tooth is to be extracted, provisions for temporization must be made in advance if removal is an esthetic issue, or a decision must be made to close the flap and schedule the extraction in the future.

BOX 17-3

Indications for Periapical Surgery

- Anatomic problems preventing complete débridement/obturation
- Restorative considerations that compromise treatment
- Horizontal root fracture with apical necrosis
- Irretrievable material preventing canal treatment or retreatment
- Procedural errors during treatment
- Large periapical lesions that do not resolve with root canal treatment

Anatomic Problems

Calcifications or other blockages, severe root curvatures, or constricted canals (i.e., calcific metamorphosis) may compromise root canal treatment, that is, prevent instrumentation, obturation, or both (Fig. 17-4). A nonobturated and cleaned canal may lead to failure because of continued apical leakage.

Although the outcome may be questionable, it is preferable to attempt conventional root canal treatment or retreatment before apical surgery. If this is not possible, removing or resecting the uninstrumented and unfilled portion of the root and placing a root end filling may be necessary.

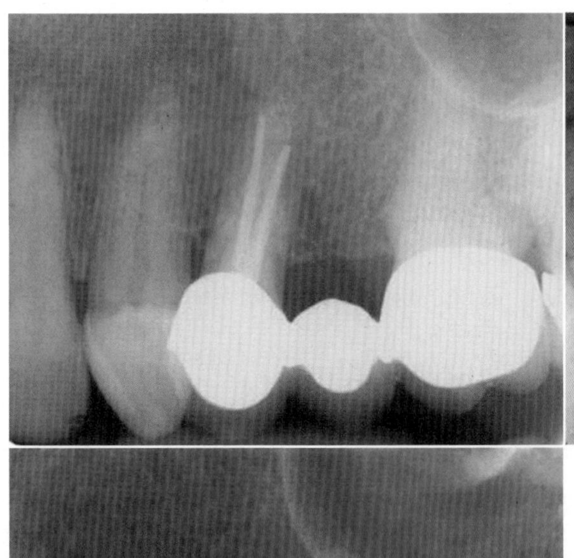

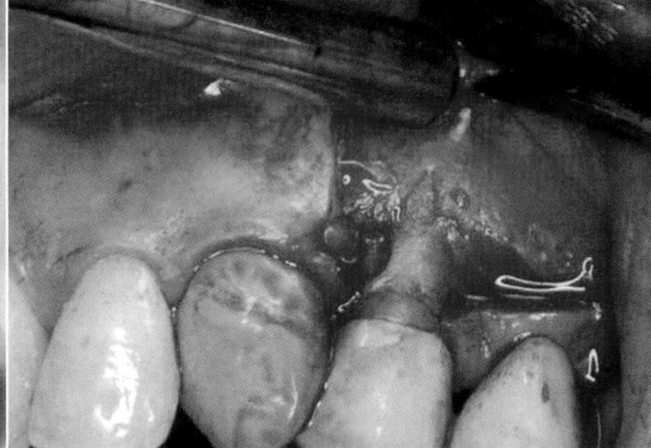

FIGURE 17-2 Surgical exploration. A, Patient had persistent pain over the midroot region following what appears to be successful endodontic treatment. B, Surgical exploration reveals perforation of the buccal root during the endodontic treatment with displaced gutta-percha. C, Postoperative periapical film of surgical removal of the extruded gutta-percha and mineral trioxide aggregate seal.

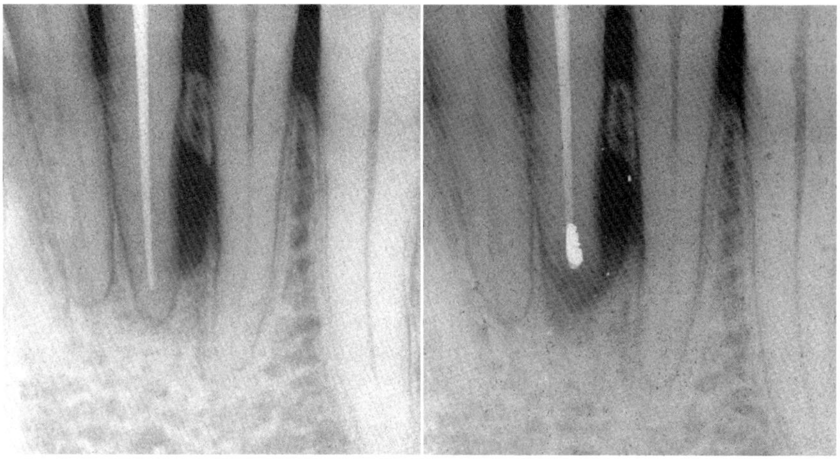

FIGURE 17-3 Surgical removal of pathosis. A, Patient was referred for surgery because of an increasing size of the radiolucent area following conventional endodontic treatment. Note the atypical nature of the radiolucent lesion, which would indicate tissue submission should be done in conjunction with the apical surgery. B, Treatment by apical surgery with amalgam retrograde seal, along with a biopsy of the associated tissue. Final diagnosis was cystic ameloblastoma.

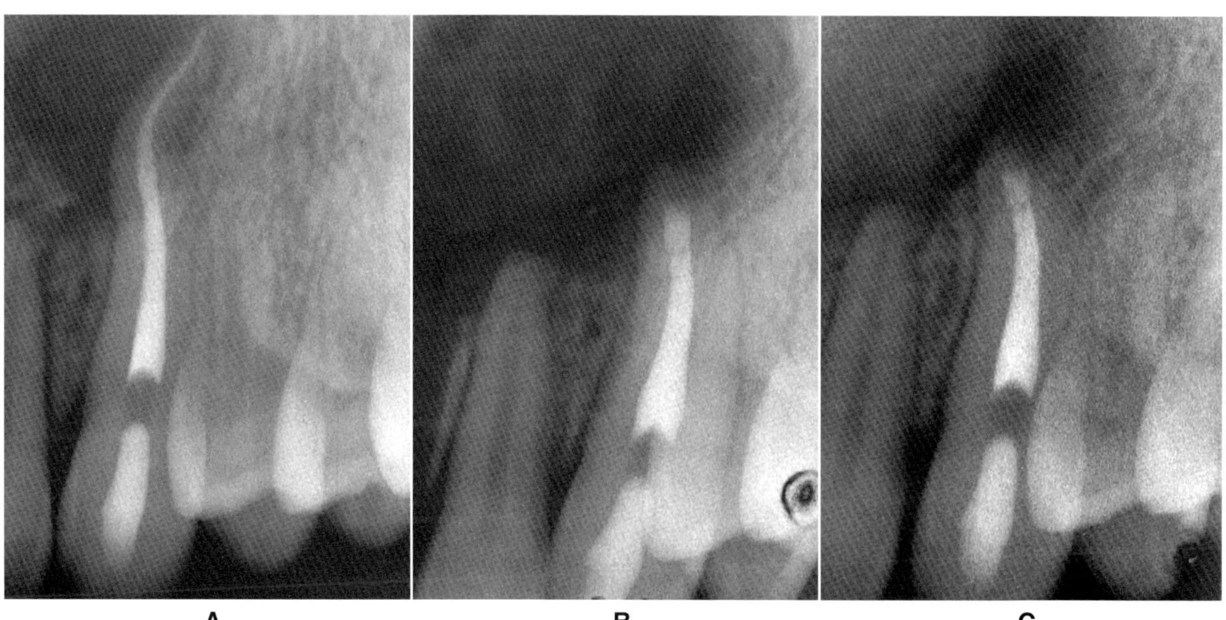

FIGURE 17-4 A, Anatomic problem of a severe root curvature for which surgery is indicated. B, Apical resection and root end retrograde mineral trioxide aggregate seal. C, Four months postoperatively shows regeneration of bone.

Restorative Considerations

Root canal retreatment may be risky because of problems that may occur from attempting access through a restoration, such as through a crown on a mandibular incisor. An opening could compromise retention of the restoration or perforate the root. Rather than attempt the root canal retreatment, root resection and root end filling may successfully eliminate the symptoms associated with the tooth.

A common requirement for surgery is failed treatment on a tooth that has been restored with a post and core (Fig. 17-5). Many posts are difficult to remove or may cause root fracture if an attempt at removal is made to re-treat the tooth.

Horizontal Root Fracture

Occasionally, after a traumatic root fracture, the apical segment undergoes pulpal necrosis. Because pulpal necrosis cannot be predictably treated from a coronal approach, the apical segment is removed surgically after root canal treatment of the coronal portion (Fig. 17-6).

Irretrievable Material in Canal

Canals are occasionally blocked by objects such as broken instruments (Fig. 17-7), restorative materials, segments of posts, or other foreign objects. If evidence of apical pathosis is found, those materials can be removed surgically, usually with a por-

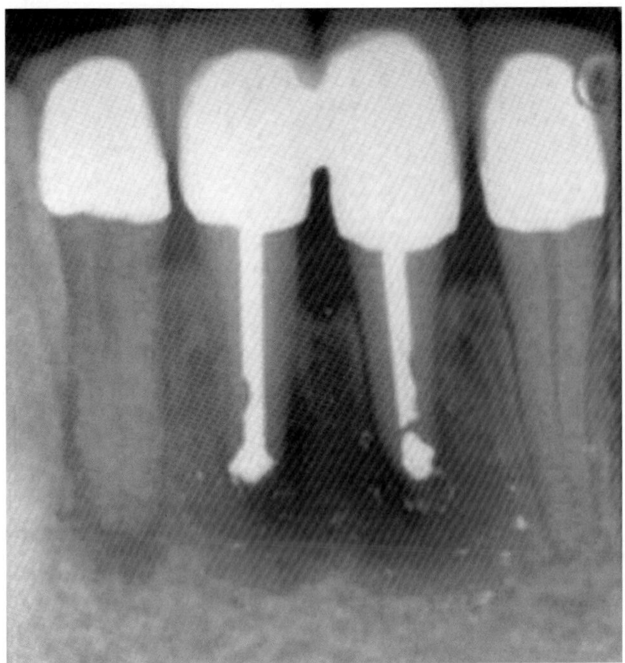

FIGURE 17-5 Irretrievable posts and apical pathosis. Root end resection and filling with amalgam to seal in irritants, likely from coronal leakage.

tion of the root (Fig. 17-8). A broken file can be left in the root canal system if the tooth remains asymptomatic.

Procedural Error

Broken instruments, ledging, gross overfills, and perforations may result in failure (Figs. 17-9 and 17-10). Although overfilling is not in itself an indication for removal of the material, surgical correction is beneficial in these situations if the tooth becomes symptomatic. Because the obturation of the canal is often dense in these situations, surgical treatment has an excellent prognosis.

Large, Unresolved Lesions After Root Canal Treatment

Occasionally, very large periradicular lesions may enlarge after adequate débridement and obturation. These lesions are generally best resolved with decompression and limited curettage to avoid damaging adjacent structures such as the mandibular nerve (Fig. 17-11). The continued apical leakage is the nidus for this expanding lesion, and root resection with the placement of an apical seal can resolve the lesion.

BOX 17-4

Contraindications (or Cautions) for Periapical Surgery

- Unidentified cause of root canal treatment failure
- When conventional root canal treatment is possible
- Combined coronal treatment/apical surgery
- When retreatment of a treatment failure is possible
- Anatomic structures (e.g., adjacent nerves and vessels) are in jeopardy
- Structures interfere with access and visibility
- Compromise of crown/root ratio
- Systemic complications (e.g., bleeding disorders)

Contraindications (or Cautions)

If other options are available, periapical surgery may not be the preferred choice (Box 17-4).

Unidentified Cause of Treatment Failure

Relying on surgery to try to correct all root canal treatment failures could be labeled indiscriminate. An important consideration is, *first,* to identify the cause of failure, and then *second,* to design an appropriate corrective treatment plan. Often, orthograde retreatment is indicated and gives the best

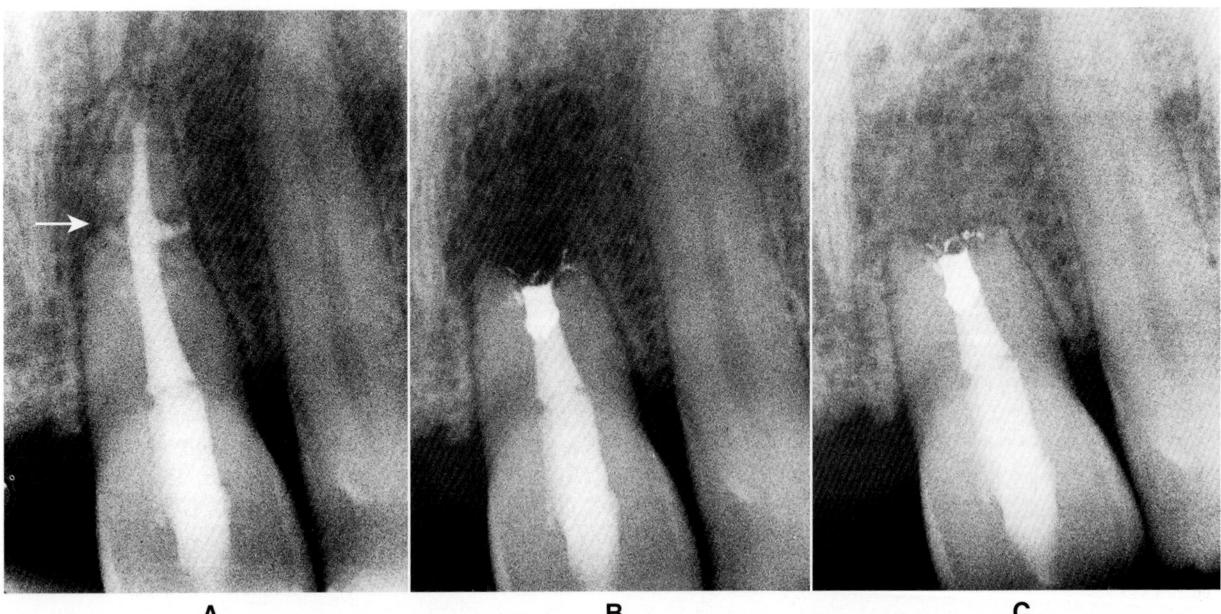

FIGURE 17-6 A, Horizontal root fracture, with failed attempt to treat both segments. B, Apical segment is removed surgically and retrograde amalgam is placed. C, Healing is complete after 1 year.

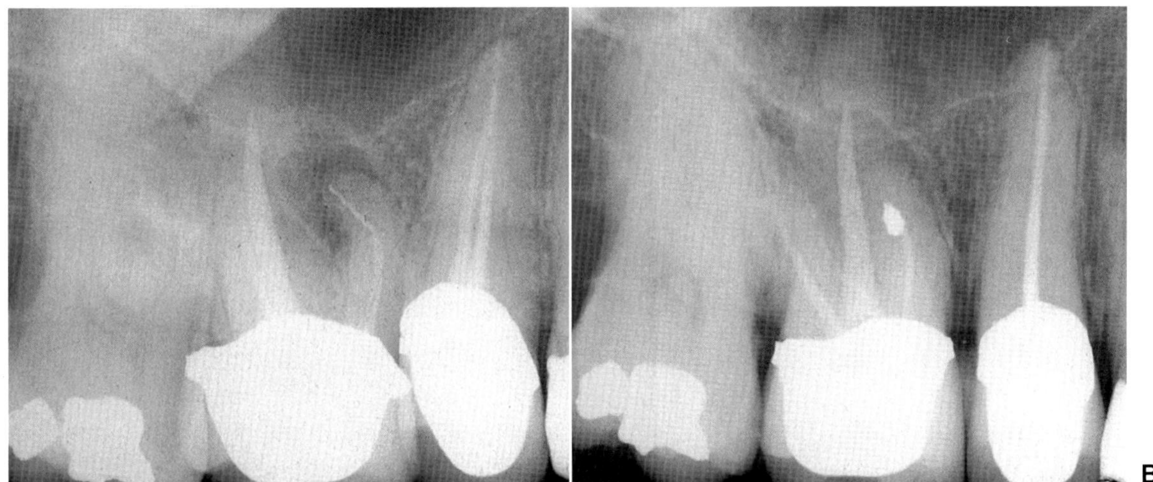

FIGURE 17-7 A, Irretrievable separated instruments in mesial-buccal canal. A separated instrument only requires surgical intervention if the tooth becomes symptomatic. B, Following resection of root with fractured instrument and placement of amalgam seal.

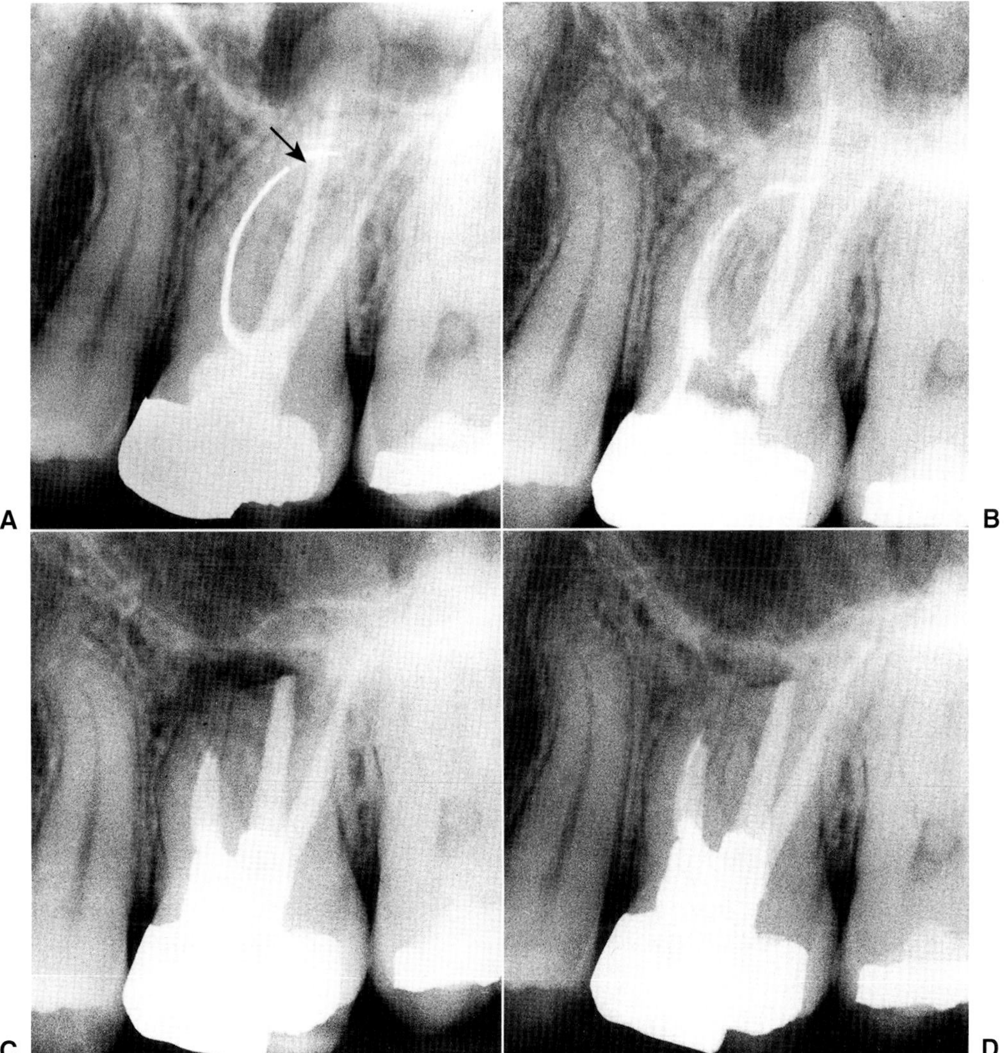

FIGURE 17-8 A, Irretrievable material in mesial and lingual canals and apical pathosis. B, Canals are re-treated, but there is failure. C, Treatment is root end resection to level of gutta-percha in the mesial and lingual aspects. D, After 2 years, healing is complete.

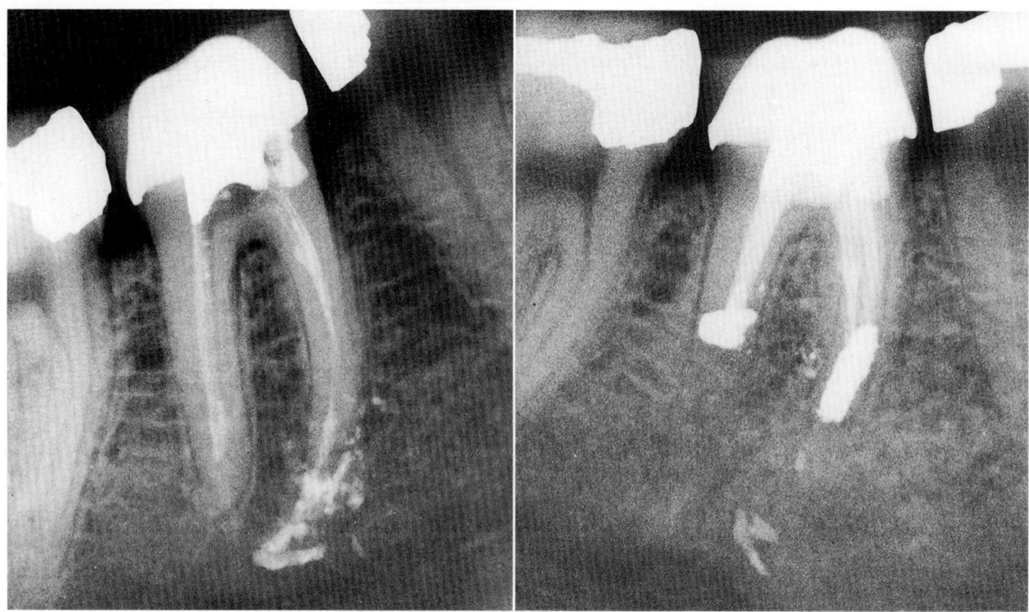

FIGURE 17-9 A, Overfill of injected obturating material has resulted in pain and paresthesia as a result of damage to inferior alveolar nerve. B, Corrected by retreatment, then apicectomy, curettage, and a root end amalgam fill.

chance of success. Surgery to correct a treatment failure for which the cause cannot be identified is often unsuccessful. Surgical management of all periapical pathoses, large periapical lesions, or both is often not necessary because they will resolve after appropriate root canal treatment. This includes lesions that may be cystic; these also usually heal after root canal treatment.

When Conventional Endodontic Treatment Is Possible

In most situations, orthograde conventional endodontic treatment is preferred (Fig. 17-12). Surgery is not indicated just because débridement and obturation are in the same visit, although there has been a long-held, incorrect notion that single-visit treatment should be accompanied by surgery, particularly if a periradicular lesion is present.

Simultaneous Root Canal Treatment and Apical Surgery

Few situations occur in which simultaneous root canal therapy and apical surgery are indicated. Usually, an approach that includes both of these as a single procedure has no advantages. It is preferable, and likely will result in better success, to perform only the conventional treatment without the adjunctive apical surgery. Another consideration is posttreatment symptoms. The level and incidence of pain after apical surgery is higher compared with root canal treatment. In some patients the conventional root canal procedure is ineffective at eliminating the symptoms. In this scenario, in spite of adequate instrumentation and antibiotics, there still is purulent exudate from the tooth or a vestibular swelling. A combined orthograde obturation with a simultaneous periapical surgery to curette the apical region and seal the tooth can successfully be coordinated and the symptoms resolved.

Anatomic Considerations

Most oral structures do not interfere with a surgical approach but must be considered. Expertise in operating around a structure such as the maxillary sinus or mental nerve region is imperative before undertaking surgery in these regions. Exposure of the maxillary sinus, which occurs in most molar apical surgeries, is in itself not a complication but a known consequence of the surgery (Fig. 17-13). Creating a sinus opening is neither unusual nor dangerous. However, caution is necessary not to introduce foreign objects into the opening and to remind the patient not to exert pressure by forcibly blowing the nose until the surgical wound has healed (for 2 weeks). Correct flap design is also crucial to prevent the development of an oral-antral communication. The sulcular flap keeps the incision line far from the sinus opening, thereby allowing spontaneous healing.

Surgical procedures around the mental foramen require caution to avoid stretch injury or direct damage to the nerve. In my opinion, exposure of the mental nerve is safer than attempting to estimate its position. Careful, subperiosteal reflection of the flap with adequate release allows the surgeon to identify the nerve where it exits from the bone. Once identified, staying a safe distance above and/or anterior is crucial to preventing an injury. Important to note is that the nerve may have an anterior loop of 2 to 4 mm, so that distance should be accounted for anteriorly.

When molar apical surgery is performed, the midroot of the molar should be identified by slow removal of bone, and then the bone removal should be carried inferiorly (Fig. 17-14, *A* to *C*). Once reaching the apical region, cautious curettage of the soft tissue lesion is carried out to avoid mechanical injury of the inferior alveolar nerve as it passes under the molar roots (Fig. 17-14, *D* to *G*). As mentioned before, it is not necessary to remove the entire area of periapical granulation tissue or cyst, if present, because the treatment of the apical lesion and sealing of the root canal with the retrograde filling causes the apical lesion to heal.

Poor Crown/Root Ratio

Teeth with very short roots have compromised bony support and are poor candidates for surgery; root end resection in such

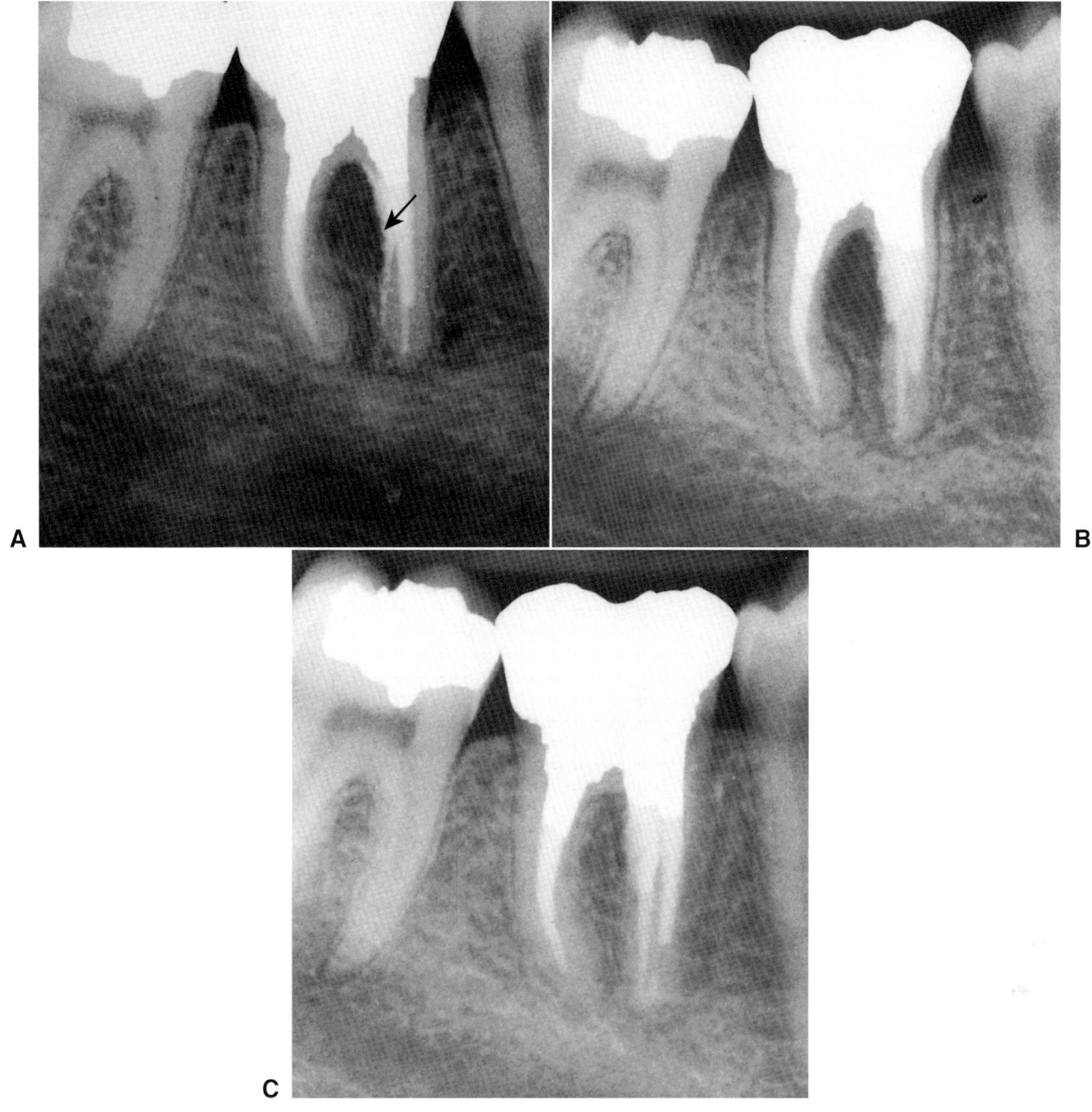

FIGURE 17-10 Repair of perforation. A, Furcation perforation results in extrusion of material (*arrow*) and pathosis. B, After flap reflection and exposure, the defect is repaired with mineral trioxide aggregate. C, Evaluation at 2 years shows successful healing. (Courtesy Dr. L. Baldassari-Cruz, University of Iowa.)

cases may compromise stability. However, shorter roots may support a relatively long crown if the surrounding cervical periodontium is healthy (see Fig. 17-6).

Medical (Systemic) Complications

The general health and condition of the patient are always essential considerations. No specific contraindications for endodontic surgery exist that would not be similar to those for other types of oral surgical procedures.

Surgical Procedure

Antibiotics

Almost without exception, periapical surgery is performed in an area with mixed acute and chronic infection. Due to the nature of the surgery and potential spread of the infection into adjacent spaces, preoperative prophylactic administration of antibiotics is indicated. A risk of infection of the hematoma exists because of the amount of edema expected after the procedure. In addition, inadvertent opening of adjacent structures such as the maxillary sinus is expected to occur with molar surgeries. As discussed elsewhere in the text, the basics of antibiotic prophylaxis are that antibiotics are to be administered before surgery to have any protective benefit. A preoperative dose of penicillin V potassium (2.0 g) or clindamycin (600 mg) 1 hour before surgery should be considered by the surgeon. The need for postoperative dosing has not been clearly defined and may not be of benefit to the patient. Other adjuncts, such as the use of corticosteroids perioperatively, may reduce edema and speed recovery.

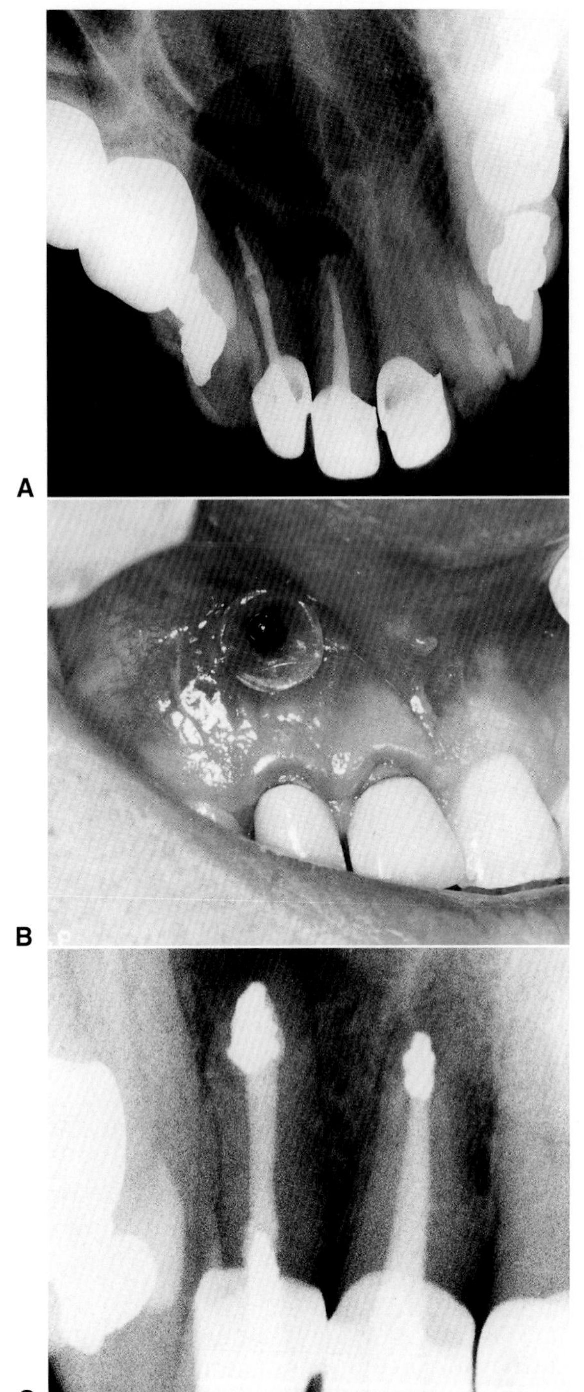

FIGURE 17-11 Decompression of large lesion. A, Extensive periradicular lesion failed to resolve. Coronal leakage in either treated tooth is possible. B, Surgical opening is created to defect; polyethylene tube extends into lesion to promote drainage. C, After partial resolution, root end resection and filling with amalgam are performed.

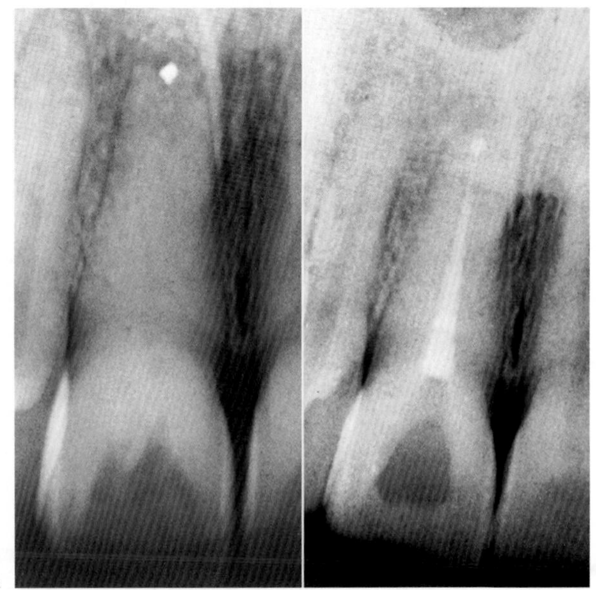

FIGURE 17-12 A, Inadequate root end resection and root end filling does not seal apex. B, Root canal treatment is readily accomplished, with good chance of success.

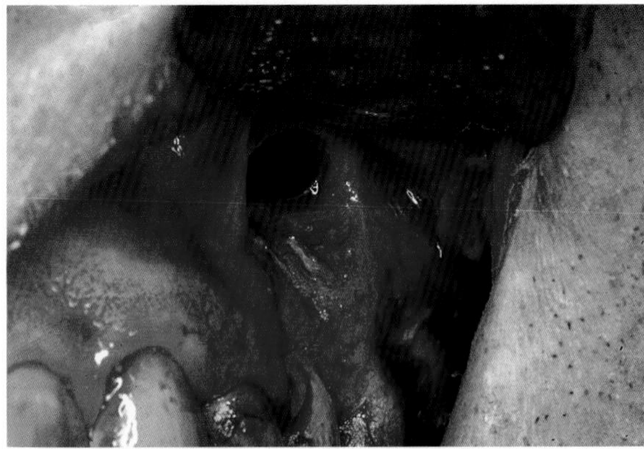

FIGURE 17-13 Sinus communication during root apical surgery of an upper molar. The closure with the sulcular incision is far away and unlikely to lead to an oral-antral communication.

Flap Design

Surgical access is a compromise between the need for visibility of the surgical site and the potential damage to adjacent structures. A properly designed and carefully reflected flap results in good access and uncomplicated healing. The basic principles of flap design should be followed; these are detailed in Chapter 8. Although several possibilities exist, the three most common incisions are (1) submarginal curved (i.e., semilunar), (2) submarginal, and (3) full mucoperiosteal (i.e., sulcular). The submarginal and full mucoperiosteal incision has either a three-corner (i.e., triangular) or four-corner (i.e., rectangular) design.

Semilunar Incision

Although the semilunar incision is a popular incision to among practitioners, the limitations and potential complications with this type of incision should lead one to abandon its use. This is a slightly curved half-moon horizontal incision in the alveolar mucosa (Fig. 17-15). Although the location allows easy reflection and quick access to the periradicular structures, it limits the clinician in providing full evaluation of the root surface. If a fracture is noted, performing a root resection through this incision or extracting the tooth is impractical.

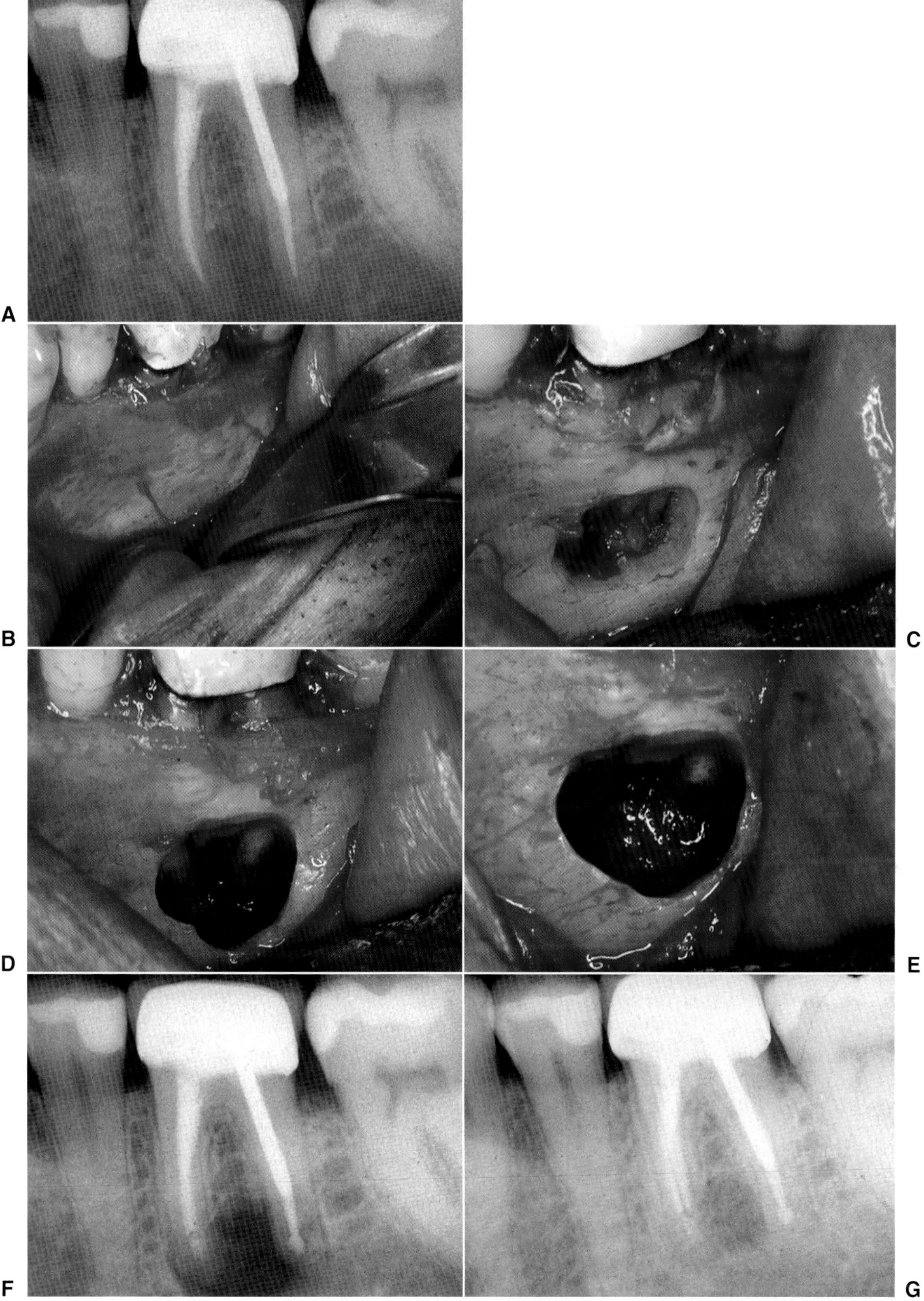

FIGURE 17-14 A, Preoperative radiographic film showing periapical pathologic condition amenable to apical surgery. B, Full-thickness mucoperiosteal flap to expose lateral border of mandible. As is typical, there is no obvious bony perforation. C, Careful removal of the thick buccal bone to expose the apical portion. D, Apical one third exposed before resection of root. E, Both roots resected and mineral trioxide aggregate seal placed following ultrasonic preparation. F, Immediate postoperative film with mineral trioxide aggregate seal visible. G, Five months postoperatively there is evidence of bone fill.

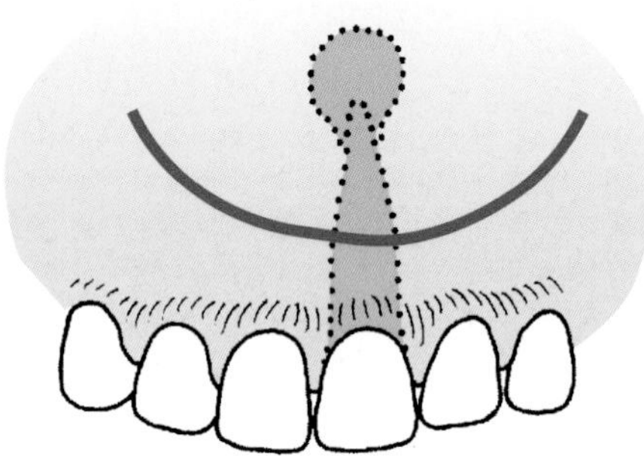

FIGURE 17-15 Semilunar flap incision, primarily horizontal and in alveolar mucosa. Because of limitations of access and poorer healing, this design is contraindicated.

The incision is based primarily in the unattached or alveolar mucosa, which heal more slowly with a greater chance of dehiscence than a flap based primarily in attached or keratinized tissue. In addition, the flap design carries the flap over the inflamed surgical site, and this inflamed mucosa is at a high risk of breakdown. Other disadvantages to this incision include excessive hemorrhage, delayed healing, and scarring; this design is therefore contraindicated for most endodontic surgery.

Submarginal Incision

The horizontal component of the submarginal incision is in attached gingiva with one or two accompanying vertical incisions (Fig. 17-16). Generally, the incision is scalloped in the horizontal line, with obtuse angles at the corners. The incision is used most successfully in the maxillary anterior region or, occasionally, with maxillary premolars with crowns. Because of the design, prerequisites are at least 4 mm of attached gingiva and good periodontal health.

The major advantage is esthetics. Leaving the gingiva intact around the margins of crowns is less likely to result in bone resorption with tissue recession and crown margin exposure. Compared with the semilunar incision, the submarginal provides less risk of incising over a bony defect and provides better access and visibility. Disadvantages include hemorrhage along the cut margins into the surgical site and occasional healing by scarring, compared with the full mucoperiosteal sulcular incision. The incision also provides limited access should a fracture be noted or other situation in which extraction or root resection is indicated.

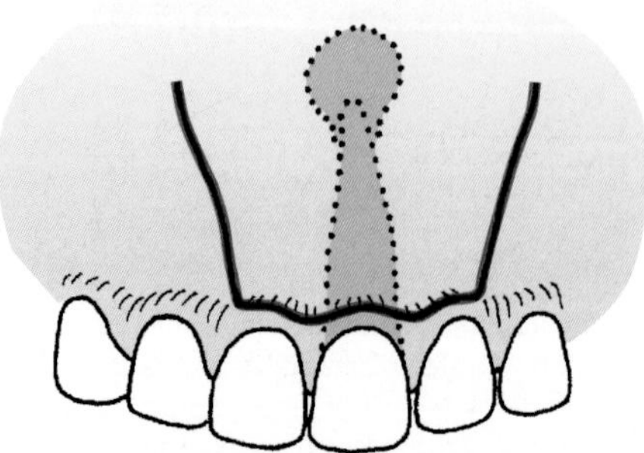

FIGURE 17-16 Submarginal incision is a scalloped horizontal line in attached gingiva, with one or two vertical components. This incision is usually confined to maxillary anterior region.

Full Mucoperiosteal Incision

The full mucoperiosteal incision is made into the gingival sulcus, extending to the gingival crest (Fig. 17-17). This procedure includes elevation of interdental papilla, free gingival margin, attached gingiva, and alveolar mucosa. One or two vertical relaxing incisions may be used, creating a triangular or rectangular design.

The full mucoperiosteal design is preferred over the other two techniques. The advantages include maximum access and visibility, not incising over the lesion or bony defect, fewer tendencies for hemorrhage, complete visibility of the root, allowance of root planing and bone contouring, and reduced likelihood of healing with scar formation. The disadvantages are that the flap is more difficult to replace and to suture; also, gingival recession can develop if the flap is not reapproximated well, exposing crown margins or cervical root surfaces (or both).

A common misconception is that flaps should be designed that are trapezoidal, having a broader base than edge (Fig. 17-17, *A*). A trapezoidal flap design creates a longer component in the nonkeratinized tissue that heals more slowly and with more discomfort. As the vertical release tends to broaden out apically, the incision crosses more bony prominences over the roots of teeth and across the muscle frenum, further delaying

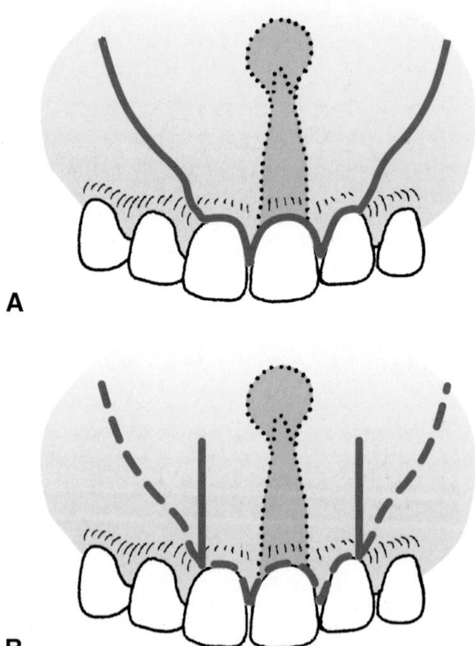

FIGURE 17-17 **A**, Full mucoperiosteal (i.e., sulcular) incision. Horizontal incision is into sulcus, accompanied by one (i.e., three-corner) or two (i.e., four-corner) vertical components. This represents the classic trapezoidal flap with the base broader than the peripheral edge. **B**, In comparison, by making the vertical-releasing incision(s) along the long axis of the adjacent teeth, the length of the flap in the nonkeratinized tissue is decreased, which reduces pain and accelerates the healing.

the healing process. The dental papilla just adjacent to the released flap actually ends up having a compromised blood supply and the potential for recession.

In contrast, by making the vertical release more perpendicular to the sulcus, a shorter length in the nonkeratinized tissue may permit the same amount of flap release (Fig. 17-17, *B*). The vertical incision should parallel the long axis of the teeth and should be made between two teeth where the tissue is the thickest and has the best blood supply. The direct vertical incision makes sense because the blood supply to the gingiva follows the long axis and is oriented longitudinally.

Anesthesia

For most surgical procedures, anesthetic approaches are conventional. In most mandibular regions a block is administered; then local infiltration of an anesthetic with epinephrine is given to enhance hemostasis. Frequently, the patient is sensitive to curettage of the inflammatory tissue, particularly toward the lingual aspect. Some of the sensitivity may be decreased by a preemptive periodontal ligament or intraosseous injection, using a device specifically designed for this purpose. Placing a cotton pellet soaked with local anesthetic solution can also reduce this discomfort.

A long-acting anesthetic agent is recommended, such as bupivacaine, for the inferior alveolar nerve block. Bupivacaine 0.5% with epinephrine 1:200,000 has been shown to give long-lasting anesthesia and, later, provide a lingering analgesia. Long-acting local anesthetic agents such as bupivacaine do not diffuse well through the tissue because they are so highly protein bound, so their effectiveness for an infiltration-type injection is limited.

Some patients request sedation because of their concern about having a surgical procedure. If there is active infection in the region, profound local anesthesia may not be able to be achieved, and these patients may be candidates for intravenous sedation or general anesthesia.

Incision and Reflection

A firm incision should be made through periosteum to bone. Incision and reflection of a full-thickness flap is important to minimize hemorrhage and to prevent tearing of the tissue. Reflection is with a sharp periosteal elevator beginning in the vertical incisions and then raising the horizontal component. To reflect the periosteum, the elevator must firmly contact bone while the tissue is raised (Fig. 17-18). Reflection is to an apical level adequate for access to the surgical site, although still allowing a retractor to have contact with bone. Enough width and vertical release of the flap must be included to prevent the flap from being stretched, which can lead to tearing and slower healing.

Periapical Exposure

Frequently, the cortical bone overlying the apex has been resorbed, exposing a soft tissue lesion. If the opening is small, it is enlarged using a large surgical round bur, until approximately half the root and the lesion are visible (Fig. 17-19).

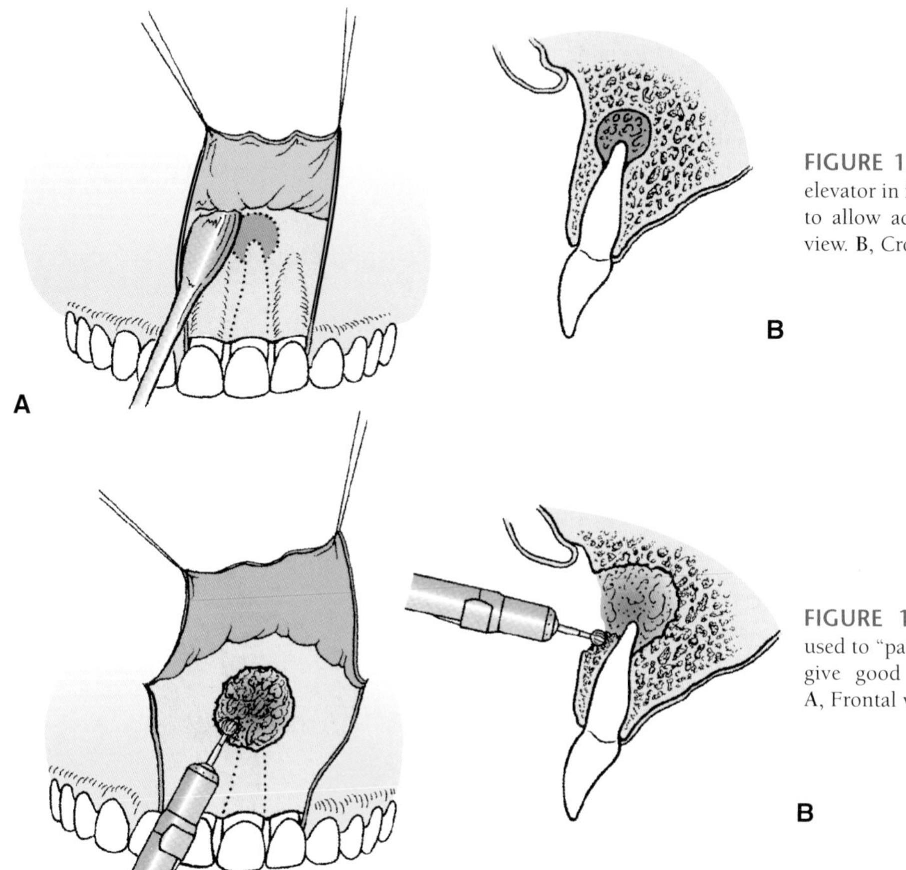

FIGURE 17-18 Full-thickness flap is raised with sharp elevator in firm contact with bone. Enough tissue is raised to allow access and visibility to apical area. **A**, Frontal view. **B**, Cross section.

FIGURE 17-19 Apical exposure. Large round bur is used to "paint" bony window. Enough bone is removed to give good visibility and access to lesion and apex. **A**, Frontal view. **B**, Cross section.

With a limited bony opening, radiographs are used in conjunction with root and bone topography to locate the apex. A measurement may be made with a periodontal probe on the radiograph and then transferred to the surgical site to determine the apex location.

To avoid air emphysema, handpieces that direct pressurized air, water, and abrasive particles (or combinations) into the surgical site must not be used. Vented high-speed handpieces or electrical surgical handpieces are preferred during osseous entry and root end resection. Sealed-end air-pressurized handpieces also direct air away from the surgical site, and handpieces that use nitrogen gas also prevent air emphysema. Regardless of the handpiece used, there should be copious irrigation with a syringe or through the handpiece with sterile saline solution. Enough overlying bone should be removed to expose the area around the apex and at least half the length of the root. Good access and visibility are important; the bony window must be adequate. The clinician should not be concerned about the bone removal because once the infection resolves, the bone will reform.

The exposure of the root is done before resecting the root to avoid the potential of blending the root in with the bone and losing surgical orientation. This is especially critical in the mandible where the bone is dense. Lower incisor roots are carefully exposed because the proximity with adjacent teeth could lead to treatment of the wrong apex. The curvature of the root, particularly the maxillary lateral incisor, demands close attention to avoid surgical misadventures.

Curettage

Most of the granulomatous, inflamed tissue surrounding the apex should be removed (Fig. 17-20) to gain access and visibility of the apex, to obtain a biopsy for histologic examination (when indicated), and to minimize hemorrhage.

If possible, the tissue should be enucleated with a suitably sized sharp curette, although total lesion removal usually does not occur. A cleaner bony cavity has the least hemorrhage and the best visibility. Often there is extensive debris that has been forced out the apex of the tooth during the initial endodontic therapy. Cleaning this out this debris removes what may have been the nidus for the acute and chronic infection. Tissue removal should not jeopardize the blood supply to an adjacent tooth. In addition, some areas of the lesion may be inaccessible to the curettes, such as on the lingual aspect of the root. Portions of inflamed tissue or epithelium may be left, without compromising healing; total removal is not necessary. As noted before, it is better to leave a small portion of this tissue than to damage the inferior alveolar nerve.

If hemorrhage from soft or hard tissue is excessive to the extent that visibility is compromised, homeostatic agents or other control techniques are useful. These agents should be removed after use. Hemorrhage control can be achieved by holding direct pressure over a bleeding site with gauze soaked in local anesthetic solution with epinephrine and by minimizing suction at the site of a bleeder.

Root End Resection

Root end resection is indicated because it removes the region that most likely had the poorest obturation because of the distance from the coronal portion of the tooth. The presence of accessory canals increases at the apex as well, which may have not been initially cleaned and débrided, thereby leaving a source of continued infection.

Before sectioning, a trough is created around the apex with a tapered fissure bur to expose and isolate the root end. The resection is done with the same tapered fissure bur. Depending on the location, a bevel of varying degrees is made in a faciolingual direction (Fig. 17-21). With the use of ultrasonic instruments to prepare the apex, a minimal bevel is needed, especially in maxillary anterior teeth. By minimizing the length of the bevel, fewer dentinal tubules are exposed, thereby reducing leakage into the apical region.

The amount of root removed depends on the reason for performing the resection. Sufficient root apex must be removed to provide a larger surface and to expose additional canals. In general, approximately 2 to 3 mm of the root is resected—more if necessary for apical access or if an instrument is lodged in the apical region; less if too much removal would further compromise stability of an already short root.

Root End Preparation and Restoration

A retrograde filling should be placed in cases unless technical aspects prohibit it. The filling seals the canal system, preventing further leakage. The depth of the preparation must be at

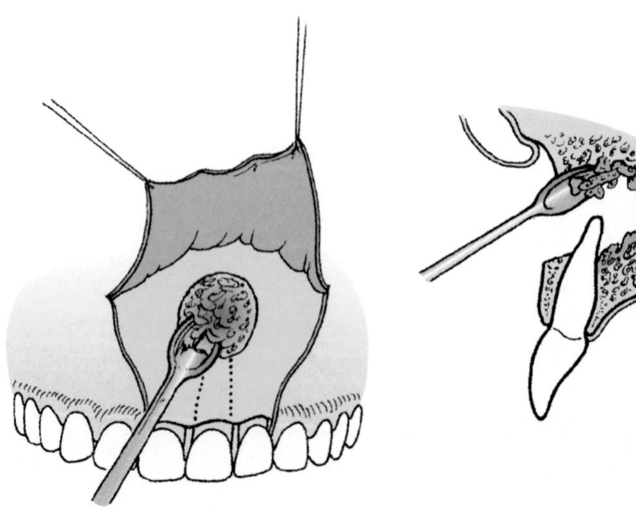

FIGURE 17-20 Curettage. Much of lesion that is accessible is removed with large curettes. Usually, remnants of tissue remain, which is not a problem. A, Frontal view. B, Cross section.

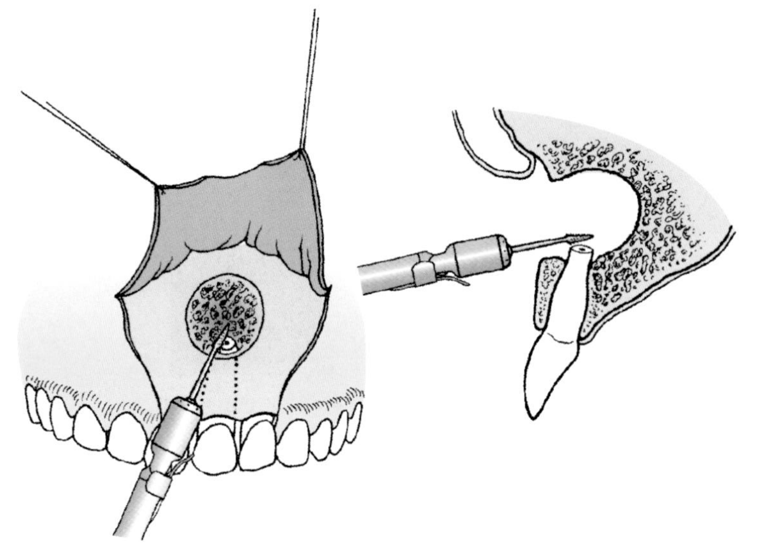

FIGURE 17-21 Root end resection. Approximately one third of apex is removed with tapered bur. Amount removed and degree of bevel varies according to situation. **A**, Frontal view. **B**, Cross section.

least 1 mm deeper than the length of the bevel to seal the apex adequately. In the past, root end preparation was done by slow-speed, specially designed microhandpieces (Fig. 17-22). The rotary instruments are too complicated to follow the root canal system, occasionally leading to misaligned preparations. Contemporary apical preparation uses ultrasonic tips (Fig. 17-23).

Ultrasonic instruments offer the advantages of control and ease of use; they also permit less apical root removal in certain situations (Fig. 17-24). Another advantage of the ultrasonic tips, particularly when diamond coated, is the formation of cleaner, better-shaped preparation. Evidence suggests that success rates are significantly improved with ultrasonic preparation. The ultrasonic tip can prepare the isthmus between the two canals of the mesiobuccal roots of upper first molars, which is a significant cause of conventional endodontic failure on these teeth. While preparing the apex with the ultrasonic instruments, constant saline irrigation is needed to avoid overheating, which causes fracture of these fine instruments. Various designs and shapes of tips are available to access different apices of each tooth in the oral cavity. The ease of use and special angulations require less of a bony opening and less beveling of the apical region and permit a deeper, denser fill.

Root End–Filling Materials

The root end–filling material is placed into the cavity preparation (Fig. 17-25). These materials should seal well and should be tissue tolerant, easily inserted, minimally affected by moisture, and visible radiographically. Importantly, the root end–filling material must be stable and nonresorbable indefinitely.

Amalgam (preferably zinc free), intermediate restorative material, and super ethoxy benzoic acid (Super-EBA) cement have been commonly used materials. Gutta-percha, composite resin, glass ionomer cement, intermediate restorative material, Cavit, and different luting cements have also been recommended; these materials have less clinical documentation of success. Mineral trioxide aggregate (MTA) has shown favorable biologic and physical properties and ease of handling; it has become a widely used material. MTA has been shown to be conducive to bone growth over the apical region. MTA is a hydrophilic material, similar to Portland cement. MTA has a working time of about 10 minutes, although it takes 2 to 3 hours to reach final set, which is not an issue because the root apex is not a load-bearing region, at least not until bone fills in the defect. The surgeon must be careful not to irrigate

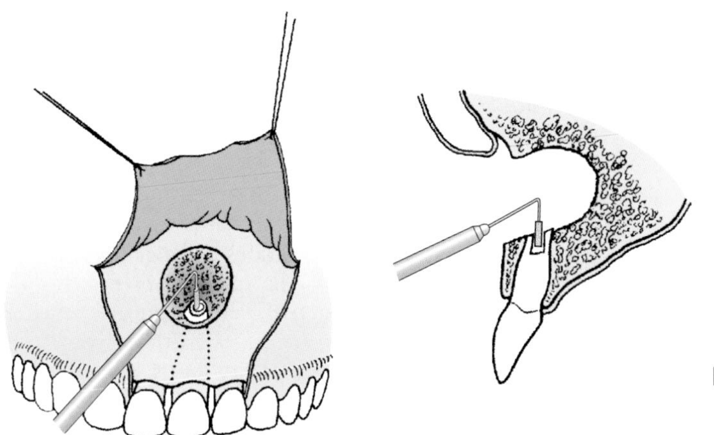

FIGURE 17-22 Root end preparation and retrograde filling material (mineral trioxide aggregate) placement. **A**, Piezoelectric unit with 3-mm long tip to prepare the apical end. **B**, Special carriers for delivering the mineral trioxide aggregate retrograde filling material.

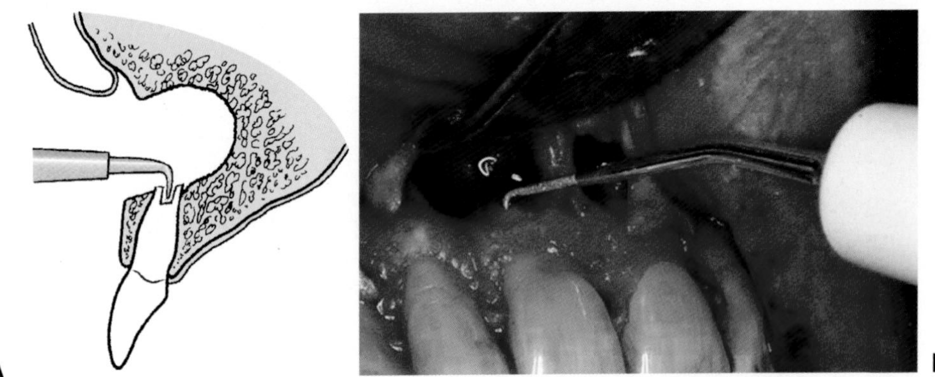

FIGURE 17-23 A, Ultrasonic tips are good alternative for root end preparation. B, These tips permit preparation with better control and less root removal and the need for less bevel, which exposes fewer dentinal tubules.

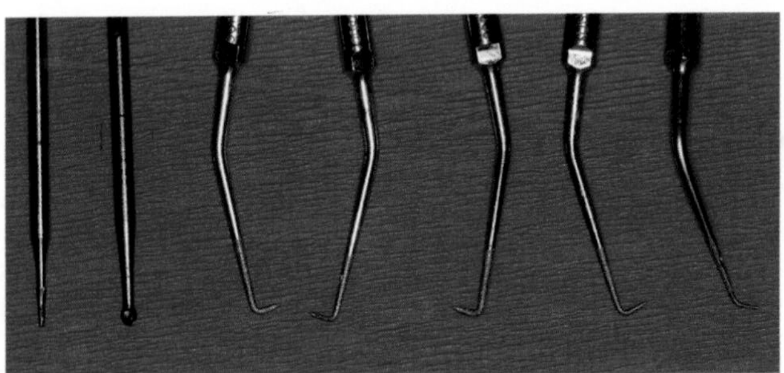

FIGURE 17-24 Ultrasonic preparation tips are available in different shapes for accessing different teeth in the oral cavity. Note in comparison the diameter of the conventionally used rotary burs.

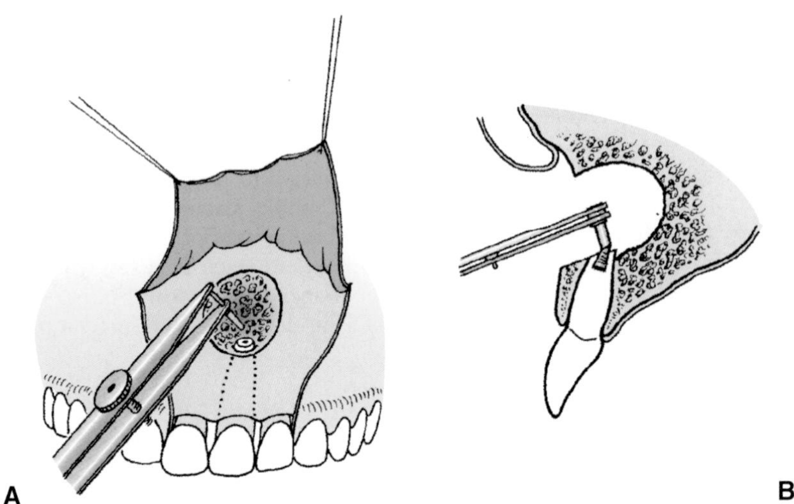

FIGURE 17-25 Special small carriers are used to place material, which is then packed with small condensers. Other cement type of materials are carried and compacted with paddles and burnishers. A, Frontal view. B, Cross section.

MTA out after placement, so irrigation is done before placing the filling, and any excess is wiped with a just dampened cotton pellet.

No single, all-purpose, superior root end–filling material exists. Those that demonstrate the best combination of physical and biologic properties, as well as documentation of clinical success, are amalgam, MTA, composite resin, and reinforced zinc oxide cements (e.g., intermediate restorative material and Super-EBA). One of these materials should be selected, according to the conditions. Amalgam should not be used if the field is bloody, if the root end preparation is less than 3 mm, or if access is limited. Patients are also reluctant to have amalgam implanted in their bone, although studies have shown no increase in serum mercury levels when amalgam is used for this purpose. Composite resin with a bonding agent must be placed in a perfectly dry field, which is complicated because of the nature of the surgery. This material may be used in a shallow, concave preparation and has been shown to be successful in molar root end surgeries. MTA, with its good properties, may be placed in a field in which some hemorrhage has occurred; the final set is not adversely affected by blood contamination.

Each of these root end–filling materials has different, unique mixing and placement characteristics. The clinician should practice with each before placement in a patient. Special carriers for MTA have been designed and work well to deliver the material. A metal carrier with a disposable plastic sleeve contains the material and keeps it from contacting additional moisture as it is carried to the surgical site. MTA can be condensed and added to so that the fill is complete.

Irrigation

The surgical site is flushed with copious amounts of sterile saline to remove soft and hard tissue debris, hemorrhage, blood clots, and excess root end–filling material. As mentioned with MTA, the irrigation is done before the MTA is placed to avoid washing the filler out of the apical preparation.

Radiographic Verification

Before suturing, a radiograph is made to verify that the surgical objectives are satisfactory. If corrections are needed, these are made before suturing.

Flap Replacement and Suturing

Just before closure, the cervical region of the exposed teeth is gently scaled to remove any debris, preexisting calculus, and granulation tissue. This brief intervention speeds the reattachment and reduces greatly the chance for recession. The flap is returned to its original position and is held with moderate digital pressure and moistened gauze. This expresses hemorrhage from under the flap and gives initial adaptation and more accurate suturing. Absorbable monofilament sutures are typically used to permit ease of removal if needed and are associated with less wicking and retention of surface bacteria. A sling suture is ideal in the esthetic zone to avoid gingival recession (Fig. 17-26). After suturing, the flap should again be compressed digitally with moistened gauze for several minutes to express more hemorrhage. This limits postoperative swelling and promotes more rapid healing.

Postoperative Instructions

Oral and written information should be supplied in simple, straightforward language. The wording should minimize anxiety arising from normal postoperative sequelae by describing the ways in which the patient can promote healing and comfort. Instructions inform the patient of what to expect (e.g., swelling, discomfort, possible discoloration, and some oozing of blood) and the ways in which these sequelae can be prevented, managed, or both. The surgical site should not be disturbed, and pressure should be maintained (cold packs over the surgical area until bedtime might help). Oral hygiene procedures are indicated everywhere except the surgical site; careful brushing and flossing may begin after 24 hours. Proper nutrition and fluid intake are important but should not traumatize the area.

A chlorhexidine rinse, twice daily, reduces bacterial count at the surgical site. This minimizes inflammation and enhances soft tissue healing.

Analgesics are recommended, although pain is frequently minimal; strong analgesics are usually not required. No category of pain medication is preferred; selection depends on the clinician and the patient. Analgesics for moderate pain usually suffice and are most effective if administered before the surgery or at least before the anesthetic wears off.

The patient is instructed to call if excessive swelling or pain is experienced. Postoperative complications are a response to injury from the procedure; infection after this type of surgical procedure is rare. However, the patient should be evaluated in person if there are difficulties. Occasionally, sutures have torn loose, a foreign body (e.g., a cotton pellet) is under the flap, or an overreaction of the soft tissues takes place. Again, antibiotics are not indicated; palliative or corrective treatment usually suffices.

Suture Removal and Evaluation

Sutures ordinarily are removed in 5 to 7 days if still present, with shorter periods being preferred to enhance healing. After 3 days, swelling and discomfort should be decreasing. In addition, there should be evidence of primary wound closure; tissues that were reflected should be in apposition. Occasionally, a loose or torn suture may result in nonadapted tissue. In these cases the margins are only readapted and resutured if in the maxillary anterior esthetic zone.

CORRECTIVE SURGERY

Corrective surgery is the management of defects that have occurred by a biologic response (i.e., resorption) or iatrogenic (i.e., procedural) error. These defects may be anywhere on the root, from cervical margin to apex. Many defects are accessible; others are difficult to reach or are in virtually inaccessible areas. Usually, an injury or defect has occurred on the root. In response to the injury, there may be an inflammatory lesion, or one may develop in the future. A corrective procedure is necessary. Generally, the procedure involves exposing, preparing, and then sealing the defect. Usually included are removal of irritants and rebuilding of the root surface (Box 17-5).

Indications

Procedural Errors

Procedural errors are openings through the lateral root surface created by the operator, typically during access, canal instrumentation, or after space preparation (Fig. 17-27). The result is perforation, which presents a difficult surgical challenge, more so than repairing damage to a root end. Perforations

BOX 17-5

Corrective Surgery

INDICATIONS
- Procedural errors (e.g., perforations)
- Resorptive defects

CONTRAINDICATIONS
- Anatomic impediments
- Inaccessible defect
- Repair would create periodontal defect

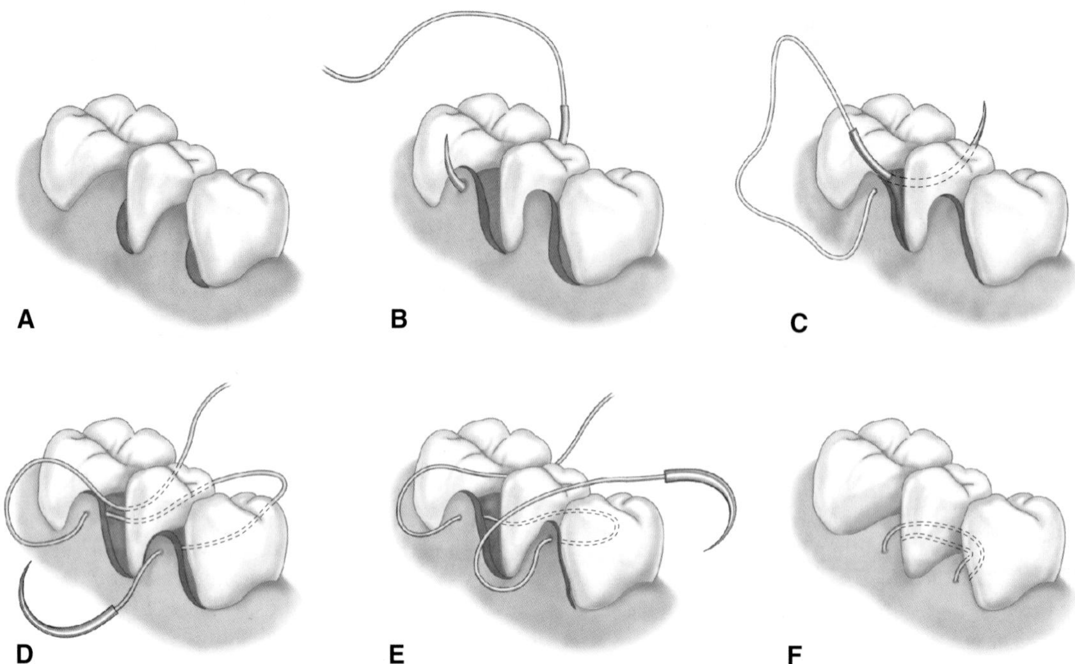

FIGURE 17-26 Schematic of sling suture for reapproximating a gingival flap. This type of suture is helpful to prevent recession around teeth and existing crowns. (Adapted from Cohen ES: Sutures and suturing. In *Atlas of cosmetic reconstructive periodontal surgery,* ed 2, Philadelphia, 1994, Lea and Febiger.)

often require restorative management and completion of the endodontic treatment, usually in conjunction with the surgical phase. The location of the perforation influences success; some are virtually inaccessible. If the defect is on the interproximal, in the furcation, or close to adjacent teeth or to the lingual, adequate repair may not be possible or is compromised. Defects that are too far posterior (particularly on the distal or lingual aspects) may be difficult to reach. The nature and location of the perforation should be determined with angled radiographs before the decision is made whether to repair surgically, to remove the involved root, or to extract.

Resorptive Perforations

Resorptive perforations may originate internally or externally (Fig. 17-28), resulting in a communication between pulp and periodontium. A more serious defect is one that extends to include cervical exposure to the oral cavity.

Resorption occurs for several reasons, but most cases include inflammation from an irritant. These irritants include sequelae to trauma, internal bleaching procedures, orthodontic tooth movement, restorative procedures, or other factors causing pulp or periradicular inflammation. Occasionally, resorptions are idiopathic, with no demonstrable cause.

As with procedural errors, the considerations as to treatability and surgical approach are similar.

Contraindications

Anatomic Considerations

Consideration must be given to structural impediments to a surgical approach. Few impediments exist, and most can be managed or avoided. Included are various nerve and vessel bundles and bony structures, such as the external oblique ridge.

Location of Perforation

As mentioned previously, the defect must be accessible surgically. This means the clinician must be able to locate and, ideally, readily visualize the surgical area.

Accessibility

A handpiece or an ultrasonic instrument generally is necessary to prepare the defect. Therefore the defect must be reachable, without impedance by structures or by lack of visibility.

Considerations

Surgical Approach

Repair presents a unique set of problems. The defect may wrap from facial to proximal to lingual, creating not only difficulties in visualization but also problems with access and hemostasis and material placement. A general guideline is that the defect is larger and more complex than it appears on a radiograph.

Generally, the defect must be enlarged to provide a sound cavosurface margin and to avoid knife-edge margins. Occasionally, the repair is internal (from inside the canal), with material being extruded through the defect. The excess is removed and contoured with burs or sharp instruments. The objective is to seal and stabilize the defect with a restorative material. If a post or other material is perforating the root, it must be reduced with burs to within root structure and a cavity prepared. Then the defect is restored with one of the materials mentioned previously.

Repair Material

External repair is often with amalgam or, if the field is dry, glass ionomer or dentin-bonding agent with composite resin. Other materials are suitable, such as MTA or Super-EBA; these have not had the test of time but are promising materials. MTA,

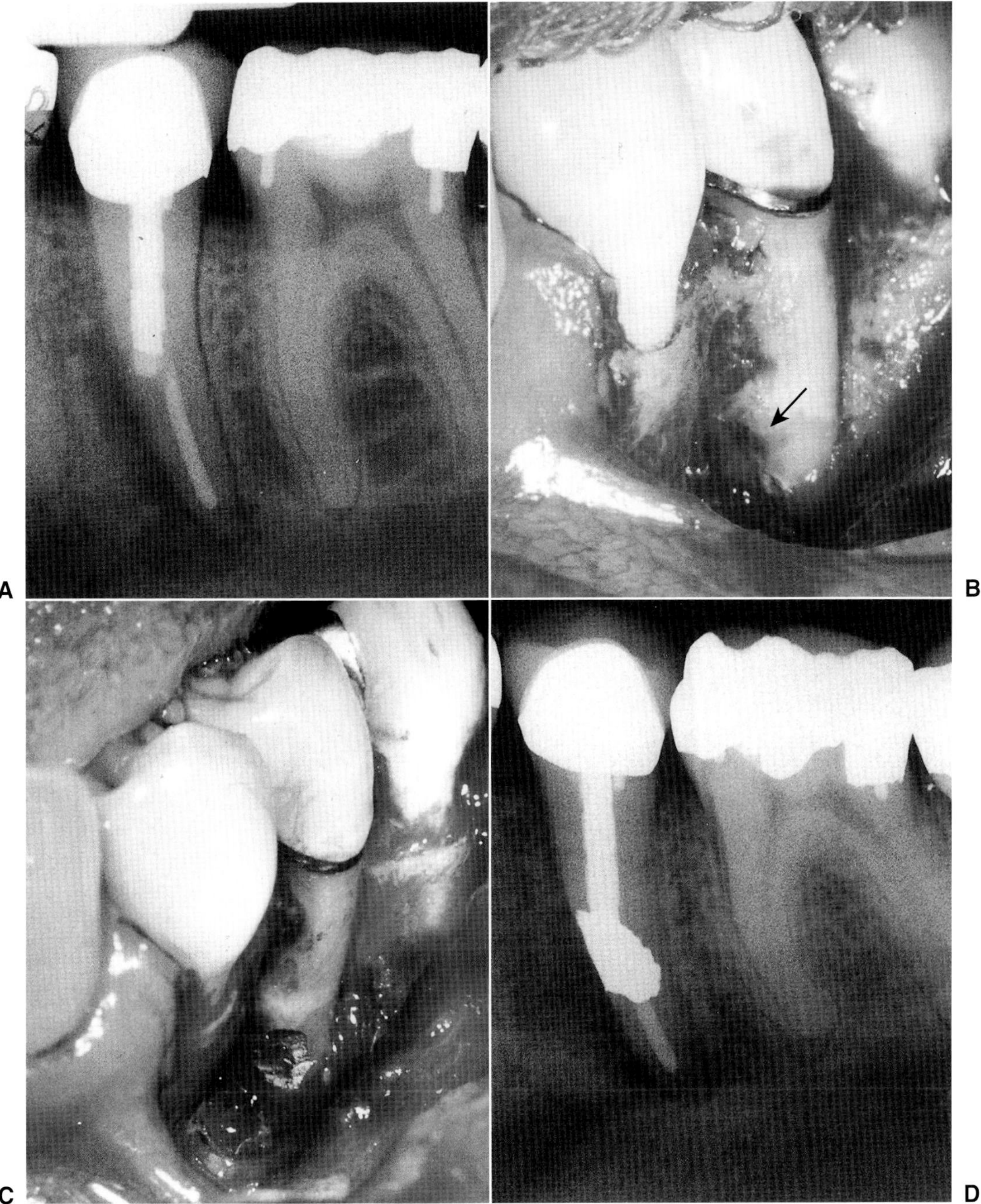

FIGURE 17-27 Postperforation repair. A, Lesion developing lateral to off-centered post suggests perforation that (B) is identified (*arrow*) on flap reflection. C, Post is reduced to within root and cavity filled with amalgam (D).

in particular, shows favorable biologic properties. The same considerations of physical and biologic properties, as just described, apply. One major difference is in the repair of a defect that will be exposed to oral fluids; Super-EBA or MTA are contraindicated because they gradually wash out of the cavity. More stable materials—composite resins, amalgam, or glass ionomers—are preferred. Certain glass ionomers have promise and have indicated the possibility of tissue attachment to the material, although long-term studies are lacking.

Prognosis

Repairs in the cervical third or furcation in particular have the poorest prognosis. Communication often is eventually established with the junctional epithelium, which results in periodontal breakdown, loss of attachment, and pocket formation. This means that a periodontal procedure (e.g., crown lengthening) would be required in conjunction with the defect repair.

A defect in the middle or apical third that is properly prepared and sealed has a very good long-term prognosis.

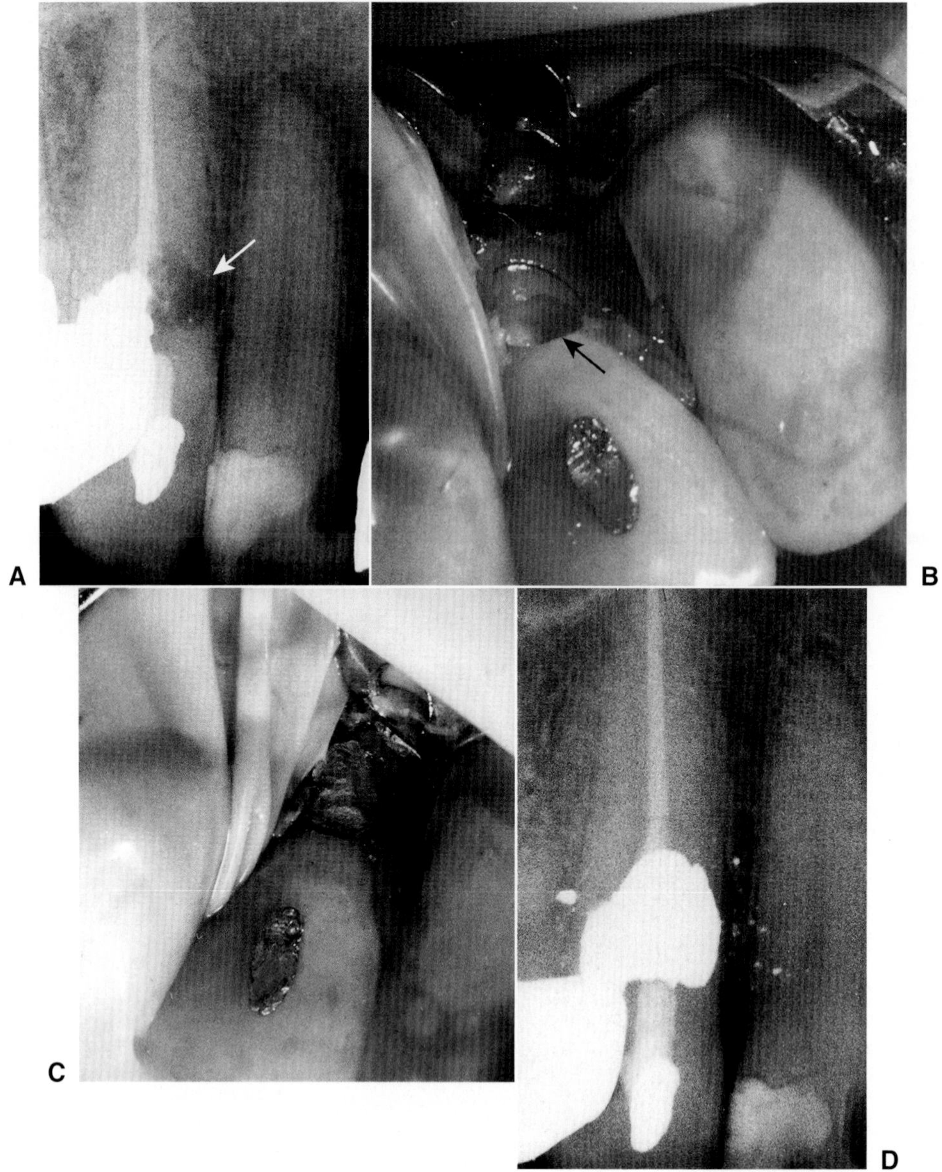

FIGURE 17-28 External resorption repair. A, Mesially angled radiograph shows defect (*arrow*) to be lingual. B, After flap reflection, crestal bone reduction, and rubber dam isolation, defect is prepared (*arrow*). Margins must be in sound tooth structure. C, Cavity is filled with amalgam, and flap is apically positioned. D, Long-term radiographic and clinical evaluation is necessary; at times, resorption recurs.

Surgical Procedure

After the basic approaches with periapical surgery, the next step is to perform corrective surgery. Flap designs are similar but are more limited. A sulcular incision is usually required, with at least one vertical incision to form a three-cornered flap. A full-thickness flap is reflected, and bone is removed to expose the defect (Fig. 17-29). Bone removal must be adequate to allow maximal visualization and access. If possible, a rim of cervical bone should be retained to support the flap and possibly to enhance reattachment; this is frequently not possible with cervical defects.

The preparation of a facial or lingual defect is similar to that of a class 1 cavity preparation (Fig. 17-30). An interproximal defect resembles a class 2 preparation, with an opening from the facial (or lingual) aspect and including the interproximal wall but leaving a lingual wall (if possible).

The facial or lingual cavity is then filled by direct placement of the material. A class 2 (i.e., interproximal, or furcation) cavity requires a matrix. For example, an amalgam matrix band is held in position with fingers or a wedge, and then material is packed into the cavity preparation. This matrix is less critical if amalgam is not used. The material is carved flush with the cavity margins. Flap replacement, suturing, and digital pressure are as described before. Suture removal should be within 3 to 6 days. Postoperative instructions are similar to those after periapical surgery.

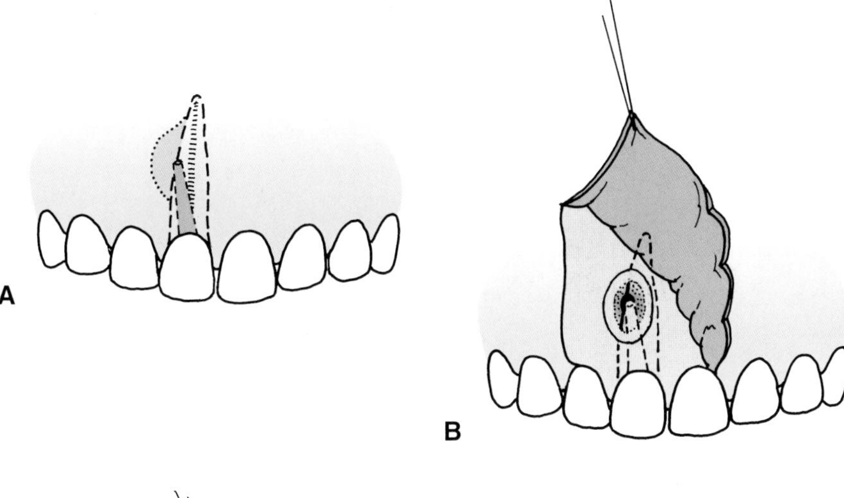

FIGURE 17-29 A, Misdirected post is perforating distally. B, Full mucoperiosteal (i.e., sulcular incision) three-corner flap is raised, and bone is removed to expose defect.

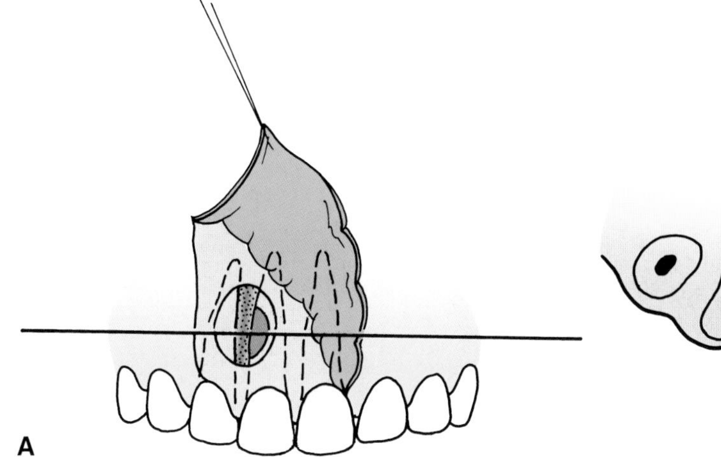

B

FIGURE 17-30 A, Post is reduced to well within root, and cavity is prepared. B, In this cross section through defect, a lingual wall to the preparation is evident.

FRACTURED TEETH

Preoperative radiographs and a careful clinical examination should be done with a high index of suspicion of a vertical root fracture before undertaking surgery. Mandibular molars and maxillary premolars are the most frequent teeth to have occult vertical root fractures. Although surgical exploration may be needed to show the presence of a fracture definitively (Fig. 17-31), subtle radiographic signs may alert the surgeon that a fracture is present and the surgery is unlikely to be successful. Tamse et al.[1] looked at radiographs of maxillary premolars for comparison with the clinical findings at the time of surgery. Very few (1 out of 15) teeth with an isolated, well corticated periapical lesion had a vertical root fracture. In contrast, halo-type radiolucency was almost always associated with a vertical root fracture (Fig. 17-32). This type of radiolucency is also known as a "J" type, in which a widened periodontal ligament space connects with the periapical lesion creating the J pattern.

In patient discussions it is critical to review the exploratory nature of the surgery, and I routinely use that as a descriptor of the planned surgery. In cases of root fracture, a decision during surgery may need to be made either to resect a root or extract a tooth if a fractured root is found. Obtaining the appropriate preoperative consent and determining how the extracted tooth site will be managed (with or without a temporary removable partial denture) must be established before surgery commences.

HEALING

Healing after endodontic surgery is rapid because most tissues being manipulated are healthy, with a good blood supply, and tissue replacement enables repair by primary intention. Soft tissues (e.g., periosteum, gingiva, alveolar mucosa, and periodontal ligament) and hard tissues (e.g., dentin, cementum, and bone) are involved. Time and mode of healing varies with each, but involve similar processes. The specifics of short-term healing of soft and hard tissues are discussed in Chapter 4.

RECALL

Recall evaluations to assess long-term healing are important. Some failures after surgery are evidenced only by radiographic findings. A 1-year follow-up is generally a good indicator. If, after 1 year, radiographic evidence shows no decrease in lesion size or the lesion size increases, it generally indicates a failure and persistent inflammation. A decrease in lesion size (indicating hard tissue formation) may lead to complete healing and requires evaluation at 6 to 12 months. Of course, persistent symptoms—such as pain or swelling (or both), presence of sinus tract, deep probing defects, or other adverse findings—also indicate failure. Healing by scar tissue after surgery occurs primarily in the maxillary incisors (Fig. 17-33). This is unusual and has a unique radiographic appearance with

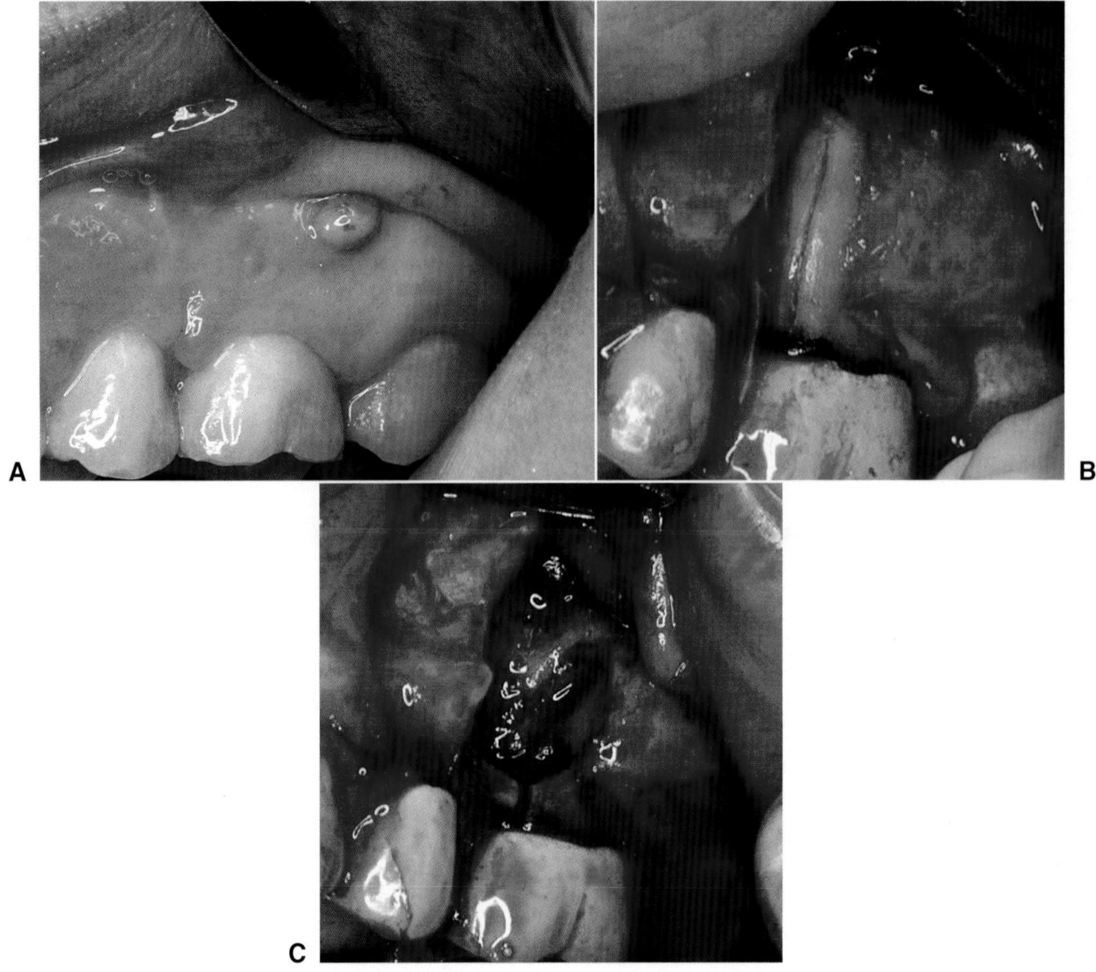

FIGURE 17-31 A, Fistula on midbuccal portion of the mesiobuccal root of a molar. B, Full-thickness sulcular incision reveals an unsuspected vertical root fracture C, Resection of the mesiobuccal root can be accomplished because a sulcular incision was used, as opposed to a semilunar type.

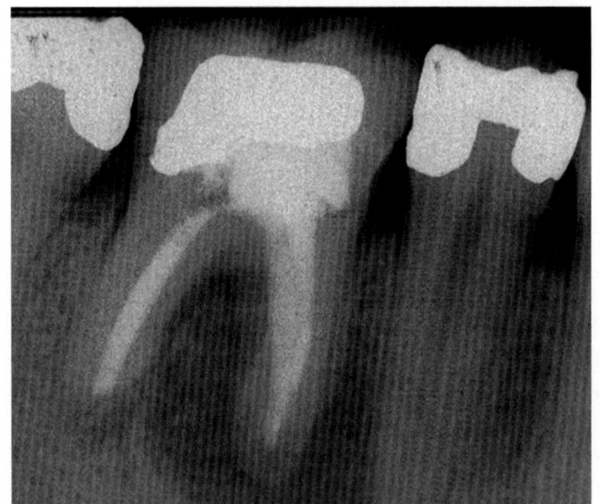

FIGURE 17-32 The halo radiolucency involving the entire length of the root is often pathognomonic for a vertical root fracture.

an irregular distinct outline, often separated from the root end. Healing by scar tissue is considered to be a successful outcome.

Frequently, structures over the apex do not regenerate to a normal appearance. At times, connective tissue or bony arrangements leave a slightly "widened" periodontal ligament space. This should have relatively distinct, corticated margins and not be diffuse (which indicates inflammation and a failure).

TO PERFORM A BIOPSY OR NOT

A clinical controversy has ensued over the consideration as to whether all periapical lesions treated surgically should have soft tissue removed and submitted for histologic evaluation. An editorial by Walton[2] questioned the rationale of submitting all soft tissue recovered for histologic examination, which then ignited a series of letters to the editor. Organizations such as the American Association of Endodontists have stated in their standards that if soft tissue can be recovered from the apical surgery, it must be submitted for pathologic evaluation.

On cursory review, it seems that it is easier to make this recommendation than to have the surgeon determine whether there is anything unusual about the case that warrants histologic examination. Walton[2] makes a convincing argument against the submission of all tissues because similar-appearing

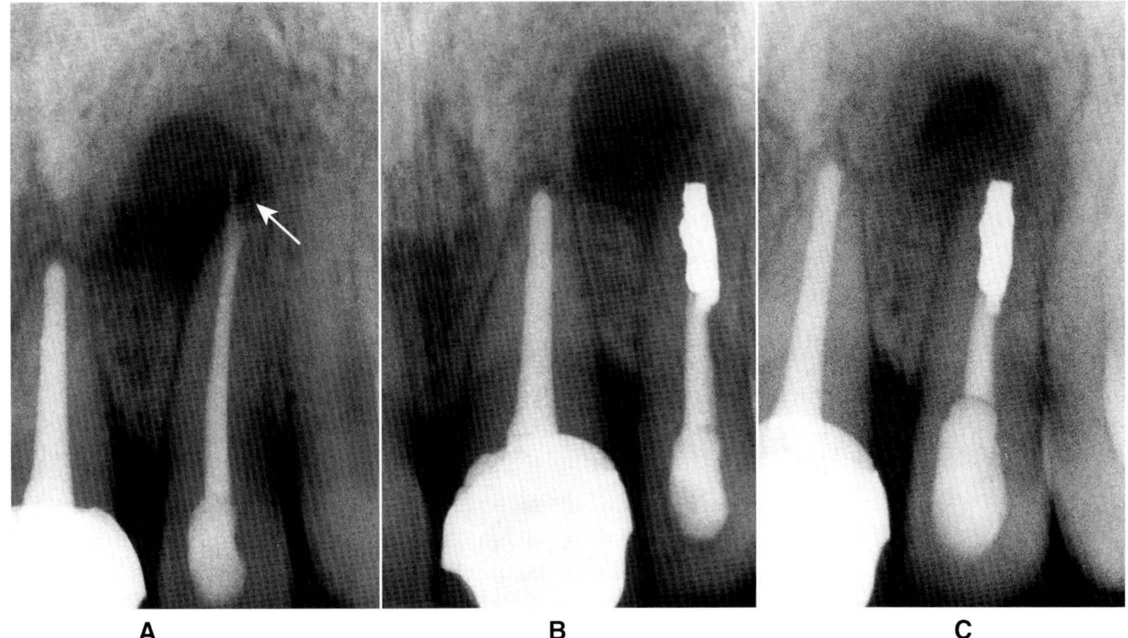

FIGURE 17-33 Healing by scar tissue. A, Failed treatment because of transportation and perforation, leaving area of canal (*arrow*) undébrided and unobturated. B, Root end resection, curettage, and root-end filling. C, After 2 years, an area of radiolucency is seen. Sharp border, separation from apex, and distinct radiolucency show this to be a scar.

radiolucencies that are not treated surgically do not have tissue retrieved for pathologic identification. It also is accepted that the differentiation between a periapical granuloma or periapical cyst has no direct bearing on clinical outcomes and therefore cannot be used as a rationalization for the submission of tissue.

The dilemma falls back to the surgeon that if a rare lesion should present itself in the context of a periapical lesion and a biopsy is not performed in a timely manner, the surgeon may have exposure in a potential malpractice suit. Many surgeons have a case or two in their careers that have "surprised" them based on the final pathologic diagnosis. However, careful review of these cases usually depicts a clinical situation inconsistent with a typical periapical infection.

An approach more logical than purely defensive is to set up guidelines upon which to determine that submission of tissue is not indicated. These guidelines are listed in Box 17-6. It is recommended that the surgeon have documented in the record the rationale for electing not to submit tissue in each specific case. At a recent meeting of the American Association of Oral and Maxillofacial Surgeons, only 8% of those attending a symposium on endodontic surgery "always" submit tissue for histologic examination.

BOX 17-6

Rationale Decision for Biopsy of Periapical Lesions

If all of the following criteria are met, the surgeon may decide not to submit routinely collected periapical tissue:

- Was there evidence of preendopulpal necrosis?
- Is the characteristic of the radiolucency "classic"?
- Will the patient return for follow-up radiographs?

ADJUNCTS

Some of the newer devices and materials have enhanced and, in some cases, improved surgical procedures. These include the light and magnification devices and techniques of guided tissue regeneration.

Light and Magnification Devices

Surgical Microscope

Recently, the microscope has been adapted and used for surgery, as well as for other diagnostic and treatment procedures in endodontics (Fig. 17-34). Advantages of the microscope include magnification and in-line illumination. Microscopes also can be adapted for videotaping and to transmit the image

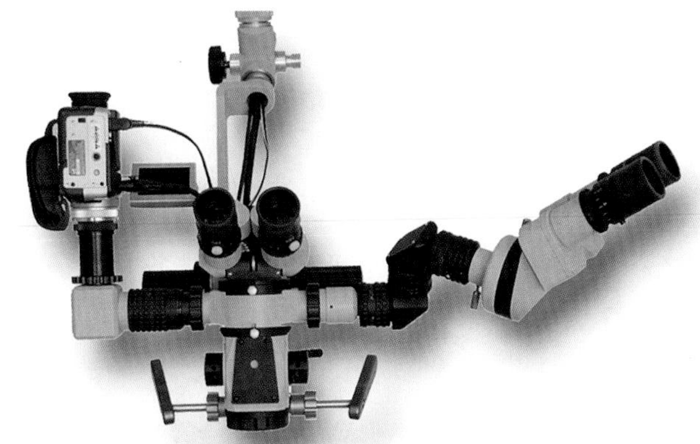

FIGURE 17-34 Surgical microscope has been adapted for endodontic procedures, including surgery. Magnification and in-line illumination enhance visualization for diagnosis and treatment. Add-on binoculars for dental assistant are useful adjunct. (From Johnson WT: *Color atlas of endodontics*, Philadelphia, 2002, WB Saunders.)

to a television monitor for direct viewing or recording. These adaptations enhance the view of the surgical field, help identify previously undetected structures, and facilitate surgical procedures. Although some clinicians advocate and are excited about the use of these microscopes, as yet there have not been demonstrated substantial clinical benefits through long-term controlled studies. However, some evidence suggests that the microscope use improves surgical techniques and short-term outcomes.

Fiberoptics

A new system, known as *endoscopy,* is available that uses a very small, flexible fiber bundle that contains a light and an optic system. The optics are connected to a monitor that permits visualization of precise details of the surgical site. This system also gives the clinician the option of videotaping and recording procedures.

Guided Tissue Regeneration

Originally intended for periodontal surgery, guided tissue regeneration also has been applied to endodontic surgery. The membranes used in this procedure are applied where defects have extended to cervical margins or as a covering of large defects surrounded by bone. These membranes, particularly those that are resorbable, may prove useful in selected situations. Yet evidence indicating their long-term effectiveness in endodontic surgery is incomplete, and studies have not shown an increase in bone density when a membrane is used. Whether use of membranes results in long-term, substantial benefits has not been demonstrated. My opinion is that the elimination of the source of infection permits regeneration of the junctional epithelium and healing without the use of membranes.

Bone Augmentation

Various substances have been placed in the periradicular surgical cavities in the attempt to enhance bony healing. Because of the location of the cavity and because most of the periphery is encased in bone or periosteum, bone regeneration is predictable. Such augmentation materials are of minimal to no benefit and need not be placed. Because the materials are being placed in a site with active infection, these adjuncts may then act as a nidus for infection.

WHEN TO CONSIDER REFERRAL

Although many of the procedures presented in this chapter appear relatively straightforward, endodontic surgery is often complex and difficult to perform. Clinicians should carefully consider the problems before undertaking such surgeries.

Training and Experience

Most generalists do not have the advanced training, including didactic and clinical experience, necessary to perform surgical procedures. These procedures are a unique discipline and require special skills in diagnosis, treatment planning, and management; they also require a special armamentarium. Also important are skill in long-term evaluation and resolution of failures or other complications. With increased emphasis on standards of care and litigation problems, coupled with the availability of experienced specialists, general dentists should consider their own expertise as it relates to case difficulty. These procedures are often the last hope of tooth retention. Lack of training may result in inadequate or inappropriate surgery and loss of a particular tooth and possible damage to other structures.

Determining the Cause of Root Canal Treatment Failure

Two steps are critical to success, particularly if surgery is being considered: (1) *identification of the cause of failure* and (2) *design of the treatment plan.* Frequently, surgery is not the best choice but when necessary must be done appropriately. A specialist is better able to identify these causes and approach their resolution. If the cause of the failure cannot be identified, these cases must be considered for referral.

Surgical Difficulties

In many situations, surgical accessibility is limited and even hazardous. For example, the neurovascular bundle near mandibular posterior teeth and maxillary palatal root apices presents the potential for creating paresthesia, excessive hemorrhage, or both. Complicating structures include overlying bone throughout the mandible and in the palate, the frena and other muscle attachments, fenestrations of cortical bone, and sinus cavities. These structures require care and the proper use of instruments and surgical skill.

In summary, most of the procedures discussed in this chapter require greater training and experience than are provided in an undergraduate dental education program. If the clinician has not had additional postgraduate training and experience, referral should be considered.

REFERENCES

1. Tamse A, Fuss Z, Lustig J et al: Radiographic features of vertically fractured, endodontically treated maxillary premolars, *Oral Surg Oral Med Oral Pathol Oral Radiol Endod* 88:348-352, 1999.
2. Walton RE: Routine histopathologic examination of endodontic periradicular surgical specimens: is it warranted? *Oral Surg Oral Med Oral Pathol Oral Radiol Endod* 86(5):505, 1998.

Bibliography

Andreassen J, Rud J: Correlation between histology and radiography in the assessment of healing after endodontic surgery in 70 cases, *Int J Oral Surg* 1:161, 1972.

Danin J, Linder LE, Lundqvist G et al: Outcomes of periradicular surgery in cases with apical pathosis and untreated canals, *Oral Surg Oral Med Oral Pathol Oral Radiol Endod* 87:227, 1999.

El Deeb ME, Tabibi A, Jensen MR Jr: An evaluation of the use of amalgam, Cavit and calcium hydroxide in the repair of furcation perforations, *J Endod* 8:459, 1982.

El-Swiah JM, Walker RT: Reasons for apicectomies: a retrospective study, *Endod Dent Traumatol* 12:185, 1996.

Forbes G: Apical microsurgery for failed endodontics, *Atlas Oral Maxillofac Surg Clin North Am* 8:1, 2000.

Garrett KK, Kerr MM, Hartwell G: The effect of a bioresorbable matrix barrier in endodontic surgery on the rate of periapical healing: an in vivo study, *J Endod* 28:503-506, 2002.

Gray G, Hatton JF, Holtzmann DJ et al: Quality of root-end preparations using ultrasonic and rotary instrumentation in cadavers, *J Endod* 26:281, 2000.

Gutmann JL, Dumsha TC, Lovdahl PE: *Problem solving in endodontics: prevention, identification, and management,* ed 4, St Louis, 2006, Mosby.

Gutmann JL, Harrison JW: Posterior endodontic surgery: anatomical consideration and clinical techniques, *Int Endod J* 18:8, 1985.

Gutmann JL, Harrison JW: *Surgical endodontics*, Boston, 1994, Blackwell Scientific.

Harrison JW, Jurosky KA: Wound healing in the periodontium following endodontic surgery. 1. The incisional wound, *J Endod* 17:425, 1991.

Harrison JW, Jurosky KA: Wound healing in the periodontium following endodontic surgery. 2. The dissectional wound, *J Endod* 17:544, 1991.

Harrison JW, Jurosky KA: Wound healing in the periodontium following endodontic surgery. 3. The osseous excisional wound, *J Endod* 18:76, 1992.

Iqblal M, Kim S: For teeth requiring endodontic treatment, what are the differences in outcomes of restored endodontically treated teeth compared to implant supported restorations? *Int J Oral Maxillofac Implants* 22(suppl):96-116, 2007.

Lieblich SE: Periapical surgery: clinical decision making, *Oral and Maxillofacial Clinics of North America* 14:179-186, 2002.

Lieblich SE, McGivenin WE: Ultrasonic retrograde preparation, *Oral and Maxillofacial Clinics of North America* 14:167-172, 2002.

Lubow RM, Wayman BE, Cooley RL: Endodontic flap design: analysis and recommendation for current usage, *Oral Surg Oral Med Oral Pathol* 58:207, 1984.

McDonald N, Torabinejad M: Surgical endodontics. In Walton R, Torabinejad M, editors: *Principles and practice of endodontics*, ed 3, Philadelphia, 2002, WB Saunders.

Morgan LA, Marshall JG: A scanning electron microscopic study of in vivo ultrasonic root-end preparations, *J Endod* 25:567, 1999.

Pantschev A, Carlsson AP, Andersson L: Retrograde root filling with EBA cement or amalgam: a comparative clinical study, *Oral Surg Oral Med Oral Pathol* 78:101, 1994.

Sauveur G, Roth F, Sobel M et al: The control of haemorrhage at the operative site during periradicular surgery, *Int Endod J* 32:225, 1999.

Shabahang S: State of the art and science of endodontics, *J Am Dent Assoc* 136:41, 2005.

Skoner JR, Wallace JA, Fochtman F et al: Blood mercury levels with amalgam retroseals: a longitudinal study, *J Endod* 22:140, 1996.

Stromberg T, Hasselgren G, Bergstedt H: Endodontic treatment of traumatic root perforations in man: a clinical and roentgenological follow-up study, *Sven Tandlak Tidskr* 65:457, 1972.

Tamse A, Fuss Z, Lustig J et al: Radiographic features of vertically fractured, endodontically treated maxillary premolars, *Oral Surg Oral Med Oral Pathol Oral Radiol Endod* 88:348-352, 1999.

Torabinejad M, Chivian N: Clinical applications of mineral trioxide aggregate, *J Endod* 25:197, 1999.

Von Arx T: Failed root canals: the case for apicoectomy (periradicular surgery), *J Oral Maxillofac Surg* 63:832, 2005.

Von Arx T, Walker WA III: Microsurgical instruments for root-end cavity preparation following apicoectomy: a literature review, *Endod Dent Traumatol* 16:47, 2000.

Walton RE: Routine histopathologic examination of endodontic periradicular surgical specimens: is it warranted? *Oral Surg Oral Med Oral Pathol Oral Radiol Endod* 86(5):505, 1998.

Witherspoon D, Gutmann J: Haemostasis in periradicular surgery, *Int Endod J* 29:135, 1996.

Zuolo ML, Ferreira MOF, Gutmann JL: Prognosis in periradicular surgery: a clinical prospective study, *Int Endod J* 33:91, 2000.

CHAPTER 18

Management of the Patient Undergoing Radiotherapy or Chemotherapy

EDWARD ELLIS III

CHAPTER OUTLINE

DENTAL MANAGEMENT OF PATIENTS UNDERGOING RADIOTHERAPY TO THE HEAD AND NECK

Radiotherapy (i.e., radiation therapy and x-ray treatment) is a common therapeutic modality for malignancies of the head and neck. Approximately 30,000 cases of head and neck cancer occur each year. Many of these are managed by therapeutic irradiation. The use of therapeutic irradiation is *ideally* predicated on the ability of the radiation to destroy neoplastic cells while sparing normal cells. In practice, however, this is never actually achieved, and normal tissues experience some undesirable effect. Any neoplasm can be destroyed by radiation if the dose delivered to the neoplastic cells is sufficient. The limiting factor is the amount of radiation that the surrounding tissues can tolerate.

Radiotherapy destroys neoplastic (and normal) cells by interfering with nuclear material necessary for reproduction, cell maintenance, or both. The faster the cellular turnover, the more susceptible the tissue is to the damaging effects of radiation. Thus neoplastic cells, which are usually reproducing at higher rates than normal tissue, are selectively destroyed (relatively). In practice, normal tissues with rapid turnover rates are also affected to some degree. Therefore, hematopoietic cells, epithelial cells, and endothelial cells are affected soon after radiotherapy begins.

Early in the course of radiotherapy, the oral mucosa shows the effects of treatment. Most notable to dentistry are the changes in and around the oral cavity as the result of destruction of the fine vasculature. Salivary glands and bone are relatively radioresistant, but because of the intense vascular compromise resulting from radiotherapy, these tissues bear a considerable hardship in the long run.

Radiation Effects on Oral Mucosa

The initial effect of radiotherapy on the oral mucosa, which is seen in the first 1 or 2 weeks, is an erythema that may progress to a severe mucositis with or without ulceration. Pain and dysphagia may be severe and make adequate nutritional intake difficult. These mucosal reactions begin to subside after completion of the course of radiotherapy. The taste buds, also composed of epithelial cells, show similar reactions. Loss of taste is a prominent complaint early in treatment and gradually returns, depending on the quantity and quality of saliva that remains after treatment.

Relief from mucositis is not predictable. Antibiotic lozenges containing amphotericin, tobramycin, and neomycin may be of some benefit.[1] When symptoms are severe, viscous lidocaine can be useful.

The long-term effects of radiotherapy to the oral mucosa are characterized by a predisposition to breakdown and delayed healing, even after minor insult. The epithelium is thin and less keratinized, and the submucosa is less vascular, which gives a pale appearance to the tissue. Radiotherapy induces submucosal fibrosis, which makes the mucosal lining of the oral cavity less pliable and less resilient. Minor trauma may create ulcerations that take weeks or months to heal. These ulcerations are often difficult to differentiate from recurrent malignant disease.

Radiation Effects on Mandibular Mobility

When irradiated, the pterygomasseteric sling and periarticular connective tissues become inflamed. Irradiated muscle becomes fibrotic and tends to contract, and the articular surfaces degenerate.[2] These factors herald the onset of trismus. The decrease in ability to open the mouth may be insidious in onset, usually occurring over the first year after radiation therapy, and is painless. When the interincisal opening decreases to 20 mm, feeding becomes difficult. Additionally, inability to open the mouth wide makes it difficult to perform dental work and to provide a general anesthetic.

Radiation Effects on Salivary Glands

Salivary gland epithelium has a slow turnover rate; therefore the salivary glands might be expected to be radioresistant. However, because of the destruction of the fine vasculature by the radiation, the salivary glands show considerable damage, with resultant atrophy, fibrosis, and degeneration. This damage manifests clinically as xerostomia (the decreased production of saliva) and gives the patient a "dry mouth." The severity of xerostomia depends on which salivary glands were within the field of radiation. A dry mouth may be the patient's most significant complaint.

Loss of salivary function leads to a plethora of adverse sequelae, including difficulty with tasting, chewing, and swallowing; difficulty sleeping; esophageal dysfunction, including chronic esophagitis; nutritional compromises; higher frequency of intolerance to medications; increased incidence of glossitis, candidiasis, angular cheilitis, halitosis, and bacterial sialadenitis; decreased resistance to loss of tooth structure from attrition, abrasion, and erosion; loss of buffering capacity; increased susceptibility to mucosal injury; inability to wear dental prostheses; and rampant caries.

The effects of xerostomia on the oral cavity are devastating. Because saliva is the principal protector of the oral tissues, absence results in serious complications. Salivary proteins such as peroxidase, lysozyme, and lactoferrin are antibacterial and limit the growth of cariogenic bacteria. The film of salivary mucins on the teeth and mucosal surfaces is believed to protect these oral structures from wear. Histatins, a family of salivary proteins, have potent antifungal properties that limit the growth of oral yeast. These salivary components, in conjunction with the mucosal tissues, form part of the innate immune system that continually protects the human body from infection. The oral cavity also is protected by secretory immunoglobulins A and M, which are produced locally by B cells within the salivary glands. These antibodies include those with specificity against oral cariogenic bacteria. When salivary volume is reduced significantly, patients are at risk for serious oral complications.

The xerostomia makes it difficult for patients to eat a normal diet because of dysphagia. Patients therefore may adopt a more cariogenic diet. Rampant "radiation caries" can swiftly destroy the remaining dentition and predispose the patient to severe infections of the jaws (Fig. 18-1). Teeth thus affected exhibit decay around the entire circumference of the cervical portion (Fig. 18-2). Periodontitis is also accelerated in the absence of saliva. Dysgeusia, dysphonia, and dysphagia are also caused by xerostomia. Another sequela of low salivary flow is an increase in oral infections such as candidiasis.

Treatment of Xerostomia

After radiotherapy, patients often complain of chronic dry mouth. At present, no general agreement exists concerning how to prevent these changes. Unfortunately, in many cases, xerostomia never improves substantially, and exogenous replacement of saliva is necessary. For the simplest form of replacement, water can be sipped throughout the day. Sipping water during meals aids in chewing, swallowing, and taste perception. In addition, several saliva substitutes can be obtained without a prescription at the pharmacy. These substitutes contain several of the ions in saliva and other ingredients (e.g., glycerin) to mimic the lubricating action of saliva. Patients should be advised not to use products containing alcohol or strong flavors, which may irritate the mucosa. Patients should avoid sugar-containing products because of their increased susceptibility to dental caries. Many of the salivary substitutes available in the United States contain carboxymethylcellulose, whereas animal-derived mucin-based products are available in other countries. Studies have shown that the use of these products reduces the severity of symptoms associated with xerostomia.[3,4]

Unfortunately, artificial salivas on the market do not possess the protective proteins that are present in the salivary secretions. The patients are therefore still prone to the problems induced by xerostomia. For comfort, however, many patients seem to be just as satisfied with plain water as artificial salivas and keep small quantities available at all times to sip.

Efforts to stimulate the patient's residual saliva have met with some success. Sugar-free chewing gum stimulates saliva production as long as there is some saliva being produced.[5] The Food and Drug Administration has now approved the use of two medications to stimulate the flow of saliva: (1) pilocarpine hydrochloride and (2) cevimeline hydrochloride, which have been shown to relieve symptoms of xerostomia for patients with xerostomia.[6] Both drugs are parasympathomimetic agents that function primarily as muscarinic agonists, causing stimulation of exocrine gland secretion. This stimulation can increase the production of saliva, even in patients whose salivary glands have been exposed to radiation. An oral dose of 5 mg of

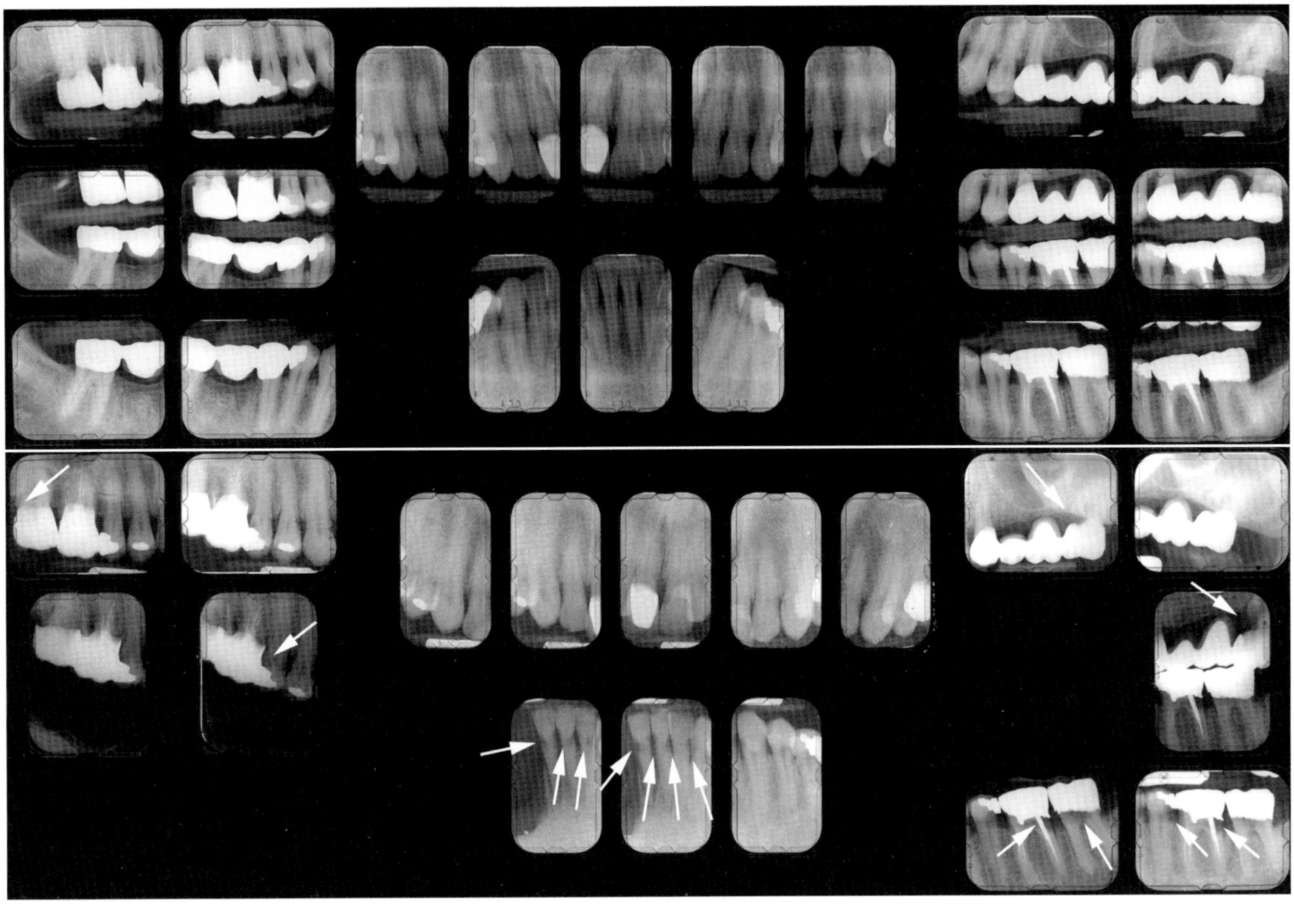

FIGURE 18-1 Radiographs illustrating the rapidity with which dental caries can occur in an irradiated patient. A, Periapical radiographs taken just before radiation therapy. B, Periapical radiographs taken 16 months after radiation therapy. Note the prevalence and severity of dental caries that have occurred throughout the dentition (*arrows*).

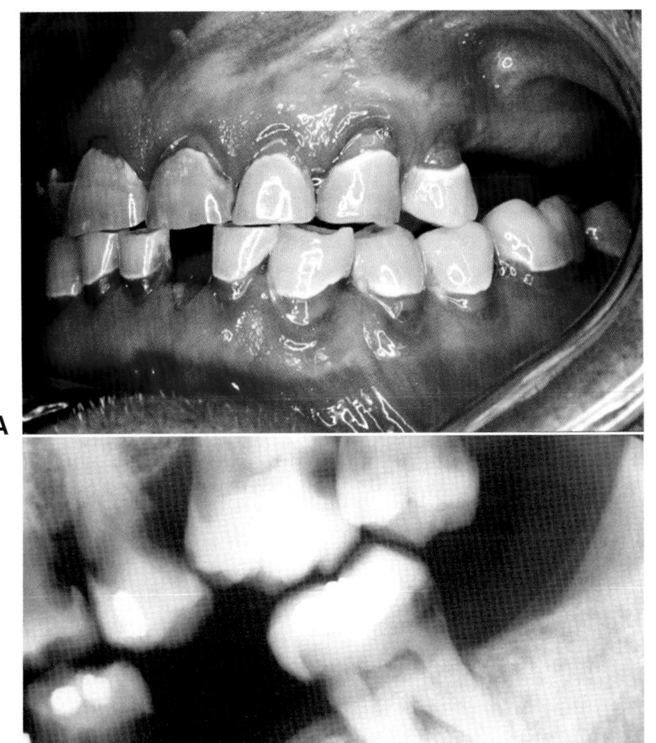

FIGURE 18-2 A, Typical clinical appearance of radiation caries. B, Typical radiographic appearance of radiation caries. Note the erosion around the cervical portion of the teeth.

pilocarpine 4 times each day or 30 mg of cevimeline 3 times a day has been shown to improve many symptoms of xerostomia without significant drug-related side effects.[7-12] The administration of these medications may prove to be beneficial for some patients with postradiation xerostomia.

Radiation Effects on Bone

One of the most severe and complicating sequelae of radiotherapy for patients with head and neck cancer is osteoradionecrosis (Fig. 18-3). Basically, osteoradionecrosis is devitalization of the bone by cancericidal doses of radiation. The bone within the radiation beam becomes virtually nonvital from an endarteritis that results in elimination of the fine vasculature within the bone. The turnover rate of any remaining viable bone is slowed to the point of being ineffective in self-repair. The continual process of remodeling normally found in bone does not occur, and sharp areas on the alveolar ridge will not smooth themselves, even with considerable time (Fig. 18-4). The bone of the mandible is denser and has a poorer blood supply than that of the maxilla. Thus the mandible is the jaw most commonly affected with nonhealing ulcerations and osteoradionecrosis.

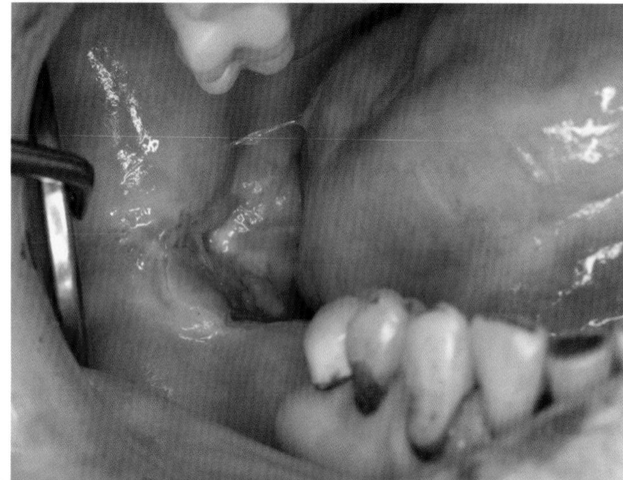

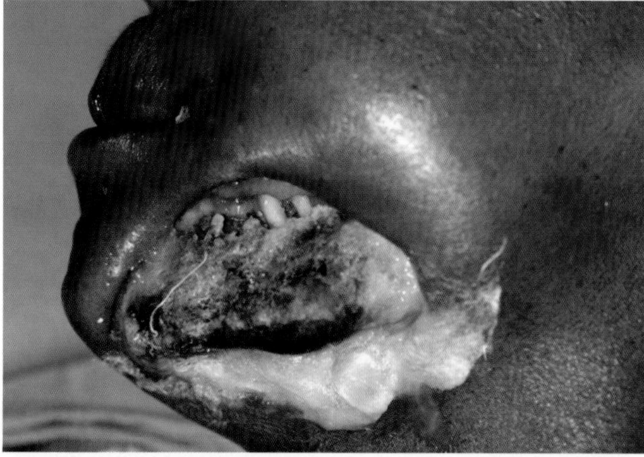

FIGURE 18-3 Two cases of osteoradionecrosis of the mandible. **A**, Bone exposure occurred 3 weeks after tooth extraction. **B**, Severe osteoradionecrosis of the mandible with dehiscence of the facial soft tissues, exposing the necrotic bone externally.

Other Effects of Radiation

Patients undergoing radiotherapy may have an alteration in the normal oral flora, with overgrowth of anaerobic species and fungi. Most researchers feel that oral flora colonizing the mucous membranes play an important role in the severity of mucositis and subsequent healing process.[13,14] *Candida albicans* commonly thrives in the oral cavities of patients who have been irradiated. Whether the alteration in the flora is caused by the radiation itself or the resultant xerostomia is not known. Patients frequently require the application of topical antifungal agents, such as nystatin, to help control the number of *Candida* organisms present. Another oral rinse frequently prescribed is 0.1% chlorhexidine (Peridex). This agent has been shown to have potent in vitro antibacterial and antifungal effects. When used throughout the course of radiation treatment, it has been shown in at least one study to reduce greatly the prevalence and symptoms associated with radiation-induced mucositis.[15] The use of chlorhexidine in other studies has been equivocal.[13,16]

Evaluation of Dentition Before Radiotherapy

The most feared side effect of radiotherapy is osteoradionecrosis. Most patients who have this complication have residual teeth throughout the course of radiotherapy. Thus the clinician may wonder what to do with the teeth before irradiation. Should teeth be extracted? This question has no categoric answer; however, several factors must be considered.[17-20]

Condition of Residual Dentition

All teeth with a questionable or poor prognosis should be extracted before radiotherapy. The more advanced the periodontal condition, the more likely the patient is to have caries and continued periodontitis. Although this may not be in keeping with usual dental principles, *if in doubt, extract.* Extraction in these cases may spare the patient months or years of suffering from osteoradionecrosis.

Patient's Dental Awareness

The present state of the dentition and periodontium is a good clue to the past care they have received. In patients with excellent oral hygiene and oral health, the clinician should retain as many of the teeth as possible. Conversely, in patients who have neglected oral health for years, the chances are that they will continue to do so, especially in the face of severe xerostomia and oral pain, which will make oral hygiene even more difficult. Preradiotherapy patient preparation is similar to preorthodontic patient preparation. If an individual cannot or will not care for his or her mouth before the application of the braces, it will be impossible for him or her to do so when faced with future obstacles.

Immediacy of Radiotherapy

If the radiotherapist feels that therapy must be instituted urgently, there may not be time to perform the necessary extractions and allow for initial healing of the extraction sites. In this instance, the dentist may elect to maintain the dentition but must work closely with the patient throughout the course of radiotherapy and thereafter in an attempt to maintain oral health as optimally as possible.

Radiation Location

The more salivary glands and bone involved in the field of radiation, the more severe the resultant xerostomia and vascular

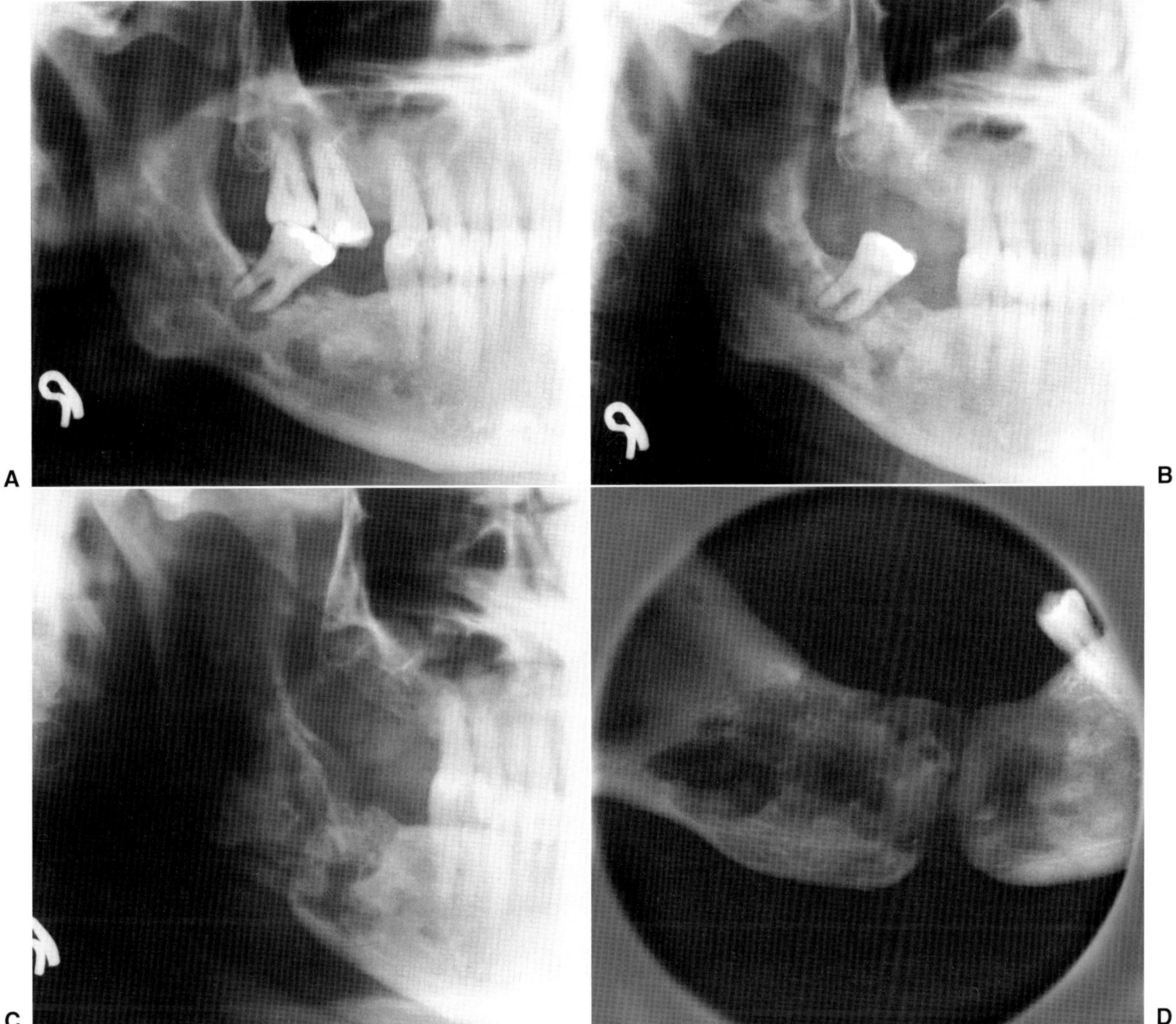

FIGURE 18-4 Progressive course of osteoradionecrosis. **A**, Radiograph showing radiolucencies in right mandible and around apex of molar tooth. **B**, Six months later, during which time antibiotics and local irrigations were used, radiolucent process is spreading into ramus. Molar was removed at this time. **C**, Five months after tooth removal, extraction site did not heal and destructive process spread, resulting in pathologic fracture of mandible. **D**, Radiograph after removal of devitalized bone, showing extent of process. (Courtesy Dr. Richard Scott, Ann Arbor, Mich.)

compromise of the jaws. Thus the dentist should discuss with the radiotherapist the locations of the radiation beams and should estimate the severity of the probable xerostomia and bone changes. Xerostomia by itself may not result in severe problems if the dentition can be maintained because the bone is still healthy. The combination of xerostomia and irradiated bone usually causes the problem. In individuals who will have radiation to the major salivary glands *and* a portion of the mandible, preirradiation extractions should be considered. Frequently, the radiotherapist agrees to delay the institution of irradiation for 1 to 2 weeks if the dentist feels that time is necessary to allow the extraction sites to begin to heal.

Radiation Dose

The higher the radiation dose, the more severe the normal tissue damage. The radiotherapist should discuss with the dentist the amount of radiation planned for the individual. Frequently, the dose is not maximal, and tissue damage may be minimized. This allows the dentist to be more conservative in preirradiation extraction considerations.

Squamous cell carcinomas of the oral cavity make up approximately 90% of malignant tumors for which radiation therapy is used. Unfortunately, this cancer requires a large dose of radiation (greater than 6000 rad [60 Gy]) to effect a result. Other malignancies, such as lymphoma, require much less radiation for a response, and the oral cavity therefore is less affected. When the total dose falls below 5000 rad (50 Gy), long-term side effects, such as xerostomia and osteoradionecrosis, are dramatically decreased.

Preparation of Dentition for Radiotherapy and Maintenance After Irradiation

Every tooth to be maintained must be carefully inspected for pathologic conditions and restored to the best state of health obtainable. A thorough prophylaxis and topical fluoride application should be performed before radiotherapy. Oral hygiene measures and instructions should be demonstrated and reinforced. Any sharp cusps should be rounded to prevent mechanical irritation. Impressions for dental casts should be obtained for fabrication of custom fluoride trays to be used during and after treatment. Because tobacco use and alcohol consumption irritate the mucosa, the patient should be encouraged to stop these before commencement of radiation therapy.

During radiation treatment the patient should rinse the mouth at least 10 times a day with saline rinses. The patient should be placed on chlorhexidine mouth rinses twice a day to help minimize the bacterial and fungal levels within the mouth. The dentist should see the patient each week during the radiotherapy for observation and oral hygiene evaluations. If an overgrowth of *C. albicans* occurs, nystatin or clotrimazole topical applications will bring this under control relatively rapidly. The ability of the patient to open the mouth should be carefully monitored throughout the course of radiation treatment. Radiation causes a progressive fibrosis within the muscles of mastication that makes it difficult for the patient to open the mouth adequately. Patients should be instructed in physiotherapy exercises to maintain the preirradiation treatment interincisal dimension. All patients must be weighed weekly to determine whether they are maintaining an adequate nutritional status. The combination of mucositis and xerostomia makes oral intake extremely uncomfortable. However, malnutrition causes further difficulties by delaying healing of the oral tissues and giving the patient an overall feeling of generalized illness. In severe cases, it may be necessary to feed the patient via nasogastric tube to maintain a reasonable nutritional status.

After radiation treatment the dentist should see the patient every 3 to 4 months. A prophylaxis is performed during these postirradiation visits, and topical fluoride applications are made. The patient should be fitted with custom trays to deliver topical fluoride applications. The patient should be instructed in the use of the trays and in *daily* self-administration of topical fluoride applications. The use of a 1% fluoride rinse for 5 minutes each day has been found to decrease the incidence of radiation caries.[21] Over-the-counter fluoride rinses currently available can be used without a customized delivery splint with good success and seem to have better patient acceptance.

All patients should also be monitored for the possible onset of trismus. It is easier to prevent trismus than to treat it. The patient should perform mouth-opening exercises when there is any decrease in the maximum interincisal dimension. For more established cases, the patient can use jaw exercising (i.e., Therabyte).

Method of Performing Preirradiation Extractions

If the decision has been made to extract some or all teeth before radiotherapy, the question becomes "How should the teeth be extracted?" In general, the principles of atraumatic exodontia apply. However, the concepts of bone preservation are disregarded, and an attempt is made to remove a good portion of the alveolar process along with the teeth and achieve a primary soft tissue closure. With the onset of radiotherapy, the normal remodeling process is inhibited; if any sharp areas of bone exist, ulceration occurs with bone exposure. Thus the teeth are usually removed in a surgical manner, with flap reflection and generous bone removal.

Atraumatic handling of the mucoperiosteal flaps is necessary to ensure a rapid soft tissue healing. Burs or files should be used to smooth the bony edges under copious irrigation because the remodeling capability of the tissues is greatly decreased after radiotherapy. Prophylactic antibiotics are indicated under these circumstances. *Note: The dentist is in a race against time. If the wound fails to heal, the radiotherapy will be delayed. If the radiation is delivered before the wound heals, healing will take months or even years.*

Interval Between Preirradiation Extractions and Beginning of Radiotherapy

No categoric answer exists to the question of how much time should be allowed after extractions before beginning radiotherapy. Obviously, the sooner radiotherapy is begun, the more beneficial it may be for treating the malignancy. Thus when the soft tissues have healed sufficiently, radiotherapy may begin. Traditionally, 7 to 14 days between tooth extraction and radiotherapy have been suggested.[17,22,23] Most authors base their recommendations on the clinical impression that reepithelialization has occurred in this period. However, radiotherapy should be delayed for 3 weeks after extraction, if possible. This helps to ensure that sufficient soft tissue healing has occurred. The radiotherapy should be delayed further, if possible, if a local wound dehiscence has occurred. In this instance, daily local wound care with irrigations and postoperatively administered antibiotics are mandatory until the soft tissues have healed.

Impacted Third Molar Removal Before Radiotherapy

If the patient has a partially erupted mandibular third molar, removal may be prudent to prevent pericoronal infection. In general, however, allowing a tooth that is totally impacted within the bone of the mandible to remain in place is more expeditious than removing it and waiting for it to heal.

Methods of Managing Carious Teeth After Radiotherapy

Teeth that develop postradiotherapy caries must be immediately cared for in an attempt to prevent further spread of infection. Composites and amalgam are the materials of choice to repair the defects caused by caries. Full crowns are probably not warranted because recurrent caries is more difficult to detect under such restorations. Oral hygiene measures, including fluoride application, must be reinforced in any patient who has postirradiation caries.

If a tooth has a necrotic pulp, endodontic intervention with systemic antibiotics can be carefully performed and the tooth can be ground out of occlusion and maintained. Frequently, root canal treatment is difficult because of a progressive sclerosis of the pulp chamber that occurs in irradiated teeth. In such instances, the tooth can simply be amputated above the gingiva and left in place.

Tooth Extraction After Radiotherapy

Can teeth be extracted after radiotherapy, and if so, how? These are probably the most difficult questions to answer. Each dentist has a view on this subject, and the literature is contradictory. Postirradiation extractions are also the most undesirable extractions the dentist will ever perform because the outcome is always uncertain.

The answer to the question of whether extractions *can* be done after radiotherapy is certainly yes. The more important question is, How? If the tooth is to be extracted, the dentist can perform a routine extraction without primary soft tissue closure or a surgical extraction with alveoloplasty and primary closure. Either of these techniques yields similar results, with a certain concomitant incidence of osteoradionecrosis. The use of systemic antibiotics is recommended.

Another technique that has been shown to be effective and that is gaining in popularity is the use of hyperbaric oxygen (HBO) *before* and *after* tooth extraction. HBO therapy is the administration of oxygen under pressure to the patient. HBO has been shown to increase the local tissue oxygenation and vascular ingrowth into the hypoxic tissues.[24,25] The usual protocol for such treatments is to have between 20 and 30 HBO dives before extraction and 10 more dives immediately after extractions. HBO chambers are not available in all communities and, when present, are usually in select hospitals. A physician that is experienced in hyperbaric medicine manages patients referred to these facilities. The patient usually undergoes one HBO session each day. Therefore, it takes 4 to 6 weeks to get the 20 to 30 treatments before surgery, and 2 weeks of treatment after surgery. In a prospective clinical trial comparing this regimen with the use of prophylactically administered antibiotics before dental extraction without hyperbaric oxygenation, Marx et al.[26] found a significant decrease in the incidence of osteoradionecrosis (5.4% compared with 30%).

Because considerable controversy exists over how to manage an extraction surgically in a patient who has undergone irradiation, because few hyperbaric oxygenation chambers are available for use, and because the incidence of severe complications is relatively high, it is recommended that an oral and maxillofacial surgeon manage the patient who has received irradiation and requires extractions.

Denture Wear in Postirradiation Edentulous Patients

Patients who were edentulous before radiotherapy manage nicely with well-constructed dentures. However, patients rendered edentulous just before or after radiotherapy exhibit more problems with mucosal ulcerations and subsequent osteoradionecrosis. The normal remodeling process of the alveolar bone cannot smooth even the most minor irregularities left by extraction. With denture wear, these minor irregularities cause ulceration of the mucosa.

Soft denture liners might seem an ideal solution for patients who have received irradiation. However, the silicone soft liners proved to be not particularly useful for several reasons. At present, patients are probably best served with ordinary dentures.

Denture fabrication for patients who were previously edentulous can proceed once the acute effects of irradiation have subsided. For patients who underwent extractions just before or after radiotherapy, it is prudent to see them frequently after delivery of their dentures to make adjustments for sore spots that develop before they cause mucosal breakdown and bone exposure.

When dentures are constructed, the dentist must be certain that the denture base and occlusal table are designed so that forces are distributed evenly throughout the alveolar ridge and that lateral forces on the denture are eliminated.

Use of Dental Implants in Irradiated Patients

The dental rehabilitation of the edentulous patient who has received radiation therapy is one of the greatest challenges facing the reconstructive dentist. Many patients who have had ablative surgery for malignancy do not have the normal anatomy that makes denture wear possible. There may be no vestibules to accommodate a denture flange.

Often, portions of the tongue have been removed. The patient may have hard and soft tissue defects and deficits. When reconstructed, the bone may have poor form for support of a tissue-borne prosthesis. Frequently, such patients have thick, nonpliable soft tissue flaps that have been grafted from distant areas and are not adherent to the underlying bone. All of these combine to make conventional denture fabrication challenging. In such instances, the use of implant-borne prostheses are preferred from a functional standpoint.

For years, however, a history of irradiation has been a relative contraindication to the placement of dental implants.[27] The effects of radiation on bone and soft tissue present a formidable challenge to the use of implanted metallic devices. It has been demonstrated that there is a 19% reduction of bone-to-implant contact of a cylindric titanium plasma–sprayed implants in rabbit tibiae after 4050 cGy irradiation during the initial healing time.[28] Not surprising, numerous clinical studies evaluating the success rates of intraoral endosseous implants placed in previously irradiated bone beds with and without adjunct HBO treatment have demonstrated success rates slightly to substantially less than in nonirradiated patients.[29-37]

However, the benefits that can accrue from providing this group of patients with a functional and esthetic dental reconstruction are great. Such patients have been through a great deal of hardship. They have lost portions of their anatomy, are frequently deformed, and feel the uncomfortable effects of the radiation therapy, such as xerostomia, dysphagia, and dysgeusia. They relish the thought of being able to chew solid food with a functional dentition. Implant-borne prostheses can help achieve this goal in these difficult situations. However, the unpredictable reaction of soft and hard tissue in an irradiated patient and the surgical trauma of treatment have combined to promote caution in such cases.

Many variables must be evaluated when considering placement of dental implants into irradiated bone, including the radiation type, dose, sites, elapsed time since the treatment, protection provided to the bone during treatment, and the patient's own physiologic responses (which themselves are affected by age, sex, genetics, smoking, and other systemic considerations). Other critical factors are whether the implants will be placed into irradiated host mandibular bone, irradiated bone grafts, or bone that has been transplanted after the radiation therapy. In the latter instance, if the mandible was reconstructed using a microvascular graft in which the blood supply to the bone is brought in from a distant source and has not been altered by the previous radiation therapy, no adverse tissue reaction should be expected after placement of dental implants.

When dental implants are to be placed into irradiated host or grafted bone, the dentist must proceed with caution. Consultation with the radiotherapist is recommended to determine the amount of radiation that has been delivered to the area of the jaws where the proposed implants will be placed. Studies have provided insight into the use of implants in irradiated bone. In general, they have shown the following:

1. The more radiation delivered, the higher the failure rate for endosseous implants.[30,36]
2. The longer the duration between radiation treatment and implantation, the higher the failure rate.[36]
3. When implants in irradiated patients fail, they usually fail early, before prosthetic reconstruction, indicating a failure of osseointegration.[36]
4. The combination of radiation and chemotherapy has a particularly negative effect on the outcome for osseointegration.[36]
5. Implant survival in irradiated patients tends to be higher in the maxilla than in the mandible.[35,36,38,39]
6. Shorter implants have the worst prognosis.[36]
7. HBO treatment reduces implant failure rates.[36]

It has been demonstrated that the success of implant retention is directly and positively correlated with the amount of radiation to which the bone was exposed.[30,36] If the amount of radiation is less than approximately 4500 rad (45 Gy), implants may be placed with care. When the amount of radiation exceeds this amount, preoperative (20 to 30) and postoperative (10) HBO treatments should be considered. HBO treatments have been shown to be beneficial in such patients.[36,40]

The time required for osseointegration will be prolonged in irradiated patients because of the lower metabolic activity in the bone, so the implants should not be loaded for at least 6 months after placement. The dentist must pay particular attention to oral hygiene in such patients because their tissues will not be as able to resist bacterial invasion as tissues in patients who have not been irradiated. The prosthetic design should therefore be made as cleanable as possible, with frequent use of overdentures. However, prostheses that do not allow contact of denture flanges with the oral soft tissues help prevent ulceration. No matter what type of prosthesis is fabricated, these patients require more careful follow-up and hygiene measures.

In spite of the fear that implants placed into irradiated bone will lead to osteoradionecrosis, the condition is uncommonly reported in the literature (Fig. 18-5).[41,42] However, there has been an insufficient duration of experience to predict the long-term outcome of implant prosthetics in the patient who has undergone radiation.

Management of Patients Who Have Osteoradionecrosis

Most mucosal breakdown and subsequent osteoradionecrosis occur in the mandible (Fig. 18-4). These conditions occur most often in mandibles that have received radiation in excess of 6500 rad (65 Gy) and do not usually occur in mandibles that have received radiation doses less than 4800 rad (48 Gy).[43-45] Severe pain may follow. The patient should discontinue wearing any prosthesis and try to maintain a good state of oral health. Irrigations should be instituted to remove necrotic debris. Only occasionally are systemic antibiotics necessary because osteoradionecrosis is not an infection of the bone but rather a nonhealing hypoxic wound.[24] Because of the decreased vascularity of the tissues, systemic antibiotics do not gain ready access to the area to perform the function for which they are intended. However, in acute secondary infections, antibiotics may be useful to help prevent spread of the infection. Any loose sequestra are removed, but no attempt is made initially to close the soft tissues over the exposed bone. Most wounds smaller than 1 cm eventually heal, although it may take weeks to months.

For nonhealing wounds or extensive areas of osteoradionecrosis, surgical intervention may be indicated. In this instance, resection of the exposed bone and a margin of unexposed bone and primary soft tissue closure can be attempted (Fig. 18-6). This treatment is successful in many cases. Greatly improved results have recently been obtained by the use of HBO therapy in conjunction with surgical intervention.[24]

Reconstructive efforts with bone grafts used for continuity defects can also be undertaken successfully in many patients who have undergone irradiation. Free microvascular grafting techniques are becoming more popular for restoring continuity defects in patients who have received radiotherapy. These bone grafts have their own blood supply from a reconnection of blood vessels and are therefore less dependent on the local tissues for incorporation and healing.

DENTAL MANAGEMENT OF PATIENTS RECEIVING SYSTEMIC CHEMOTHERAPY FOR MALIGNANT DISEASE

Destruction of malignant cells by tumoricidal chemotherapeutic drugs has proved an effective treatment for a variety of malignancies. Like radiotherapy, the antitumor effect of cancer chemotherapeutic agents is based on their ability to destroy or retard the division of rapidly proliferating cells, such as tumor cells, nonspecifically. Unfortunately, normal host cells that have a high mitotic index are also adversely affected. Normal cells most affected are the epithelium of the gastrointestinal tract (including oral cavity) and the cells of the bone marrow. The commonest oral side effects are altered taste sensation, xerostomia, and mucositis.[46]

Effects on Oral Mucosa

Many chemotherapeutic agents reduce the normal turnover rate of oral epithelium, which results in atrophic thinning of the oral mucosa manifested clinically as painful, erythematous, and ulcerative mucosal surfaces in the mouth. The effects are most noted on the unattached mucosa and are rarely seen on gingival surfaces. These changes are seen within 1 week of the onset of the administration of the antitumor agents. The effects are usually self-limiting, and spontaneous healing occurs in 2 to 3 weeks after cessation of the agent.

Effects on Hematopoietic System

Myelosuppression—as manifested by leukopenia, neutropenia, thrombocytopenia, and anemia—is a common sequela of

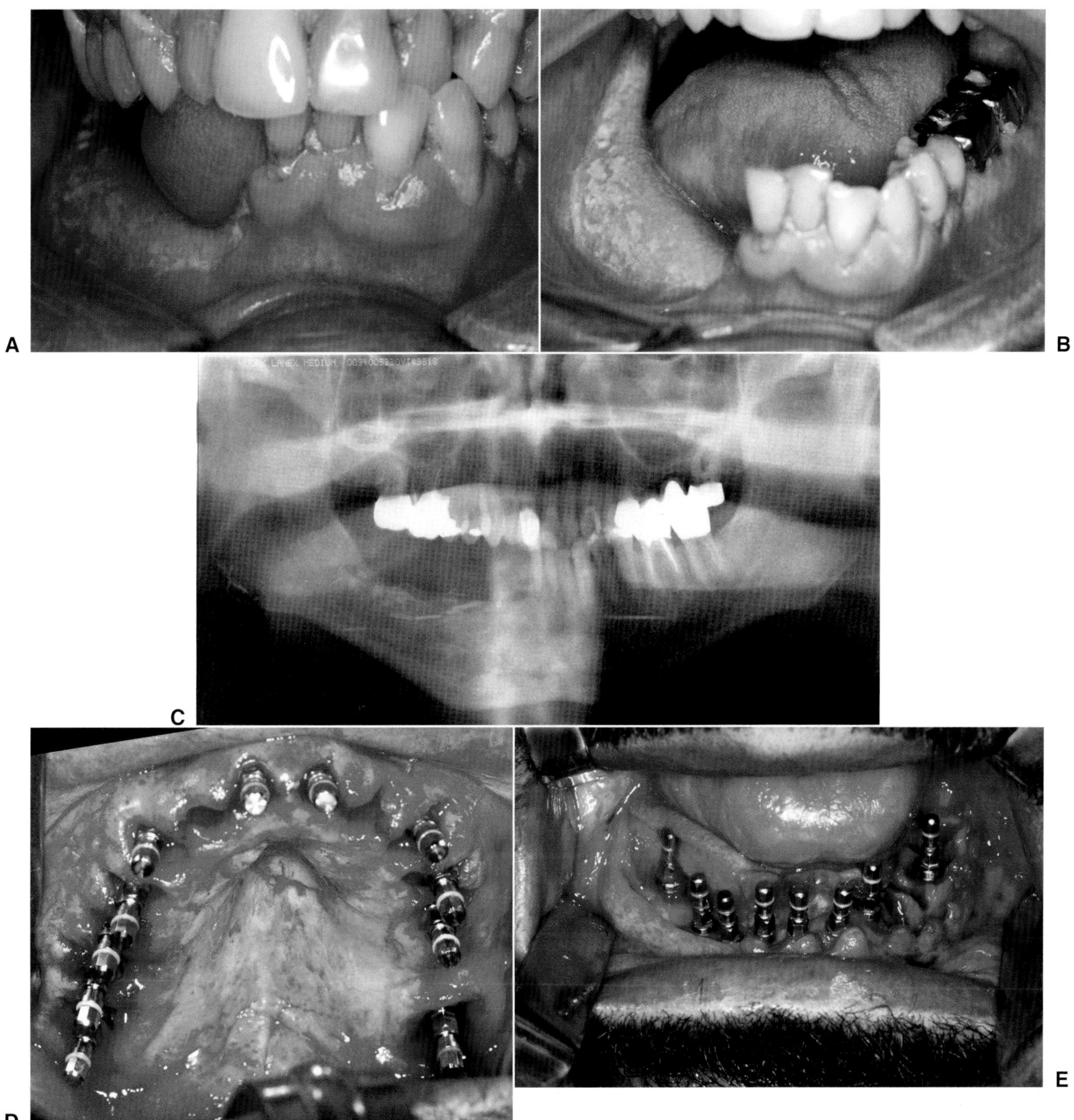

FIGURE 18-5 Photographs of a case of dental implant reconstruction in a patient who had full-course radiation treatment for squamous cell carcinoma. His existing dentition developed rampant dental caries (A to C) within a year after radiation therapy. After hyperbaric oxygen treatment, his teeth were extracted and implanted (D and E). After a waiting period of 6 months, full-fixed prosthetic restorations (crowns and bridges) were fabricated.

Continued

several forms of cancer chemotherapy. Within 2 weeks of the beginning of chemotherapy administration, the white blood cell count falls to an extremely low level. The effect of myelosuppression in the oral cavity is marginal gingivitis. Mild infections may develop, and bleeding from the gingiva is common. If the neutropenia is severe and prolonged, severe infections may develop. The microorganisms involved in these infections may be overgrowths of the usual oral flora, especially fungi; however, other microorganisms may be causative. Thrombocytopenia can be significant, and spontaneous bleeding may occur. This is especially common in the oral cavity after oral hygiene measures. Recovery from myelosuppression is usually complete 3 weeks after cessation of chemotherapy.

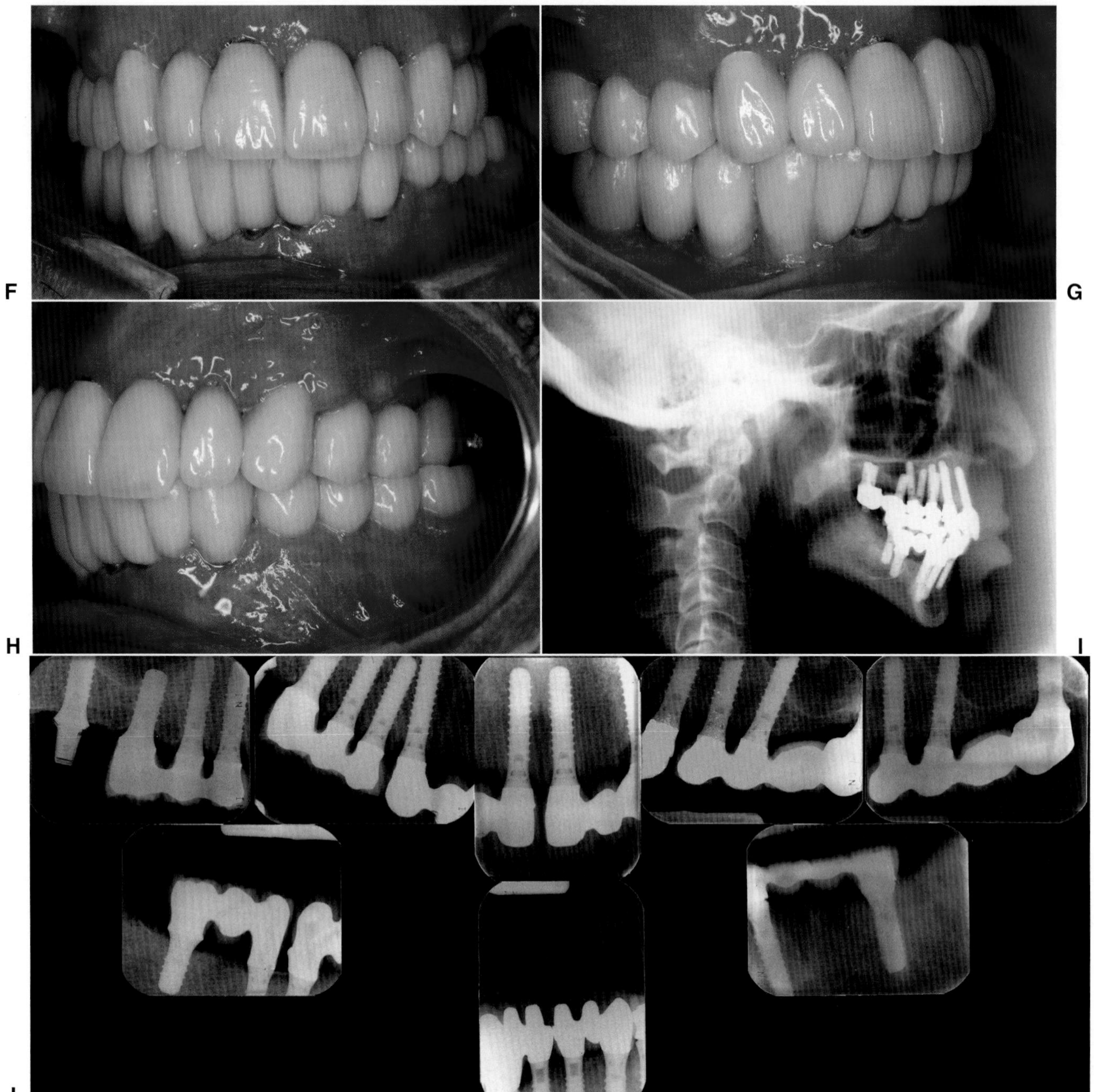

FIGURE 18-5, cont'd His prosthesis (F, G, and H) and lateral cephalometric radiograph (I) 1 year after placement of his prostheses. J, The bone levels have been maintained around all of the implants.

The type of neoplasm for which the patient is being treated is important to determine. The type of neoplasm dictates the type of chemotherapeutic agents to be used. Many hematologic neoplasms (e.g., leukemia) are treated with chemotherapeutic agents that result in profound alterations in the function and number of bone marrow elements. Comparatively, chemotherapeutic management of some nonmarrow solid tumors may not be associated with as severe a marrow aplasia as is found in patients with hematologic neoplasms.

Effects on Oral Microbiology

Chemotherapeutic agents, because of their immunosuppressive side effect, cause profound changes in the oral flora. For example, overgrowth of indigenous microbes, superinfection with gram-negative bacilli, and opportunistic infections are common sequelae and lead to patient discomfort and morbidity. Systemic infections are responsible for about 70% of the deaths in patients receiving myelosuppressive cancer chemotherapy.[47,48] *Oral* microorganisms have been shown to be a common source

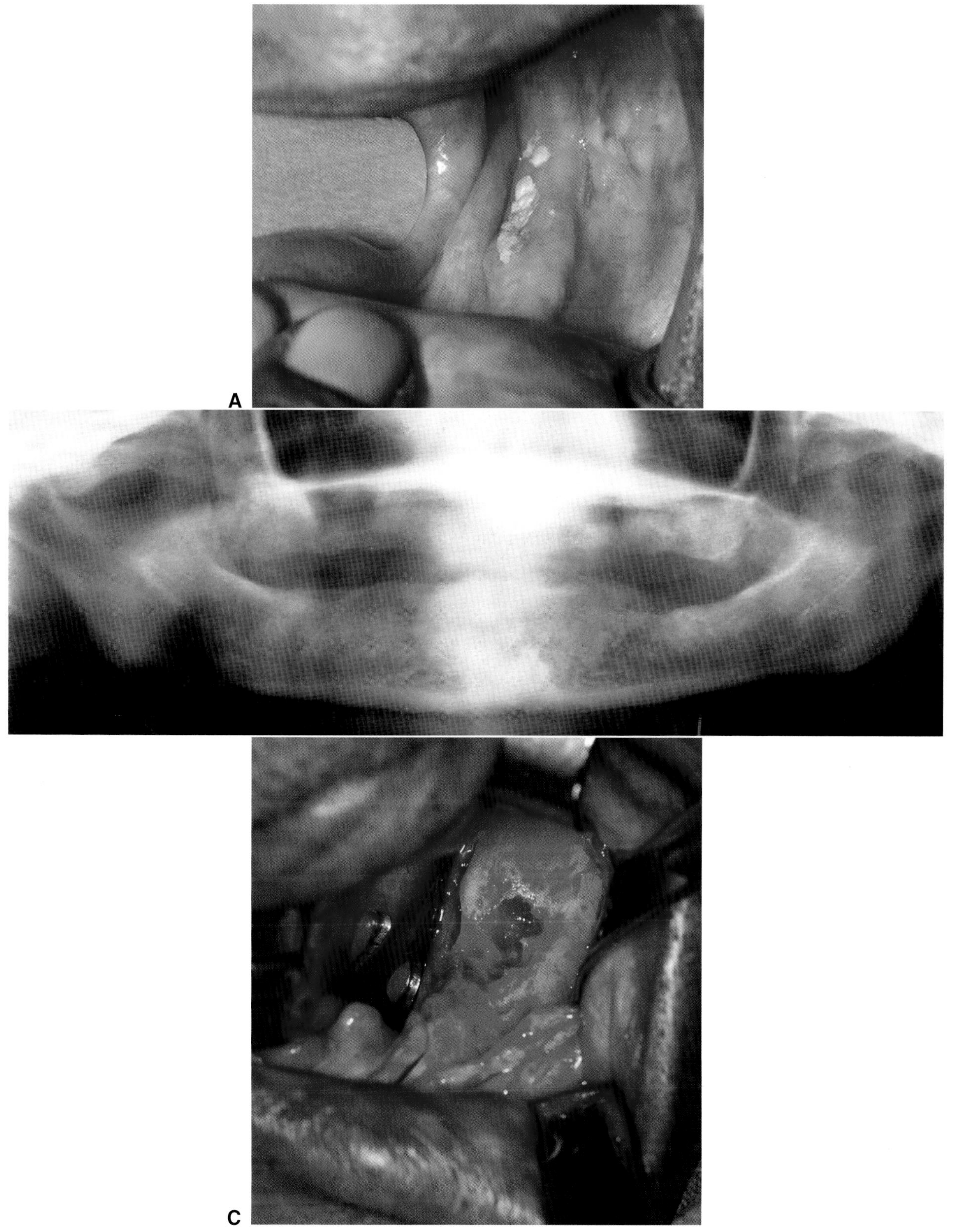

FIGURE 18-6 Osteoradionecrosis of the left mandible. This patient had a full course of tumoricidal radiotherapy for squamous cell carcinoma. The dentition was removed at the time of the cancer resection. This patient was prepared for treatment of the osteoradionecrosis with preoperative and postoperative hyperbaric oxygen treatments. A, Exposed devitalized bone along alveolar ridge of left mandible. B, Panoramic radiograph showing diffuse irregularity without good cortication of alveolar crest. C, Surgical exposure of the area shows devital bone margins and a central crater devoid of bone.

Continued

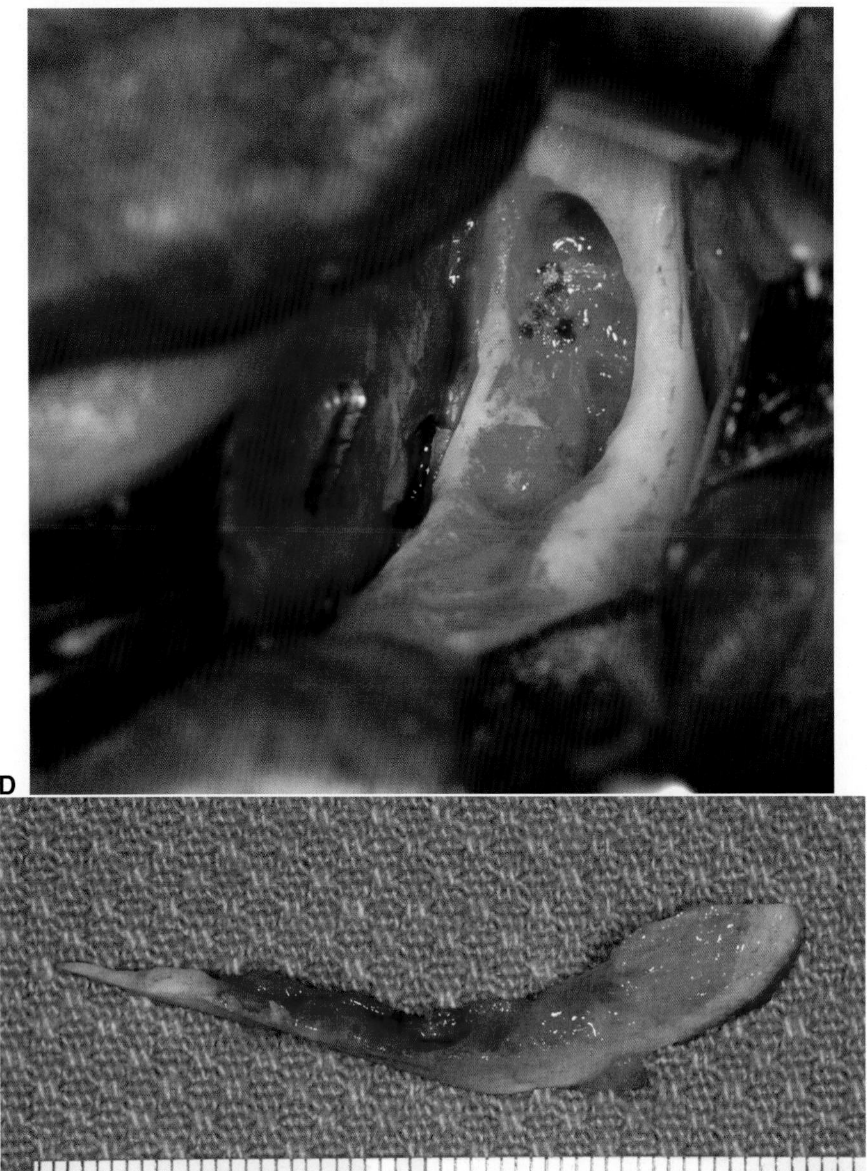

FIGURE 18-6, cont'd Osteoradionecrosis of the left mandible. This patient had a full course of tumoricidal radiotherapy for squamous cell carcinoma. The dentition was removed at the time of the cancer resection. This patient was prepared for treatment of the osteoradionecrosis with preoperative and postoperative hyperbaric oxygen treatments. **D**, The bone of the alveolar crest is removed, and the remainder is smoothed with a bur until bleeding bone is encountered. The central crater is similarly burred out. **E**, Resected specimen of alveolar crest.

of bacteremia in these patients.[47] Thus most patients who are receiving chemotherapy are treated concomitantly with systemic antimicrobial agents. However, in spite of these regimens, patients frequently have overgrowth of some organisms, most commonly the *Candida* species.[49-51]

General Dental Management

In general, the principles of dental management for the patient who has had or will have radiotherapy apply equally well to the patient who has had or will have chemotherapy.[52,53] However, because of the intermittent nature of the chemotherapy delivered in many instances, the minimal effects on the vasculature, and the almost normal state of the individual between chemotherapeutic administrations, dental management can be much easier. The effects of the chemotherapy are almost always temporary, and with the passage of time, systemic health improves to optimal levels, which allows almost routine dental management.

Primary concerns for the dentist should be the severity and duration of bone marrow suppression. The dentist must be aware of the dates of chemotherapy and the hematologic status of the patient before beginning dental care. If the patient is being treated for a hematologic neoplasm (e.g., leukemia), *both*

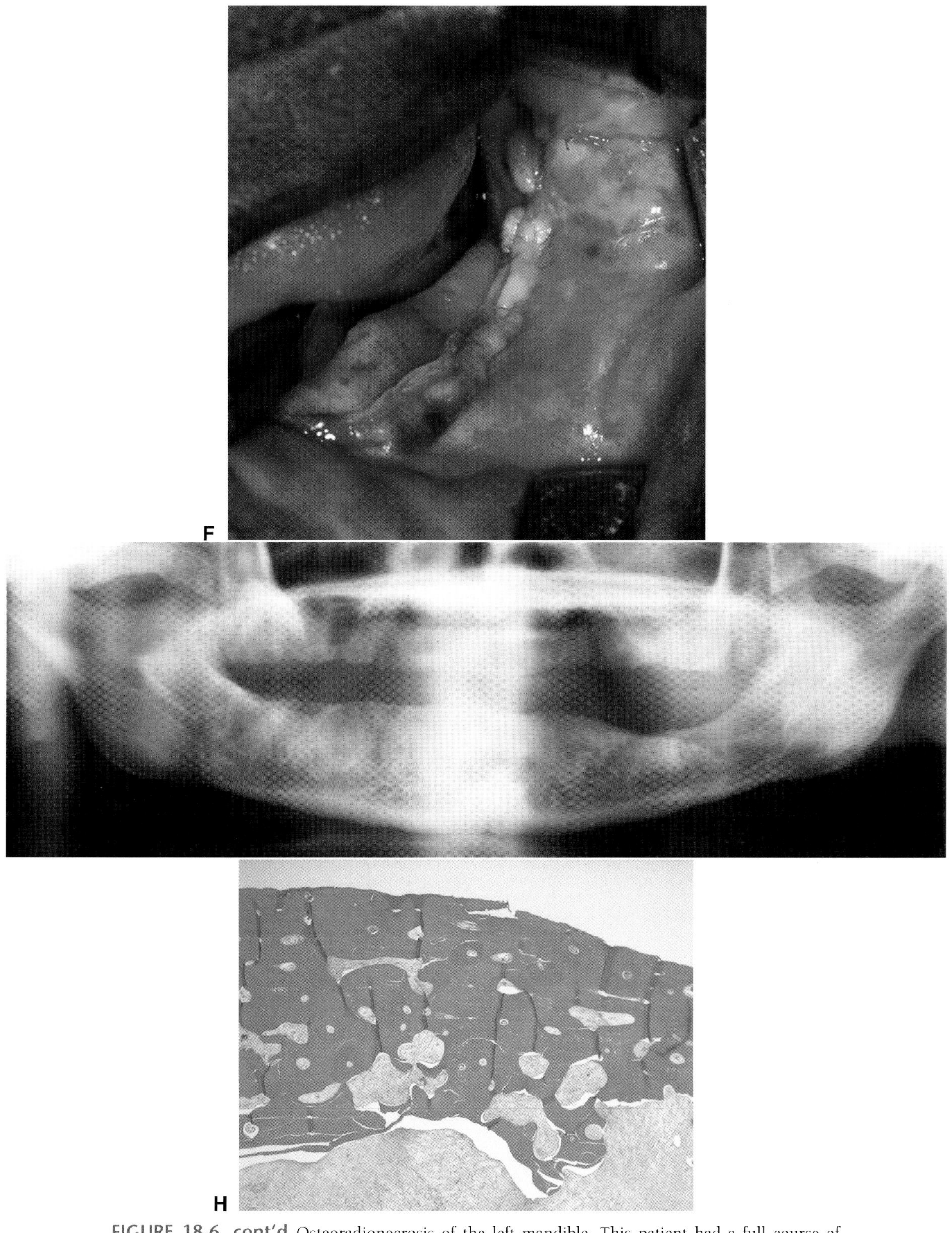

FIGURE 18-6, cont'd Osteoradionecrosis of the left mandible. This patient had a full course of tumoricidal radiotherapy for squamous cell carcinoma. The dentition was removed at the time of the cancer resection. This patient was prepared for treatment of the osteoradionecrosis with preoperative and postoperative hyperbaric oxygen treatments. F, Closure of soft tissues. G, Panoramic radiograph 8 months after surgery showing slight remodeling and healing of the bone. H, Histology of the resected specimen showed osteoradionecrosis and fibrosis in marrow area of haversian systems.

the disease *and* the chemotherapy lead to decreases in the functional blood elements. Therefore, these patients may be at great risk for infection and hemorrhage at any time in the course of their disease. Consultation with the patient's physician in these instances is mandatory. In most cases of nonhematopoietic neoplasm, the patient is at risk for infection and hemorrhage only during the course of the chemotherapy, after which recovery of the blood elements occurs.

The decision of when to extract teeth before treatment is based on the condition of the residual dentition, the patient's past dental hygiene practices, the immediacy of the need for chemotherapy, and the overall prognosis of the malignant disease.

Prechemotherapy dental measures that should routinely be performed are a thorough prophylaxis, fluoride treatment, and any necessary scaling. Unrestorable teeth should be removed before chemotherapy begins.

Patients who have begun chemotherapy must maintain scrupulous oral hygiene. This is difficult in the face of mucositis and ulceration, which frequently occur. No dental procedures should be performed on any patient receiving chemotherapy whose white blood cell and platelet status is unknown. In general, patients who have a white blood cell count greater than or equal to 2000/mm^3, with at least 20% polymorphonuclear leukocytes and a platelet count greater than or equal to 50,000/mm^3, can be treated in routine fashion. Antibiotics should be administered prophylactically if the patient has had chemotherapy within 3 weeks of dental treatment. If the white blood cell count and platelet levels fall below those specified, minimal oral care should be practiced because infection, severe bleeding, or both can occur. The patient may even need to avoid flossing and to use an extremely soft toothbrush during these periods. Any removable dental appliance should be left out at these times to prevent ulceration of the fragile mucosa.

Treatment of Oral Candidiasis

Initial treatment of candidiasis is with topical application of an antifungal medication.[49] The advantage of using topical medication is that systemic side effects are minimized. Similarly, in patients with persistent infection, advantage can be gained by continuing topical agents in addition to systemic medications. The use of this combination may allow a reduced dose and duration of systemic administration of the antifungal medication and also may reduce the potential side effects.

Topical agents are available as oral rinses, oral tablets, and creams. In general, oral rinses provide a short contact time for the drug and are therefore of less efficacy. The tablets are one of the most accepted forms of topically treating candidiasis because they can be dissolved slowly in the mouth and provide increased exposure time of the drug with the oral flora. The cream forms of topical antifungals are helpful for *Candida* of the oral commissures or for application to the oral surfaces of prosthetic devices to prolong medication exposure.

The two most commonly administered topical medications for oropharyngeal *Candida* infections are clotrimazole and nystatin. Clotrimazole and nystatin are available in several forms and should be applied 4 times daily. Therapy should continue 2 weeks after cessation of clinical signs and symptoms. Clotrimazole troches are available and are dissolved in the mouth 4 or 5 times a day.

For more stubborn cases, ketoconazole or fluconazole (i.e., systemic antifungal medications) can be prescribed. However, the dentist must be careful with systemic administration of these antifungal medications because of their toxic side effects. These vary widely with the type of medication and can be serious.

Another widely prescribed medication for oral candidiasis is chlorhexidine mouth rinse. Chlorhexidine (Peridex) has been shown to have potent antibacterial and antifungal properties in vitro. The in vivo effects of chlorhexidine are less well documented, especially for use against *Candida* spp. in immunosuppressed individuals.[13,54] However, chlorhexidine is used in most of such patients on the basis that it probably does no harm and may prove beneficial in many instances.

DENTAL MANAGEMENT OF PATIENTS WITH BISPHOSPHONATE-ASSOCIATED OSTEONECROSIS OF THE JAWS (BOJ)

Recently, a new oral complication of cancer treatment has been identified that looks similar to osteoradionecrosis, with exposure of devital areas of bone of the jaws. However, the complication is seen in patients who have not had any radiation treatment, and the methods used to treat osteoradionecrosis do not seem to be effective for the treatment of these lesions. This new oral lesion is called bisphosphonate-associated osteonecrosis of the jaws (BOJ)[55] because what patients with these lesions have in common is that they are taking a bisphosphonate medication, usually as an adjunct to chemotherapy for malignant disease.

BOJ is a condition of chronically exposed necrotic bone; it is usually painful and often primarily or secondarily infected. Bone exposure might occur spontaneously or more commonly following an invasive dental procedure.[56] Patients complain of halitosis and have difficulty eating and speaking.

Clinically, the lesions appear as oral mucosal ulcerations that expose the underlying bone and frequently are extremely painful. The lesions are persistent and do not respond to conventional treatment modalities such as débridement, antibiotic therapy, or HBO therapy.

Bisphosphonates

Bisphosphonates are a class of agents used to treat osteoporosis and malignant bone metastases. Bisphosphonates inhibit bone resorption and thus bone renewal by suppressing the recruitment and activity of osteoclasts, thus shortening their life span. Millions of postmenopausal women are taking bisphosphonates to stabilize bone loss caused by osteoporosis, decreasing their risk of pathologic fracture.[57] Besides osteoporosis, bisphosphonates are used to manage Paget's disease of bone and hypercalcemia of malignancy. Bisphosphonates are given to patients with cancer to help control bone loss resulting from metastatic skeletal lesions.[58,59] The mechanism of action of bisphosphonates is by binding to bone mineral, where they are concentrated and accumulate over time. Bisphosphonates are potent inhibitors of osteoclastic activity,[6] and this is why they are usually prescribed. Depending on the duration of the treatment and the specific bisphosphonate prescribed, the drug may remain in the body for years.[8] Physiologic bone deposition and remodeling are severely compromised in patients receiving bisphosphonate therapy.[60,61] Bisphosphonates also have antiangiogenic properties and may be directly tumoricidal, making them an important agent in cancer therapy.[62,63]

TABLE 18-1

Bisphosphonates in Clinical Usage in the United States

Genetic Name	Brand Name	Manufacturer	Route of Administration
Alendronate	Fosamax	Merck Co, West Point, Va.	Oral
Clodronate	Bonefos	Schering AG, Montville, N.J.	Intravenous
Etidronate	Didronel	Procter and Gamble, Cincinnati, Ohio	Oral
Ibandronate	Boniva	GlaxoSmith Kline, Philadelphia, Pa.	Oral
Pamidronate	Aredia	Novartis Pharmaceuticals, East Haven, N.J.	Intravenous
Risedronate	Actonel	Procter and Gamble, Cincinnati, Ohio	Oral
Tiludronate	Skelid	Sanofi-Synthe Lab Inc, N.Y.	Oral
Zoledronate	Zometa	Novartis Pharmaceuticals, East Haven, N.J.	Intravenous

Many bisphosphonate medications are available, some given intravenously (pamidronate, zoledronic acid, clodronate) and some orally (alendronate; etidronate, risedronate, tiludronate, ibandronate; Table 18-1). The decision on which to be prescribed varies with the type of medical condition being treated and the potency of the drug required. For example, orally administered bisphosphonates often are used in patients with osteoporosis, whereas the injectable bisphosphonates are used in patients with cancer who have primary lesions of bone or skeletal metastasis.

Mechanism of BOJ

The exact mechanism that leads to the induction of BOJ is unknown. Bisphosphonates bind to bone and incorporate in the osseous matrix. During bone remodeling, the drug is taken up by osteoclasts and internalized in the cell cytoplasm, where it inhibits osteoclastic function and induces apoptotic cell death.[64] Bisphosphonates also inhibit osteoblast-mediated osteoclastic resorption and have antiangiogenic properties.[58,65,66] As a result, bone turnover becomes profoundly suppressed, and over time the bone shows little physiologic remodeling.[61,67] The bone becomes brittle and unable to repair physiologic microfractures that occur in the human skeleton with daily activity.[68,69] The need for repair and remodeling is increased greatly when there is infection in the maxilla or mandible and/or when an extraction is performed. Therefore, BOJ results from a complex interplay of bone metabolism, local trauma, increased demand for bone repair, infection, and hypovascularity.

Patients receiving bisphosphonates intravenously clearly are more susceptible to BOJ than are those receiving the drug orally. Thus, it is not common to see BOJ in patients taking bisphosphonates orally for prevention or treatment of osteoporosis; however, beginning in 2006, cases began to appear in the literature and now number around 200. Other metabolic factors may play a role in the development of BOJ, such as diabetes mellitus, as might the concomitant use of steroids, anticancer chemotherapeutic agents, and smoking.

Clinical Signs and Symptoms of BOJ

Apparently, BOJ exclusively affects the jaws.[70] The most common clinical presentation associated with BOJ is an ulcer with exposed bone in a patient who has had a dental extraction (Fig. 18-7).[55,56,71-74] An ulcer from a ill-fitting prosthetic device has also been implicated in the initiation of this pathologic process. However, spontaneous bone exposures that cannot be associated with any injury or infection occur in many cases.[74] Similar to osteoradionecrosis, in the early stages of oral BOJ, no radiographic manifestations can be seen. Patients may be asymptomatic but may have severe pain because of the necrotic bone becoming infected secondarily after it is exposed to the oral environment. The osteonecrosis often is progressive and may lead to extensive areas of bony exposure and dehiscence (Fig. 18-8).

In cancer patients taking intravenous forms of bisphosphonates, the median time from starting therapy to developing necrosis of bone in the jaws was 25 months.[75] In addition, the elderly (over 65 years) also may have increased risk.[76,77] The most common dental comorbidity in these patients reportedly is clinically and radiographically apparent

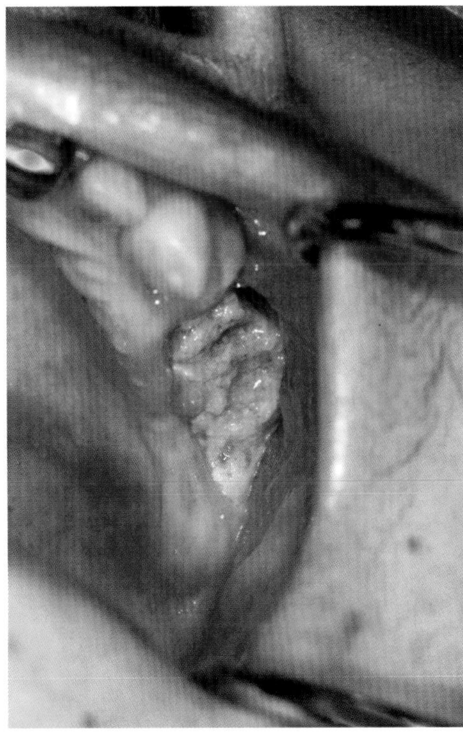

FIGURE 18-7 Bisphosphonate-related osteonecrosis of the maxilla. This area of exposed bone occurred 2 weeks after extractions. Sharp areas were débrided, but the wound had not healed after several months.

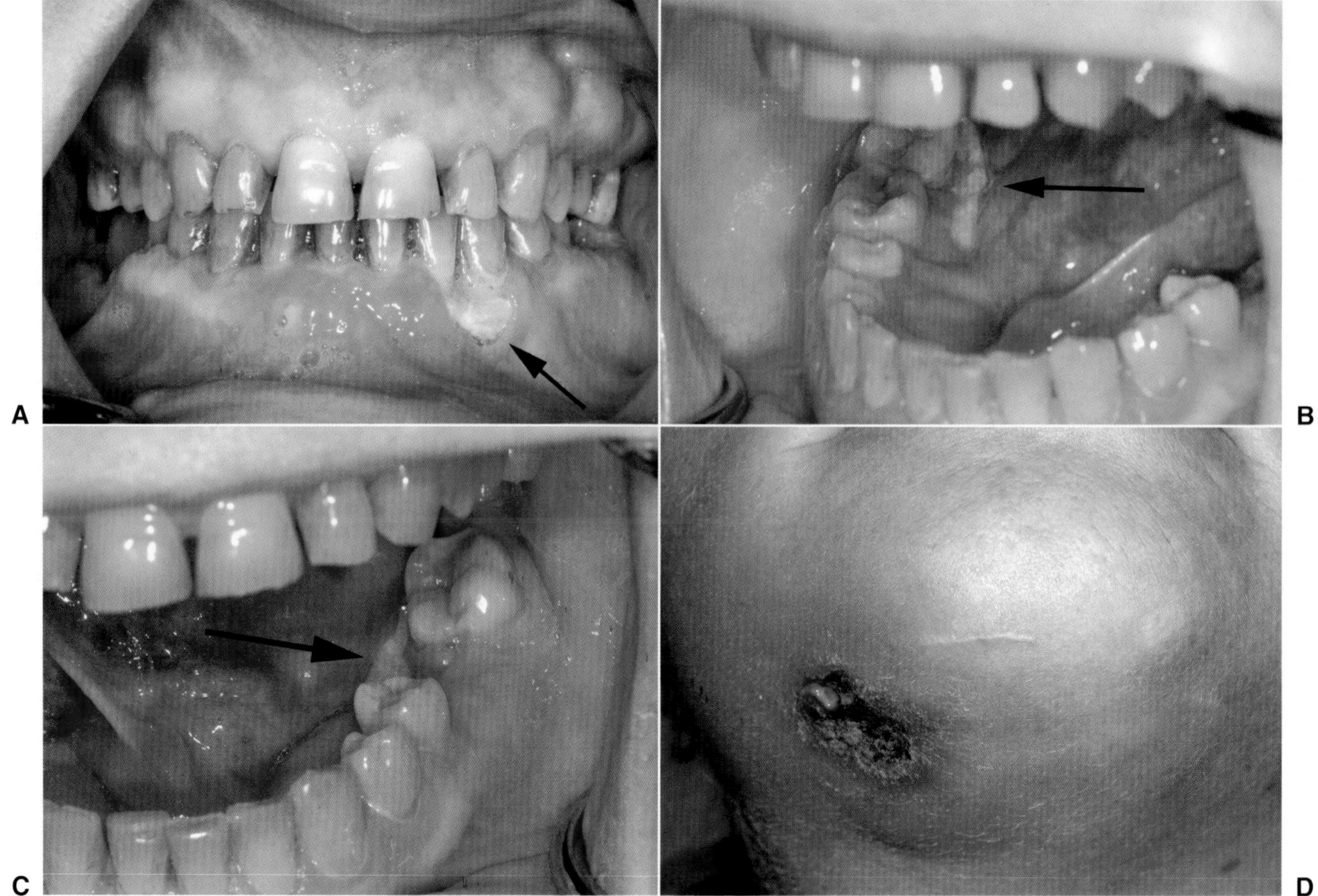

FIGURE 18-8 A progressive case of bisphosphonate-related osteonecrosis of the mandible. At initial presentation, areas of bone exposure occurred along the anterior teeth (A) and along the mylohyoid ridges bilaterally (B and C). Minor débridements were performed, but an infection of the right mandible developed, with spontaneous breakdown of the skin in the submental region (D).

periodontitis.[74] Other local factors associated with BOJ are infected teeth, dental abscesses, previous endodontic treatments, and tori.

In patients in whom BOJ develops spontaneously, the most common initial complaint is the sudden presence of intraoral discomfort and the presence of roughness of the exposed bone that may progress to traumatize the oral soft tissues surrounding the area of necrotic bone.

Often a purulent discharge and local swelling occur in the adjacent soft tissues, with trismus and regional lymphadenopathy. One must differentiate BOJ from simple cases of transient mucosal ulcerations (in patients who have not been taking bisphosphonates) associated with ill-fitting prosthetic appliances, traumatic dental extractions, or spontaneously occurring denudation of bone in areas where the overlying mucosa is thin and prone to abrasion (e.g., mylohyoid ridge and tori). These areas heal spontaneously once the irritation has been removed. Lesions of BOJ will not.

Dental Care for Patients Who Are About to Start Taking Bisphosphonates

Because BOJ is a newly documented oral complication, consistently effective therapeutic measures have not yet been identified. Although several reports of this drug-associated complication have been published, there is no concensus on treatment strategies that yield predictable resolution and healing of BOJ. This presents a dilemma for the patient and the clinicians. The inability to manage lesions of BOJ worsens the patient's medical status as the patient becomes more and more nutritionally compromised. Prevention of this condition is therefore critical for these patients so that they can receive the anticancer therapies they require for their neoplastic disease.

Similar to the management of patients who will receive radiation treatment, the dentist should see all patients before intravenous bisphosphonate therapy begins. The main emphasis at this time should be to minimize the risk of occurrence of BOJ. Most reports of BOJ occur after the patient has been taking bisphosphonates for 6 months or more,[55,74] so it may be possible to provide dental care early in the treatment without unduly risking the development of BOJ from dental treatment. Although a small percentage of patients receiving bisphosphonates have BON spontaneously, the majority of affected patients experience this complication following routine dentoalveolar surgery (i.e., extraction, dental implant placement, or apical surgery). Therefore, teeth with a poor prognosis should be removed before bisphosphonate administration or as early as possible after institution of treatment. If possible, institution of bisphosphonate therapy should be delayed for approximately 4 to 6 weeks after invasive procedures such as dental extractions to give the bone a chance to recover.[74]

Dental prophylaxis, caries control, and conservative restorative dentistry are critical to maintaining functionally sound teeth. This level of care must be continued indefinitely. Patients with full or partial dentures should be examined for areas of mucosal trauma, especially along the lingual flange region. It is critical that patients be educated as to the importance of dental hygiene and regular dental evaluations and specifically instructed to report any pain, swelling, or exposed bone that would predict or characterize BOJ.

Dental Care for Patients Who Are Taking Bisphosphonates

The treatment of patients receiving oral or intravenous bisphosphonate therapy is principally preventive. Dentists should contact the patient's physician to find out why the patient is taking the bisphosphonate, the type the patient is taking, and expected duration of treatment. It is recommended that dentists follow existing guidelines for a dental consultation for the prevention of oral complications of cancer therapy (chemotherapy, radiation therapy). Elimination of all potential sites of infection must be the primary objective of this consultation. Restorative dentistry should be performed to eliminate caries and defective restorations. Crowns and more extensive fixed prosthodontic work may not be appropriate for some patients. Prosthodontic appliances should be evaluated for fit, stability, and occlusion. Necessary adjustments should be made. Extraction of teeth should be avoided when possible. The goal of therapy should be to attain a state of good oral and dental health to prevent the need for invasive dental procedures in the future. Prophylaxis should be performed and oral hygiene instructions given. The patient also should be given information about BOJ and be made aware of the early signs of development of this condition. Once the active dental treatment is over, frequent periodic follow-up visits should be scheduled to reinforce the importance of oral hygiene maintenance and to conduct a new oral examination.

Role of Orally Administered Alendronate

It is unclear whether patients taking alendronate and having BOJ had other systemic or local comorbid factors.[55,56,71,74] Because of the vast numbers of patients taking alendronate (Fosamax) for osteoporosis (approximately 22 million),[78] a frequently asked question is whether such individuals can safely have invasive procedures such as dental extractions and dental implants placed to restore missing teeth. The risk of developing BOJ after dental extractions, implant placement, and periodontal and other surgical procedures for patients taking oral bisphosphonates such as alendronate is unknown. The duration of the physiologic effect of these drugs is variable. Evidence shows that severe suppression of bone remodeling may occur during long-term alendronate therapy[61] and that bone resorption and formation markers may remain suppressed for the time during which the patient is taking the medication.[60,67] At this time, it appears that the incidence of BOJ manifesting in patients taking alendronate for osteoporosis is low.[79] However, the longer a patient takes this medication, the higher the risk for BOJ.

Dental Care for Patients with BOJ

For patients with established lesions of BOJ, the goal is to get the patient comfortable because it is likely the patient will have to live with the exposed bone. Treatment should be directed at eliminating or controlling pain, and preventing progression of the exposed bone. If the exposed bone has sharp edges that are irritating the adjacent soft tissues, eliminating sharp edges of bone may be performed using a rotating diamond bur. This is particularly important when the lingual aspect of the posterior mandibular arch is involved. However, superficial débridements should only be performed as a last resort. Attempts to cover the exposed bone with flaps may cause more bone exposure and worsening of symptoms, with risk of pathologic fracture. Several treatment modalities for BOJ are reported in the literature and include minor débridement under local anesthesia, major surgical sequestrectomies, marginal and segmental mandibular resections, partial and complete maxillectomies, and HBO therapy. Unfortunately, none of these therapeutic modalities have proved routinely successful. Despite the "appearance" of vascularized bone at the surgical margins, healing may not occur in the patients[56,77] because the entire bone is affected, making it impossible to débride to "normal" bone. Many cases have a very poor outcome in spite of therapy, progressing to extensive dehiscence and exposure of bone.[56,74,77]

Patients should be closely followed up to reevaluate the areas and to ensure that they have not become suppurative. If the area around the exposed bone exhibits painful erythema and suppuration and/or sinus tracts, the patient should be treated with antibiotics until the areas resolve. Use of chlorhexidine mouth rinse 3 or 4 times a day also is recommended to reduce bacterial load and colonization.

The dentist can discuss the care of the patient with the patient's oncologist. Because of the extremely long half-life of bisphosphonates (years), it is not reasonable to discontinue the medication in an attempt to facilitate healing of the BOJ. Further, patients taking bisphosphonates for metastatic cancer need their medication. However, if there is no cancer-related indication for continued bisphosphonate therapy or the original indication has resolved, it might be reasonable to discontinue the medication, although it will be present in the patient's bone for a long time.

Routine restorative care may be provided to patients with BOJ. Local anesthetic can be used as necessary. Scaling and prophylaxis should be done as atraumatically as possible, with gentle soft tissue management. If the tooth is nonrestorable because of caries, root canal treatment and amputation of the crown may be a better option than removing the tooth unless it is very loose. One should try to avoid dental extractions if possible and, if necessary, should perform them as atraumatically as possible. Patients should be followed closely for the first several weeks afterward, then monthly until the sockets are completely closed and healed. If there is an indication for antibiotic use, penicillin V, amoxicillin, or clindamycin may help to reduce the incidence of local infection.

Any existing prosthetic appliances should be reevaluated to ensure that they fit well. Relining a denture with a soft liner to promote a better fit and to minimize soft tissue trauma and pressure points is recommended.

Odontogenic infections should be treated aggressively with systemic antibiotics. Although penicillin is the first-choice antibiotic in dentistry, amoxicillin and/or clindamycin provide better bone penetration and a wider spectrum of coverage.

REFERENCES

1. Okuno SH, Foote RL, Loprinzi CL et al: A randomized trial of a nonabsorbable antibiotic lozenge given to alleviate radiation-induced mucositis, *Cancer* 79:2193-2199, 1997.
2. Sciubba JJ, Goldenberg D: Oral complications of radiotherapy, *Oncology* 7:175-183, 2006.
3. Sweeney MP, Bagg J, Baxter WP et al: Clinical trial of a mucin-containing oral spray for treatment of xerostomia in hospice patients, *Palliat Med* 11:225-232, 1997.
4. Davies AN: A comparison of artificial saliva and chewing gum in the management of xerostomia in patients with advanced cancer, *Palliat Med* 14:197-203, 2000.
5. Risheim H, Amegerg P: Salivary stimulation by chewing gum and lozenges in rheumatic patients with xerostomia, *Scand J Dent Res* 101:40-43, 1993.
6. Grisius M: Salivary gland dysfunction: a review of systemic therapies, *Oral Surg Oral Med Oral Pathol* 92:156, 2001.
7. Greenspan D, Daniels TE: Effectiveness of pilocarpine in post-radiation xerostomia, *Cancer* 59:1123-1125, 1987.
8. Johnson JT, Ferretti GA, Nethery WJ et al: Oral pilocarpine for post-irradiation xerostomia in patients with head and neck cancer, *N Engl J Med* 329:390-395, 1993.
9. LeVeque FG, Montgomery M, Potter D et al: A multicenter, randomized, double-blind, placebo-controlled, dose-titration study of oral pilocarpine for treatment of radiation-induced xerostomia in head and neck cancer patients, *J Clin Oncol* 11:1124-1131, 1993.
10. Khan Z, Jacobsen CS: Oral pilocarpine HCl for post-irradiation xerostomia in head and neck cancer patients. In *Proceedings of the First International Congress on Maxillofacial Prosthetics,* New York, 1995, Memorial Sloan-Kettering Cancer Center.
11. Atkinson JC, Baum BJ: Salivary enhancers, *J Dent Educ* 65:1096-1101, 2001.
12. Leek H, Albertsson M: Pilocarpine treatment of xerostomia in head and neck patients, *Micron* 33:153-155, 2002.
13. Spijkervet FK: *Irradiation mucositis,* Copenhagen, 1991, Munksgaard.
14. Spijkervet FK, Van Saene HK, Van Saene JJ et al: Effect of selective elimination of the oral flora on mucositis in irradiated head and neck cancer patients, *J Surg Oncol* 46:167, 1991.
15. Matheis MJ, Esposito SJ, Sherman T: Evaluation of oral mucositis in patients receiving radiation therapy for head and neck cancer: a pilot study of 0.12% chlorhexidine gluconate oral rinse. In *Proceedings of the First International Congress on Maxillofacial Prosthetics,* New York, 1995, Memorial Sloan-Kettering Cancer Center.
16. Ferretti GA, Raybould TP, Brown AT et al: Chlorhexidine prophylaxis for chemotherapy- and radiation-induced stomatitis: a randomized double-blind trial, *Oral Surg Oral Med Oral Pathol* 70:331, 1990.
17. Beumer J, Brady F: Dental management of the irradiated patient, *Int J Oral Surg* 7:208, 1978.
18. Beumer J, Curtis T, Harrison RE: Radiation therapy of the oral cavity. I. Sequelae and management, *Head Neck Surg* 1:301, 1979.
19. Beumer J, Curtis T, Harrison RE: Radiation therapy of the oral cavity. II. Sequelae and management, *Head Neck Surg* 1:392, 1979.
20. Beumer J, Curtis TA, Morrish RB: Radiation complications in edentulous patients, *J Prosthet Dent* 36:193, 1976.
21. Dreizen S, Brown LR, Daly TE et al: Prevention of xerostomia-related dental caries in irradiated cancer patients, *J Dent Res* 56:99, 1977.
22. Bedwinek JM, Shukovsky LJ, Fletcher GH et al: Osteonecrosis in patients treated with definitive radiotherapy for squamous cell carcinomas of the oral cavity and naso- and oropharynx, *Radiology* 119:665, 1976.
23. Starcke EN, Shannon IL: How critical is the interval between extractions and irradiation in patients with head and neck malignancy? *Oral Surg Oral Med Oral Pathol* 43:333, 1977.
24. Marx RE: A new concept in the treatment of osteoradionecrosis, *J Oral Maxillofac Surg* 41:351, 1983.
25. Marx RE: Osteoradionecrosis: a new concept in its pathophysiology, *J Oral Maxillofac Surg* 41:283, 1983.
26. Marx RE, Johnson RP, Kline SN: Prevention of osteoradionecrosis: a randomized prospective clinical trial of hyperbaric oxygen versus penicillin, *J Am Dent Assoc* 111:49, 1985.
27. Hobo S, Ichida E, Garcia LT: *Osseointegration and occlusal rehabilitation,* Tokyo, 1989, Quintessence.
28. Hum S, Larsen P: The effect of radiation at the titanium-bone interface. In Laney W, Tolman D, editors: *Tissue integration in oral, orthopedic and maxillofacial reconstruction,* Chicago, 1990, Quintessence.
29. Granström G, Tjellstrom A, Branemark PI, et al: Bone-anchored reconstruction of the irradiated head and neck cancer patient, *Otolaryngol Head Neck Surg* 108:334, 1993.
30. Visch LL, Levendag PC, Denissen HW: Five-year results of 227 HA-coated implants in irradiated tissues. In *Proceedings of the First International Congress on Maxillofacial Prosthetics,* New York, 1995, Memorial Sloan-Kettering Cancer Center.
31. Esser E, Wagner W: Dental implants following radical oral cancer surgery and adjuvant radiotherapy, *Int J Oral Maxillofac Implants* 12:552-557, 1997.
32. Franzen L, Rosenquist JB, Rosenquist KI et al: Oral implant rehabilitation of patients with oral malignancies treated with radiotherapy and surgery without adjunctive hyperbaric oxygen, *Int J Oral Maxillofac Implants* 10:183-187, 1995.
33. Watzinger F, Ewers R, Henninger A et al: Endosteal implants in the irradiated lower jaw, *J Craniomaxillofac Surg* 24:237-244, 1996.
34. Keller E, Tolman DE, Zuck SL et al: Mandibular endosseous implants and autogenous bone grafting in irradiated tissue: a ten-year retrospective study, *Int J Oral Maxillofac Implants* 12:800-813, 1997.
35. Nimi A, Ueda M, Keller EE et al: Experience with osseointegrated implants placed in irradiated tissues in Japan and the United States, *Int J Oral Maxillofac Implants* 13:407-411, 1998.
36. Granstrom G: Osseointegration in irradiated cancer patients: an analysis with respect to implant failures, *J Oral Maxillofac Surg* 63:579-585, 2005.
37. Moy PK, Medina D, Shetty V et al: Dental implant failure rates and associated risk factors, *Int J Oral Maxillofac Implants* 20:569-577, 2005.
38. Nimi A, Fujimoto T, Nosaka Y et al: A Japanese multicenter study of osseointegrated implants placed in irradiated tissues: a preliminary report, *Int J Oral Maxillofac Implants* 12:259, 1997.
39. Weischer T, Mohr C: Ten-year experience in oral implant rehabilitation of cancer patients: treatment concept and proposed criteria for success, *Int J Oral Maxillofac Implants* 14:521, 1999.
40. Granström G, Jacobsson M, Tjellström A: Titanium implants in the irradiated tissue: benefits from hyperbaric oxygen, *Int J Oral Maxillofac Implants* 7:15, 1992.
41. Albrektsson T: A multicenter report on osseointegrated oral implants, *J Prosthet Dent* 60:75, 1988.
42. Taylor TD, Worthington P: Osseointegrated implant rehabilitation of the previously irradiated mandible: results of a limited trial at 3 to 7 years, *J Prosthet Dent* 69:60, 1993.
43. Murray CG, Herson J, Daly TE, Zimmerman S: Radiation necrosis of the mandible: a 10-year study. I. Factors influencing the onset of necrosis, *Int J Radiat Oncol Biol Phys* 6:543, 1980.
44. Murray CG, Herson J, Daly TE, Zimmerman S: Radiation necrosis of the mandible: a 10-year study. II. Dental factors: onset, duration, and management of necrosis, *Int J Radiat Oncol Biol Phys* 6:549, 1980.
45. Beumer J 3rd, Harrison R, Sanders B et al: Postradiation dental extractions: a review of the literature and a report of 72 episodes, *Head Neck Surg* 6:581, 1983.
46. Wilson J, Rees JS: The dental treatment needs and oral side effects of patients undergoing outpatient cancer chemotherapy, *Eur J Prosthodont Restor Dent* 13:129-134, 2005.
47. Greenberg MS, Cohen SG, McKitrick JC, et al: The oral flora as a source of septicemia in patients with acute leukemia, *Oral Surg Oral Med Oral Pathol* 53:32, 1982.
48. McElroy TH: Infection in the patient receiving chemotherapy: oral considerations, *J Am Dent Assoc* 109:454, 1984.

49. Epstein JB: Antifungal therapy in oropharyngeal mycotic infections, *Oral Surg Oral Med Oral Pathol* 69:32, 1990.
50. Heimdahl A, Nord CE: Oral yeast infections in immunocompromised and seriously diseased patients, *Acta Odontol Scand* 48:77, 1990.
51. Odds FC, Kibbler CC, Walker E et al: Carriage of *Candida* species and *C. albicans* biotypes in patients undergoing chemotherapy or bone marrow transplantation for haematological disease, *J Clin Pathol* 42:1259, 1989.
52. DePaola LG, Peterson DE, Overholser CD Jr et al: Dental care for patients receiving chemotherapy, *J Am Dent Assoc* 112:198, 1986.
53. Wright WE, Haller JM, Harlow SA, et al: An oral disease prevention program for patients receiving radiation and chemotherapy, *J Am Dent Assoc* 110:43, 1985.
54. Thurmond JM, Brown AT, Sims RE et al: Oral *Candida albicans* in bone marrow transplant patients given chlorhexidine rinses: occurrence and susceptibilities to the agent, *Oral Surg Oral Med Oral Pathol* 72:291, 1991.
55. Migliorati CA, Casiglia J, Epstein J et al: Managing the care of patients with bisphosphonate-associated osteonecrosis: an American Academy of Oral Medicine position paper, *J Am Dent Assoc* 136:1658, 2005.
56. Ruggiero SL, Mehrotra B, Rosenberg TJ et al: Osteonecrosis of the jaws associated with the use of bisphosphonates: a review of 63 cases, *J Oral Maxillofac Surg* 62:527-534, 2004.
57. Watts NB: Treatment of osteoporosis with bisphosphonates, *Endocrinol Metab Clin North Am* 27:419-439, 1998.
58. Rogers MJ, Watts DJ, Russell RG: Overview of bisphosphonates, *Cancer* 80(suppl 8):1652-1660, 1997.
59. Licata AA: Discovery, clinical development, and therapeutic uses of bisphosphonates, *Ann Pharmacother* 39:668-677, 2005.
60. Ensrud KE, Barrett-Connor EL, Schwartz A et al: Randomized trial of effect of alendronate continuation versus discontinuation in women with low BMD: results from the Fracture Intervention Trial long-term extension, *J Bone Miner Res* 19:1259-1269, 2004.
61. Odvina CV, Zerwekh JE, Rao DS et al: Severely suppressed bone turnover: a potential complication of alendronate therapy, *J Clin Endocrinol Metab* 90:1294-1301, 2005.
62. Wood J, Bonjean K, Ruetz S et al: Novel antiangiogenic effects of the bisphosphonate compound zoledronic acid, *J Phamacol Exp Ther* 302(3):1055-1061, 2002.
63. Fournier P, Boissier S, Filleur S et al: Bisphosphonates inhibit angiogenesis in vitro and testosterone-stimulated vascular regrowth in the ventral prostate in castrated rats, *Cancer Res* 62:6538-6544, 2002.
64. Russell RG, Rogers MJ, Frith JC et al: The pharmacology of bisphosphonates and new insights into their mechanisms of action, *J Bone Miner Res* 14(suppl 2):53-65, 1999.
65. Fleisch H: Development of bisphosphonates, *Breast Cancer Res* 4(1):30-34, 2002.
66. Sietsema WK, Ebetino FH, Salvagno AM et al: Antiresorptive dose-dependent relationship across three generations of bisphosphonates, *Drugs Exp Clin Res* 15:389-396, 1989.
67. Ott SM: Long-term safety of bisphosphonates, *J Clin Endocrinol Metab* 90:1897-1899, 2005.
68. Whyte MP, Wenkert D, Clements KL et al: Bisphosphonate-induced osteopetrosis, *N Engl J Med* 349:457-463, 2003.
69. Marini JC: Do bisphosphonates make children's bones better or brittle? *N Engl J Med* 349:423-426, 2003.
70. Ruggiero SL, Fantasia J, Carlson E: Bisphosphonate-related osteonecrosis of the jaw: background and guidelines for diagnosis, staging and management, *Oral Surg Oral Med Oral Pathol Oral Radiol Endod* 102:433-441, 2006.
71. Marx RE: Pamidronate (Aredia) and zoledronate (Zometa) induced avascular necrosis of the jaws: a growing epidemic, *J Oral Maxillofac Surg* 61:1115-1157, 2003.
72. Melo MD, Obeid G: Osteonecrosis of the jaws in patients with a history of receiving bisphosphonate therapy: strategies for prevention and early recognition, *J Am Dent Assoc* 136:1675-1681, 2005.
73. Migliorati CA, Schubert MM, Peterson DE et al: Bisphosphonate-associated osteonecrosis of mandibular and maxillary bone: an emerging oral complication of supportive cancer therapy, *Cancer* 104:83-93, 2005.
74. Marx RE, Sawatari Y, Fortin M et al: Bisphosphonate-induced exposed bone (osteonecrosis/osteopetrosis) of the jaws: risk factors, recognition, prevention and treatment, *J Oral Maxillofac Surg* 63:1567-1575, 2005.
75. Bagan JV, Murillo J, Jimenez Y et al: Avascular jaw osteonecrosis in association with cancer chemotherapy: series of 10 cases, *J Oral Pathol Med* 34:120-123, 2005.
76. Markiewicz MR, Margarone JE, Campbell JH et al: Bisphosphonate-associated osteonecrosis of the jaws: a review of current knowledge, *J Am Dent Assoc* 136:1669-1674, 2005.
77. Bagan JV, Jimenez Y, Murillo J et al: Jaw osteonecrosis associated with bisphosphonates: multiple exposed areas and its relationship to teeth extractions: study of 20 cases, *Oral Oncol* 42:327-329, 2006.
78. Sachs HC: One year post exclusivity adverse event review: alendronate. *Center for Drug Evaluation and Research, Food and Drug Administration*: http://www.fda.gov/ohrms/dockets/ac/04/slides/2004-4067s1_07_Sachs%202%20Final.pdf. Accessed August 25, 2006.
79. Jeffcoat MK: Safety of oral bisphosphonates: controlled studies on alveolar bone, *Int J Oral Maxillofac Implants* 21:349-353, 2006.

CHAPTER 19

Odontogenic Diseases of the Maxillary Sinus

MYRON R. TUCKER AND STERLING R. SCHOW

CHAPTER OUTLINE

EMBRYOLOGY AND ANATOMY

The maxillary sinuses are air-containing spaces that occupy the maxillary bone bilaterally. The maxillary sinuses are the first of the paranasal sinuses (e.g., maxillary, ethmoid, frontal, and sphenoid) to develop embryonically and begin in the third month of fetal development as mucosal invaginations or pouching of the ethmoid infundibula. The initial maxillary sinus development, also termed *primary pneumatization,* progresses as the invagination expands into the cartilaginous nasal capsule.[1] Secondary pneumatization begins in the fifth month of fetal development as the initial invaginations expand into the developing maxillary bone.

After birth the maxillary sinus expands by pneumatization into the developing alveolar process and extends anteriorly and inferiorly from the base of the skull, closely matching the growth rate of the maxilla and the development of the dentition. As the dentition develops, portions of the alveolar process of the maxilla, vacated by the eruption of teeth, become pneumatized.[2] By the time a child reaches age 12 or 13, the sinus will have expanded to the point at which its floor will be on the same horizontal level as the floor of the nasal cavity. In adults the apices of the teeth may extend into the sinus cavity and can be identified in anatomic specimens or through computed tomography imaging.[3] Expansion of the sinus normally ceases after the eruption of the permanent teeth, but on occasion the sinus will pneumatize further, after the removal of one or more posterior maxillary teeth, to occupy the residual alveolar process. In many of the cases the sinus often extends virtually to the crest of the edentulous ridge. The maxillary sinus is significantly larger in adult patients who are edentulous in the posterior maxilla compared with patients with complete posterior dentition.[4]

The maxillary sinus is the largest of the paranasal sinuses. The maxillary sinus is also known as the antrum or the antrum of Highmore. *Antrum* is derived from the Greek word meaning cave. Dr. Nathaniel Highmore, an English physician in the 1600s, described a sinus infection associated with a maxillary tooth, and his name has long been associated with sinus nomenclature.

The maxillary sinus is described as a four-sided pyramid, with the base lying vertically on the medial surface and forming the lateral nasal wall. The apex extends laterally into the zygomatic process of the maxilla. The upper wall, or roof, of the sinus is also the floor of the orbit. The posterior wall extends the length of the maxilla and dips into the maxillary tuberosity. Anteriorly and laterally the sinus extends to the region of the first bicuspid or cuspid teeth. The floor of the sinus forms the base of the alveolar process (Figs. 19-1 and 19-2). The adult maxillary sinus averages 34 mm in anteroposterior direction, 33 mm in height, and 23 mm in width. The volume of the sinus is approximately 15 to 20 mL.

The sinuses are primarily lined by respiratory epithelium, a mucus-secreting, pseudostratified, ciliated, columnar epithelium. The cilia and mucus are necessary for the drainage of the sinus because the sinus opening, or ostium, is not in a dependent (inferior) position but lies two thirds the distance up the medial wall and drains into the nasal cavity (Figs. 19-1 and 19-2). The maxillary sinus opens into the posterior, or inferior, end of the semilunar hiatus, which lies in the middle meatus of the nasal cavity, between the inferior and middle nasal conchae. Beating of the cilia moves the mucus produced by the lining epithelium and any foreign material contained within the sinus toward the ostium, from which it drains into the nasal cavity. The cilia beat at a rate of up to 1000 strokes per minute and can move

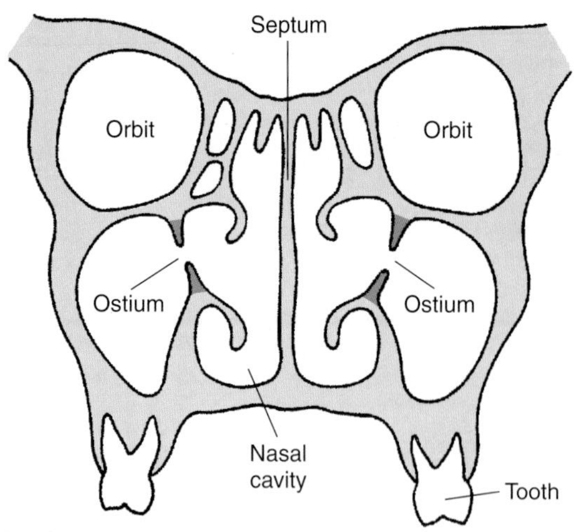

FIGURE 19-1 Frontal diagram of midface at ostium or opening of maxillary sinuses into middle meatus of nasal cavity. Ostium is in upper third of sinus cavity.

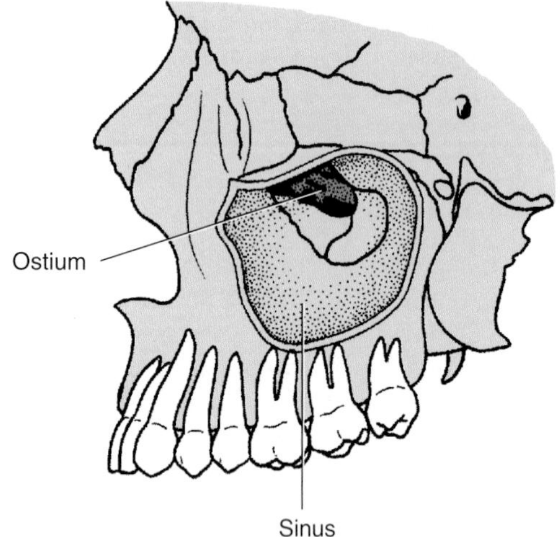

FIGURE 19-2 Lateral diagram of left maxillary sinus with zygoma removed. Medial sinus wall (i.e., lateral nasal wall) is seen in depth of sinus, as is the ostium. Maxillary sinus is pyramidal, with its apex directed into base of zygoma.

mucus a distance of 6 mm per minute.[5] The environment within the sinus is a constantly moving thin layer of mucus that is transported along the walls of the sinus, through the ostium and into the nasopharynx.

CLINICAL EXAMINATION OF THE MAXILLARY SINUS

Clinical evaluation of a patient with suspected maxillary sinusitis should begin with a careful visual examination of the patient's face and intraoral vestibule for swelling or redness. Nasal discharge may be evident during the initial evaluation. The examination of the patient with suspected maxillary sinus disease should also include tapping of the lateral walls of the sinus externally over the prominence of the cheek bones and palpation intraorally on the lateral surface of the maxilla between the canine fossa and the zygomatic buttress. The affected sinus may be very tender to gentle tapping or palpation. In some cases, there may be erosion of the lateral wall of the sinus/maxilla with a palpable defect. Patients with maxillary sinusitis frequently complain of dental pain, and pain to percussion of several maxillary posterior teeth is often indicative of an acute sinus infection.

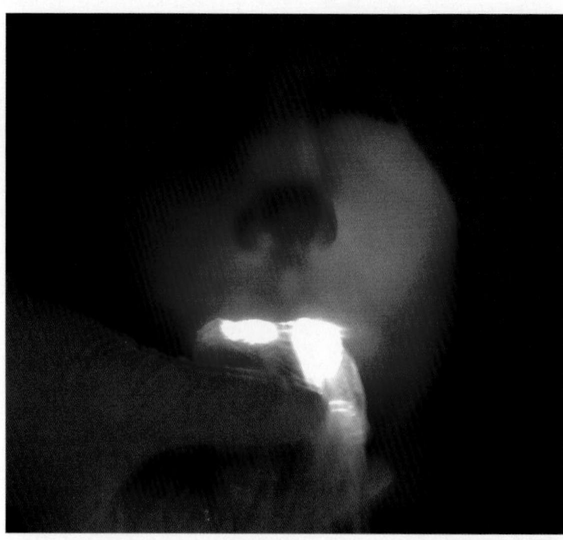

FIGURE 19-3 Transillumination of the maxillary sinus with a fiberoptic light source. Left maxillary sinus is normal and transilluminates from fiberoptic light source in palate. Right maxillary sinus is filled with fluid/pus from infection with decreased transillumination.

Further examination may include transillumination of the maxillary sinuses. Transillumination of the maxillary sinus is done by placing a bright fiberoptic light against the mucosa on the palatal or facial surfaces of the sinus and observing the transmission of light through the sinus in a darkened room (Fig. 19-3). In unilateral disease, one sinus may be compared with the sinus on the opposite side. The involved sinus shows decreased transmission of light because of the accumulation of fluid, debris, or pus and the thickening of the sinus mucosa. These simple tests may help to distinguish sinus disease, which may cause pain in the upper teeth, from abscess or other pain of dental origin associated with the molar and premolar teeth.

RADIOGRAPHIC EXAMINATION OF THE MAXILLARY SINUS

Radiographic examination of the maxillary sinus may be accomplished with a wide variety of exposures readily available in the dental office or radiology clinic. Standard dental radiographs that may be useful in evaluating the maxillary sinus include periapical, occlusal, and panoramic views. A periapical radiograph is limited in that only a small portion of the inferior aspect of the sinus can be visualized. In some cases the apices of the roots of the posterior maxillary teeth may be seen to project into the sinus floor (Fig. 19-4). Panoramic radiographs may provide a "screening" view of the maxillary sinuses (Fig. 19-5). This projection is the best radiograph available in most dental offices to provide a view of both maxillary sinuses for comparison. Because a panoramic radiograph provides a focused image within a limited focal trough, structures outside of this area may not be clearly delineated.

Periapical, occlusal, and occasionally panoramic radiographs are of value in locating and retrieving foreign bodies within the

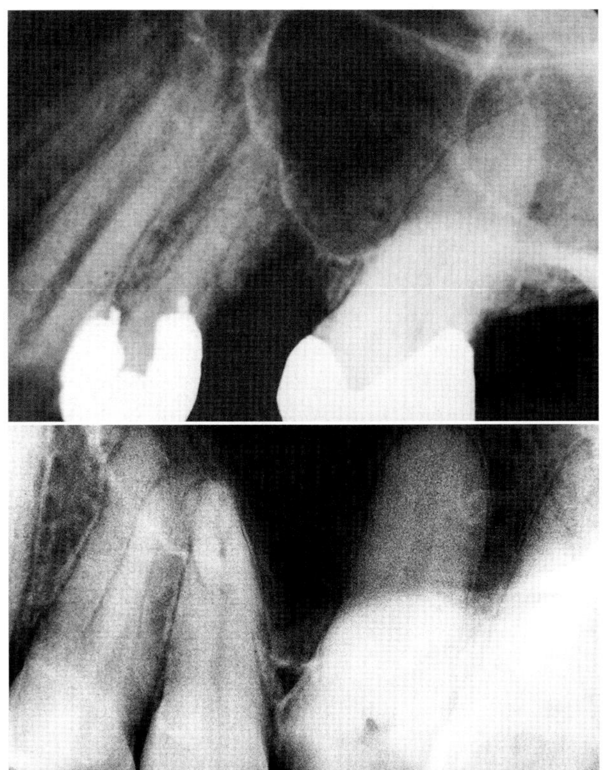

FIGURE 19-4 Periapical radiographs showing inferior portion of pneumatized maxillary sinus. Molar roots appear to be protruding into the sinus because sinus has pneumatized around roots.

sinus—particularly teeth, root tips, or osseous fragments—that have been displaced by trauma or during tooth removal (Fig. 19-6). These radiographs should also be used for the careful planning of surgical removal of teeth adjacent to the sinus.

If additional radiographic information is required, the Waters' and lateral views are two plain film radiographs that are frequently useful.[6] The Waters' view is taken with the head tipped 37 degrees to the central beam (Fig. 19-7). This projection places the maxillary sinus area above the petrous portion of the temporal bones, allowing for a clearer view of the sinuses than a standard posterior-anterior view of the skull. The lateral view can be obtained in a standard cephalometric machine with the patients head tipped slightly toward the cassette (Fig. 19-8). Tipping of the patient's head avoids superimposition of the walls of the sinus.

Computed tomography is a useful technique for imaging of the maxillary sinuses and other facial bony structures.[7] The decreased cost and more accessibility combined with clear, easily visualized images has made computed tomography scans increasingly popular for evaluating all types of facial bone pathologic conditions including abnormalities of the maxillary sinus (Fig. 19-9).

Interpretation of radiographs of the maxillary sinus is not difficult. The findings in the normal antrum are those to be expected of a rather large, air-filled cavity surrounded by bone and dental structures. The body of the sinus should appear radiolucent and should be outlined in all peripheral areas by a well-demarcated layer of cortical bone. Comparison of one side with the other is helpful when examining the radiographs. One should not see evidence of thickened mucosa on the bony walls, air-fluid levels (caused by accumulation of mucus, pus, or blood), or foreign bodies lying free. Partial or complete opacification of the maxillary sinus may be caused by the mucosal hypertrophy and fluid accumulation of sinusitis, by filling with blood following trauma, or by neoplasia. Radiographic changes are to be expected with acute maxillary sinusitis. Mucosal thickening caused by infections may obstruct the ostium of the sinus and allow accumulation of mucus, which will become infected and produce pus. The characteristic radiographic changes may include an air-fluid level in the sinus (Fig. 19-7), thickened mucosa on any or all of the sinus walls (Fig. 19-10), or complete opacification of the sinus cavity. The radiographic changes indicative of chronic maxillary sinusitis include mucosal thickening, sinus opacification, and nasal or antral polyps. Air-fluid levels in the sinuses are more characteristic of acute sinus disease

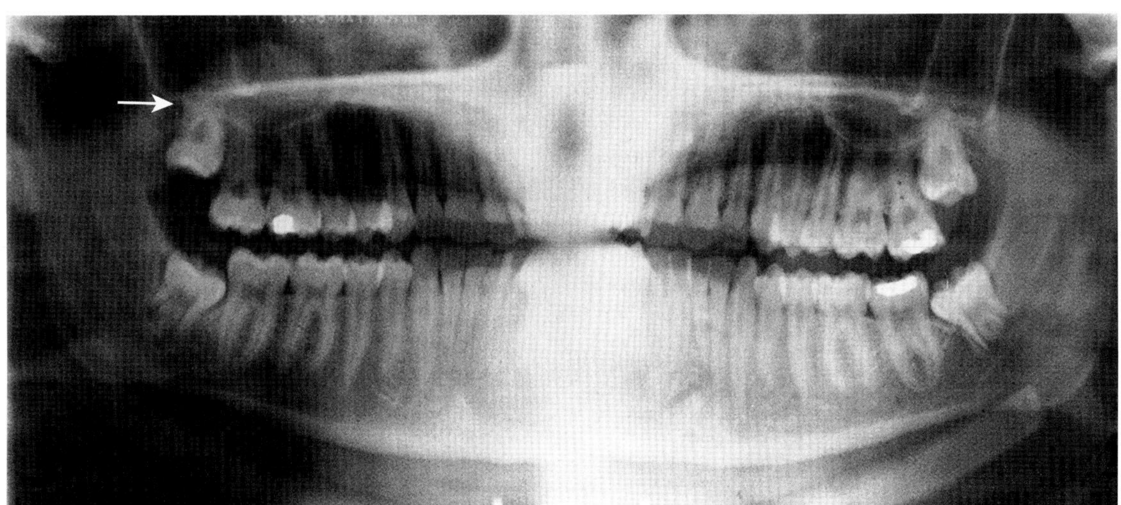

FIGURE 19-5 Panoramic radiograph showing mucous retention phenomenon on the floor of the right maxillary sinus *(arrow)*.

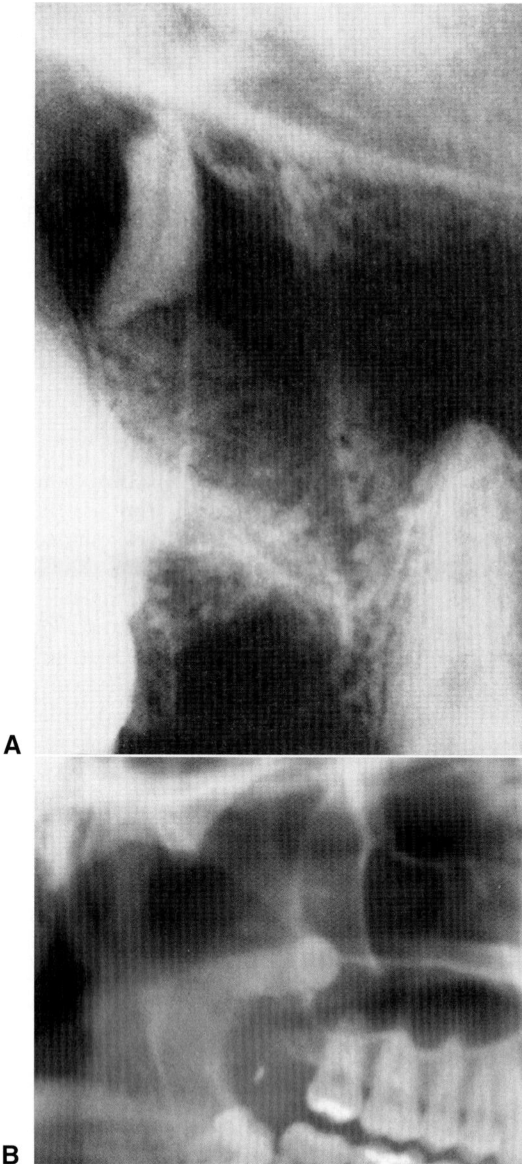

FIGURE 19-6 A, Periapical radiograph showing apical one third of palatal root of maxillary first molar, which was displaced into maxillary sinus during removal of the tooth. B, Close-up view of panoramic view of right maxillary sinus with third molar displaced superiorly, lying against the posterior wall of the sinus.

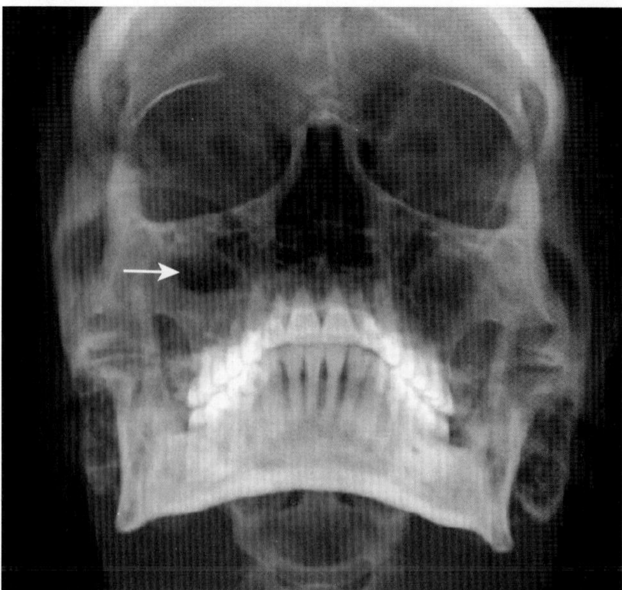

FIGURE 19-7 Waters' view radiograph demonstrating right maxillary sinus with air-fluid level (*arrow*) and increased opacity of the left sinus because of fluid, significant thickening of the mucosa, or both.

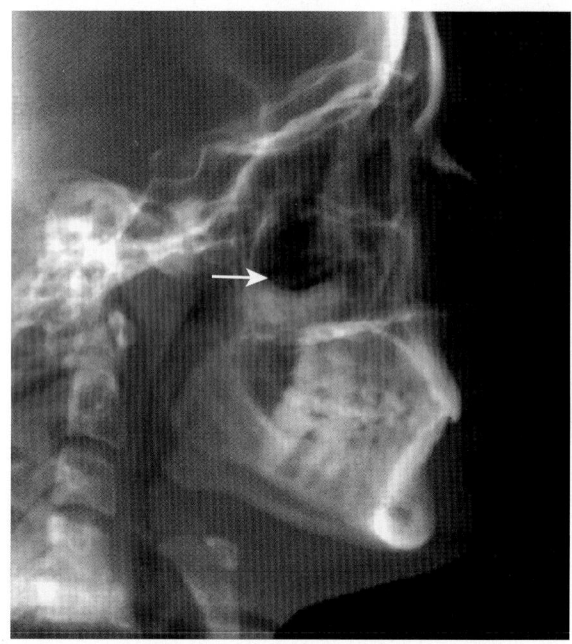

FIGURE 19-8 Lateral radiograph demonstrates air-fluid levels in maxillary sinus (*arrow*).

but may be seen in chronic sinusitis in periods of acute exacerbation.

Disruption of the cortical outline may be a result of trauma, tumor formation, an infectious process with abscess and fistula formation (Fig. 19-11), or a surgical procedure that violates the sinus walls. Expansion of the bony walls may also be apparent (Fig. 19-12). Dental pathologic conditions such as cysts or granulomas may produce radiolucent lesions that extend into the sinus cavity. These conditions may be distinguished from normal sinus anatomy by their association with the tooth apex, the clinical correlation with the dental examination, and the presence of a cortical osseous margin on the radiograph, which generally separates the area in question from the sinus itself.

NONODONTOGENIC INFECTIONS OF THE MAXILLARY SINUS

Historically, the consensus has been that the maxillary sinus is usually not colonized by any bacteria and is essentially sterile.[8] More recent studies using updated techniques have occasionally shown that some bacteria may be cultured from a healthy paranasal sinus.[9] Even though there may be some microorganisms present in the normal sinus, this appears to be minimal, and the dynamic nature of the sinus with active epithelium

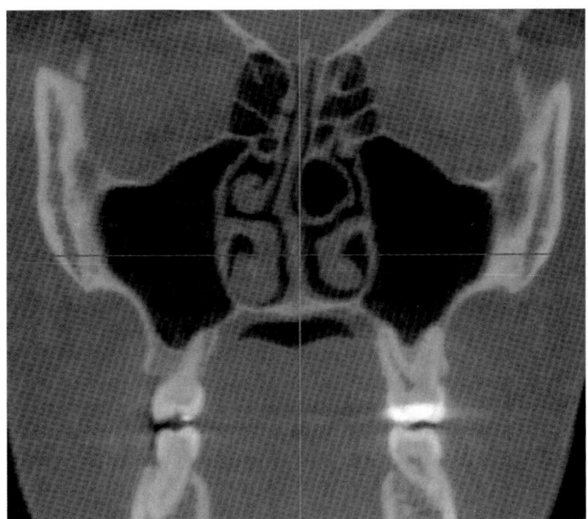

FIGURE 19-9 Computed tomography scan, coronal view, showing normal maxillary sinus anatomy with thin bony walls without any thickening of the mucosal lining, masses, or fluid.

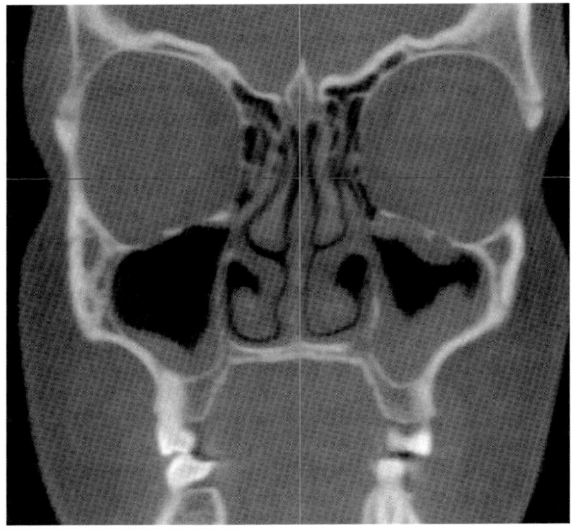

FIGURE 19-10 Computed tomography scan showing right maxillary sinus with thickened mucosa at the inferior portion of the sinus. The patient's left side has significant mucosal thickening along the entire lining of the sinus.

and a constant moving mucus layer prevents any significant colonization.

The mucosa of the sinus is susceptible to infectious, allergic, and neoplastic diseases. Inflammatory diseases of the sinus, such as infection or allergic reactions, cause hyperplasia and hypertrophy of the mucosa and may cause obstruction of the ostium. If the ostium becomes obstructed, the mucus produced by the secretory cells lining the sinus is collected over long periods. Bacterial overgrowth may then produce an infection resulting in the signs and symptoms of sinusitis, as well as the radiographic changes seen with these conditions.

When inflammation develops in any of the paranasal sinuses, whether caused by infection or allergy, the condition is described as *sinusitis*. Inflammation of most or all of the paranasal sinuses simultaneously is known as *pansinusitis* and is usually caused

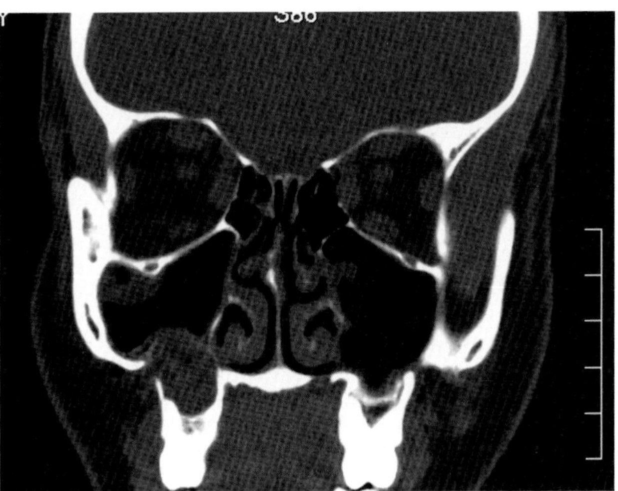

FIGURE 19-11 Perforation of the lateral wall of the right sinus as a result of an odontogenic infection associated with a molar tooth. The abscess expanded into the floor of the sinus and eroded the lateral wall of the sinus.

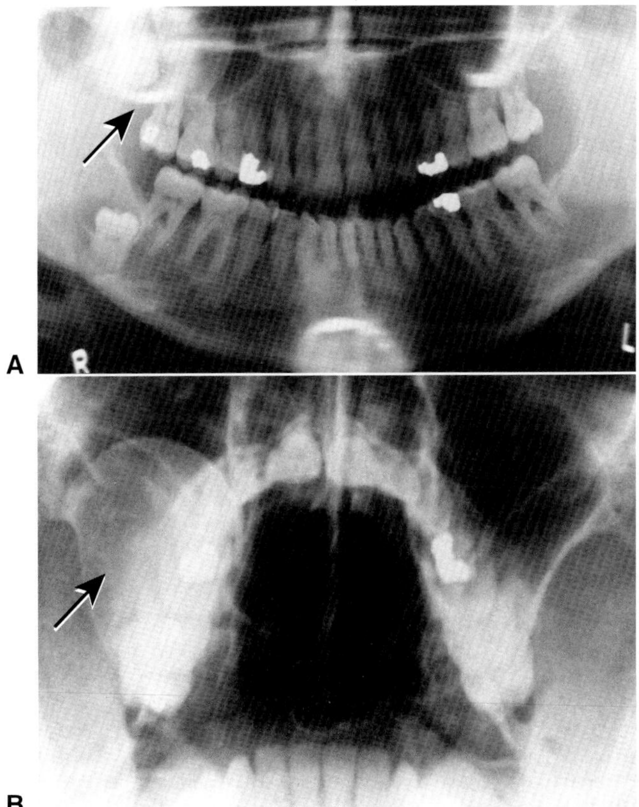

FIGURE 19-12 A, Panoramic radiograph shows large odontogenic keratocyst associated with impacted right maxillary third molar tooth (*arrow*). Cyst has impinged on right maxillary sinus as it expanded. Sinus cavity is almost totally obstructed by lesion. Another odontogenic keratocyst is seen associated with impacted right mandibular third molar. B, Waters' view radiograph demonstrates the odontogenic keratocyst (seen in A). Lesion is also seen to have expanded lateral wall of right maxillary sinus (*arrow*).

by infection. Similar conditions of individual sinuses are known, for example, as *maxillary sinusitis* or *frontal sinusitis*.

Acute maxillary sinusitis may occur at any age. The onset is usually described by the patient as a rapidly developing sense of pressure, pain, and/or fullness in the vicinity of the affected sinus. The discomfort rapidly increases in intensity and may be accompanied by facial swelling and erythema, malaise, fever, and drainage of foul smelling mucopurulent material into the nasal cavity and nasopharynx.

Chronic maxillary sinusitis is usually a result of bacterial or fungal infections that are low grade and recurrent, obstructive nasal disease or allergy. Chronic maxillary sinusitis is characterized by episodes of sinus disease that respond initially to treatment, only to return, or that remain symptomatic in spite of treatment.

Aerobic, anaerobic, or mixed bacteria may cause infections of the maxillary sinuses. The organisms usually associated with maxillary sinusitis of nonodontogenic origin include those organisms usually found within the nasal cavity. Mucostasis that occurs within the sinus allows for colonization of these organisms. The causative bacteria are primarily aerobic, with a few anaerobes. The important aerobes are *Streptococcus pneumoniae, Haemophilus influenzae,* and *Branhamella catarrhalis.* Anaerobes include *Streptococcus viridans, Staphylococcus aureus,* Enterobacteriaceae, *Porphyromonas, Prevotella, Peptostreptococcus, Veillonella, Propionibacterium, Eubacterium,* and *Fusobacterium.*

ODONTOGENIC INFECTIONS OF THE MAXILLARY SINUS

Maxillary sinusitis is occasionally a result of odontogenic sources because of the anatomic juxtaposition of the teeth and the maxillary sinus (Fig. 19-13). Odontogenic sources account for approximately 10% to 12% of all maxillary sinusitis.[10] This condition may readily spread to involve the other paranasal sinuses if left untreated or inadequately treated. In rare cases, these infections become life threatening and can include orbital cellulitis, cavernous sinus thrombosis, meningitis, osteomyelitis, intracranial abscess, and death.

Sources of odontogenic infections that involve the maxillary sinus include acute and chronic periapical disease and periodontal disease. Infection and sinusitis may also result from trauma to the dentition or from surgery in the posterior maxilla, including removal of teeth, alveolectomy, tuberosity reduction, sinus lift grafting and implant placement, or other procedures that create an area of communication between the oral cavity and the maxillary sinus.

Maxillary sinus infections of odontogenic origin are more likely to be caused by anaerobic bacteria, as is the usual odontogenic infection. Rarely does *H. influenzae* or *S. aureus* cause odontogenic sinusitis. The predominant organisms are aerobic and anaerobic streptococci and anaerobic *Bacteroides,* Enterobacteriaceae, *Peptococcus, Peptostreptococcus, Porphyromonas, Prevotella,* and *Eubacterium.*

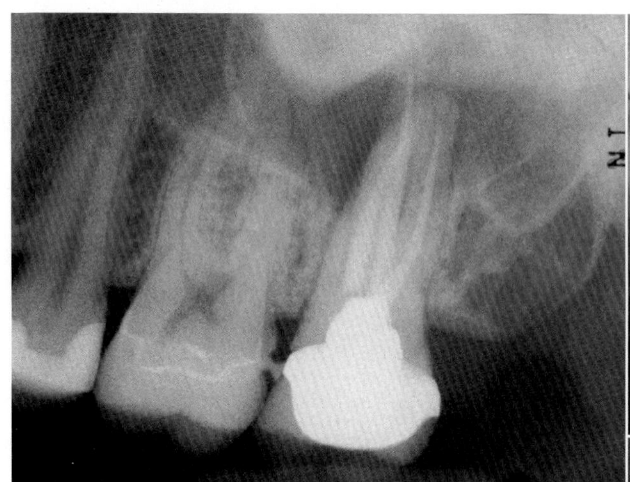

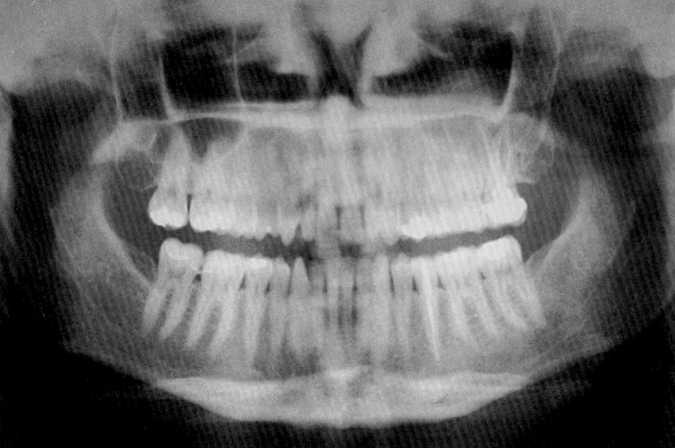

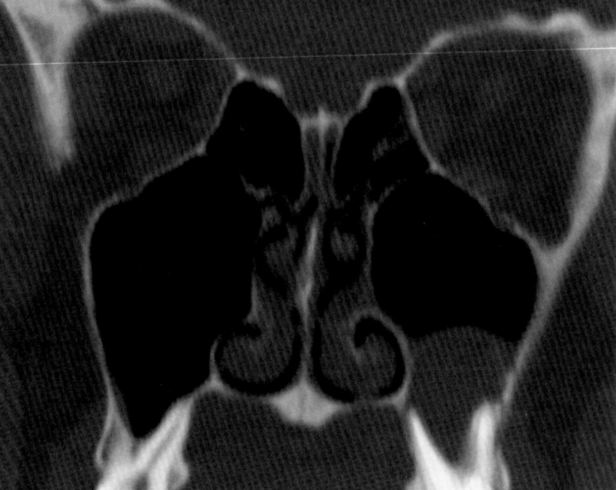

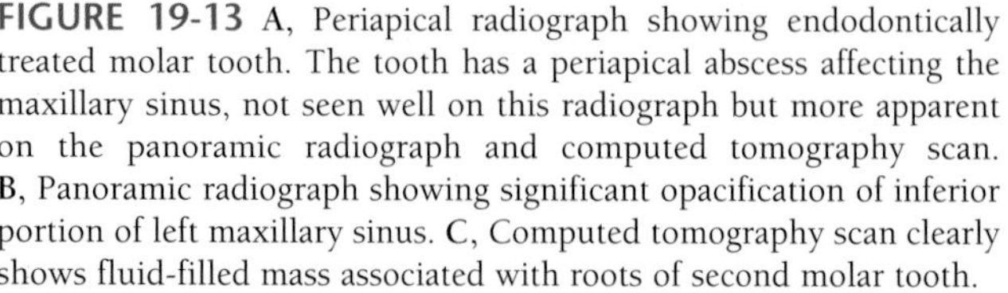

FIGURE 19-13 A, Periapical radiograph showing endodontically treated molar tooth. The tooth has a periapical abscess affecting the maxillary sinus, not seen well on this radiograph but more apparent on the panoramic radiograph and computed tomography scan. B, Panoramic radiograph showing significant opacification of inferior portion of left maxillary sinus. C, Computed tomography scan clearly shows fluid-filled mass associated with roots of second molar tooth.

TREATMENT OF MAXILLARY SINUSITIS

Early treatment of maxillary sinusitis consists of humidification of inspired air to loosen and aid in the removal of dried secretions from the nasal passage and the sinus ostium. Systemically administered decongestants such as pseudoephedrine (Sudafed) and nasal spray containing vasoconstrictors, such as 2% ephedrine or 0.25% phenylephrine, decrease nasal and sinus congestion and help facilitate normal drainage. Patients with sinus infections often experience moderate to severe pain, and prescribing a nonsteroidal or narcotic analgesic may be appropriate.[11]

Many cases of sinusitis are caused by allergies that result in congestion and altered natural drainage of the sinus. Allergic sinusitis often responds to the measures described before. However, when sinusitis is a result of an infectious process, the use of antibiotics is indicated. Knowledge of the bacteria most likely to be isolated in sinusitis is important in selecting an antibiotic. In cases of nonodontogenic sinusitis, the most likely organisms are *H. influenzae* and *S. aureus, Streptococcus pneumonia,* and a variety of anaerobic streptococci. Antibiotic choices for treatment of nonodontogenic maxillary sinusitis include amoxicillin, trimethoprim-sulfamethoxazole, amoxicillin/clavulanate, azithromycin, and cefuroxime.

Odontogenic sinusitis usually involves organisms that are associated with common odontogenic infections, including aerobic and anaerobic streptococci and anaerobes such as *Bacteroides* and Enterobacteriaceae. Therefore, antibiotics generally effective for odontogenic infections such as penicillin, clindamycin, and metronidazole are effective for sinusitis of odontogenic origin.

Because of the wide variety of microorganisms that can contribute to infections of the maxillary sinus, it is important to obtain purulent material for culture and sensitivity testing whenever possible. Sensitivity testing may suggest a change to another antibiotic if resistant organisms are cultured from the sinus and if the infection is failing to respond to appropriate initial treatment.

If the patient fails to respond to this initial treatment regimen within 72 hours, it is necessary to reassess the treatment and the antibiotic. If the cause of the problem has not been identified and eliminated, this must be carefully reevaluated. The results of the culture and sensitivity tests should be evaluated, and changes should be made if indicated. As many as 25% of the organisms cultured from acute sinus infections are β-lactamase producers, and many may be anaerobic, especially if the infection is odontogenic.[11] If the organism or organisms causing the infection are β-lactamase producers, another antibiotic, such as the combination agent trimethoprim-sulfamethoxazole (Bactrim, Septra), may be effective. Cefaclor or a combination of amoxicillin and clavulanate potassium (Augmentin) has also been shown to be effective.

Acute maxillary sinusitis is a painful, potentially serious condition that requires immediate attention and aggressive medical and surgical care. Patients suspected of having maxillary sinusitis should be referred to an oral and maxillofacial surgeon or another specialist, such as an otolaryngologist. The referring clinician should send radiographs, the results of clinical procedures, the results of culture and sensitivity tests of purulent drainage, and any other pertinent diagnostic information to the surgeon.

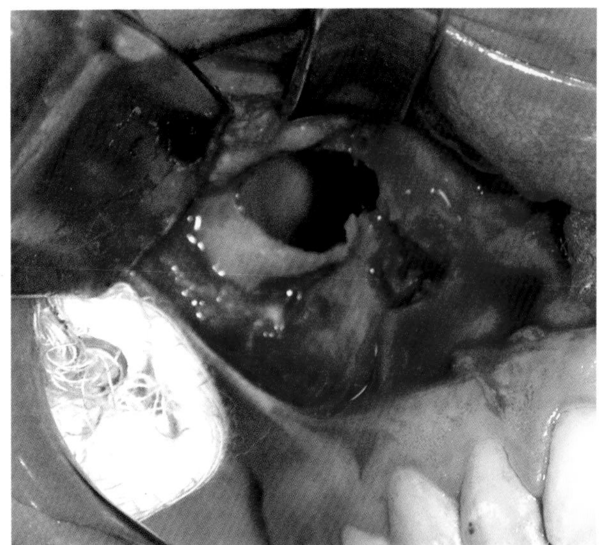

FIGURE 19-14 Caldwell-Luc exposure of the maxillary sinus through a vestibular incision and bony window created in the anterior maxillary wall.

Diagnosis and treatment of chronic maxillary sinusitis is difficult and may include allergy testing, nasal or septal surgery, and surgical débridement of the sinuses. The goal of sinus surgery is to remove abnormal tissue from within the sinus cavity and restore normal drainage through the ostium. Traditionally, this was accomplished with an open approach to the sinus known as a Caldwell-Luc procedure (Fig. 19-14).[12] In this technique the anterior wall of the sinus is accessed in the area of the canine fossa through a vestibular approach. The sinus is opened, and abnormal tissue or foreign bodies can be removed. The ostiomeatal area can be evaluated and opened, or a new opening for more dependent drainage into the nose (termed an *antrostomy*) can be created near the floor of the sinus. Newer techniques allow exploration and surgical treatment of the sinus with less invasive endoscopic approaches (Fig. 19-15).[12,13]

Sinus lift procedures, done primarily as preprosthetic surgical procedures to improve the posterior maxillary alveolar base for secondary or simultaneous endosseous implant placement, occasionally contribute to sinus infections. In most cases, careful elevation of the schneiderian (i.e., sinus) membrane creates a space into which particulate grafts of autologous bone, allogeneic bone, alloplastic materials, or combinations of these can be placed. If the procedure is done carefully, complications resulting from sinus lift operations are rare. Complications became more frequent in at least two instances: (1) when the sinus membrane is severely lacerated or avulsed or (2) when the sinus is overfilled.

Significant disruption of the sinus membrane allows exposure of the graft material to the open sinus and possible contamination by nasal bacteria. Disruption also allows particulate material from the sinus grafts or implants to become free foreign bodies within the sinus, which can cause foreign-body rejection responses from the sinus mucosa or outright infection. Lacerated sinus membranes may also interfere with normal nasal epithelial ciliary motility and thereby impede physiologic sinus drainage. Finally, fragments of sinus mucosa or graft material may obstruct the sinus ostium, further preventing normal sinus drainage.

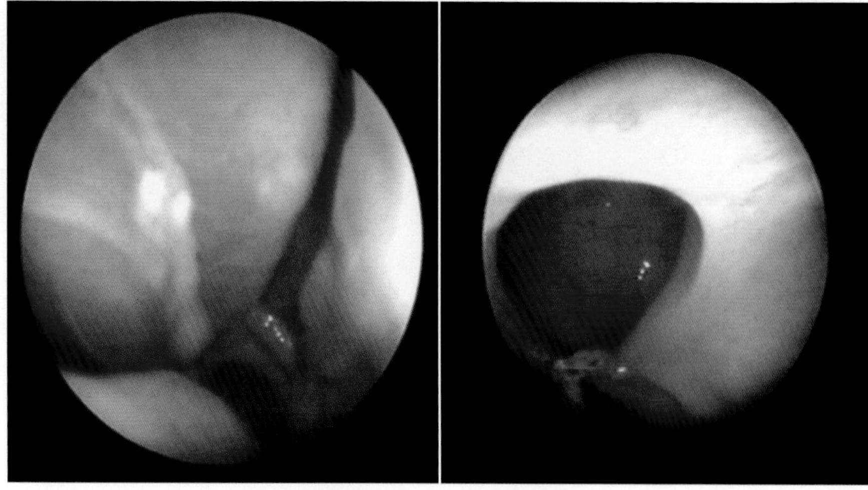

FIGURE 19-15 A, View of ostium and surrounding inflamed mucosa as seen through the endoscope. B, Ostium and surrounding healthy sinus mucosa. (From Costa F, Emanuelli E, Robiony M et al: Endoscopic surgery for maxillary sinusitis, *J Oral Maxillofac Surg* 65: 225-226, 2007, with permission.)

When these situations occur, treatment consists of infection control and removal of contaminated or devitalized graft materials. This treatment also includes removal of foreign-body free segments and debulking of overly extended grafts. These procedures are usually accomplished through a Caldwell-Luc lateral sinus wall surgical approach or, rarely, with nasal access endoscopic sinus surgery. Antibiotic therapy alone may temporarily improve the acute problem, but the ultimate treatment will require sinus exploration and débridement.

ANTRAL PSEUDOCYSTS

Pseudocysts, mucoceles, and retention cysts are benign accumulations of fluid underneath or surrounded by sinus epithelium. The term *mucocele* has often been used to describe any type of localized fluid accumulation, but this is not accurate.[14] Although each of these may appear as a round, faint radiopacity within the sinus, the cause of each is different, as is the histology.

The antral pseudocyst is seen in 2% to 10% of panoramic radiographs. This pseudocyst is a result of accumulation of serum (not sinus mucus) under the sinus mucosa. The cause of these accumulations is not clear but may be related to inflammation of the sinus lining. These lesions are of no clinical consequence, require no treatment, and often disappear over time.

Sinus mucoceles are actually cystic lesions in that they are lined by epithelium. One of the most common causes of true mucoceles is surgery on the sinus that results in separation of a portion of the sinus lining from the main portion of the sinus. This area can then become filled with mucus and walled off, forming a separate cystic lesion. These lesions are termed *surgical ciliated cysts* or *postoperative maxillary cysts.* These lesions can become expansile and may expand or erode walls of the sinus and must be differentiated, usually through removal and biopsy, from more aggressive and even malignant lesions of the sinus.

Retention cysts in the maxillary sinus result from blockage of ducts within the mucus-secreting glands within the sinus. The accumulated mucin becomes surrounded by epithelium, forming a true cystic lesion. These lesions are usually so small as not to be seen on radiographic images.

COMPLICATIONS OF ORAL SURGERY INVOLVING THE MAXILLARY SINUS

The most common dental complications of oral surgical procedures that subsequently involve the maxillary sinus include displacement of teeth, roots, or instrument fragments into the sinus or the creation of a communication between the oral cavity and the sinus during surgery of the posterior maxilla. Retrieval of a tooth, root fragment, or broken instrument can be accomplished in several ways. In many cases the opening created during initial displacement can be enlarged slightly, and the tooth or other object can be visualized and retrieved with small forceps or with the use of suction. Irrigating or flooding the sinus followed by suction can often accomplish retrieval or position the object close to the opening for easy recovery. In some cases, however, the sinus needs to be opened through a Caldwell-Luc approach and the object retrieved.

A sinus perforation resulting from a tooth extraction most commonly occurs when a maxillary molar with widely divergent roots that is adjacent to edentulous spaces requires extraction. In this instance the sinus is likely to have become pneumatized into the edentulous alveolar process surrounding the tooth, which weakens the entire alveolus and brings the tooth apices into a closer relationship with the sinus cavity. Other causes of perforation into the sinus include abnormally long roots, destruction of a portion of the sinus floor by periapical lesions, perforation of the floor and sinus membrane with injudicious use of instruments, forcing a root or tooth into the sinus during attempted removal, and removal of large cystic lesions that encroach on the sinus cavity.

In many cases the opening is small and primary closure can be easily accomplished with adequate healing. In some cases a larger perforation or communication is apparent, and routine closure is not possible or not adequate to cover the opening.

The treatment of oroantral communications is accomplished immediately, when the opening is created, or later, as in the instance of a long-standing fistula or failure of an attempted primary closure.

Oroantral Communications: Immediate Treatment

The best treatment of a potential sinus exposure is avoiding the problem through careful observation and treatment planning. Evaluation of high-quality radiographs before surgery usually reveals the presence or absence of an excessively pneumatized sinus or widely divergent or dilacerated roots, which have the potential of having a communication with the sinus or causing fractures in the bony floor of the antrum during removal. If this observation is made, surgery may be altered to section the tooth and remove it one root at a time (see Chapter 8).

When exposure and perforation of the sinus result, the least invasive therapy is indicated initially. If the opening to the sinus is small and the sinus is disease free, efforts should be made to establish a blood clot in the extraction site and preserve it in place. Additional soft tissue flap elevation is not required. Sutures are placed to reposition the soft tissues, and a gauze pack is placed over the surgical site for 1 to 2 hours. The patient is instructed to use nasal precautions for 10 to 14 days. These include opening the mouth while sneezing, not sucking on a straw or cigarettes, and avoiding nose blowing and any other situation that may produce pressure changes between the nasal passages and oral cavity. The patient is placed on an antibiotic, usually a penicillin; an antihistamine; and a systemic decongestant for 7 to 10 days to prevent infection, to shrink mucous membranes, and to lessen nasal and sinus secretions. The patient is seen postoperatively at 48- to 72-hour intervals and is instructed to return if an oroantral communication becomes evident by leakage of air into the mouth or fluid into the nose or if symptoms of maxillary sinusitis appear.

The majority of patients treated in this manner heal uneventfully if there is no evidence of preexisting sinus disease. If larger perforations occur, it may be necessary to cover the extraction site with some type of flap advancement to provide primary closure in an attempt to cover the sinus opening. The most commonly used flap procedure involves elevating a buccal flap, releasing the periosteum and advancing the flap to cover the extraction site (Fig. 19-16). The most important aspects of flap advancement for closure include elevating a broad-based flap with adequate width to cover the communication with margins of the flap positioned over bone rather than directly over the defect of area of communication. The flap must be free of any tension. To accomplish this, the periosteum usually must be incised and released at the height of the dissection. Following closure, the patient is instructed to follow the sinus precautions as described previously.

Oroantral Fistulae: Delayed Treatment

Successful treatment and closure of the oroantral fistula requires more extensive medical and surgical treatment. Before closure of an oroantral fistula, it is imperative to eliminate any acute or chronic infection within the sinus. This may require frequent irrigation of the fistula and sinus combined with the use of antibiotics and decongestants. It may also be helpful to construct a temporary appliance to cover the fistula to prevent food and other oral contaminants from getting into the sinus. If sinus disease persists, it may be necessary to remove diseased tissues from the sinus using a Caldwell-Luc procedure through the lateral maxillary wall above the apices of the remaining teeth.

Adjacent teeth must be carefully evaluated for possible involvement. If the fistula has developed in approximation to the root of an adjacent tooth, closure is further complicated; and to be successful, removal of the tooth may be necessary.

Methods of closing oroantral fistulae include buccal flap advancement (Fig. 19-17), palatal flap advancement (Fig. 19-18), and advancement of palatal and facial flaps over a membrane of alloplastic material (Fig. 19-19). The buccal flap procedure is performed in a manner similar to the buccal advancement described before for immediate closure of an oroantral communication.[15] In the case of a chronic fistula, however, the fistulous tract will be lined with epithelium that must be excised or elevated from the bony walls of the fistula, sutured together if possible, and inverted into the sinus cavity (Fig. 19-17). This should be accomplished before elevating the buccal flap so that the actual size of the bony defect can be inspected and the size of the flap designed appropriately to allow the flap to cover the entire defect with the margins lying over bone. The flap is elevated, the periosteum is released, and the flap is then extended over the defect and carefully sutured in place. A similar technique has been described of elevating a larger buccal flap but then using a pedicled portion of the buccal fat pad to cover the defect directly with partial closure of the mucoperiosteal flap.[16] Regardless of the technique used, one must remember that the osseous defect surrounding the fistula is always much larger than the clinically apparent soft tissue deformity.[17] Surgical planning of closure technique must be adjusted accordingly.

Rotation of a palatal flap is often used to close an oroantral fistula.[18] The advantages of using a full-thickness palatal flap are that a large amount of tissue can be elevated with good blood supply from palatal vessels and the thickness and keratinized nature of palatal tissue more closely resemble crestal ridge tissue than thinner, less keratinized tissue in the buccal vestibule. The disadvantage of this flap is the large area of exposed bone that results from elevation of the flap. The size of the flap must allow for passive rotation of the flap to cover the entire defect with flap margins extending past the bony margins of the defect. Once the fistula is excised and the flap is elevated, rotated, and sutured in place, the palatal defect will eventually heal with granulation and secondary epithialization (Fig. 19-18). In some cases the defect can be covered with a temporary obturator with some type of soft tissue conditioning liner; however, it is important that no pressure be applied over the flap area because this may decrease blood supply and cause tissue necrosis.

Another technique for fistula closure uses excision of the fistula, elevation of flaps on the facial and palatal aspect of the defect, covering of the defect with some type of alloplastic material, and approximation of the flaps as closely as possible over the alloplast. Thin metallic foil such as gold foil or thin titanium has been used for this purpose and must be closely adapted to the contour of the bony surface.[19] The sinus lining and in some cases crestal bone heals over the superior surface of the metal. In some cases the foil remains permanently, but more frequently a small portion of the metal eventually becomes exposed and the material is gradually exfoliated. An identical closure technique may also be performed using material such as a collagen membrane that is eventually resorbed.[20,21]

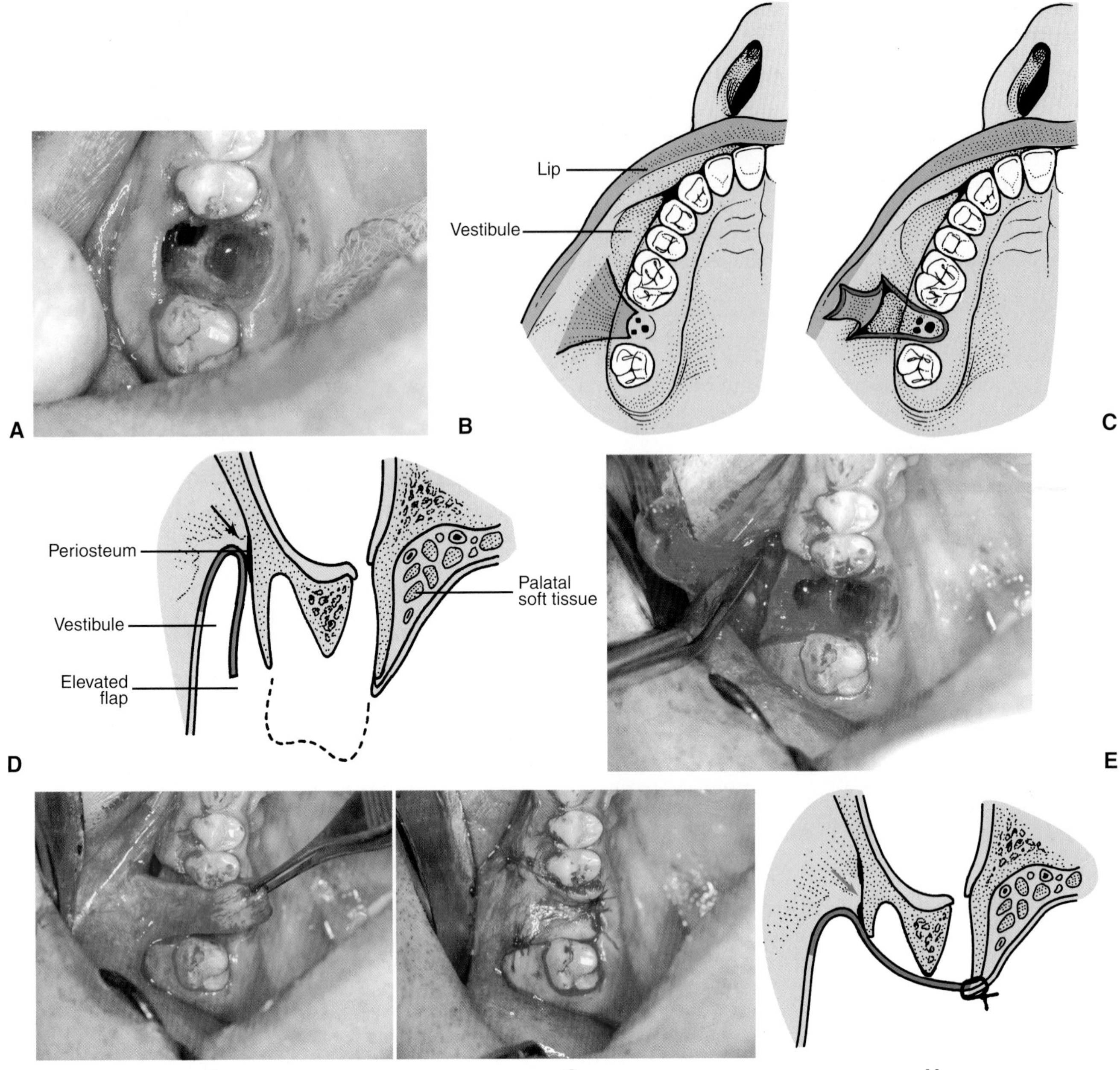

FIGURE 19-16 Closure of large oroantral communication. A, Clinical photograph of large oroantral fistula in molar region of right maxilla. B, Diagram of flap design. C, Illustration of flap elevated to depth of vestibule. D, Cross-section view of flap elevation. Periosteum must be incised in at the height of dissection (*arrow*) in the vestibule, releasing flap attachment in this area to allow tissue flap to be positioned without tension across extraction site. E, Clinical photograph showing elevation and flap. Scissors used to incise periosteum at height of dissection. F, Passive repositioning of flap across extraction site. G, Flap sutured in position. Note flap margins extend well beyond extraction site and communication defect. H, Cross section of closure. In some cases a small amount of bone reduction may be necessary over the facial aspect to facilitate flap closure.

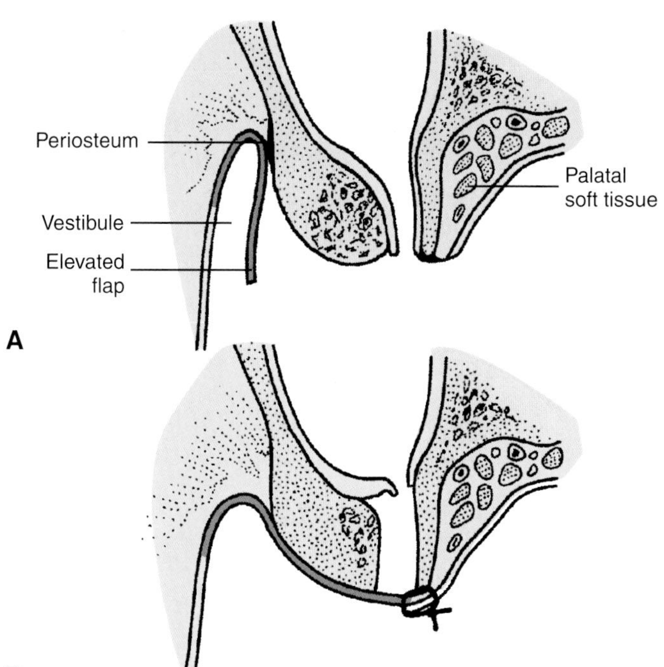

FIGURE 19-17 Buccal flap closure of oroantral fistula. **A**, Cross-section illustration of oroantral fistula in molar region. Buccal flap has been elevated. **B**, Epithelium lining the fistula has been excised, the periosteum has been released at the vestibular height of the dissection, and the tension-free flap has been closed across the defect with margins of the flap resting over bone.

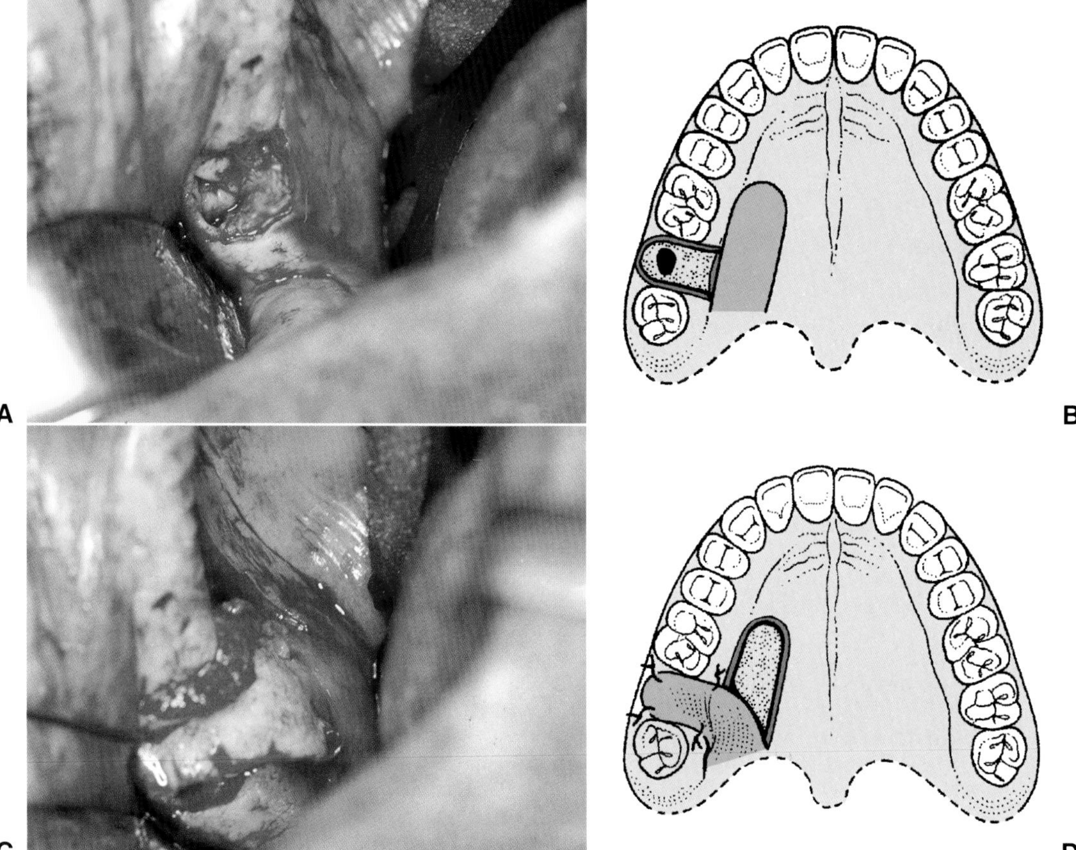

FIGURE 19-18 Palatal flap closure of oroantral fistula. **A**, Clinical photograph of fistula resulting from removal of lone standing molar in posterior maxilla where sinus was pneumatized. **B**, Soft tissues surrounding oroantral opening are excised, exposing underlying alveolar bone around osseous defect. Full-thickness palatal flap is outlined, incised, and elevated from anterior to posterior. Flap should be full thickness of mucoperiosteum, should have broad posterior base, and should include the palatine artery. Flap width should be sufficient to cover entire defect around oroantral opening, and its length must be adequate to allow rotation of flap and repositioning over defect without placing undue tension on flap. **C**, Flap rotated to cover to ensure that there is no tension on flap when positioned to cover osseous defect. **D**, Illustration of flap rotation and closure.

Continued

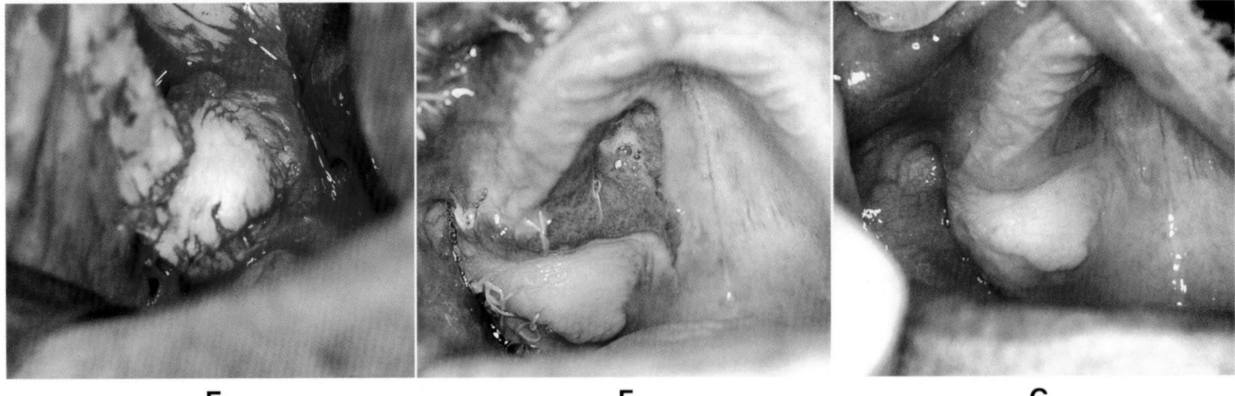

FIGURE 19-18, cont'd E, Clinical photograph of closure. F, Healing at 1 week postoperatively. G, Three weeks postoperatively.

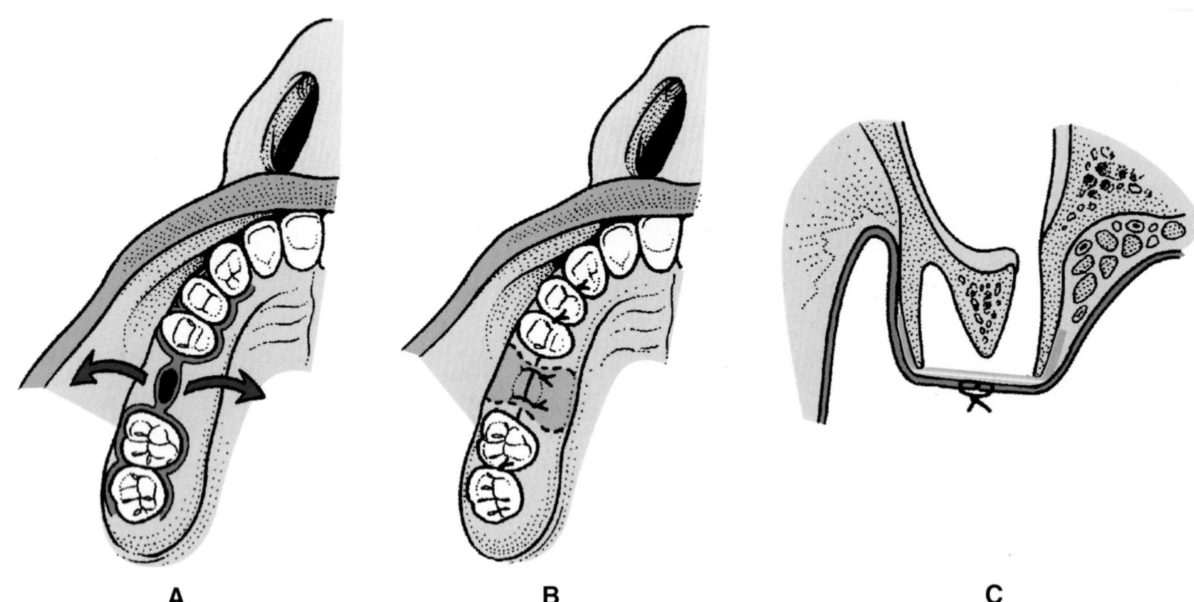

FIGURE 19-19 Membrane-assisted closure of oroantral communications. **A**, Diagrammatic illustration of oroantral fistula in right maxillary alveolar process in region of missing first molar tooth, which is to be closed with subperiosteal placement of alloplastic material such as gold or titanium foil or a resorbable collagen membrane. Facial and palatal mucoperiosteal flaps are developed. Extension of the flaps along the gingival sulcus one or two teeth anterior and posterior allows some stretching of the flap to facilitate advancement for closure over the defect. Fistulous tract is excised. Osseous margins must be exposed 360 degrees around bony defect to allow placement of membrane beneath mucoperiosteal flaps. Flap is supported on all sides by underlying bone. **B**, Diagram of closure. Ideally, the flaps can be approximated over the defect. In some small cases a small gap between the flaps will heal over the membrane by secondary intention. Even if the intraoral mucosa does not heal primarily, the sinus lining usually heals and closes, and the membrane is then exfoliated or resorbed and mucosal healing progresses. **C**, Cross-sectional diagram of membrane closure technique. Buccal and palatal mucoperiosteal flaps are elevated to expose osseous defect and large area of underlying alveolar bone around oroantral communication. Membrane overlaps all margins of the defect, and the facial and palatal flaps are sutured over the membrane.

In rare cases, larger defects, particularly those resulting from surgical removal of pathologic lesions, may require larger flaps to accomplish closure and may include the use of pedicle flaps from the tongue or temporalis muscle.

REFERENCES

1. Moss-Salentijn L: Anatomy and embryology. In Blitzer A, Lawson W, Friedman WH, editors: *Surgery of the paranasal sinuses*, Philadelphia, 1991, WB Saunders.

2. Anon JB, Rontal M, Zinreich SJ: Maxillary sinus anatomy. In Anon JG, Rontal MK, Zinreich SJ, editors: *Anatomy of the paranasal sinuses,* New York, 1996, Thieme.
3. Eberhardt JA, Torabinejad M, Christiansen EL: A computed tomographic study of the distances between the maxillary sinus floor and the apices of the maxillary posterior teeth, *Oral Surg Oral Med Oral Pathol Oral Radiol Endod* 73:345, 1992.
4. Harorh A, Bacutoglu O: The comparison of vertical height and width of maxillary sinus by means of Waters' view radiograms taken from dentate and edentulous cases, *Ann Dent* 54:47, 1995.
5. McCafferey TF, Kern EB: Clinical evaluation of nasal obstruction, *Arch Otolaryngol Head Neck Surg* 105:542, 1979.
6. Som PM, Brandwein M: Anatomy, physiology, and plain film normal anatomy. In Som P, Curtin HD, editors: *Head and neck imaging,* ed 3, St Louis, 1996, Mosby.
7. Zinreich SJ, Benson JL, Oliverio PJ: Sinonasal cavities: CT normal anatomy, imaging of the osteomeatal complex and functional endoscopic surgery. In Som P, Curtin HD, editors: *Head and neck imaging,* ed 3, St Louis, 1996, Mosby.
8. Gwaltney JM Jr: Acute community-acquired sinusitis, *Clin Infect Dis* 23:1209-1225, 1996.
9. Weymouth LA: Microbiology of the maxillary sinus, *Oral and Maxillofacial Clinics of North America* 11:21-33, 1999.
10. Brook I: Sinusitis of odontogenic origin, *Otolaryngol Head Neck Surg* 135:349-355, 1006.
11. Okeson J, Falace D: Nonodontogenic toothache, *Dent Clin North Am* 41:367, 1997.
12. Nariki-Makela M, Qvarnberg Y: Endoscopic sinus surgery or Caldwell-Luc operation in the treatment of chronic and recurrent maxillary sinusitis, *Acta Otolaryngol* 529:177, 1997.
13. Costa F, Emanuelli E, Robiony M et al: Endoscopic surgical treatment of chronic maxillary sinusitis of dental origin, *J Oral Maxillofac Surg* 65:223-228, 2007.
14. Gardner DG, Gullane PJ: Mucoceles of the maxillary sinus, *Oral Surg Oral Med Oral Pathol Oral Radiol Endod* 62:538-543, 1986.
15. Killey H, Kay LW: An analysis of 250 cases of oroantral fistula treated by the buccal flap operation, *J Oral Surg* 24:726, 1967.
16. Hanazawa Y, Itoh K, Mabashi T et al: Closure of oroantral communications using a pedicled buccal fat pad graft, *J Oral Maxillofac Surg* 53:771, 1995.
17. Juselius H, Katollio K: Closure of antroalveolar fistulae, *J Laryngol Otol* 85:387, 1991.
18. Awang MN: Closure of oroantral fistula, *Int J Oral Maxillofac Surg* 17:110, 1988.
19. Mainous EG, Hammer DD: Surgical closure of oroantral fistula using the gold foil technique, *J Oral Surg* 32:528, 1974.
20. Mitchell R, Lamb J: Immediate closure of oroantral communications with a collagen implant: a preliminary report, *Br Dent J* 154:171, 1983.
21. Van Minnen B, Stegenga B, vanLeeuwen MBM et al: Nonsurgical closure of oroantral communications with a biodegradable polyurethane foam: a pilot study in rabbits, *J Oral Maxillofac Surg* 65:218, 2007.

CHAPTER 20

Diagnosis and Management of Salivary Gland Disorders

MICHAEL MILORO

CHAPTER OUTLINE

The clinician is frequently confronted with the need to assess and treat salivary gland disorders. A thorough knowledge of the embryology, anatomy, and pathophysiology is necessary to manage patients appropriately. This chapter examines the causes, diagnostic methods, radiographic evaluation, and management of a variety of salivary gland disorders, including sialolithiasis and obstructive phenomena (e.g., mucocele and ranula), acute and chronic salivary gland infections, traumatic salivary gland disorders, Sjögren's syndrome, necrotizing sialometaplasia, and benign and malignant salivary gland tumors.

EMBRYOLOGY, ANATOMY, AND PHYSIOLOGY

The salivary glands can be divided into two groups: the major and minor glands. All salivary glands develop from the embryonic oral cavity as buds of epithelium that extend into the underlying mesenchymal tissues. These epithelial ingrowths, or anlages, are apparent at 8 weeks' gestation (Fig. 20-1) and then branch to form a primitive ductal system that eventually becomes canalized to provide a structural salivary gland unit for drainage of salivary secretions (Fig. 20-2). This unit consists of a myoepithelial cell, intercalated duct, striated duct, and excretory duct. The minor salivary glands begin to develop around the fortieth day in utero, whereas the larger major glands begin to develop slightly earlier, at about the thirty-fifth day in utero. At around the seventh or eighth month in utero, secretory cells called *acini* begin to develop around the ductal system. The acinar cells of the salivary glands are classified as *serous cells,* which produce a thin, watery serous secretion, or *mucous cells,* which produce a thicker, more viscous mucous secretion. The minor salivary glands are well developed and functional in the newborn infant. The acini of the minor salivary glands primarily produce mucous secretions, although some are made up of serous cells as well, thus classifying these minor glands as mixed. Between 800 and 1000 minor salivary glands are found throughout the portions of the oral cavity that are covered by mucous membranes, with a few exceptions, such as the anterior third of the hard palate, the attached gingiva, and the dorsal surface of the anterior third of the tongue. The minor salivary glands are referred to as the *labial, buccal, palatine, tonsillar* (Weber's glands), *retromolar (Carmalt's glands),* and *lingual glands,* which are divided into three groups: (1) inferior apical (glands of Blandin and of Nuhn), (2) taste buds (Ebner's glands), and (3) posterior lubricating glands (Table 20-1).

The major salivary glands are paired structures and are the parotid, submandibular, and sublingual glands. The parotid glands contain primarily serous acini with few mucous cells. Serous cells are cuboidal cells with eosinophilic secretory granules and produce thin, watery secretions with a low viscosity (1.5 Pa • s). Conversely, the sublingual glands are for the most part composed of mucous cells, which are clear low columnar cells with nuclei polarized away from the lumen of the acini, and produce a thick secretion with high viscosity (13.4 Pa • s). The submandibular glands are mixed glands, made up of approximately equal numbers of serous and mucous acini, and produce a secretion with an intermediate viscosity of 3.4 Pa • s.

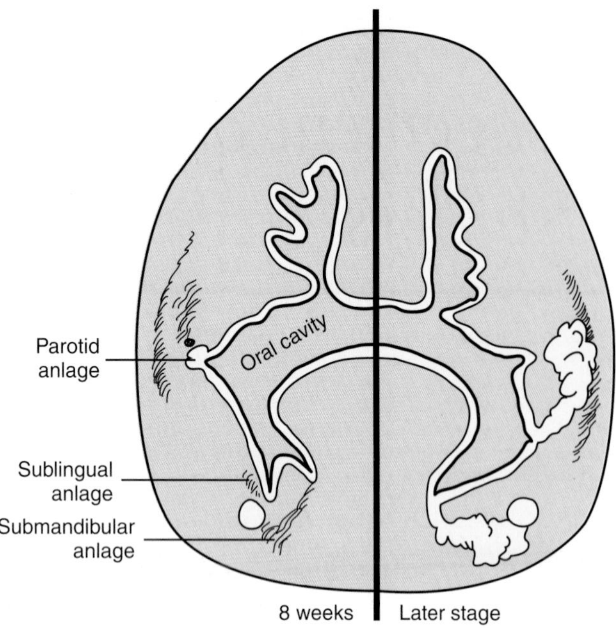

FIGURE 20-1 Embryologic development of the major salivary glands.

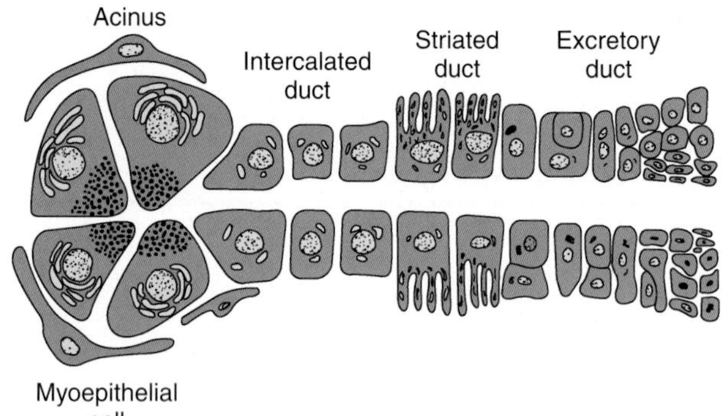

FIGURE 20-2 Basic salivary gland unit.

TABLE 20-1

Salivary Gland Embryology and Anatomy

	Minor Salivary Glands	Major Salivary Glands
In utero development:	Day 40	Day 35
Number:	800-1000	6
Types:	Labial	Parotid
	Buccal	Submandibular
	Palatine	Sublingual
	Tonsillar	
	◆ Weber's glands	
	Retromolar	
	◆ Carmalt's glands	
	Lingual	
	◆ Inferior apical (glands of Blandin and of Nuhn)	
	◆ Taste buds (Ebner's glands)	
	◆ Posterior lubricating glands	

The parotid glands, the largest salivary glands, lie superficial to the posterior aspect of the masseter muscle and the ascending ramus of the mandible. Peripheral portions of the parotid gland extend to the mastoid process, along the anterior aspect of the sternocleidomastoid muscle, and around the posterior border of the mandible into the pterygomandibular space (Fig. 20-3). The major branches of the seventh cranial (facial) nerve roughly divide the parotid gland into a superficial lobe and a deep lobe while coursing anteriorly from their exit at the stylomastoid foramen to innervate the muscles of facial expression. Small ducts from various regions of the gland coalesce at the anterosuperior aspect of the parotid gland to form Stensen's duct, which is the major duct of the parotid gland. Stensen's duct is about 1 to 3 mm in diameter and 6 cm in length.

Occasionally, a normal anatomic variation occurs in which an accessory parotid duct may aid Stensen's duct in drainage of salivary secretions. Additionally, an accessory portion of the parotid gland may be present somewhere along the course of Stensen's duct. The duct runs anteriorly from the gland and is superficial to the masseter muscle. At the location of the anterior edge of the masseter muscle, Stensen's duct turns sharply medial and passes through the fibers of the buccinator muscle. The duct opens into the oral cavity through the buccal mucosa, usually adjacent to the maxillary first or second molar. The parotid gland receives innervation from the ninth cranial (glossopharyngeal) nerve via the auriculotemporal nerve from the otic ganglion (see Fig. 20-7).

The submandibular glands are located in the submandibular triangle of the neck, which is formed by the anterior and posterior bellies of the digastric muscles and the inferior border of the mandible (Fig. 20-4). The posterosuperior portion of the gland curves upward around the posterior border of the mylohyoid muscle and gives rise to the major duct of the submandibular gland known as *Wharton's duct.* This duct passes forward along the superior surface of the mylohyoid muscle in the sublingual space, adjacent to the lingual nerve. The anatomic relationship is such that the lingual nerve loops under Wharton's duct, from lateral to medial, in the posterior floor of the mouth. Wharton's duct is about 5 cm in length, and the diameter of its lumen is 2 to 4 mm. Wharton's duct opens into the floor of the mouth via a punctum located close to the incisors at the most anterior aspect of the junction of the lingual frenum and the floor of the mouth. The punctum is a constricted portion of the duct, and it functions to limit retrograde flow of bacteria-laden oral fluids. This particularly limits those bacteria that tend to colonize around the ductal orifices.

The sublingual glands lie on the superior surface of the mylohyoid muscle, in the sublingual space, and are separated from the oral cavity by a thin layer of oral mucosa (Fig. 20-5). The acinar ducts of the sublingual glands are called *Bartholin's ducts* and in most instances coalesce to form 8 to 20 ducts of Rivinus. These ducts of Rivinus are short and small in diameter. The ducts open individually directly into the anterior floor of the mouth on a crest of mucosa, known as the *plica sublingualis,* or they open indirectly through connections to the submandibular duct and then into the oral cavity via Wharton's duct. The sublingual and submandibular glands are innervated by the facial nerve through the submandibular ganglion via the chorda tympani nerve (see Fig. 20-8).

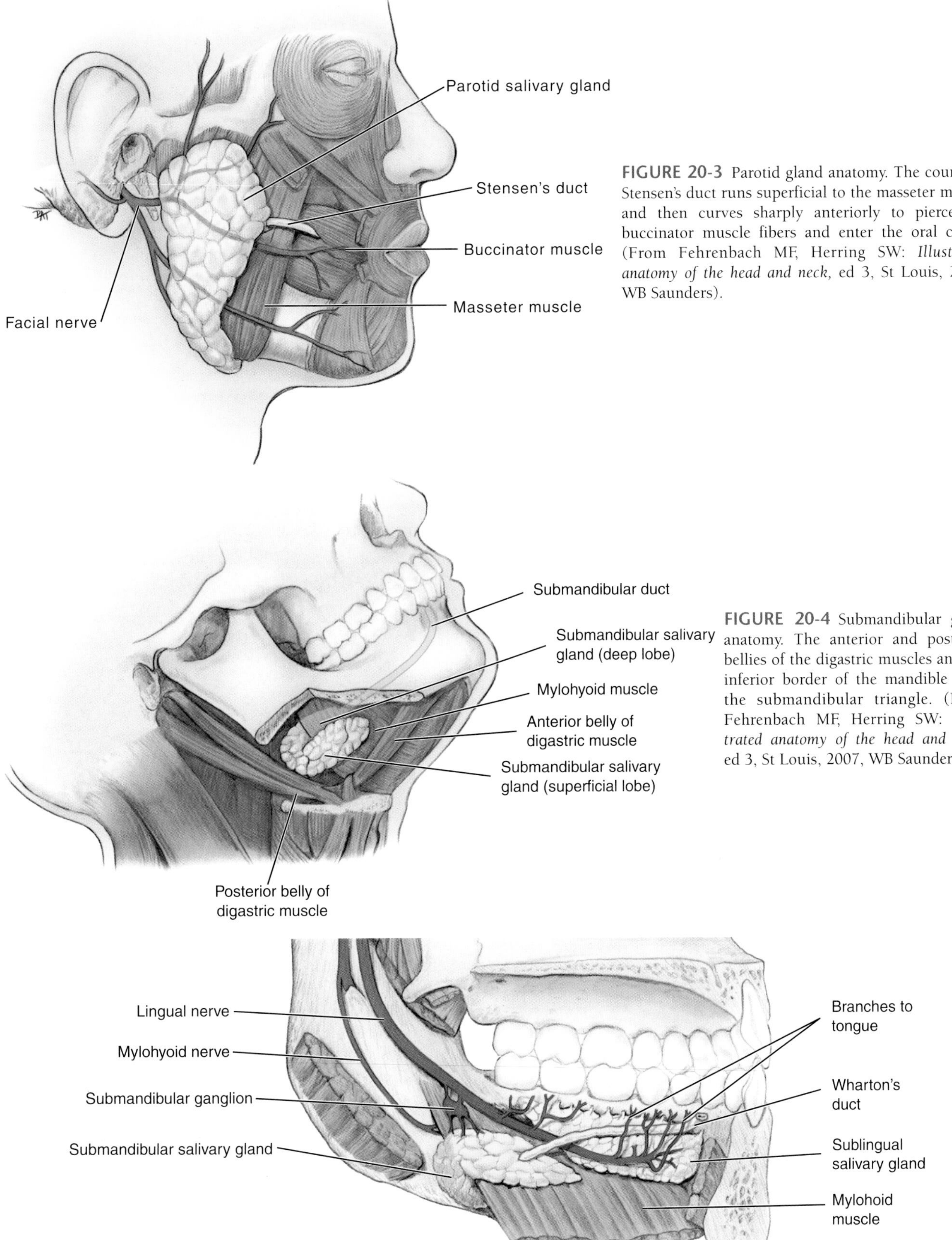

FIGURE 20-3 Parotid gland anatomy. The course of Stensen's duct runs superficial to the masseter muscle and then curves sharply anteriorly to pierce the buccinator muscle fibers and enter the oral cavity. (From Fehrenbach MF, Herring SW: *Illustrated anatomy of the head and neck,* ed 3, St Louis, 2007, WB Saunders).

FIGURE 20-4 Submandibular gland anatomy. The anterior and posterior bellies of the digastric muscles and the inferior border of the mandible form the submandibular triangle. (From Fehrenbach MF, Herring SW: *Illustrated anatomy of the head and neck,* ed 3, St Louis, 2007, WB Saunders).

FIGURE 20-5 Sublingual gland anatomy. The interrelationships between the ductal systems of the submandibular and the sublingual glands and the relationship of the lingual nerve to Wharton's duct are demonstrated. (From Fehrenbach MF, Herring SW: *Illustrated anatomy of the head and neck,* ed 3, St Louis, 2007, WB Saunders).

The functions of saliva are to provide lubrication for speech and mastication, to produce enzymes for digestion, and to produce compounds with antibacterial properties (Table 20-2). The salivary glands produce approximately 1000 to 1500 mL of saliva per day, with the highest flow rates occurring during meals. The relative contributions of each salivary gland to total daily production varies, with the submandibular gland providing 70%, the parotid gland 25%, the sublingual gland 3% to 4%, and the minor salivary glands contributing only trace amounts of saliva (Box 20-1). The electrolyte composition of saliva also varies between salivary glands, with parotid gland concentrations generally higher than the submandibular gland, except for submandibular calcium concentration, which is approximately twice the concentration of parotid calcium. The relative viscosities of saliva vary according to gland and correspond to the percentage of mucous and serous cells; therefore the highest viscosity is in the sublingual gland composed of mostly mucous cells, followed by the submandibular gland (mixed mucous and serous cells), and lastly, the parotid gland, which is composed mainly of serous cells (Fig. 20-6). Interestingly, the daily production of saliva begins to decrease gradually after the age of 20.

The control of salivary production is derived from sympathetic and parasympathetic stimulation. The sympathetic innervation is from the superior cervical ganglion to the glands via the arterial plexus of the face. The parasympathetic innervation to the parotid gland originates from the tympanic branch of the glossopharyngeal nerve (IX), which then travels via the lesser petrosal nerve to the otic ganglion. Postganglionic parasympathetic nerves then travel via the auriculotemporal nerve to the parotid gland (Fig. 20-7). The parasympathetic control of the submandibular and sublingual glands originates in the superior salivatory nucleus, which travels via the facial nerve (chorda tympani branch) to the submandibular ganglion. Postganglionic parasympathetic nerves then travel directly to the submandibular gland or with the lingual nerve to the sublingual gland (Fig. 20-8).

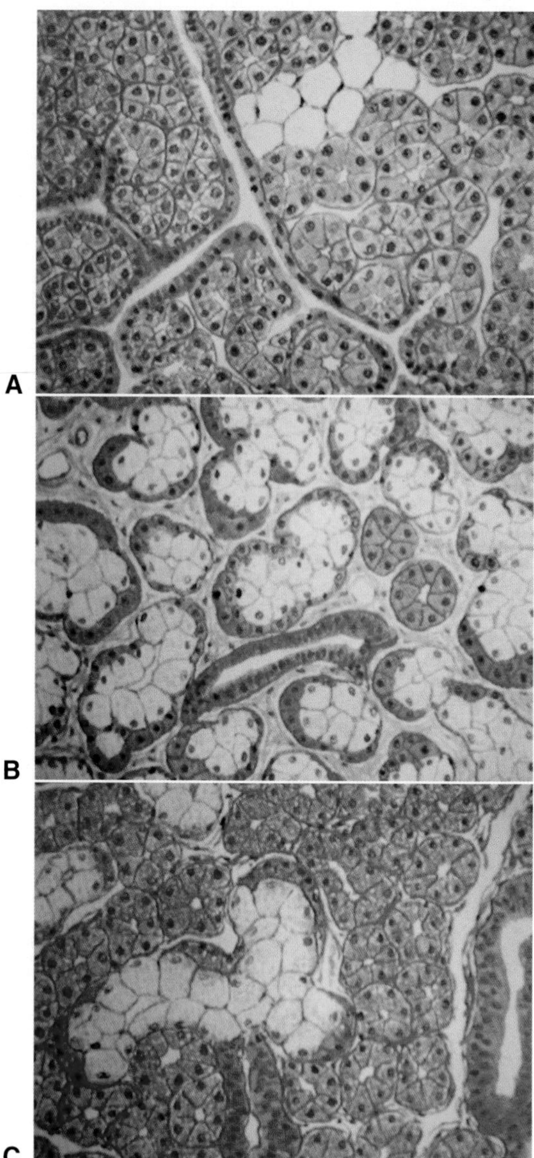

FIGURE 20-6 A, Parotid gland histology (serous cells). B, Sublingual gland (mucous cells). C, Submandibular gland (mixed mucous and serous cells).

TABLE 20-2

Composition of Normal Adult Saliva

	Parotid Gland	Submandibular Gland
Amino acids	1.5 mg/dL	<1.0 mg/dL
Ammonia	0.3 mg/dL	0.2 mg/dL
Bicarbonate	20.0 mEq/L	18.0 mEq/L
Calcium	2.0 mEq/L	3.6 mEq/L
Chloride	23.0 mEq/L	20.0 mEq/L
Cholesterol	<1.0 mg/dL	<1.0 mg/dL
Fatty acids	1.0 mg/dL	<1.0 mg/dL
Glucose	<1.0 mg/dL	<1.0 mg/dL
Magnesium	0.2 mEq/L	0.3 mEq/L
Phosphate	6.0 mEq/L	4.5 mEq/L
Potassium	20.0 mEq/L	17.0 mEq/L
Proteins	250.0 mg/dL	<150.0 mg/dL
Sodium	23.0 mEq/L	21.0 mEq/L
Urea	15.0 mg/dL	7.0 mg/dL
Uric acid	3.0 mg/dL	2.0 mg/dL

BOX 20-1

Daily Saliva Production by Salivary Gland

Submandibular gland	70%
Parotid gland	25%
Sublingual gland	3% to 4%
Minor glands	Trace

DIAGNOSTIC MODALITIES

History and Clinical Examination

The most important component of diagnosis in salivary gland disorders, as with most other disease processes, is the patient history and the clinical examination. In most cases the patient will guide the doctor to the diagnosis merely by relating the events that have occurred in association with the presenting

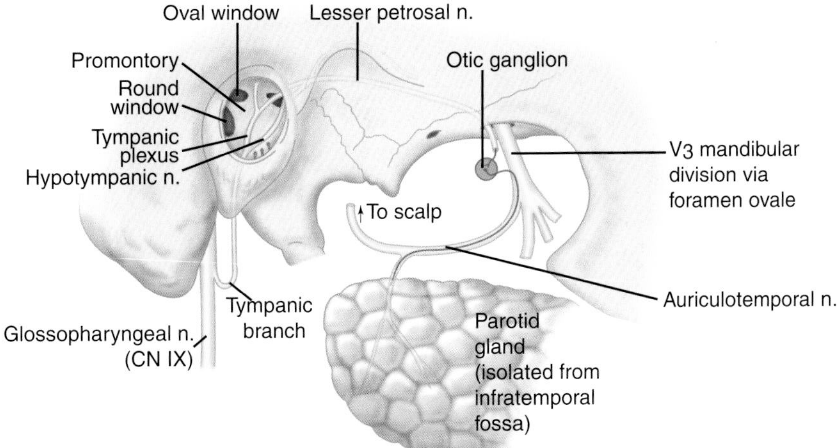

FIGURE 20-7 Parotid gland innervation.

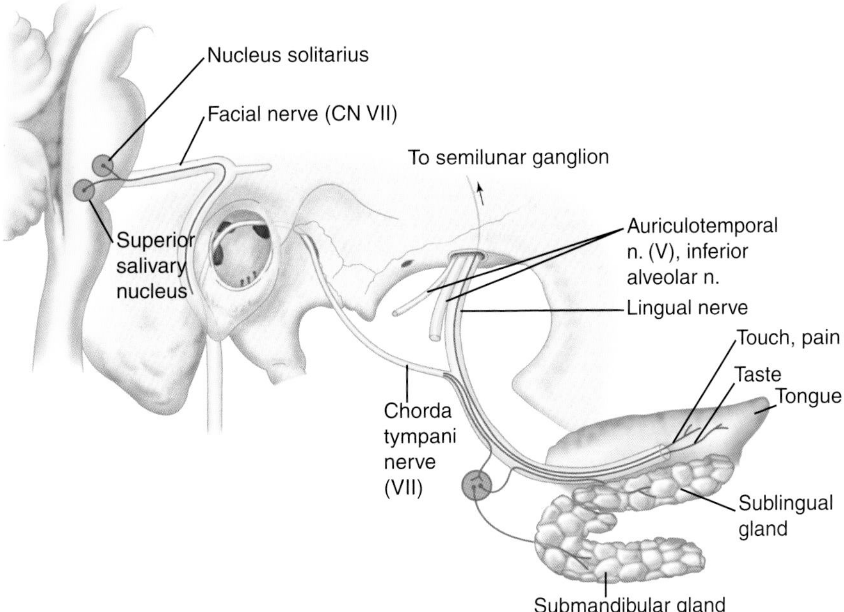

FIGURE 20-8 Submandibular and sublingual gland innervation.

complaint. The astute clinician must perform a thorough evaluation, and in many instances the diagnosis can be determined without the necessity of further diagnostic evaluation. At the very least the clinician may be able to categorize the problem as reactive, obstructive, inflammatory, infectious, metabolic, neoplastic, developmental, or traumatic and guide further diagnostic testing. Occasionally, the clinician may find it necessary to use any of several diagnostic modalities.

Salivary Gland Radiology

Plain Film Radiographs

The primary purpose of plain films in the assessment of salivary gland disease is to identify salivary stones (calculi), although only 80% to 85% of all stones are radiopaque and therefore visible radiographically. The incidence of radiopaque stones varies, depending on the specific gland involved (Box 20-2). A mandibular occlusal film is most useful for detecting sublingual and submandibular gland calculi in the anterior floor of the mouth (Fig. 20-9). Periapical radiographs can show calculi in each salivary gland or duct, including minor salivary glands, depending on film placement. A "puffed cheek view," in which the patient forcibly blows the cheek laterally to distend the soft tissues overlying the lateral ramus, may demonstrate radiopaque parotid stones. In most instances the radiographic image corresponds in size and shape to the actual stone. Panoramic radiographs can reveal stones in the parotid gland and posteriorly located submandibular stones (Fig. 20-10).

BOX 20-2

Incidence of Radiopaque Stones

Submandibular gland	80%
Parotid gland	40%

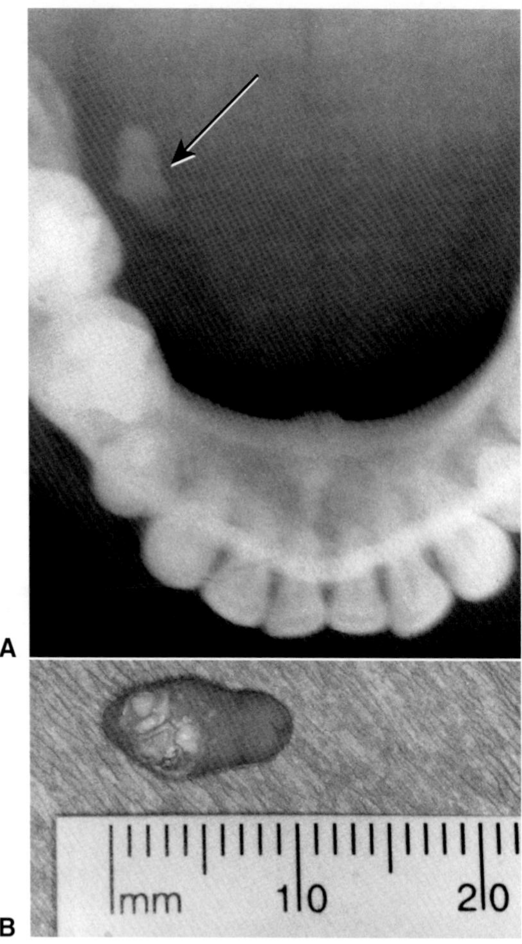

FIGURE 20-9 A, Mandibular occlusal radiograph showing a radiopaque sialolith (*arrow*). B, Submandibular sialolith (1.0 cm) after intraoral removal is demonstrated.

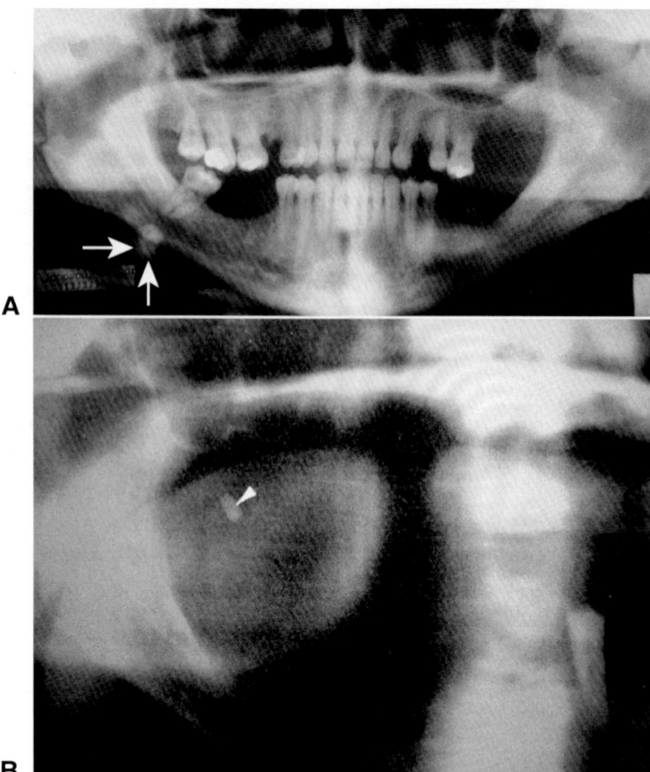

FIGURE 20-10 A, Panoramic radiograph demonstrates a right submandibular sialolith (*arrows*). B, Panoramic radiograph showing right parotid stone (*arrowhead*).

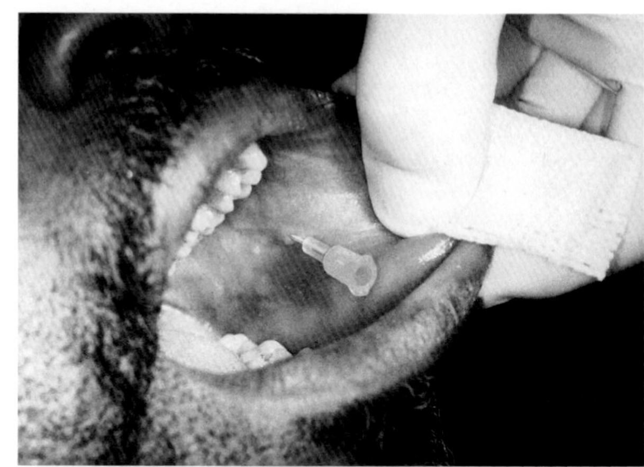

FIGURE 20-11 Cannulation of Stensen's duct with a plastic catheter.

Sialography

The gold standard in diagnostic salivary gland radiology may be the sialogram. Sialography is indicated as an aid in the detection of radiopaque stones. In addition, when 15% to 20% of stones are radiolucent, sialography is also useful in the assessment of the extent of destruction of the salivary duct or gland or both as a result of obstructive, inflammatory, traumatic, and neoplastic diseases. In addition to its diagnostic role, sialography may be used as a therapeutic maneuver because the ductal system is dilated during the study, and small mucous plugs or necrotic debris may be cleared during injection of contrast medium.

Sialography is a technique in which the salivary duct (Stensen's or Wharton's duct) is cannulated with a plastic or metal catheter (Fig. 20-11), a radiographic contrast medium is injected into the ductal system and the substance of the gland, and a series of radiographs are obtained during this process. Approximately 0.5 to 1 mL of contrast material can be injected into the duct and gland before the patient begins to experience pain. The two types of contrast media available for sialographic studies are water-soluble and oil-based. Both types of contrast material contain relatively high concentrations (25% to 40%) of iodine. Most clinicians prefer to use water-soluble media, which are more miscible with salivary secretions, more easily injected into the finer portions of the ductal system, and more readily eliminated from the gland after the study is completed by drainage through the duct or systemic absorption from the gland and excretion through the kidneys. The oil-based media are more viscous and require a higher injection pressure to visualize the finer ductules than do the water-soluble media. As a result, oil-based media usually produce more discomfort to the patient during injection. Oil-based media are poorly eliminated from the ductal system and may cause iatrogenic ductal obstruction. Residual oil-based contrast medium is not absorbed by the gland and may produce severe foreign-body reactions and glandular necrosis. Additionally, if the patient has ductal disruption resulting from chronic inflammatory changes, the extravasation of oil-based media may cause significantly more soft tissue damage than water-soluble material.

A complete sialogram consists of three distinct phases, depending on the time at which the radiograph is obtained after injection of the contrast material:

1. Ductal phase (Fig. 20-12), which occurs almost immediately after injection of contrast material and allows visualization of the major ducts
2. Acinar phase (Fig. 20-13), which begins after the ductal system has become fully opacified with contrast medium and the gland parenchyma becomes filled subsequently
3. Evacuation phase (Fig. 20-14), which assesses normal secretory clearance function of the gland to determine whether any evidence remains of retention of contrast medium in the gland or ductal system after the sialogram

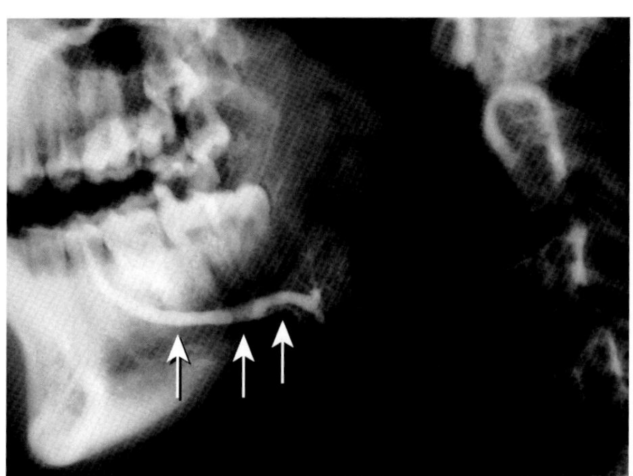

FIGURE 20-12 Ductal phase of a submandibular sialogram. Contrast medium is contained only within the main salivary ducts (*arrows*).

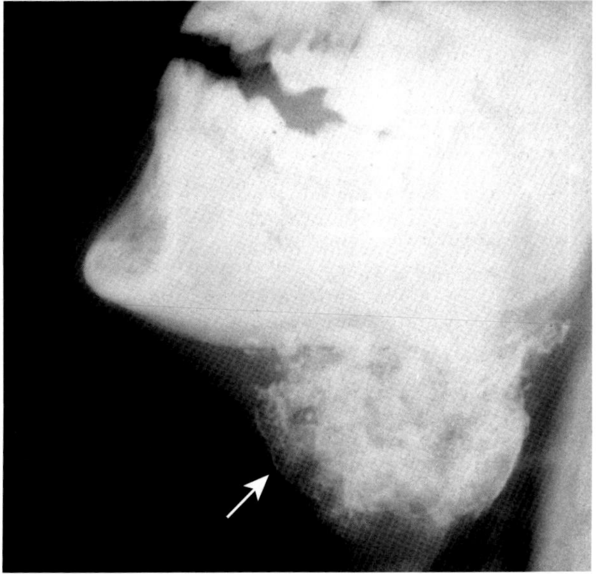

FIGURE 20-13 Acinar phase of a submandibular sialogram. Normal arborization of the entire ductal system of the gland (*arrow*) is demonstrated.

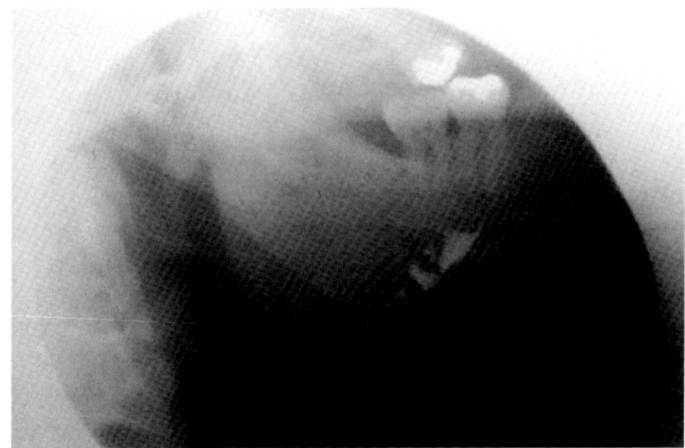

FIGURE 20-14 Evacuation phase of a submandibular sialogram with some abnormal retention of contrast medium in the ductal system after 5 minutes.

The retention of contrast medium in the gland or ductal system beyond 5 minutes is considered abnormal. A normal sialogram shows a large primary duct branching gradually and smoothly into secondary and terminal ductules. Evenly distributed contrast medium results in opacification of the acinoparenchyma that outlines the gland and its lobules. When a stone obstructs a salivary duct, continued secretion by the gland produces distention of the ductal system proximal to the obstruction and finally leads to pressure atrophy of the parenchyma of the gland (Fig. 20-15).

Sialodochitis is a dilation of the salivary duct resulting from epithelial atrophy as a result of repeated inflammatory or infectious processes, with irregular narrowing caused by reparative fibrosis (i.e., "sausage link" pattern; Fig. 20-16). Sialadenitis represents inflammation mainly involving the acinoparenchyma of the gland. Patients with sialadenitis experience saccular dilation of the acini of the gland resulting from acinar atrophy and infection, which results in "pruning" of the normal arborization of the small ductal system of the gland (Fig. 20-17). Centrally located lesions or tumors that occupy a part of the gland or impinge on its surface displace the normal ductal anatomy. On sialography, ducts adjacent to the lesion are curvilinearly draped and stretched around the mass, producing a characteristic ball-in-hand appearance (Fig. 20-18).

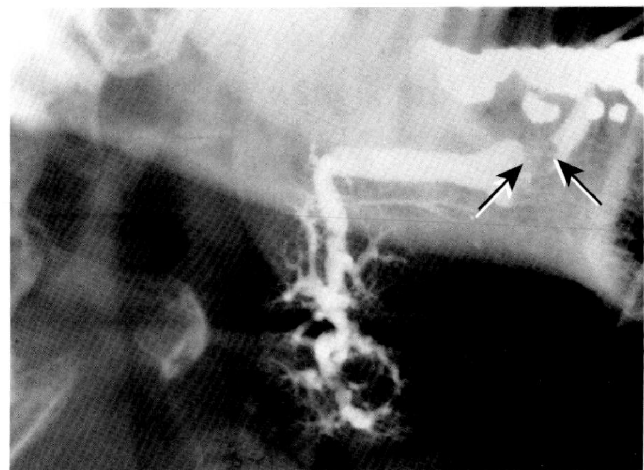

FIGURE 20-15 Sialogram of right submandibular gland. Obstruction of duct by a radiolucent sialolith (*arrows*) has caused dilation of the duct and loss of normal parenchyma of the gland.

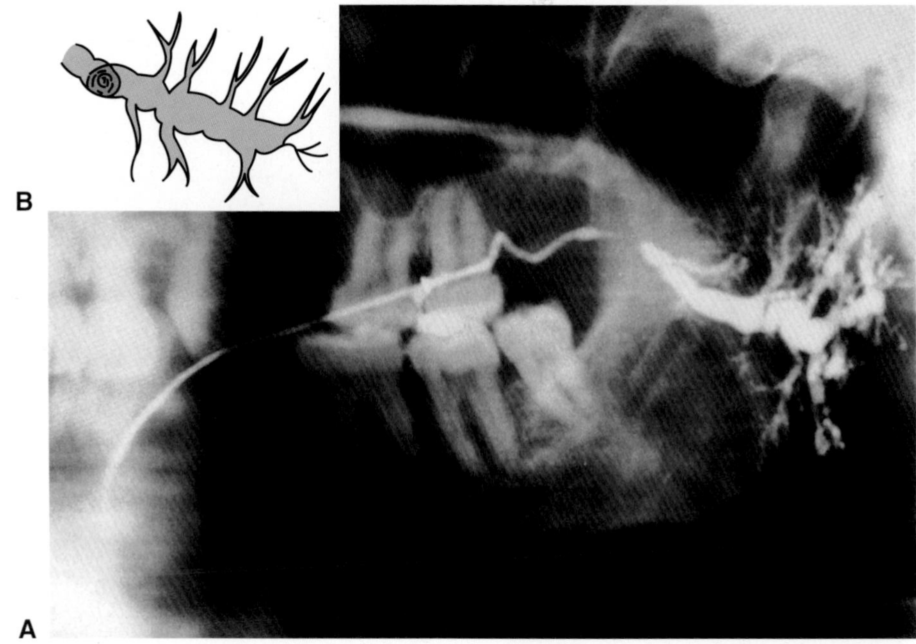

FIGURE 20-16 A, Sialogram of right parotid gland. The characteristic "sausage link" appearance of the duct is demonstrated, which indicates ductal damage from obstructive disease with irregular narrowing of duct caused by reparative fibrosis. B, Diagram of obstruction with proximal dilatation of the ductal system.

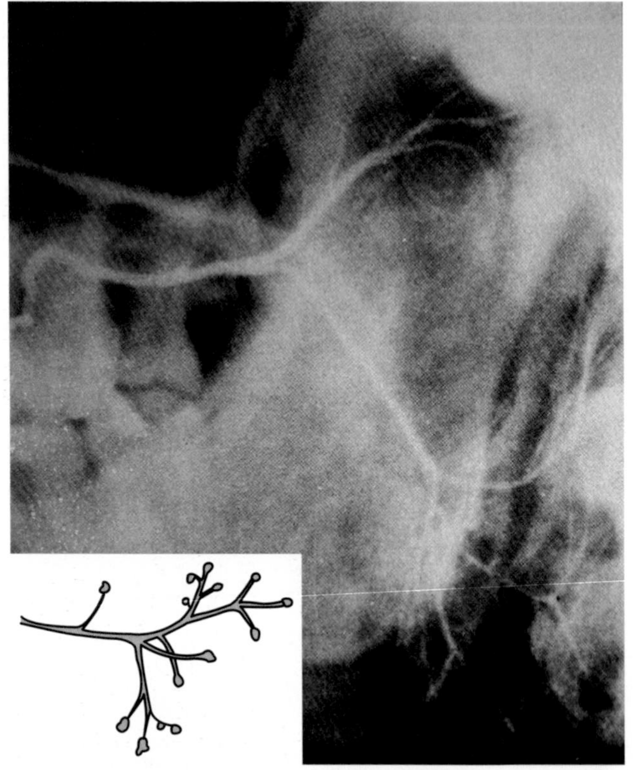

FIGURE 20-17 A, Parotid sialadenitis with acinar destruction from chronic disease. B, Diagram of "pruning of the tree" due to acinar destruction.

Sialograms are specialized radiologic studies performed by oral and maxillofacial surgeons and some interventional radiologists trained in the technique. Those inexperienced in performance of or proper interpretation of the sialogram should not attempt this examination. The three contraindications to performing a sialogram are (1) acute salivary gland infections, because a disrupted ductal epithelium may allow extravasation of contrast medium into the soft tissues and cause severe pain and possibly a foreign-body reaction; (2) patients with a history of iodine sensitivity, especially a severe allergic reaction after a previous radiologic examination using contrast medium; and (3) before a thyroid gland study, because retained iodine in the salivary gland or ducts may interfere with the thyroid scan.

Computed Tomography, Magnetic Resonance Imaging, and Ultrasound

The use of computed tomography (CT) has been generally reserved for the assessment of mass lesions of the salivary glands. Although CT scanning results in radiation exposure to patients, it is less invasive than sialography and does not require the use of contrast material. Additionally, CT scanning can demonstrate salivary gland calculi, especially submandibular stones that are located posteriorly in the duct, at the hilum of the gland, or in the substance of the gland itself (Fig. 20-19). Three-dimensional CT scanning now allows a much better delineation of the stone and of the ductal system in a noninvasive fashion (Fig. 20-20).

Magnetic resonance imaging is superior to CT scanning in delineating the soft tissue detail of salivary gland lesions, specifically tumors, with no radiation exposure to the patient or the necessity of contrast enhancement.

Ultrasonography is a relatively simple, noninvasive imaging modality but provides images with poor detail resolution. The primary role of ultrasonography is in the assessment of super-

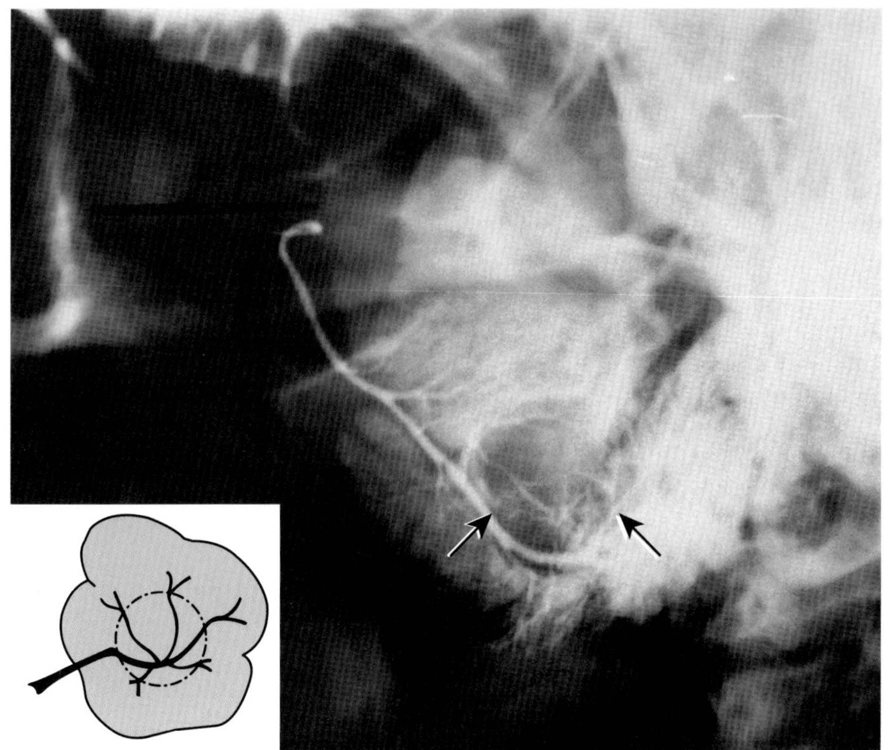

FIGURE 20-18 A, Sialogram of right parotid gland illustrates ball-in-hand phenomenon (*arrows*). The filling defect in this sialogram locates a tumor of the gland with displacement of normal surrounding ductal anatomy. B, Diagram of ball-in-hand phenomenon due to tumor displacement of acini.

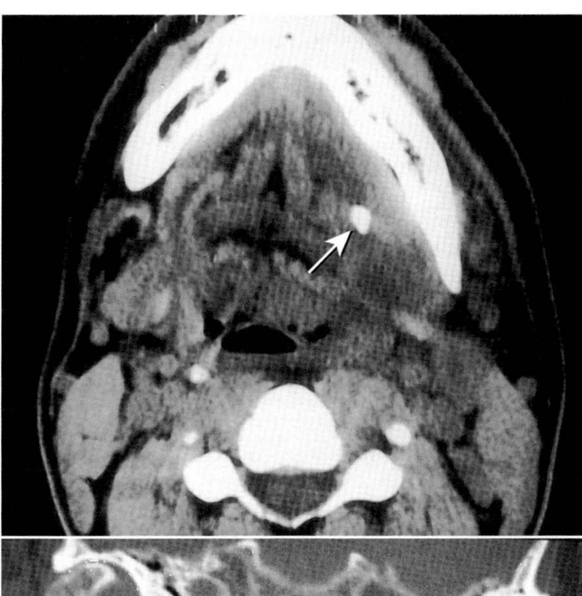

FIGURE 20-19 A, Computerized axial tomographic scan of the mandible and floor of mouth shows a posterior submandibular sialolith (*arrow*). B, Coronal computed tomography scan showing a multisegment submandibular duct stone.

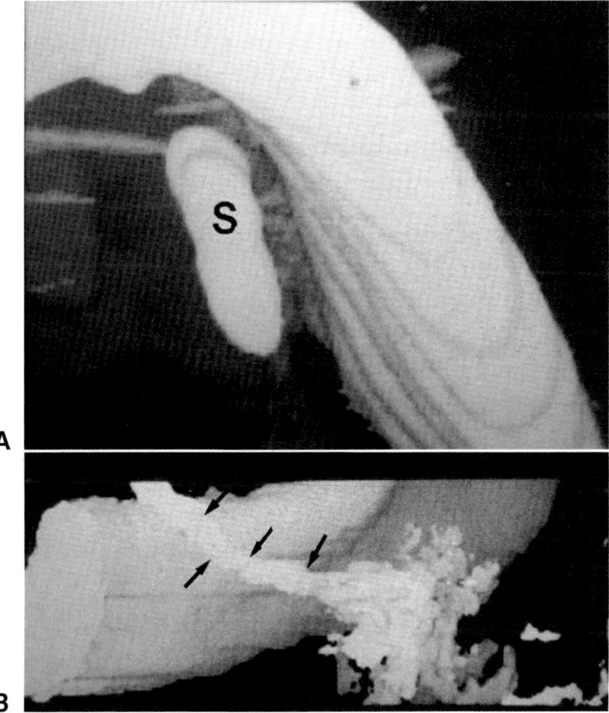

FIGURE 20-20 A, Three-dimensional computed tomography scan showing a submandibular stone (*S*). B, Destruction of the submandibular duct (*arrows*).

ficial structures to determine whether a mass lesion that is being evaluated is solid or cystic (fluid-filled).

Salivary Scintigraphy (Radioactive Isotope Scanning)

The use of nuclear imaging in the form of radioactive isotope scanning, or salivary scintigraphy, allows a thorough evaluation of the salivary gland parenchyma with respect to the presence of mass lesions and the function of the gland itself. This study uses a radioactive isotope (usually, technetium-99m) injected intravenously, which is distributed throughout the body and taken up by a variety of tissues, including the salivary glands. The major limitation of this study, aside from patient radiation exposure, is the poor resolution of the images obtained. Salivary gland scintigraphy may demonstrate increased uptake of radioactive isotope in an acutely inflamed gland or decreased uptake in a chronically inflamed gland, as well as the presence of a mass lesion, benign or malignant.

Salivary Gland Endoscopy (Sialoendoscopy)

Minimally invasive modalities of diagnosis and treatment have recently been applied to the major salivary glands. Salivary gland endoscopy (sialoendoscopy) is a specialized procedure that uses a small video camera (endoscope) with a light at the end of a flexible cannula, which is introduced into the ductal orifice. The endoscope can be used diagnostically and therapeutically. Salivary gland endoscopy can demonstrate strictures and kinks in the ductal system, as well as mucous plugs and calcifications. The endoscope may be used to dilate small strictures and flush clear, small mucous plugs from the salivary gland ducts. Specialized devices such as small balloon catheters (similar to those used for coronary angioplasty procedures) may be used to dilate sites of ductal constriction, and small metal baskets may be used to retrieve stones in the ductal system (Fig. 20-21).

Sialochemistry

An examination of the electrolyte composition of the saliva (Table 20-2) of each gland may indicate a variety of salivary gland disorders. Principally, the concentrations of sodium and potassium, which normally change with salivary flow rate, are measured. Certain changes in the relative concentrations of these electrolytes are seen in specific salivary gland diseases. For example, an elevated sodium concentration with a decreased potassium concentration may indicate an inflammatory sialadenitis.

Fine-Needle Aspiration Biopsy

The use of fine-needle aspiration biopsy in the diagnosis of salivary gland tumors has been well documented. This procedure has a high accuracy rate for distinguishing between benign and malignant lesions in superficial locations. Fine-needle aspiration biopsy is performed using a syringe with a 20-gauge or smaller needle. After local anesthesia administration, the needle is advanced into the mass lesion, the plunger is activated to create a vacuum in the syringe, and the needle is moved back and forth throughout the mass, with pressure maintained on the plunger (Fig. 20-22). The pressure is then released, the needle is withdrawn, and the cellular material and fluid are expelled onto a slide and fixed for histologic examination. This allows an immediate determination of benign versus malignant disease; examination also offers the possibility of providing a tissue diagnosis, especially if the oral surgeon and oral pathologist are experienced in performing and interpreting this examination and its results.

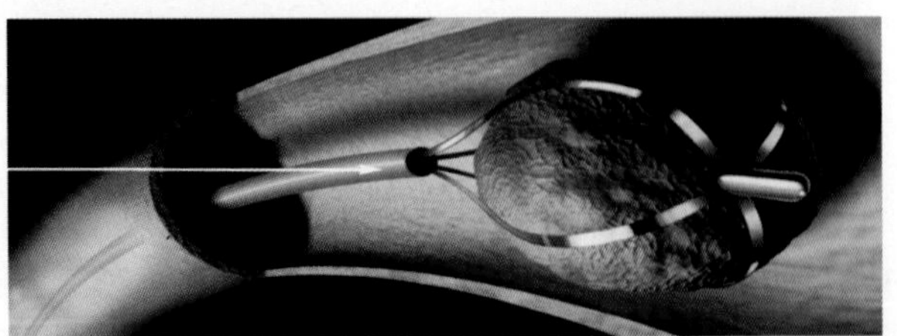

FIGURE 20-21 Diagram of an endoscopic retrieval of a stone with the basket technique (*arrow*).

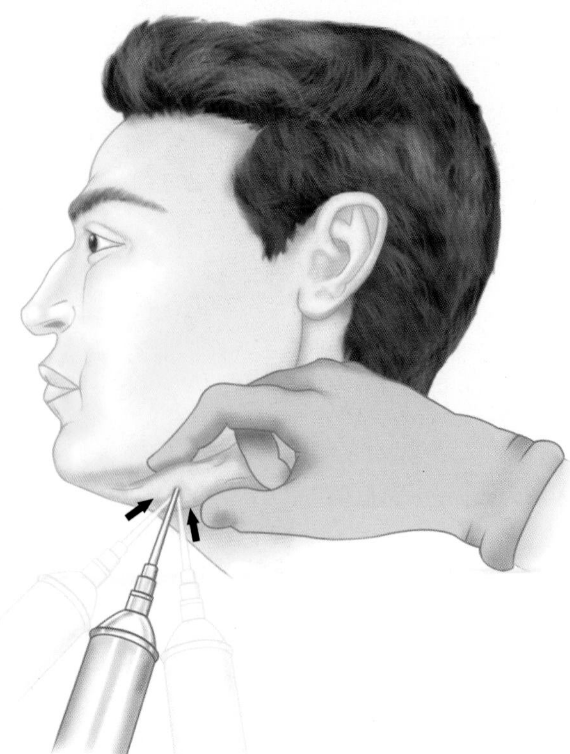

FIGURE 20-22 Fine-needle aspiration biopsy technique of a submandibular gland mass lesion with multiple redirectional passes of the needle in the lesion.

Salivary Gland Biopsy

A salivary gland biopsy, incisional or excisional, can be used to diagnose a tumor of one of the major salivary glands, but it is usually performed as an aid in the diagnosis of Sjögren's syndrome (SS). The lower lip labial salivary gland biopsy has been shown to demonstrate certain characteristic histopathologic changes that are seen in the major glands in SS. The procedure is performed using local anesthesia, and approximately 10 minor salivary glands are removed for histologic examination (Fig. 20-23). The labial minor salivary glands are then examined histologically, and they are assigned a "focus score." A "focus" represents an aggregate of 50 or more lymphocytes, histiocytes, and plasma cells per 4 mm^2 of salivary gland tissue at high power (Fig. 20-24). The diagnosis of SS is supported by the presence of one or more foci in the minor salivary gland tissue.

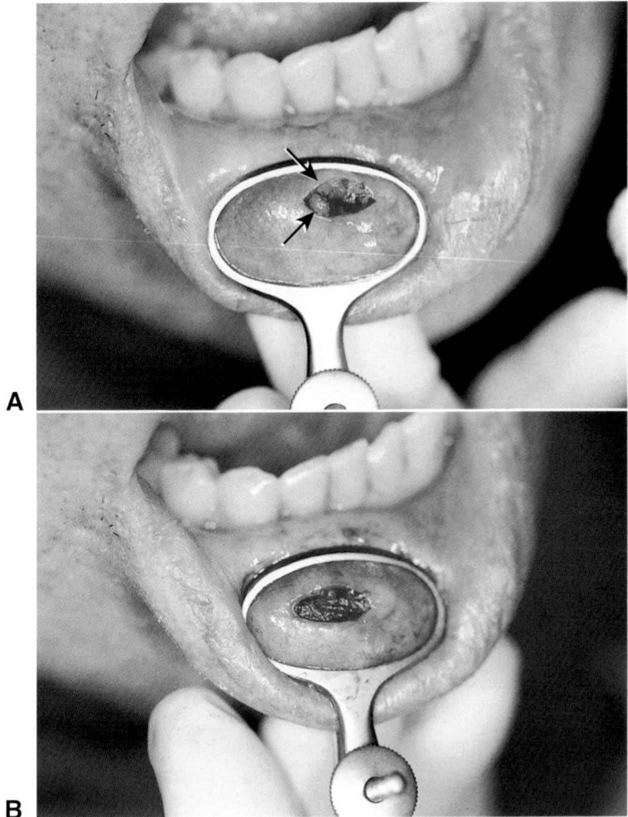

FIGURE 20-23 A, Labial salivary gland biopsy. The lower lip is everted and controlled with a Chalazion clamp. An incision through mucosa permits visualization of the minor salivary glands (*arrows*). B, The minor salivary glands are removed and submitted for histopathologic assessment.

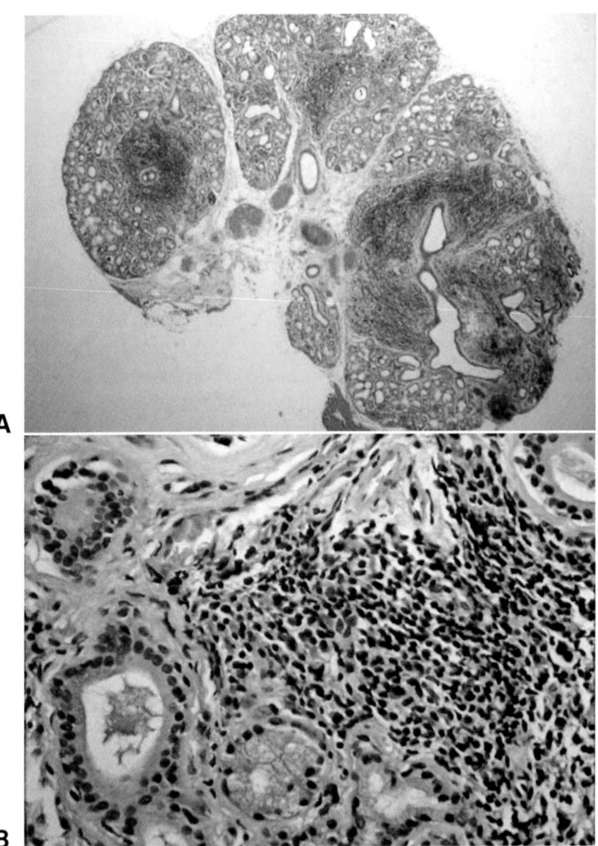

FIGURE 20-24 A, Labial salivary gland biopsy specimen in a patient with Sjögren's syndrome (note the presence of three foci of lymphocytes at low power). B, A high-power view of a specimen of labial salivary gland showing one focus (>50 lymphocytes) and normal adjacent acinar tissue.

OBSTRUCTIVE SALIVARY GLAND DISEASE: SIALOLITHIASIS

The formation of stones, or calculi, may occur throughout the body, including the gallbladder, urinary tract, and salivary glands. The occurrence of salivary gland stones is twice as common in men, with a peak incidence between ages 30 and 50. Multiple stone formation occurs in approximately 25% of patients. The pathogenesis of salivary calculi progresses through a series of stages beginning with an abnormality in calcium metabolism and salt precipitation, with formation of a nidus that subsequently becomes layered with organic and inorganic material, to form a calcified mass.

The incidence of stone formation varies, depending on the specific gland involved (Box 20-3). The submandibular gland is involved in 85% of cases, which is more common than all other glands combined. A variety of factors contribute to the higher incidence of submandibular calculi. Salivary gland secretions contain water, electrolytes, urea, ammonia, glucose, fats, proteins, and other substances; in general, parotid secretions are more concentrated than those of the other salivary glands. The main exception is the concentration of calcium, which is about twice as abundant in submandibular saliva as in parotid saliva (Table 20-2). In addition, the alkaline pH of submandibular saliva may further support stone formation. In addition to salivary composition, several anatomic factors of the submandibular gland and duct are important. Wharton's duct is the longest salivary duct; therefore, saliva has a greater distance to travel before being emptied into the oral cavity. In addition, the duct of the submandibular gland has two sharp curves in its course: The first occurs at the posterior border of the mylohyoid muscle, and the second is near the ductal opening in the anterior floor of the mouth. Finally, the punctum of the submandibular duct is smaller than the opening of Stensen's duct. These features contribute to a slowed salivary flow and provide potential areas of stasis of salivary flow, or obstruction, which is not found in the parotid or sublingual ductal systems. Precipitated material, mucus, and cellular debris are more easily trapped in the tortuous and lengthy submandibular duct, especially when its small orifice is its most elevated location, and its flow therefore occurs against the force of gravity. The

BOX 20-3

Incidence of Sialolithiasis

Submandibular gland	85%
Parotid gland	10%
Sublingual gland	5%
Minor glands	Rare

precipitated material forms the nidus of mucous plugs and radiopaque or radiolucent sialoliths that may eventually enlarge to the point of obstructing the flow of saliva from the gland to the oral cavity.

The clinical manifestations of the presence of submandibular stones become apparent when acute ductal obstruction occurs at mealtime, when saliva production is at its maximum and salivary flow is stimulated against a fixed obstruction. The resultant swelling is sudden and is usually very painful (Box 20-4; Fig. 20-25). Gradual reduction of the swelling follows, but swelling reoccurs repeatedly when salivary flow is stimulated. This process may continue until complete obstruction, infection, or both occur. Obstruction, with or without infection, causes atrophy of the secretory cells of the involved gland. Infection of the gland manifests itself by swelling in the floor of the mouth, erythema, and an associated lymphadenopathy. Palpation of the gland and simultaneous examination of the duct and its opening may reveal the total absence of salivary flow or the presence of purulent material.

Sialolithiasis in children is rare. Boys are more commonly affected than girls, and the left submandibular gland is most commonly affected. The diagnosis can be made clinically and confirmed radiographically by plain films, ultrasound, sialography, or sialoendoscopy.

BOX 20-4

Sialolithiasis for the General Dentist

CLASSIC SIGNS AND SYMPTOMS OF SIALOLITHIASIS

- Pain and swelling are exacerbated at mealtimes.
- Check for flow from Wharton's duct.
- Check for tenderness of submandibular gland.
- Palpate for stone in floor of mouth.
- Check mandibular occlusal radiograph.

TREATMENT

Anterior Stone

- Attempt to dilate Wharton's duct with lacrimal probes.
- Be careful not to dislodge stone posteriorly.
- "Milk" the gland to express stone.
- If successful, prescribe salivary stimulants.

Posterior Stone or No Stone Visualized

- Refer to oral maxillofacial surgeon.

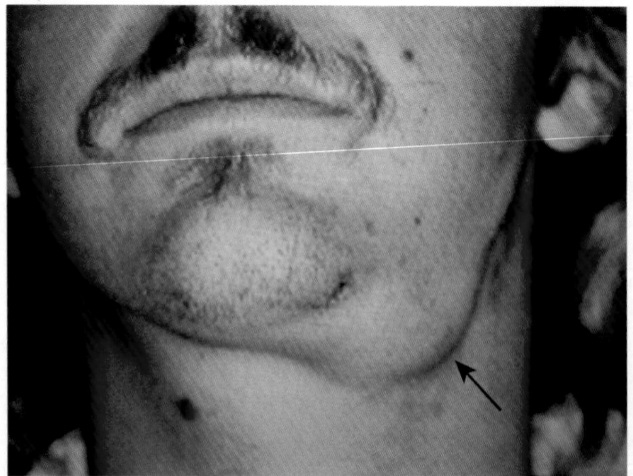

FIGURE 20-25 Clinical photograph demonstrates a left submandibular swelling (*arrow*) caused by obstruction from a submandibular sialolith.

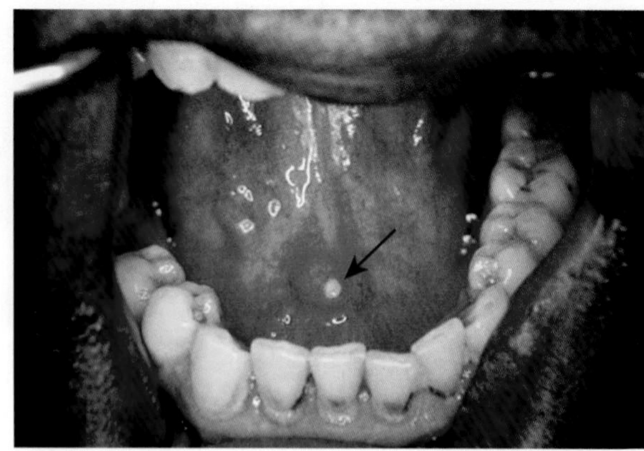

FIGURE 20-26 Stone at the orifice of Wharton's duct that is amenable to intraoral removal (*arrow*).

The management of submandibular gland calculi depends on the duration of symptoms, the number of repeated episodes, the size of the stone, and perhaps most importantly, the location of the stone. Submandibular stones are classified as *anterior* or *posterior* stones in relation to a transverse line between the mandibular first molars. Stones that occur anterior to this line are generally well visualized on a mandibular occlusal radiograph and may be amenable to intraoral removal. Small anteriorly located stones may be retrieved through the ductal opening after dilation of the orifice (Fig. 20-26).

Occasionally, it becomes necessary to remove submandibular stones via an incision made in the floor of the mouth to expose the duct and the stone (Fig. 20-27, *A*). A longitudinal incision is then made in the duct, the stone is retrieved, and the ductal lining is sutured to the mucosa of the floor of the mouth (Fig. 20-27, *B*). Saliva then flows out of the revised duct. This procedure, known as a *sialodochoplasty* (i.e., revision of the salivary duct), eliminates many of the factors that contributed to formation of the stone. The entire length of the duct is decreased, the opening created is now larger, and gravity contributes less to salivary stasis. Regardless of the procedure performed, patients are encouraged to maintain ample salivary flow by using salivary stimulants, such as citrus fruits, flavored candies, or glycerin swabs. Posterior stones occur in up to 50% of cases and may be located at the hilum of the gland or within the substance of the gland itself. A routine occlusal film will likely not demonstrate the stone, and a panoramic radiograph or a CT scan may be necessary to localize the stone. In cases of posterior stones that cannot be palpated intraorally and in many instances of repeated chronic stone formation and symptoms, the submandibular gland and the stone should be removed by an extraoral approach (Fig. 20-28).

Clinical trials using extracorporeal shock wave lithotripsy have been successful in treating small salivary gland stones. This technology uses transcutaneous electromagnetic waves to break the calculus apart into smaller calcified debris particles, which can be flushed from the ductal system by the normal flow of saliva. This procedure has few reported complications

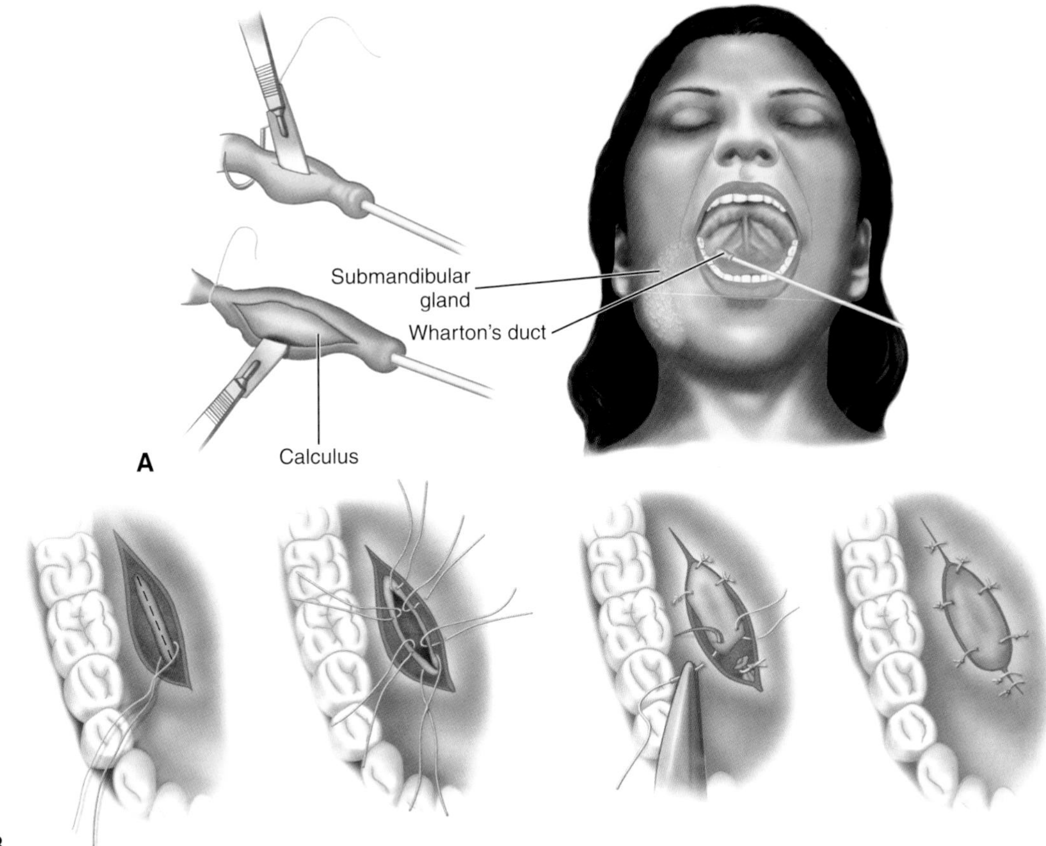

FIGURE 20-27 A, Surgical opening of the submandibular duct (sialodochotomy) and removal of the stone (sialolithectomy). B, This is followed by a ductal revision sutured to the floor of mouth mucosa (sialodochoplasty).

but is limited by the size of the salivary gland stone (usually less than 3 mm), the number of stones (usually fewer than three), and the location of the stone (intraglandular stones may be less amenable to extracorporeal shock wave lithotripsy).

Salivary gland calculi occur much less commonly in the parotid gland. The parotid gland is examined by inspection and palpation of the gland extraorally over the ascending mandibular ramus. Stensen's duct and its orifice can be examined intraorally. Palpation of the gland and simultaneous observation of the duct allow observation of salivary flow or the production of other material, such as purulence, from the punctum of the duct. Parotid sialoliths found in the distal third of Stensen's duct that can be palpated intraorally may be removed after dilation of the duct orifice or, if slightly more proximal, may require surgical exposure to gain access to the stone. On rare occasions the presence of a parotid stone at the hilum of the gland or in the gland itself may necessitate an extraoral approach to remove the stone and the superficial lobe of the parotid gland.

Obstruction of the sublingual gland as a result of stone formation is unusual, but if it occurs, it is usually the result of obstruction of Wharton's duct on the same side of the oral cavity. Although stone formation is rare in the sublingual and minor salivary glands, the treatment is simple excision of the stone and associated gland. The sublingual gland is examined by observation and bimanual palpation of the anterior third of the floor of the mouth.

MUCOUS RETENTION AND EXTRAVASATION PHENOMENA

Mucocele

Salivary ducts, especially those of the minor salivary glands, are occasionally traumatized, commonly by lip biting, and severed beneath the surface mucosa. Subsequent saliva production may then extravasate beneath the surface mucosa into the soft tissues. Over time, secretions accumulate within the tissues and produce a pseudocyst (without a true epithelial lining) that contains thick, viscous saliva. These lesions are most common in the mucosa of the lower lip and are known as *mucoceles* (Fig. 20-29). The second most common site of mucocele formation is the buccal mucosa. Mucocele formation results in an elevated, thinned, stretched overlying mucosa that appears as a vesicle filled with a clear or blue-gray mucus. The patient frequently relates a history of the lesion filling with fluid, rupture of the fluid collection, and refilling of these lesions. Some instances of mucocele formation regress spontaneously without surgery. For persistent or recurrent lesions, the preferred treatment consists of excision of the mucocele and the associated minor salivary glands that contributed to its formation (Fig. 20-30). Usually, local anesthesia is administered via a mental nerve block, and an incision is made through the mucosa. Careful dissection around the mucocele may permit its complete removal; however, in many cases the thin lining ruptures and decompresses the mucocele before removal. The

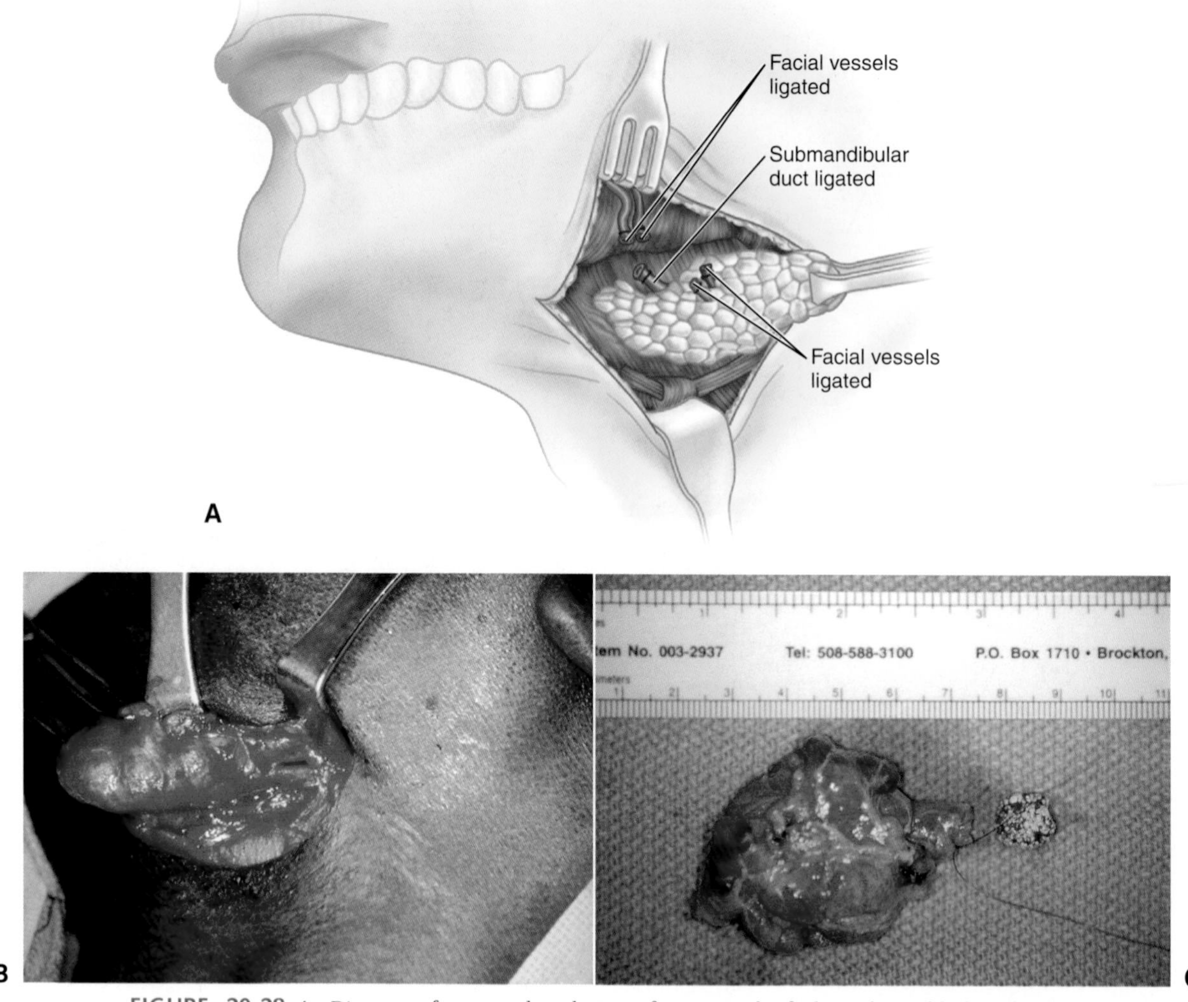

FIGURE 20-28 A, Diagram of extraoral technique for removal of the submandibular gland. B, Submandibular gland removal (sialoadenectomy). C, Specimen of submandibular gland and associated stone.

regional associated minor salivary glands are removed as well and sent for histopathologic evaluation. The recurrence rates of mucoceles may be as high as 15% to 30% after surgical removal, possibly caused by incomplete removal or repeat trauma to the minor salivary glands.

Ranula

The most common lesion of the sublingual gland is the ranula, which may be considered a mucocele of the sublingual salivary gland. Ranulas result from mucous retention in the sublingual gland ductal system or mucous extravasation as a result of ductal disruption. The two types of ranulas are the simple ranula and the plunging ranula. The simple ranula is confined to the area occupied by the sublingual gland in the sublingual space, superior to the mylohyoid muscle (Fig. 20-31). The progression to a plunging ranula occurs when the lesion extends beyond the level of the mylohyoid muscle into the submandibular space (Fig. 20-32). Ranulas may reach a larger size than mucoceles because their overlying mucosa is thicker and because trauma that would cause their rupture is less likely in the floor of the mouth. As a result, a plunging ranula has the potential to extend through the mylohyoid muscle into the neck and to compromise the airway, resulting in a medical emergency. The differential diagnosis of a floor of mouth swelling includes ranula, lymphoepithelial cyst, epidermoid or dermoid cyst, salivary gland tumors (e.g., mucoepidermoid carcinoma), and mesenchymal tumors (e.g., lipoma, neurofibroma, or hemangioma). The differential diagnosis of a midline neck mass includes thyroid enlargement (i.e., goiter or tumor), thyroglossal duct cyst, dermoid cyst, and plunging ranula. The differential diagnosis of a lateral neck mass includes lymphadenopathy, epidermoid cyst, lipoma, infectious mononucleosis, metastatic carcinoma, lymphoma, salivary gland tumors (e.g., submandibular gland or tail of the parotid gland), submandibular gland sialadenitis, lymphoepithelial cyst, sarcoidosis, tuberculosis, cat-scratch disease, cystic hygroma, carotid body tumor, or plunging ranula. The usual treatment of the ranula is marsupialization, in which a portion of the oral mucosa of the floor of the mouth is excised, along with the superior wall of the ranula (Fig. 20-33). Subsequently, the ranula wall is sutured to the oral mucosa of the floor of the mouth and allowed to heal by secondary intention. The preferred treat-

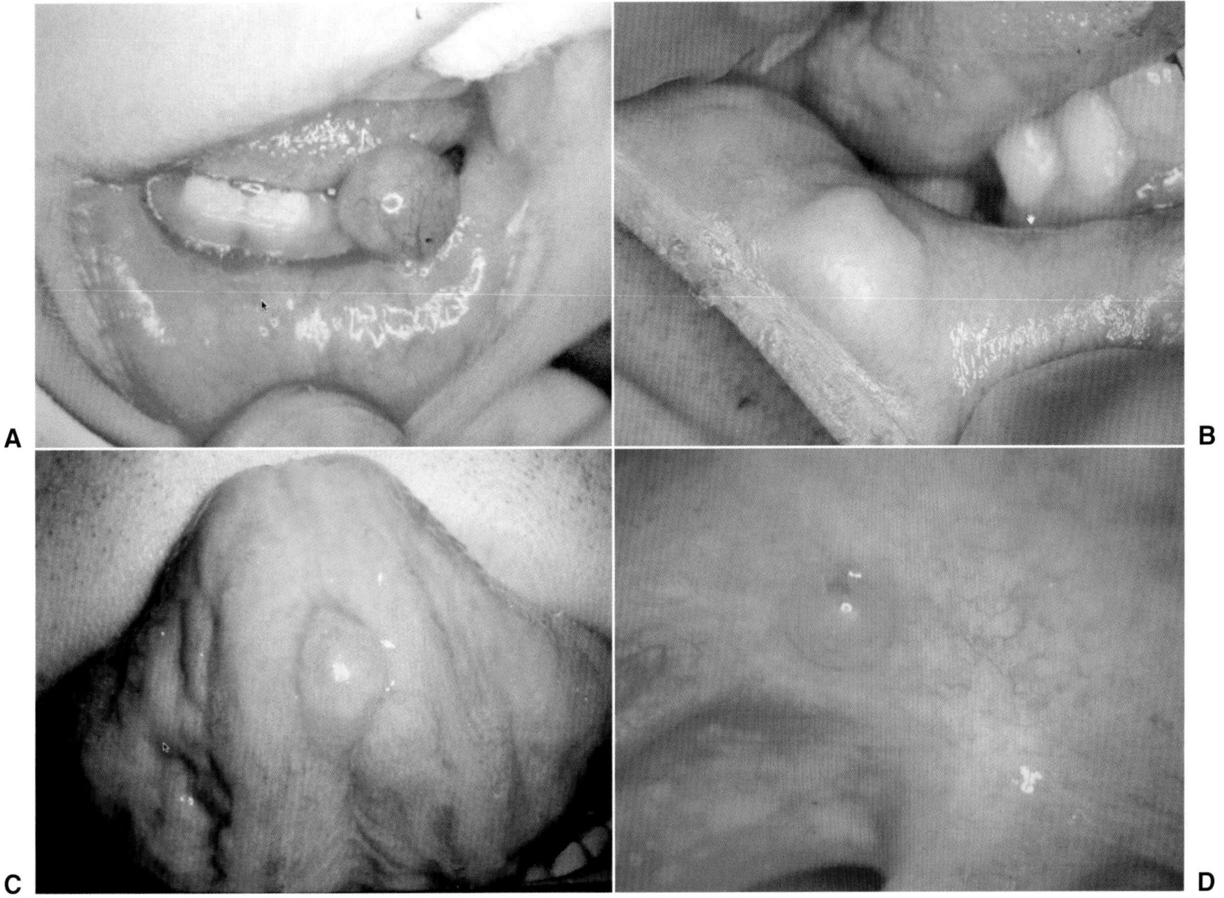

FIGURE 20-29 Mucoceles of (**A**) lower lip, (**B**) buccal mucosa, (**C**) ventral tongue, and (**D**) soft palate.

ment for recurrent or persistent ranulas is excision of the ranula and sublingual gland via an intraoral approach (Fig. 20-34); several recent studies have indicated that this might be appropriate for initial therapy.

SALIVARY GLAND INFECTIONS

Infections of the major salivary glands can be acute or chronic and are commonly, but not always, related to obstructive disease, especially in the submandibular gland (obstruction leads to infection). The cause of acute suppurative sialadenitis of the parotid gland usually involves a change in fluid balance that is likely to occur in patients who are elderly, debilitated, malnourished, dehydrated, or plagued with chronic illness. In these cases, gland infections are usually bilateral. The mean age of occurrence of infections is 60 years, with a slight male predilection. Salivary gland infections may be caused by a variety of organisms, including aerobic and anaerobic bacteria, viruses, fungal organisms, and mycobacteria. In most cases, mixed bacterial flora is responsible for sialadenitis. The single most common organism implicated in salivary gland infection is *Staphylococcus aureus* because this organism normally colonizes around ductal orifices. In addition, during instances of decreased or slowed salivary flow (i.e., obstruction or dehydration), retrograde influx of *S. aureus* into the ductal system and gland occurs and results in infection.

The clinical characteristics of acute bacterial salivary gland infections include rapid onset of swelling in the preauricular (parotid gland) or submandibular regions, with associated erythema and pain (Fig. 20-35). Palpation of the involved gland reveals no flow or elicits a thick, purulent discharge from the orifice of the duct (Fig. 20-36).

Treatment of bacterial salivary gland infections includes symptomatic and supportive care, including intravenous fluid hydration, antibiotics, and analgesics. Initial empirical antibiotics should be aimed at the most likely causative organism, *S. aureus*, and should include a cephalosporin (first generation) or antistaphylococcal semisynthetic penicillin (oxacillin or dicloxacillin). Culture and sensitivity studies of purulent material should be obtained to aid in selecting the most appropriate antibiotic for each patient.

Antibiotics should be administered intravenously in high doses for the majority of these patients, who ordinarily require hospitalization. On most occasions, surgery consisting of incision and drainage becomes necessary in the management of salivary gland infections. Untreated infections may progress rapidly and can cause respiratory obstruction, septicemia, and eventually, death. In some instances of recurrent salivary gland infection, the repeated insults result in irreversible functional impairment of gland function, and excision of the gland may be indicated.

Viral parotitis, or mumps, is an acute, nonsuppurative communicable disease. Before routine vaccination (e.g., measles, mumps, and rubella vaccine) against the disease began, viral parotitis occurred in epidemics during the winter and spring. Differentiation of viral from bacterial salivary gland infection is

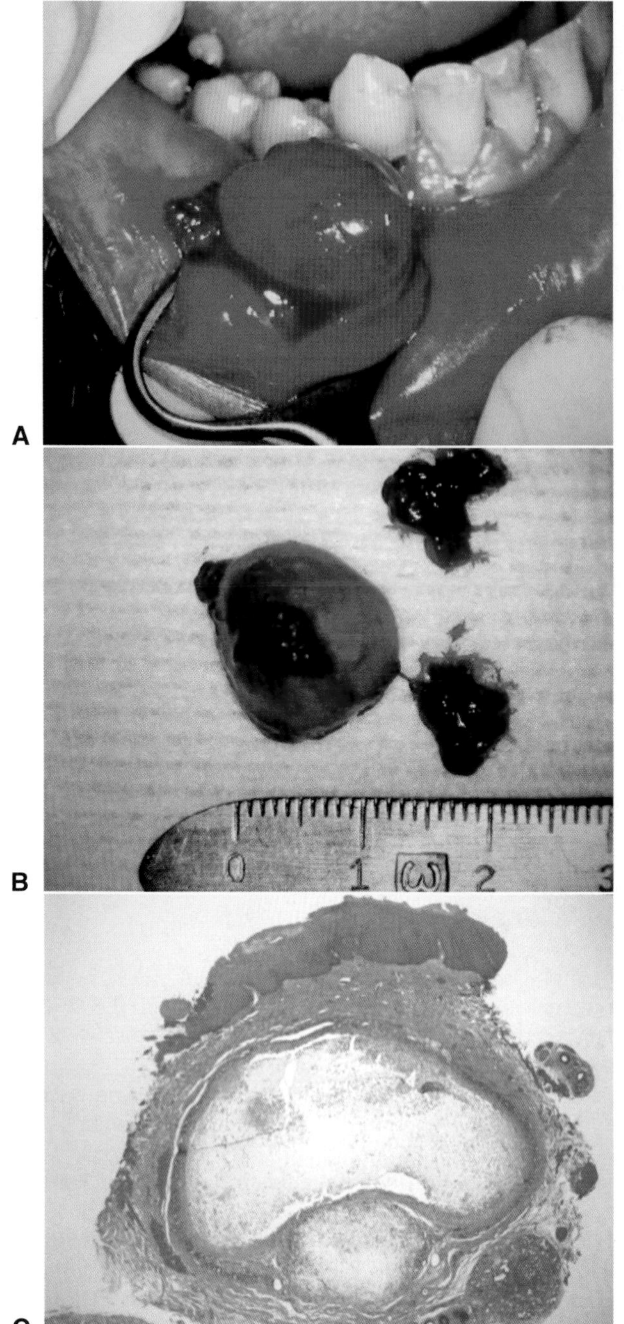

FIGURE 20-30 A, Excision of mucocele of right lower lip. B, Gross specimen of intact mucocele is demonstrated. C, Histologic specimen of a mucocele and associated minor salivary glands.

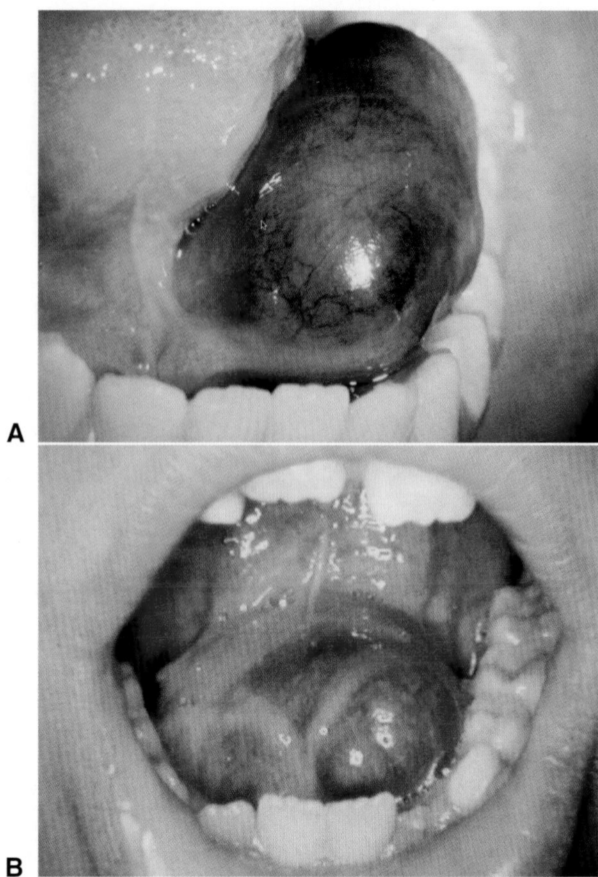

FIGURE 20-31 A, Left floor of mouth ranula. B, Bilateral floor of mouth ranula.

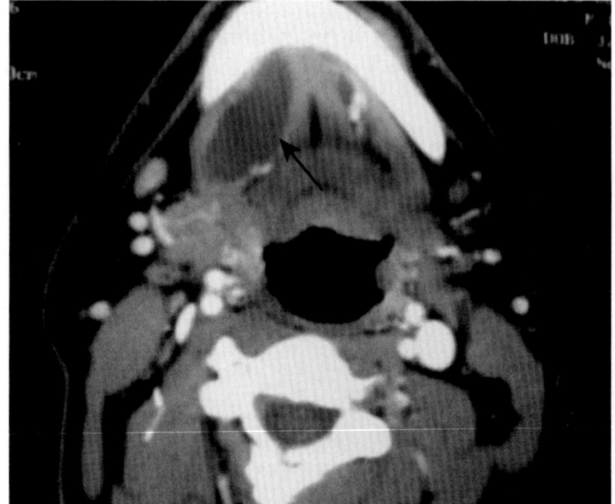

FIGURE 20-32 Right plunging ranula through the mylohyoid muscle seen on computed tomography scan *(arrow)*.

important because viral infections are not the result of obstructive disease and require different treatment, not including antibiotics.

Mumps is characterized by a painful, nonerythematous swelling of one or both parotid glands that begins 2 to 3 weeks after exposure to the virus (incubation period). This disease occurs most commonly in children between ages 6 and 8. The signs and symptoms of mumps include preauricular pain and swelling, fever, chills, and headache.

Viral parotitis usually resolves in 5 to 12 days after its onset. Supportive and symptomatic care for fever, headache, and malaise with antipyretics, analgesics, and adequate hydration treats viral parotitis. Complications of the disease include meningitis, pancreatitis, nephritis, orchitis, testicular atrophy, and sterility in approximately 20% of young males affected.

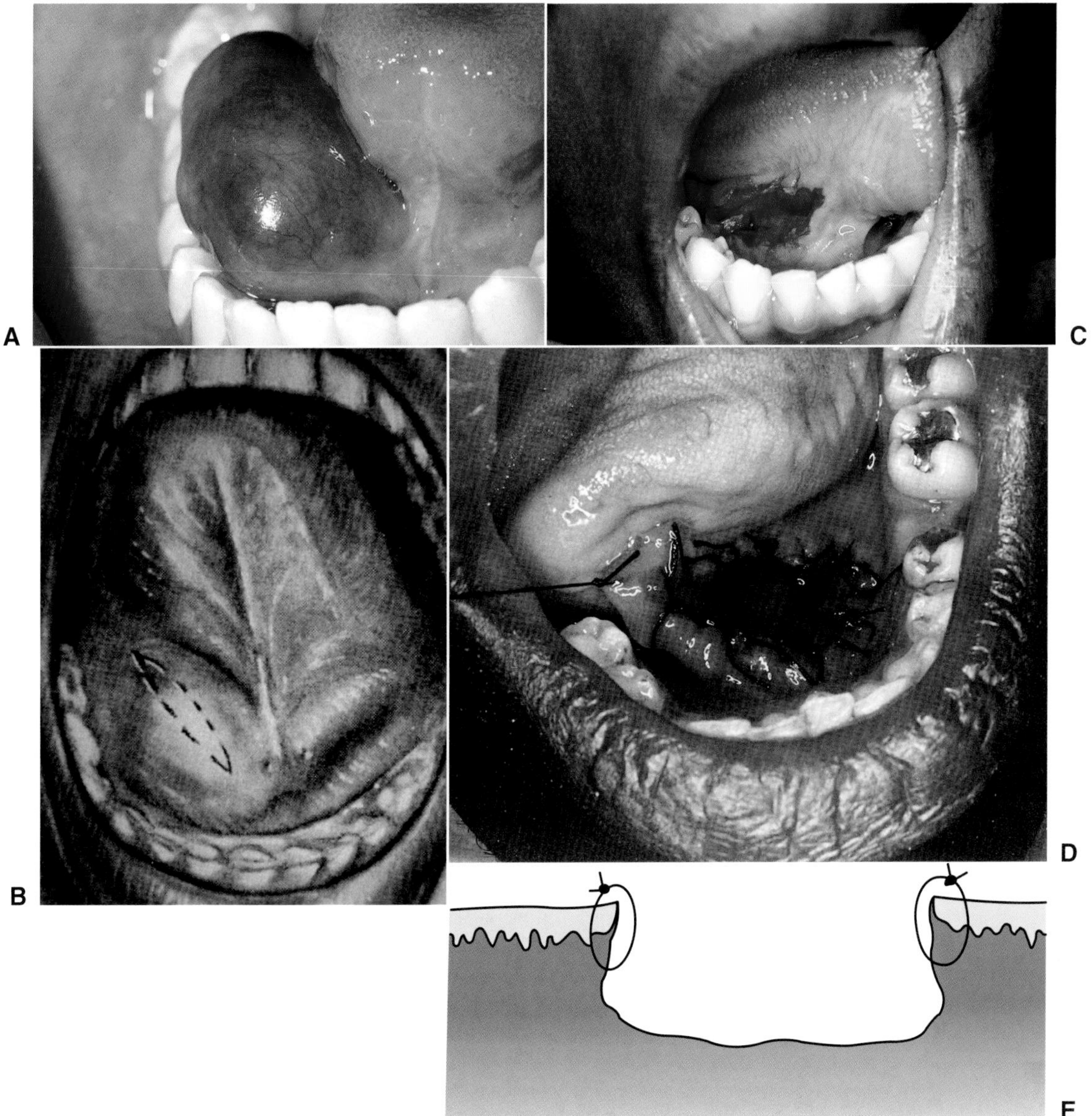

FIGURE 20-33 A, Ranula in the right floor of mouth caused by accumulation of sublingual gland secretions in soft tissues resulting from rupture of salivary duct. B, Diagram of marsupialization incision. C, Marsupialization of ranula, with excision of oral mucosa and superior wall of ranula. D, Completion of marsupialization of left floor of mouth ranula with placement of circumferential sutures. E, Diagram of completed marsupialization.

NECROTIZING SIALOMETAPLASIA

Necrotizing sialometaplasia is a reactive, nonneoplastic inflammatory process that usually affects the minor salivary glands of the palate. However, it may involve minor salivary glands in any location. Necrotizing sialometaplasia is of unclear origin but is thought to result from vascular infarction of the salivary gland lobules. Potential causes of diminished blood flow to the affected area include trauma, local anesthetic injection, smoking, diabetes mellitus, vascular disease, and pressure from a denture prosthesis. The usual age range of affected patients is between 23 and 66 years.

Lesions usually appear as large (1 to 4 cm), painless or painful, deeply ulcerated areas lateral to the palatal midline and near the junction of the hard and soft palate (Fig. 20-37, *A*). Although lesions are usually unilateral, bilateral involvement may occur. Some patients may report a prodromal flulike illness before the onset of the ulceration.

This condition is of considerable concern because, clinically and histologically (Fig. 20-37, *B*), it resembles a malignant carcinoma (squamous cell or mucoepidermoid carcinoma). The appropriate diagnosis and management of this disease relies on evaluation by an oral maxillofacial surgeon and pathologist who

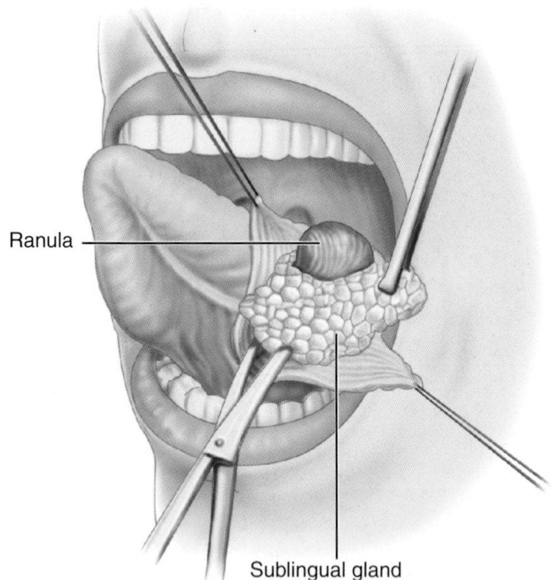

FIGURE 20-34 Intraoral sublingual gland and ranula removal.

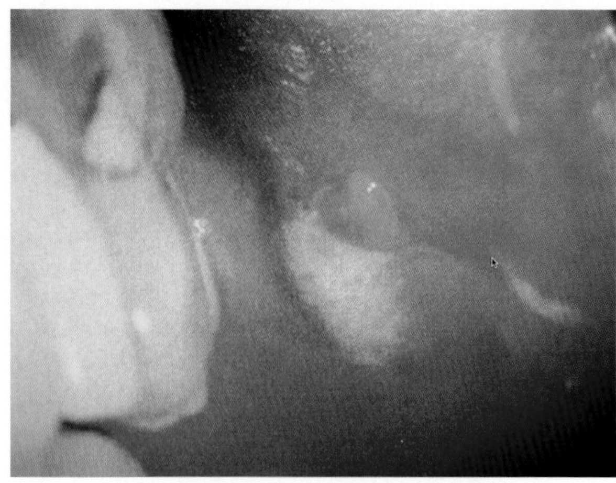

FIGURE 20-36 Purulent discharge from left parotid duct is demonstrated in patient with an infection involving parotid gland.

are familiar with this entity because the result of a misdiagnosis may be extensive, unwarranted surgical resection. Helpful histologic criteria for distinguishing necrotizing sialometaplasia from a malignant process include the maintenance of the overall salivary lobular morphology, the generally nondysplastic appearance of the squamous islands or nests, and evidence of residual ductal lumina within the epithelial nests. The ulcerations of necrotizing sialometaplasia usually heal spontaneously within 6 to 10 weeks after their onset and require no surgical management.

SJÖGREN'S SYNDROME

Sjögren's syndrome (SS) is a multisystem disease process with a variable presentation. The two types of SS are (1) primary SS, or sicca syndrome, characterized by xerostomia (dry mouth) and keratoconjunctivitis sicca (dry eyes; Fig. 20-38); and (2) secondary SS, which is composed of primary SS and an associated connective tissue disorder, most commonly rheumatoid arthritis. Although the cause of SS is unknown, there appears to be a strong autoimmune influence. SS shows a female predilection of 9:1, with more than 80% of affected individuals being females with a mean age of 50 years.

Generally, the first symptoms to appear are arthritic complaints, followed by ocular symptoms, and late in the disease process, salivary gland symptoms. The involvement of the salivary and lacrimal glands results from a lymphocytic replacement of the normal glandular elements. The xerostomia results from a decreased function of the major and minor salivary glands, with the parotid gland being the most sensitive. The diagnosis of SS is suggested by the patient's complaints and by a variety of abnormal immunologic laboratory tests. The

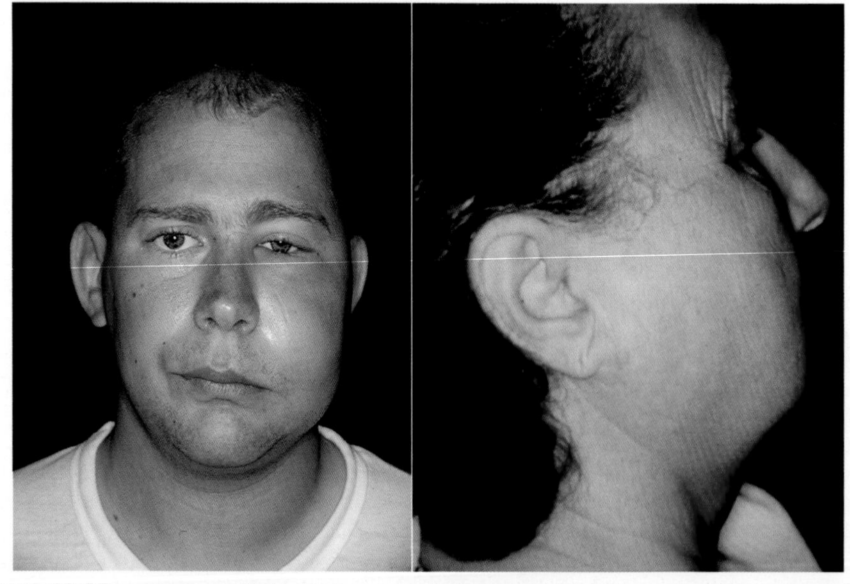

FIGURE 20-35 A, Left parotid gland infection. B, Right acute bacterial parotitis with erythema. This infection is extremely painful and may indicate another serious illness. Treatment requires hospitalization, intravenously administered antibiotics, and possibly surgical drainage.

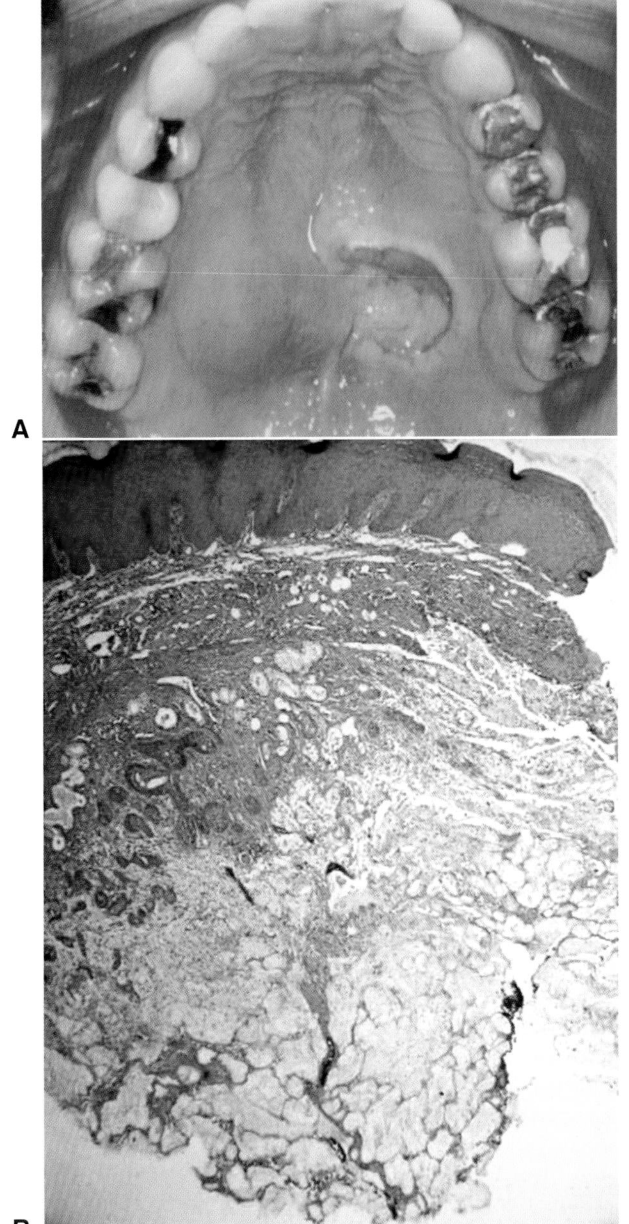

FIGURE 20-37 A, Necrotizing sialometaplasia of posterior palate with ulceration. B, Histopathologic examination of necrotizing sialometaplasia shows pseudoepitheliomatous hyperplasia that appears similar to epithelial infiltration of a squamous cell carcinoma into the underlying connective tissues.

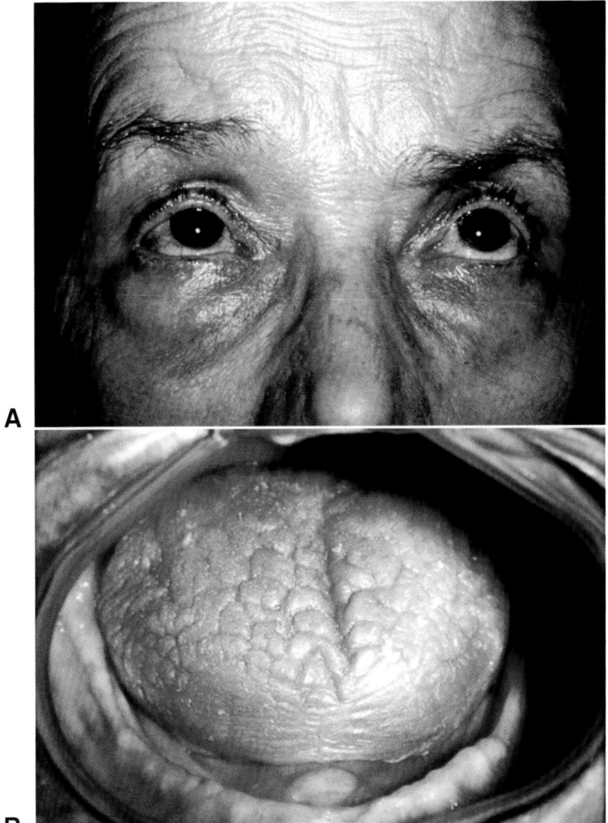

FIGURE 20-38 Sjögren's syndrome showing (A) dry eyes (keratoconjunctivitis sicca) and (B) dry mouth (xerostomia).

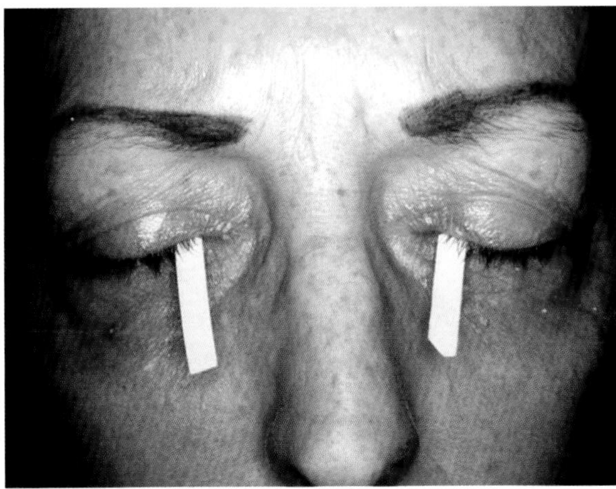

FIGURE 20-39 Schirmer's test for dry eyes in a patient with Sjögren's syndrome. Filter paper is placed in the ocular fornix and observed for "wetting" to a certain distance within a specific time limit.

oral component of SS may be diagnosed using salivary flow rate studies and sialograms that can show acinar destruction. The use of a labial minor salivary gland biopsy, as mentioned previously, currently is considered to be highly accurate in aiding the diagnosis. The histopathologic changes seen in the minor glands are similar to those in the major glands (parotid). Keratoconjunctivitis sicca is suggested by the patient's complaints and a Schirmer's test for lacrimal flow (Fig. 20-39). The treatment for SS includes symptomatic care with artificial tears for the dry eyes and salivary substitutes for the dry mouth. Additionally, the medication pilocarpine (Salagen) or the Biotene products may be useful to stimulate salivary flow from the remaining functional salivary gland tissue.

TRAUMATIC SALIVARY GLAND INJURIES

Traumatic injuries, particularly lacerations, involving the salivary glands and their ducts may accompany a variety of facial injuries, including fractures. Injuries that occur in proximity to one of the major salivary glands or ducts require careful evaluation.

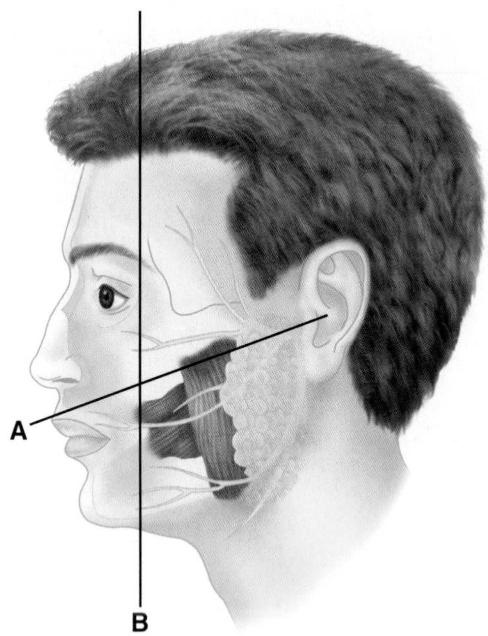

FIGURE 20-40 *A*, Diagram showing the position of Stensen's duct along a line drawn from the tragus to the middle of the upper lip. *B*, Injuries to the terminal branches of the facial nerve anterior to line do not require repair, and function usually returns.

Facial lacerations may involve not only the gland and its ductal system but also branches of the facial nerve and branches of major facial vessels. These structures require meticulous attention for appropriate diagnosis and prompt repair. Usually, facial nerve lacerations that are anterior to a vertical line from the lateral canthus of the eye to the mental foramen are not amenable to surgical repair (Fig. 20-40). Stensen's ductal repair may include ductal anastomoses, in which the proximal and distal portions of the duct are identified, a plastic or metal catheter is placed as a stent, and the duct is sutured over the stent (Fig. 20-41). The catheter usually remains in place for 10 to 14 days for epithelialization of the duct to occur. Additionally, nerve anastomoses may be required and performed by placing epineurial sutures, using magnification, to reapproximate the nerve stumps. The lacerations are closed in a usual layered fashion, after débridement of the soft tissue wounds to cleanse the site of entrapped particles, such as glass or dirt. Potential sequelae of trauma involving the major salivary glands include infection, facial paralysis, cutaneous salivary gland fistula, sialocele formation, and duct obstruction as a result of scar formation, with eventual glandular atrophy and decreased function. The involved gland may eventually require surgical removal.

NEOPLASTIC SALIVARY GLAND DISORDERS

Although a comprehensive discussion of salivary gland neoplasms is beyond the scope of this chapter and many other sources are available for this information, a brief review of several important aspects of the more common lesions is warranted. Salivary gland tumors occur much more commonly in the major glands (80% to 85%) as opposed to the minor glands (15% to 20%; Table 20-3). Additionally, between 75% and 80% of major gland tumors are benign, whereas 50% to 55% of minor gland tumors are benign. The overwhelming majority of salivary tumors occur in the parotid gland, and the majority of those are benign (mostly pleomorphic adenomas).

TABLE 20-3

Salivary Gland Tumor Distribution

Location of Tumor	Occurrence
MAJOR GLANDS	80%-85%
Parotid gland	85%-90%
Submandibular gland	5%-10%
Sublingual gland	Rare
MINOR GLANDS	15%-20%
Palate	55%
Lips	15%
Remainder	Rare

Benign Salivary Gland Tumors

The *pleomorphic adenoma*, or *benign mixed tumor*, is the most common salivary gland tumor. The mean age of occurrence is 45 years, with a male-to-female ratio of 3:2. In the major glands the parotid gland is involved in more than 80% of cases; in the minor glands the most common intraoral site is the palate (Fig. 20-42). Pleomorphic adenomas are usually slow-growing, painless masses. The histopathologic examination shows two cell types: (1) the ductal epithelial cell and (2) the myoepithelial cell, which may differentiate along a variety of cell lines (*pleomorphic* means many forms). A connective tissue capsule exists, which may be incomplete. The treatment involves complete surgical excision with a margin of normal uninvolved tissue. Parotid lesions are treated with removal of the involved lobe along with the tumor. Recurrence is possible in rare occasions, as well as a small risk (5%) of malignant transformation to a *carcinoma ex pleomorphic adenoma*.

Warthin's tumor, or *papillary cystadenoma lymphomatosum*, almost exclusively affects the parotid gland, specifically the tail of the parotid gland (Fig. 20-43). The peak incidence is in the sixth decade of life, with a male-to-female ratio of 7:1. This lesion presents as a slow-growing, soft, painless mass. Warthin's tumor is believed to be caused by entrapped salivary epithelial rests within developing lymph nodes. The histopathologic examination shows an epithelial component in a papillary pattern and a lymphoid component with germinal centers. The treatment of this lesion is simple surgical excision, and recurrence is rare.

The *monomorphic adenoma* is an uncommon solitary lesion composed of one cell type, affecting predominantly the upper lip minor glands (*canalicular adenoma*; Fig. 20-44) and the parotid gland (*basal cell adenoma*). The mean age of occurrence is 61 years, and the lesion usually presents as an asymptomatic, freely movable mass. The histopathologic examination reveals an encapsulated lesion composed of one type (monomorphic) of salivary ductal epithelial cell. The treatment is simple surgical excision.

Malignant Salivary Gland Tumors

The *mucoepidermoid carcinoma* is the most common malignant salivary gland tumor. The tumor makes up 10% of major gland tumors (mostly parotid) and 20% of minor gland tumors

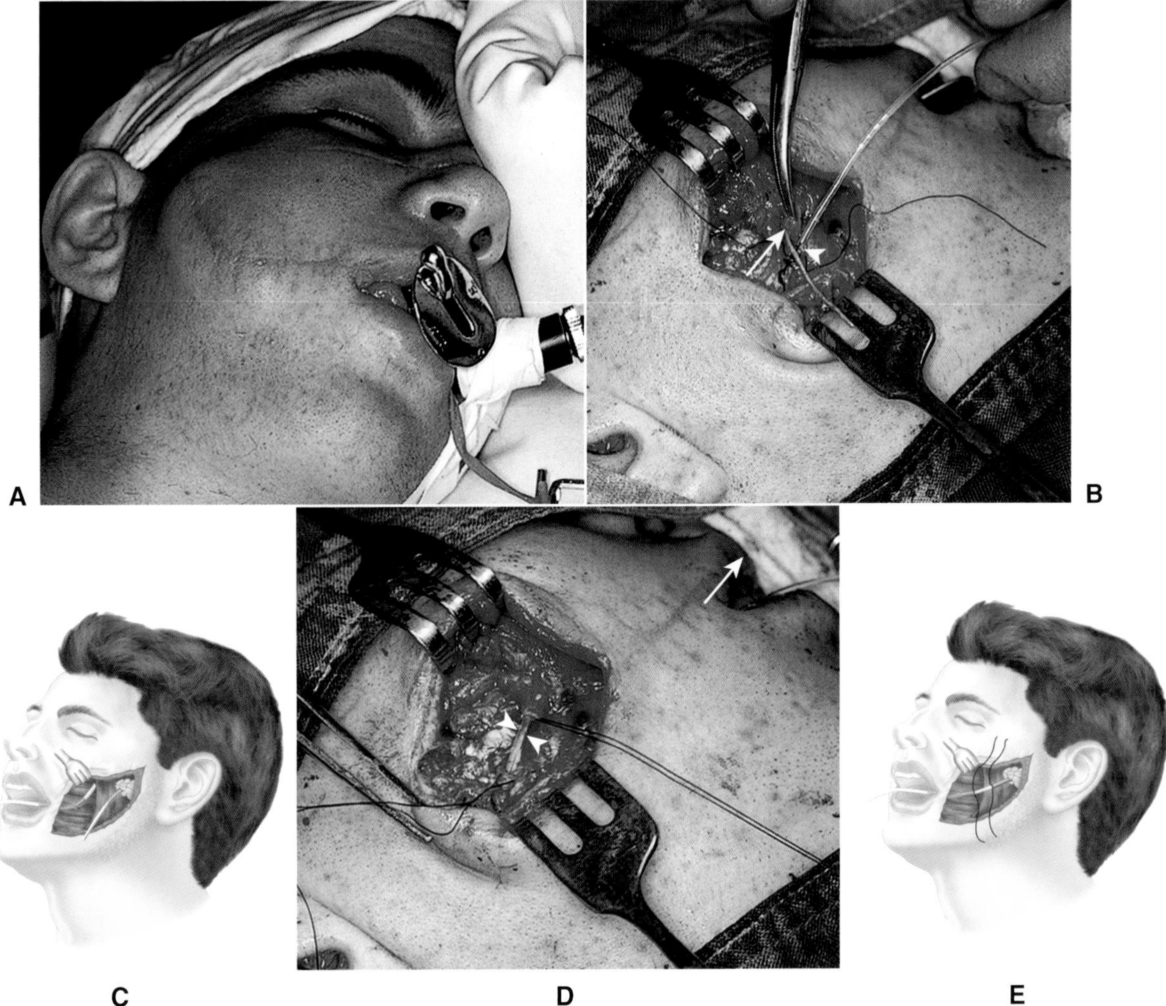

FIGURE 20-41 A, Patient who had cheek laceration repaired with failure to appreciate a Stensen's duct laceration and subsequently developed a sialocele (localized collection of saliva). B, Operative repair of Stensen's duct laceration with a metal probe in the distal duct (*arrow*) and a plastic catheter (*arrowhead*) placed into the proximal portion of the duct. C, Diagram of catheter placement for repair. D, Repair of Stensen's duct laceration via suturing over a plastic stent (*arrowheads*) placed via intraoral cannulation of Stensen's duct (*arrow*). E. Diagram of completed repair.

(mostly palatal; Fig. 20-45). This lesion may occur at any age, but the mean age is 45 years. The male-to-female ratio is 3:2. The clinical presentation is a submucosal mass that may be painful or ulcerated. The mass may appear to have a bluish tinge because of the mucous content contained within the lesion. An intraosseous form of mucoepidermoid carcinoma may present as a multilocular radiolucency of the posterior mandible (Fig. 20-46). The histopathologic examination shows three cell types: (1) mucous cells, (2) epidermoid cells, and (3) intermediate (clear) cells. The proportion of each cell type helps to grade the mucoepidermoid carcinoma as high-, intermediate-, or low-grade lesions. The higher the grade, the more predominance of epidermoid cells and pleomorphism, lack of mucous cells and cystic areas, and overall more aggressive behavior. The treatment of low-grade lesions is wide surgical excision with a margin of uninvolved normal tissue; high-grade lesions require more aggressive surgical removal with margins, and possibly, local radiation therapy. The low-grade lesions have a 95% 5-year survival rate, whereas the high-grade lesions have less than a 40% 5-year survival rate.

The *polymorphous low-grade adenocarcinoma* is the second most common intraoral salivary gland malignancy. This lesion was first described in 1983; before its identification, many cases were probably misdiagnosed as adenoid cystic carcinoma. The most common site is the junction of the hard and soft palates (Fig. 20-47). The male-to-female ratio is 3:1, with a mean age of 56 years. These tumors present as slow-growing, asymptomatic masses that may be ulcerated. The histopathologic examination shows many cell shapes and patterns (polymorphous). Patients experience an infiltrative proliferation of ductal epithelial cells in an "Indian file" pattern. This lesion shows a predilection for invasion of surrounding nerves. The treatment of this tumor is wide surgical excision, with a relatively high recurrence rate of 14%.

The *adenoid cystic carcinoma* is the third most common intraoral salivary gland malignancy, with a mean age of

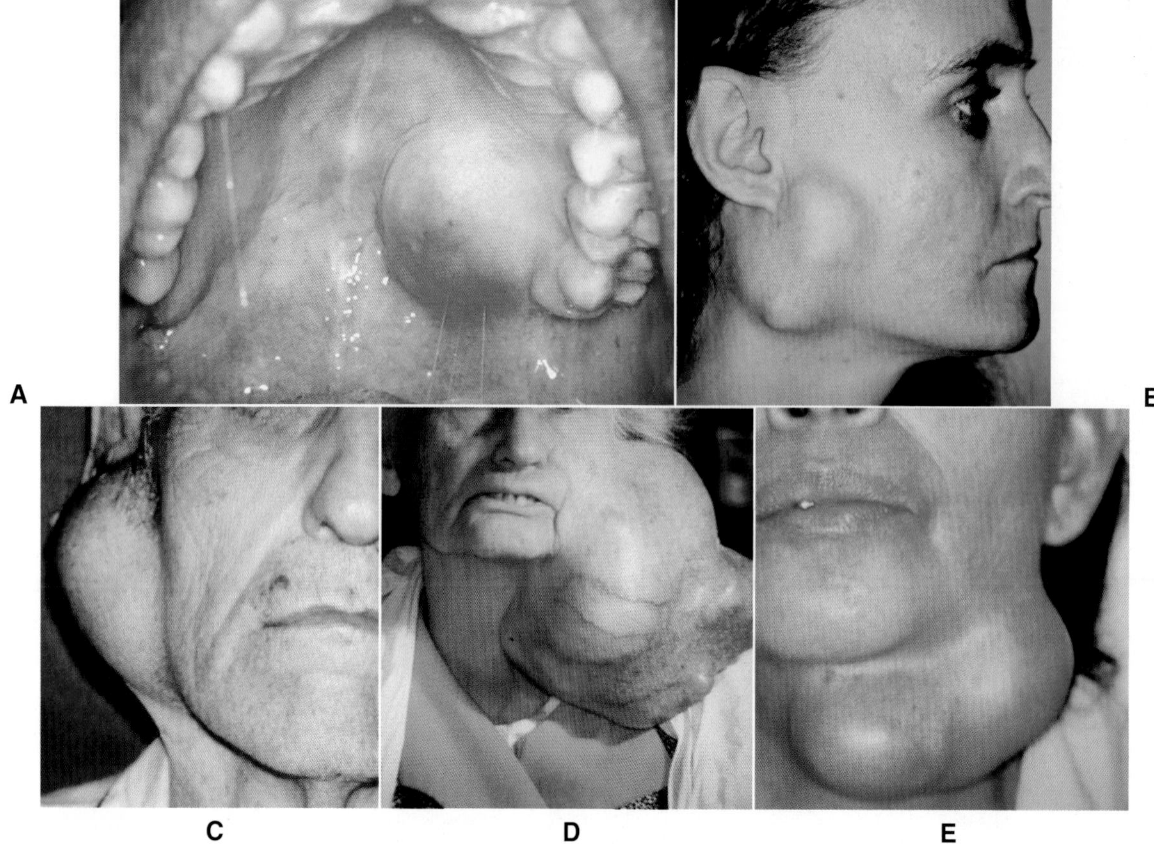

FIGURE 20-42 Pleomorphic adenomas. A, Palate. B to D, Parotid gland. E, Submandibular gland.

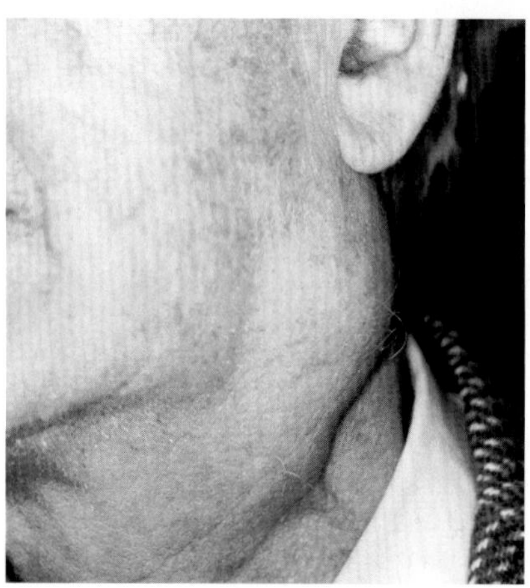

FIGURE 20-43 Warthin's tumor of the tail of the parotid gland.

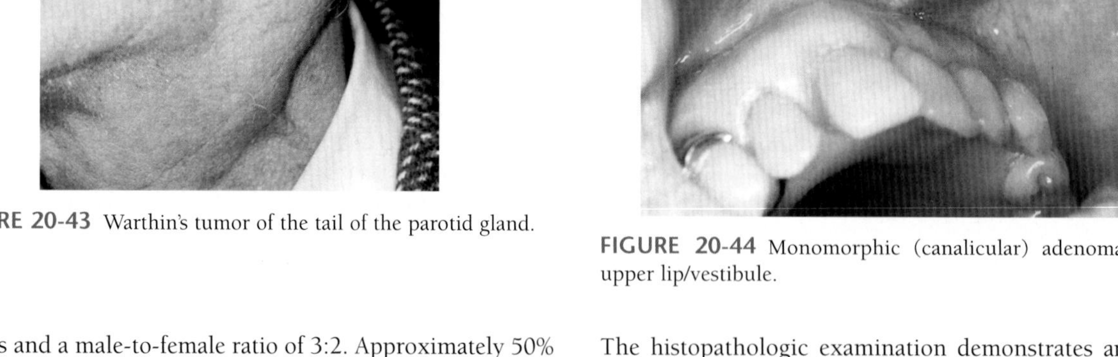

FIGURE 20-44 Monomorphic (canalicular) adenoma of the left upper lip/vestibule.

53 years and a male-to-female ratio of 3:2. Approximately 50% of these tumors occur in the parotid gland, whereas the other 50% occur in the minor glands of the palate (Fig. 20-48). These tumors present as slow-growing, nonulcerated masses, with an associated chronic dull pain. Occasionally, parotid lesions may result in facial paralysis as a result of facial nerve involvement. The histopathologic examination demonstrates an infiltrative proliferation of basaloid cells arranged in a cribriform (Swiss cheese) pattern. As seen in the polymorphous low-grade adenocarcinoma, there may be perineural invasion. The treatment is wide surgical excision, followed in some cases by radiation therapy. The prognosis is poor despite aggressive therapy.

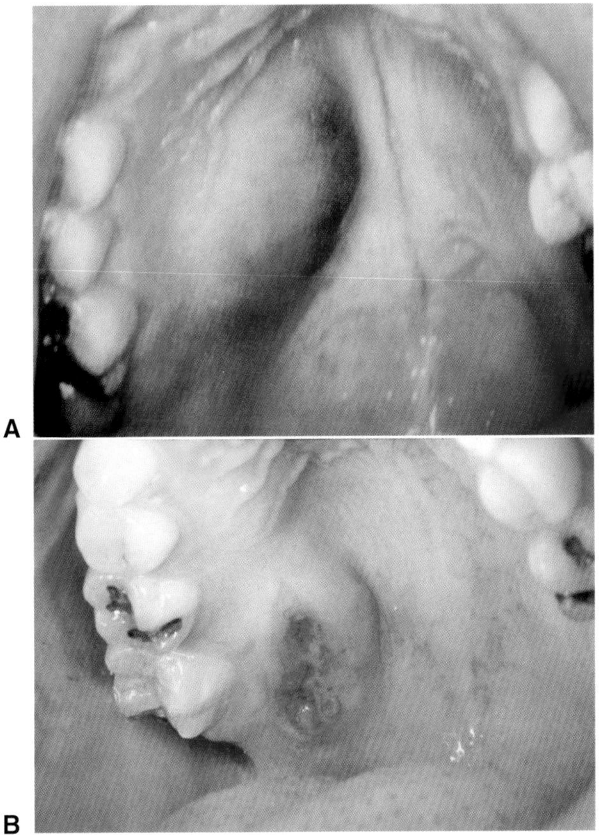

FIGURE 20-45 A, Mucoepidermoid carcinoma of the palate (note bluish tinge from mucin content). B, Mucoepidermoid carcinoma of the palate with ulceration.

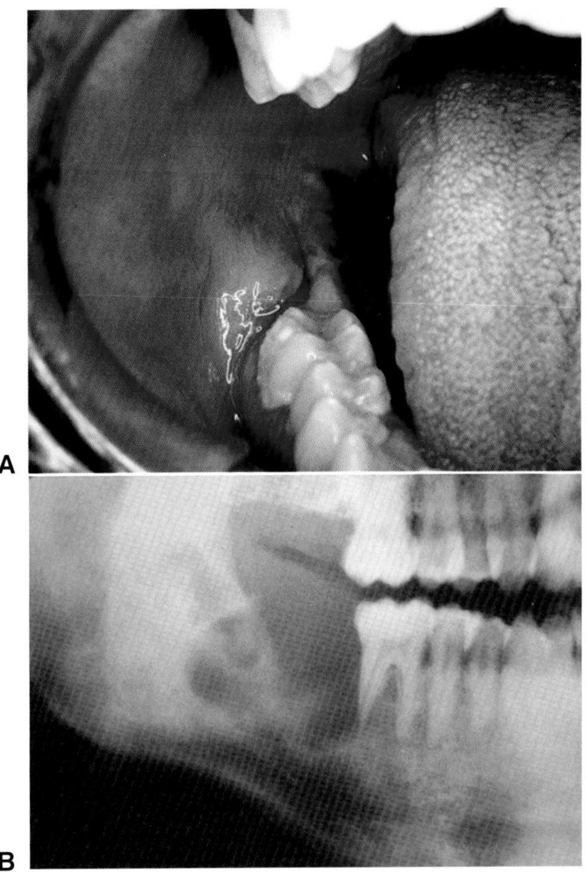

FIGURE 20-46 A, Central mucoepidermoid carcinoma of the right retromolar pad minor salivary glands. B, Panoramic radiograph showing an underlying multilocular radiolucency.

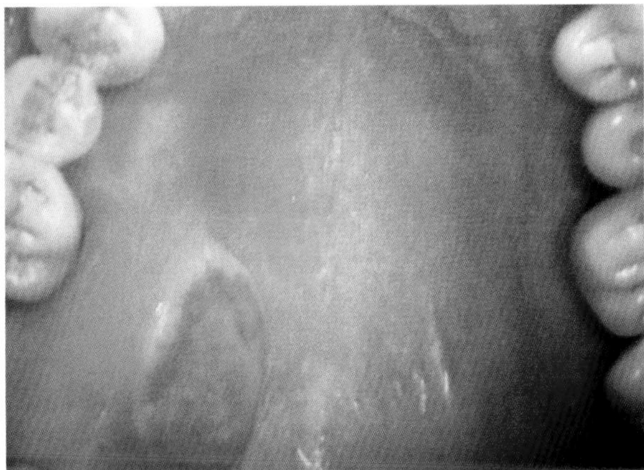

FIGURE 20-47 Polymorphous low-grade adenocarcinoma of the palate.

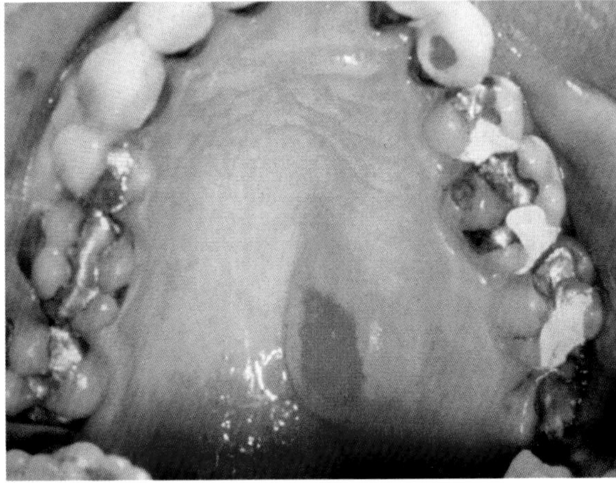

FIGURE 20-48 Adenoid cystic carcinoma of the palate.

Bibliography

Abaza N, Miloro M: The role of labial salivary gland biopsy in the diagnosis of Sjögren's syndrome: report of three cases, *J Oral Maxillofac Surg* 51:574, 1993.

Abaza NA, Miloro M: The role of fine-needle aspiration in oral and maxillofacial diagnosis, *Oral and Maxillofacial Surgery Clinics of North America* 6:401, 1994.

Baurmash HD: Marsupialization for treatment of oral ranula: a second look at the procedure, *J Oral Maxillofac Surg* 50:1274, 1992.

Berry RL: Sialadenitis and sialolithiasis: diagnosis and management, *Oral and Maxillofacial Surgery Clinics of North America* 7:479, 1995.

Carlson ER: Salivary gland tumors: classification, histogenesis, and general considerations, *Oral and Maxillofacial Surgery Clinics of North America* 7:519, 1995.

Curtin HD: Assessment of salivary gland pathology, *Otolaryngol Clin North Am* 21:547, 1988.

Dardick I, editor: *Color atlas/text of salivary gland pathology,* New York, 1996, Igaku-Shoin Medical.

Delbalso A: Salivary imaging, *Oral and Maxillofacial Surgery Clinics of North America* 7:387, 1995.

Goldberg MH, Bevilacqua RG: Infections of the salivary glands, *Oral and Maxillofacial Surgery Clinics of North America* 7:423, 1995.

Lustmann J, Regev E, Melamed Y: Sialolithiasis: a survey on 245 patients and a review of the literature, *Int J Oral Maxillofac Surg* 19:135, 1990.

Mandel ID: Sialochemistry in diseases and clinical situations affecting salivary glands, *Crit Rev Clin Lab Sci* 12:321, 1980.

Miloro M, Ghali GE, Larsen P, et al, editors: *Peterson's principles of oral and maxillofacial surgery,* ed 2, Hamilton, Ontario, Canada, 2004, BC Decker.

Nahlieli O, Eliav E, Hasson O et al: Pediatric sialolithiasis, *Oral Surg Oral Med Oral Pathol Oral Radiol Endod* 90:709, 2000.

Nahlieli O, Shacham R, Yoffe B et al: Diagnosis and treatment of strictures and kinks in salivary gland ducts, *J Oral Maxillofac Surg* 59:484, 2001.

Neville B et al, editors: *Oral and maxillofacial pathology,* Philadelphia, 1995, WB Saunders.

Regezzi JA, Sciubba JJ: Salivary gland diseases. In Regezzi JA, Sciubba JJ, editors: *Oral pathology: clinical-pathologic correlations,* ed 4, Philadelphia, 2003, WB Saunders.

Topazian RG, Goldberg MH, Hupp JR: *Oral and maxillofacial infections,* ed 4, Philadelphia, 2002, WB Saunders.

Van der Akker HP: Diagnostic imaging in salivary gland disease, *Oral Surg Oral Med Oral Pathol* 66:625, 1988.

Van Sickels JE, Alexander JM: Parotid duct injuries, *Oral Surg* 52:364, 1981.

Yoshimura Y, Obara S, Kondoh T et al: A comparison of three methods used for treatment of ranula, *J Oral Maxillofac Surg* 53:280, 1995.

Youngs RP, Walsh-Waring GP: Trauma to the parotid region, *J Laryngol Otol* 101:475, 1987.

PART V

Management of Oral Pathologic Lesions

Pathologic growths and lesions frequently develop in the mouth and adjacent structures. General dentists have a more frequent and repetitive exposure to the tissues in patients' oral cavities and contiguous structures than any other health care provider. Although most of these lesions are benign and not threatening to the patient's well-being, dentists nevertheless have a professional responsibility for the maintenance and overall health of the oral and perioral structures. Whether by referral to another health care provider or by directly assuming responsibility for the surgical management of these hard and soft tissue pathologic entities, the dentist is the "gateway" provider who initially recognizes the departure from normal, coordinates the needed definitive care, ensures adequate patient follow-up, and provides any required dental restorative support.

The unique role of general dentists as oral health experts requires them to be constantly vigilant for any abnormalities in the bony and soft tissues of the head and neck area during the routine care of patients. General dentists must be observant clinicians and astute diagnosticians and must remain knowledgeable about the natural history of the more common oral and maxillofacial disease manifestations. Early diagnosis and treatment is always the best practice for managing these pathologic entities.

The next two chapters describe the potential roles of the general dentist in the comprehensive management of a patient's pathologic conditions. The most important aspect of this care begins with performing a thorough oral, head, and neck examination; formulating a rational tentative diagnosis; and providing needed treatment or appropriate referrals when indicated. Chapter 21 covers these topics in detail, with emphasis on the role of a general dentist. Chapter 22 describes the surgical management of more complex pathologic lesions of the oral cavity and contiguous structures. Expanded details on surgical technique are provided for management of less complex lesions that might be managed by general dentists. The surgical management of more complex and difficult pathologic conditions, cysts, and tumors of the oral and maxillofacial region are also presented, with emphasis on the general dentist's supportive roles in patient management and referral to specialists.

CHAPTER 21

Principles of Differential Diagnosis and Biopsy

EDWARD ELLIS III AND ROGER E. ALEXANDER

CHAPTER OUTLINE

EXAMINATION AND DIAGNOSTIC METHODS

Lesions of the oral cavity and perioral areas *must* be identified and accurately diagnosed so that appropriate therapy can eliminate the lesions. When abnormal tissue growth is discovered, several important orderly steps should be undertaken to identify and characterize it (Fig. 21-1). These steps include a comprehensive health history, history of the identified lesion(s), clinical and radiographic examinations, and relevant laboratory testing, if indicated. These steps lead to a period of close observation, referral to another health care provider when indicated, or initiation of surgical procedures to obtain a specimen for histologic examination (biopsy), which in turn lead to appropriate treatment decisions.

When the dentist discovers or confirms the presence of a lesion, the information must be discussed with the patient in a sensitive manner that conveys the importance of urgent attention to the problem without alarming the patient. Words such as *lesion, tumor, growth,* and *biopsy* can carry terrifying connotations to many patients. The empathetic dentist can spare patients undue anxiety and emotional trauma by carefully wording the discussion relating to the lesion and reminding the patient that most discovered lesions in the head and neck region are benign, so the steps being taken are merely precautionary.

Health History

Discerning the overall medical status of the patient is important during the diagnostic stages. Recent findings have led to a growing realization that there is frequently a close interrelationship between the medical and dental health of patients, and oral lesions can be a reflection of or contribute to systemic health problems. Therefore, documentation of a detailed and annotated health history, coupled with a thorough clinical evaluation (including medical consultation when necessary), is essential for two basic reasons:

1. First, a preexisting medical problem may affect or be affected by the dentist's treatment of the patient. As outlined in Chapters 1 and 2, patients with certain medical conditions (e.g., hypertension, certain cardiac conditions, those taking potentially interactive medications, those taking anticoagulants, and those with implanted orthopedic or cardiovascular prostheses) may require special management precautions when invasive dental surgery is required. Additionally, surgical intervention may upset the delicate balance between health and disease in a fragile or poorly controlled patient, such as a diabetic or an immunocompromised patient.
2. The second reason for a thorough knowledge of the patient's overall health status is that the lesion under investigation

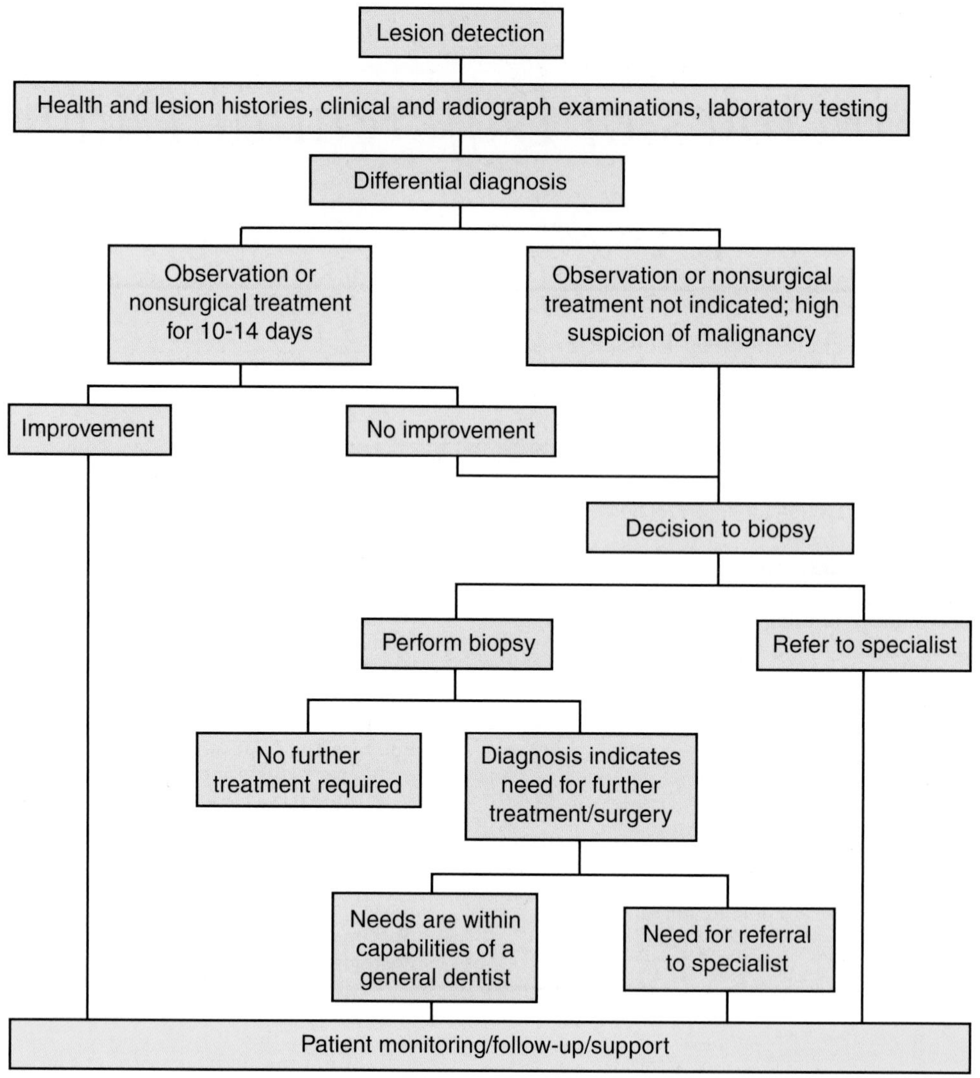

FIGURE 21-1 Decision tree for treatment of oral lesions.

may be the oral manifestation of a significant systemic disease. For instance, certain conditions (e.g., agranulocytosis, leukemia, or Crohn's disease) may often present with oral lesions. Surface ulcerations in a chronic smoker should alert the dentist to the possibility of oral or pharyngeal cancers. Literally hundreds of systemic disease processes can manifest with oral lesions, so the dentist must always maintain awareness of these relationships.

History of the Specific Lesion

An old saying in medicine is, "If you listen to the patient long enough, they will generally lead you to the diagnosis." The *art* of history taking sometimes gets lost in modern medicine in the rush to get to the next patient. A generally accepted axiom in medicine is that many systemic diseases (up to 85% to 90%) can be diagnosed by gathering a detailed, annotated medical history. The same can be true of many oral lesions when the diagnostician is familiar with the natural history of the more common diseases. Questioning of the patient who has a pathologic condition should include the following:

1. *How long has the lesion been present?* The duration of a lesion may provide valuable insight into its nature. For instance, a lesion that has been present for several years might be congenital and is more likely benign, whereas a rapidly developing lesion is considered more ominous. Although establishing the duration of a lesion provides valuable information, duration must be taken in context with other elements of the history because it is possible the lesion was present for an extended period before the patient became aware of its presence.
2. *Has the lesion changed in size?* A change in the radiographic and/or clinical size of a lesion is an important piece of information for the dentist to determine. An aggressive, enlarging lesion is more likely to be malignant, whereas a slower-growing lesion suggests a possibly benign lesion. By combining information on the growth rate with findings regarding the duration of presence, one can make a more accurate assessment of the nature of the lesion.
3. *Has the lesion changed in character or features (e.g., Did a lump become an ulcer or an ulcer start as a vesicle?)?* Noting

changes in the physical characteristics of a lesion can often assist in the diagnosis. For example, if an ulcer began as a vesicle, it could suggest a localized or systemic vesiculobullous or viral disease.

4. *What symptoms are associated with the lesion (e.g., pain, altered function, anesthesia or paresthesia, abnormal taste or odors, dysphagia, or tenderness of cervical lymph nodes)? If painful, is the pain acute or chronic, constant or intermittent? What increases or decreases the pain?* Lesions with an inflammatory component are most often associated with pain. Cancers, erroneously thought by many to be painful, actually are often painless unless secondarily infected. Sensory nerve changes, such as numbness or tingling, often occur with a malignant or inflammatory process unless other identifiable causes can be ascertained. Dysphagia can suggest changes in the floor of the mouth or in the parapharyngeal tissues. Swelling can often result from and occur with oral lesions, indicating an expansile process from any of a number of causes, including inflammation, infection, cysts, or tumor formation. The patient may indicate feeling a sensation of fullness even before the doctor can actually visualize or verify the swelling during clinical examination. Painful lymph nodes usually indicate an inflammatory or infectious cause but may also be a manifestation of malignancy.
5. *What anatomic location(s) is/are involved?* Certain lesions have a predilection for certain anatomic areas or tissues. Noting whether the lesions is confined to keratinized or nonkeratinized tissues, regions with salivary gland tissues, or areas of neural or vascular anatomy can sometimes provide clues to the diagnosis.
6. *Are there any associated systemic symptoms (e.g., fever, nausea, or malaise)? Has the patient noted any similar or concurrent changes elsewhere in the body or previously had similar lesions in the oral or perioral tissues in the past?* The dentist should look for possible relationships or manifestations from related systemic diseases or conditions. For example, many systemic viral conditions (e.g., measles, mumps, mononucleosis, herpes, and acquired immunodeficiency syndrome) can cause oral manifestations concurrent with the systemic involvement. Autoimmune conditions may also manifest with oral lesions. Many oral ulcerative conditions can also present lesions elsewhere in the body (e.g., pemphigus, lichen planus, erythema multiforme, and sexually transmitted diseases). Other factors could include drug abuse or injuries from domestic violence.
7. *Is there any historical event associated with the onset of the lesions (e.g., trauma, recent treatment, exposure to toxins or allergens, or visits to foreign countries)?* One of the initial steps the dentist should take when a lesion is noted is to seek a possible explanation based on the patient's medical, dental, family, or social histories. Frequently, oral and perioral lesions can be caused by parafunctional habits, hard or hot foods, application of medications not intended for topical use, recent trauma, conditions involving the dentition (e.g., caries, periodontal disease, or fractured teeth), or an identified event or exposure.

Clinical Examination

When a lesion is discovered, careful clinical and radiographic examinations and palpation of regional lymph nodes is mandatory. Once the examination is complete, a detailed description of all objective and subjective findings should be documented in the patient's chart. A drawing of a graphic schematic of the location, orientation, general shape, and dimensions of the lesion in the patient record is helpful. The use of standardized illustrations can simplify the documentation (Fig. 21-2). Additionally, good-quality digital photographs are useful for documentation if the dentist has the appropriate camera and accessories. Details, descriptions, and drawings allow the dentist or subsequent referral specialists to evaluate the course of the lesion over time and determine whether it is enlarging or changing its features, or appearing in new, different anatomic areas.

An examination is classically described as including inspection, palpation, percussion, and auscultation. In the head and neck region, inspection and palpation are more commonly used as diagnostic modalities, with inspection always preceding palpation. Early inspection facilitates description of the lesion before it is handled because some lesions are so fragile that manipulation of any kind may result in hemorrhage or rupture of a fluid-filled lesion or loss of loosely attached surface tissues, which would compromise any subsequent examinations. Percussion is reserved for examination of the dentition. Auscultation is infrequently used but is important when examining suspected vascular lesions. The following are some important additional points to be considered during inspection of the lesion.

1. *Anatomic location of the lesion.* Pathologic lesions can arise from any tissue within the oral cavity, including epithelium, subcutaneous and submucosal connective tissues, muscle, tendon, nerve, bone, blood vessels, lymphatic vessels, or salivary glands. The dentist should attempt to ascertain as much as possible regarding which tissues are contributing to the lesion, based on the anatomic location of the lesion. For example, if a mass appears on the dorsum of the tongue, the dentist would logically consider an epithelial, connective tissue, lymphatic, vascular, glandular, neural, or muscular origin. Similarly, a mass on the inner aspect of the lower lip would prompt the dentist to include a minor salivary gland origin in the differential diagnosis, along with connective tissue origin and other possibilities. Certain lesions may have unique anatomic characteristics, such as the linear tendencies of herpes zoster lesions as they follow neural pathways. The possible role of trauma should always be entertained as possible sources of the lesion (ill-fitting dental appliances, parafunctional habits such as cheek biting, sharp edges on teeth or restorations, and trauma from acts of domestic violence). Finally, pulpal, periapical, and periodontal pathologic or inflammatory conditions also cause a significant percentage of oral lesions.
2. *The overall physical characteristics of the lesion.* Appropriate medical terminology should always be used to describe clinical findings in the record because lay terminology can be misleading and nonspecific. Terms such as "ulcer" or "nodule" may be interpreted differently by different examiners. Good-quality digital photographs can also be printed and enclosed with the biopsy specimen or can be e-mailed separately to the pathologist. Photographs are helpful in demonstrating the clinical characteristics of the lesion. Box 21-1 lists several common physical descriptions that are useful in describing oral pathologic entities.

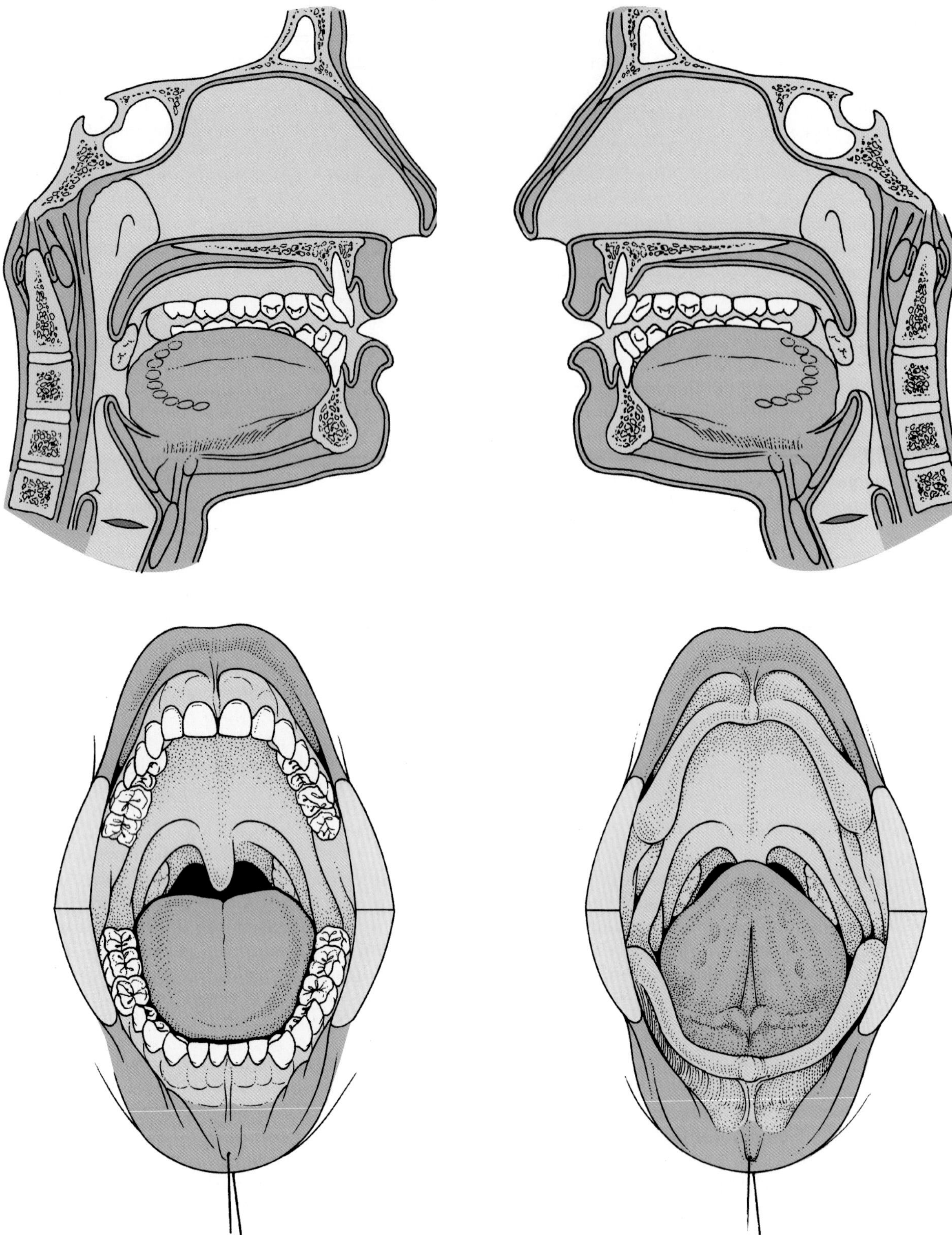

FIGURE 21-2 Illustrations of oral cavity and perioral areas, which are useful for indicating size and location of oral lesions.

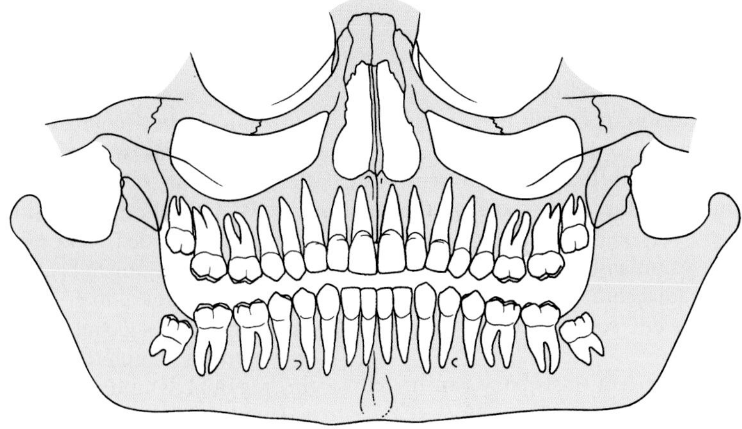

FIGURE 21-2, cont'd Illustrations of oral cavity and perioral areas, which are useful for indicating size and location of oral lesions.

BOX 21-1

Descriptive Pathology Terminology

Bulla (pl. bullae): A blister; an elevated, circumscribed, fluid-containing lesion of skin or mucosa

Crusts (crusted): Dried or clotted serum on the surface of the skin or mucosa

Dysplasia (dysplastic): Any abnormal development of cellular size, shape, or organization in tissue

Erosion: A shallow, superficial ulceration

Hyperkeratosis: An overgrowth of the cornified layer of epithelium

Hyperplasia (hyperplastic): An increased number of normal cells

Hypertrophy (hypertrophic): An increase in size caused by an increase in the size of cells, not in the number of cells

Keratosis (keratotic): An overgrowth and thickening of cornified (horned layer) epithelium

Leukoplakia: A slowly developing change in mucosa characterized by firmly attached, thickened, white patches

Macule: A circumscribed, nonelevated area of color change that is distinct from adjacent tissues

Malignant: Anaplastic; a cancer that is potentially invasive and metastatic

Nodule: A large, elevated, circumscribed, solid, palpable mass of the skin or mucosa

Papule: A small, elevated, circumscribed, solid, palpable mass of the skin or mucosa

Plaque: Any flat, slightly elevated, superficial lesion

Pustule: A small, cloudy, elevated, circumscribed, pus-containing vesicle on the skin or mucosa

Scale: A thin, compressed, superficial flake of cornified (keratinized) epithelium

Stomatitis: Any generalized inflammatory condition of the oral mucosa

Ulcer: A craterlike, circumscribed surface lesion resulting from necrosis of the epithelium

Vesicle: A small blister; a small, circumscribed elevation of skin or mucosa containing serous fluid

Terminology such as that listed in Box 21-1 should generally be used to describe the characteristics of a lesion. Lay terminology such as "swelling" and "sore" are generally not helpful and may be subject to misinterpretation.

3. *Single versus multiple lesions.* The presence of multiple lesions is an important feature. When multiple ulcerations are found within the mouth, the dentist can think of specific possibilities for the differential diagnosis. To find multiple or bilateral neoplasms in the mouth is unusual, whereas vesiculobullous, bacterial, and viral diseases commonly present such a pattern. Similarly, an infectious process can exhibit outward spread, as one lesion infects the adjacent tissues with which it has had contact.
4. *Size, shape, and growth presentation of the lesion.* Documentation of the size and shape of the lesion should be made, as noted previously. A small metric ruler made out of a material that can be disinfected (e.g., metal or plastic) is useful to have. The ruler is valuable for measuring the diameters of clinically evident lesions, which measurements can then be entered into the record with the drawing. The growth presentation should also be noted: whether the lesion is flat or slightly elevated, endophytic (growing inward) or exophytic (growing outward from the epithelial surface), sessile (broad based) or pedunculated (on a stalk).
5. *The surface appearance of the lesion.* The epithelial surface of a lesion may be *smooth, lobulated (verruciform),* or *irregular.* If ulceration is present, the characteristics of the ulcer base and margins should be recorded. Margins of an ulcer can be flat, rolled, raised, or everted. The base of the ulcer can be smooth; granulated; or covered with fibrin membrane, slough, or hemorrhagic crust (scab) or can have the fungating appearance that is characteristic of some malignancies.
6. *Lesion coloration.* The surface color(s) of a lesion can reflect various characteristics and even the origin of many lesions. A dark bluish swelling that blanches on pressure suggests a vascular lesion, whereas a lighter-colored, bluish lesion that does not blanch may suggest a mucus-retaining cyst. A pigmented lesion within the mucosa may suggest a "traumatic tattoo" of restorative material or a more ominous melanotic tumor. Keratinized white lesions can reflect a reaction to repetitive local tissue trauma or

represent potentially premalignant changes. An erythematous (or mixed red/white) lesion may represent an even more ominous prognosis for dysplastic changes than a white lesion. Inflammation can be superimposed on areas of mechanical trauma or ulceration, resulting in a varied presentation from one examination to the next.

7. *Sharpness of lesion borders and mobility.* If a mass is present, the dentist should determine whether it is fixed to the surrounding deep tissues or freely movable. Determining the boundaries of the surface lesion will aid in establishing whether the mass is fixed to adjacent bone, arising from bone and extending into adjacent soft tissues, or only infiltrating the soft tissue.
8. *Consistency of the lesion to palpation.* Consistency can be described as *soft* or *compressible* (e.g., a lipoma or abscess), *firm* or *indurated* (e.g., a fibroma or neoplasm), or *hard* (e.g., torus or exostosis). *Fluctuant* is a term used to describe the wavelike motion felt during bidigital palpation of a lesion with nonrigid walls and that contains fluid. This valuable sign can be elicited by palpating with two or more fingers in a rhythmic fashion. As one finger exerts pressure, the opposing finger feels the impulse transmitted through the fluid-filled cavity.
9. *Presence of pulsation.* Palpation of a mass may reveal a rhythmic pulsation that is suggestive of a significant vascular component. This sensation can be subtle and is especially significant when dealing with intrabony lesions. The pulsation can be accompanied by a palpable vibration, called a *thrill.* If a thrill is palpated, auscultation of the area with a stethoscope may reveal a *bruit,* or audible murmur, in the area. Invasive procedures on lesions with thrills and/or bruits should be avoided, and patients should be referred to specialists for treatment because life-endangering hemorrhage can result if surgical intervention (biopsy) is attempted.
10. *Examination of regional lymph nodes.* No evaluation of an oral lesion is complete without a thorough examination of the regional lymph nodes. This examination should be accomplished *before* any biopsy procedure. Sometimes lymphadenitis develops in the regional nodes following a surgical procedure such as biopsy, thus creating a subsequent diagnostic dilemma. It can then become difficult to differentiate between reactive lymphadenitis as a surgical sequela, coincidental regional infection or inflammation, or metastatic spread of the tumor in question. Figure 21-3 illustrates the primary lymph nodes of significance in the cervicofacial region.

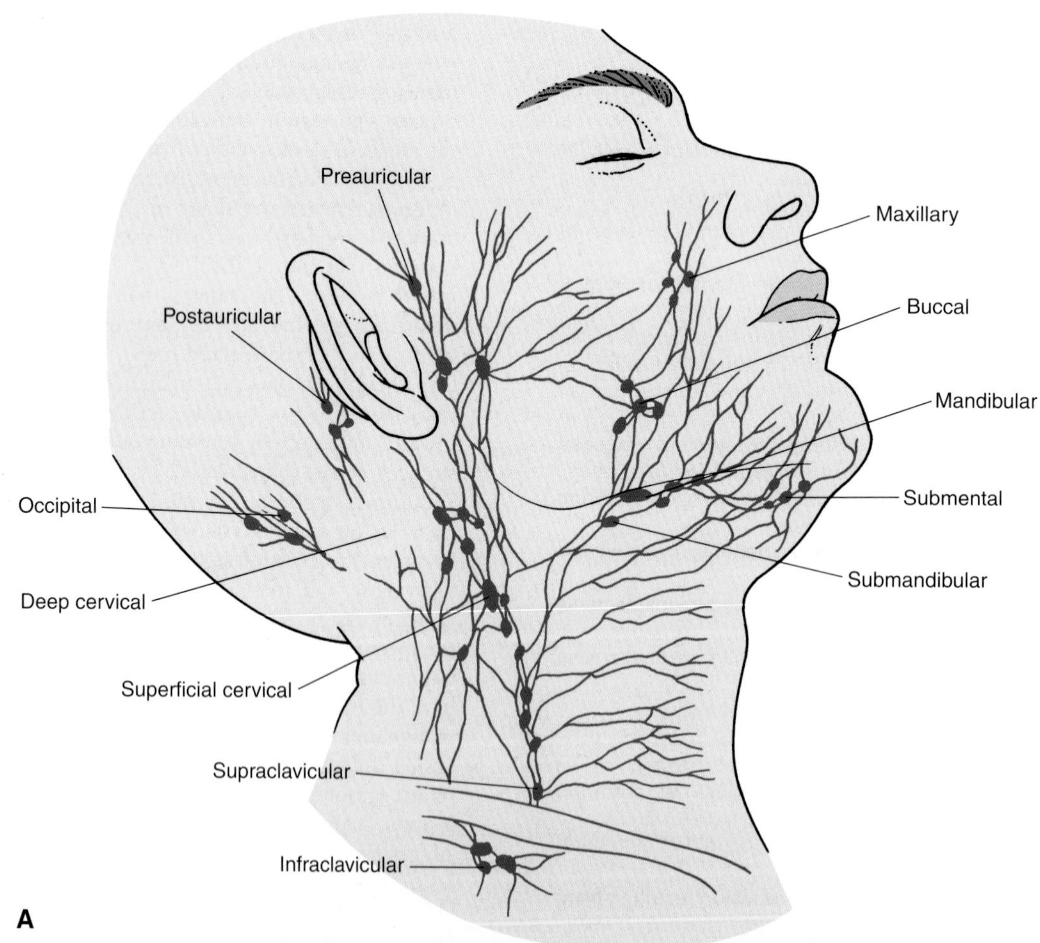

FIGURE 21-3 A, Anatomic location of cervicofacial lymph nodes.

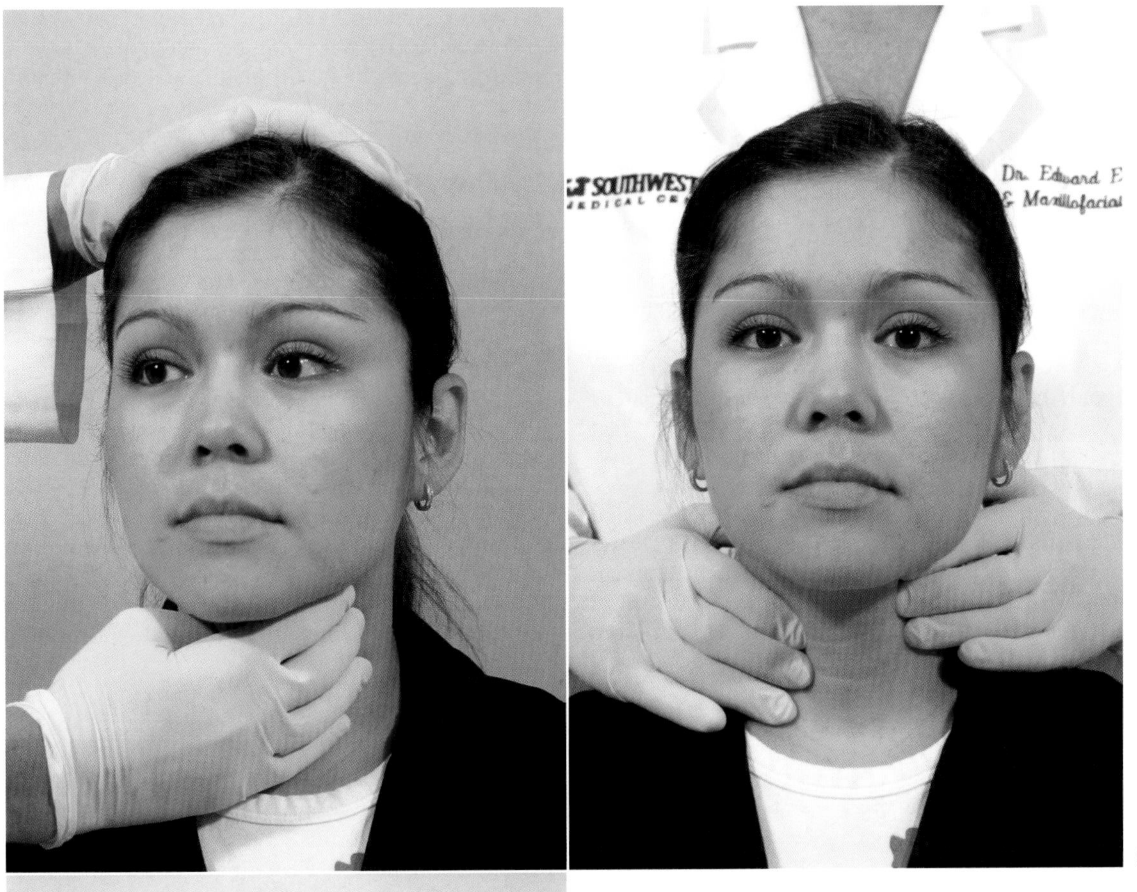

B C

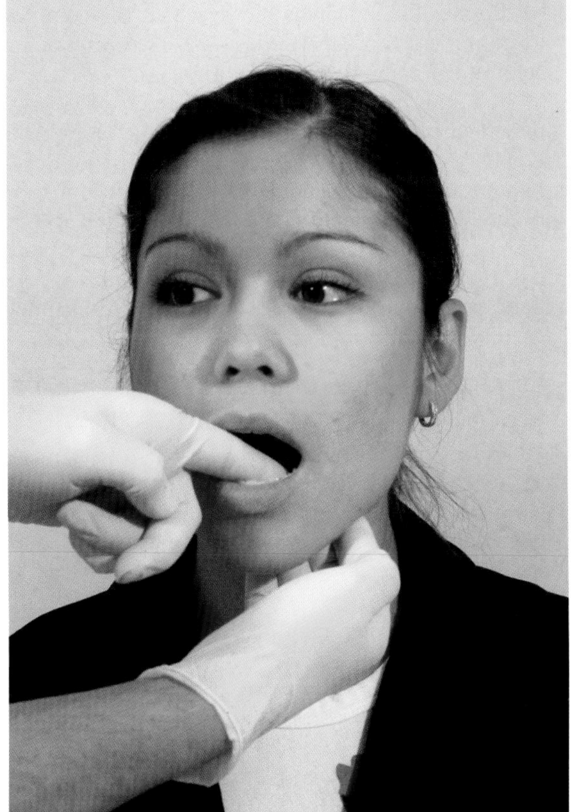

D

FIGURE 21-3, cont'd B, Anterior approach to cervical lymph node examination. Fingers are gently moved in circular motion along full length of sternocleidomastoid muscle. C, Posterior approach to cervical lymph node examination. It is generally helpful for patient to move the head from side to side and to tilt the head forward to make lymph nodes more palpable. D, Bimanual palpation of floor of mouth and submandibular lymph nodes.

The standard examination of lymph nodes requires only simple inspection and palpation. Comparison of left and right sides is often useful, using the middle three fingers for light palpation. Movements during palpation should be slow and gentle, with the fingers moving lightly across each area in vertical and horizontal directions, as well as rotary motion. In adults, normal lymph nodes are not palpable unless enlarged by inflammation or neoplasia, but cervical nodes of up to 1 cm in diameter can often be palpated in children up to the age of 12 years and are generally not considered an abnormal finding. In recording lymph node findings, the following five characteristics should be routinely documented: (1) location; (2) size (preferably recording the diameters in centimeters); (3) presence of pain or tenderness; (4) degree of fixation (fixed, matted, or movable); and (5) texture (soft, firm, or hardened). When multiple nodes are slightly enlarged but barely palpable, they can feel like bird shot and are described as "shotty nodes."

The lymph node examination should be methodical and should include the following groups: (1) occipital, (2) preauricular and postauricular; (3) mandibular, submandibular, and submental; (4) deep anterior cervical chain; (5) superficial cervical nodes (along the sternocleidomastoid muscle); (6) deep posterior cervical chain; and (7) supraclavicular nodes. Buccal lymph nodes may or may not be routinely palpable.

Light-Enhanced Adjuncts for Clinical Screening

At least two low-intensity, blue/white light systems are being marketed to the dental profession as tissue examination adjuncts. These systems claim that their lights will highlight lesions with dysplasia or abnormal cells because the emitted wavelength of light (around 490 to 510 nanometers) is absorbed and reflected differently between normal and abnormal cells. Few blinded comparison studies have been published, however, and much of the sensitivity/specificity data are extrapolated from the success of a similar technology in diagnosing lesions of the vaginal mucosa. In the oral cavity the precise role, indications, and limitations of this technology in diagnosis have yet to be fully defined. The technology appears to have the potential to become a helpful *adjunct* for screening and for clinically following up patients for abnormal oral tissue lesions after appropriate biopsy and treatment, if future studies continue to confirm the high specificity and sensitivity of the devices. One of the new technologies, ViziLite, uses a chemiluminescent method that features a disposable lightstick and has patients prerinsing with 1% acetic acid to remove the glycoprotein barrier covering the oral mucosa. The tissues are then illuminated with the light. Studies have demonstrated the utility of this technique for the detection of subclinical high-risk areas.[1-4] However, one study showed that the use of 1% acetic acid and the naked eye was as effective as using the light.[5]

Another device, VELscope (visually enhanced lesion scope), is a countertop-sized, handheld, fluorescent light–based system from Canada that functions in a manner similar to the ViziLite. Using a blue-tinted fluorescent technology, the optical device reportedly causes "normal" tissues to reflect a pale green color while abnormal tissues appear as a dark brown or black color, thus alerting the clinician to the need for closer scrutiny of the area. The dentist wears special goggles to view the tissues. Manufacturer-supported research on 44 patients showed that the device accurately diagnosed abnormal tissue 98% of the time (results were biopsy confirmed). In a multicenter study, authors report that white and mixed red/white lesions reflect the chemiluminescent light well, but red lesions are less diagnostic.[6] The high initial cost of purchase may compromise the potential of the device to become a practical adjunct in most practices.

Radiographic Examination

Radiographs are useful diagnostic adjuncts after the completion of the history and clinical examination, especially for lesions occurring within or adjacent to bone. When soft tissue lesions are proximate to bone, radiographs may indicate whether the lesion is causing an osseous reaction, eroding into the bone, or arising from an intraosseous origin. Various radiographic techniques may be used depending on the anatomic location of the lesion. Most pathologic conditions of the mandible or maxilla can be adequately viewed on routine plain views (e.g., periapical, occlusal, or panoramic), but occasionally specialized imaging techniques are needed, including computerized tomograms (including the newer cone beam computed tomography technology) or magnetic resonance imaging views, to fully delineate the exact nature and location of intrabony lesions.

The radiographic appearance may frequently give clues to the diagnosis of a lesion. For example, a cyst usually appears as a radiolucency with sharp borders (Fig. 21-4, *A* and *B*), whereas a radiolucency with ragged, irregular borders might indicate a malignant or more aggressive lesion (Fig. 21-4, *C* and *D*). When viewing a radiograph, if an intraosseous area shows a departure from normal structures or appearance, the dentist must determine whether the change is pathologic or simply an atypical presentation of a normal anatomic structure. This is particularly true when viewing certain projections of the maxilla and mandible in which the complex adjacent anatomy leads to superimpositions of contiguous structures, such as the paranasal sinus cavities.

In unique diagnostic situations, radiopaque dyes or markers may be used in conjunction with routine or specialized radiographs. For example, sialography involves the injection of radiopaque dye into glandular ducts to produce an indirect image of the gland architecture and delineate any pathologic lesions within the gland. Cysts may be injected to assist in determining the true extent of the anatomic boundaries of the cyst. Radiopaque markers, such as needles or metal spheres, can be used to localize a foreign object or pathologic lesion.

Laboratory Investigation

In certain instances, supplementary laboratory tests can assist in lesion identification. Certain oral lesions may be manifestations of a systemic disease process, such as hyperparathyroidism, multiple myeloma, leukemia, and certain lymphomas. To cite an example of the role of laboratory testing, examination of a patient with multiple lytic lesions and loss of lamina dura bone might suggest hyperparathyroidism. This diagnosis could be clarified by the dentist requesting serum calcium, phosphorus, and alkaline phosphatase tests. Guidance for requesting such tests can be found in leading oral pathology textbooks and other literature resources.

In the majority of cases, screening laboratory studies are considered unnecessary because they often have low diagnostic yield per total cost involved in performing such tests. Once the surgical biopsy has provided a definitive diagnosis, however, laboratory testing can contribute meaningful infor-

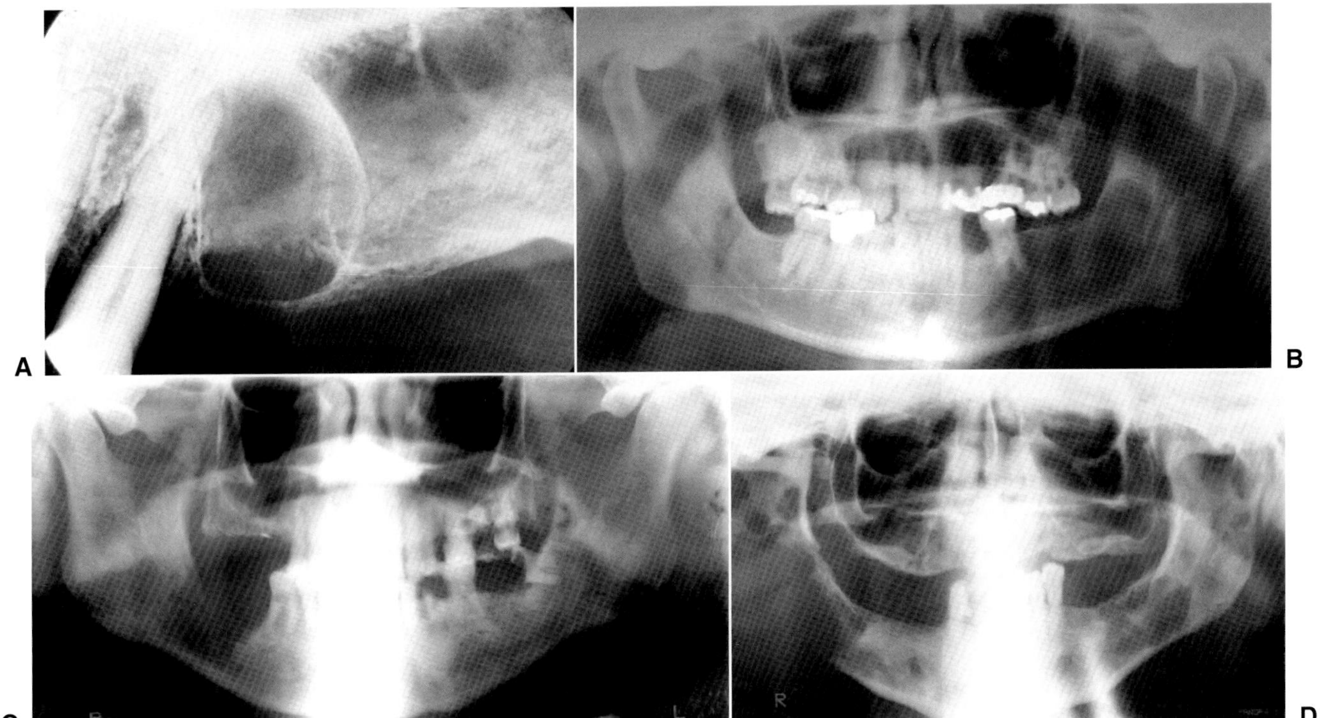

FIGURE 21-4 A and B, Radiographic appearance of cysts. A, Note peripheral condensing osteitis around radiolucent center. B, Large unilocular radiolucency in left mandible with well-defined peripheral border. C and D, Radiographic appearance of bone destruction by malignancy. C, Squamous cell carcinoma has eroded into the right mandible. Note ragged appearance. D, Intraosseous malignancy has completely destroyed the normal architecture of the right mandibular ramus and has produced a pathologic fracture.

mation that is relevant to the subsequent management of the lesion.

Presumptive Clinical Differential Diagnosis

After completing the initial dental, medical, and lesion histories and clinical, radiographic, and laboratory examinations (as indicated), the dentist next should compile a presumptive list of reasonable differential diagnoses. These diagnoses convey the clinician's impression to the pathologist regarding what the dentist feels the lesion most likely is, based on the total assessment. These diagnoses may or may not ultimately be consistent with the final histologic diagnosis but are nonetheless important because the pathologist rules out entities that may have similar clinical and pathologic presentations.

Prebiopsy Monitoring

Any undiagnosed or suspicious change in oral tissues that cannot be explained by localized trauma (and the source corrected) or other factors should be followed up in 7 to 14 days, with or without local treatment. If the lesion enlarges or expands, develops an altered appearance, or does not respond as expected to local therapy, then biopsy is usually indicated. Areas of leukoplakia (which is used as a clinical, not pathologic, term) can be problematic because up to 15% to 20% of those areas (and 100% of erythroplakia lesions) can exhibit histologic evidence of dysplasia or frank malignancy.[7] *High risk* areas of the mouth include the floor of the mouth, the lateral and ventral surfaces of the tongue, and the buccal and lower lip mucosa. Areas of redness or pebbling within areas of leukoplakia are especially troubling. Incisional biopsies from one or more of such suspicious areas are generally indicated.

During subsequent examinations, the patient record should provide details on whether the observed lesion has improved or not improved, and the dentist's plan for subsequent management (i.e., continued observation on a structured timetable, continued local treatment, biopsy, or referral).

Basic Tenets of Follow-up and Referral

Failure to diagnose and refer a patient with a possible pathologic condition in a timely manner has become one of the leading causes of professional litigation. Over the years, numerous articles and textbook chapters have provided guidance on how to obtain biopsies of lesions and to formulate differential diagnoses. Little guidance has been provided on the proper follow-up protocols for "suspicious" lesions and guidelines for appropriate referrals between practitioners. One article has attempted to provide this needed guidance without imposing a legal precedent that could be construed as a legal standard.[8]

The dentist should not delegate examination of patients for pathologic conditions to auxiliary staff, such as dental hygienists. Although most hygienists are well-trained to be observant for soft tissue changes in the oral cavity, the ultimate responsibility for detection of pathologic conditions (including oral cancer screening) rests with the dentist. Delegation of this duty is not permitted by law in most, if not all, states. If the dentist does not follow up on the hygienist's discovery of abnormal tissues, the patient record should reflect the rationale for that decision.

If the dentist decides to refer the patient for a second opinion or specialty management, the referral appointment should ideally be arranged before the patient leaves the office. If left to make the appointment themselves, many patients may fail to do so out of fear, denial, or procrastination. The arranged appointment should be followed up with a letter, fax, or computerized message from the referring general dentist to the specialist, outlining the details of the case, the concerns, and the requested procedures. A copy of this correspondence should be placed in the patient record. Copies of the specialist's findings, recommendations, procedures, and biopsy findings should also be placed in the patient record. These formal exchanges provide precise documentation that prevents miscommunications between offices and may provide some element of protection if litigation is initiated later. Returned reports from the pathologist should be acted on promptly. The patient should be notified of the results, and if the results are unexpected or positive, requiring further treatment, the patient should be counseled in person by the dentist.

Biopsy or Referral

Clinicians vary in their surgical interests, training, and skills. Some dentists may feel comfortable performing many biopsy procedures on their patients, whereas others may refer their patients. This is a personal choice and should take several points into consideration.

1. *Health of the patient.* The patient pool in the United States is getting older, and a growing number of elderly patients are seeking treatment in dental offices. Many of these patients have systemic diseases, multiple medications, or physical compromises that pose an increased surgical risk or potential hazards. These conditions are outlined and discussed in Chapters 1 and 2, and they may complicate any planned surgical procedures, including biopsy. The presence of such conditions, however, should not significantly delay biopsy or referral in most cases. Patients can be referred to specialists who are trained to deal with patients with special medical needs so that the procedure is carried out as safely as possible.
2. *Surgical difficulty.* If any of the basic surgical principles outlined in Chapter 3 (such as access, lighting, anesthesia, tissue stabilization, and instrumentation) pose a problem if the dentist were to treat the patient, then referral should be considered. Similarly, as the size of a lesion increases or its position encroaches on significant anatomic structures, the potential for significant complications (e.g., bleeding and nerve damage) increases. Each dentist should use good judgment when deciding whether the biopsy is within the dentist's surgical abilities or whether the patient would be better managed by a more highly trained specialist.
3. *Malignant potential.* The dentist who suspects that a lesion is malignant has two choices: To perform a surgical biopsy *after* completion of comprehensive diagnostic workup or to refer the patient *before* biopsy is performed to a specialist who is able to provide definitive treatment if the lesion is shown to be malignant. The latter choice usually represents better service to the patient if the referral can be executed in a prompt and timely manner. In such cases, it is better for the referral specialist to evaluate the lesion before any surgical intervention has compromised its clinical features. Biopsy can also produce reactive lymph nodes that are possibly unrelated to the original lesion. Allowing the referral specialist to evaluate the patient before biopsy allows a more accurate diagnosis and simplifies the formulation of a suitable treatment plan.

Informed Consent and Shared Risk

Some clinicians argue that *all* lesions should be removed and/or that a biopsy should be obtained. In some clinical situations, however, the patient and the dentist can jointly elect periodically to observe some innocent-appearing lesions that occur in low-risk areas in low-risk patients (e.g., nonsmokers). However, lesions demonstrating any dysplastic changes on histopathologic examination should always be removed in their entirety. One has to remember that observation over time can be a calculated risk. Many life-threatening conditions can initially masquerade as innocuous lesions, and many different lesions can present similar clinical appearances. The dentist should err on the side of caution and must always ensure that the patient is fully informed of the risks, rationales, and alternatives before deciding that a lesion should not be removed. The patient must understand that he or she is sharing responsibility for that decision, and the discussions on which the decision is based should be well documented in the patient record. If the dentist advises removal and the patient declines, that discussion and decision should likewise be thoroughly documented, reflecting the patient's understanding of the potential negative consequences of the decision.

Postbiopsy Monitoring

Following an incisional biopsy for diagnosis, a positive pathology report (indicating dysplastic changes or malignancy) generally mandates appropriate surgical excision of the lesion and contiguous tissues as indicated by the histopathologic diagnosis. This might necessitate referral to an oral and maxillofacial surgeon or other head and neck specialist, who is experienced in the management of malignancies. A negative biopsy report, however, should never be taken at face value but interpreted with clinical and historical findings in mind. If doubt exists, a second biopsy might be indicated. At the very least, plans should be developed for a structured schedule of continued close observation at appropriate intervals. Generally, it is prudent to reexamine the patient within 1 month and then at 3, 6, and 12 months during the first year. Thereafter, if clinical and radiographic findings are unchanged, the interval between follow-up visits can be increased to 6 and then 12 months, as appropriate. Patients should always be counseled to contact the dentist immediately if any clinical changes or new symptoms are noted between visits.

GENERAL PRINCIPLES OF BIOPSY

The term *biopsy* indicates the removal of tissue from a living body for microscopic diagnostic examination. Biopsy is the most precise and accurate of all diagnostic tissue procedures and should be performed whenever a definitive diagnosis cannot be obtained using less invasive procedures. The primary purpose of biopsy is to determine the diagnosis precisely so that proper treatment can be provided, for many different lesions have similar clinical or radiographic appearances. In actuality, a biopsy is more likely to rule out malignancy than to diagnose cancer because the majority of oral and odontogenic lesions are benign. Nevertheless, the term *biopsy* leads many patients to a perception that the dentist suspects malignancy, so discussions that include that word need to be carefully phrased so it will not cause the patient undue alarm or anxiety.

Indications for biopsy are summarized in Box 21-2. The typical characteristics of lesions that should raise the dentist's suspicion of malignancy are listed in Box 21-3. Figure 21-5 shows examples of lesions that should be suspect. The four major types of biopsy generally performed in and around the oral cavity include (1) cytologic biopsy, (2) incisional biopsy, (3) excisional biopsy, and (4) aspiration biopsy.

BOX 21-2

Indications for Biopsy

- Any persistent pathologic condition that cannot be clinically diagnosed
  - Lesions with no identifiable cause that persist for more than 10 to 14 days despite local therapy
  - Intrabony lesions that appear to be enlarging
  - Visible or palpable submucosal swelling beneath clinically normal mucosa
- Any lesion that is felt to have malignant or premalignant characteristics (See also Box 21-3.)
  - Any lesion that has grown rapidly for no obvious reason
  - Red, white, or pigmented mucosal lesions for which a cause or diagnosis is not evident
  - Any lesion that is firmly attached or fixed to adjacent anatomic structures
  - Any unknown lesion in high-risk areas for development of cancer (e.g., floor of mouth and tongue)
- Confirmation of clinical diagnostic suspicions
- Any lesion that does not respond to routine clinical management (i.e., removal of local irritant) over a 10- to 14-day period
  - Inflammatory signs that persist for long periods
- Any lesion that is the basis of extreme concern to the patient (cancerphobia)

Modified from Alexander RE, Wright JM, Thiebaud S: Evaluating, documenting and following up oral pathological conditions: a suggested protocol, *J Am Dent Assoc* 132:329-335, 2001.

BOX 21-3

Characteristics of Lesions that Raise Suspicion of Malignancy

Bleeding: Lesion bleeds on gentle manipulation
Duration: Lesion has persisted more than 2 weeks
Erythroplasia: Lesion is totally red or has a speckled red and white appearance
Fixation: Lesion feels attached to adjacent structures
Growth rate: Lesion exhibits rapid growth
Induration: Lesion and surrounding tissue are firm to the touch
Ulceration: Lesion is ulcerated or presents as an ulcer

Oral Cytology-based Procedures

Noninvasive, cytology-based screening tests and modalities have many pitfalls and should not be considered substitutes for surgical biopsy. These tests are generally used as screening or follow-up adjuncts to careful clinical examinations or as adjuncts to assist in clinical decision making. Three main forms of oral cytologic tests are available for use in clinical practice, depending on the method of collection or examination.

The first is *exfoliative cytologic* examination of mucosal cells, which was first described and most commonly used as a diagnostic procedure for the detection of uterine cervical cancer. Although some authors have suggested oral applications, studies have consistently shown that the results are not as reliable with keratinized oral tissues and often yield an unacceptable incidence of false-negative diagnoses, especially when the examining cytologists lack expertise in examining the unique nature of oral tissues. Furthermore, postoperative discomfort from a properly performed cytologic scraping can be more significant than if a surgical biopsy had been performed.

A second form of cytologic examination is *oral brush cytologic* examination (often imprecisely referred to as oral brush "biopsy"). This is a more recent development that is marketed heavily to general dentists. A handheld rotary wire brush is used to collect epithelial cells (Fig. 21-6, *A* and *B*), which are then fixed on a glass slide (Fig. 21-6, *C*) and submitted for evaluation. Studies have shown this technique to be superior to exfoliative oral cytologic examinations.[9,10] A few experts have raised questions concerning accuracy; however, a multicenter clinical trial of nearly 1000 patients at 35 academic centers using the technique showed that the technique was precise.[10] The test independently detected 100% of histologically confirmed oral cancers and precancers and had a statistically significant sensitivity of greater than 96% ($p < 0.05$, $n = 131$). Furthermore, the technique discovered cancer or precancer among 4.5% of lesions that clinically appeared benign to experienced examiners and that normally would not have received additional testing.

The cost of oral brush cytologic examinations is nominal and is covered as a diagnostic test in many insurance plans. If a subsequent surgical biopsy is required for diagnosis, however, it can be rejected by an insurance company as an unnecessary duplication of the original "biopsy," or it may be noted that cytologic examination is not a covered benefit. The insurance claim might be denied because it is alleged to be a duplication of the original (brush biopsy) test. The nuances of insurance coverage should be predetermined before the technique is used. The accuracy, advantages, and limitations of this adjunctive diagnostic tool are still evolving.

Another indication for oral brush cytologic examination may be as a valuable noninvasive tool for monitoring patients with chronic mucosal changes (e.g., leukoplakia, lichen planus, and irradiation damage) or may serve as an adjunct for follow-up of patients with a history of oral cancer that requires ongoing surveillance for adverse mucosal changes. Brush cytologic examinations can be implemented with more frequency than might be considered for a standard incisional or excisional surgical biopsy. Rather than simply "observing" clinical characteristics, the dentist can readily obtain a cell sample for computer-assisted analysis.

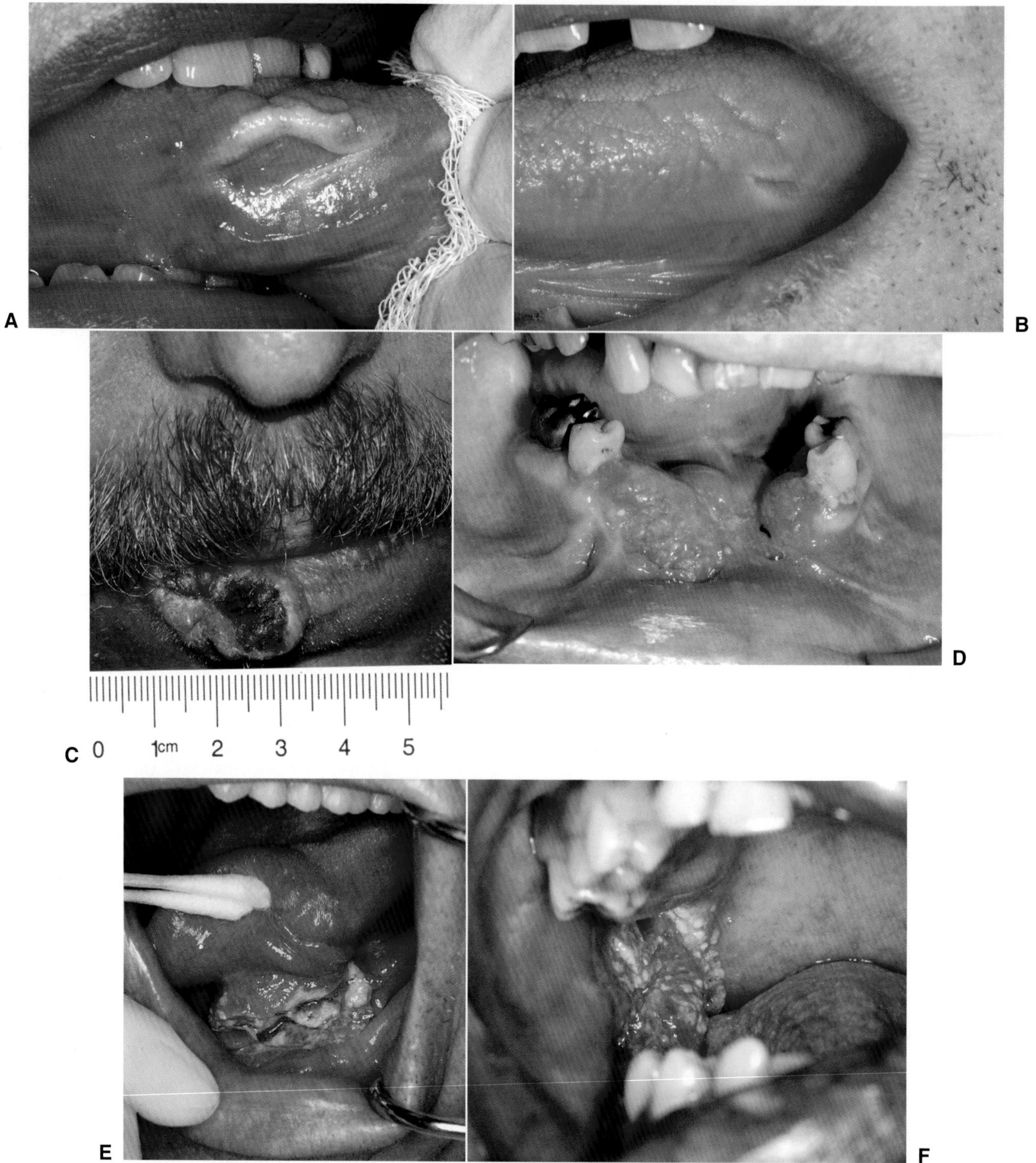

FIGURE 21-5 Examples of lesions that should considered for biopsy. A, Ulcer on lateral border of tongue. In this case, it was a traumatic ulcer from biting. B, Another ulcer on lateral border of tongue. In this case, it was from a sharp edge of a fractured tooth cusp. C, Large ulcer of the lower lip, especially if in a patient with a history of smoking. This lesion was squamous cell carcinoma. D, Typical appearance of squamous cell carcinoma of the alveolar ridge. E, Typical appearance of squamous cell carcinoma of the floor of the mouth. F, Typical appearance of squamous cell carcinoma of the retromolar area.

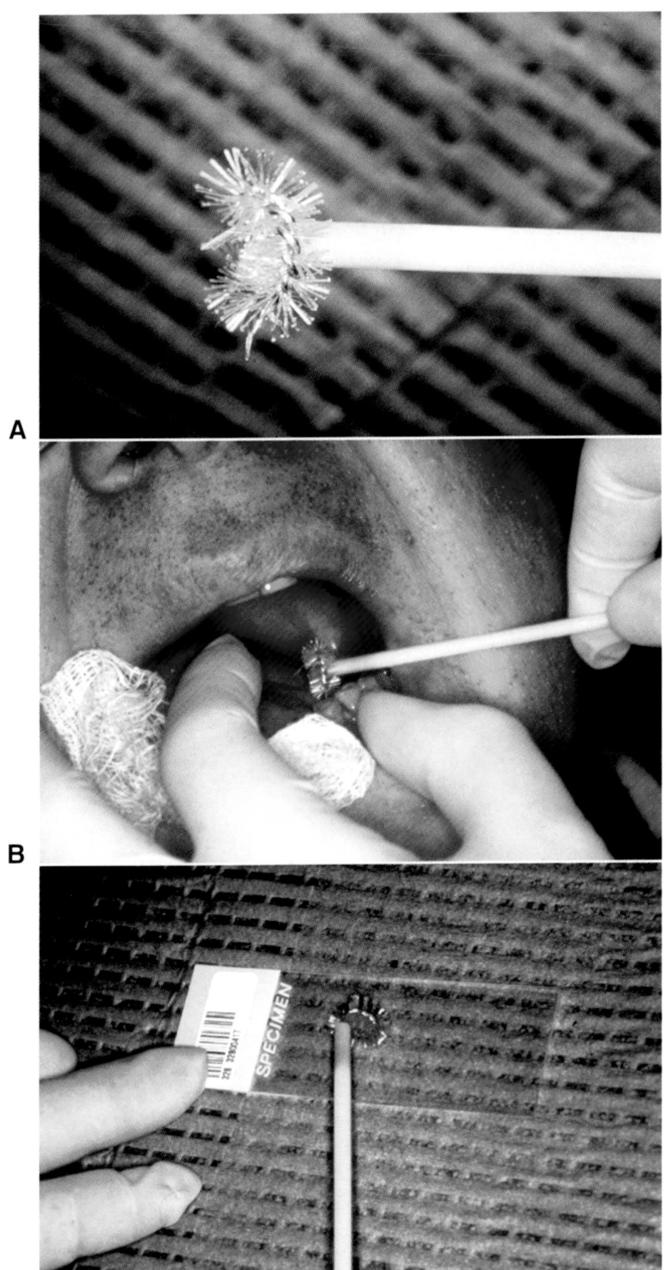

FIGURE 21-6 Technique of oral brush cytologic examination. A, Brush that is used to obtain specimen. B, Brush contacts tissue in area where cells are desired and is rotated 5 to 10 times with moderate pressure. C, The cells are then transferred to a microscopic slide, and a fixative is applied.

Technique of Oral Brush Cytologic Examination

Local or topical anesthesia is generally not required for the procedure, and postsampling sequelae are minimal. The rotary brush is placed in contact with the surface of the suspected lesion and rotated with firm pressure 5 to 10 times (Fig. 21-6, *B*). When properly performed, epithelial cells are collected by the brush from all three layers (basal, submucosal, and mucosal); however, cellular architectural information necessary to stage and grade a malignant lesion are absent. The brush with its collected cellular material is smeared on a provided glass slide and is flooded with the fixative solution (Fig. 21-6, *C*). After the slide is dry, it is mailed to a laboratory where the specimen is examined, first by computer and then by an oral and maxillofacial pathologist who is trained in computer-assisted analysis. If the specimen does not contain cells from the full-thickness of epithelium, the report will state that the sample was inadequate and a repeat procedure will be required. If the sample is adequate, a computerized scanning program prescreens each slide for dysplastic and malignant cells. Images of cells identified as atypical or abnormal are displayed on a high-resolution monitor where the trained pathologist can review them. Each specimen is then categorized into one of three categories: (1) negative (no epithelial abnormalities detected), (2) positive (definitive cellular evidence of dysplastic changes or malignancy present), or (3) atypical (abnormal epithelial changes present, not dysplastic or malignant).

A *negative* report would require the same clinical follow-up as if the dentist had received a negative biopsy report. A *positive* report would necessitate the patient being referred for excision or scalpel biopsy to grade and stage the lesion. An *atypical* report might suggest a benign inflammatory lesion (e.g., lichen planus). The dentist and the patient may elect scalpel biopsy for more definitive guidance, referral for treatment, or structured follow-up.

Incisional Biopsy

An incisional biopsy is a biopsy procedure that removes only a small portion of a lesion. If the lesion is large or demonstrates differing characteristics in different locations, then more than one area of the lesion may require sampling. Incisional sampling is used if the lesion is large (>1 cm in diameter), is located in a risky or hazardous location, or whenever a definitive histopathologic diagnosis (e.g., for suspected malignancy) is desired before planning a complex removal or other treatment.

The biopsy is generally excised as a wedge of tissues in such a manner as to include normal- and abnormal-appearing tissues in the sample (Figs. 21-7 and 21-8). Central areas of a large lesion are often necrotic and therefore of little diagnostic value to the pathologist, whereas active growth is taking place at the perimeter, and inclusion of the lesion interface with normal-appearing tissue can demonstrate many significant cellular changes. Care must be taken to include an adequate depth of tissue as well so that cellular features from the base of the lesion are included. Generally, it is better to take a narrow, deep specimen than a broad, shallow one. Care should be taken not to compromise significant adjacent anatomic structures, such as nerves and major blood vessels, unless one thinks they have a relationship with the origins or pathology of the lesion.

Excisional Biopsy

An excisional biopsy implies removal of a lesion in its entirety, to include a 2- to 3-mm perimeter of normal tissue around the lesion (Fig. 21-9). The width of the perimeter of normal tissue may vary, depending on the presumptive diagnosis. An additional 2 to 3 mm in tissues may be required for specimens suspected of malignancy, including some pigmented lesions and lesions already diagnosed as having dysplastic or malignant cells. Complete excision often constitutes definitive treatment of the lesion biopsied. Excisional biopsy is reserved for smaller lesions (<1 cm in diameter). For lesions that can be removed

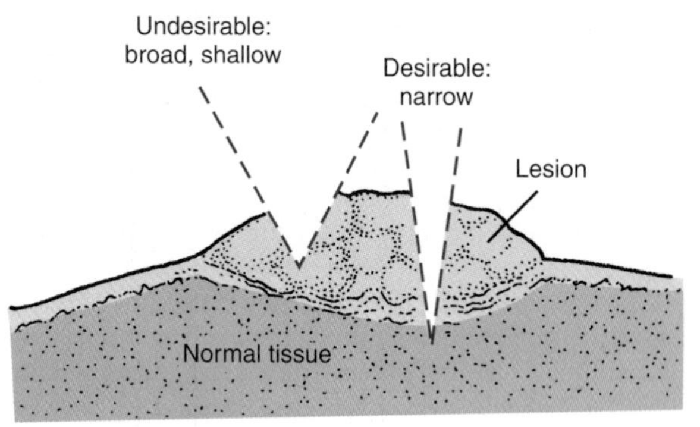

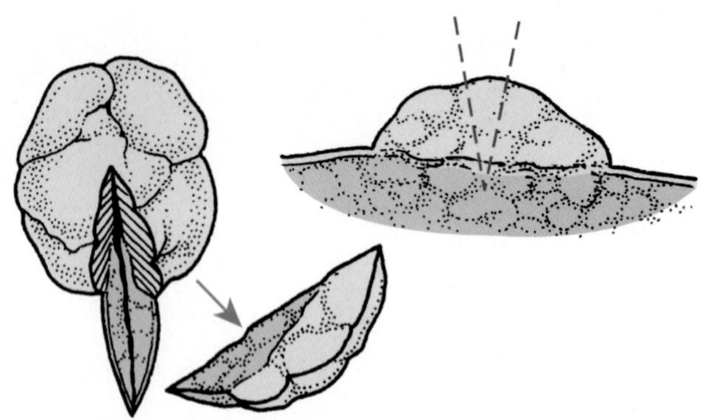

FIGURE 21-7 A, Illustration showing desirability of obtaining deep specimen rather than broad and shallow specimen when incisional biopsy is performed. If malignant cells are present only at base of lesion, broad and shallow biopsy might not obtain these diagnostic cells. B, Illustration showing desirability of obtaining incisional biopsy at margin of soft tissue lesion. Junction of lesion with normal tissue frequently provides pathologist with more diagnostic information than if biopsy were taken only from center of lesion. This is particularly important when a biopsy of an ulcer is performed.

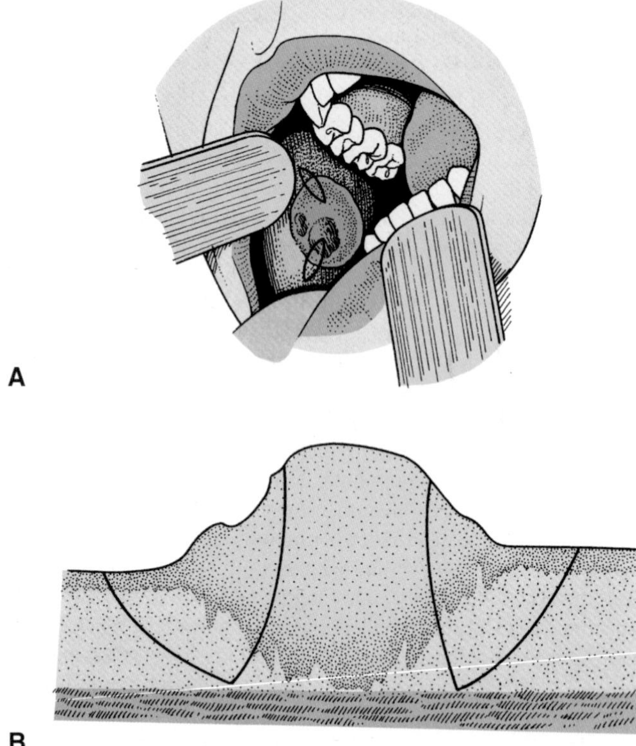

FIGURE 21-8 Illustration demonstrating desirability of obtaining more than one incisional biopsy if characteristics of lesion differ from one area to another. A, Frequently, one area of lesion appears histologically different from another. B, When obtaining biopsy on buccal or labial mucosa, incision is usually carried to depth of musculature.

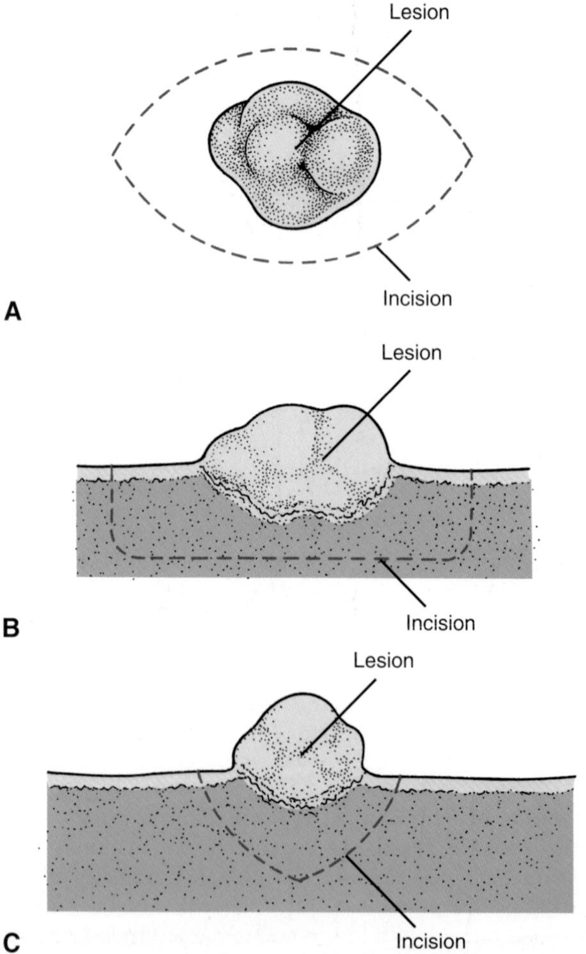

FIGURE 21-9 Illustration of excisional biopsy of soft tissue lesion. A, Surface view. Elliptical incision is made around lesion, at least 3 mm away from lesion. B, Side view. Incision is made deep enough to remove lesion completely. C, End view. Incisions are made convergent to depth of wound. Excision made in this way facilitates closure.

in toto without excessively compromising the patient's features or oral function, and lesions that *must* be removed in their entirety to remove the threat to the patient's well-being.

Aspiration Biopsy

Aspiration biopsy is performed with a needle and syringe by penetrating a suspicious lesion and aspirating its contents. Two main types of aspiration biopsy are used in clinical practice: The first is used only to explore whether a lesion contains a fluid; the second is used actually to aspirate cells for pathologic diagnosis. This latter variation is termed *fine-needle aspiration* and is often performed by pathologists trained in the technique. Fine-needle aspiration is used when a soft tissue mass is detected beneath the skin or mucosal surface and the patient wishes to avoid a scar or adjacent anatomic structures pose a risk. Fine-needle aspiration is an especially good diagnostic tool for neck masses, from which it can be difficult to obtain a biopsy surgically. Routine aspiration of intraosseous radiolucent lesions is also performed before entering into the bony defect to rule out the potential of the lesion being vascular in origin and to define whether it is cystic or solid. Details on this can be found later in this chapter. Aspiration is performed on any fluid-filled lesion, except mucocele. A 16- to 18-gauge needle connected to an aspirating syringe is used. The needle tip may have to be repositioned repeatedly in an effort to locate a suitable fluid-containing cavitation.

Soft Tissue Biopsy Techniques and Surgical Principles

Biopsy of oral soft tissues is a competency that every general dentist should possess. Properly performed, most biopsies are simple procedures that can be easily performed in the dental office under local anesthesia with minimal instrumentation (Box 21-4). The only variables of the technique relate to areas of anatomic risk or limitations imposed by the size and type of lesion. The surgical principles presented in Chapter 3 apply to biopsy, as do other surgical procedures within the oral cavity. These basic surgical principles are briefly summarized in the following sections.

Anesthesia

Block local anesthesia techniques are preferred over infiltration whenever possible so that the anesthetic solution is not inadvertently incorporated in the surgical specimen. This can cause distortion of the cellular architecture of the specimen and make pathologic diagnosis more difficult, if not impossible. Peripheral infiltration of local anesthetic with a vasoconstrictor is often helpful, and it should be injected at least 1 cm away from the lesion perimeter to prevent tissue architectural distortions. The vasoconstrictor will decrease hemorrhaging in the wound and improve the surgeon's visibility of the site during surgery.

Tissue Stabilization

Oral and perioral soft tissue biopsies frequently involve mobile surfaces and structures (e.g., lips, cheek, soft palate, and tongue). Accurate surgical incisions can be placed with greater ease when the involved tissues are first stabilized. This can be accomplished by any of several methods. The surgical assistant can grasp the lips on both sides of the biopsy site with his or her fingers, which also retracts and immobilizes the lips (Fig. 21-10, *A* to *E*). This may also help reduce bleeding by compressing area blood vessels and their tributaries. The surgeon must be careful to avoid iatrogenic scalpel injury to the assistant's stabilizing fingers (Fig. 21-10, *B*). A variety of retractors are available that can perform the same function. Towel clips, Adson (fine-tip) forceps, chalazion forceps, or a heavy retraction suture can also be used for stabilization and retraction of some mobile soft tissues (Fig. 21-10, *F* and *G;* Fig. 21-11). When used, retraction sutures should be placed deeply into the tissues, away from the planned biopsy site so that they will function without pulling through and damaging the tissues.

BOX 21-4

Instruments for Mucosal Soft Tissue Biopsy

- Local anesthesia administration equipment and supplies
- Scalpel handle with No. 15 blade
- Appropriate tissue retractor (Seldin 20, Minnesota, Chalazion, or other)
- Small, pointed, fine-tip scissors (such as curved iris or Metzenbaum)
- Fine-tip tissue pickups (such as Adson)
- Small, curved hemostat (such as mosquito)
- Suction tip and hose
- 2 × 2-, 3 × 3-, or 4 × 4-inch sterile gauze sponges
- Needle holder, suture with attached cutting or reverse cutting needle
- 3-0 or 4-0 black silk
- 4-0 Resorbable (polyglycolic acid or polyglactin 910)
- Dean suture scissors
- Irrigation syringe and sterile irrigating fluid (0.9% normal saline) in appropriate bowl/basin
- Screw-top, labeled biopsy specimen bottle containing 10% formalin
- Biopsy specimen data input sheet

ADDITIONAL INSTRUMENTS FOR INTRAOSSEOUS BIOPSY

- Soft tissue curettes (angled)
- Periosteal elevator (such as Molt No. 9 or Molt No. 4 curette)
- End-cutting rongeurs (such as Blumenthal)
- Surgical handpiece (air does not discharge around bur), No. 8 round bur
- 5- to 10-mL disposable syringe with 18-gauge Luer-Lok needle

Hemostasis

The use of a suction device for keeping the surgical field free of blood during the procedure should be minimized as much as possible, especially the high-volume suction devices found in modern dental offices. The assistant can often use gauze sponges to blot the site. Suctioning not only can increase bleeding but also increases the risk of the biopsy tissue sample being accidentally aspirated into the suction. If suction is needed, it is helpful to place a gauze over the end of the suction tip to serve as a filter.

Incisions

A sharp scalpel, usually with a No. 15 blade, should be used to incise the tissues. Two football-shaped surface incisions can be angled in such a way as to converge at the base and will yield an optimal specimen and a resulting wound that is easy to close (Figs. 21-10 and 21-12). The use of some laser devices and electrosurgical equipment for making incisions for biopsies

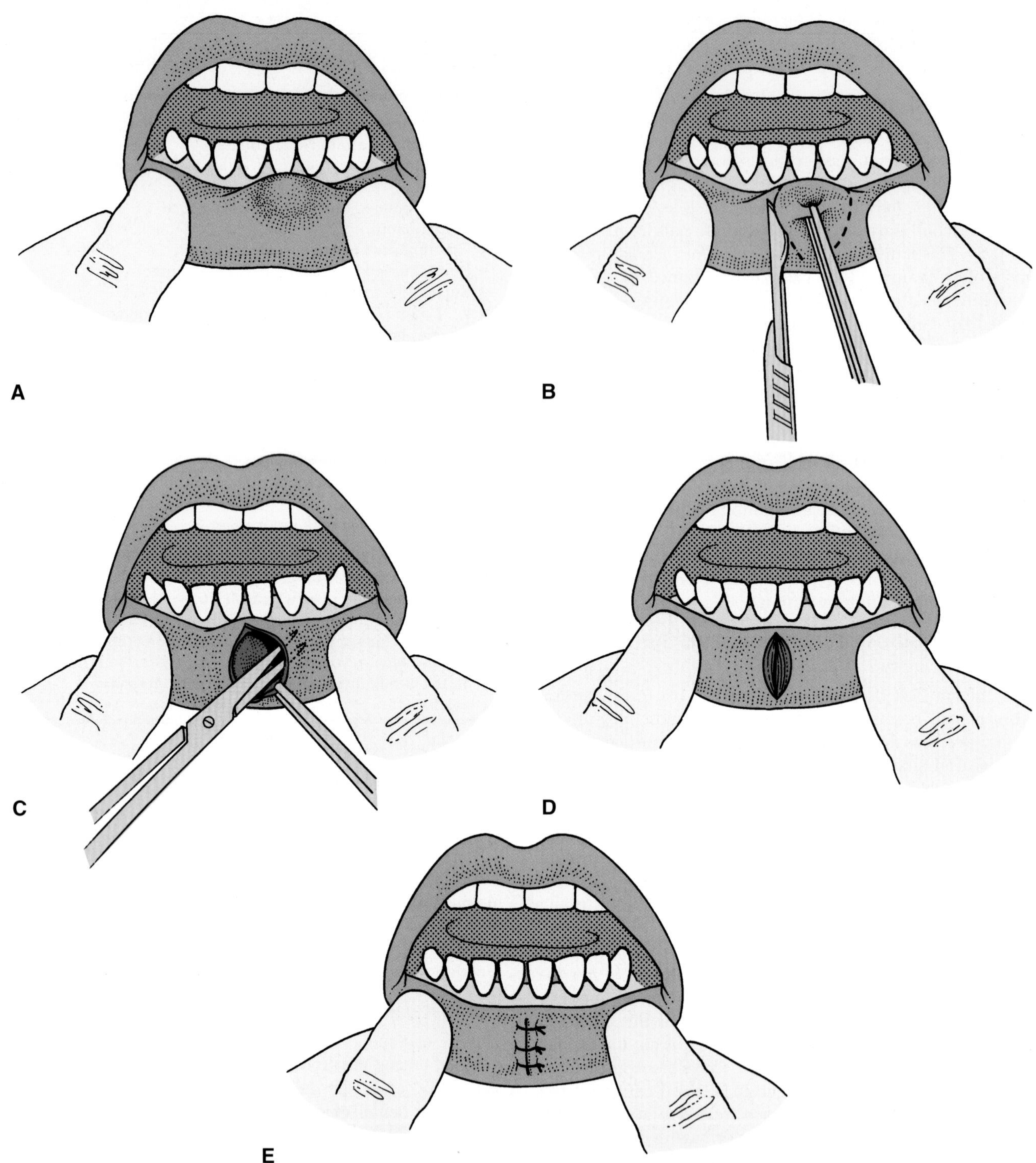

FIGURE 21-10 Examples of methods to stabilize tissue for biopsy. A, Assistant's fingers used to stabilize tissue before excisional biopsy of mucocele. B, Elliptical incision is made around lesion. C, Surgeon makes a submucosal excision of associated minor salivary glands. D and E, Mucosa is undermined and closed.

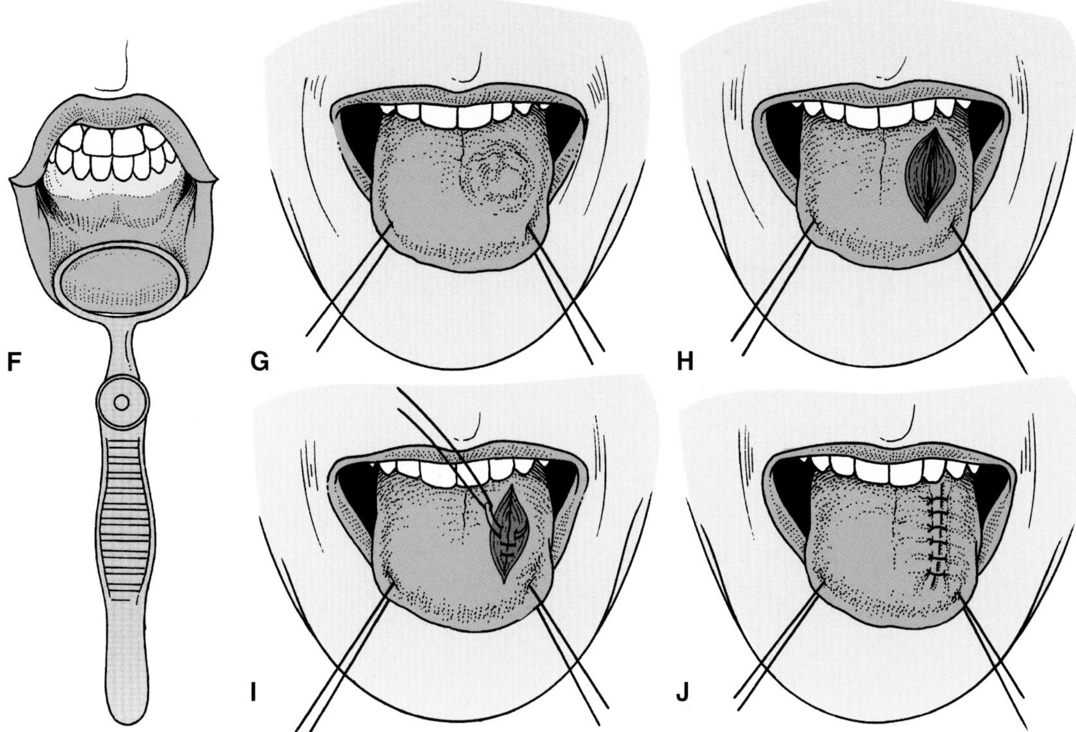

FIGURE 21-10, cont'd Examples of methods to stabilize tissue for biopsy. **F**, Stabilization of tissue with chalazion-type device. **G**, Stabilization of tissue with traction sutures. Two silk sutures are used to stabilize tongue before excisional biopsy. They are placed through substance of tongue (mucosa and muscle) to prevent pulling through tissue. **H**, Lesion is removed after elliptical incision was made around it. **I**, Resorbable sutures are placed to approximate muscle. **J**, Mucosa is closed.

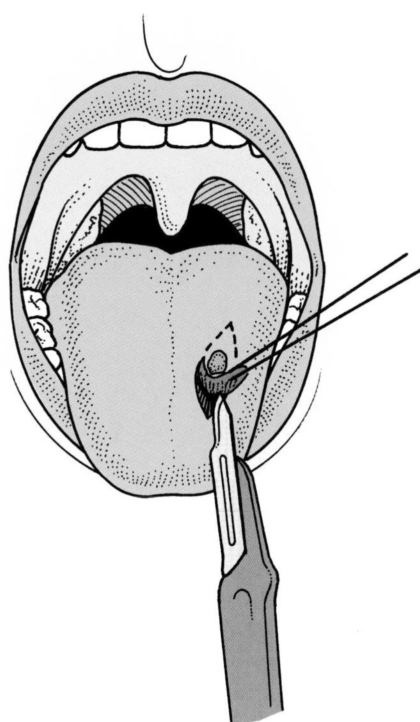

FIGURE 21-11 Illustration showing use of traction suture placed through specimen. While lesion is incised, traction suture is used to lift specimen from wound bed. Suture can then be tied and left attached to lesion to identify margin of specimen.

is *not* desirable because the tissue effects cause destruction of adjacent tissues and may distort the histologic architecture of the specimen to such a degree that definitive microscopic details are destroyed. The carbon dioxide laser in the superpulsed mode with a tight, well-focused beam can be used if necessary (e.g., for hemostasis), but the surgeon should understand that there will be a narrow zone of necrosis next to the margins of the specimen from the laser.

Variations in the size of the ellipse and degree of convergence toward the base of the lesion depend on the depth of encroachment of the lesion on normal tissues. Palpation can offer clues regarding the depth and expanse of the submucosal portions of the lesion. When performing an *excisional* biopsy, the surgeon must ensure that there is a perimeter of normal tissues beneath the lesion as well. As noted previously, in most cases thin, deep specimens are preferable to wide, shallow specimens (Fig. 21-7). To the maximal extent possible, incisions should parallel the normal course of nerves and blood vessels, as well as lines of muscular tension (i.e., smile lines and facial creases), to minimize secondary injuries and maximize esthetic results. As noted previously, a 2- to 3-mm band of normal tissue should ideally be included around the specimen during an excisional biopsy. If the lesion appears malignant, pigmented, or vascular or has diffuse borders, an *additional* 2 to 3 mm of normal-appearing peripheral tissues should be excised with the specimen.

In larger lesions with variable surface characteristics, an *incisional* biopsy may be indicated, and occasionally more than

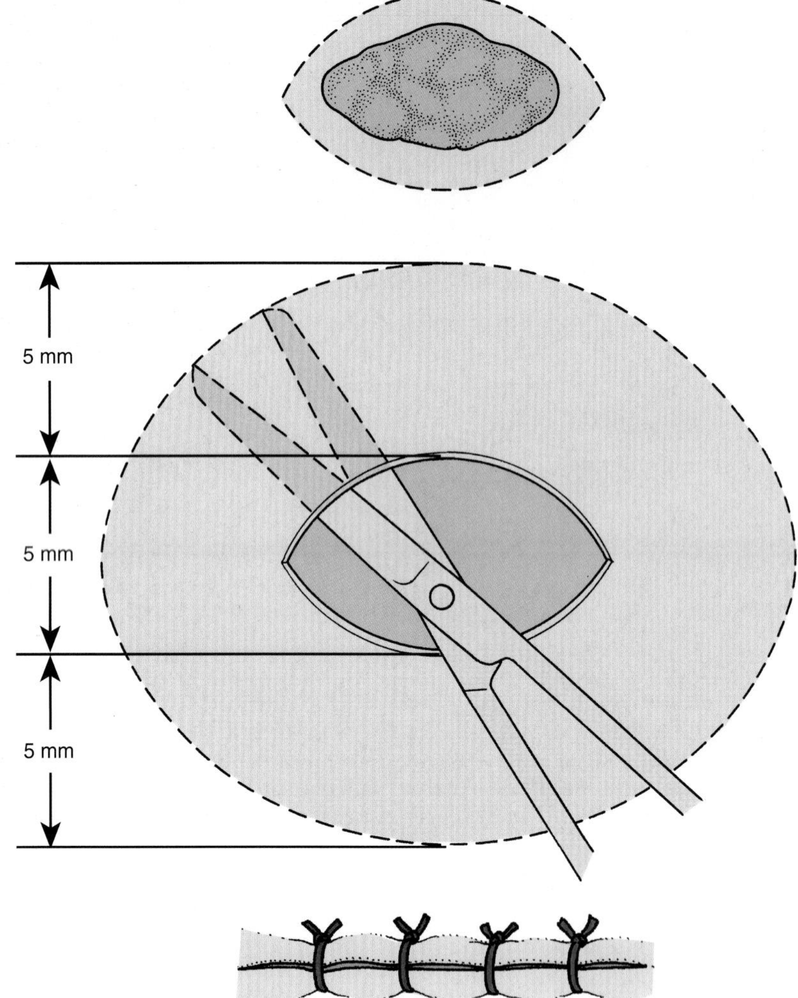

FIGURE 21-12 Illustration showing principles used in closing an elliptical biopsy wound. Mucosa should be undermined bluntly with scissors to width of original ellipse in each direction. This allows approximation of wound margins without tension.

one sample has to be taken from different areas of the lesion (Fig. 21-8).

Wound Closure

Following removal of the tissue sample, primary closure of the wound is desirable and usually possible. If the wound is deep, incorporating different tissue layers, deep closure should be carried out for each layer, using a resorbable suture material (e.g., polyglycolic acid or chromic gut; Fig. 21-10, *I*). Following excision of the specimen and any closure of deeper tissues, the mucosa (or skin) is undermined by using a spreading action of the tips of small scissors (e.g., iris or Metzenbaum scissors) to separate the mucosal from the submucosal tissues (Fig. 21-12). The submucosal layer is largely loose connective tissue that is easily dissected free from the overlying mucosa without sharp incision or snipping. This permits the mucosa to be closed as a separate layer without regard to the closure in the deeper layers. The extent to which this undermining is carried out is determined by the size of the wound and the anatomic location. In the lips, cheek, floor of mouth, and soft palate, wound margins are usually undermined in all directions by a distance that is at least the width of the defect before surface closure. Undermining permits tension-free approximation of the tissue margins. Suture materials of choice are generally black silk or a nonreactive, slowly resorbable material such as polyglycolic acid (Dexon) or polyglactin 910 (Vicryl) sutures. Wounds on attached mucosal surfaces (e.g., gingiva and hard palate) are generally not closed but are allowed to heal by secondary intention. Protective periodontal dressings or vacuum-formed or acrylic splints, lined with a tissue-conditioning liner, can be used to protect the healing area(s), enhance patient comfort, and promote healing. If necessary, these customized postsurgical splints can be secured to adjacent teeth with circumdental fine wires or heavy suture material to aid retention. Postsurgical splints are usually left in place for 7 to 10 days. Biopsy wounds on the dorsum or lateral border of the tongue require deeply placed sutures at close intervals in order to counteract the inherent muscle movements and maintain closure (Fig. 21-10, *I*). Resorbable sutures can be used, but gut sutures are not recommended because they have poor knot security (resulting in lost sutures) and undergo rapid enzymatic degradation. Examples of lip and tongue biopsy are shown in Figures 21-13 and 21-14.

Handling of Tissues; Specimen Care

Any tissue specimen must be maintained in a condition that is optimal for preserving the histologic and structural architecture of the cells of the lesion. Specimens that have been crushed, frozen, desiccated, burned, or otherwise compromised may not be microscopically diagnostic once they reach the oral and maxillofacial pathologist, necessitating a repeat biopsy (which may or may not be feasible). Extreme care should be exercised when removing surgical specimens to avoid instrument damage to the specimen during manipulation. The removed tissue sample should not be wrapped in gauze (wet or dry) because it is then at risk to get accidentally thrown away with the gauze. The specimen also should not be set on paper or linen drapes and allowed to dry out while the surgery is being completed. Rather, the specimen should be immediately placed in a glass or plastic container that can be capped and that contains a quantity of 10% formalin solution (4% formaldehyde) that is at least 20 times the volume of the specimen itself (Fig. 21-15). The specimen must be totally immersed in the preservative solution at all times, even if the container is tilted sideways during transporting. The dentist should also ensure that the tissue sample does not adhere to the container wall above the level of the formalin before turning his or her attention to wound closure. If the specimen is mailed to the pathologist, it must be labeled with a biohazard label approved by the Occupational Safety and Health Administration; if the specimen is transported internally (e.g., within a hospital), such labeling is not mandated.

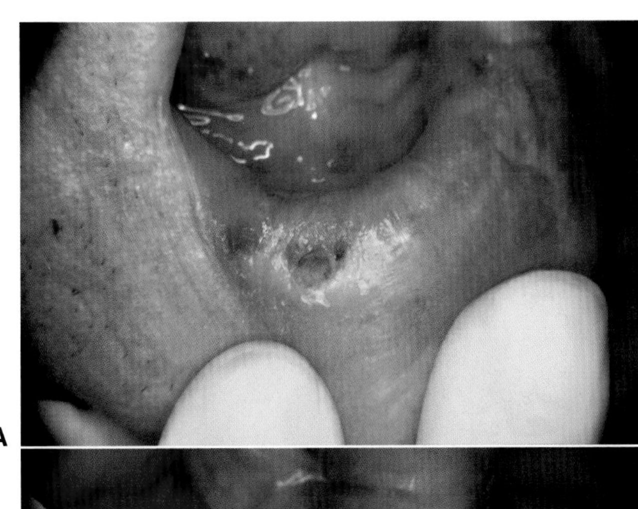

A

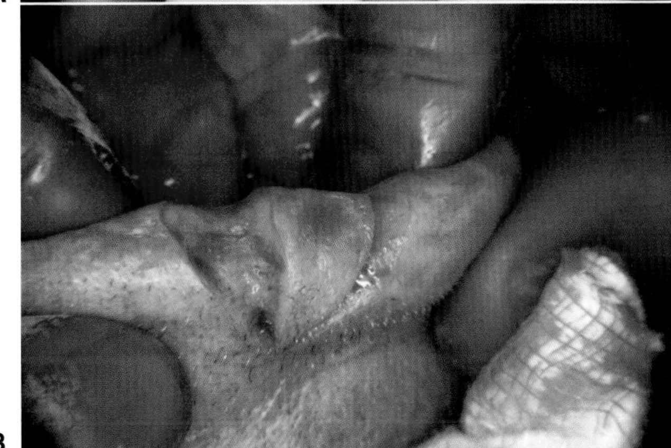

B

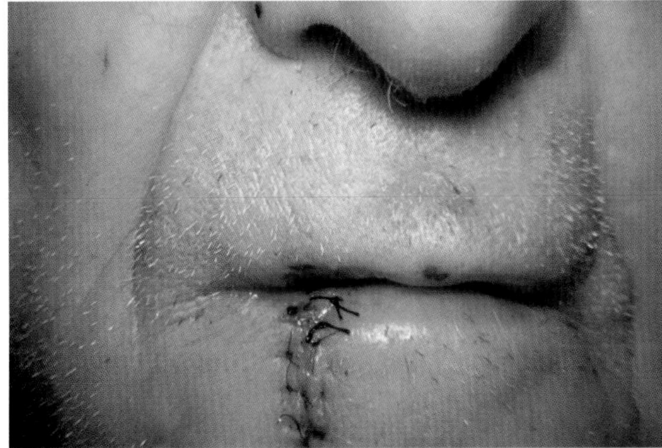

C

FIGURE 21-13 Photographs showing excisional biopsy of an ulcer (A) of the lower lip. B, V-shaped incisions made with 2- to 3-mm margin of normal tissue. C, Appearance after layered closure.

Suture Tagging of Specimens; Margin Identification

If dysplasia or malignancy is suspected, it is helpful to the pathologist if the surgeon "tags" one of the margins of a specimen with a loosely tied suture to orient the anatomic alignment of the specimen. This allows the pathologist to report precisely which specific margins or areas, if any, require wider or deeper excision. The orientation and the location of the marker suture should be illustrated and/or documented on the oral pathology service's submission form (Fig. 21-16).

Suture tagging can also be used to identify multiple specimens from one lesion when accompanied by a drawing that delineates from which area each specimen was removed and the orientation of each specimen (Fig. 21-17). The first specimen receives one tagging suture, whereas the second receives two, and so for all other specimens. Each specimen should be submitted in its own container, however.

Submission of Specimens

Every dental office should prearrange a connection with a local or regional oral pathology examination service where specimens can be submitted. Generally, it is preferable to have odontogenic tissues submitted to an oral and maxillofacial pathologist whenever possible. Highly competent, general (medical) pathologists may not be familiar with the subtleties of odontogenic cysts and tumors, which can occasionally result in incorrect diagnoses and treatment. If the city or town in which the dental office is located does not have such a service available, many dental schools and oral pathology practices in most major cities offer mail-based service and provide the dental office, upon request, with mailing kits that can be used for submissions. Mailed specimen containers should contain a form with detailed information, a capped, biohazard-labeled container (usually glass or plastic) with an appropriate amount of formalin and labeled with the address of the pathology service. The patient's name and the referring dentist's name should also be entered on the specimen bottle label in case the outer mailing container is damaged in transit and the bottle becomes separated from it (Fig. 21-18).

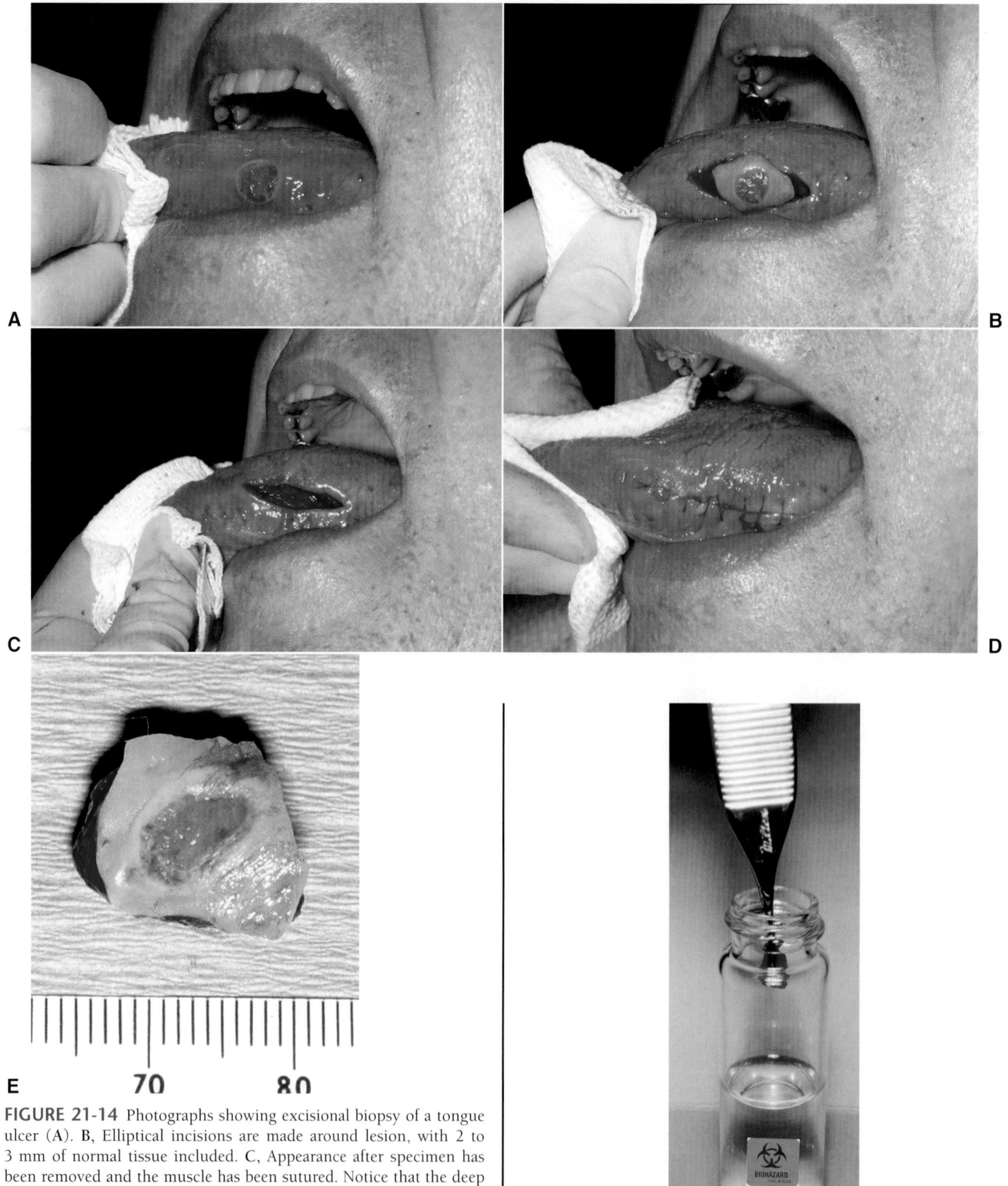

FIGURE 21-14 Photographs showing excisional biopsy of a tongue ulcer (A). B, Elliptical incisions are made around lesion, with 2 to 3 mm of normal tissue included. C, Appearance after specimen has been removed and the muscle has been sutured. Notice that the deep sutures have made an almost linear closure of the mucosa possible. D, Appearance after mucosal closure. E, Specimen.

FIGURE 21-15 Photograph of a specimen being dropped into a biopsy bottle filled with formalin.

A

LOCAL ORAL PATHOLOGY LABORATORY

1234 Main Street

Anytown, State Zip

Date: *01/02/200X* **Case Number:** _________

Patient Name: *Perry Osteum* **Gender:** *Male* **Age:** *32 yrs*

Race: *Cauc*

Address: *5678 N. 2nd Street, #401* **City/State/Zip:** *Anytown, State Zip*

Home Phone: *(777)888-9999* **Work Phone:** *(777) 888-0000*

Occupation: *Construction*

Submitting Doctor's Name: *Matt Tikulus*

Mailing Address: *8910 Anystreet, Anytown, State, Zip*

Office Phone: *(777) 888-6666* **E-mail Address:** *mtikdds@server.net*

History: *asymptomatic white plaque of unknown duration but first noticed by patient about 2 months ago, left lateral border of tongue. Not recorded at last dental visit 2 years ago. We observed area X 2 weeks, without change in size, appearance. Patient denies tobacco usage, alcohol abuse, parafunctional habits. No HIV test on record. Lesion has not been painful. No local trauma source noted (sharp edged restoration, etc.). PMH is unremarkable, no known allergies, no meds. Denies lesions elsewhere on body.*

Type of Biopsy: **Excisional** ______ **Incisional**□✓□ **Other** □□□

Clinical Description/Location: *3X5 cm white, rough surfaced plaque, left lateral border of the tongue, extending onto the dorsum of the tongue midlesion (see drawing). Texture is leather-like, nonulcerated. Uniform thickness throughout lesion. No ipsi- or contralateral lymphadenopathy noted. Excised with 1 cm clinical margin. Anteriorborder tagged with single suture. Superior border tagged with 2 sutures.*

Provisional Clinical Diagnosis/es: *Epithelial Dysplasia, CA in-situ, SCCa? (Your best guess of what the lesion might be)*

X-rays taken?: Y____ **N**__✓__ **X-rays Enclosed?Y**____**N**__✓__

Photographs Taken?: Y____**N**__✓__

Photographs Enclosed?: Y____**N**__✓__

Additional Comments or Instructions:

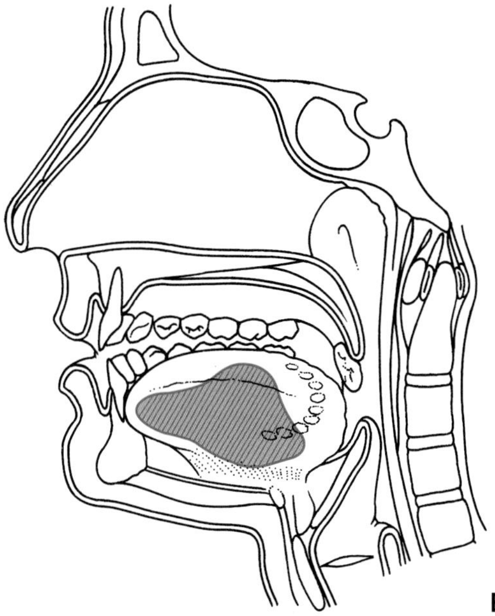

B

FIGURE 21-16 A, Biopsy data sheet. Such sheets vary from one laboratory to the next; the one here represents several. Information provided on this data sheet describes lesion shown in Figure 21-17. B, Drawing of lesion that is to be sent with the data sheet.

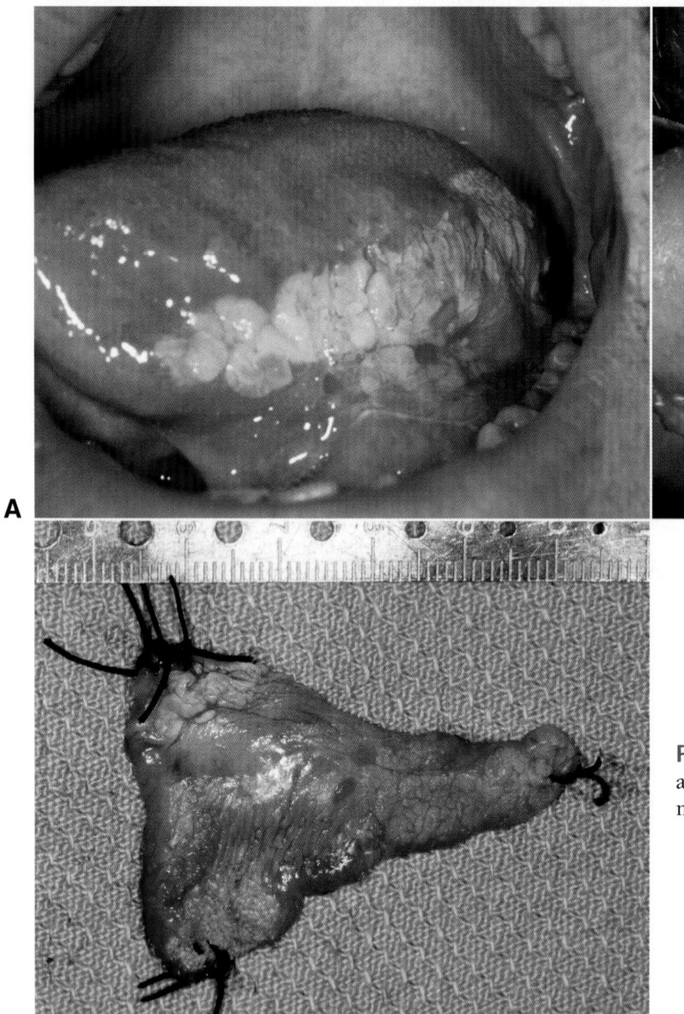

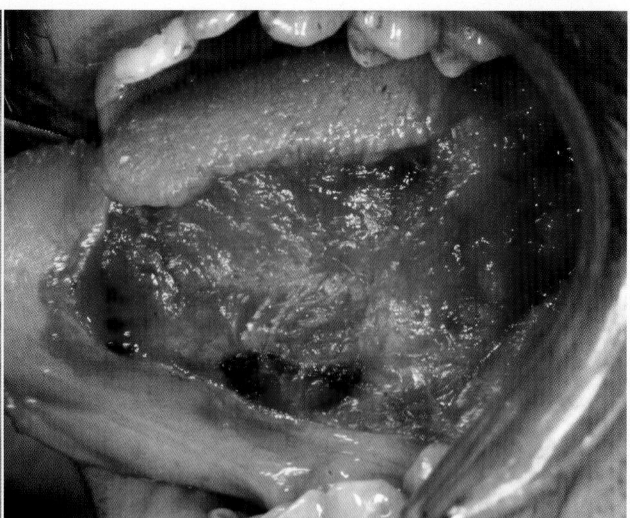

FIGURE 21-17 A, Lesion described in Figure 21-16. B, Surgical site after excision of lesion. C, Specimen after removal. Note marking of margins with sutures to orient pathologist.

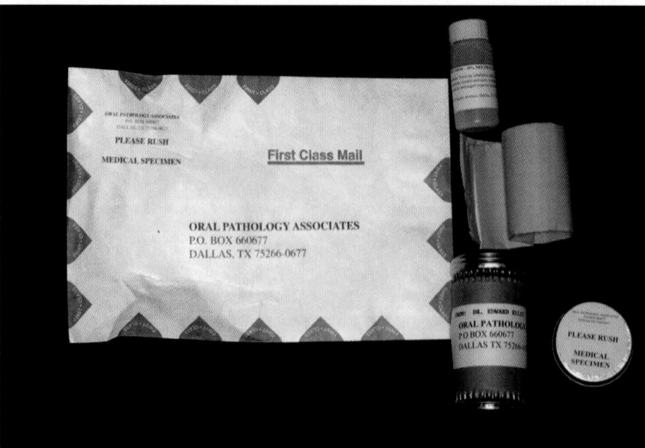

FIGURE 21-18 Typical biopsy kit that is available from a number of pathology laboratories. Kit includes a specimen bottle containing formalin, a biopsy data sheet onto which information about the patient and specimen is documented, and a mailer to send the specimen back to the laboratory.

Biopsy Submission Data Form

Pathology laboratories each have a form unique to their facility for use in submitting specimens for examination (Fig. 21-16). As noted previously, the specimen container itself must be labeled and identified with the demographic data of the patient and the name and address of the submitting dentist in the event it gets separated from the submission form and/or transporting container. Most forms are structured to gather supporting information and data that generally include the following: demographic data about the patient; name and contact information for the submitting dentist; pertinent medical, family, social, and/or lesion history; clinical description of the lesion and/or specimen; presumptive clinical differential diagnoses. When dealing with intraosseous lesions, inclusion of a diagnostic-quality radiograph can be useful to the pathologist. For soft tissue lesions, a good-quality, color printout of a digital photograph of the lesion may be useful to include with certain specimens, especially if one is suspicious of dysplasia or malignancy. The dentist must take the time to provide as much information on the submission form as possible to aid the pathologist. Insufficient information, incomplete data, or important omitted historical notes can lead to wasted time and inaccurate diagnoses.

Most pathology laboratories have the written microscopic examination report back to the referring dentist within 7 to 14 days following receipt of the specimen. The dentist should plan to see the patient in approximately 1 week to remove sutures and counsel the patient on the biopsy results, if available. If not yet received, the dentist can elect to call the patient at home (if the report is negative for malignancy, documenting the call in the patient record) or appoint the patient to return postoperatively after the second week (if the microscopic diagnosis is one of malignancy) so that the results can be discussed in person with the patient and timely referral appointments can be arranged. As noted previously, patients who must be informed of adverse diagnoses (e.g., cancer) should be counseled with great sensitivity to counteract possible anxiety or depression over the diagnosis. At the same time there is a need to impress upon the patient the importance of early treatment and close follow-up. Delays in beginning treatment (procrastination) may significantly worsen the prognosis of many lesions, so it is important to arrange *prompt* referral for such patients to specialists with the ability to manage their condition.

A negative (benign) pathology report should never be taken as a final assessment, and the dentist should not be lulled into a false sense of security by receiving one. One experienced clinician stated it this way: "Treat the patient, not the paperwork." If the clinical behavior of a lesion suggests that it is not benign, then a second biopsy of the area should be considered. Also possible is that a nondiagnostic or nonrepresentative area of the lesion was sampled and the areas of pathologic cellular changes were not included in the specimen(s). Errors in microscopic diagnosis can also occur, especially if odontogenic tissues are examined by general pathologists who may be unfamiliar with the nuances of oral and odontogenic lesions. It is not inappropriate in such cases to ask for a second pathology opinion from an oral pathologist before contemplating ablative or disfiguring surgery. General dentists who submit biopsies must also be conversant with the terminology used in reports to fully grasp the meaning of the microscopic diagnosis and the course of treatment or follow-up that is appropriate for that diagnosis. If there is any uncertainty about the contents of the report, then the dentist should seek clarifications from the pathologist.

INTRAOSSEOUS (HARD TISSUE) BIOPSY TECHNIQUES AND PRINCIPLES

Any lesion on or within the osseous tissues of the jaws mandates scrutiny of the dentist until a definitive diagnosis is obtained. Often the cause is odontogenic, and the lesion will resolve once the dental problem is addressed. If the lesion appears to be unrelated to the dentition or does not respond to treatment of the presumed odontogenic problem, then the lesion should be removed for definitive diagnosis.

The most common intraosseous lesions encountered by the dentist are periapical granulomas and odontogenic cysts. Because these are generally asymptomatic lesions with characteristic radiographic appearances, a presumptive diagnosis is frequently possible. Treatment generally involves surgical removal of the lesion by way of excisional biopsy (enucleation). When such a lesion is large, perforating into soft tissues overlying the bone, or where there is a suspicion of malignancy based on history and radiographic characteristics, then incisional biopsy is indicated so that a definitive diagnosis can be reached.

Before performing intraosseous biopsy, the dentist should carefully palpate the area of the jaw and compare it to the contralateral side. Bone that has a normal contour and feels firm and smooth suggests that the lesion has not expanded or eroded the cortical plate of bone. However, a spongy feel when the jaw is compressed with the fingers usually indicates erosion or thinning of the cortical plate, which suggests a more aggressive neoplastic lesion. Biopsy procedures and principles within hard tissues are no different than those guiding soft tissue biopsy, but some additional aspects must be considered.

Mucoperiosteal Flaps

Because of their proximity to the jaws or their location within the bone, most biopsies require an approach through a mucoperiosteal flap. Several variations of flaps are available, and the choice depends mostly on the size and location of the lesion to be removed. The basic principles of flap design outlined in Chapter 8 are the same whether the dentist is removing a tooth or performing an osseous biopsy. The location of the lesion often dictates where the incisions for the flap must be made, and optimal access may necessitate extension of the flap margins. Major neurovascular structures must be avoided whenever possible, and the flap should rest entirely on sound bone for closure—in other words, extend 4 to 5 mm beyond the surgical margins of any bony defects (Fig. 21-19). Flap elevation for any intraosseous lesion that may have eroded the cortical bone of the jaw should be approached in an area well away from the lesion margins over sound bone. This allows establishment of a proper tissue plane for subperiosteal elevation of the mucoperiosteal flap and any required dissection needed to free the overlying tissues from the lesion. All mucoperiosteal flaps for biopsies in or on the jaws should be full thickness with the incisions transecting mucosa, submucosa, and periosteum.

Precautionary Aspiration

Aspiration of all intraosseous lesions should be performed routinely before opening into the osseous defect to determine whether it contains fluid, including blood. After achieving local anesthesia in the surgical area, use a 16- or 18-gauge needle connected to a 5- or 10-mL syringe. If the cortical plate cannot be penetrated by pressing the needle firmly through the mucoperiosteum with a twisting movement, then a flap can be reflected and a large round bur, under constant irrigation, can be used cautiously to penetrate the cortical plate. The needle can then be advanced through the cortical bur hole. The needle tip may have to be repositioned if the initial effort fails to locate an area of fluid to verify that the needle placement is correct.

Inability to aspirate fluid or air suggests that the intraosseous mass is probably a solid tumor. If straw-colored fluid is aspirated, the dentist is likely dealing with a cyst, which can then be enucleated (Fig. 21-20). If pus is aspirated, an inflammatory or infectious process is likely present, whereas aspiration of air without any fluid is suggestive of a traumatic bone cavity. If blood is aspirated, several diagnoses must be entertained, the most significant of which would be a pulsatile vascular lesion within the jaw (e.g., hemangioma or arteriovenous malformation). Surgical invasion into such a lesion could produce

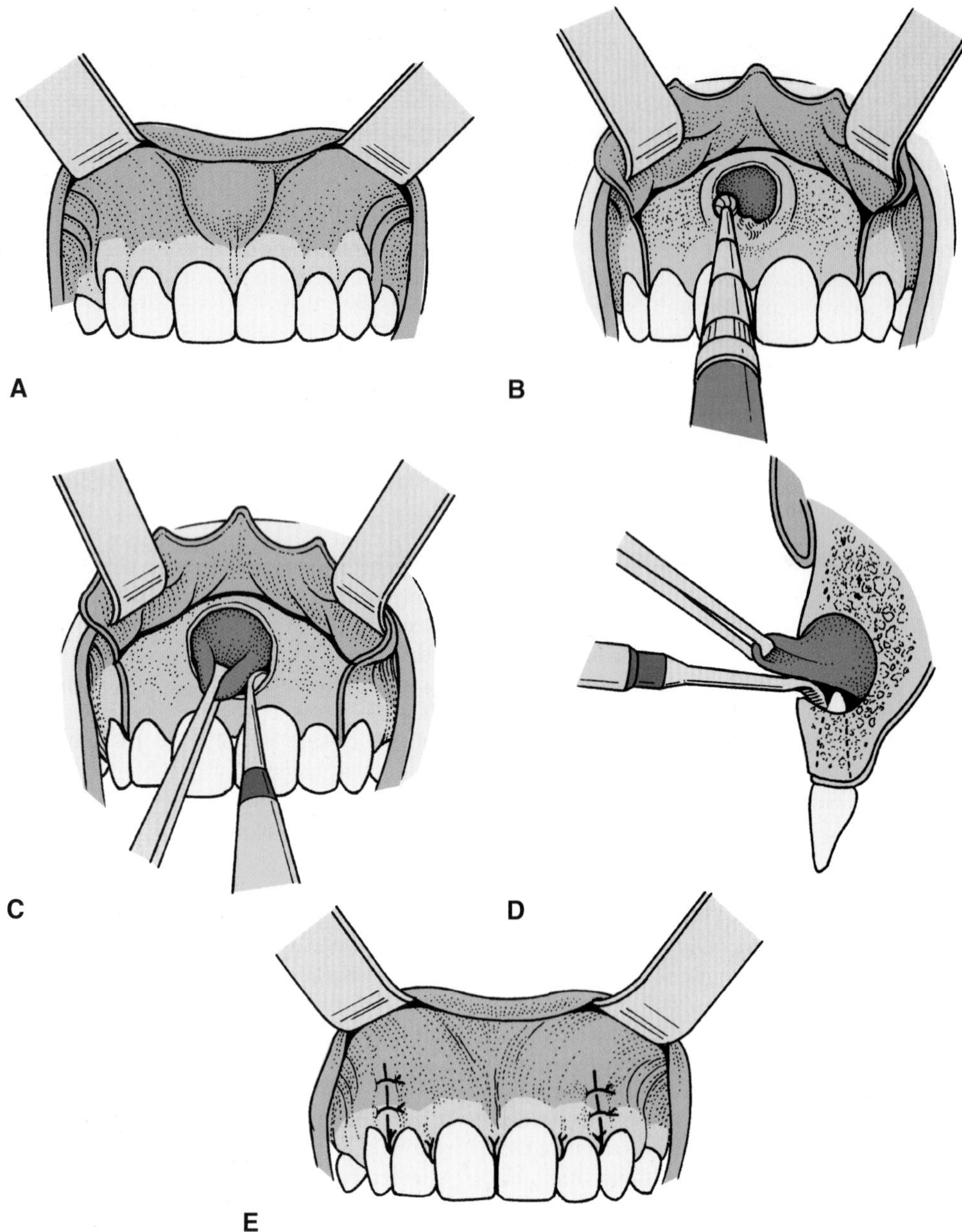

FIGURE 21-19 Illustrations demonstrating enucleation of cyst. **A**, Mild swelling in area of periapical cyst. **B**, Mucoperiosteal flap is elevated from around necks of teeth, and bur is used to remove thinned cortical bone overlying cyst. Care is taken to prevent rupturing cystic contents during this and following steps. **C** and **D**, Spoon type of curette is used to strip cyst from bone. Note concave side of curette is kept in contact with bone. Convex surface is working end of instrument. **E**, Closure.

sudden, life-threatening hemorrhage and should not be attempted by the general dentist. Other vascularized intraosseous lesions can passively (i.e., nonpulsating) produce blood upon syringe aspiration, including aneurysmal bone cysts and central giant cell lesions. Lesion aspirant can also be submitted for chemical analysis, microbiologic culturing, and even microscopic evaluation. If no aspirant is found, then incisional biopsy should be planned on the soft tissue mass within the bone to obtain a definitive microscopic diagnosis before further surgery is planned.

Osseous Window

Intraosseous lesions of the jaws generally require creation of a cortical window for access. If the cortical plate is intact, a round surgical bur under constant fluid irrigation can be used to create an osseous window over the lesion site (see Fig. 21-19, *B*). If expansion has caused erosion of the cortical plate, and an osseous defect is noted when the surgical flap is elevated, then that pathologic defect can be enlarged with rongeurs or a round surgical bur to create the osseous window. The size of the window depends on the size of the lesion and the proximity

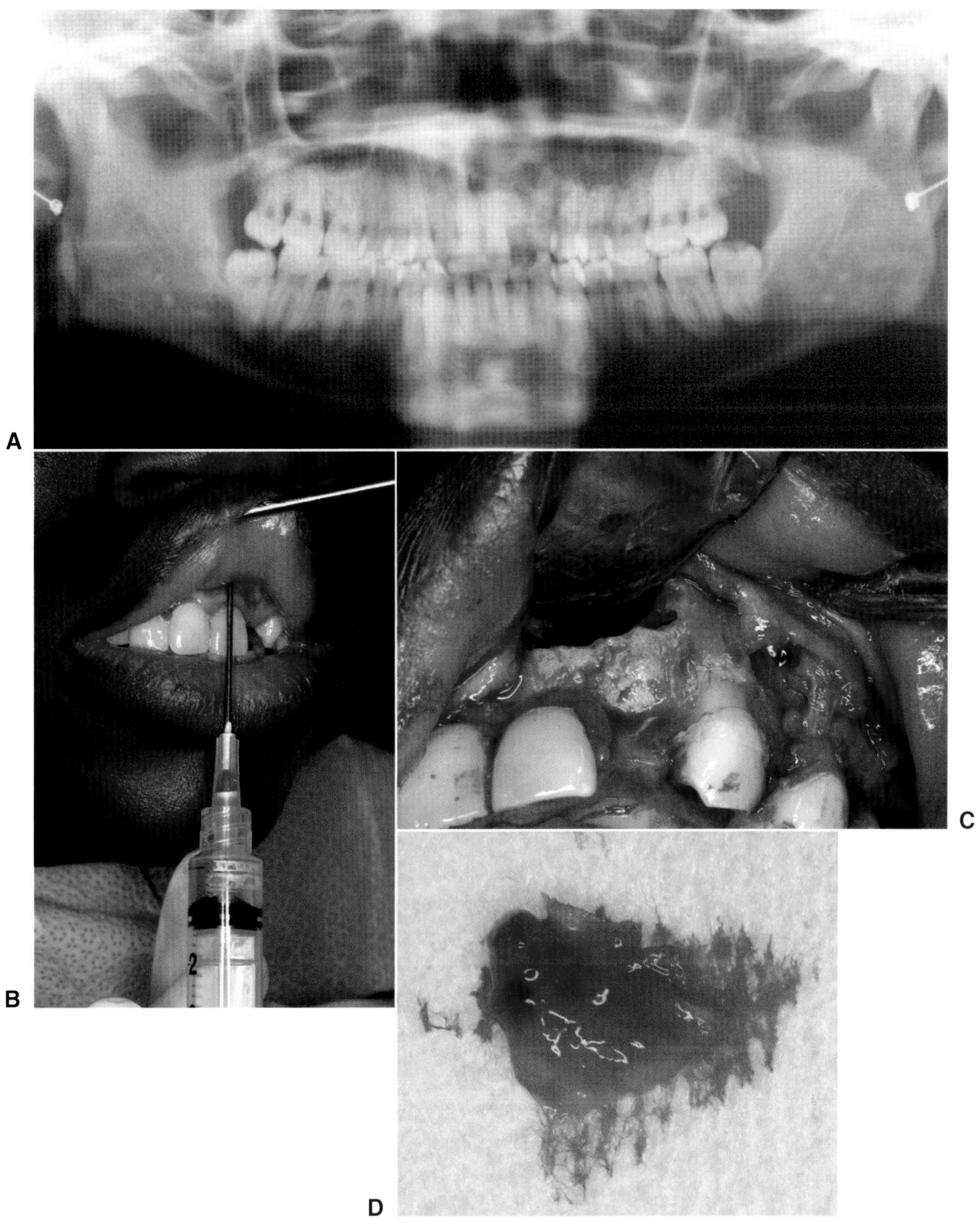

FIGURE 21-20 Incisional biopsy of an intraosseous lesion. A, Panoramic radiograph showing large radiolucency in left maxilla. B, Aspiration of lesion by penetration of a needle through the mucosa and thin bone over lesion reveals straw-colored fluid. C, After raising a soft tissue flap and removal of bone in area of lesion and removal of a specimen for pathologic examination (D).

of significant anatomic structures, such as tooth roots and neurovascular structures. Once the window is created, it can be progressively enlarged with a rongeur as necessary for access. The removed bone that composed the window should be submitted along with the primary specimen if the lesion is a solid tumor.

Specimen Management

The technique for removal of the specimen depends on whether an incisional or excisional biopsy is planned and the consistency of the tissue encountered. Most small lesions that have a connective tissue capsule (e.g., cysts) can be enucleated in their entirety. A dental curette is used progressively to peel the specimen away from the surrounding bone and dentition, keeping the instrument constantly in contact with the osseous surface of the bone cavity (Fig. 21-19, *C* and *D*). Once the lesion is completely freed from attachment, it can be removed and placed immediately into the formalin preservative. If resistance to enucleation is noted and the lesion does not separate from the bone easily, that detail should be noted on the specimen submission form, along with the exact location(s) of adherence. The resulting bone cavity should then be irrigated, suctioned, and examined for any residual fragments of soft tissue. If any are noted, they should be curetted out so that the cavity is devoid of any residual pathologic tissues. Following final irrigation, the mucoperiosteal flap is repositioned and sutured.

If the dentist encounters a solid soft tissue lesion of small size that separates readily from the surrounding bone, it can be curetted and enucleated in the same manner as the cystic lesion and submitted as a specimen. If resistant to curettage is noted during removal, the dentist should try to remove a millimeter of adjacent osseous tissue after the bulk of the lesion is removed. Tooth root surfaces within the bone defect should be thoroughly curetted. If incisional biopsy is indicated, then a section of tissue is removed and the remaining lesion is left undisturbed until the pathologic diagnosis is available.

Whenever possible, diagnostic radiographs should be included with the intraosseous specimen or digitally transmitted to the pathology facility. As previously noted, the pathologist should be provided with as much clinical information as possible when the accompanying specimen submission data form is filled out. Also important is to note whether the specimen contains hard (osseous) and soft tissues. The pathology report may take 2 weeks or longer, if decalcification of osseous tissues is required before microscopic evaluation.

Postbiopsy Follow-up

If the lesion is though to be benign, then routine follow-up is carried out, with periodic radiographs to monitor osseous healing. If an incisional biopsy was performed, once the microscopic diagnosis becomes available, the patient should be reevaluated and plans should be formulated for any required definitive treatment and/or referral for additional treatment.

REFERENCES

1. Kerr AR, Sirois DA: Clinical evaluation of a new adjunctive technique for oral mucosal examinations, *OS OM OP* 97:451, 2004 (abstract).
2. Ram S, Siar CH: Chemiluminescence as a diagnostic aid in the detection of oral cancer and potentially malignant epithelial lesions, *Int J Oral Maxillofac Surg* 34:521-527, 2005.
3. Epstein JB Gorsky M, Lonky S et al: The efficacy of oral lumenoscopy (Vizlite) in visualizing oral mucosal lesions, *Spec Care Dentist* 26:171-174, 2006.
4. Poh CF, Zhang L, Anderson DW et al: Fluorescence visualization detection of field alterations in tumor margins of oral cancer patients, *Clin Cancer Res* 12:6716-6722, 2007.
5. Oh ES, Laskin DM: Efficacy of the ViziLite system in the identification of oral lesions, *J Oral Maxillofac Surg* 65:424-426, 2007.
6. Kerr AR, Sirols DA, Epstein JB: Clinical evaluation of chemiluminescent lighting: an adjunct for oral mucosal examination, *J Clin Dent* 17:59-63, 2006.
7. Wright JM: A review and update of oral precancerous lesions, *Tex Dent J* 115:15-19, 1998.
8. Slater LJ: Oral brush biopsy: false positives redux, *Oral Surg Oral Med Oral Pathol Oral Radiol Endod* 97:419, 2004.
9. Nichols ML, Quinn FB Jr, Schnadig VJ et al: Interobserver variability in the interpretation of brush cytologic studies from head and neck lesions, *Arch Otolaryngol Head Neck Surg* 117:1350, 1991.
10. Sciubba JJ: Improving detection of precancerous and cancerous oral lesions, *J Am Dent Assoc* 130:1445, 1999.

CHAPTER 22

Surgical Management of Oral Pathologic Lesions

EDWARD ELLIS III

CHAPTER OUTLINE

The specific surgical techniques for treatment of oral pathologic lesions can be as varied as those for surgical management of any other entity. Each clinician surgically treats patients using techniques based on previous training, biases, experience, personal skill, intuition, and ingenuity. The purpose of this chapter is not to describe the specifics of surgical techniques for management of individual oral pathologic lesions but to present basic principles that can be applied to a variety of techniques to treat patients satisfactorily. Discussion of this topic is made easier by the fact that many different lesions can be treated in much the same manner, as is outlined later.

BASIC SURGICAL GOALS

Eradication of Pathologic Condition

The therapeutic goal of any ablative surgical procedure is to remove the entire lesion and leave no cells that could proliferate and cause a recurrence of the lesion. The methods used to achieve this goal vary tremendously and depend on the nature of the pathologic condition of the lesion. Excision of an oral carcinoma necessitates an aggressive approach that must sacrifice adjacent structures in an attempt to thoroughly remove the lesion. Using this approach on a simple cyst would be a tragedy. Therefore, it is imperative to identify the lesion histologically with a biopsy before undertaking any major ablative surgical procedure. Only then can the appropriate surgical procedure be chosen to eradicate the lesion with as little destruction of adjacent normal tissue as is feasible.

Functional Rehabilitation of Patient

As just noted, the primary goal of surgery to remove a pathologic condition is total removal of the lesion. Although eradication of disease may be the most important goal of treatment, by itself it is frequently inadequate in the comprehensive treatment of patients. The second goal of any treatment used for eradication of disease is an allowance for the functional rehabilitation of the patient. After the primary objective of eradicating a lesion has been achieved, the most important consideration is dealing with the residual defects resulting from the ablative surgery. These defects can range from a mild obliteration of the labial sulcus resulting from the elimination of an area of denture epulis to a defect in the alveolus after removal of a benign odontogenic tumor to a hemimandibulectomy defect resulting from carcinoma resection. The best results are obtained when future reconstructive procedures are considered before excision of lesions. Methods of grafting, fixation principles, soft tissue deficits, dental rehabilitation, and patient preparation must be thoroughly evaluated and adequately handled preoperatively.

SURGICAL MANAGEMENT OF CYSTS AND CYSTLIKE LESIONS OF THE JAWS

Surgical management of oral pathologic lesions can best be discussed by broadly classifying pathologic lesions into the following major categories: cysts and cystlike lesions of the jaws, benign tumors of the jaws, malignant tumors, and benign lesions of oral soft tissues.

A cyst is defined generally as an epithelium-lined sac filled with fluid or soft material. The prevalence of cysts in the jaws can be related to the abundant epithelium that proliferates in bone during the process of tooth formation and along lines where the surfaces of embryologic jaw processes fuse. Cysts of the jaws may be divided into two types: (1) those arising from odontogenic epithelium (i.e., odontogenic cysts) and (2) those arising from oral epithelium that is trapped between fusing processes during embryogenesis (i.e., fissural cysts). The stimulus that causes resting epithelial cells to proliferate into the surrounding connective tissue has not been determined. Inflammation seems to play a major role in those cysts arising in granulomas from infected dental pulps.

Residual fragments of cystic membrane tend to produce recurrent cysts, which necessitates complete excision of the epithelial lining of the cyst at the time of operation. Some cysts (e.g., keratocysts) behave more aggressively in destructive characteristics and recurrence rates. Cysts have been known to destroy large portions of the jaws and to push teeth into remote areas of the jaws (i.e., mandibular condyle or angle and coronoid process; Fig. 22-1). Enlargement of cysts is caused by a gradual expansion, and most are discovered on routine dental radiographs. Cysts are usually asymptomatic unless they are secondarily infected. The overlying mucosa is normal in color and consistency, and no sensory deficits from encroachment on nerves are found.

If the cyst has not expanded or thinned the cortical plate, normal contour and firmness are noted. Palpation with firm pressure may indent the surface of an expanded jaw with characteristic rebound resiliency. If the cyst has eroded through the cortical plate, fluctuance may be noted on palpation.

The radiographic appearance of cysts is characteristic and exhibits a distinct, dense periphery of reactive bone (i.e., condensing osteitis) with a radiolucent center (Fig. 22-2). Most cysts are unilocular; however, multilocular forms are often seen in some keratocysts and cystic ameloblastomas (Fig. 22-3). Cysts do not usually cause resorption of the roots of teeth; therefore, when resorption is seen, the clinician should suspect a neoplasm. The epithelial lining of cysts on rare occasions undergoes ameloblastic or malignant changes. Therefore, all excised cystic tissue must be submitted for pathologic examination.

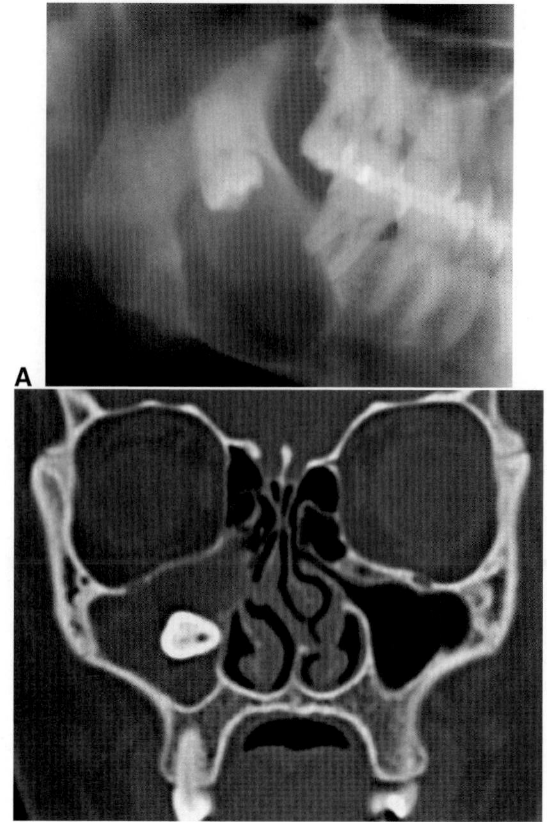

FIGURE 22-1 Two examples of dentigerous cysts that have displaced teeth. A, Mandibular third molar is displaced into the ramus by cyst. B, Maxillary molar is displaced into the maxillary sinus by a cyst that fills the entire sinus.

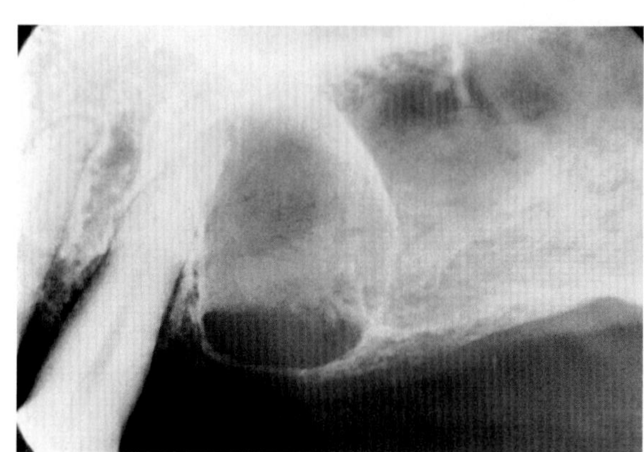

FIGURE 22-2 Typical radiographic appearance of cyst. Radiolucent center is surrounded by zone of reactive bone (condensing osteitis).

Although cysts are broadly classified as odontogenic and fissural, this classification is not relevant to the discussion of surgical techniques to remove cysts. The surgical treatment of cysts is discussed without regard to type of cyst, except for types that warrant special consideration. The principles of

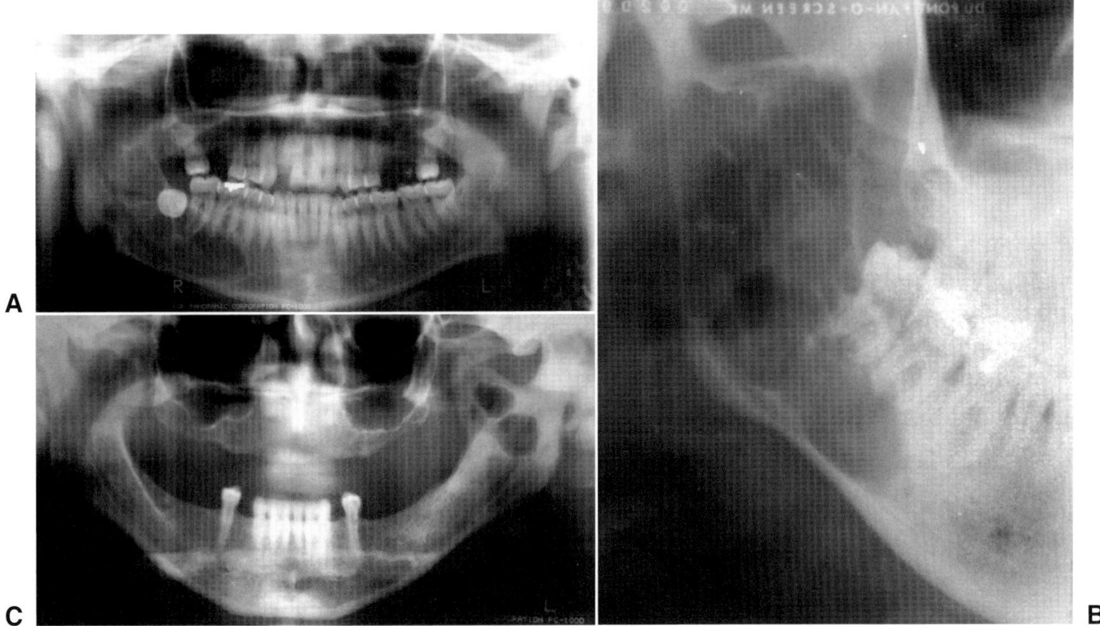

FIGURE 22-3 Multilocular appearance of cysts. A, Right mandibular cyst associated with an impacted tooth. B, Right mandibular cyst not associated with an impacted tooth. C, Left ramus cyst not associated with teeth. All of these lesions were diagnosed histologically as odontogenic keratocysts.

surgical management of cysts are also important for managing the more benign odontogenic tumors and other oral lesions.

Cysts of the jaws are treated in one of the following four basic methods: (1) enucleation, (2) marsupialization, (3) a staged combination of the two procedures, and (4) enucleation with curettage.

Enucleation

Enucleation is the process by which the total removal of a cystic lesion is achieved. By definition, it means a *shelling-out of the entire cystic lesion without rupture.* A cyst lends itself to the technique of enucleation because of the layer of fibrous connective tissue between the epithelial component (which lines the interior aspect of the cyst) and the bony wall of the cystic cavity. This layer allows a cleavage plane for stripping the cyst from the bony cavity and makes enucleation similar to stripping periosteum from bone.

Enucleation of cysts should be performed with care in an attempt to remove the cyst in one piece without fragmentation, which reduces the chances of recurrence by increasing the likelihood of total removal. In practice, however, maintenance of the cystic architecture is not always possible, and rupture of the cystic contents may occur during manipulation.

Indications

Enucleation is the treatment of choice for removal of cysts of the jaws and should be used with any cyst of the jaw that can be safely removed without unduly sacrificing adjacent structures.

Advantages

The main advantage to enucleation is that pathologic examination of the entire cyst can be undertaken. Another advantage is that the initial excisional biopsy (i.e., enucleation) has also appropriately treated the lesion. The patient does not have to care for a marsupial cavity with constant irrigations. Once the mucoperiosteal access flap has healed, the patient is no longer bothered by the cystic cavity.

Disadvantages

If any of the conditions outlined under the section on indications for marsupialization exist, enucleation may be disadvantageous. For example, normal tissue may be jeopardized, fracture of the jaw could occur, devitalization of teeth could result, or associated impacted teeth that the clinician may wish to save could be removed. Thus each cyst must be addressed individually, and the clinician must weigh the pros and cons of enucleation versus marsupialization (with or without enucleation; see Enucleation After Marsupialization).

Technique

The technique for enucleation of cysts was described in Chapter 21; however, the clinician must address special considerations. The use of antibiotics is unnecessary unless the cyst is large or the patient's health condition warrants it (see Chapters 1 and 2).

The periapical (i.e., radicular) cyst is the most common of all cystic lesions of the jaws and results from inflammation or necrosis of the dental pulp. Because it is impossible to determine whether a periapical radiolucency is a cyst or a granuloma, removal at the time of the tooth extraction is recommended. If, however, the tooth is restorable, endodontic treatment followed by periodic radiographic follow-up allows assessment of the amount of bone fill. If none occurs or the lesion expands, the lesion probably represents a cyst and should be removed by periapical surgery. When extracting teeth with periapical radiolucencies, enucleation via the tooth socket can be readily accomplished using curettes when the cyst is small (Fig. 22-4). Caution is used in teeth with apices

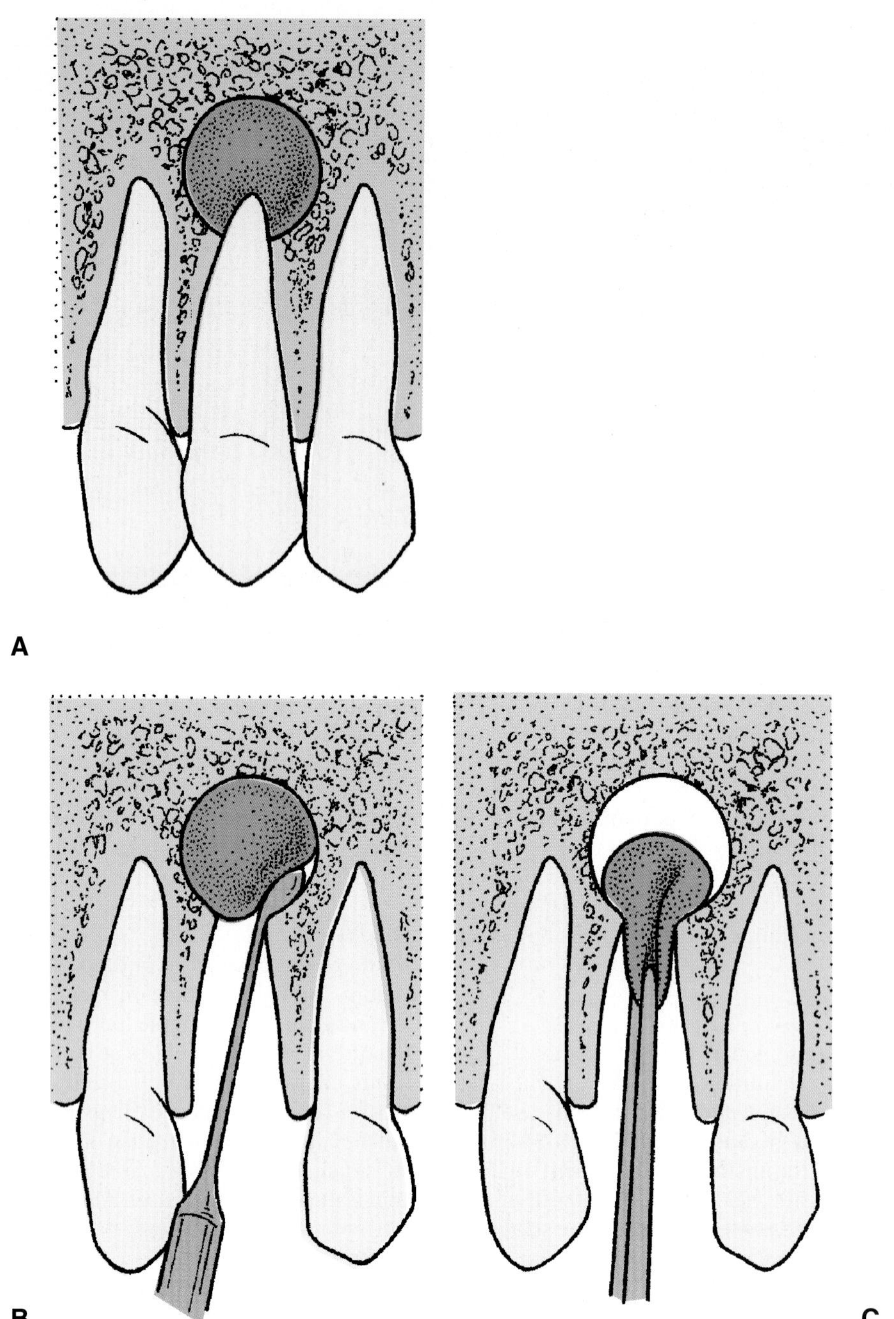

FIGURE 22-4 Apical cystectomy performed at time of tooth removal. A to C, Removal with curette via tooth socket is visualized. An apical cystectomy must be performed with care because of proximity of apices of teeth to other structures, such as maxillary sinus and inferior alveolar canal.

that are close to important anatomic structures, such as the inferior alveolar neurovascular bundle or the maxillary sinus, because the bone apical to the lesion may be very thin or nonexistent. With large cysts, a mucoperiosteal flap may be reflected and access to the cyst obtained through the labial plate of bone, which leaves the alveolar crest intact to ensure adequate bone height after healing (Fig. 22-5).

Once access to a cyst has been achieved through the use of an osseous window, the dentist should begin to enucleate the cyst. A thin-bladed curette is a suitable instrument for cleaving the connective tissue layer of the cystic wall from the bony cavity. The largest curette that can be accommodated by the size of the cyst and of the access should be used. The concave surface should always be kept facing the bony cavity; the edge of the convex surface performs the stripping of the cyst. Care must be exercised to avoid tearing the cyst and allowing the cystic contents to escape because margins of the cyst are easier to define if the cystic wall is intact. Furthermore, the cyst separates more readily from the bony cavity when the intracystic pressure is maintained.

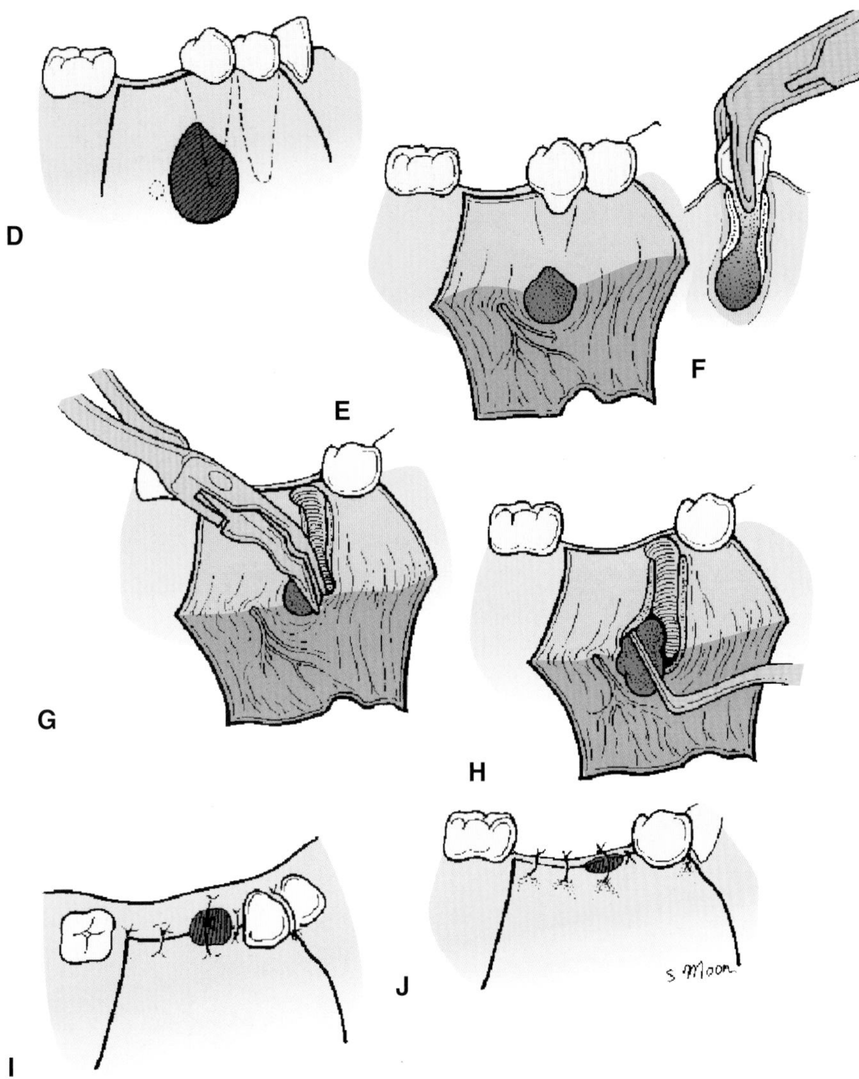

FIGURE 22-4, cont'd Apical cystectomy performed at time of tooth removal. **D** to **J**, Removal of apical cyst by flap reflection and creation of osseous window is demonstrated at the time of tooth removal.

In large cysts or cysts proximal to neurovascular structures, nerves and vessels are usually found pushed to one side of the cavity by the slowly expanding cyst and should be avoided or handled as atraumatically and as little as possible. Once the cyst has been removed, the bony cavity should be inspected for remnants of tissue. Irrigating and drying the cavity with gauze aids in visualizing the entire bony cavity. Residual tissue is removed with curettes. The bony edges of the defect should be smoothed with a file before closure.

Cysts that surround tooth roots or are in inaccessible areas of the jaws require aggressive curettage, which is necessary to remove fragments of cystic lining that could not be removed with the bulk of the cystic wall. Should obvious devitalization of teeth occur during a cystectomy, endodontic treatment of the teeth may be necessary in the near future, which may help to prevent odontogenic infection of the cystic cavity from the necrotic dental pulp.

After enucleation, a watertight primary closure should be obtained with appropriately positioned sutures. The bony cavity fills with a blood clot, which then organizes over time. Radiographic evidence of bone fill will take 6 to 12 months. Jaws that have been expanded by cysts slowly remodel to a more normal contour.

If the primary closure should break down and the wound open, the bony cavity should then be packed open to heal by secondary intention. The wound should be irrigated with sterile saline, and an appropriate length of strip gauze lightly impregnated with an antibiotic ointment should be gently packed into the cavity. This procedure is repeated every 2 to 3 days, gradually reducing the amount of packing until no more is necessary. Granulation tissue is seen on the bony walls in 3 to 4 days and slowly obliterates the cavity and obviates the need for packing. The oral epithelium then closes over the top of the opening, and osseous healing progresses.

Marsupialization

Marsupialization, decompression, and the Partsch operation refer to creating a surgical window in the wall of the cyst, evacuating the contents of the cyst, and maintaining continuity between the cyst and the oral cavity, maxillary sinus, or nasal

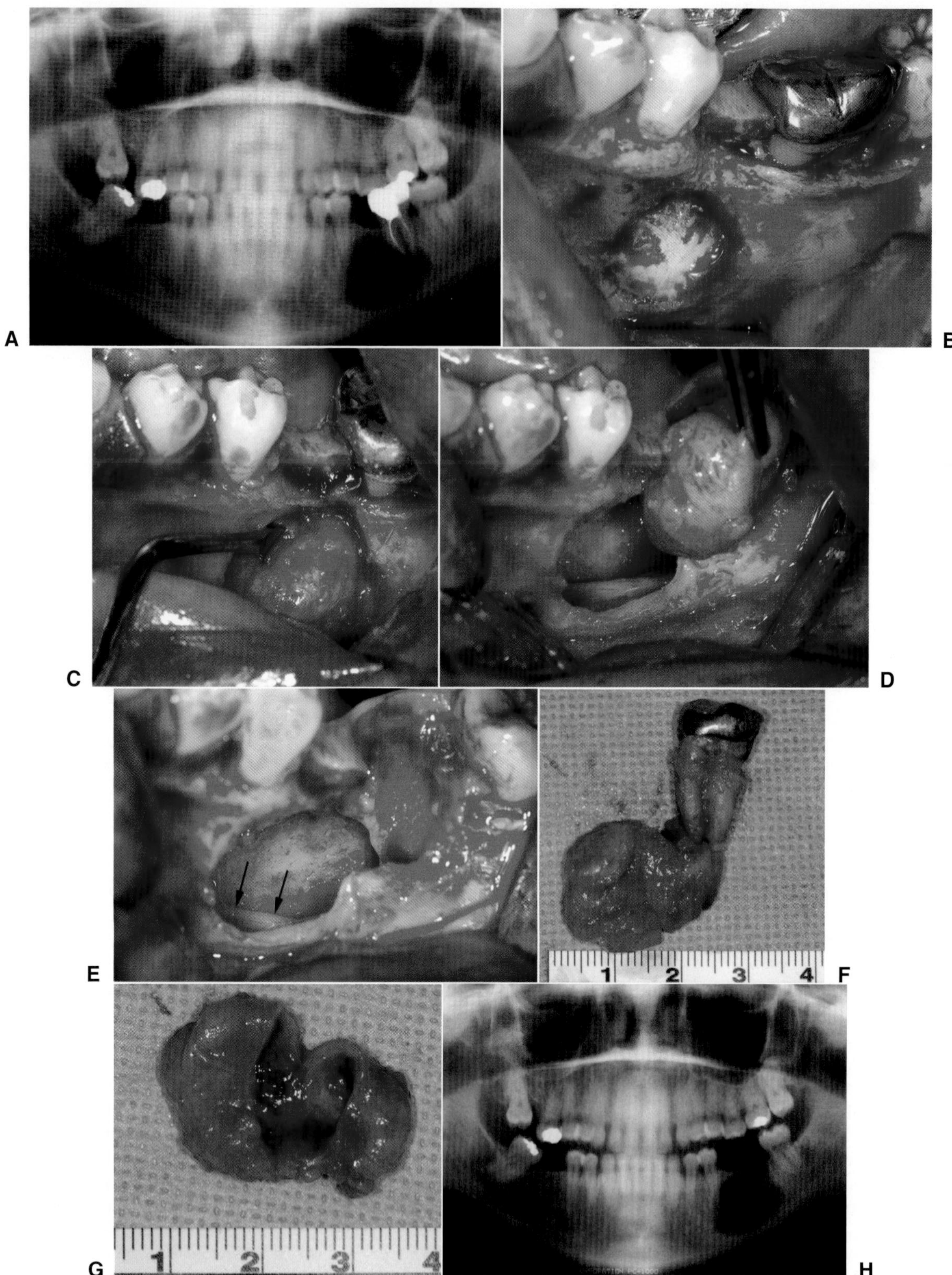

FIGURE 22-5 Photographs of a clinical case of apical cystectomy performed at time of tooth extraction. **A**, Pretreatment panoramic radiograph showing large radiolucent lesion at the apices of teeth No. 18 and 20. **B**, Appearance of lesion after buccal flap elevated. Note that the lesion has eroded the bone. **C**, Curette used to elevate the lesion from the bony walls. **D**, Cyst being removed. Note the inferior alveolar neurovascular bundle passing along the inferior aspect of the bony cavity (**E**). **F**, Surgical specimen, which when opened (**G**) appeared to be cystic. **H**, Postoperative panoramic radiograph showing defect. The patient should be monitored with periodic radiographs to ensure bone fill and no recurrence of the lesion.

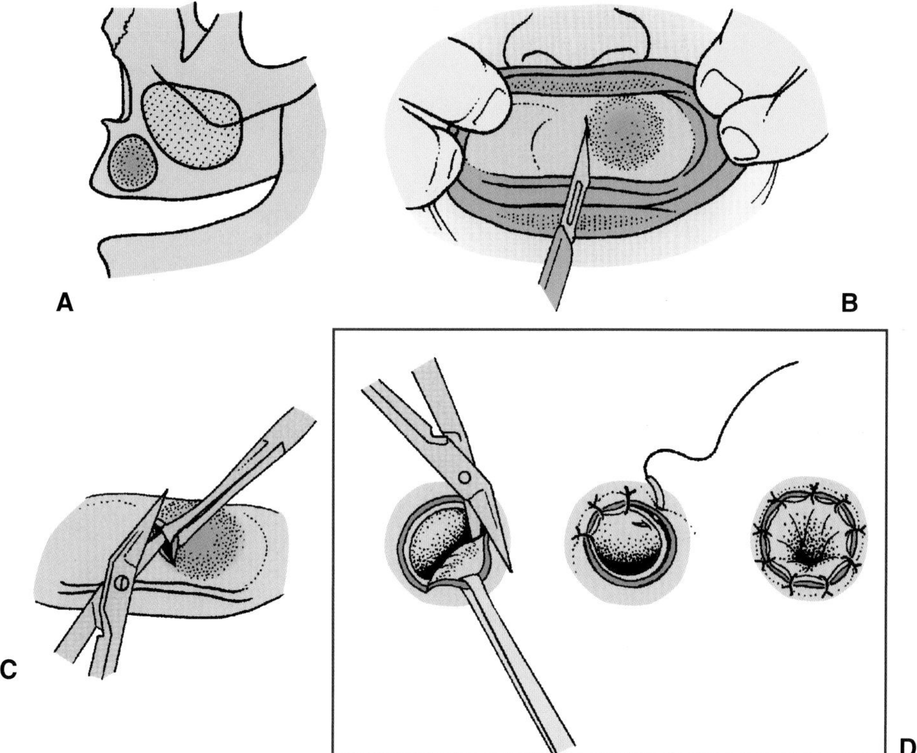

FIGURE 22-6 Marsupialization technique. A, Cyst within maxilla. B, Incision through oral mucosa and cystic wall into center of cyst. C, Scissors used to complete excision of window of mucosa and cystic wall. D, Oral mucosa and mucosa of cystic wall sutured together around periphery of opening.

cavity (Fig. 22-6). The only portion of the cyst that is removed is the piece removed to produce the window. The remaining cystic lining is left in situ. This process decreases intracystic pressure and promotes shrinkage of the cyst and bone fill. Marsupialization can be used as the sole therapy for a cyst or as a preliminary step in management, with enucleation deferred until later.

Indications

The following factors should be considered before deciding whether a cyst should be removed by marsupialization:

1. *Amount of tissue injury.* Proximity of a cyst to vital structures can mean unnecessary sacrifice of tissue if enucleation is used. For example, if enucleation of a cyst would create oronasal or oroantral fistulae or cause injury to major neurovascular structures (e.g., the inferior alveolar nerve) or devitalization of healthy teeth, marsupialization should be considered.
2. *Surgical access.* If access to all portions of the cyst is difficult, portions of the cystic wall may be left behind, which could result in recurrence. Marsupialization should therefore be considered.
3. *Assistance in eruption of teeth.* If an unerupted tooth that is needed in the dental arch is involved with the cyst (i.e., a dentigerous cyst), marsupialization may allow its continued eruption into the oral cavity (Fig. 22-7).
4. *Extent of surgery.* In an unhealthy or debilitated patient, marsupialization is a reasonable alternative to enucleation because it is simple and may be less stressful for the patient.
5. *Size of cyst.* In very large cysts, a risk of jaw fracture during enucleation is possible. It may be better to perform marsupialization of the cyst and defer enucleation until after considerable bone fill has occurred.

Advantages

The main advantage of marsupialization is that it is a simple procedure to perform. Marsupialization may also spare vital structures from damage should immediate enucleation be attempted.

Disadvantages

The major disadvantage of marsupialization is that pathologic tissue is left in situ, without thorough histologic examination. Although the tissue taken in the window can be submitted for pathologic examination, a more aggressive lesion may be present in the residual tissue. Another disadvantage is that the patient is inconvenienced in several respects. The cystic cavity must be kept clean to prevent infection because the cavity frequently traps food debris. In most instances, this means that the patient must irrigate the cavity several times every day with a syringe. This may continue for several months, depending on the size of the cystic cavity and the rate of bone fill.

Technique

Prophylactic administration of systemic antibiotics is not usually indicated in marsupialization, although antibiotics should be used if the patient's health condition warrants it (see Chapters 1 and 2). After anesthetization of the area, the cyst is aspirated as discussed in Chapter 20. If the aspirate confirms the presumptive diagnosis of a cyst, the marsupialization procedure may proceed (Fig. 22-8). The initial incision is usually

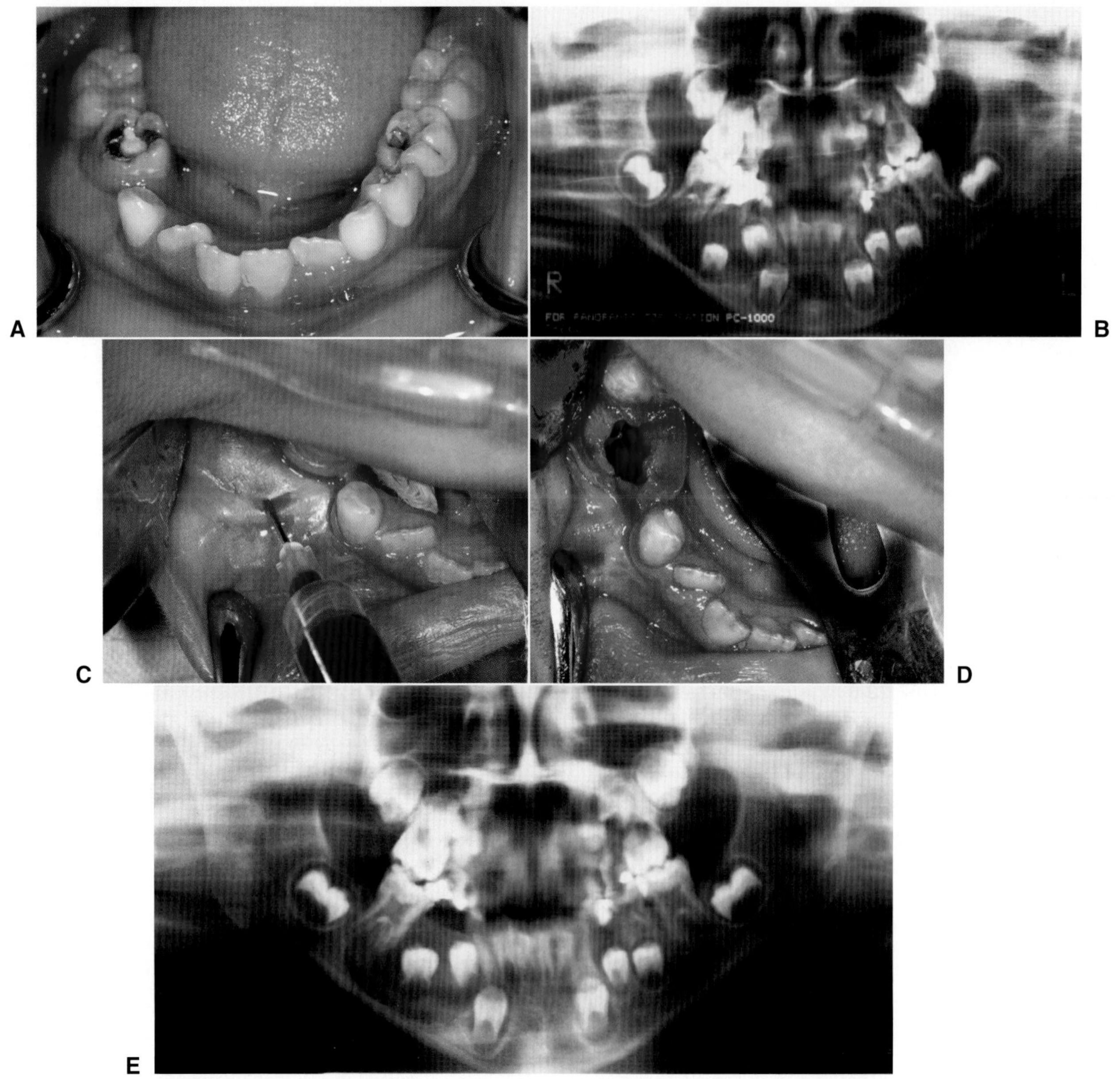

FIGURE 22-7 Marsupialization of cyst in right mandible associated with unerupted teeth. **A**, Photograph showing swelling around right second deciduous molar. **B**, Radiographic appearance before marsupialization. Note the large radiolucent lesion and displacement of the second right premolar toward the inferior border (compare to opposite side). Cystectomy would probably injure or necessitate the removal of the premolars, so it was decided to perform marsupialization of the cyst instead. **C**, Aspiration performed to determine whether the lesion was fluid filled (cystic). **D**, The lower right deciduous second molar was removed and the cyst was opened through the socket (decompressed). **E**, Panoramic radiograph taken 5 months after surgery showing bone fill and eruption of the premolars.

circular or elliptical and creates a large (1 cm or larger) window into the cystic cavity. If the bone has been expanded and thinned by the cyst, the initial incision may extend through the bone into the cystic cavity. If this is the case, the tissue contents of the window are submitted for pathologic examination. If the overlying bone is thick, an osseous window is removed carefully with burs and rongeurs. The cyst is then incised to remove a window of the lining, which is submitted for pathologic examination. The contents of the cyst are evacuated, and if possible, visual examination of the residual lining of the cyst is undertaken. Irrigation of the cyst removes any residual fragments of debris. *Areas of ulceration or thickening of the cystic wall should alert the clinician to the possibility of dysplastic or neoplastic changes in the wall of the cyst.* In this instance, enucleation of the entire cyst or incisional biopsy of the suspicious area or areas should be undertaken. If the cystic lining is thick enough and if access permits, the perimeter of the cystic wall around the window can be sutured to the oral mucosa.

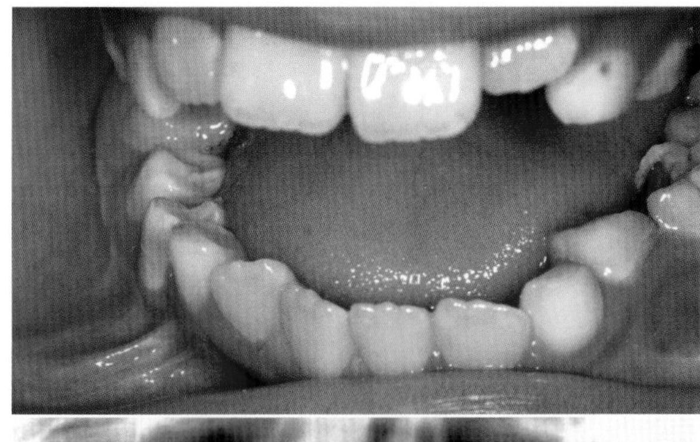

F

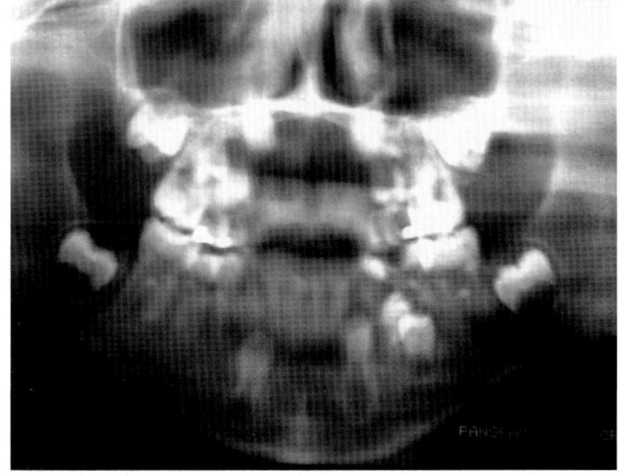

G

FIGURE 22-7, cont'd Marsupialization of cyst in right mandible associated with unerupted teeth. F, Clinical photograph taken 1 year after surgery. Both premolars have erupted. G, Panoramic radiograph taken at 1 year showing the complete fill of the bone defect and eruption of the premolars.

Otherwise, the cavity should be packed with strip gauze impregnated with tincture of benzoin or an antibiotic ointment. This packing must be left in place for 10 to 14 days to prevent the oral mucosa from healing over the cystic window. By 2 weeks the lining of the cyst should be healed to the oral mucosa around the periphery of the window. Careful instructions to the patient regarding cleansing of the cavity are necessary.

With marsupialization of cysts of the maxilla, the clinician has two choices of where the cyst will brought to the exterior: (1) the cyst may be surgically opened into the oral cavity, as just described, or (2) into the maxillary sinus or nasal cavity. For cysts that have destroyed a large portion of the maxilla and encroached on the antrum or nasal cavity, the cyst may be approached from the facial aspect of the alveolus, as just described. Once a window into the cyst has been made, a second unroofing can be widely performed into the adjacent maxillary antrum or nasal cavity. (If access permits, the entire cyst can be enucleated at this point, which allows the cystic cavity to become lined with respiratory epithelium that migrates from the adjoining maxillary sinus or nasal cavity.) The oral opening is then closed and permitted to heal. The cystic lining is thereby continuous with the lining of the antrum or nasal cavity.

Marsupialization is rarely used as the sole form of treatment for cysts. In most instances, enucleation is done after marsupialization. In the case of a dentigerous cyst, however, there may not be any residual cyst to remove once the tooth has erupted into the dental arch. In addition, if further surgery is contraindicated because of concomitant medical problems, marsupialization may be performed without future enucleation. The cavity may or may not obliterate totally with time. If it is kept clean, the cavity should not become a problem.

Enucleation After Marsupialization

Enucleation is frequently done (at a later date) after marsupialization. Initial healing is rapid after marsupialization, but the size of the cavity may not decrease appreciably past a certain point. The objectives of the marsupialization procedure have been accomplished at this time, and a secondary enucleation may be undertaken without injury to adjacent structures. The combined approach reduces morbidity and accelerates complete healing of the defect.

Indications

The indications for this combined modality of surgical therapy are the same as those listed for the technique of marsupialization. These indications are predicated on a thorough evaluation of the amount of tissue injury enucleation would cause, the degree of access for enucleation, whether impacted teeth associated with the cyst would benefit from eruptional guidance with marsupialization, the medical condition of the patient, and the size of the lesion. However, if the cyst does not totally obliterate after marsupialization, enucleation should be considered. Another indication for enucleation of a cyst after marsupialization is a cystic cavity that the patient is finding difficult to cleanse. The clinician may also desire to examine the entire lesion histologically.

Advantages

The advantages of combined marsupialization and enucleation are the same as those listed for marsupialization *and* enucleation. In the marsupialization phase the advantage is that this is a simple procedure that spares adjacent vital structures. In the enucleation phase the entire lesion becomes available for histologic examination. Another advantage is the development of a thickened cystic lining, which makes the secondary enucleation an easier procedure.

Disadvantages

The disadvantages of this modality of surgical intervention are the same as those for marsupialization. The total cyst is not removed initially for pathologic examination. However, subsequent enucleation may then detect any occult pathologic condition.

Technique

First, marsupialization of the cyst takes place, and osseous healing is allowed to progress. Once the cyst has decreased to a size that makes it amenable to complete surgical removal, enucleation is performed as the definitive treatment. The appropriate time for enucleation is when bone is covering adjacent vital structures, which prevents their injury during enucleation, and when adequate bone fill has provided enough strength to the jaw to prevent fracture during enucleation.

The initial incisions for enucleation of the cyst differ, however, from those when marsupialization of the cyst does not take place first. The cyst has a common epithelial lining with the oral cavity after marsupialization. The window initially made into the cyst contains the epithelial bridge between the cystic cavity and the oral cavity. This epithelium *must* be

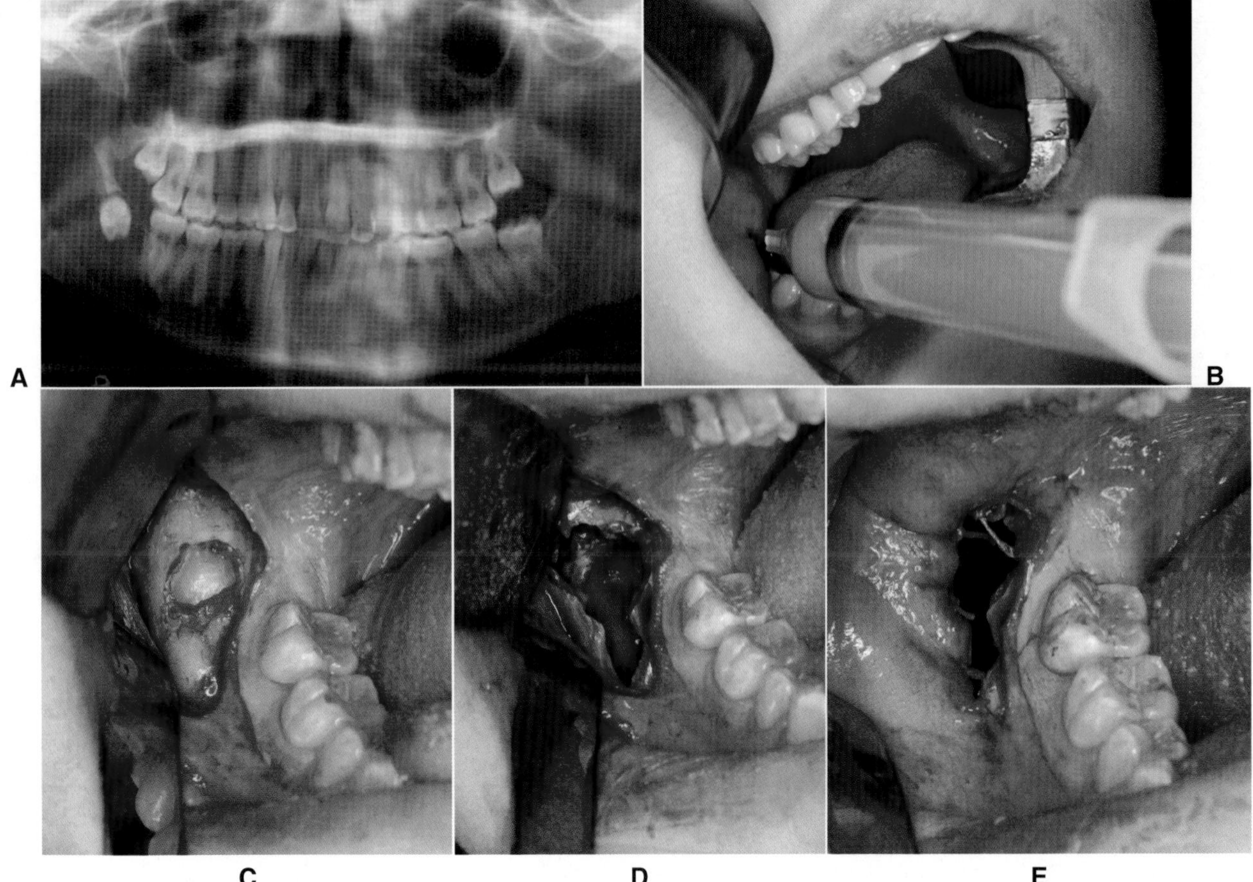

FIGURE 22-8 Marsupialization of an odontogenic keratocyst in right mandible associated with an impacted third molar. A, Panoramic radiograph showing large multilocular radiolucent lesion associated with tooth No.32. B, Aspiration of the lesion reveals creamy liquid (keratin). C, Exposure and removal of bone behind second molar reveals the impacted third molar crown. The impacted tooth was removed and additional bone was removed to provide a large window into the lesion (D). A portion of the lining was excised and sent for pathologic examination. The cavity was inspected through the opening to ensure there was no solid mass that might indicate tumor. E, Holes were drilled around the periphery of the bony opening to pass sutures from the oral mucosa, through the holes in the bone, and through the cyst lining. This provided a stable opening from the oral cavity into the cyst.

removed completely with the cystic lining; an elliptical incision completely encircling the window must be made down to sound bone. The clinician then has the opportunity to begin stripping the cyst from the window into the cystic cavity. The plane of dissection is easily established with this approach, and the cyst can be enucleated without difficulty.

Once the cyst has been enucleated, the oral soft tissues must be closed over the defect, if possible, which may require the development and mobilization of soft tissue flaps that can be advanced and sutured in a watertight manner over the osseous window. If complete closure of the wound cannot be achieved, packing the cavity with strip gauze impregnated with an antibiotic ointment is acceptable. This packing must be changed repeatedly with cleansing of the cavity until granulation tissue has obliterated the opening and epithelium has closed over the wound.

Enucleation with Curettage

Enucleation with curettage means that after enucleation a curette or bur is used to remove 1 to 2 mm of bone around the entire periphery of the cystic cavity. This is done to remove any remaining epithelial cells that may be present in the periphery of the cystic wall or bony cavity. These cells could proliferate into a recurrence of the cyst.

Indications

The clinician should perform curettage with enucleation in two instances: The first instance is if the clinician is removing an odontogenic keratocyst. In this case the more aggressive approach of enucleation with curettage should be used because odontogenic keratocysts exhibit aggressive clinical behavior and a considerably high rate of recurrence.[1] Reported recurrence rates have been between 20% and 60%.[2] Reasons for locally aggressive behavior are based on the increased mitotic activities and cellularity of the epithelium of the odontogenic keratocyst.[3-5] Daughter, or satellite, cysts found in the periphery of the main cystic lesion may be incompletely removed, which contributes to the increased rate of recurrence. The cystic lining is usually very thin and readily fragmented, making thorough enucleation difficult. Therefore, when an odontogenic keratocyst is clinically suspected, the minimal treatment should be careful enucleation with aggressive curettage of the bony cavity.

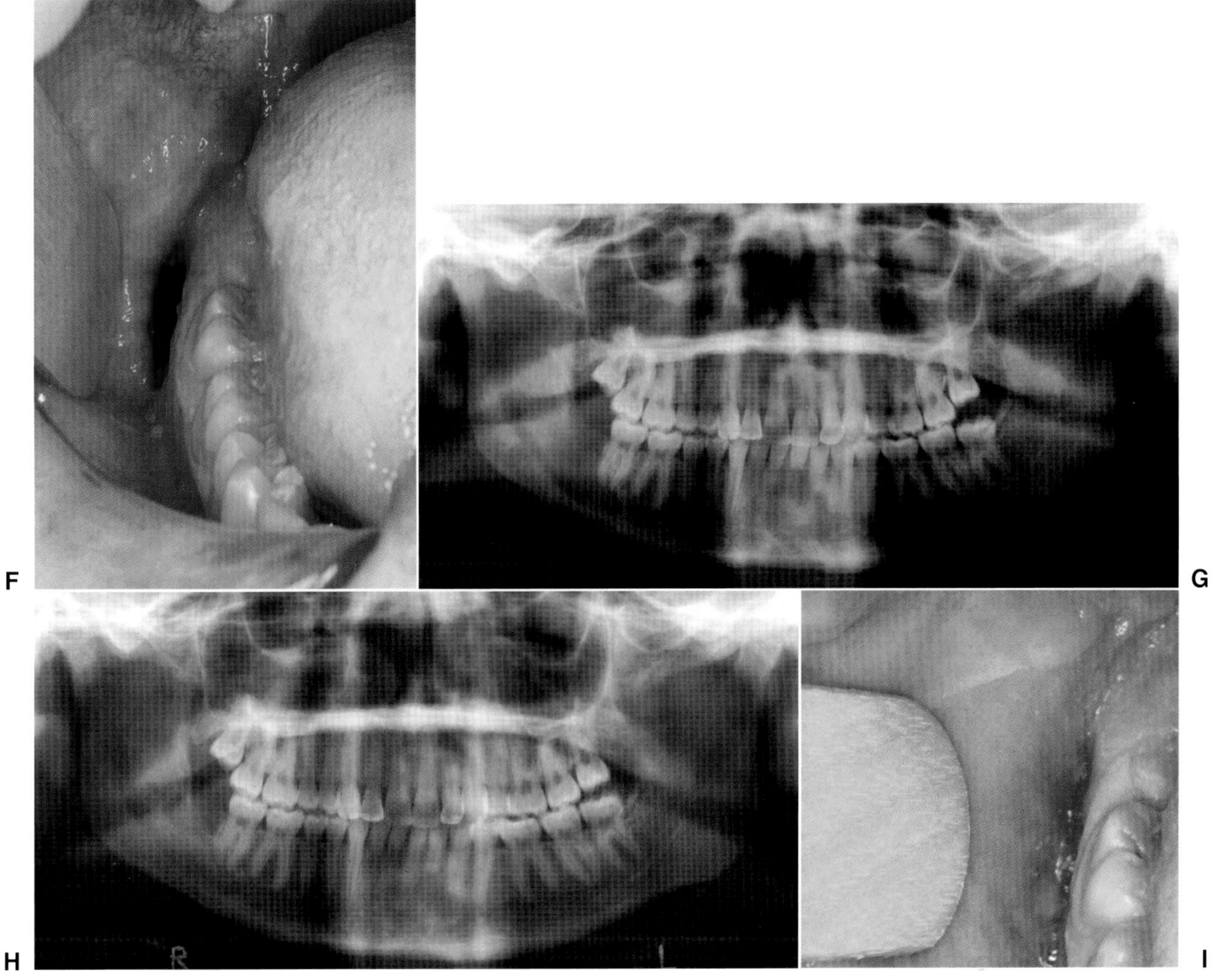

FIGURE 22-8, cont'd Marsupialization of an odontogenic keratocyst in right mandible associated with an impacted third molar. **F**, Patent opening into the cavity 1 month after surgery. Panoramic radiographs taken at 5 (**G**) and 10 (**H**) months after surgery show bone fill. **I**, By 10 months, the opening into the cyst has completely closed.

Should the lesion recur, treatment must be predicated on the following factors: If the area is accessible, another attempt at enucleation could be undertaken; if inaccessible, bony resection with 1-cm margins should be considered. Whatever the treatment, the patient must be followed closely for recurrence because odontogenic keratocysts have recurred years after treatment.

The second instance in which enucleation with curettage is indicated is with any cyst that recurs after what was deemed a thorough removal. The reasons for curettage in this case are the same as those outlined previously.

Advantages

If enucleation leaves epithelial remnants, curettage may remove them, thereby decreasing the likelihood of recurrence.

Disadvantages

Curettage is more destructive of adjacent bone and other tissues. The dental pulps may be stripped of their neurovascular supply when curettage is performed close to the root tips. Adjacent neurovascular bundles can be similarly damaged. Curettage must always be performed with great care to avoid these hazards.

Technique

After the cyst has been enucleated and removed, the bony cavity is inspected for proximity to adjacent structures. A sharp curette or a bone bur with sterile irrigation can be used to remove a 1- to 2-mm layer of bone around the complete periphery of the cystic cavity. This should be done with extreme care when working proximal to important anatomic structures. The cavity is then cleansed and closed.

PRINCIPLES OF SURGICAL MANAGEMENT OF JAW TUMORS

A discussion of the surgical management of jaw tumors is made easier by the fact that many tumors behave similarly and therefore can be treated in a similar manner. The three main modalities of surgical excision of jaw tumors are (1)

BOX 22-1

Types of Surgical Operations Used for the Removal of Jaw Tumors

A. Enucleation and/or curettage: Local removal of tumor by instrumentation in direct contact with the lesion; used for very benign types of lesions
B. Resection: Removal of a tumor by incising through uninvolved tissues around the tumor, thus delivering the tumor without direct contact during instrumentation (also known as en bloc resection)
   1. Marginal (i.e., segmental) resection: Resection of a tumor without disruption of the continuity of the bone
   2. Partial resection: Resection of a tumor by removing a full-thickness portion of the jaw (In the mandible, this can vary from a small continuity defect to a hemimandibulectomy. Jaw continuity is disrupted.)
   3. Total resection: Resection of a tumor by removal of the involved bone (e.g., maxillectomy and mandibulectomy)
   4. Composite resection: Resection of a tumor with bone, adjacent soft tissues, and contiguous lymph node channels (This is an ablative procedure used most commonly for malignant tumors.)

enucleation (with or without curettage), (2) marginal (i.e., segmental) or partial resection, and (3) composite resection (Box 22-1). Many benign tumors behave nonaggressively and are therefore treated conservatively with enucleation, curettage, or both (Table 22-1).

Another group of benign oral tumors behaves more aggressively and requires margins of uninvolved tissue to lessen the chance of recurrence. Marginal (i.e., segmental) or partial resection is used for removal of these lesions (Fig. 22-9). The last group of tumors includes the malignant varieties. These tumors require more radical intervention, with wider margins of uninvolved tissue. Surgery may include the removal of adjacent soft tissues and dissection of lymph nodes. Radiotherapy, chemotherapy, or both, alone or in addition to surgery, may be used.

Besides cysts, the most common jaw lesions the dentist encounters, are inflammatory or are benign neoplasms. Most of these cysts lend themselves to removal by simple excisional biopsy techniques. However, more aggressive lesions are occasionally encountered, and several factors must be used to determine the most appropriate type of therapy. The most important of these factors is the aggressiveness of the lesion. Other factors that must be evaluated before surgery are the anatomic location of the lesion, its confinement to bone, the duration of the lesion, and the possible methods for reconstruction after surgery.

Aggressiveness of Lesion

Surgical therapy of oral lesions ranges from enucleation or curettage to composite resection. Histologic diagnosis positively identifies and therefore directs the treatment of the lesion. Because of the wide range in behavior of oral lesions, the prognosis is related more to the histologic diagnosis, which indicates the biologic behavior of the lesion, than to any other single factor.

TABLE 22-1

Types of Jaw Tumors and Primary Treatment Modalities

Enucleation and/or Curettage	Marginal or Partial Resection	Composite Resection*
ODONTOGENIC TUMORS		
Odontoma	Ameloblastoma	Malignant ameloblastoma
Ameloblastic fibroma	Calcifying epithelial odontogenic tumor	Ameloblastic fibrosarcoma
Ameloblastic fibroodontoma		Ameloblastic odontosarcoma
Adenomatoid odontogenic tumor	Myxoma	Primary intraosseous carcinoma
Calcifying odontogenic cyst	Ameloblastic odontoma	
Cementoblastoma	Squamous odontogenic tumor	
Central cementifying fibroma		
FIBROOSSEOUS LESIONS		
Central ossifying fibroma	Benign chondroblastoma	Fibrosarcoma
Fibrous dysplasia (if necessary)		Osteosarcoma
Cherubism (if necessary)		Chondrosarcoma
Central giant cell granuloma		Ewing's sarcoma
Aneurysmal bone cyst		
Osteoma		
Osteoid osteoma		
Osteoblastoma		
OTHER LESIONS		
Hemangioma	Hemangioma	Lymphomas
Eosinophilic granuloma		Intraosseous salivary gland malignancies
Neurilemmoma		Neurofibrosarcoma
Neurofibroma		Carcinoma that has invaded jaw
Pigmented neuroectodermal tumor		

Note: These are generalities. Treatment is individualized for each patient and each lesion.
*These lesions are malignancies and may be treated variably. For lesions totally within the jaw, partial resection may be performed without adjacent soft tissue and lymph node dissections. Radiotherapy and chemotherapy may also play a role in the overall therapy.

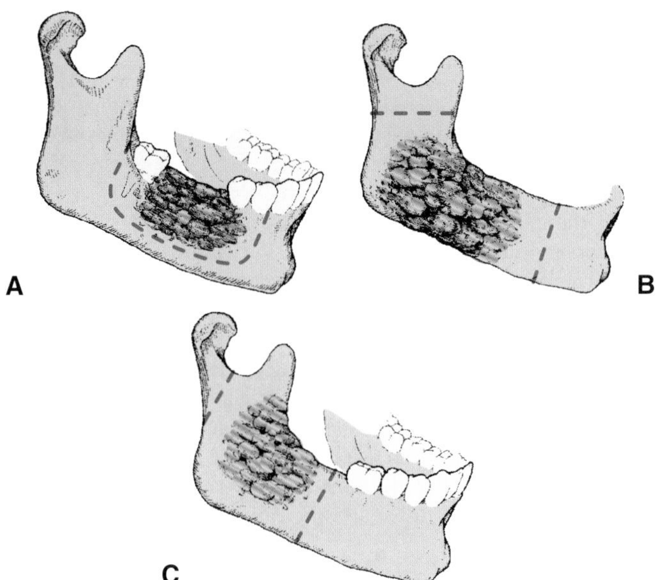

FIGURE 22-9 Common types of mandibular resection. A, Marginal or segmental resection, which does not disrupt mandibular continuity. B and C, Partial mandibular resections, which disrupt mandibular continuity. Attempts to leave mandibular condyle to facilitate reconstruction are demonstrated.

Anatomic Location of Lesion

The location of a lesion within the mouth or perioral areas may severely complicate surgical excision and therefore jeopardize the prognosis. A nonaggressive, benign lesion in an inaccessible area, such as the pterygomaxillary fissure, presents an obvious surgical problem. Conversely, a more aggressive lesion in an easily accessible and resectable area, such as the anterior mandible, often offers a better prognosis.

Maxilla Versus Mandible

Another important consideration with some oral lesions, such as the more aggressive odontogenic tumors and carcinomas, is whether they are within the mandible or the maxilla. The adjacent maxillary sinuses and nasopharynx allow tumors of the maxilla to grow asymptomatically to large sizes, with symptoms occurring late. Thus maxillary tumors produce a poorer prognosis than those within the mandible.

Proximity to Adjacent Vital Structures

The proximity of benign lesions to adjacent neurovascular structures and teeth is an important consideration because preservation of these structures should be attempted. Frequently, the apices of adjacent tooth roots are completely uncovered during a surgical procedure. The dental pulps are stripped of their blood supply. These teeth should be considered for endodontic treatment to prevent an odontogenic infection, which would complicate healing and jeopardize the success of bone grafts placed in an adjacent area.

Size of Tumor

The amount of involvement within a particular site, such as the body of the mandible, has a bearing on the type of surgical procedure necessary to obtain a cure with the more aggressive lesions. When possible, the inferior border of the mandible is left intact to maintain continuity. This can be accomplished by marginal resection of the involved area. When the tumor extends through the entire thickness of the involved jaw, a partial resection becomes mandatory.

Intraosseous Versus Extraosseous Location

An aggressive oral lesion confined to the interior of the jaw, without perforation of the cortical plates, offers a better prognosis than one that has invaded surrounding soft tissues. Invasion of soft tissues indicates a more aggressive tumor, which, because of its presence in soft tissues, makes complete removal more difficult and sacrifices more normal tissues. In the latter case the soft tissue in the area of the perforation should be locally excised. A supraperiosteal excision of the involved jaw should be undertaken if the cortical plate has been thinned to the point of being eggshell thick without obvious perforation.

Duration of Lesion

Several oral tumors exhibit slow growth and may become static. The odontomas, for example, may be discovered in the second decade of life, and their size may remain unchanged for many years. The slower-growing lesions seem to follow a more benign course, and treatment should be individually tailored to each case.

Reconstructive Efforts

As previously noted, the goal of any surgical procedure to remove a pathologic lesion should be not only the eradication of disease but also the facilitation of the patient's functional well-being. Thus reconstructive procedures should be planned and anticipated *before* initial surgery is performed. Frequently, the goals of reconstruction dictate a surgical technique that is just as effective as another technique in the removal of the disease but more optimal for facilitating future reconstructive efforts.

Jaw Tumors Treated with Enucleation, Curettage, or Both

Most jaw tumors with a low rate of recurrence can be treated with enucleation or curettage: for example, most of the odontogenic tumors, including odontomas, ameloblastic fibromas, ameloblastic fibroodontomas, keratinizing and calcifying odontogenic cysts, adenomatoid odontogenic tumors, cementoblastomas, and central cementifying (i.e., ossifying) fibromas. Table 22-1 lists other lesions that are treated in this manner.

Technique

The technique for enucleation or curettage of jaw tumors is not unlike that described for cysts. However, additional procedures, such as sectioning large calcified masses with burs in odontomas and cementomas, may be required. In these instances, the principles discussed in Chapter 9 for the removal of impacted teeth are used.

Jaw Tumors Treated with Marginal or Partial Resection

When the lesion is known to be aggressive, by histopathologic determination or by its clinical behavior, or it is of such a consistency that total removal by enucleation, curettage, or both would be difficult, removal may be facilitated by resecting the lesion with adequate bony margins. Odontogenic lesions treated in this manner are the ameloblastoma, the odontogenic myxoma (i.e., fibromyxomas), the calcifying epithelial odontogenic tumor (i.e., Pindborg), the squamous odontogenic tumor, and the ameloblastic odontoma. Table 22-1 lists other lesions treated in this manner.

Technique

As a general principle the resected specimen should include the lesion and 1-cm bony margins around the radiographic boundaries of the lesion. If this can be achieved with the inferior border of the mandible left intact, marginal resection is the preferred method. Reconstruction then is limited to replacing the lost osseous structure, including the alveolus (Fig. 22-10). If the lesion is close to the inferior border, the full thickness of the mandible must be included in the specimen, which disrupts mandibular continuity (Fig. 22-11). Reconstruction in this instance is much more difficult because the remaining mandibular fragments must be secured in their proper relationship to one another for proper function and symmetry to be restored.

The surgical technique for marginal (i.e., segmental) resection is straightforward. A full-thickness mucoperiosteal flap is developed and stripped from the bone to be removed. Air-driven surgical saws or burs are then used to section the bone in the planned locations, and the segment is removed. Whenever marginal or partial resection is used, the clinician must determine whether the tumor has perforated the cortical plates and invaded adjacent soft tissues, in which case it is necessary to sacrifice a layer of soft tissue to eradicate the tumor, and a supraperiosteal dissection of the involved bone is performed. Immediate reconstruction is more difficult because there may not be enough remaining soft tissues to close over bone grafts.

If the clinician is concerned about the adequacy of the soft tissue surgical margins around a lesion when surgery is being performed in a hospital setting, specimens along the margins can be removed and sent immediately to the pathologist for histopathologic examination. This process is performed in approximately 20 minutes by freezing the tissue in liquid carbon dioxide or nitrogen and then sectioning and staining the tissue for immediate examination. The accuracy of frozen-section examination is good when used for detecting adequacy of surgical margins. However, such examination is less accurate when trying to diagnose a lesion histopathologically for the first time.

MALIGNANT TUMORS OF THE ORAL CAVITY

Malignancies of the oral cavity may arise from a variety of tissues, such as salivary gland, muscle, and blood vessels, or may even present as metastases from distant sites. Most common, however, are epidermoid carcinomas of the oral mucosa, which are the form of cancer that the dentist is in a position to discover first by doing thorough oral examinations. The

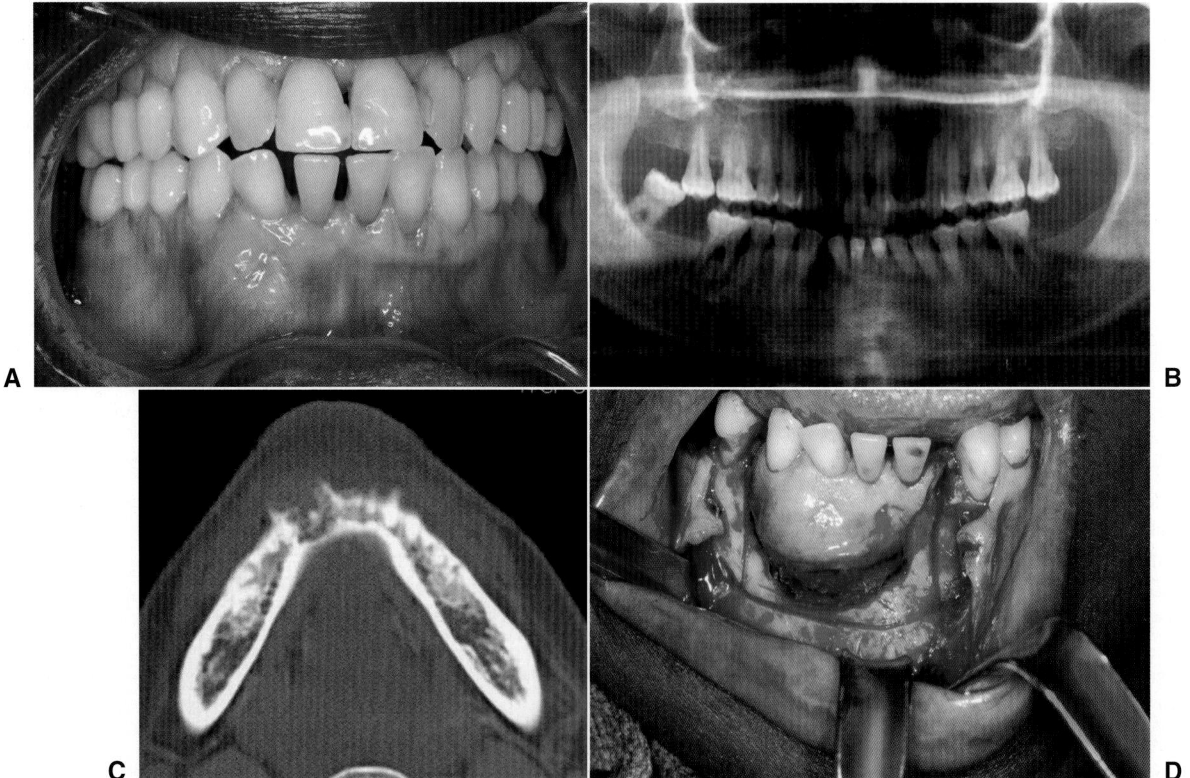

FIGURE 22-10 Marginal (or segmental resection) of ameloblastoma. **A**, Preoperative photograph showing swelling of anterior mandible around roots of teeth. Panoramic radiograph (**B**) shows spacing of the roots from an ill-defined radiolucency. **C**, Computed tomographic scan shows an exophytic lesion that seems to be coming out of bone. **D**, Intraoral exposure of mandible and osseous cuts made around lesion. The inferior border was left intact.

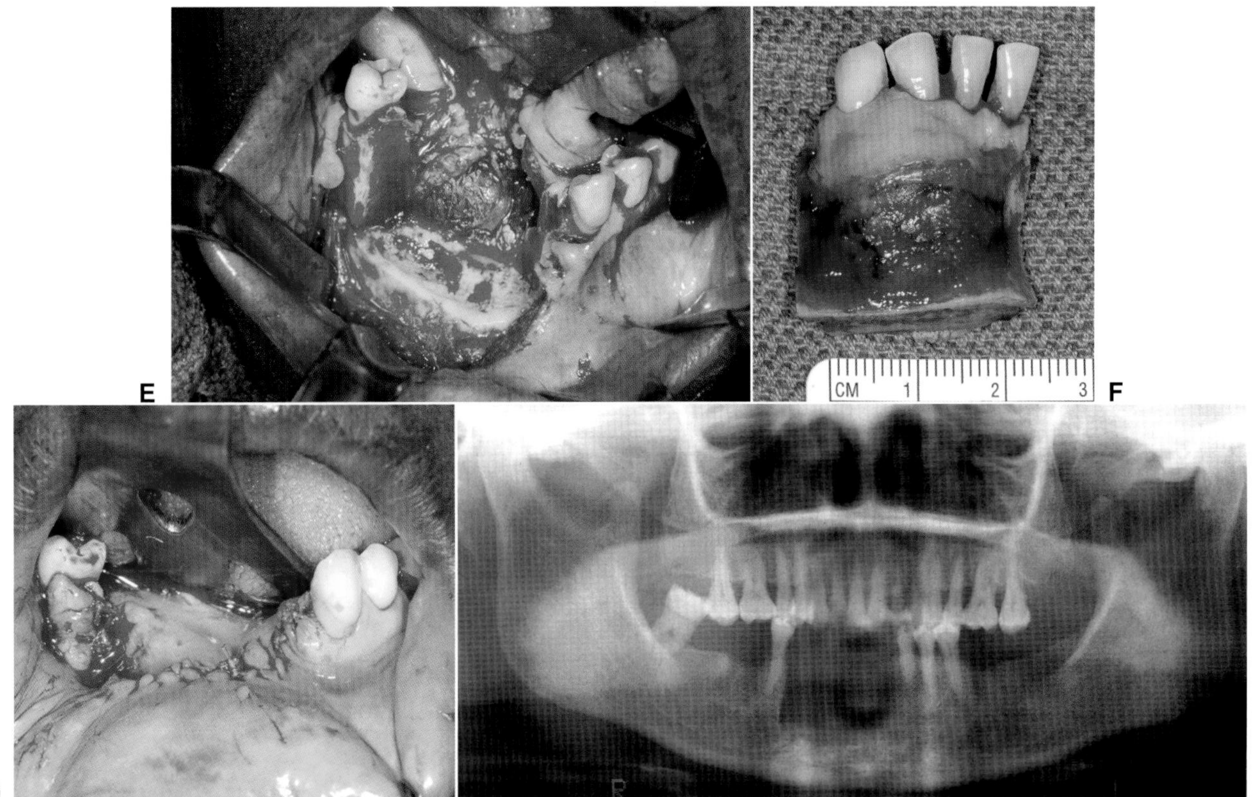

FIGURE 22-10, cont'd E, Intraoral defect after removal of lesion. Height of bone along the inferior border was sufficient to maintain continuity of the mandible. Bony reconstruction of the alveolar process was delayed until a later date. F, Surgical specimen. G, Appearance of the defect after soft tissue closure. H, Panoramic radiograph taken after surgery.

seriousness of an oral malignancy can vary from the necessity for a simple excisional biopsy to composite jaw resection with neck dissection (i.e., removal of the lymph nodes and other visceral structures adjacent to lymph node channels in neck) to affect a cure. Because of the variation in clinical presentation, *clinical staging* is usually undertaken before a treatment plan is formulated.

Clinical staging refers to assessing the extent of the disease before undertaking treatment and has as two purposes: (1) selection of the best treatment, and (2) meaningful comparison of the end results reported from different sources. Clinical staging of the lesion is performed for several varieties of oral malignancies, including epidermoid carcinomas and oral lymphomas. Staging is performed differently for each type of malignancy and may involve extensive diagnostic tests, such as radiographs, blood tests, and even surgical exploration of other body areas to evaluate the extent of possible tumor metastasis. Once the tumor is staged, treatment is formulated. Several types of malignancies have well-defined treatment protocols that have been designed by surgeons and oncologists in an effort to study the effectiveness of treatment regimens more carefully.

Treatment Modalities for Malignancies

Malignancies of the oral cavity are treated with surgery, radiation, chemotherapy, or a combination of these modalities. The treatment for any given case depends on several factors, including the histopathologic diagnosis, the location of the tumor, the presence and degree of metastasis, the radiosensitivity or chemosensitivity of the tumor, the age and general physical condition of the patient, the experience of the treating clinicians, and the wishes of the patient. In general, if a lesion can be completely excised without mutilating the patient, this is the preferred modality. If spread to regional lymph nodes is suspected, radiation may be used before or after surgery to help eliminate small foci of malignant cells in the adjacent areas. If widespread systemic metastasis is detected or if a tumor, such as a lymphoma, is especially chemosensitive, chemotherapy is used with or without surgery and radiation.

Currently, malignancies are often treated in an institution where several specialists evaluate each case and discuss treatment regimens. These "tumor boards" include at least a surgeon, a chemotherapist, and a radiotherapist. Most head and neck tumor boards also include a general dentist, a maxillofacial prosthodontist, a nutritionist, a speech pathologist, and a sociologist or psychiatrist.

Radiotherapy

Radiotherapy for treatment of malignant neoplasms is based on the fact that tumor cells in stages of active growth are more susceptible to ionizing radiation than adult tissue. The faster the cells are multiplying or the more undifferentiated the tumor cells, the more likely that radiation is to be effective. Radiation prevents the cells from multiplying by interfering with their nuclear material. Normal host cells are also affected by radiation and must be protected as much as possible during treatment.

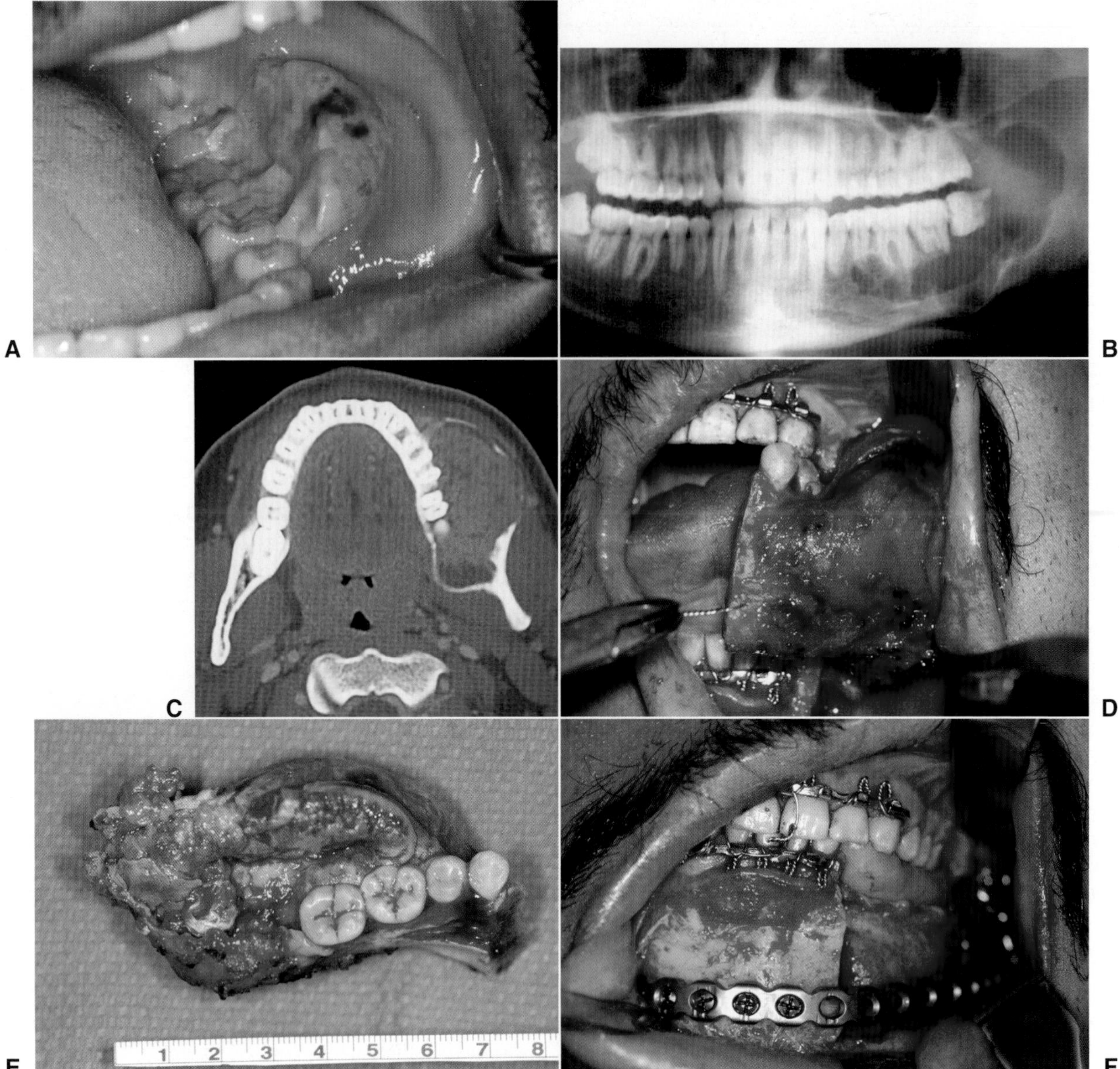

FIGURE 22-11 Partial mandibular resection for ameloblastoma. **A**, Photograph of lesion in the left mandibular molar area. **B**, Panoramic radiographic appearance on initial presentation showing multilocular radiolucency associated with an impacted tooth. Incision biopsy proved lesion to be an ameloblastoma. **C**, Computed tomographic scan showing extent of lesion. **D**, Photograph of intraoral resection of tumor. **E**, Surgical specimen. **F**, Reconstruction of the mandible with a large bone plate.

Radiation can be delivered to the patient in several forms, including implantation of radioactive material into the tumor. Most commonly, however, radiation is delivered externally by the use of large x-ray generators. The amount of radiation that a person may normally tolerate is not exceeded, and adjacent uninvolved areas are spared by the use of protective shielding. Two mechanisms of delivery, fractionation and multiple ports, spare the patient's host tissues in the immediate area of the tumor.

Fractionation of the delivery of radiation means that instead of giving the maximal amount of radiation a person can withstand at one time, smaller increments of radiation (i.e., fractions) are given over several weeks, which allows the healthier normal tissues time to recover between doses. The tumor cells, however, are less able to recover between doses. The other delivery method uses *multiple ports* for radiation exposure. Instead of delivering the entire dose through one beam (i.e., port), multiple beams are used. All beams are focused on the tumor but from different angles. Thus the tumor is exposed to the entire dose of radiation. However, because different beams are used, the normal tissues in the path of the x-ray beams are spared maximal exposure and instead receive only a fraction of the tumor dose.

Chemotherapy

Chemicals that act by interfering with rapidly growing tumor cells are used for treating many types of malignancies. As with

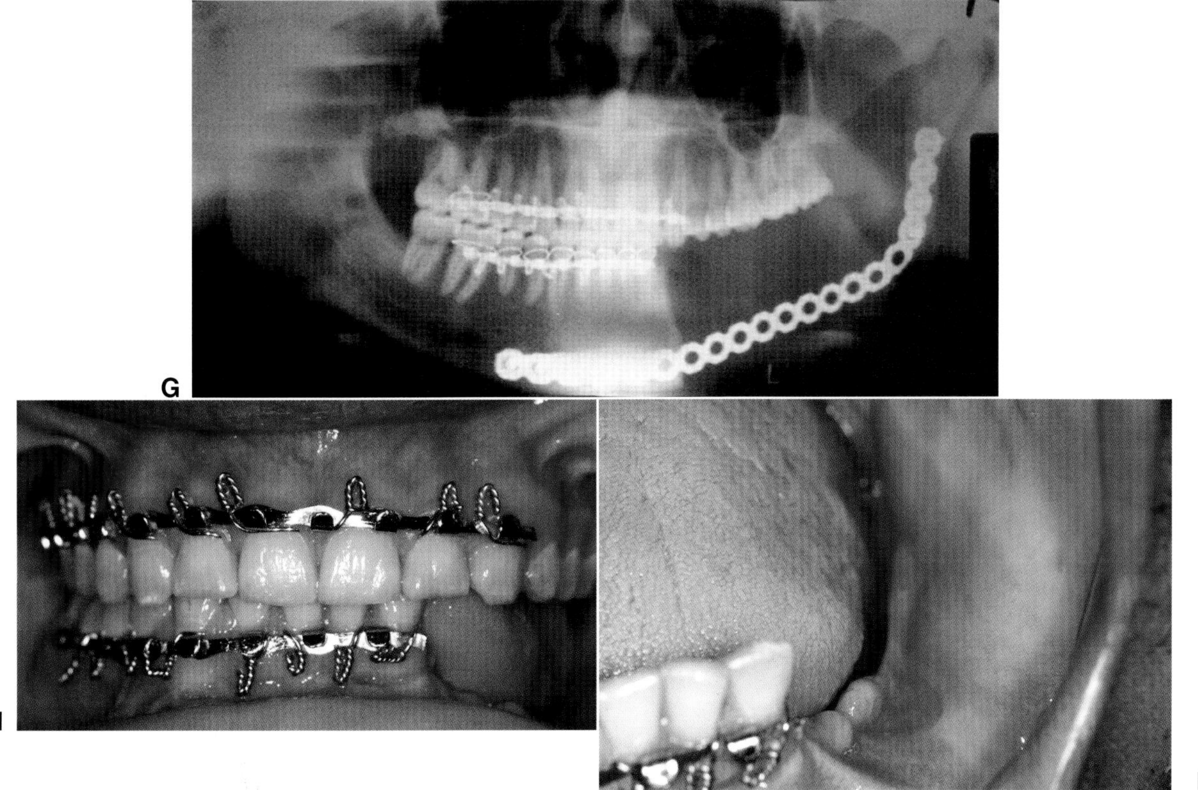

FIGURE 22-11, cont'd G, Panoramic radiograph taken after surgery showing resection margins and bone plate reconstruction. H, Occlusion and (I) intraoral appearance of patient 6 weeks postoperatively. Bony reconstruction was performed later.

radiation the chemicals are not totally selective but affect normal cells to some extent. Most of these agents are given intravenously; however, recently injections into the arteries feeding the tumor have been used. Because the agents are delivered systemically, they adversely affect many body systems; most notable is the hematopoietic system, which is considerably affected because of its rapid rate of cellular turnover. Thus patients who are undergoing chemotherapy are in a delicate balance between effectiveness in killing the tumor cells and anemia, neutropenia, and thrombocytopenia (see Chapter 18). Infections and bleeding are therefore common complications in these patients.

To reduce the toxicity of a single agent given in large quantities, multiple-agent therapy is frequently administered. Many patients are given three to five agents at the same time. Each may work at a different point in the life cycle of the tumor cell, thus increasing effectiveness with less toxicity to the host.

Surgery

The surgical procedures for excision of oral malignancies vary with the type and extent of the lesion. Small epidermoid carcinomas that are in accessible locations (e.g., the lower lip) and are not associated with palpable lymph nodes can be excised (Fig. 22-12). A larger lesion associated with palpable lymph nodes or a similar lesion in the area of the tonsillar pillar may require extensive surgery to remove it adequately with its local metastases.

Malignancies of the oral cavity that have suspected or proven lymph node involvement are candidates for composite resection in which the lesion, surrounding tissues, and lymph nodes of the neck are totally removed. This procedure may produce large defects of the jaws and extensive loss of soft tissues, which make functional and esthetic rehabilitation a long, involved process.

SURGICAL MANAGEMENT OF BENIGN LESIONS IN ORAL SOFT TISSUES

Superficial soft tissue lesions of the oral mucosa are usually benign and in most instances lend themselves to simple surgical removal using biopsy techniques (see Chapter 21). These lesions include fibromas, pyogenic granulomas, papillomas, peripheral giant cell granulomas, verruca vulgaris, mucoceles (i.e., mucous extravasation phenomena), and epulis fissurata. All of these lesions are overgrowths of the normally present histologic elements in the oral mucosa and submucosa. The principles of removal are the same as those outlined previously and include the use of elliptical, wedge type of incisions during removal. In the case of lesions that appear associated with the dentition (i.e., pyogenic granuloma), the associated tooth or teeth should be thoroughly curetted and polished to remove any plaque, calculus, or foreign material that may have played a role in the development of the lesion and that may cause a recurrence if not removed.

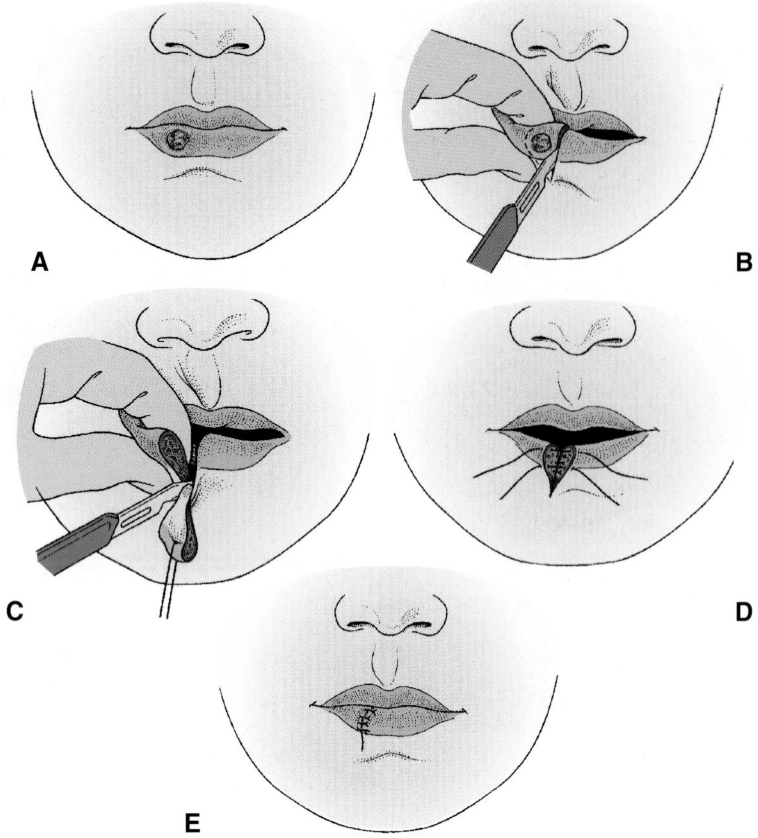

FIGURE 22-12 Local excision of lip carcinoma. A to E, Full-thickness V excision of lip.

RECONSTRUCTION OF JAW AFTER REMOVAL OF ORAL TUMORS

Osseous defects may occur after removal of oral tumors. These defects may range from loss of alveolar bone to loss of major portions of the jaw and may cause the patient concern on a functional or cosmetic basis. The treatment of oral pathologic entities should always include immediate or future plans for reconstruction that have been made *before* the surgical procedure to remove the lesion to afford the patient optimal reconstructive results.

The general dentist plays a crucial role in the functional and cosmetic rehabilitation of the patient by providing dental replacements for teeth that have been surgically removed. However, before dental rehabilitation is pursued, the underlying skeleton of the jaws should be reconstructed, if necessary. Frequently, surgical removal of a lesion involves removal of a portion of the alveolus, which presents the dentist with an obvious problem: Any bridge across the site or any complete or partial denture will have no osseous base on which to rest. In these cases the patient would be well served to undergo ridge augmentation before dental restorative treatment. This augmentation can be in the form of bone grafts, synthetic bone grafts, or a combination of these materials. Optimal dental restorations can then be completed.

When the patient has lost a portion of the maxilla, the maxillary sinuses or nasal cavity may be continuous with the oral cavity, which presents great difficulties for the patient in speaking and eating. Defects of the maxilla can be managed in one of two ways: The first is with surgery. Defects that are not excessive may be closed with available soft tissues of the buccal mucosa and palate. Bone grafts may also be used to provide the patient with a functional alveolar process. Very large defects or defects in patients who are poor surgical risks may require prosthetic obliteration in which a partial or complete denture extends into the maxillary sinus or nasal cavities and effectively partitions the mouth from these structures (Fig. 22-13).

The reconstruction of a defect caused by resection of the mandible or a portion thereof can be performed immediately (i.e., at the time of the surgical removal of the lesion) or may be delayed until a later date. In general, benign processes of the jaws are reconstructed immediately, whereas malignancies are reconstructed later. Reconstruction after the surgical removal of a malignancy is performed for several reasons. Radiation is frequently used adjunctively with surgery and may jeopardize the survival of bone grafts. Another reason for delay is that soft tissue deficits may result after removal of the malignancy, and additional soft tissues may be required before osseous reconstruction can be performed. An important reason, however, is that recurrence of the malignancy may require further ablative surgery that will negate the reconstructive efforts.

Several surgeons also delay reconstruction of defects caused by removal of benign tumors. They suggest that the presence of a simultaneous intraoral and extraoral defect, which frequently is necessary to remove the tumor, contraindicates an immediate reconstruction of the mandible. Instead, a space-

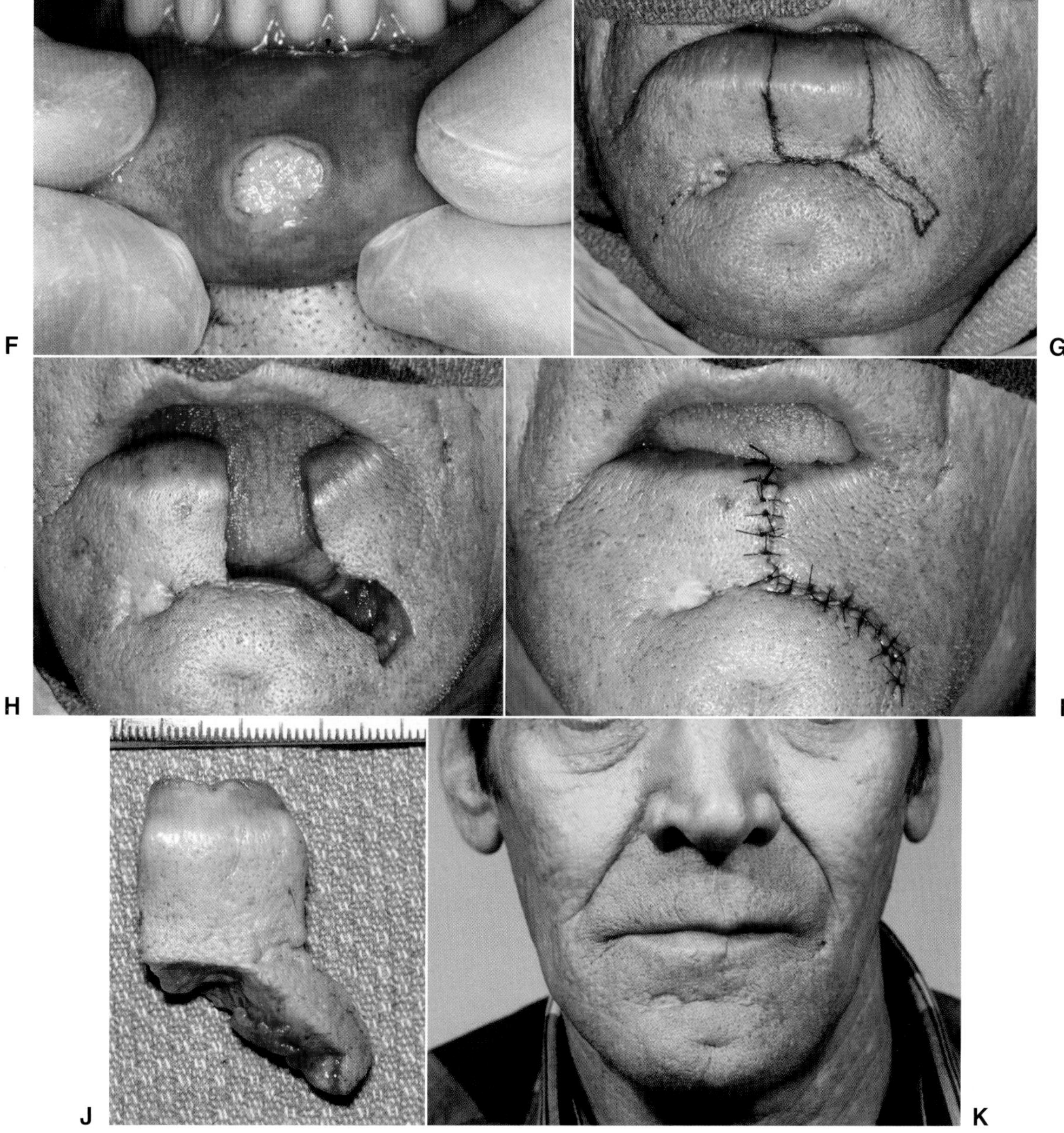

FIGURE 22-12, cont'd Local excision of lip carcinoma. F, Carcinoma of lower lip. G, Surgical incisions outlined. H, Lip after excision of specimen. I, Closure. J, Specimen. K, Appearance after healing.

maintaining device is placed at the time of resection, and a secondary reconstruction is performed weeks to months later.[6,7]

When delayed reconstruction is decided upon, consideration should be given to maintaining the residual mandibular fragments in their normal anatomic relationship with intermaxillary fixation, external pin fixation, splints, internal fixation, or a combination of these modalities. This technique prevents cicatricial and muscular deformation and displacement of the segments and simplifies secondary reconstructive efforts.

Clinical results have shown that immediate reconstruction is a viable option and has the advantages of requiring a single surgical procedure and having an early return to function with a minimal compromise to facial esthetics.[6] A possible disadvantage is loss of the graft from infection. The risk of infection may be higher when a graft is placed transorally or in an extraoral wound that was orally contaminated during the ablative surgery. Because the recurrence rate is substantial in some tumors, prudent planning and meticulous surgery are mandatory before reconstruction is attempted. These measures minimize the risk of failure as a result of recurrence. Three choices for immediate reconstruction are possible:

1. The entire surgical procedure is performed intraorally by first removing the tumor and then grafting the defect.
2. The tumor is removed by a combined intraoral and extraoral route. A watertight oral closure is obtained, which is followed immediately by grafting the defect through the extraoral incision.
3. When the tumor has not destroyed the alveolar crestal bone and when no extension of the tumor into oral soft tissues has occurred, the involved teeth are extracted. A waiting

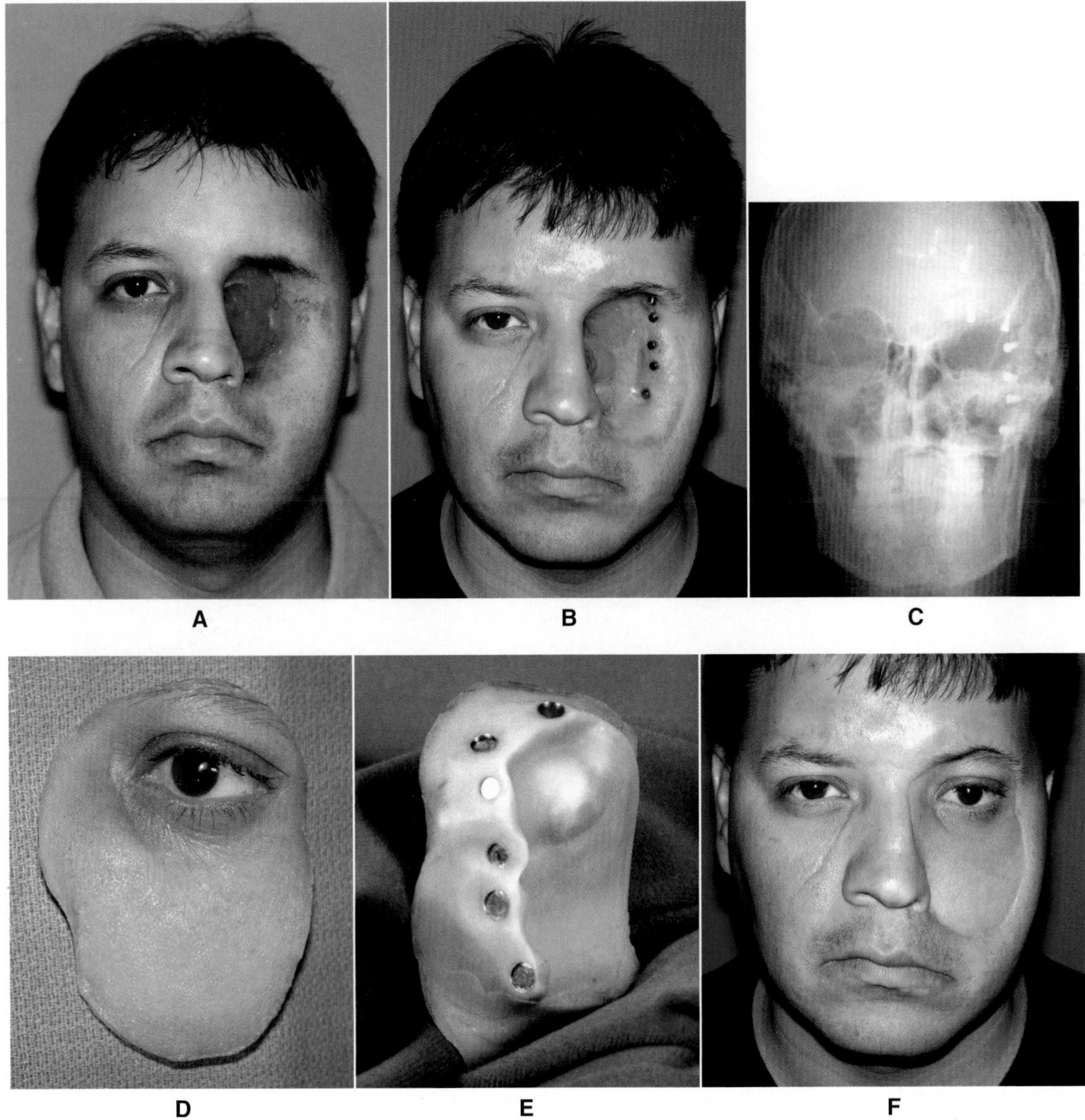

FIGURE 22-13 Maxillofacial prosthetic reconstruction of patient who had left eye and palate removed because of tumor. **A**, Photograph shows defect in palate and loss of eye. **B** and **C**, Denture with obturator. **D**, Prosthetic eye. **E**, Prosthetic denture. **F**, Patient with prosthetic eye and denture in place.

period of 6 to 8 weeks is allowed for healing of the gingival tissues. The tumor is then removed and the defect is grafted through an extraoral incision, with care taken to avoid perforation of the oral soft tissues. This procedure is the only type of *immediate* reconstruction by which oral contamination can be avoided.

REFERENCES

1. Eversole LR, Sabes WR, Rovin S: Aggressive growth and neoplastic potential of odontogenic cysts with special reference to central epidermoid and mucoepidermoid carcinomas, *Cancer* 35:270, 1975.
2. Shafer WG, Hine MK, Levy BM: *A textbook of oral pathology*, ed 4, Philadelphia, 1983, WB Saunders.
3. Main DMG: Epithelial jaw cysts: a clinicopathological reappraisal, *Br J Oral Surg* 8:114, 1970.
4. Toller PA: Autoradiography of explants from odontogenic cysts, *Br Dent J* 131:57, 1971.
5. Wysocki GP, Sapp JP: Scanning and transmission electron microscopy of odontogenic keratocysts, *Oral Surg Oral Med Oral Pathol* 40:494, 1975.
6. Adekeye EO: Reconstruction of mandibular defect by autogenous bone grafts: a review of 37 cases, *J Oral Surg* 36:125, 1978.
7. Kluft O, Van Dop F: Mandibular ameloblastoma (resection with primary reconstruction): a case report with concise review of the literature, *Arch Chir Neerl* 28:289, 1976.

PART VI

Oral and Maxillofacial Trauma

One of the most rewarding and demanding aspects of dental and surgical practice is the management of the patient who has suffered facial trauma. The abruptness of the injury can cause intense emotional distress, even when only minor injuries are present. The perception of the injury by the patient or family and their reaction to the trauma may seem out of proportion to the degree of injury. The patient and family may be anxious and fearful, and they depend heavily on the clinician to make an accurate diagnosis, communicate that diagnosis to them, offer hope for a successful outcome, and perform the treatment necessary to repair the injury. Therefore the clinician must effectively deal with the patient's physical injuries and the patient's emotional state. Few conditions in clinical practice demand such compassion, competence, and attention to detail.

Whenever a maxillofacial injury is sustained, the patient goes abruptly from a normal state to one of tissue disruption. Patients usually expect that the treatment of the injury will make them appear as they did before the trauma. Unfortunately, this is rarely achieved. The most the clinician can do is provide the individual with the most favorable physical circumstances for optimal healing. The clinician accomplishes this by cleaning, débriding, and replacing tissues into their former positions. The resulting appearance therefore depends on the site, type, and degree of injury; the ability of the clinician performing tissue repair; and the ability of the patient's tissues to heal the wounds. The dentist's approach with the patient should be hopeful yet realistic.

The next two chapters discuss the diagnosis and management of injuries to the maxillofacial region. In Chapter 23 the injuries that dentists see with some frequency are discussed in detail. These include injuries to the teeth, alveolar process, and surrounding soft tissues. Chapter 24 presents an overview of the management of more severe maxillofacial injuries.

CHAPTER 23

Soft Tissue and Dentoalveolar Injuries

EDWARD ELLIS III

CHAPTER OUTLINE

SOFT TISSUE INJURIES

The types of soft tissue injuries the dentist may see in practice vary considerably. However, it is fair to assume that given the current availability of other health care providers, the dentist will probably not be involved in the management of severe soft tissue injuries around the face. Those injuries seen with some frequency are the ones associated with concomitant dentoalveolar trauma or those that the dentist may inadvertently cause in practice.

In the following descriptions of the wounds the dentist may see in practice and their management, one must remember that patients may have combinations of these injuries; therefore, management may be more complicated.

Abrasion

An abrasion is a wound caused by friction between an object and the surface of the soft tissue. This wound is usually superficial, denudes the epithelium, and occasionally involves deeper layers. Because abrasions involve the terminal endings of many nerve fibers, they are painful. Bleeding is usually minor because it is from capillaries and responds well to application of gentle pressure.

The type of abrasions most commonly seen by laypersons are the scrapes that children sustain on their elbows and knees from rough play. If the abrasion is not particularly deep, reepithelialization occurs without scarring. When the abrasion extends into the deeper layers of the dermis, healing of the deeper tissues occurs with the formation of scar tissue, and some permanent deformity can be expected.

The dentist may see abrasions on the tip of the nose, lips, cheeks, and chin in patients who have sustained dentoalveolar trauma (Fig. 23-1). The abraded areas should be thoroughly cleansed to remove foreign material. Surgical hand soap and copious saline irrigation are useful for this purpose. All particles of foreign matter must be removed. If these particles are allowed to remain within the tissue, a difficult to treat permanent "tattoo" results. In deep abrasions that are contaminated with dirt or other material, it may be necessary to anesthetize the area and use a surgical scrub brush (or toothbrush) to remove the debris completely.

Once the wound is free of debris, topical application of an antibiotic ointment is adequate treatment. A loose bandage can be applied if the abrasion is deep but is unnecessary in superficial abrasions. Systemic antibiotics are not usually indicated. Over the next week, reepithelialization will occur under the eschar, which is a crust of dried blood and serum that develops after an injury to soft tissue (e.g., a scab). The eschar will then drop off.

If a deep abrasion on the skin surface is discovered after wound cleansing, referral to an oral and maxillofacial surgeon is indicated because skin grafting may be necessary to prevent excessive amounts of scar formation.

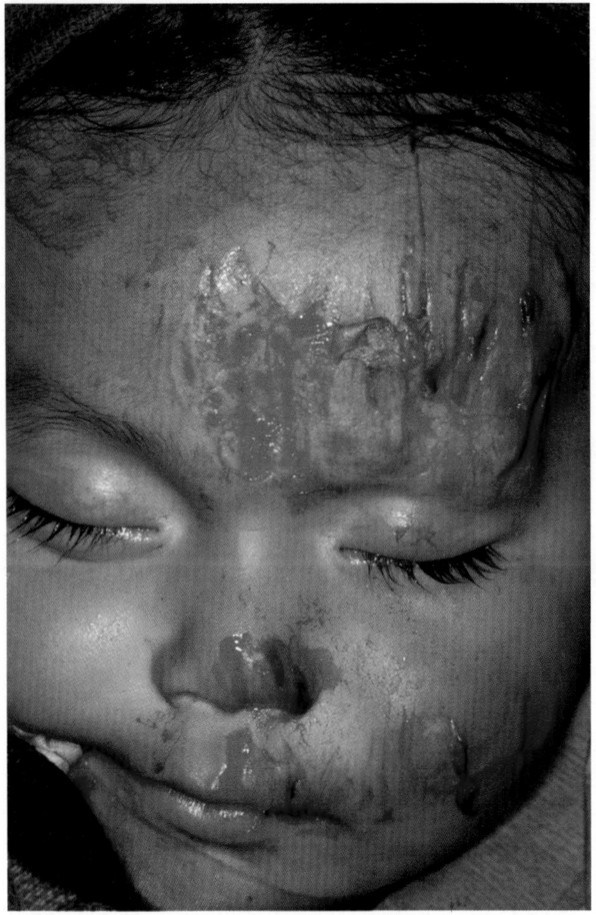

FIGURE 23-1 Patient with abrasions to the tip of nose, cheek, and forehead. Some of the abrasions are superficial, and some are deeper with peeling off of the epithelium.

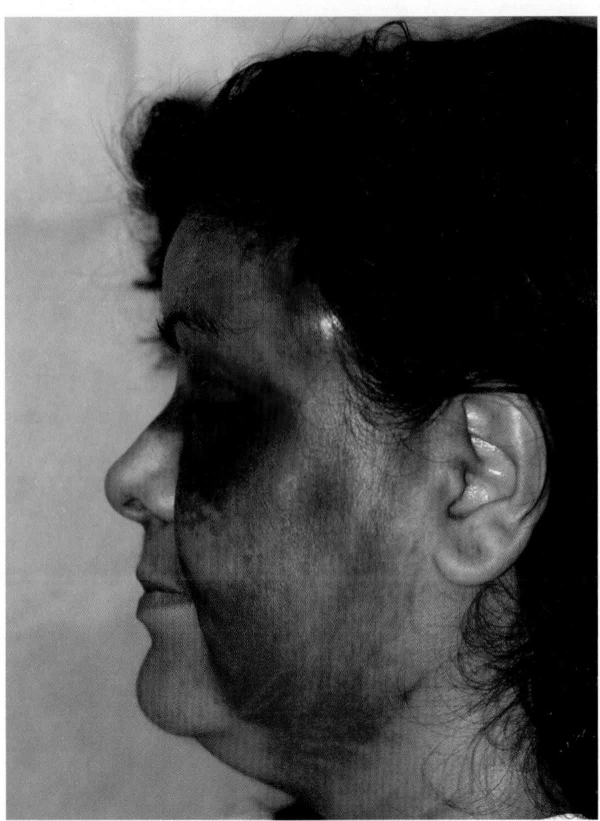

FIGURE 23-2 Soft tissue contusions caused by blunt injury with no underlying facial fractures.

The dentist may create abrasions iatrogenically, as occurs when the shank of a rotating bur touches the oral mucosa or when a gauze pack or other fabric (e.g., absorbent triangular pads) abrades the mucosa during removal from the mouth. Fortunately, the oral epithelium regenerates rapidly, and no treatment other than routine oral hygiene is indicated.

Contusion

A contusion is more commonly called a *bruise* and indicates that some amount of tissue disruption has occurred within the tissues, which resulted in subcutaneous or submucosal hemorrhage without a break in the soft tissue surface (Fig. 23-2).

Contusions are usually caused by trauma inflicted with a blunt object but are also frequently found with concomitant dentoalveolar injuries or facial bone fractures. In this instance, the trauma to the deeper tissues (e.g., floor of mouth or labial vestibule) has occurred from the disrupting effect of the fractured bones. The importance of contusions from a diagnostic point of view is that when they occur, one should search for osseous fractures.

A contusion generally requires no surgical treatment. Once the hydrostatic pressure within the soft tissues equals the pressure within the blood vessels (usually capillaries), bleeding ceases. If a contusion is seen early, the application of ice or pressure dressings may help constrict blood vessels and therefore decrease the amount of hematoma that forms. If a contusion does not stop expanding, a hemorrhaging artery within the wound is likely. The hematoma may require surgical exploration and ligation of the vessel.

Because there has been no disruption of the soft tissue surfaces, the body in time resorbs the hemorrhage formed within a contusion, and the normal contour is reestablished. In the next several days, however, the patient can expect areas of ecchymosis (i.e., purplish discoloration caused by extravasation of blood into the skin or mucosa; a "black-and-blue mark"), which turns a variety of colors (i.e., blue, green, and yellow) before fading. These areas may extend down below the clavicles and cause alarm, but they are innocuous.

When there has been no break in the surface of the soft tissue, infection is unlikely and systemic antibiotics are not indicated. If, however, the contusion results from dentoalveolar trauma, it is likely that communication may exist between the oral cavity and the submucosal hematoma. In this case, systemic antibiotics are warranted because coagulated blood represents an ideal culture medium.

Laceration

A laceration is a tear in the epithelial and subepithelial tissues. A laceration is perhaps the most frequent type of soft tissue injury and is caused most commonly by a sharp object, such as a knife or a piece of glass. If the object is not sharp, the lacerations created may be jagged because the tissue is literally torn by the force of the blow (Fig. 23-3). As with abrasions, the depth of a laceration can vary. Some lacerations involve the

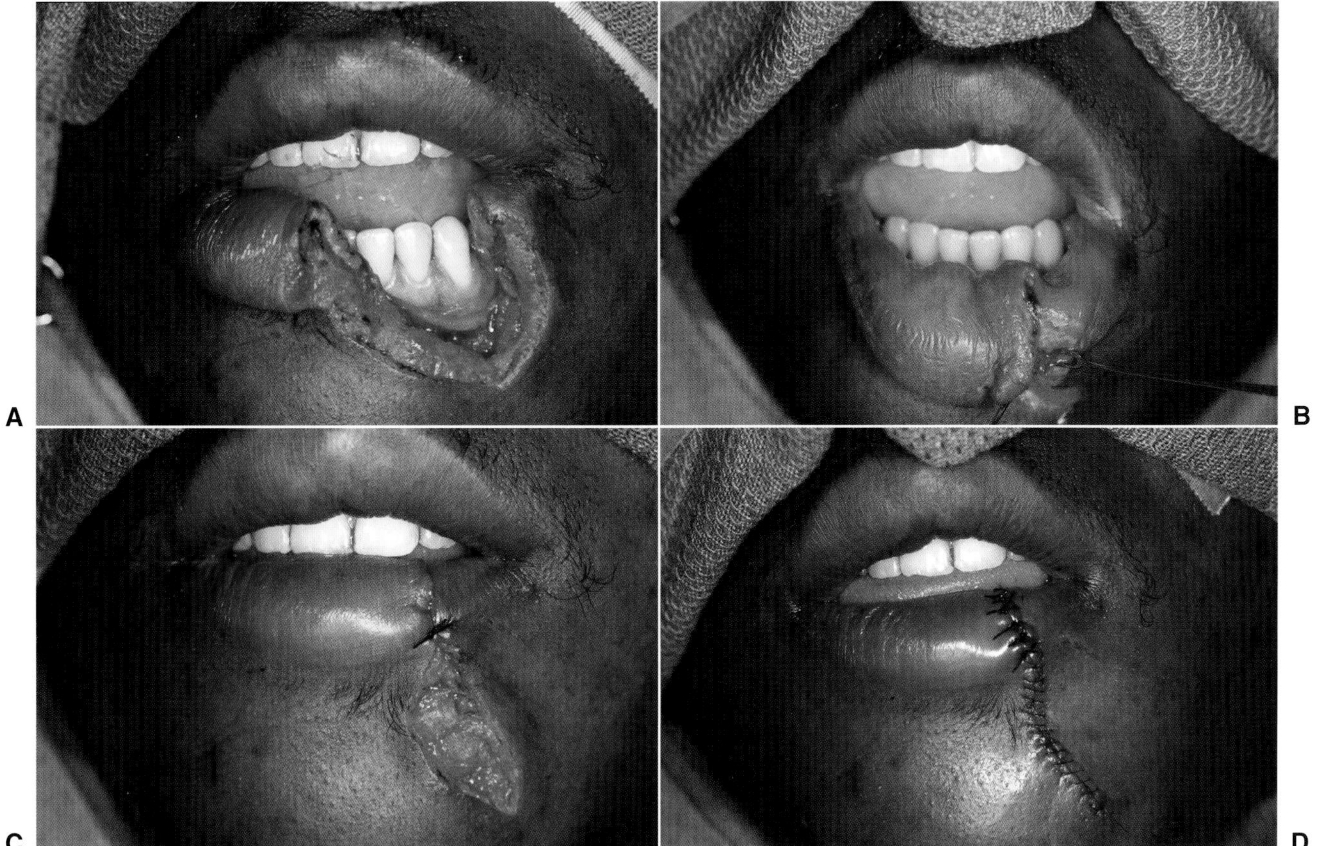

FIGURE 23-3 Photographs showing the repair of a full-thickness laceration of the lower lip. **A**, Tissues have been cleaned and hemostasis has been obtained. **B**, Muscle has been closed with interrupted 3-0 chromic catgut sutures. These sutures are the ones that primarily pull the tissues back together. The sutures should make it possible to close the skin without any tension. **C**, A 4-0 silk suture is placed at the mucocutaneous junction. This suture is critical because it aligns the vermilion border. If not done carefully, after healing a noticeable step or notch will show from misalignment. **D**, Skin and mucosal sutures are placed. Silk sutures were used to close the vermilion of the lip while nylon sutures were used to close the skin surface.

external surface only, but others extend deeply into the tissue, disrupting nerves, blood vessels, muscle, and other major anatomic cavities and structures.

The dentist frequently encounters lacerations of the lips, floor of mouth, tongue, labial mucosa, buccolabial vestibule, and gingiva caused by trauma. One should explore the oral cavity thoroughly to identify ones that are not gaping. For instance, lacerations within the vestibule can be overlooked unless the lips are retracted, allowing a laceration to gape. Lip lacerations are commonly seen with dentoalveolar trauma, but in many instances of trauma the teeth are uninjured because the soft tissues have absorbed the force of the blow.

Soft tissue wounds associated with dentoalveolar trauma are always treated *after* the management of the hard tissue injury. If the soft tissue is sutured first, time is wasted because the sutures are likely to be stressed too much and pulled out of the tissue during the intraoral manipulation necessary to replant an avulsed tooth or treat a dentoalveolar fracture. Furthermore, once sutures have been pulled out of the tissues, the tissues will be more difficult to close on the second attempt.

After adequate anesthesia is provided, the surgical management of lacerations involves four major steps: (1) cleansing, (2) débridement, (3) hemostasis, and (4) closure. These steps apply to lacerations anywhere in the body, including the oral cavity and perioral areas.

Cleansing of Wound

Mechanical cleansing of the wound is necessary to prevent debris from remaining. Cleansing can be performed with surgical soap and may necessitate the use of a brush. An anesthetic is usually necessary. Copious saline irrigation is then used to remove all water-soluble material and to flush out particulate matter. Pulsed irrigation has been shown to be more effective in removing debris than is a constant flow of irrigation.

Débridement of Wound

Débridement refers to the removal of contused and devitalized tissue from a wound and the removal of jagged pieces of surface tissue to enable linear closure. In the maxillofacial region, which enjoys a rich blood supply, the amount of débridement should be kept to a minimum. Only tissue that is obviously not vital is excised. For most of the lacerations a dentist encounters, no débridement is necessary, except for minor salivary gland tissue (discussed later).

Hemostasis in Wound

Before closure, hemostasis must be achieved. Continued bleeding might jeopardize the repair by creating a hematoma within the tissues that can break the tissues open once they are sutured closed. If any bleeding vessels are identified, they should be clamped and tied with ligatures or cauterized with an electrocoagulation unit. The largest vessel the dentist will probably encounter is the labial artery, which runs horizontally across the lip just beneath the labial mucosa. Because of its position, the labial artery is frequently involved in vertical lip lacerations. This artery is approximately 1 mm in diameter and usually can be clamped and tied, or clamped and cauterized.

Closure of Wound

Once the wound has been cleansed, débrided, and hemostasis achieved, the laceration is ready to be closed with sutures. However, not every laceration in the oral cavity must be closed with sutures. For example, a small laceration in the palatal mucosa caused by falling on an object extending from the mouth need not be closed. Similarly, a small laceration on the inner aspect of the lip or tongue caused by entrapment between the teeth during a fall usually does not require closure. These small wounds heal well by secondary intention and are best left to do so.

If closure of a laceration is deemed appropriate, the goal during closure is proper positioning of all tissue layers. The manner in which closure proceeds depends totally on the location and depth of the laceration.

When lacerations of the gingiva and alveolar mucosa (or floor of mouth) are noted, they are simply closed in one layer. If a patient has a laceration of the tongue or lip that involves muscle, resorbable sutures should be placed to close the muscle layer or layers, after which the mucosa is sutured. Minor salivary gland tissue protruding into a wound can be judiciously trimmed to allow for a more favorable closure.

In lacerations extending through the entire thickness of the lip, a triple-layered closure is necessary (Fig. 23-4). If the laceration involves the vermilion border, the first suture placed should be at the mucocutaneous junction. Perfect alignment of this junction of skin and mucosa is imperative, or it can result in a noticeable deformity that can be seen from a distance. Once this suture is placed, the wound is closed in layers *from the inside out.* The oral mucosa is first closed with silk or resorbable suture. The orbicularis oris muscle is then sutured with interrupted resorbable sutures. Finally, the dermal surface of the lip is sutured with 5-0 or 6-0 nylon sutures. The wound will look as good at the completion of suturing as it ever will. If the alignment of tissues appears poor, consideration should be given to removing the sutures and replacing them in a more favorable manner. The dermal surface should then be covered with an antibiotic ointment.

Once a laceration is closed, the clinician must consider what supportive therapy can be instituted to bring about uneventful healing. Systemic antibiotics (e.g., penicillin) should be considered whenever a laceration extends through the full substance of the lip. In superficial lacerations, antibiotics are not indicated. The patient's tetanus status should be ascertained; if in doubt, patients should be referred to their physicians. Patients should also be instructed in postsurgical diet and wound care.

Generally, facial skin sutures should be removed 4 to 6 days postoperatively. When removing a suture, it should be cut and

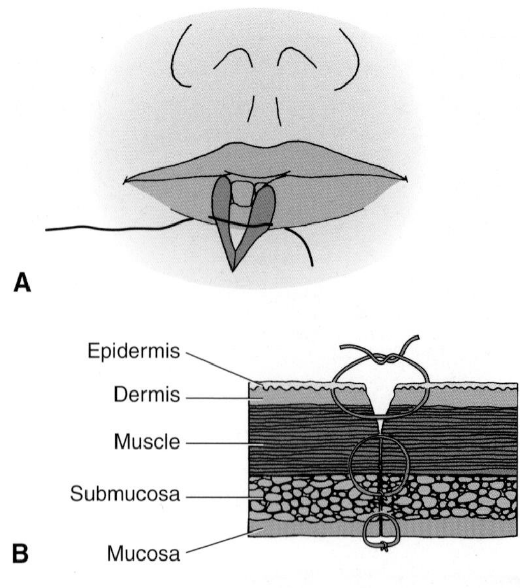

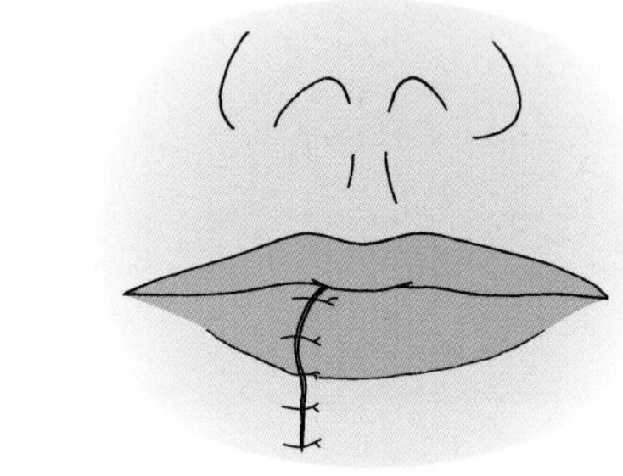

FIGURE 23-4 Illustrations showing the closure of a lip laceration or incision. A, Critical suture is placed at mucocutaneous junction. Realign of mucocutaneous junction is critical; otherwise, cosmetic deformity will be noticeable. B and C, Lip is closed in three layers: (1) oral mucosa, (2) muscle, and (3) dermal surface. Choice of suture for oral and dermal surfaces varies with surgeon; however, muscle layer should be closed with chromic or plain catgut (resorbable) suture.

then pulled in a direction that does not cause the wound to gape. Adhesive strips can be placed at the time of suture removal to give external support to the healing wound.

DENTOALVEOLAR INJURIES

Dentoalveolar and perioral soft tissue injuries frequently occur and are caused by many types of trauma. The most common causes are falls, motor vehicle accidents, sports injuries, altercations, child abuse, and playground accidents. Falling causes many injuries, which starts when a child begins to walk and peaks just before school age.[1] The dentist is likely to be called by a frantic parent whose child has just fallen and is bleeding from the mouth. Dentists must be familiar with dentoalveolar injuries so that they can effectively manage them when they occur.

A force directly on a tooth or an indirect force, most commonly transmitted through overlying soft tissues (e.g., the lip), may cause dentoalveolar injuries. Injuries of the surrounding soft tissues almost always accompany injuries to the dentoalveolus. For example, gingival tissues may be torn; the lower lip may have been caught between the teeth during the injury, creating a full-thickness laceration; or the floor of the mouth may be lacerated. Knowledge of management techniques for injuries to the dentoalveolus and the soft tissues is necessary to allow the dentist to treat these injuries effectively.

Management of Dentoalveolar Injuries

Injuries to the teeth and alveolar process are common and should be considered emergency conditions because a successful outcome depends on prompt attention to the injury. Because proper treatment can be given only after an accurate diagnosis, the diagnostic process should commence immediately.

History

The first step in any diagnostic process should be to secure an accurate history. A comprehensive history of the injury should be obtained from the patient, incorporating information on who, when, where, and how. The dentist must ask the following questions of the patient, parent, or a reliable respondent:

1. *Who is the patient?* Included in the answer should be the patient's name, age, address, telephone number, and other pertinent demographic data. It is imperative that this data be obtained quickly and that time not be wasted.
2. *When did the injury occur?* This is one of the most important questions to ask because studies have shown that the sooner an avulsed tooth can be repositioned, the better the prognosis.[2] Similarly the results of treating displaced teeth, crown fractures (with and without exposed dental pulps), and alveolar fractures may be influenced by a delay in treatment.[1,3]
3. *Where did the injury occur?* This question may be important because the possibility and degree of bacterial or chemical contamination should be ascertained. For example, if a child falls on the playground and gets dirt in the wound, a tetanus prophylaxis history should be carefully established. However, if an injury occurs from a clean object held in the mouth, gross bacterial contamination from external sources is not expected.
4. *How did the injury occur?* The nature of the trauma provides valuable insight into what the resultant tissue injury is likely to be. For example, an unrestrained car passenger who is thrown forward into the dashboard with sufficient force to damage several teeth may also have sustained occult injuries to the neck. The manner in which the injury occurred is valuable information and should make the clinician investigate the possibility of further injuries. Additional information that can be gained from this question may relate to the cause of the injury. If a patient cannot remember what happened, a preexisting medical condition, such as a seizure disorder, may have caused the accident producing the injury. Injuries caused by possible negligence by others are open for litigation. These considerations should caution the clinician to document the findings carefully and word any discussions with the patient thoughtfully. One other thought that must be kept in the clinician's mind when examining children whose injuries do not seem to be a likely result of the injury described by the parent is child abuse.

Unfortunately, child abuse has become more prevalent in recent years, and a high degree of suspicion may be the only manner by which it can be discovered by health care providers.

5. *What treatment has been provided since the injury (if any)?* This question elicits important information regarding the original condition of the injured area. Did the patient or parent replant a partially avulsed tooth? How was the avulsed tooth stored before presentation to the dentist?
6. *Did anyone note teeth or pieces of teeth at the site of the accident?* Before an accurate diagnosis and treatment plan are made, it is imperative that each tooth the patient had before the accident be accounted for. If, during the clinical examination a tooth or crown is found missing and no history suggests that it was lost at the scene, radiographic examination of the perioral soft tissues, the chest, and the abdominal region is necessary to rule out the presence of the missing piece within the tissues or other body cavities (Fig. 23-5).
7. *What is the general health of the patient?* A succinct medical history is essential; it should not be ignored in the dentist's haste to replant an avulsed tooth. The history, however, can be performed concomitantly with treatment or immediately thereafter. A history that touches on drug allergy, heart murmur, bleeding disorder, other systemic disease, and current medications should be taken before treatment because their existence affects the treatment the dentist will provide.
8. Did the patient have nausea, vomiting, unconsciousness, amnesia, headache, visual disturbances, or confusion after the accident? An affirmative answer to any of these questions may indicate intracranial injury and direct the dentist to obtain medical consultation immediately after completing treatment. Immediate referral should be made if the patient is still having any of the symptoms or if the patient does not feel or look well. The patient's life should not be jeopardized to save an avulsed tooth.
9. Is there a disturbance in the bite? An affirmative answer to this question may indicate tooth displacement or dentoalveolar or jaw fracture.

Clinical Examination

The clinical examination is perhaps the most important part of the diagnostic process. A thorough examination of a patient who has had injury to the dentoalveolar structures should not focus only on that structure. Concomitant injuries may also be present; the history may direct the dentist to examine other areas for signs of injury. Vital signs such as pulse rate, blood pressure, and respiration should be measured. Such tests can usually be obtained during the taking of the history. The mental state of the patient is also assessed throughout the taking of the history and while performing the clinical examination by observation of the manner in which the patient reacts to the examination and responds to the questioning. During the clinical examination, the following areas should be examined routinely:

1. *Extraoral soft tissue wounds.* Lacerations, abrasions, and contusions of the skin are common with dentoalveolar injuries and should be noted. If a laceration is present, the depth of it should also be determined. Does the laceration extend through the entire thickness of the lip or cheek? Are there any vital structures, such as the parotid duct or facial nerve, crossing the line of the laceration? An oral and maxillofacial surgeon best treats major lacerations such as these.

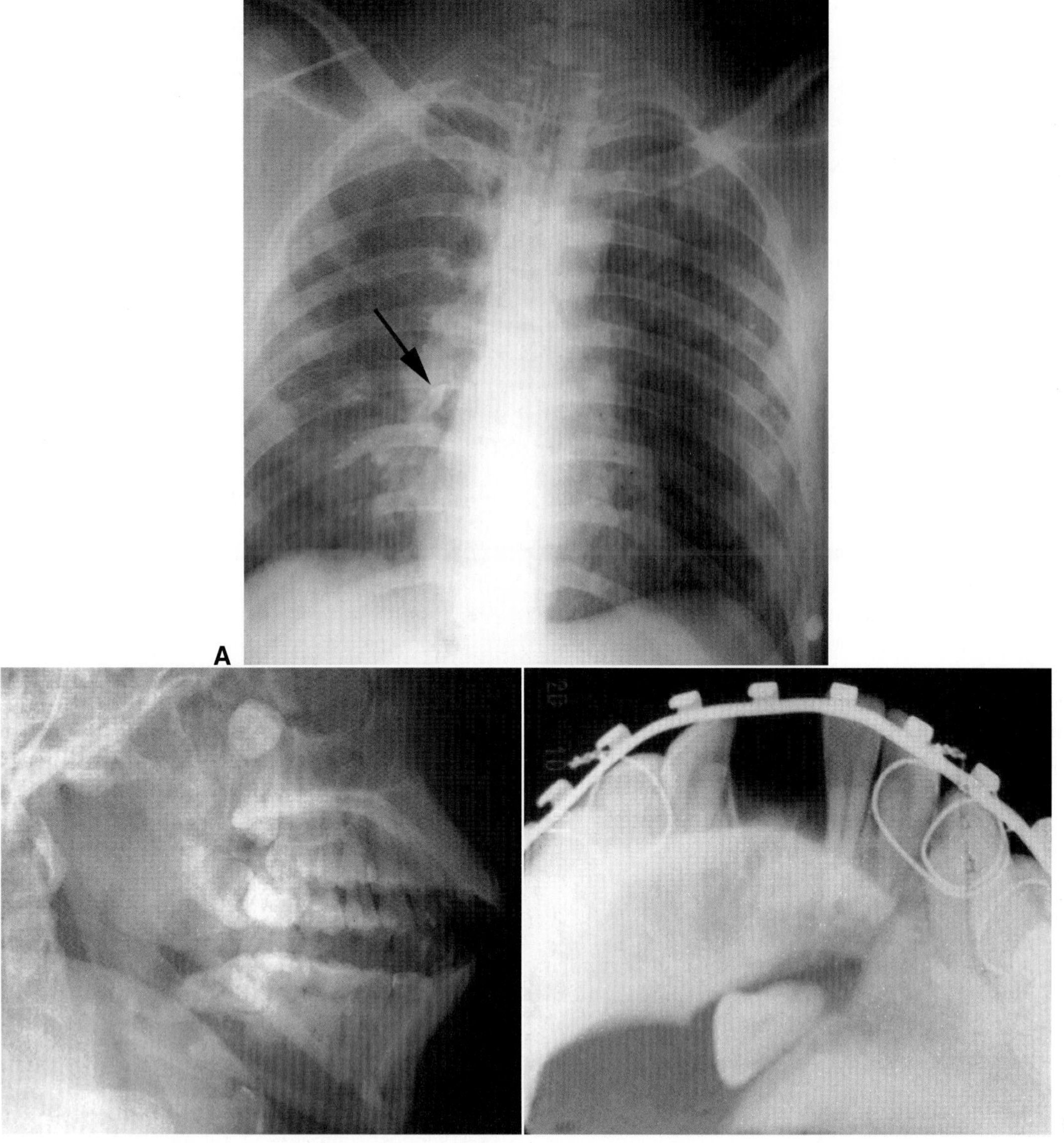

FIGURE 23-5 Teeth displaced into abnormal locations. A, Chest radiograph showing maxillary canine tooth in right main stem bronchus after traumatic displacement. B, Molar displaced into the maxillary sinus from maxillary fracture. C, Incisor tooth in line of fracture preventing anatomic reduction.

2. *Intraoral soft tissue wounds.* Injuries to the oral soft tissues are commonly associated with dentoalveolar injuries. Before a thorough examination, it may be necessary to remove blood clots, irrigate with sterile saline, and cleanse the oral cavity. Areas of bleeding usually respond to pressure applied through gauze sponges. Soft tissue injuries should be noted, and an examination should ascertain whether any foreign bodies, such as tooth crowns or teeth, remain within the substance of the lips, floor of mouth, cheeks, or other areas. The dentist should also note areas of extensive loss of soft tissues; blood supply to a segment of tissue may thereby be lost.
3. *Fractures of the jaws or alveolar process.* Fractures of the jaws are most readily found on palpation. However, because pain may be severe after the injury, examination can be difficult. Bleeding into the floor of the mouth or into the labial vestibule may indicate a fracture of the jaw. Segments of alveolar process that have been fractured are readily detected by visual examination and palpation.
4. *Examination of the tooth crowns for the presence of fractures or pulp exposure.* For adequate examination, the teeth should be cleansed of blood. Any fractures should be noted. The depth of the fracture is important to note. Does it extend into dentin or into the pulp?
5. *Displacement of teeth.* Teeth can be displaced in any direction. Most commonly they are displaced in a buccolingual direction, but they may also be extruded or intruded. In the most severe type of displacement, the teeth are avulsed, that is, totally displaced out of their alveolar process. Observation of the dental occlusion may provide assistance in determining minimal degrees of tooth displacement.

6. *Mobility of teeth.* All teeth should be checked for mobility in the horizontal and vertical directions. A tooth that does not appear to be displaced but that has considerable mobility may have sustained a root fracture. If adjacent teeth move with the tooth being tested, a dentoalveolar fracture (in which a segment of alveolar bone and teeth are separated from the remainder of the jaw) should be suspected.
7. *Percussion of teeth.* When a tooth does not appear to be displaced but pain is felt in the region, percussion determines whether the periodontal ligament has undergone some injury.
8. *Pulp testing of teeth.* Although rarely used in acute injuries, vitality tests (which induce a reaction from the teeth) may direct the type of treatment the teeth will receive once the injury has healed. False-negative results may occur, so the teeth should be retested several weeks later and before endodontic therapy is performed.

Radiographic Examination

A host of radiographic techniques are available to evaluate dentoalveolar trauma. Most techniques can be readily performed in the dental office with available equipment. Most commonly a combination of occlusal and periapical radiographs is used. The radiographic examination should provide the following information[4]:

1. Presence of root fracture
2. Degree of extrusion or intrusion
3. Presence of preexisting periapical disease
4. Extent of root development
5. Size of the pulp chamber and root canal
6. Presence of jaw fractures
7. Tooth fragments and foreign bodies lodged in soft tissues

A single radiograph may not be sufficient to demonstrate a root fracture.[1] For a radiograph to demonstrate a fractured root, the central beam of the x-ray device must be parallel to the line of fracture; otherwise, the fracture may not be clearly seen (Fig. 23-6). Multiple views with differing vertical and horizontal angulations of the central ray may be necessary.

Displaced teeth may show a widening of the periodontal ligament space or displacement of the lamina dura. Extruded teeth may demonstrate a conic periapical radiolucency (Fig. 23-7). Intruded teeth may show minimal radiographic findings because of the continued close adaptation of the lamina dura and the root surface. Frequently, however, intruded teeth show an absence of the periodontal ligament space.

Radiographic evaluation for foreign bodies within the soft tissues of the lips or cheeks are taken with the radiographic film placed inside the soft tissues to be examined, labial to the alveolus (Fig. 23-8, *A*). A reduced radiographic exposure time is used (approximately one third of normal). Foreign bodies in the floor of the mouth are viewed with cross-sectioned occlusal radiographs, also with reduced radiographic exposure time (Fig. 23-8, *B*).

Classification of Traumatic Injuries to the Teeth and Supporting Structures

Many systems are used for the description of dentoalveolar injuries, all of which have advantages and disadvantages. A relatively simple yet useful classification was presented by Sanders et al.[4] (Box 23-1). Their method is based entirely on a description of the injury sustained during the traumatic episode, describing the tooth structures involved, the type of displacement, and the direction of crown or root fracture.

BOX 23-1

Classification of Dentoalveolar Injuries

CROWN CRAZE OR CRACK (I.E., INFRACTION; FIG. 23-9)
Crack or incomplete fracture of the enamel without a loss of tooth structure

HORIZONTAL OR VERTICAL CROWN FRACTURE (FIG. 23-10)
Confined to enamel
Enamel and dentin involved
Enamel, dentin, and exposed pulp involved
Horizontal or vertical
Oblique (involving the mesioincisal or distoincisal angle)

CROWN-ROOT FRACTURE (FIG. 23-11)
No pulp involvement
Pulp involvement

HORIZONTAL ROOT FRACTURE (FIG. 23-12)
Involving apical third
Involving middle third
Involving cervical third
Horizontal or vertical

SENSITIVITY (I.E., CONCUSSION)
Injury to the tooth-supporting structure, resulting in sensitivity to touch or percussion but without mobility or displacement of the tooth

MOBILITY (I.E., SUBLUXATION OR LOOSENESS)
Injury to the tooth-supporting structure, resulting in tooth mobility but without tooth displacement

TOOTH DISPLACEMENT (FIG. 23-13)
Intrusion (displacement of tooth into its socket—usually associated with compression fracture of socket)
Extrusion (partial displacement of tooth out of its socket—possibly no concomitant fracture of alveolar bone)
Labial displacement (alveolar wall fractures probable)
Lingual displacement (alveolar wall fractures probable)
Lateral displacement (displacement of tooth in mesial or distal direction, usually into a missing tooth space—alveolar wall fractures probable)

AVULSION
Complete displacement of tooth from its socket (may be associated with alveolar wall fractures)

ALVEOLAR PROCESS FRACTURE
Fracture of alveolar bone in the presence or absence of a tooth or teeth

Modified from Sanders B, Brady FA, Johnson R: Injuries. In Sanders B, editor: *Pediatric oral and maxillofacial surgery,* St Louis, 1979, Mosby.

Treatment of Dentoalveolar Injuries

After conducting a thorough history and clinical and radiologic examinations, the dentist should be able to determine whether the treatment plan for the patient's type of injury is within the clinician's range of expertise. Several circumstances may render an otherwise minor injury untreatable by the dentist alone. A problem the dentist frequently encounters is the uncooperative

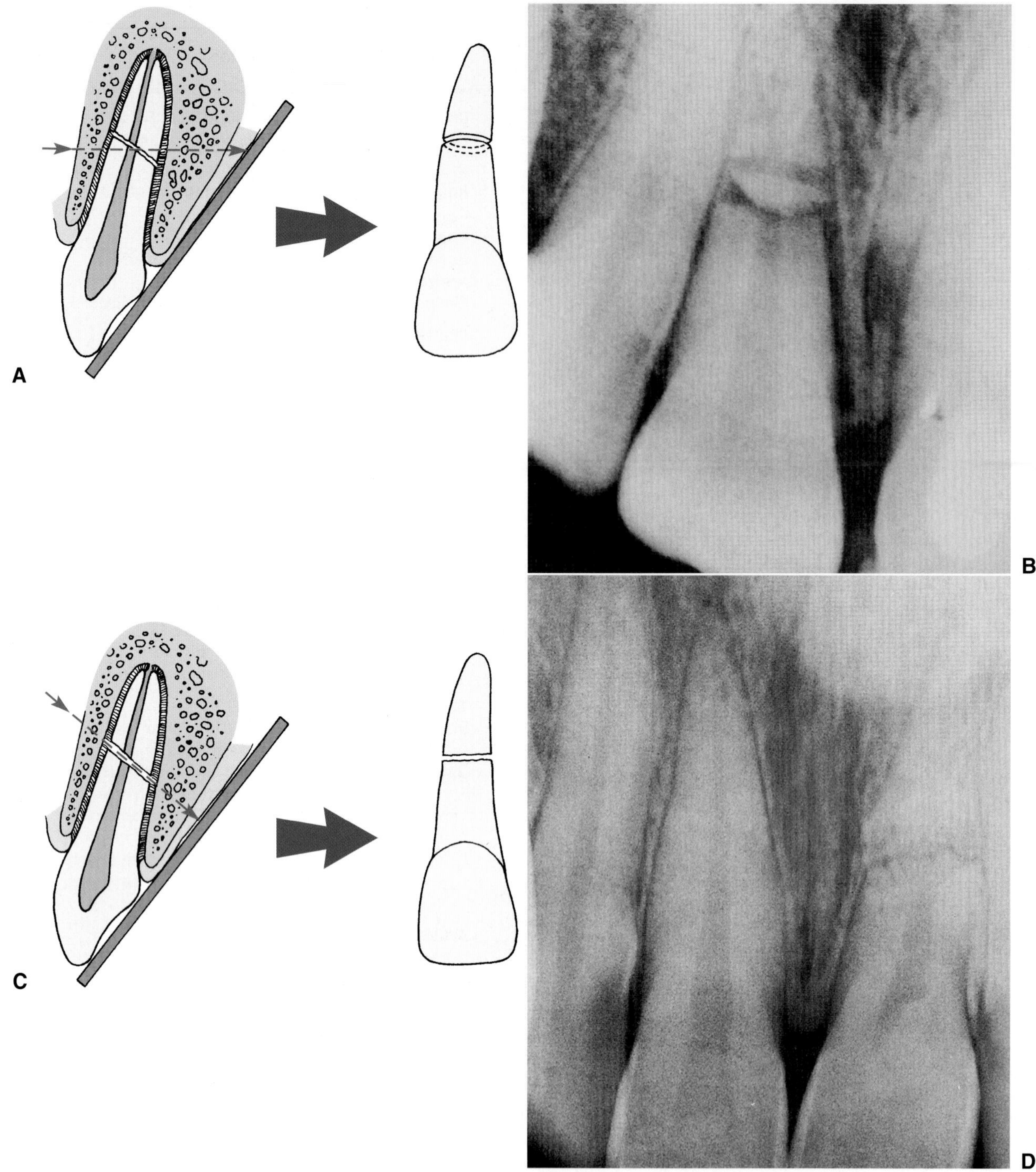

FIGURE 23-6 Effect of vertical angulation of central x-ray beam on the detection of horizontal root fracture. When central ray is not parallel to fracture (**A**), either a double fracture (**B**) or no fracture at all may be observed on radiograph. When central ray is parallel to fracture (**C**), fracture appears on radiograph (**D**).

patient, most commonly a child. The combination of the traumatic episode and the child's fear of the dentist may render a simple surgical procedure impossible without general anesthesia. Another difficulty is the patient with multiple medical problems. When dentists do not think that they can effectively manage a patient because of surgical difficulty, anesthesia requirement, concomitant medical problems, or other reasons, an oral and maxillofacial surgeon should immediately be consulted for assistance with treatment.

The goal in the treatment of dentoalveolar injuries is reestablishing normal form and function of the masticatory apparatus. When the pulp is directly involved, treatment differs

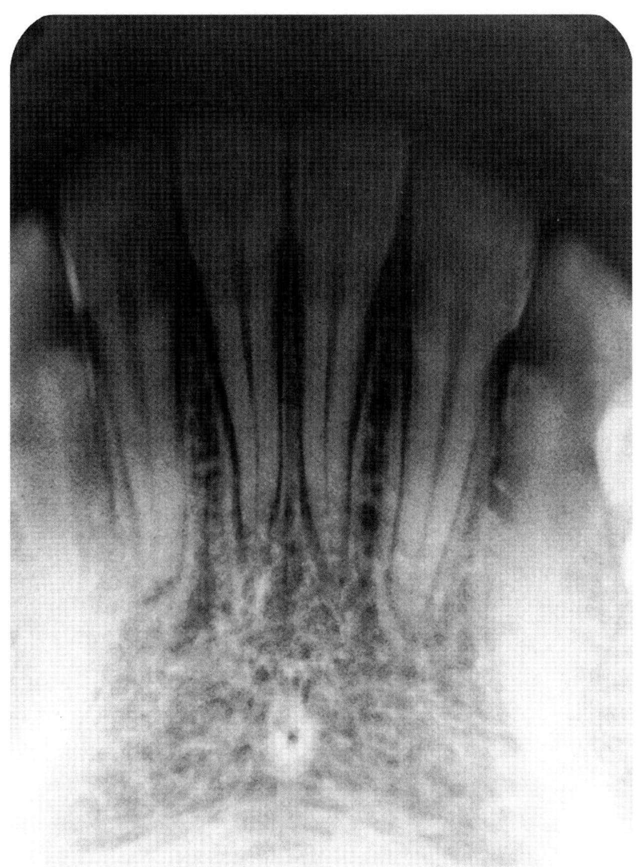

FIGURE 23-7 Radiograph showing widened periodontal ligament spaces around several teeth that are displaced coronally.

from that of tooth injuries in which the pulp is not involved. Because of the training in operative dentistry and endodontics, a dentist has the knowledge, the instrumentation, and the medications routinely available to manage cases of tooth fracture. The treatment regimen for these injuries is therefore outlined only briefly. More severe injuries, such as tooth dislocations, avulsions, or dentoalveolar fractures, are fields in which the dentist may have had little training; these are presented in greater detail.

Primary teeth that have been injured are generally treated in a manner similar to that for permanent teeth. However, in many instances, the lack of cooperation by the child results in treatment compromises and, frequently, extraction of the damaged tooth. If this occurs, the dentist should consider space maintenance measures in the near future where indicated.

Crown Craze or Crack

Because the cracks are limited to the enamel (i.e., enamel infraction) and usually stop before reaching the dentinoenamel junction, no treatment is usually indicated. However, because any force to the tooth can result in injury to the pulp and periodontal tissues, periodic follow-up examinations are valuable (Fig. 23-9). Multiple cracks may be sealed with an unfilled resin to prevent their becoming stained.

Crown Fracture

The depth of tooth tissue involvement determines the treatment of crown fractures.[5] For fractures that are only through the enamel or those with minimal amounts of dentin involvement, no acute treatment other than smoothing off the sharp edges is warranted. If reshaping the teeth would leave a noticeable deformity, replacement of the missing enamel by acid-etched composite resin techniques is indicated. The sooner the teeth are treated, the better the prognosis, because inflammatory hyperemia of the pulp is decreased. Periodic follow-up examinations are necessary to monitor pulp and periodontal health (Fig. 23-10).

If a considerable amount of dentin is exposed, the pulp must be protected. Measures to seal the dentinal tubules and promote secondary dentin deposition by the pulp can be undertaken. Calcium hydroxide has been the traditional material applied to the exposed dentin before the fractured part is covered with a suitable restoration, most commonly a composite with or without acid etching. Current recommendations are the placement of a dentin-bonding agent or glass ionomer cement over the exposed dentin, followed by the placement of a resin composite restoration.[6] Glass ionomer cements chemically bind to dentin, facilitating placement and restoration. The status of pulp vitality at periodic follow-up visits dictates what the final treatment plan will be. If pulp and periodontal health are satisfactory, no more intervention is necessary other than for esthetic reasons.

If the pulp is exposed, the aim of treatment is to preserve it in a vital, healthy state. This can usually be accomplished by pulp capping if five conditions are present: (1) the exposure is small, (2) the patient is seen soon after injury, (3) the patient had no root fractures, (4) the tooth has not been displaced, and (5) no large or deep fillings exist that might indicate chronic inflammation within the pulp. The most common injury for which pulp capping is instituted is in a tooth in which a single pulp horn was exposed with a crown fracture.

The more apically immature the tooth, the more favorable is the response the dentist can expect from pulp capping. As with any operative procedure on the dental pulp, isolation with a rubber dam is recommended. After application of calcium hydroxide on the exposed pulp, glass ionomer cement is placed over the exposed dentin and a watertight acid-etch composite restoration is placed (Fig. 23-14).

A pulpotomy involves aseptic removal of damaged and inflamed pulp tissue to the level of clinically healthy pulp, after which calcium hydroxide is applied. A pulpotomy is usually implemented in larger exposures in which the apex is not closed. In these instances a pulpotomy should be only a temporary measure to maintain the vitality of the radicular pulp until the apex is closed. Endodontic therapy should then be instituted.

Periodic follow-up examinations are mandatory after any pulpal procedure. The final restorative decision is based on the pulpal health of the tooth. Because the prognosis is guarded, endodontic treatment may be necessary if the pulp degenerates.

Another technique that can be used to restore the tooth is by replacing the original fractured tooth fragment using the acid-etch technique or with the newer enamel and dentin adhesives.[7] This technique is particularly useful for large fractures.

Crown-Root Fracture

The treatment of crown-root fractures depends on the location of the fracture and local anatomic variance. If the coronal fragment is still in place, it must be removed to assess the depth to

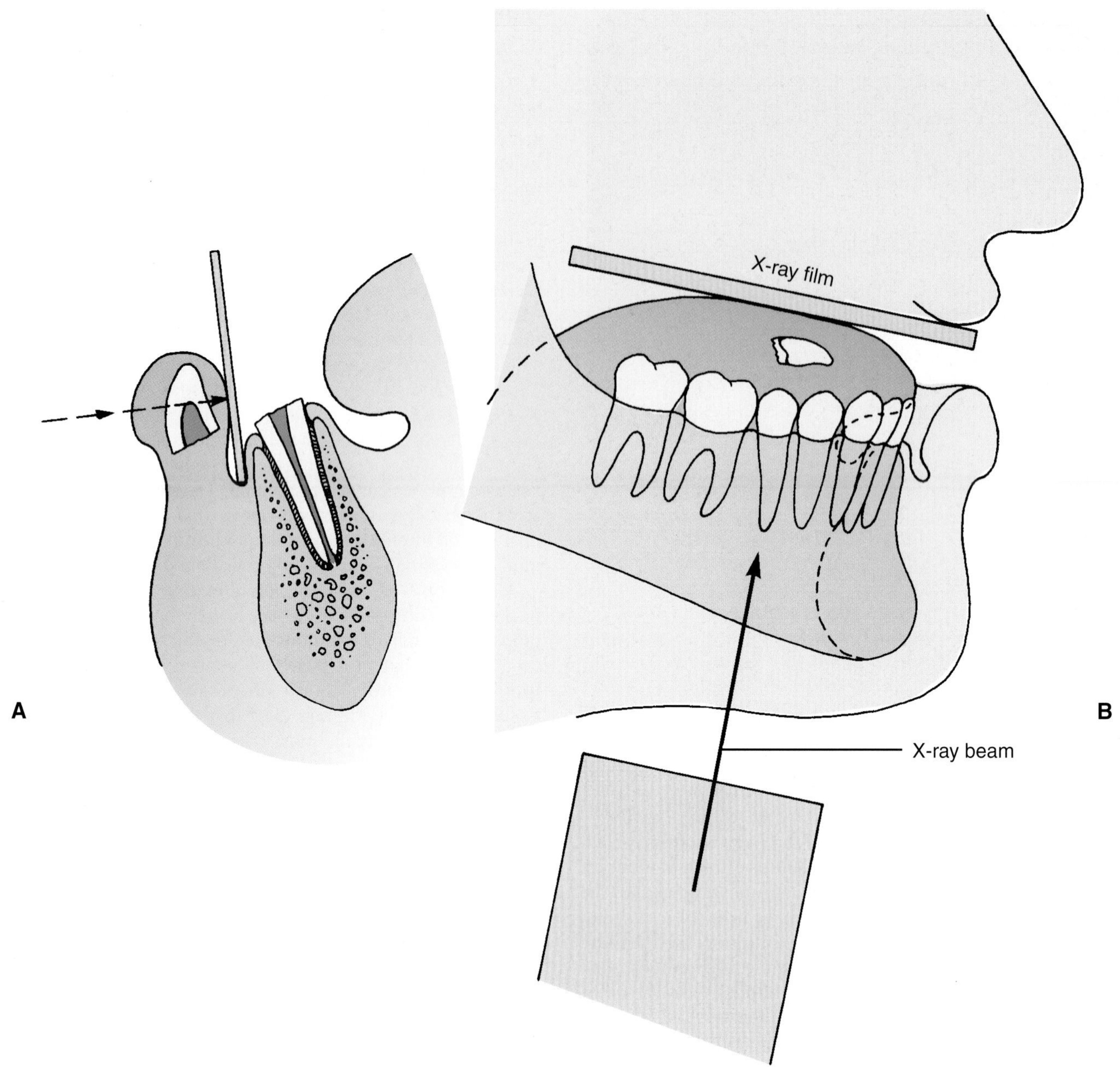

FIGURE 23-8 Radiographic technique to detect foreign bodies within lip (A) and tongue (B). The clinician should use one half to one third of normal exposure for soft tissue radiography.

which the fracture has gone. If the fracture does not descend too far apically (and the tooth is therefore restorable) and if the pulp has not been exposed, the tooth is treated as already discussed for crown fracture.

Depending on the apical extent of the fracture, it may be necessary to perform periodontal procedures to make the apical margin of the fracture accessible for restorative procedures. Alternatively, orthodontic extrusion of the root can make it accessible for restorative procedures. If the pulp is involved and the tooth is restorable, endodontic treatment is implemented. If, however, the tooth is not restorable, removal is indicated. If a concomitant alveolar fracture is found, the extraction may be delayed for several weeks to permit the fracture to heal and thus prevent undue loss of alveolar bone at the time of extraction (Fig. 23-11).

Horizontal Root Fracture

When a horizontal or oblique fracture of the root occurs, the main factor in determining the prognosis and therefore in directing treatment is the position of the fracture in relation to the gingival crevice. If the fracture is above or close to the gingival crevice, the tooth should be removed or the coronal fragment should be removed and endodontic treatment performed on the root. The root can then be restored with a post and core restoration. Fractures in the middle to apical one third of the root have a good prognosis for survival of the pulp

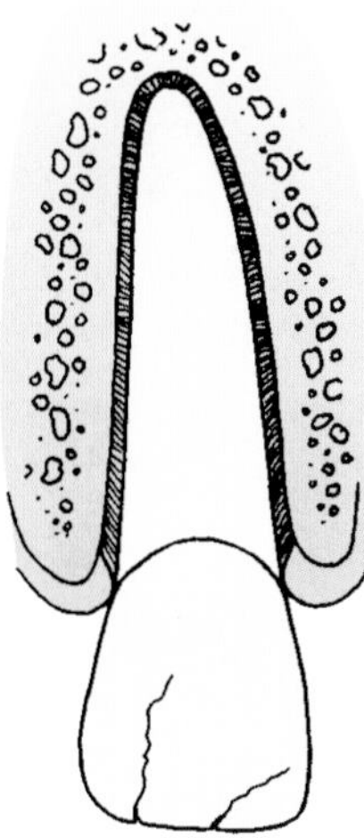

FIGURE 23-9 Crown cracks or crazes. These injuries usually extend only into enamel.

and healing of the root fragments to one another. These fractures should be treated with repositioning (if any mobility is detectable) and firm immobilization for 2 to 3 months (these techniques are described later). During this time, bridging of the fracture with calcified tissue usually occurs, and the tooth remains vital (Figs. 23-6 and 23-12).

Sensitivity

No acute treatment is recommended for sensitivity (i.e., concussion) other than symptomatic relief, such as relieving the tooth from occlusal contact. This is easiest to perform by grinding the occlusal contacts from the opposing tooth. Follow-up examinations should be instituted to monitor periodontal and pulpal health.

Mobility

If the tooth is only mildly mobile, relieving the occlusal contact is effective treatment. Most mobile teeth stabilize (i.e., "tighten up") with time. If the tooth is extremely mobile, splinting it to adjacent teeth is recommended (described later). Periodic observation is then necessary.

Intrusion

Traumatic intrusion of teeth indicates that the alveolar socket has sustained a compression fracture to permit the new tooth position. On percussion the tooth emits a metallic sound similar to an ankylosed tooth, distinguishing it from a partially erupted or unerupted tooth. The intrusion may be so severe that the tooth actually appears to be missing on clinical examination. Traumatic tooth intrusion is less frequent than lateral displacements; when seen, intrusion usually involves maxillary teeth. This type of nonavulsive tooth displacement has the worst prognosis (Fig. 23-13).

The treatment of intruded teeth is controversial. Some clinicians favor surgically repositioning and splinting the teeth; however, this treatment has resulted in serious periodontal and pulpal consequences. Others think that, if left alone, many intruded teeth will reerupt. Others use orthodontic forces to assist reeruption of the tooth (Fig. 23-15).

When orthodontic assisted eruption is used, the tooth should be extruded slowly, over a 3- to 4-week period. Once the tooth is in position within the dental arch, it is splinted for 2 to 3 months. Recent evidence suggests that *immediate* application of orthodontic force is necessary to prevent ankylosis in the intruded position.[8] The decision to perform endodontic treatment is based on the follow-up findings of each case.

However, if the intrusion occurred in an apically mature tooth, pulpal degeneration is likely and endodontic treatment should be performed as described later.

If a deciduous tooth has been intruded to the point that it is touching the follicle of a succedaneous tooth, the deciduous tooth should be removed as atraumatically as possible. If the deciduous tooth is not in direct proximity to the succedaneous tooth, a period of observation should be followed because reeruption is common. If the dentist is in doubt about the position of a deciduous tooth, removal is a sound prophylactic approach that helps to ensure the health of the succedaneous tooth.

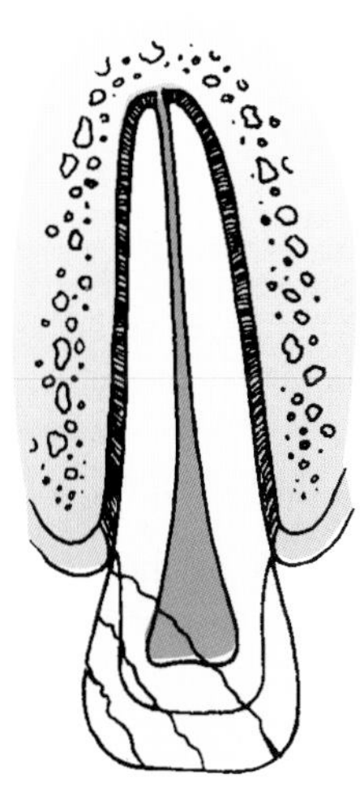

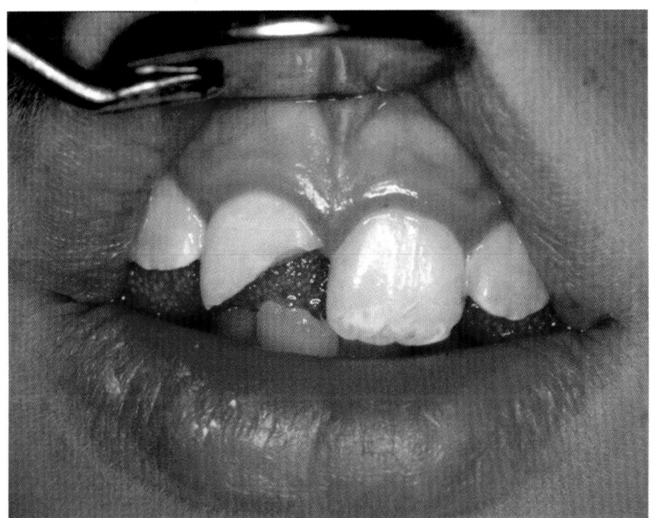

FIGURE 23-10 A, Coronal fractures involving enamel, dentin, and pulp. B, Photograph of a coronal fracture that involved enamel and dentin.

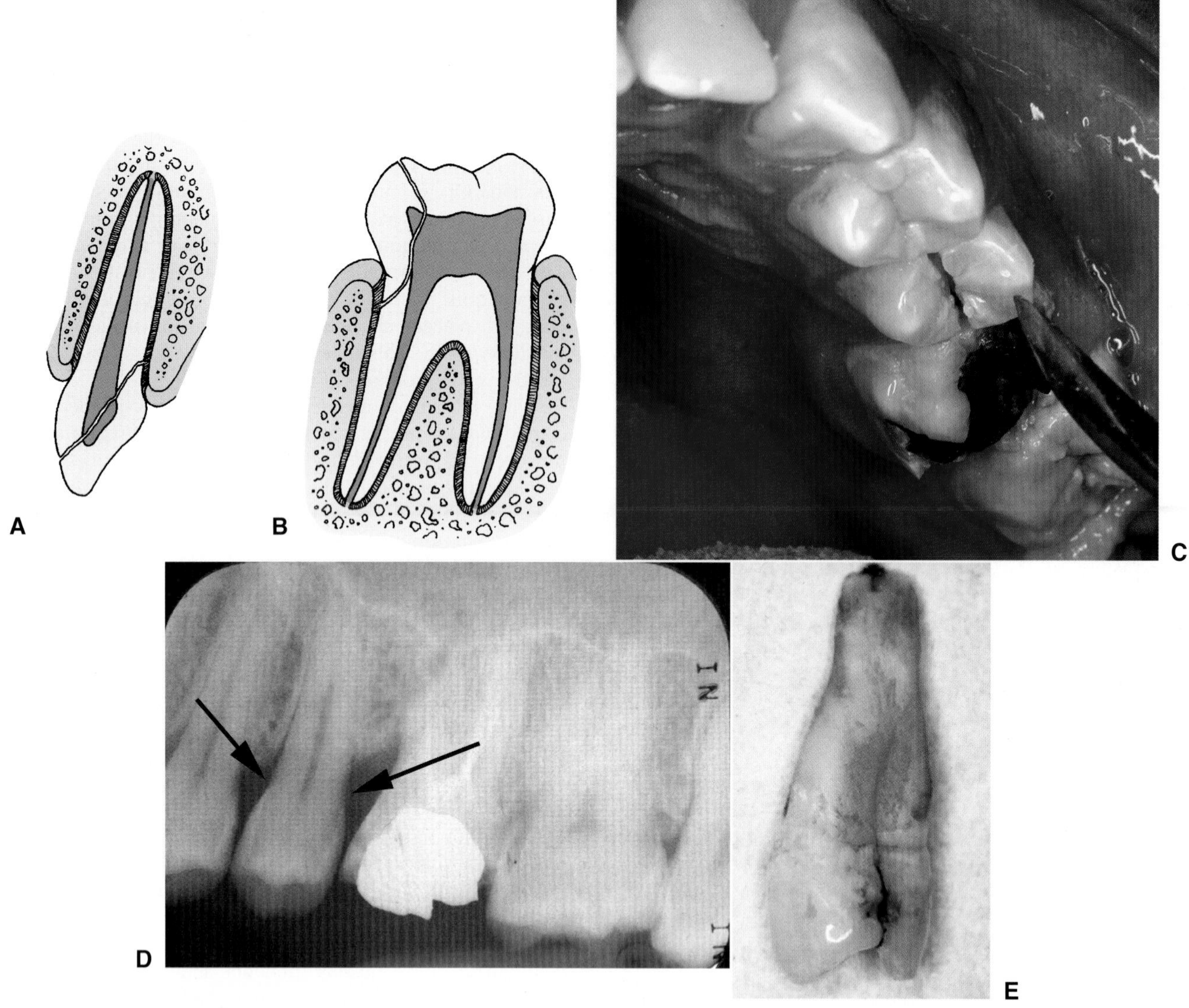

FIGURE 23-11 Crown-root fractures. **A** and **B**, Illustrations of crown-root fractures in incisor and molar, respectively. Fractures extend below alveolar crest of bone. **C**, Clinical photograph of crown-root fracture in premolar. This tooth is commonly fractured in this manner, especially when there is a restoration extending across the occlusal surface (i.e., MOD). **D**, Radiograph of this premolar showing no obvious fracture because the fracture is in the mesiodistal direction. **E**, Tooth after extraction showing the fracture extending apically.

Extrusion

Extruded teeth can usually be manually seated back into their sockets if the injury was recent. After replacement of the tooth within the socket, splinting for 1 to 3 weeks is usually necessary, as is endodontic treatment (discussed later; Figs. 23-13, *B*, and 23-16).

Lateral Displacement

If a tooth is minimally displaced, the accompanying alveolar wall fractures may not be grossly displaced. In this case, manual repositioning of the tooth and splinting for several weeks is indicated. When substantial tooth displacement has occurred, displaced alveolar bone fractures have also been sustained (Fig. 23-13, *C* and *D*). Gingival lacerations frequently accompany this type of injury. The tooth and the alveolar bone must be manually repositioned, the tooth splinted, and soft tissues sutured (Fig. 23-17).

Postsurgical follow-up examinations will determine the state of the pulp and periodontal damage.

Avulsion

Total avulsion from its socket is the gravest situation for a tooth because the health of the pulp and the periodontal tissues is in severe jeopardy. The factors most important for determining how successful treatment measures will be are the length of time the tooth has been out of the socket, the state of the tooth and periodontal tissues, and the manner in which the tooth was preserved before replantation. The sooner the tooth can be replanted, the better the prognosis.[2]

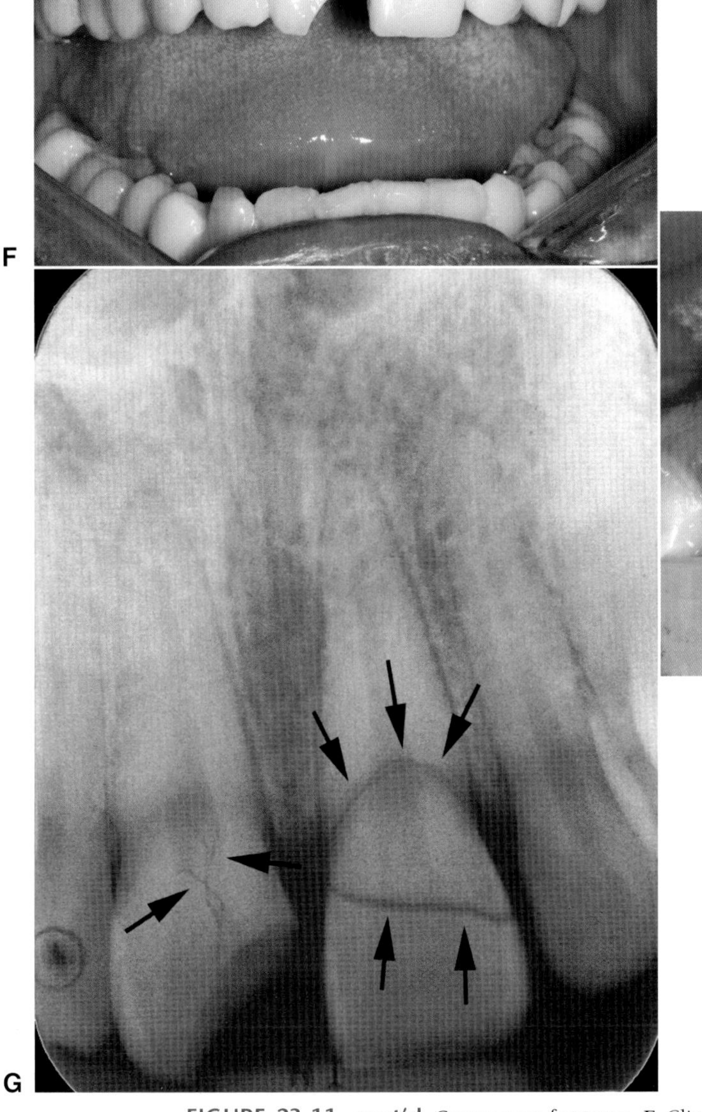

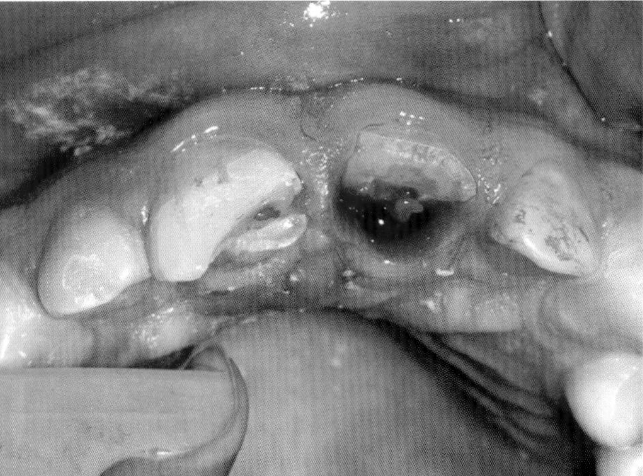

FIGURE 23-11, cont'd Crown-root fractures. F, Clinical photograph of two incisors with crown-root fractures. Tooth No. 8 appears to have only a fracture of the crown, but the radiograph (G) shows that there are fracture lines extending into the root. Similarly, the clinical examination does not reveal the depth of the fracture on tooth No. 9, but the radiograph (G) shows it extends apical to the cementoenamel junction. After the loose crown portion was removed, the fracture was found to involve the pulp and to extend well above the cementoenamel junction (H). Both of these teeth were removed and replaced with dental implants.

Therefore, when the dentist receives a call from a patient, parent, teacher, or other responsible person regarding a totally avulsed tooth, the dentist should direct the caller to rinse the tooth immediately with the patient's saliva, tap water, or saline solution and to replant the tooth. The patient should hold the tooth by the crown, while trying to not touch the root, and then hold the tooth in place and go immediately to the dentist. If the patient cannot replace the tooth, it should be placed into an appropriate medium until care by a dentist can be delivered. Many storage mediums have been recommended, including water, the vestibule of the mouth, physiologic saline, milk, and cell culture media in specialized containers. Water is the least desirable because it is hypotonic and causes cell lysis. Saliva keeps the tooth moist but is not ideal because of incompatible osmolality and pH and the presence of bacteria. The most ideal storage medium is Hanks balanced salt solution, which can be

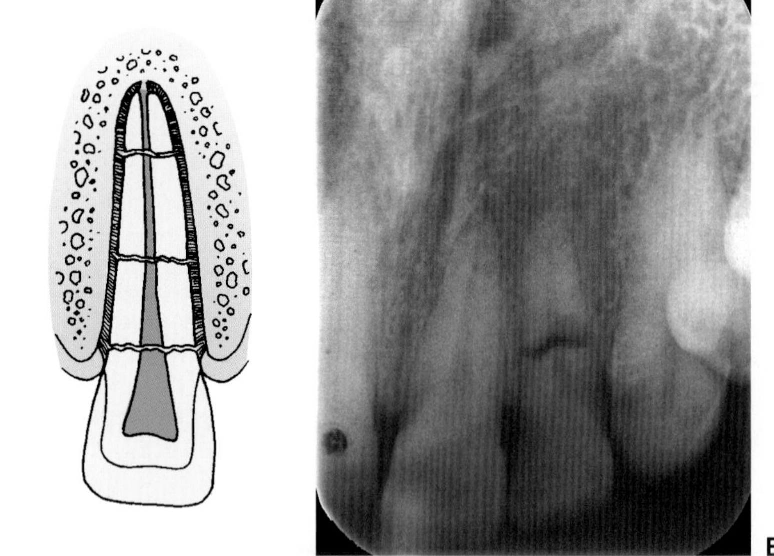

FIGURE 23-12 A, Illustration showing horizontal root fractures at apical, middle, and coronal levels of root (*top, middle,* and *bottom,* respectively). B, Radiograph of a horizontal root fracture at the junction of the coronal and middle thirds. This tooth was extremely mobile, so it was removed and replaced with an immediate dental implant. Figure 23-6, *B,* shows a radiograph of a horizontal root fracture at the junction of the apical and middle thirds. This tooth had slight mobility but was stabilized, and it healed.

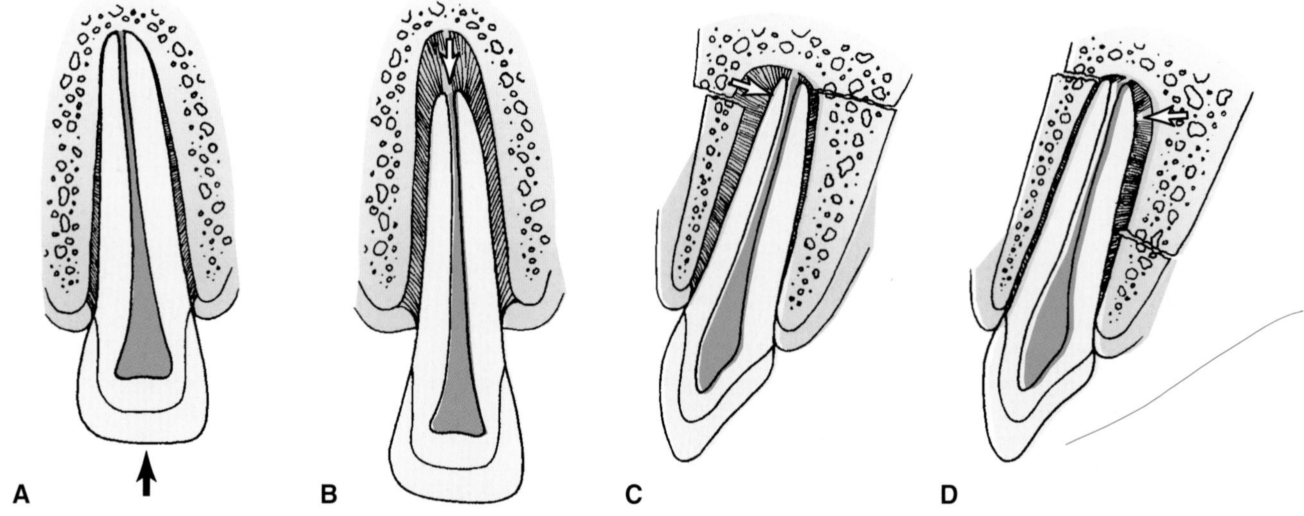

FIGURE 23-13 Tooth displacement. A, Intruded tooth. The absence of periodontal ligament space along apex is demonstrated. B, Tooth displaced from its socket in coronal direction (i.e., extruded). C and D, Displacement of incisor tooth crown buccally and lingually, respectively. Associated alveolar wall fractures, which are frequently present, are visualized.

purchased as part of a commercial tooth-preserving system (Save-A-Tooth, Biologic Rescue Products, Conshohocken, Pennsylvania). Many schools, sporting venues, and ambulances have these kits on hand for use in cases of tooth avulsion. If this solution is not available, milk is considered the best alternative storage medium because it is readily available at or near an accident site, it has a pH and osmolarity compatible with vital cells, and it is relatively free of bacteria. Milk has been shown effectively to maintain the vitality of periodontal ligament cells.[9]

When the patient gets to the dentist's office, the dentist must decide whether the tooth is salvageable. If the tooth has already been replanted and seems to be in good position, it should be radiographed and then splinted for 7 to 10 days. If the tooth is carried into the office and it has been out of its socket less than 20 minutes, it should be immediately rinsed in saline and replanted by the dentist. Removal of all of the blood clot from within the socket is not necessary; however, careful suctioning and gentle irrigation with sterile saline will remove the bulk of the clot. The root surface and tooth socket should

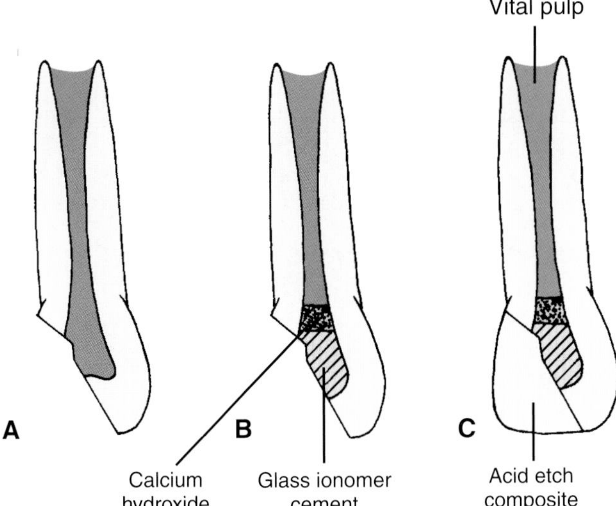

FIGURE 23-14 Pulpotomy technique. **A**, Apically immature tooth with coronal fracture involving pulp. **B**, Coronal pulp removed aseptically, after which calcium hydroxide solution is applied over exposed pulp. Glass ionomer cement can then be used to fill remainder of coronal pulp chamber, and temporary or permanent (i.e., composite) filling is placed (**C**).

never be scraped, "sterilized," or manipulated before replantation because this destroys viable periodontal tissue.

If the tooth has been out of the socket for more than 20 minutes, it should not be replanted until after it has been placed into Hanks balanced salt solution for 30 minutes and then in doxycycline (1 mg/20 mL saline) for 5 minutes. The tooth should then be replanted and splinted. Soaking the tooth in Hanks solution seems to reduce the incidence of ankylosis by improving the survival of periodontal cells on the root. The solution also helps cleanse debris from the root and dilutes bacteria. The doxycycline helps inhibit bacteria in the pulpal lumen, which reduces a major obstacle to revascularlization. Even teeth that were stored in milk or saline should undergo this regimen before implantation.

Stabilization of an avulsed tooth can be achieved using a variety of materials, such as wires, arch bars, and splints. However, several factors must be considered: The stabilizing device should be as hygienic as possible and should be positioned away from the gingiva and tooth roots, if possible. During the healing response, inflammation must be kept to a minimum or inflammatory root resorption will be favored, which is one of the drawbacks to interdental wiring and cold-cured acrylic splints. Patients have difficulty cleansing teeth that are covered with wires or splints. Furthermore, wire can slip apically around the cervical aspect and damage the cementum. The stabilization applied to the tooth need not be absolutely rigid because this may predispose to ankylosis and external root resorption. Physiologic movements of the tooth are thought by some to promote fibrous (i.e., desired) instead of osseous (i.e., tending toward ankylosis) attachment of the root to the alveolar bone. The stabilization device should also be easy to apply and remove with readily available instruments.

A technique that serves admirably for the stabilization of avulsed teeth is the use of an acid-etched composite system (Figs. 23-17 and 23-18). A wire of moderate stiffness but that still has some flexibility, such as braided orthodontic wire, is adapted to the facial surfaces of one or two teeth on each side of the avulsed tooth. The fewer teeth required to stabilize the avulsed tooth, the more physiologic movement that can be imparted to the replanted tooth during function. If braided orthodontic wire is unavailable, any wire—even a paper clip—will suffice. The facial surfaces of the avulsed and the adjacent teeth are acid-etched, and the wire is cemented to them with composite. This technique makes cleansing the teeth easy because the wire is away from the gingiva. The wire can be readily removed, and most dentists have the necessary supplies and instrumentation available for its use.

TABLE 23-1

Stabilization Periods for Dentoalveolar Injuries

Dentoalveolar Injury	Duration of Immobilization
Mobile tooth	7-10 days
Tooth displacement	2-3 weeks
Root fracture	2-4 months
Replanted tooth (mature)	7-10 days
Replanted tooth (immature)	3-4 weeks

The duration of stabilization (Table 23-1) should be as short a time as necessary for the tooth to become reattached, usually 7 to 10 days. Studies have shown that the more rigid and the longer the stabilization, the more root resorption that can be expected.[1,10]

On removal of the stabilization device, the tooth will still be mobile. Therefore, it is important that the stabilization device be removed with great care and that the patient be instructed to avoid this region during mastication. If, however, the apical foramen is wide open, pulp may survive and revascularize. To promote this possibility, the tooth is usually stabilized for 3 to 4 weeks instead of the shorter time for apically mature teeth.

Patients who have no recollection of a tetanus booster within the past 5 to 10 years should be referred to their physician for one. The use of antibiotics (e.g., penicillin) for 7 to 10 days is appropriate.

The patient should be told that several outcomes are possible after replantation. The best result to be expected is a relatively normal, functional tooth that in most instances will require endodontic therapy (described later). However, varying amounts of root resorption and ankylosis may occur. The development of these signs determines the prognosis of the tooth. Although acute dental infection is rare, it can lead to loss of the replanted tooth. These patients must be followed carefully at regular and frequent intervals for some time after replantation. Andreasen and Hjorting-Hansen[3] list the following five factors to be considered before replanting avulsed teeth:

1. The avulsed tooth should have no advanced periodontal disease.
2. The alveolar socket should be reasonably intact to provide a seat for the avulsed tooth.
3. There should be no orthodontic contraindications, such as significant crowding of teeth.
4. The extraalveolar period should be considered; periods exceeding 2 hours are usually associated with poor results. If the tooth is replanted within the first 30 minutes, excellent results can be expected.

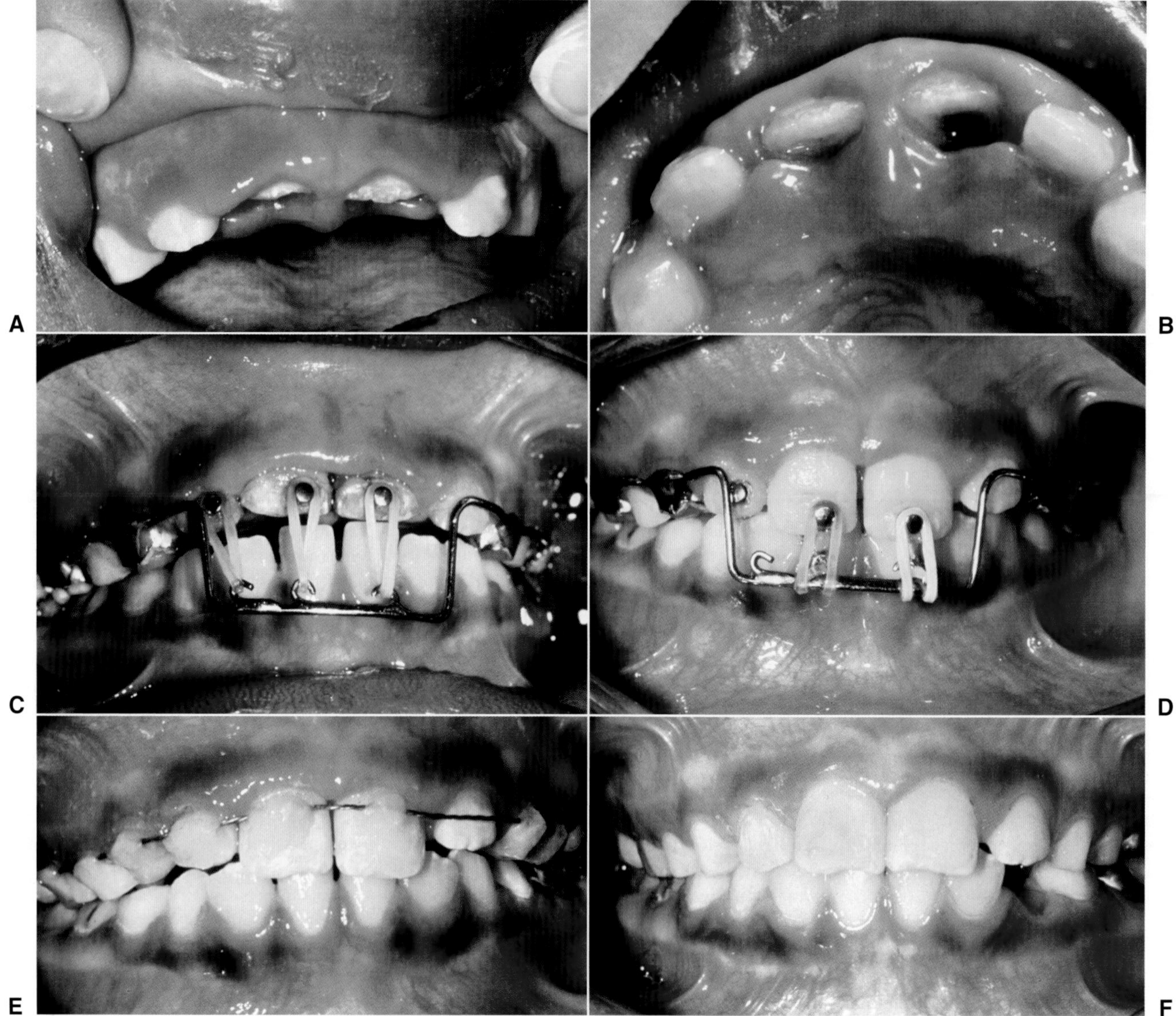

FIGURE 23-15 Treatment of intruded maxillary incisors with immature apices. Buccal (**A**) and palatal (**B**) views of intruded maxillary incisor teeth. **C**, Orthodontic traction instituted to extrude teeth a few weeks after traumatic episode. **D**, Appearance after 6 weeks of traction. **E**, Stabilization of teeth after orthodontic-guided reeruption with acid-etch technique for 11 weeks. **F**, Appearance after 1 year. This patient had calcium hydroxide pulpectomies and apexification during period of orthodontic extrusion and subsequently had root canals. (From Spalding PM, Fields HW Jr, Torney D et al: The changing role of endodontics and orthodontics in the management of traumatically intruded permanent incisors, *Pediatr Dent* 7:104, 1985.)

5. The stage of root development should be evaluated. Survival of the pulp is possible in teeth with incomplete root formation if replantation is accomplished within 2 hours after injury.

If the tooth to be replanted is not favorable for replantation, as determined by these factors, the patient should be made aware that the prognosis will be worse. One should keep in mind the alternatives to replantation in cases where the factors involved are unfavorable, such as teeth with existing periodontal disease, large restorations, alveolar disruption, and long extra-alveolar duration. Today the use of dental implants can offer patients who suffered tooth avulsion an option that was not available in the past. In hopeless cases, one might elect to defer tooth replantation for placement of a dental implant once the alveolus has healed.

Alveolar Fractures

Small fractures through the alveolar process, as mentioned previously, frequently accompany injuries to the teeth. However, injuries to the alveolar process often occur independently and can be challenging to manage. In most instances the segment of bone contains at least one tooth but more frequently several.

Concomitant injuries, such as crown fractures, root fractures, and soft tissue injuries, may have occurred. These injuries

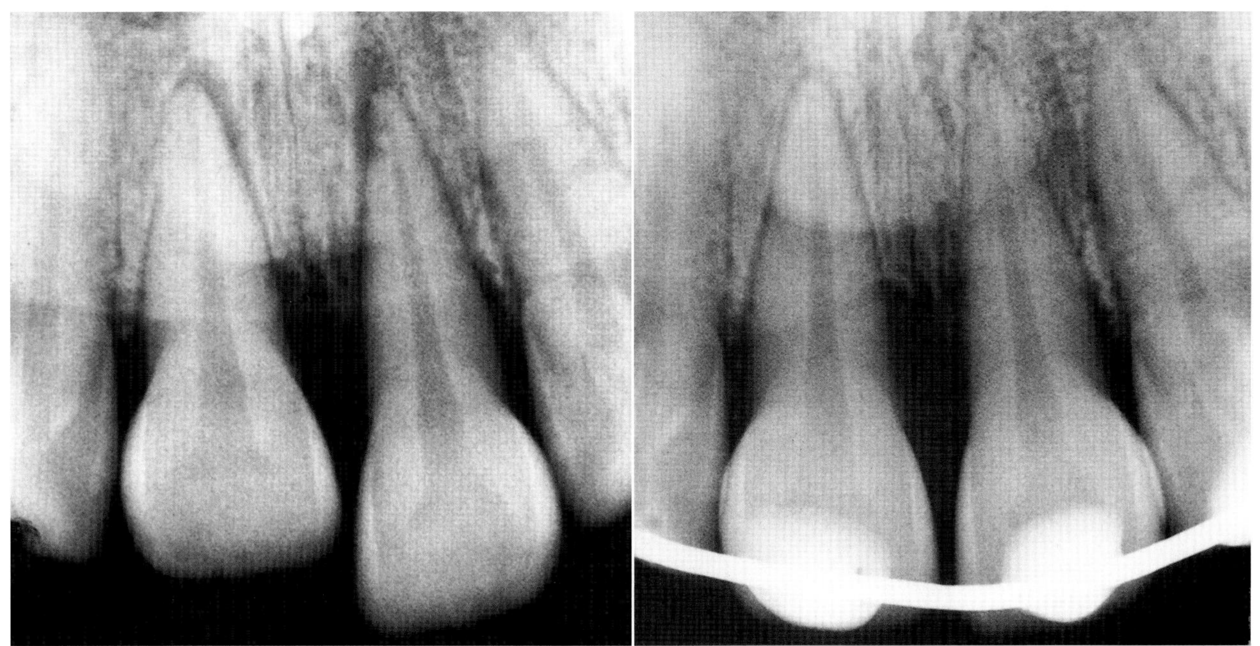

FIGURE 23-16 Radiographs of extruded tooth before (**A**) and after (**B**) repositioning and stabilization with acid-etch composite technique.

may best be managed by referral to an oral and maxillofacial surgeon because management may involve open surgical treatment to reposition the bony segments.

The treatment of this type of injury, as for any fracture, is first to place the segment into its proper position and then to stabilize it until osseous healing occurs. This procedure may be simply performed with digital pressure applied after an appropriate anesthetic is administered (Fig. 23-19). Frequently, however, splintering of the dentoosseous segment margins makes repositioning difficult, and open surgical treatment might then be required.

Teeth with root apices that are denuded within a dentoalveolar fracture should undergo endodontic treatment within 1 to 2 weeks to help prevent inflammatory root resorption and infection. The dentoosseous segment must be stabilized for approximately 4 weeks to allow osseous healing. Several acceptable methods can be used to stabilize the segment: The simplest is to ligate an arch bar to the teeth both mesial and distal to the segment and within the fractured alveolar segment. The teeth immediately adjacent to the fracture are frequently not wired to the arch bar, so these teeth are more amenable to oral hygienic measures. Not wiring them also helps to prevent their loosening from the forces placed by the wire. The use of an acid-etched arch wire, as just described, is also acceptable. A cold-cured acrylic splint can be made in situ or on casts obtained by taking an impression immediately after repositioning the alveolar segment. The splint can be wired to adjacent teeth and to teeth within the fractured segment.

Treatment of Pulp

The dental pulp may be damaged during any of the tooth injuries just described, as a result of direct exposure, the inflammatory response of near exposure, concussive effects, or disruption of the nutrient artery of the pulp. In any injury to the tooth, the possibility for pulpal degeneration is real, and early detection is imperative. If a pulp degenerates, an inflammatory response occurs that leads to tooth resorption and ankylosis (Fig. 23-20). Therefore, for all injuries described, the status of the pulp must be ascertained. Because it is difficult to establish the health status of the pulp immediately after injury, the dentist must assume that if the apex of a mature tooth has moved more than 1 mm in any direction, pulpal degeneration will occur.

Root canal treatment should not be performed at the time of tooth repositioning or replantation because the extra time necessary to perform this treatment is not warranted and exposes the tooth to more chance of external damage. However, in all teeth with closed apical foramina, endodontic treatment should be instituted after approximately 2 weeks. This treatment helps minimize inflammatory root resorption by eliminating nonvital tissue from the pulp. A standard biomechanical preparation of the root canal system is then performed. However, instead of filling the root canal with gutta-percha, the clinician treats the canal in a manner similar to an apexification technique; that is, a 1:1 mixture of calcium hydroxide and barium sulfate is placed within the canal for 6 to 12 months. The barium sulfate allows radiographic evaluation of the amount of calcium hydroxide present because it slowly dissipates within the root canal after placement. Periodic radiographic evaluations should be performed, and the calcium hydroxide should be replaced every 3 months if noted to be absent from the root canal system. A conventional root canal can be performed when successive radiographs indicate no further root resorption. This regimen should be used instead of placing a permanent endodontic filling soon after biomechanical preparation because it appears to minimize inflammatory root resorption.

In teeth with apical foramina that are wide open, endodontic treatment may be delayed for several weeks while careful follow-up examinations, including pulp vitality tests,

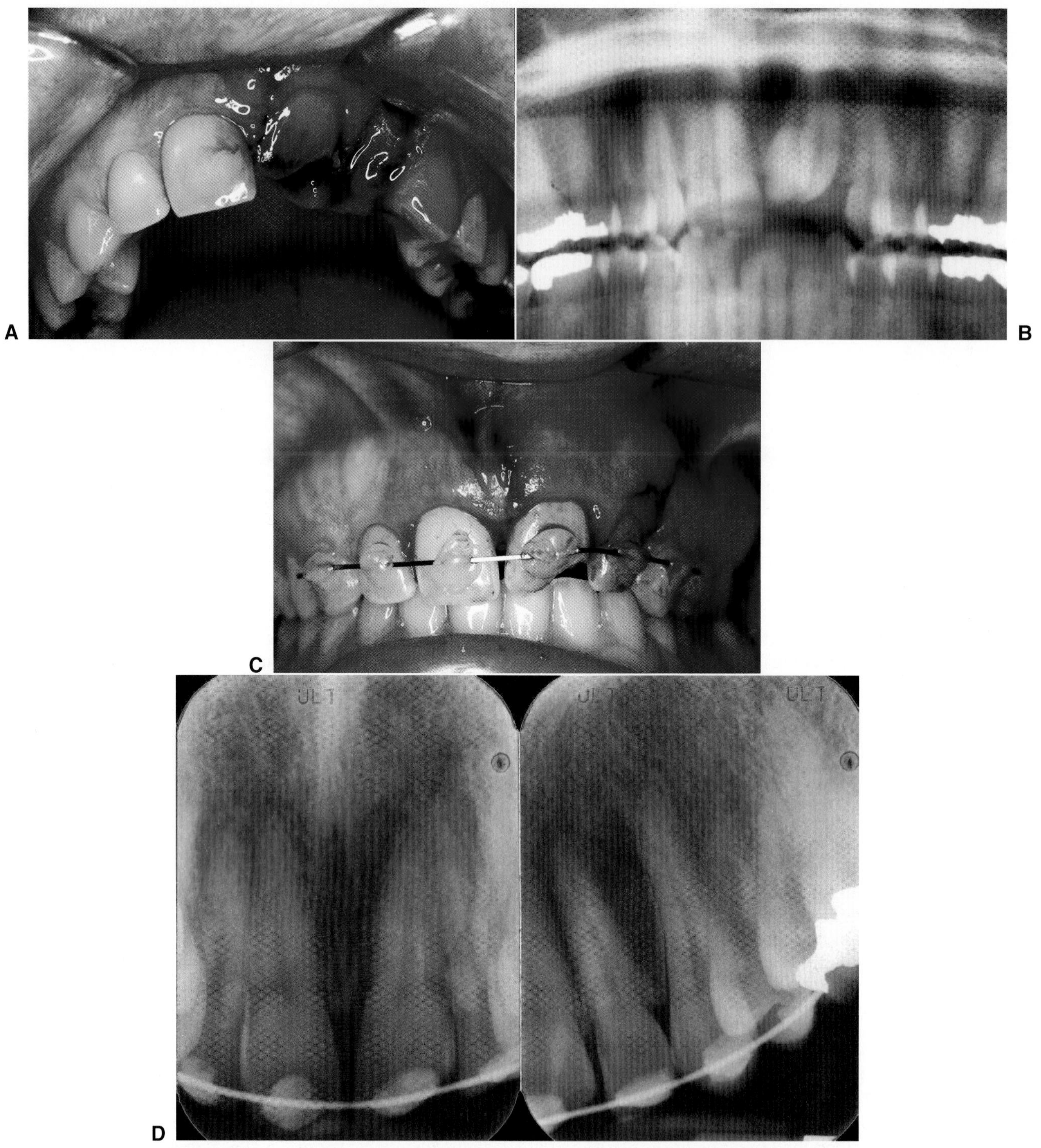

FIGURE 23-17 Treatment of lingually displaced central and lateral incisors in apically mature tooth. A, Appearance on presentation. B, Radiograph showing position of the teeth and the lack of root fracture(s). C, Position of teeth after digital reduction and stabilization with an arch wire bonded to the teeth with composite resin. D, Immediate postreduction radiograph showing that the teeth have been replaced into their sockets.

determine its necessity. When the apices are open, it is likely that revascularization of the root canal system will occur. If root canal therapy appears necessary, apexification procedures with use of calcium hydroxide can be used before filling of the root canal system with a permanent filling material. The technique of apexification is illustrated in Figure 23-21.

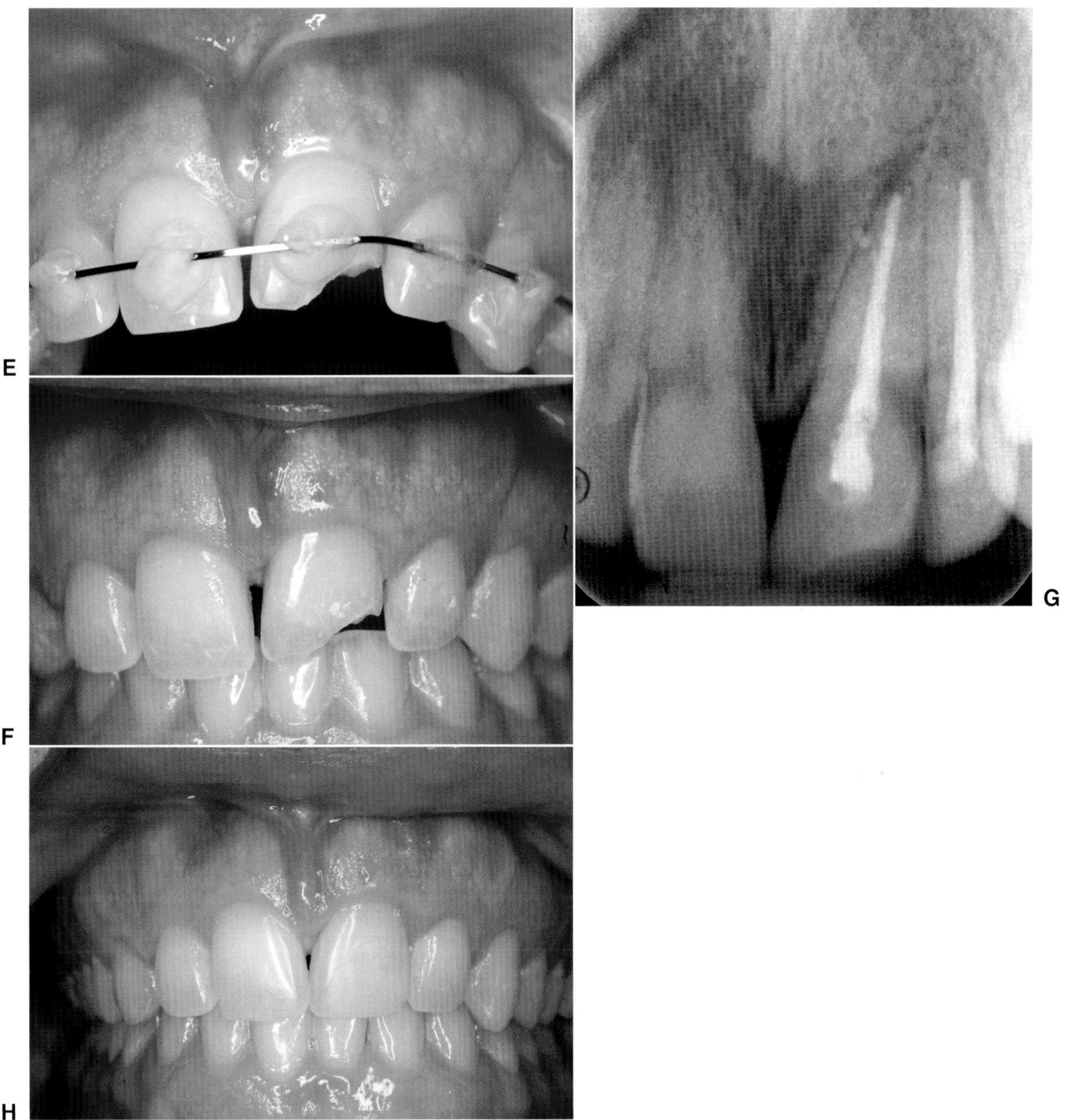

FIGURE 23-17, cont'd Treatment of lingually displaced central and lateral incisors in apically mature tooth. E, Clinical appearance at 3 weeks just before the arch wire was removed. F, Clinical appearance 1 week after arch wire removed. The patient was sent for endodontic therapy (G), and composite was used to reconstruct the missing portion of the crown of tooth No. 9 (H).

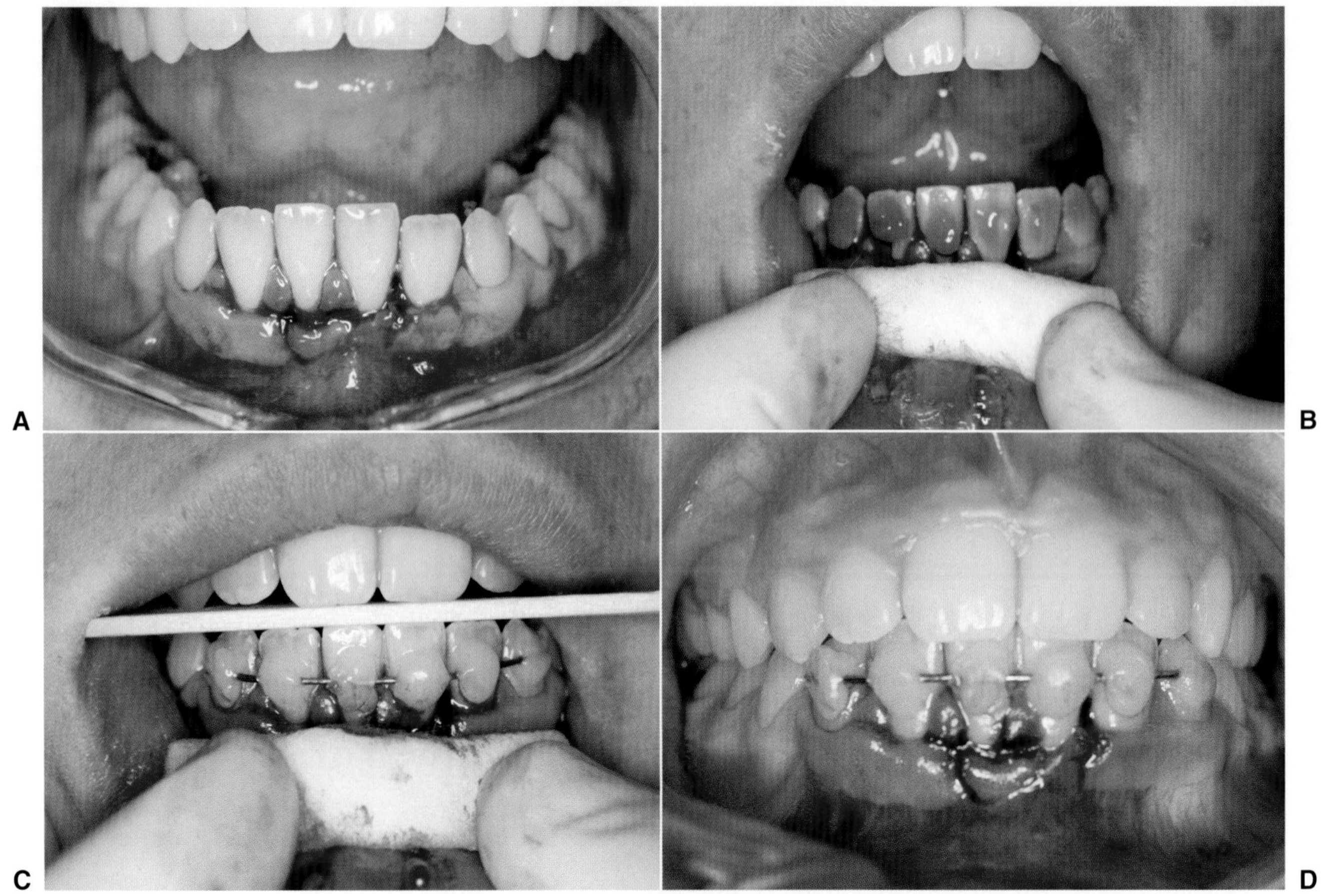

FIGURE 23-18 Technique of acid-etch composite stabilization of displaced teeth. A, Lower incisor teeth displaced lingually. B, After digital repositioning, acid is applied to facial surfaces of displaced incisors and one or two teeth on each side after isolation and drying. C, Composite material and wire applied. D, Occlusion checked during and after stabilization.

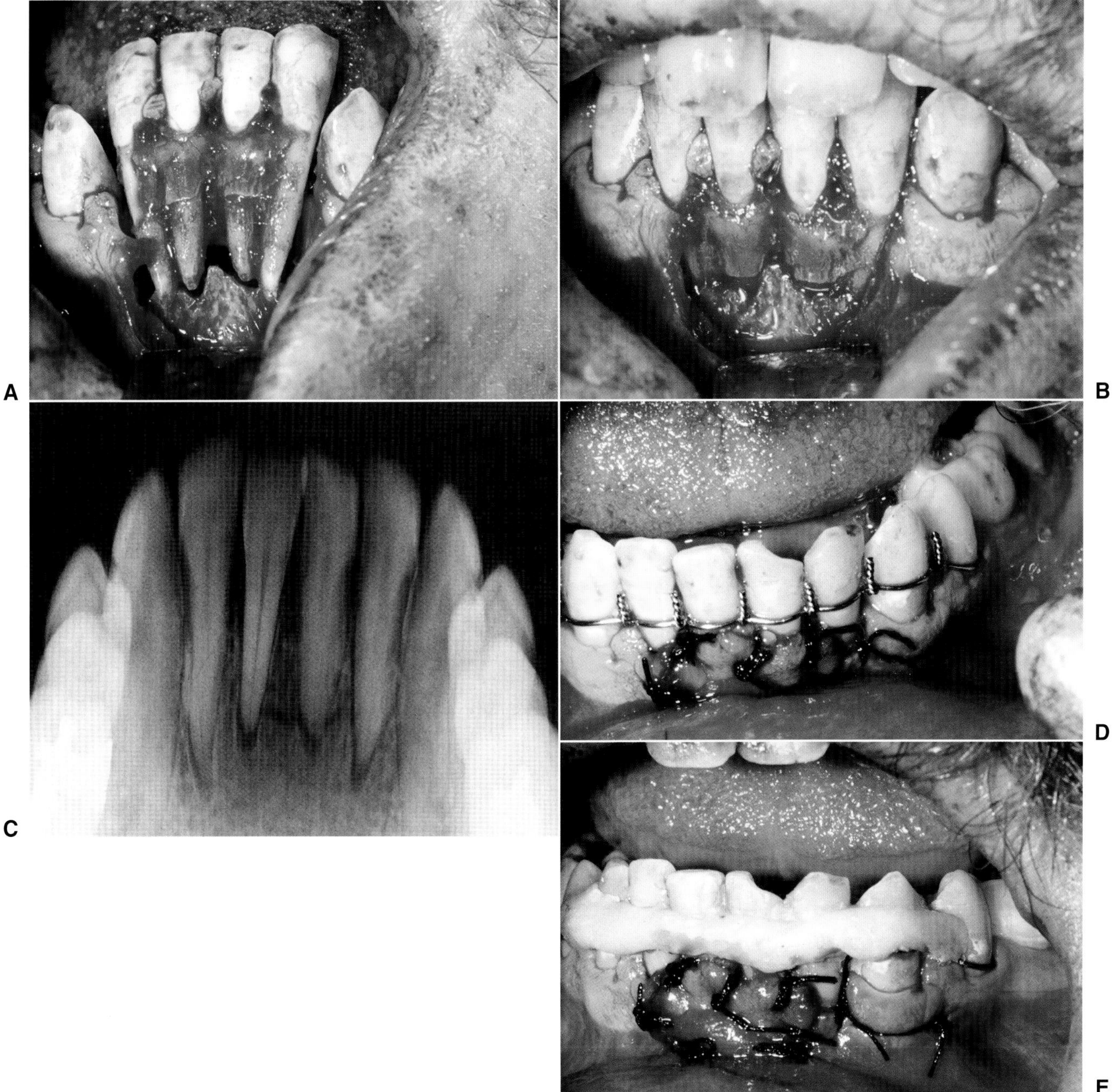

FIGURE 23-19 Treatment of dentoalveolar fracture. A, Clinical appearance of fracture involving four mandibular incisors. The teeth are apically mature and have minimal bone around lateral and apical areas. B, Clinical appearance after digital reduction of fracture. Occlusal relationship is verified before stabilization of these teeth. C, Radiographic appearance of teeth after digital reduction. D, Appearance after application of Essig wire and suturing of mucosa. E, Cold-curing acrylic added for rigidity (Note: Bonding an arch wire to the teeth with the acid-etch composite technique demonstrated in Figure 23-18 would be preferable). Because of maturity of apices, root canal treatment should be performed on these teeth in 1 to 2 weeks after trauma. (B Courtesy Dr. Stephen Feinberg, University of Michigan, Ann Arbor.)

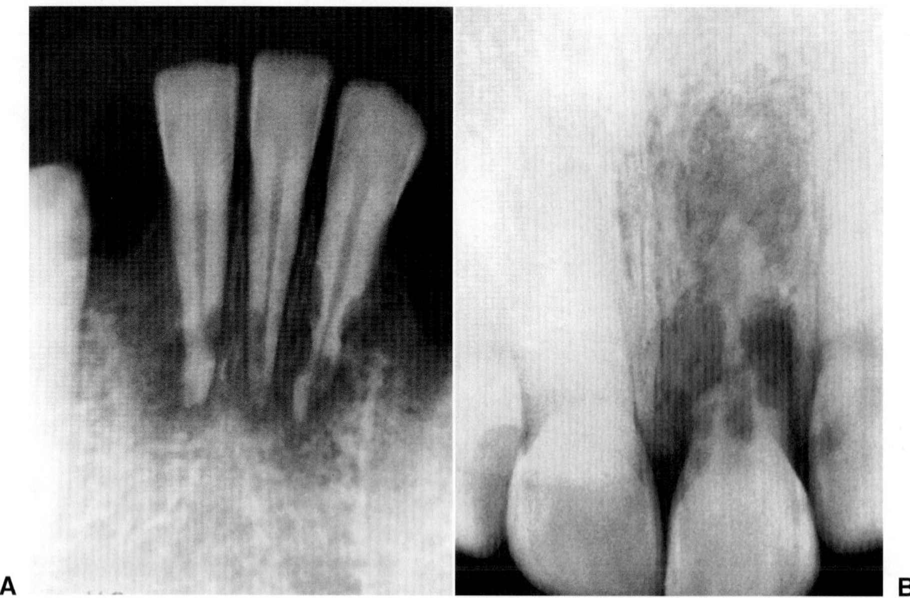

FIGURE 23-20 A and B, Two cases of inflammatory root resorption that occurred several months after dentoalveolar trauma without root canal treatment.

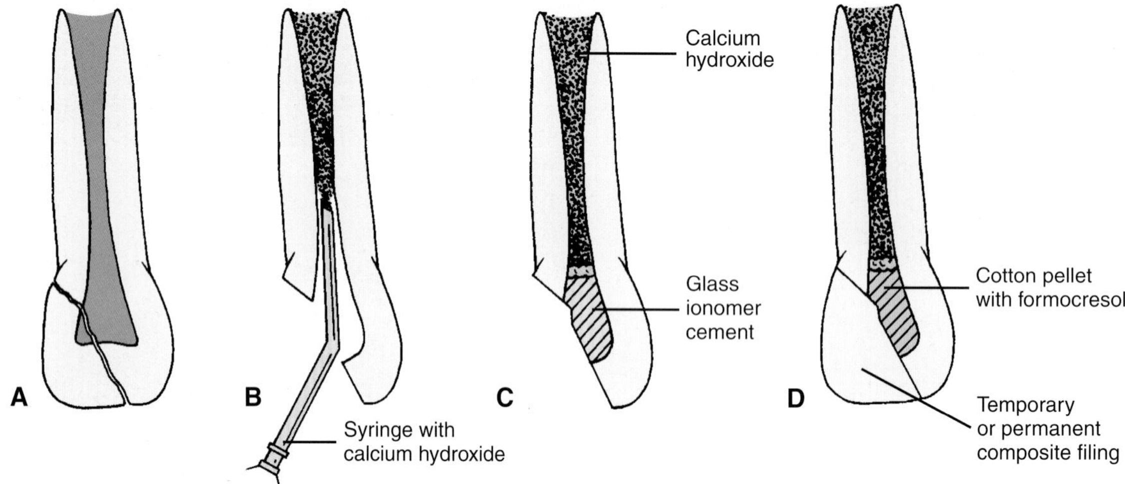

FIGURE 23-21 Apexification procedure. A, Coronal fracture involving pulp of apically immature tooth. B, Removal of entire pulp and filling with calcium hydroxide solution. Calcium hydroxide can be injected from syringe or spun in with spiral on rotating instrument. C, Cotton pledget (with or without formocresol) is then placed, after which coronal pulp chamber is filled with glass ionomer cement. D, Temporary or permanent composite filling is then placed. Calcium hydroxide solution may require replacing every 3 months until apex is closed.

REFERENCES

1. Andreasen JO: The effect of splinting upon periodontal healing after replantation of permanent incisors in monkeys, *Acta Odontol Scand* 33:313, 1975.
2. Andreasen JO, Andreasen FM: *Textbook and color atlas of traumatic injuries to the teeth,* ed 3, Copenhagen, 1994, Munksgaard.
3. Andreasen JO, Hjorting-Hansen E: Replantation of teeth. I. Radiographic and clinical study of 110 human teeth replanted after accidental loss, *Acta Odontol Scand* 24:263, 1966.
4. Sanders B, Brady FA, Johnson R: Injuries. In Sanders B, editor: *Pediatric oral and maxillofacial surgery,* St Louis, 1979, Mosby.
5. Donley KJ: Management of sports-related crown fractures, *Dent Clin North Am* 44:85, 2000.
6. Rauschenberger CR, Hovland EJ: Clinical management of crown fractures, *Dent Clin North Am* 39:25, 1995.
7. Pagliarini A, Rubini R, Rea M et al: Crown fractures: effectiveness of current enamel-dentin adhesives in reattachment of fractured fragments, *Quintessence Int* 31:133, 2000.
8. Turley PK, Joiner MW, Hellstrom S: The effect of orthodontic extrusion on traumatically intruded teeth, *Am J Orthod* 85:47, 1984.
9. Trope M: Clinical management of the avulsed tooth, *Dent Clin North Am* 39:93, 1995.
10. Andreasen JO: Etiology and pathogenesis of traumatic dental injuries, *Scand J Dent Res* 78:339, 1970.

CHAPTER 24

Management of Facial Fractures

MARK W. OCHS and MYRON R. TUCKER

CHAPTER OUTLINE

Trauma to the facial region frequently results in injuries to soft tissue, teeth, and major skeletal components of the face, including the mandible, maxilla, zygoma, nasoorbital-ethmoid (NOE) complex, and supraorbital structures. In addition, these injuries frequently occur in combination with injuries to other areas of the body.[1] Participation in the treatment and rehabilitation of the patient with facial trauma involves a thorough understanding of the types of, principles of evaluation for, and surgical treatment of facial injuries. This chapter outlines the fundamental principles for treatment of the patient with facial trauma.

EVALUATION OF PATIENTS WITH FACIAL TRAUMA

Immediate Assessment

Before completing a detailed history and physical evaluation of the facial area, critical injuries that may be life threatening must be addressed. The first step in evaluating a trauma patient is to assess the patient's cardiopulmonary stability by ensuring that the patient has a patent airway and that the lungs are adequately ventilated. Vital signs, including respiratory and pulse rates and blood pressure, should be taken and recorded. During this initial assessment (i.e., primary survey), other potentially life-threatening problems, such as excessive bleeding, should also be addressed. Immediate measures, such as pressure dressings, packing, and clamping of briskly bleeding vessels, should be accomplished as quickly as possible. An assessment of the patient's neurologic status and an evaluation of the cervical spine should be completed next. Forces severe enough to cause fractures of the facial skeleton are often transmitted to the cervical spine. The neck should be temporarily immobilized until neck injuries have been ruled out. Careful palpation of the neck to assess possible areas of tenderness and a cervical spine radiographic series should be completed as soon as possible.

Treatment of head and neck injuries generally should be deferred until a thorough evaluation, assessment, and stabilization of the patient has been accomplished. However, some initial treatment is often necessary to stabilize the patient. Management of the patient's airway is of vital importance. Frequently, fractures of the facial bones severely compromise the patient's ability to maintain the airway, particularly when the patient is unconscious or completely supine. Severe mandible fractures, especially bilateral or comminuted fractures, can cause posterior displacement of the mandible and tongue, which results in obstruction of the upper airway (Fig. 24-1).

Simply grasping, repositioning, and stabilizing the mandible into a more anterior position may alleviate this obstruction. Placement of a nasopharyngeal or an oropharyngeal airway may also be sufficient to temporarily maintain a patent airway. In some cases, endotracheal intubation may be necessary. Any prosthetic devices, avulsed teeth, pieces of completely avulsed bone, or other debris may also contribute to airway occlusion and must be removed immediately. Any areas of bleeding should be quickly examined and managed with packing, pressure dressings, or clamping. All excess saliva and blood must be suctioned from the pharynx to avoid aspiration and laryngospasm.

Injuries to the facial region may involve not only bones of the face but also soft tissue, such as the tongue or upper neck areas, or they may be associated with injuries such as a fractured larynx.[2] In some cases an emergency tracheostomy may be necessary to provide an adequate airway. In trauma patients who have complete upper airway obstruction, a cricothyrotomy is the most rapid way to access the trachea (Fig. 24-2).

History and Physical Examination

After the patient has been initially stabilized, as complete a history as possible should be obtained. This history should be obtained from the patient; however, because of loss of

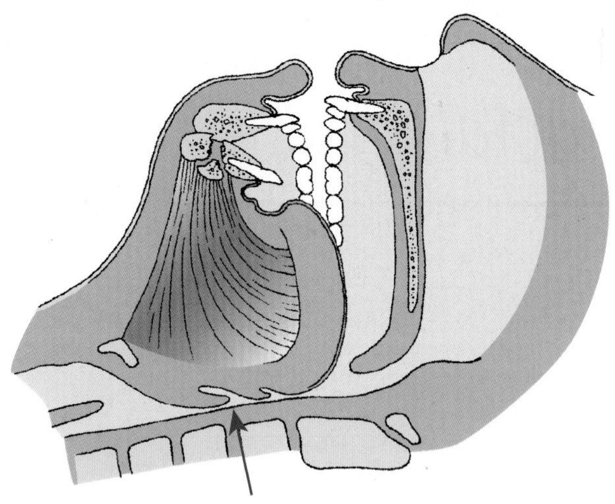

FIGURE 24-1 Posterior displacement of tongue and occlusion of upper airway resulting from bilateral mandibular fractures.

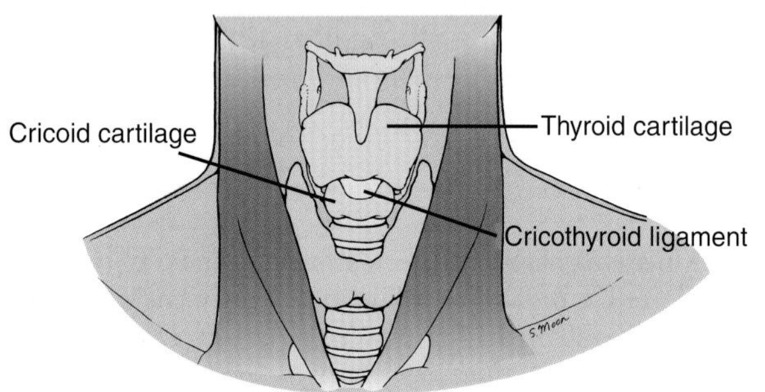

FIGURE 24-2 Tracheostomy and cricothyrotomy sites with landmarks for emergency surgical airway access.

consciousness or impaired neurologic status, information must often be obtained from witnesses or accompanying family members. Five important questions should be considered: (1) How did the accident occur? (2) When did the accident occur? (3) What are the specifics of the injury, including the type of object contacted, the direction from which contact was made, and similar logistic considerations? (4) Was there a loss of consciousness? (5) What symptoms are now being experienced by the patient, including pain, altered sensation, visual changes, and malocclusion? A complete review of systems, including information about allergies, medications, and previous tetanus immunization, medical conditions, and prior surgeries should be obtained.

Physical evaluation of the facial structures should be completed only after an overall physical assessment that addresses cardiopulmonary and neurologic functions and other areas of potential trauma, including the chest, abdomen, and pelvic areas. Because patients with multiple severe injuries frequently require evaluation and treatment by several specialists, *trauma teams* have become standard in the emergency departments of major hospitals. These teams usually include general surgeons and specialists in cardiothoracic surgery, vascular surgery, orthopedic surgery, neurosurgery, and anesthesiology; these specialists are on call to provide immediate attention to emergency department patients. Other trauma team specialists include oral and maxillofacial surgeons, ophthalmologists, otolaryngologists, plastic surgeons, and urologists. The combined efforts of these

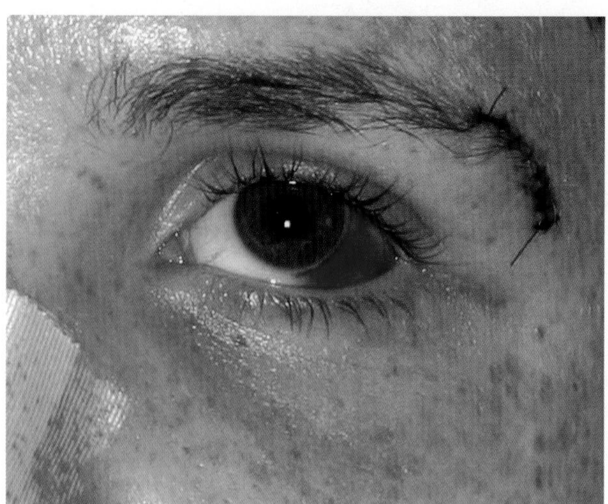

FIGURE 24-3 Periorbital ecchymosis and lateral subconjunctival hemorrhage associated with zygomatic complex fracture.

specialists are frequently required to assess and treat the patient's injuries properly.

Evaluation of the facial area should be performed in an organized and sequential fashion. The face and cranium should be carefully inspected for evidence of trauma, including lacerations, abrasions, contusions, areas of edema or hematoma formation, and possible contour defects. Areas of ecchymosis should be carefully evaluated.

Periorbital ecchymosis, especially with subconjunctival hemorrhage, is often indicative of orbital rim or zygomatic complex fractures (Fig. 24-3). Bruises behind the ear, or Battle's sign, suggest a basilar skull fracture. Ecchymosis in the floor of the mouth usually indicates an anterior mandibular fracture.

A neurologic examination of the face should include careful evaluation of all cranial nerves. Vision, extraocular movements, and pupillary reaction to light should be carefully evaluated. Visual acuity or pupillary changes may suggest intracranial (cranial nerve II or III dysfunction) or direct orbital trauma. Uneven pupils (anisocoria) in a lethargic patient suggest an intracranial bleed (subdural or epidural hematoma or intraparenchymal bleed) or injury. An asymmetric or irregular (not round) pupil is most likely caused by a globe (eyeball) perforation. Abnormalities of ocular movements may also indicate central neurologic problems (cranial nerves III, IV, or VI) or mechanical restriction of the movements of the eye muscles resulting from fractures of the orbital complex (Fig. 24-4). Motor function of the facial muscles (cranial nerve VII) and muscles of mastication (cranial nerve V) and sensation over the facial area (cranial nerve V) should be evaluated. Any lacerations should be carefully cleaned and evaluated for possible transection of major nerves or ducts, such as the facial nerve or Stensen's duct.

The mandible should be carefully evaluated by extraorally palpating all areas of the inferior and lateral borders and the temporomandibular joint, paying particular attention to areas of point tenderness. The occlusion should be examined, and step deformities along the occlusal plane and lacerations of gingival areas should be assessed (Fig. 24-5). Bimanual palpation of the suspected fracture area should be performed by placing firm pressure over the mandible posterior and anterior to the fracture area in an attempt to manipulate and elicit mobility in this area. The occlusion should be reexamined after

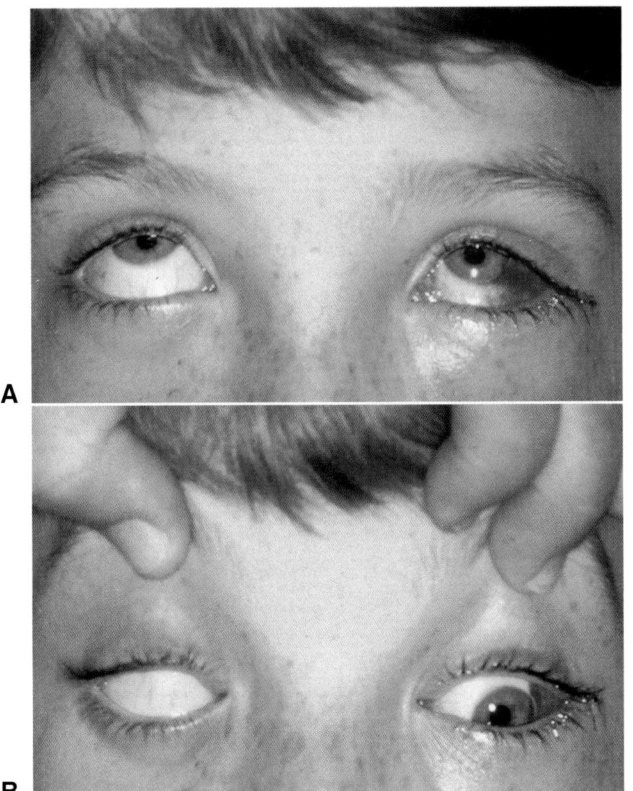

FIGURE 24-4 A, 14-year-old patient with a left orbital floor fracture in upward gaze. B, Entrapment of inferior rectus muscle is the result of impingement in area of linear orbital floor fracture. In down gaze, patient is unable to rotate the left eye inferiorly, whereas the right eye is fully rotated inferiorly.

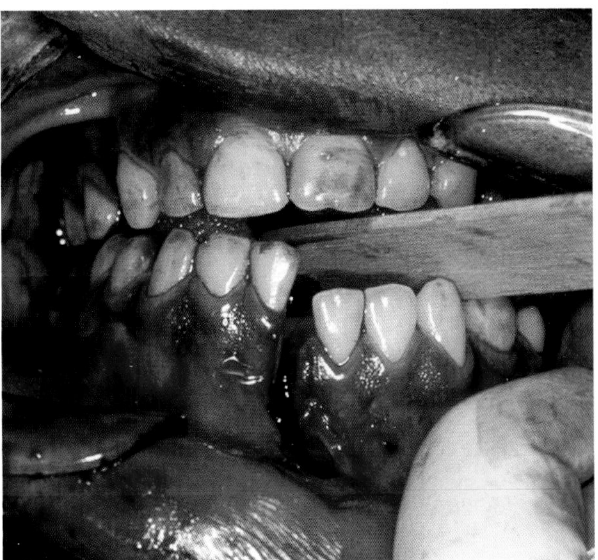

FIGURE 24-5 Irregularity of plane of occlusion and laceration in gingiva and mucosa between the mandibular central incisors, indicating a likelihood of mandibular fracture in this area.

this maneuver. Mobility of the teeth in the area of a possible fracture should also be noted.

The evaluation of the midface begins with an assessment of the mobility of the maxilla as an isolated structure or in combination with the zygoma or nasal bones. To assess maxillary mobility, the patient's head should be stabilized by using pressure over the forehead with one hand. With the thumb and forefinger of the other hand, one grasps the maxilla; firm pressure should be used to elicit maxillary mobility (Fig. 24-6).

The upper facial and midfacial regions should be palpated for step deformities in the forehead, orbital rim, or nasal or zygoma areas. Firm digital pressure over these areas is used to carefully evaluate the bony contours and may be difficult when these areas are grossly edematous. In checking for a zygomatic complex or arch fracture, an index finger can be inserted in the maxillary vestibule adjacent to the molars while palpating and applying pressure superolaterally. Bony crepitus (the ability to feel the vibration as fractured bone edges are rubbed against one another) or extreme tenderness warrants a further work-up. An evaluation of the nose and paranasal structures includes measurement of the intercanthal distance between the innermost portions of the left and right medial canthus. Frequently, nasoorbital ethmoid injuries cause spreading of the nasal bones and displacement of the medial canthal ligaments, resulting in traumatic telecanthus (widening of the medial intercanthal distance; Fig. 24-7). Normally, the medial intercanthal distance should equal the alar base width. The nose should also be evaluated for symmetry. The bony anatomy of the nose should be evaluated by palpation. A nasal speculum is used to visualize internal aspects of the nose to locate excessive bleeding or hematoma formation, particularly in the area of the nasal septum.

Intraoral inspection should include an evaluation of areas of mucosal laceration or ecchymosis in the buccal vestibule or along the palate and an examination of the occlusion and areas of loose or missing teeth. These areas should be assessed before, during, and after manual manipulation of the mandible and midface. Unilateral occlusal prematurities with contralateral open bites are highly suspicious for some type of jaw fracture.

Radiographic Evaluation

After a careful clinical assessment of the facial area, radiographs should be taken to provide additional information about facial injuries.[3] In cases of severe facial trauma, cervical spine injuries should be ruled out with a complete cervical spine series (i.e., cross-table, odontoid, and oblique views) before any manipulation of the neck. The facial radiographic examination should depend to some degree on the clinical findings and the suspected injury. Haphazard or excessive radiographic examination is generally not warranted. In the patient with facial trauma, the purpose of radiographs should be to confirm the suspected clinical diagnosis, obtain information that may not be clear from the clinical examination, and more accurately determine the extent of the injury. Radiographic examination should also document fractures from different angles or perspectives.

Radiographic evaluation of the mandible generally requires two or more of the following four radiographic views: (1) panoramic view, (2) open-mouth Towne's view, (3) posteroanterior view, and (4) lateral oblique views (Fig. 24-8). Occasionally, even these radiographs do not provide adequate information; therefore, supplemental radiographs, including occlusal or periapical views, may be helpful.[3] Computed tomography (CT) scans, axial views without intravenous contrast medium, may provide information not obtainable from plain radiographs or when cervical spine precautions or other injuries do not permit standard facial films. Because many patients with facial

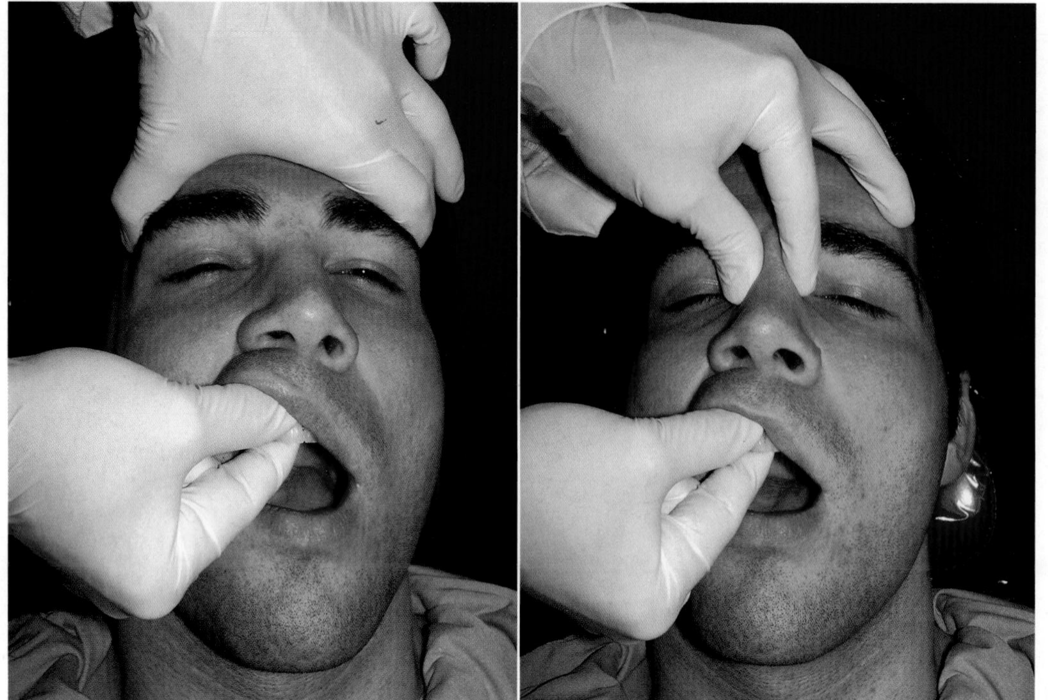

FIGURE 24-6 Examination of maxilla for mobility. A, Firm pressure on forehead is used to stabilize patient's head. Pressure is placed on maxilla in attempt to elicit mobility. B, Stabilizing hand can also evaluate mobility in area of nasal bones.

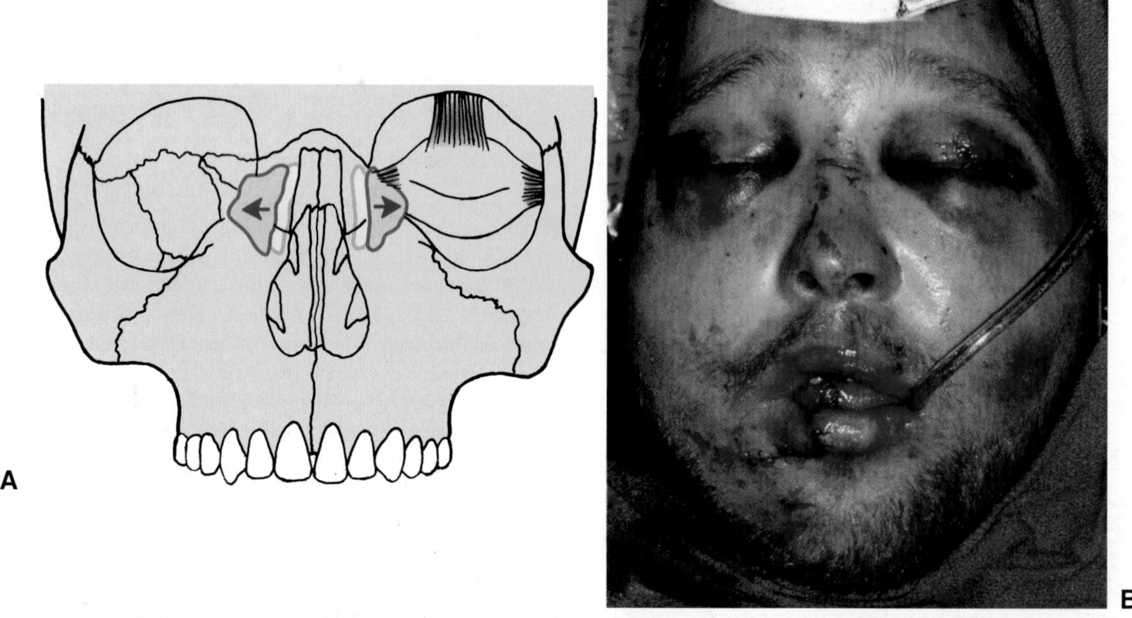

FIGURE 24-7 Injury to nasoorbital-ethmoid (NOE) complex, which resulted in the displacement of medial canthal ligaments and a widening of the intercanthal distance (i.e., traumatic telecanthus). A, Diagram of bony fractures and medial canthal ligament displacement. B, Clinical photograph.

trauma often receive a CT scan to rule out neurologic injury, this scan can also be used to supplement the radiographic evaluation.

Evaluation of midface fractures was often supplemented with radiographic views, including Waters' view, lateral skull view, posteroanterior skull view, and submental vertex view (Fig. 24-9). However, because of the difficulty of interpreting plain radiographs of the midface, more sophisticated techniques are generally used. These techniques often include CT scans done in several planes of space (e.g., axial and coronal) or, frequently with three-dimensional reconstruction (Fig. 24-10).[4]

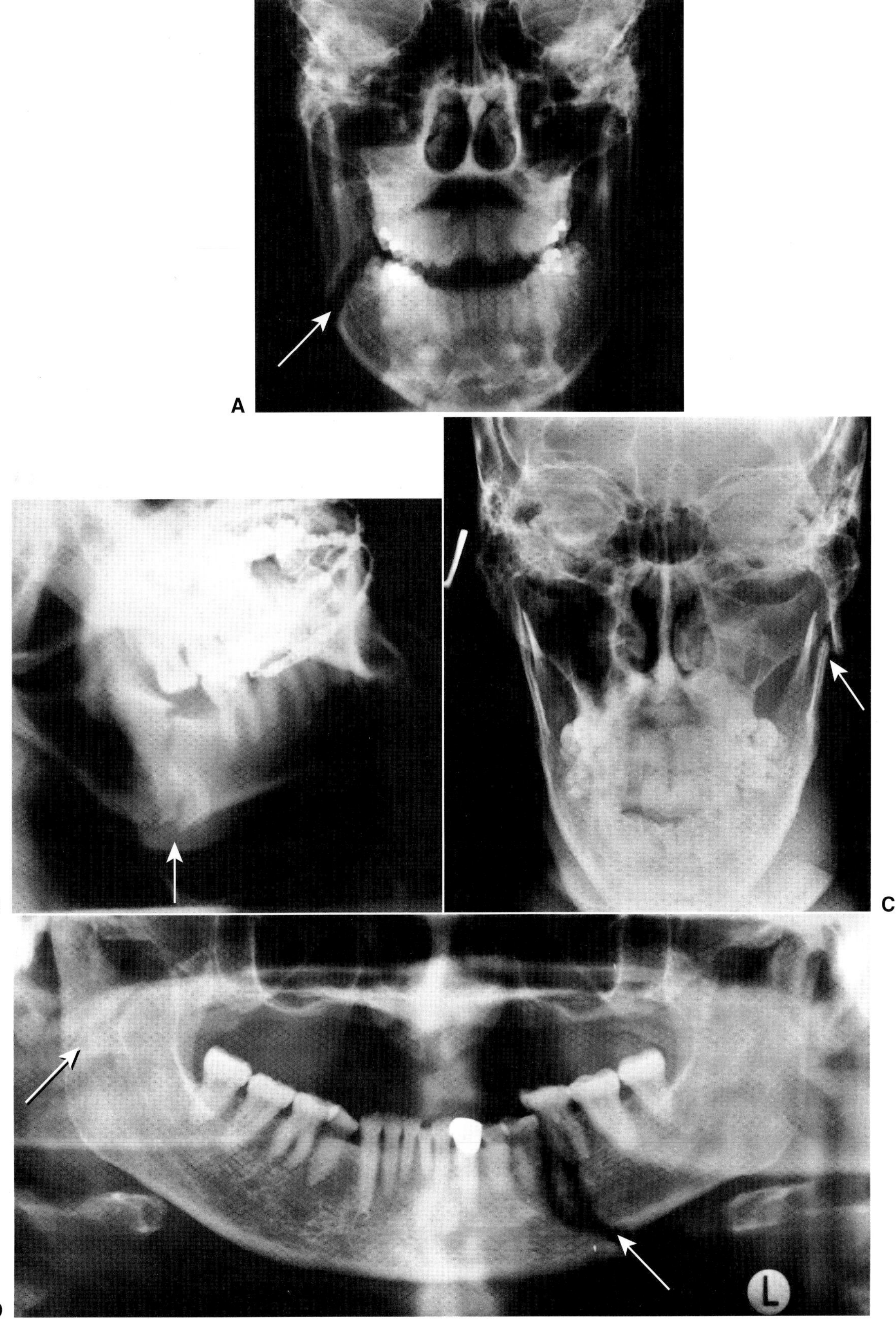

FIGURE 24-8 A, Posterior-anterior view demonstrates a fracture in the angle area of the mandible (*arrow*). B, Lateral oblique view shows a fracture in the angle area (*arrow*). C, Towne's view shows a displacement of condylar fracture (*arrow*). D, Panoramic view shows a displaced fracture of the left mandibular body and right subcondylar fracture (*arrows*).

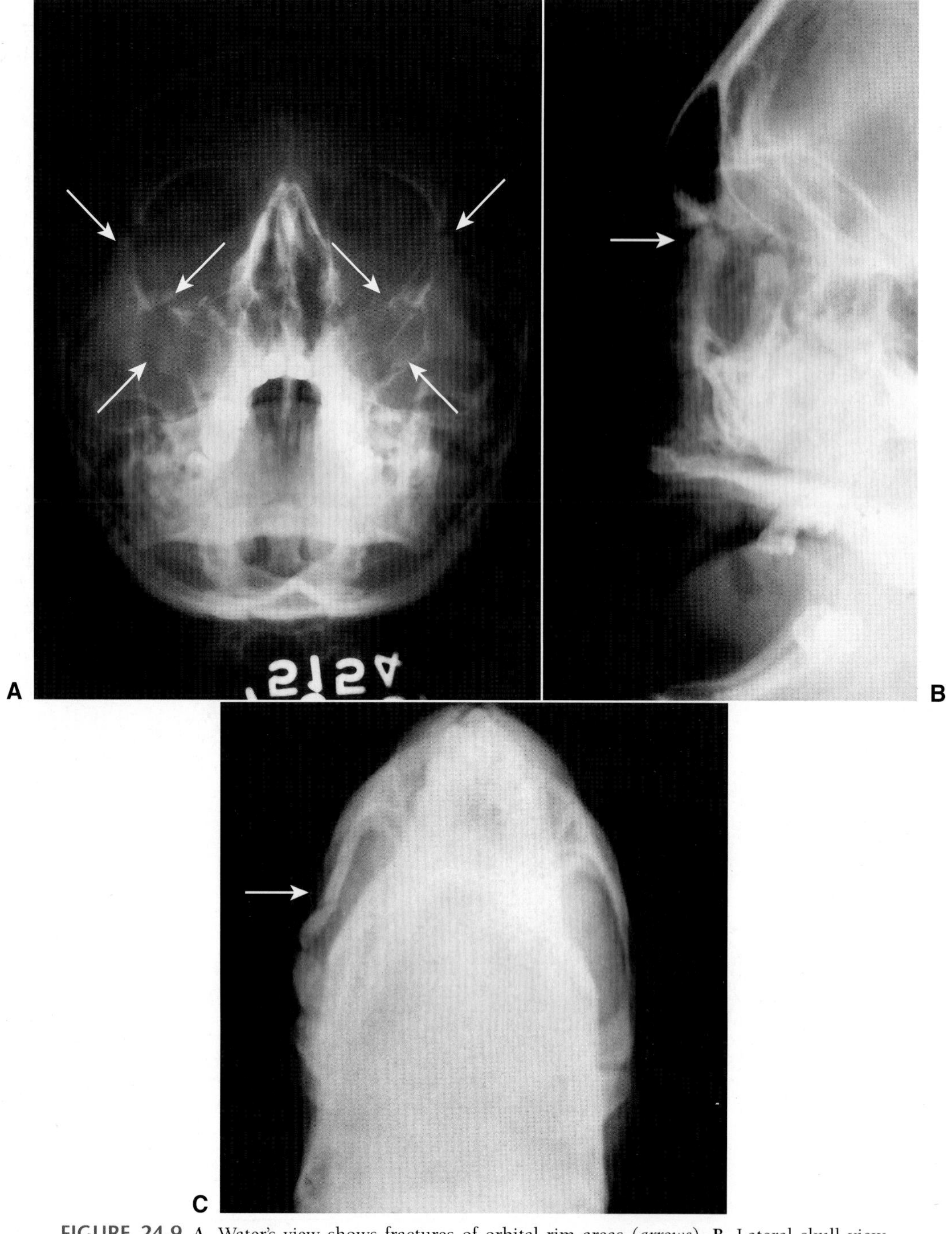

FIGURE 24-9 A, Water's view shows fractures of orbital rim areas (*arrows*). B, Lateral skull view illustrates a Le Fort III fracture or craniofacial separation. The fracture line (*arrow*) separates the midface from the cranium. C, Submental vertex demonstrates a zygomatic arch fracture (*arrow*).

CAUSE AND CLASSIFICATION OF FACIAL FRACTURES

Causes of Facial Fractures

The major causes of facial fractures include motor vehicle accidents and altercations. Other causes of injuries include falls, sports-related incidents, and work-related accidents.[5,6] Facial fractures resulting from motor vehicle accidents are far more frequent in persons who were not wearing restraints at the time of the accident.

Mandibular Fractures

Depending on the type of injury and the direction and force of the trauma, fractures of the mandible commonly occur in several locations. One classification of fractures describes mandibular fractures by anatomic location. Fractures are designated as occurring in the condylar, ramus, angle, body, symphyseal, alveolar, and, rarely, coronoid process areas. Figure 24-11 illustrates the location and frequency of different types of mandibular fractures.[7]

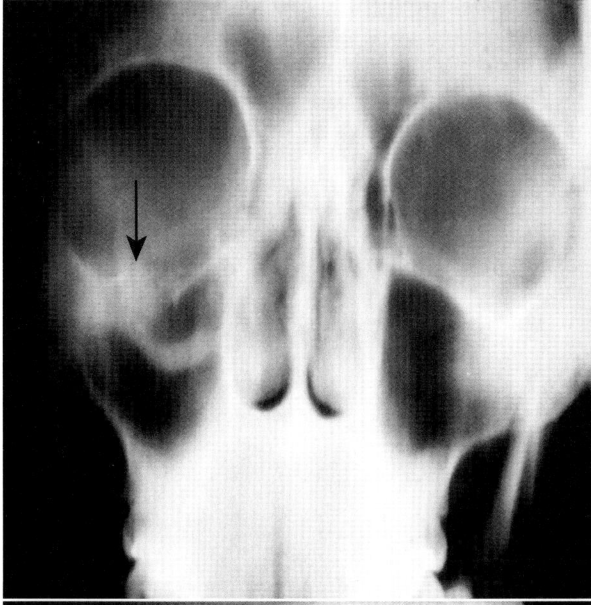

A

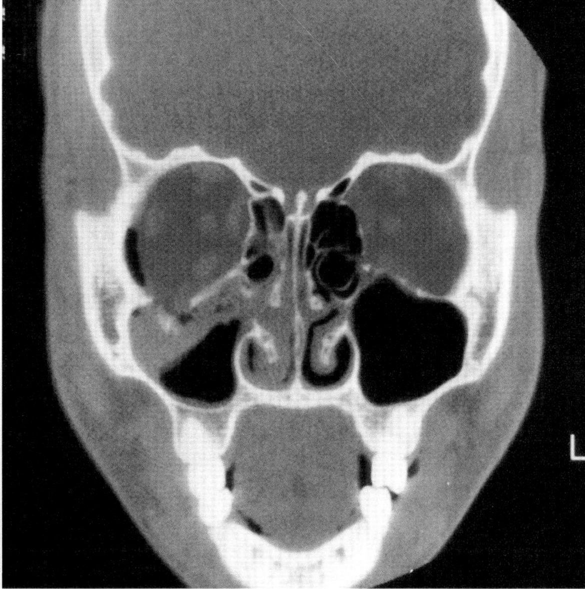

B

C

FIGURE 24-10 A, Tomographic view demonstrates a disruption of orbital floor (*arrow*). B, Computed tomography scan shows disruptions of the medial wall and floor of the right orbit. C, Three-dimensional reconstruction of shotgun wound that resulted in avulsion of the mandible and midface structures.

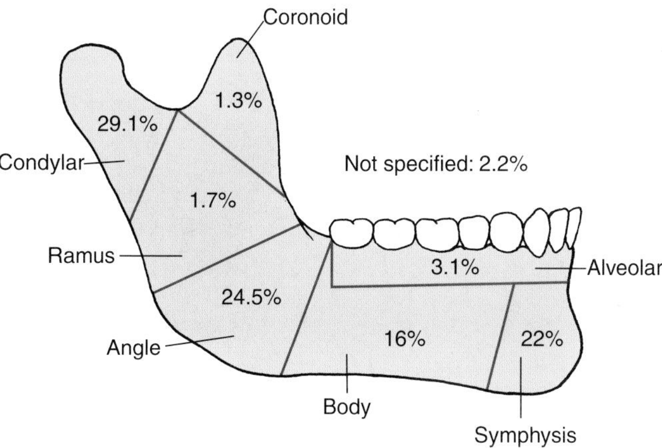

FIGURE 24-11 Anatomic distribution of mandibular fractures. (From Olson RA, Fonseca RJ, Zeitler DL et al: Fractures of the mandible: a review of 580 cases, *J Oral Maxillofac Surg* 40:23, 1982.)

Another system of classification of mandibular fractures categorizes the type of fracture as *greenstick, simple, comminuted,* and *compound* fractures (Fig. 24-12). These categories describe the condition of the bone fragments at the fracture site and possible communication with the external environment. Greenstick fractures are those involving incomplete fractures with flexible bone. Greenstick fractures generally exhibit minimal mobility when palpated and the fracture is incomplete. A simple fracture is a complete transection of the bone with minimal fragmentation at the fracture site. In a comminuted fracture the fractured bone is left in multiple segments. Gunshot wounds, penetrating objects, and other high-impact injuries to the jaws frequently result in comminuted fractures. A compound fracture results in communication of the margin of the fractured bone with the external environment. In maxillofacial fractures, communication with the oral or external environment may result from mucosal tears, perforation through the gingival sulcus and periodontal ligament, communication with sinus linings, and lacerations in the overlying skin. By definition, any jaw fracture within a tooth-bearing segment is an open or compound fracture.

Fractures of the mandible are referred to as *favorable* or *unfavorable,* depending on the angulation of the fracture and the force of the muscle pull proximal and distal to the fracture. In a favorable fracture, the fracture line and the muscle pull resist displacement of the fracture (Fig. 24-13). In an unfavorable fracture, the muscle pull results in displacement of the fractured segments.

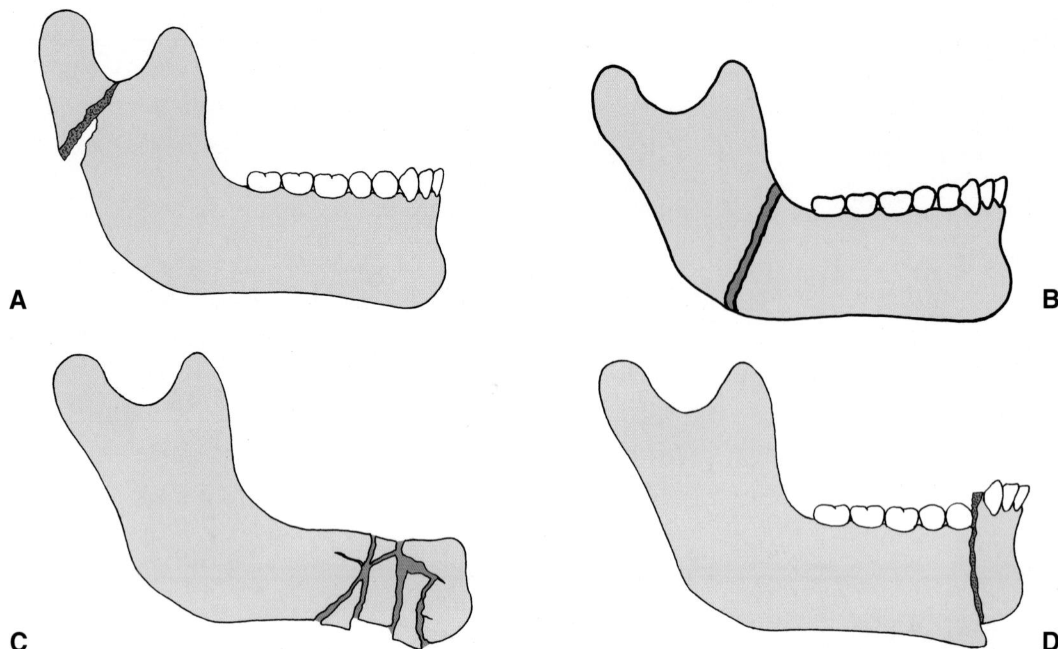

FIGURE 24-12 Types of mandible fractures classified according to extent of injury in area of fracture site. **A**, Greenstick. **B**, Simple. **C**, Comminuted. **D**, Compound. Bone would be exposed through mucosa near teeth.

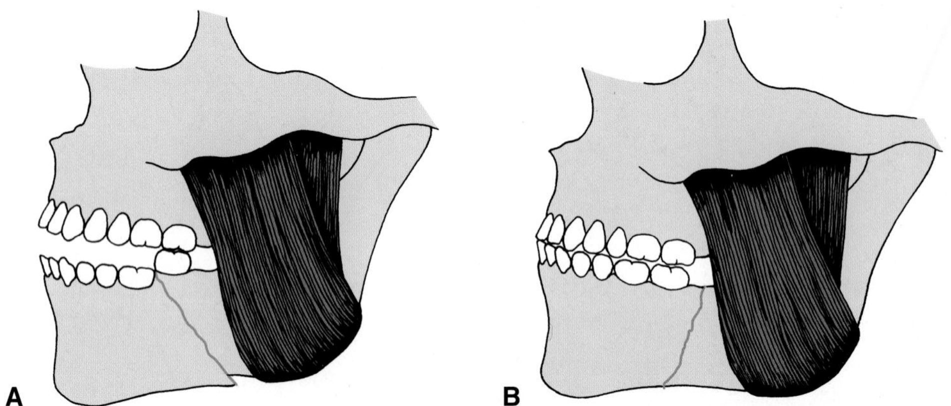

FIGURE 24-13 Favorable and unfavorable fractures of mandible. **A**, Unfavorable fractures resulting in displacement at fracture site caused by pull of masseter muscle. **B**, Favorable fracture in which direction of fracture and angulation of muscle pull resists displacement.

Midface Fractures

Midfacial fractures include fractures affecting the maxilla, the zygoma, and the nasoorbital-ethmoid (NOE) complex. Midfacial fractures can be classified as *Le Fort I, II,* or *III fractures, zygomaticomaxillary complex fractures, zygomatic arch fractures,* or *NOE fractures.* These injuries may be isolated or occur in combination.[8]

The Le Fort I fracture frequently results from the application of horizontal force to the maxilla, which fractures the maxilla through the maxillary sinus and along the floor of the nose. The fracture separates the maxilla from the pterygoid plates and nasal and zygomatic structures (Fig. 24-14, *A*). This type of trauma may separate the maxilla in one piece from other structures, split the palate, or fragment the maxilla. Forces that are applied in a more superior direction frequently result in Le Fort II fractures, which is the separation of the maxilla and the attached nasal complex from the orbital and zygomatic structures (Fig. 24-14, *B*). A Le Fort III fracture results when horizontal forces are applied at a level superior enough to separate the NOE complex, the zygomas, and the maxilla from the cranial base, which results in a so-called craniofacial separation (Fig. 24-14, *C*). Invariably, midfacial fractures are hybrids or combinations of the previously mentioned injuries.

The most common type of midfacial fracture treated in the operating room setting is the zygomatic complex fracture (Fig. 24-15, *A*). This type of fracture results when an object, such as a fist or a baseball, strikes the lateral aspect of the cheek. Similar trauma can also result in isolated fractures of the nasal bones, the orbital rim, or the orbital floor areas. Blunt trauma to the eye can result in compression of the globe and subsequent

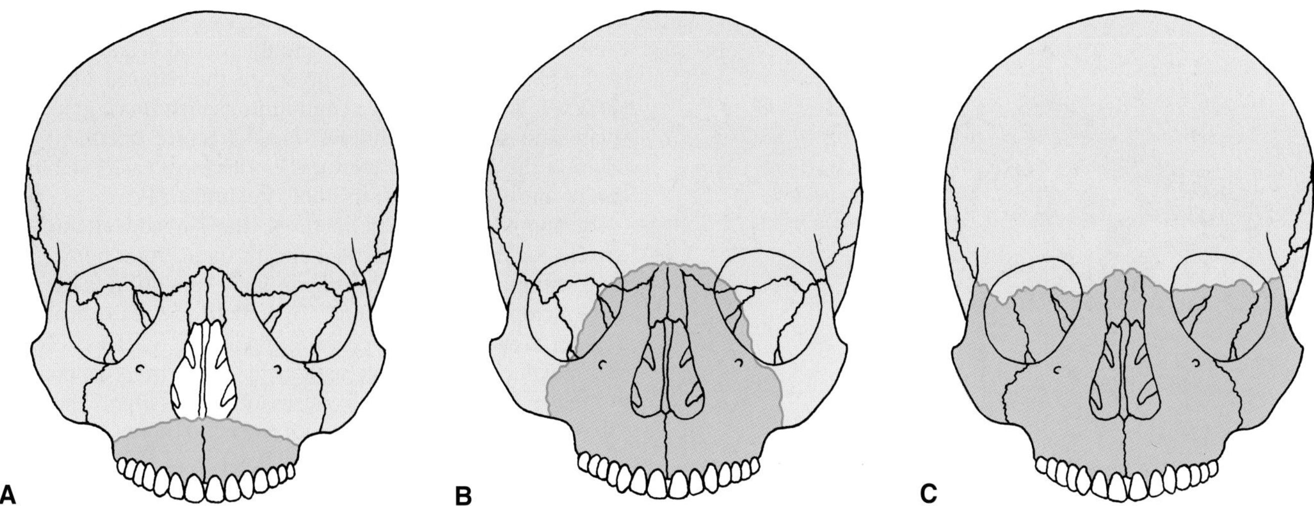

FIGURE 24-14 Le Fort midfacial fractures. **A**, Le Fort I fracture separating inferior portion of maxilla in horizontal fashion, extending from piriform aperture of nose to pterygoid maxillary suture area. **B**, Le Fort II fracture involving separation of maxilla and nasal complex from cranial base, zygomatic orbital rim area, and pterygoid maxillary suture area. **C**, Le Fort III fracture (i.e., craniofacial separation) is complete separation of midface at level of nasoorbital-ethmoid complex and zygomaticofrontal suture area. Fracture also extends through orbits bilaterally.

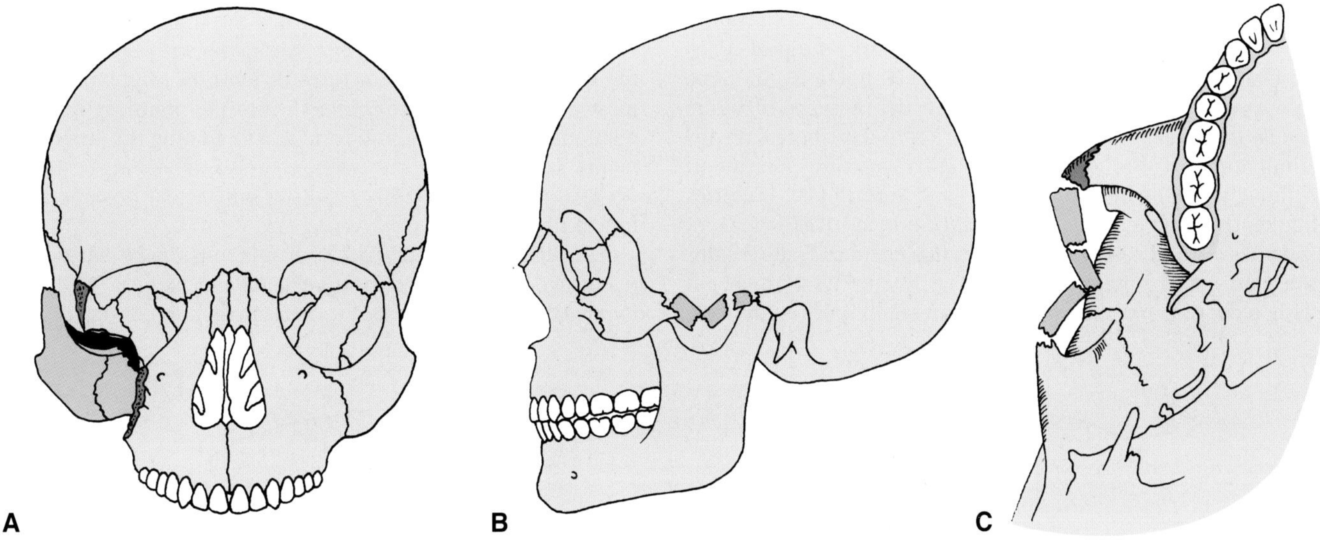

FIGURE 24-15 **A**, Zygomatic complex fracture. **B**, Lateral view. Isolated zygomatic arch fracture. **C**, Submental vertex view showing zygomatic arch fracture in different view. (**A** and **C** modified from Kruger E, Schilli W: *Oral and maxillofacial traumatology,* vol 1, Chicago, 1982, Quintessence.)

blow-out facture of the orbital floor (Fig. 24-16). The zygomatic arch may also be affected, alone or in combination with other injuries (Fig. 24-15, *B* and *C*).

TREATMENT OF FACIAL FRACTURES

Whenever facial structures are injured, treatment must be directed toward maximal rehabilitation of the patient. For facial fractures, treatment goals include rapid bone healing; a return of normal ocular, masticatory, and nasal function; restoration of speech; and an acceptable facial and dental esthetic result. During the treatment and healing phases, it is also important to minimize the adverse effect on the patient's nutritional status and achieve treatment goals with the least amount of discomfort and inconvenience possible.

To achieve these goals, the following basic surgical principles should serve as a guide for treatment of facial fractures: reduction of the fracture (i.e., restoration of the bony segments to their proper anatomic location) and fixation of the bony segments to immobilize segments at the fracture site. In addition, the preoperative occlusion must be restored, and any infection in the area of the fracture must be eradicated or prevented.

The timing of treatment of facial fractures depends on many factors. In general, it is always better to treat an injury as soon as possible. Evidence shows that the longer open or compound wounds are left untreated, the greater is the incidence of infection and malunion. In addition, a delay of several days or weeks makes an ideal anatomic reduction of the fracture difficult if not impossible. Additionally, edema progressively

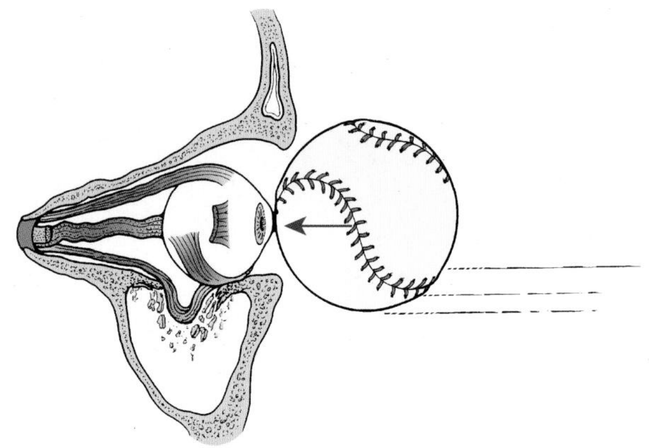

FIGURE 24-16 Blunt-force trauma from a baseball, causing an orbital floor blow-out fracture, with bony fragments and orbital contents sagging into the maxillary sinus below.

worsens over 2 to 3 days after an injury and frequently makes treatment of a fracture more difficult.

However, treatment of facial fractures is frequently delayed for several reasons. In many cases, patients have other injuries that demand more immediate treatment. An injury such as severe neurologic trauma that precludes presurgical stabilization of the patient and increases anesthetic and surgical risks should obviously be managed before facial fractures. In some cases a delay of 1 or 2 days results in the presence of tissue edema that makes a further wait of 3 to 4 days necessary for elimination of the edema and easier fracture treatment. Although treatments of maxillary and mandibular fractures frequently have many aspects in common, these types of fractures are addressed separately in this chapter. Traditionally, the plan for treatment of most facial fractures was to begin with reduction of mandibular fractures and work superiorly through the midface. The rationale was that the mandible could be most easily stabilized, and the occlusion and remainder of the facial skeleton could be set to the reduced mandible. However, with the advent of and improvement in rigid fixation (plate and screw) techniques, facial fracture treatment may begin in the area where fractures can be most easily stabilized and progress to the most unstable fracture areas.

In approaching facial fractures, the surgeon attempts to rebuild the face based on the concept that certain bony structures within the face provide the primary support in the vertical and anteroposterior directions. Three buttresses exist bilaterally that form the primary vertical supports of the face: (1) the nasomaxillary, (2) the zygomatic, and (3) the pterygomaxillary buttresses (Fig. 24-17).[9] The structures that support the facial projection in an anterior-posterior direction include the frontal bar, zygomatic arch and zygoma complex, maxillary alveolus and palate, and the basal segment of the mandible.[10] Regardless of the type of facial fracture or the surgical approach used, the initial procedure should be to place the teeth in the proper occlusion and then appropriately reduce the bony fractures. Bony repair should also precede soft tissue repair.

Mandibular Fractures

The first and most important aspect of surgical correction is to reduce the fracture properly or place the individual segments of the fracture into the proper relationship with each other. In the proper reduction of fractures of tooth-bearing bones, it is most important to place the teeth into the preinjury occlusal relationship. Merely aligning and interdigitating the bony fragments at the fracture site without first establishing a proper occlusal relationship rarely results in satisfactory postoperative functional occlusion.

Establishing a proper occlusal relationship by wiring the teeth together is termed *maxillomandibular fixation* (MMF) or *intermaxillary fixation* (IMF). Several techniques have been

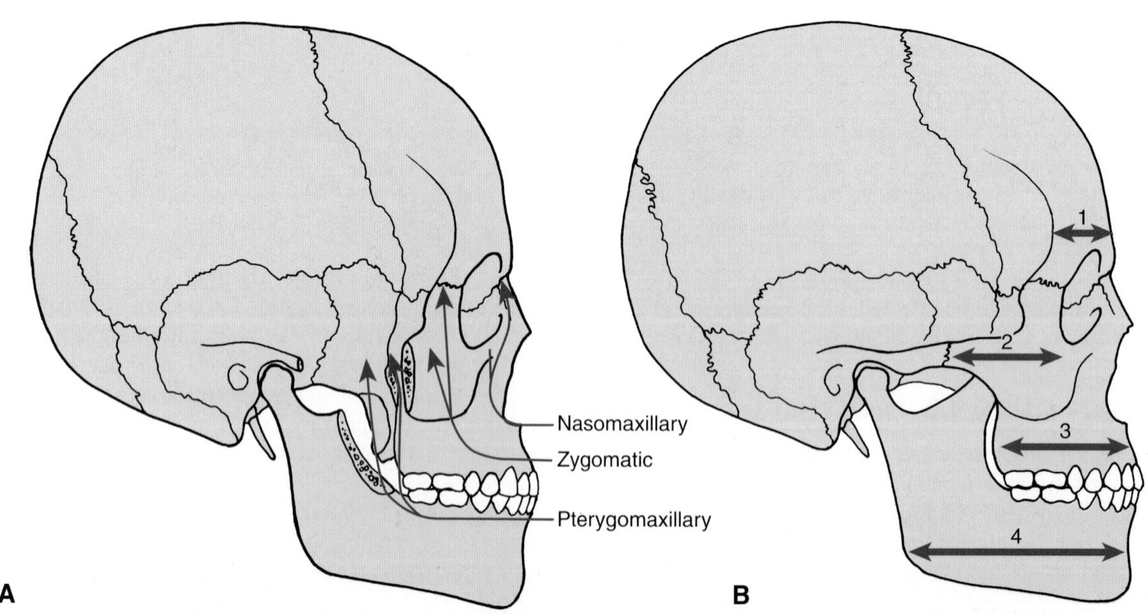

FIGURE 24-17 A, Facial buttresses responsible for vertical support: nasomaxillary, zygomatic, and pterygomaxillary. B, Anteroposterior buttresses: frontal (*1*), zygomatic (*2*), maxillary (*3*), and mandibular (*4*).

advocated for IMF (Fig. 24-18). The most common technique includes the use of a prefabricated arch bar that is adapted and circumdentally wired to teeth or acid-etch bonded in each arch; the maxillary arch bar is wired to the mandibular arch bar, thereby placing the teeth in their proper relationship. Other wiring techniques, such as Ivy loops or continuous loop wiring, have also been used for the same purpose. When fractures have not been treated for several days or are grossly displaced, it may be difficult to place the fractured segments immediately into their proper position and into adequate IMF. Heavy elastic traction can be used to pull the bony segments into their proper positions gradually over several hours or a few days (Fig. 24-19). Treatment of fractures using only IMF is called *closed reduction* because it does not involve direct opening, exposure, and manipulation of the fractured area.

In the case of a fracture of an edentulous patient, the mandibular dentures can be wired to the mandible with circummandibular wiring, and the maxillary denture can be secured to the maxilla using wiring techniques or bone screws to hold the denture in place. The maxillary and mandibular dentures can then be wired together, which produces a type of IMF. In many instances, the totally edentulous fracture patient

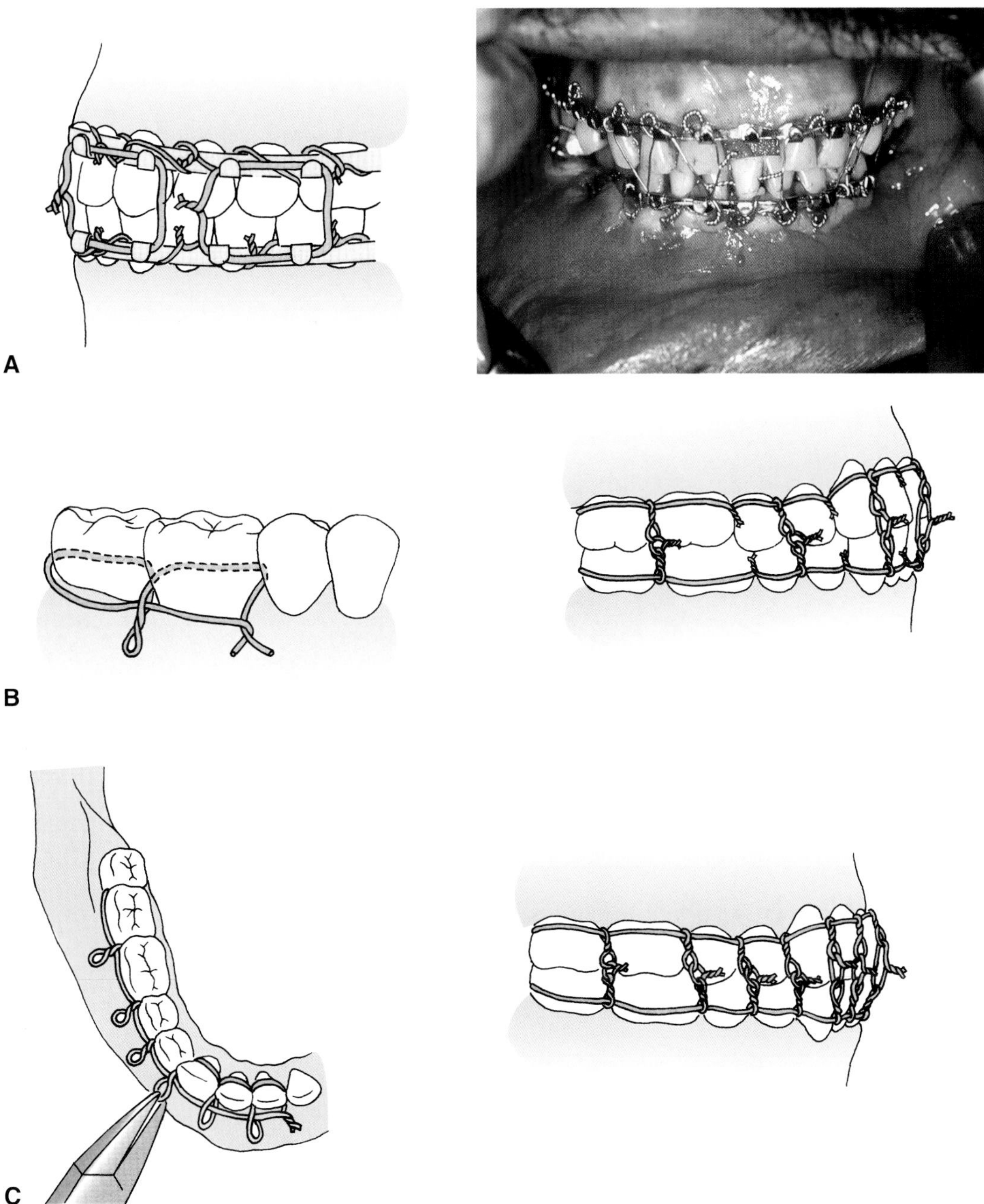

FIGURE 24-18 Intermaxillary fixation wiring techniques. **A**, Arch bar intermaxillary fixation. **B**, Ivy loop wiring technique. **C**, Continuous loop wiring technique. (Modified from Kruger E, Schilli W: *Oral and maxillofacial traumatology*, vol 1, Chicago, 1982, Quintessence.)

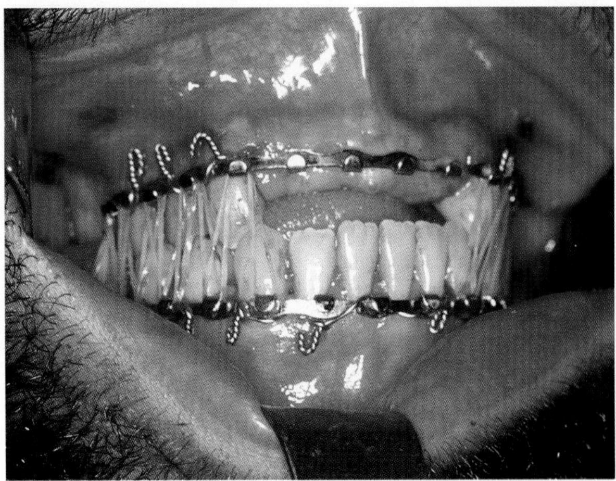

FIGURE 24-19 Arch bars used in combination with heavy elastic traction to pull bones gradually into proper alignment and to establish preinjury occlusion. Once the closed reduction had been achieved, maxillomandibular wires replace the elastics and are maintained for 6 weeks.

undergoes open reduction and internal fixation with anatomic alignment (Fig. 24-20). After an appropriate period of healing (minimum of 4 to 6 weeks), new dentures can be fabricated.

A splinting technique that can be used for dentate patients involves the use of a lingual or occlusal splint (Fig. 24-21). This technique is particularly useful in treatment of mandibular fractures in children in whom placement of arch bars and bone plates is difficult because of the configuration of the deciduous teeth, because of developing permanent teeth, and because patient understanding and cooperation is difficult to obtain. After a complete clinical and radiographic examination, all fractures and soft tissue injuries should be identified and categorized. Then, with input from the patient and the patient's family, a treatment plan should be developed as to method and sequencing of surgery. Discussion regarding closed versus open reduction, any period of IMF, and anticipated morbidity should lead to a decision, and surgical consent should be obtained.

After completing a closed reduction of the mandible and placing the dental component or alveolar process into the proper relationship with the maxilla, the necessity for an open reduction (i.e., direct exposure and reduction of the fracture through a surgical incision) must be determined. If adequate bony reduction has occurred, IMF may provide adequate stabilization during the initial bony healing phase of approximately 6 weeks. Indications for open reduction include continued displacement of the bony segments or an unfavorable fracture, such as in an angle fracture (Fig. 24-13), in which the pull of the masseter and medial pterygoid muscles can cause distraction of the proximal segment of the mandible. With rigid fixation techniques, patients can be allowed to heal without undergoing IMF or at least a decreased time of IMF. This alone may be an important factor in the decision to perform an open reduction. In most instances, patients opt to undergo open reduction and internal fixation, which allows an earlier return to more normal function without IMF.

In some cases it is not be necessary to achieve an ideal anatomic reduction of the fracture area. This is especially true

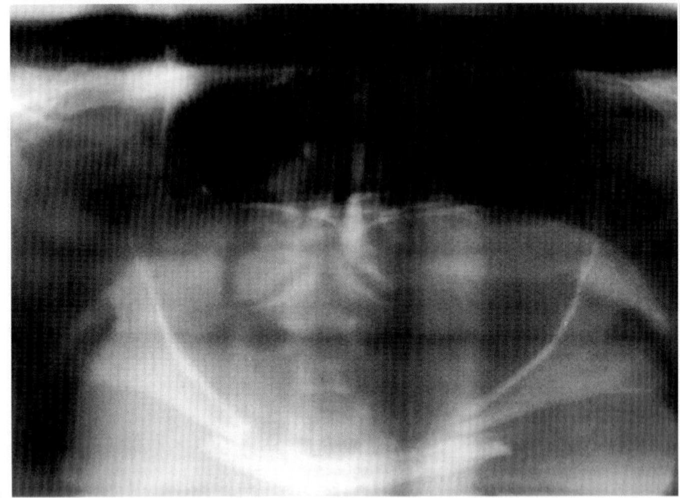

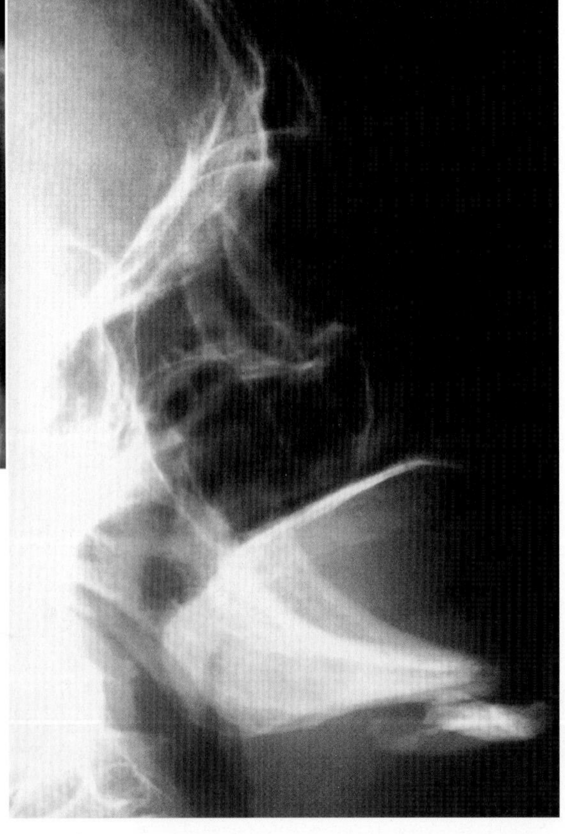

FIGURE 24-20 A, Panoramic radiograph demonstrating bilateral body fractures of an edentulous atrophic mandible. B, Lateral cephalogram showing inferior displacement of the anterior mandibular segment as a result of the suprahyoid muscle pull.

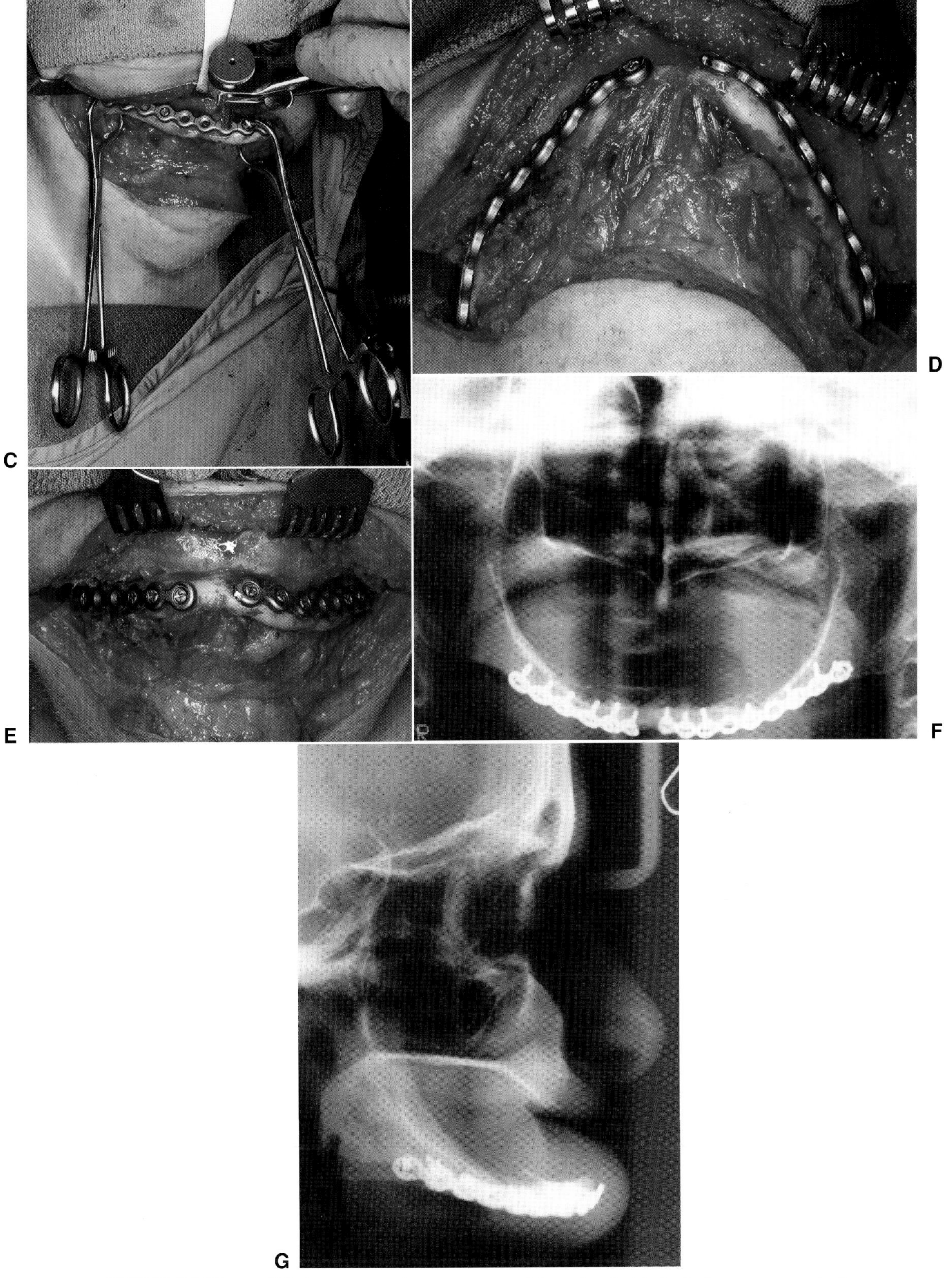

FIGURE 24-20, cont'd C, Intraoperative appearance of the reduced right body fracture approached by a submandibular skin incision. Self-retaining bone clamps are used to hold the rigid fracture plate while a drill guide is used to ensure properly centered drilling within the plate holes. D, Intraoperative submental view of separate rigid plate fixation of the bilateral body fractures. E, Frontal view. F, Postoperative panoramic radiograph and, G, lateral cephalogram with restored anatomic alignment.

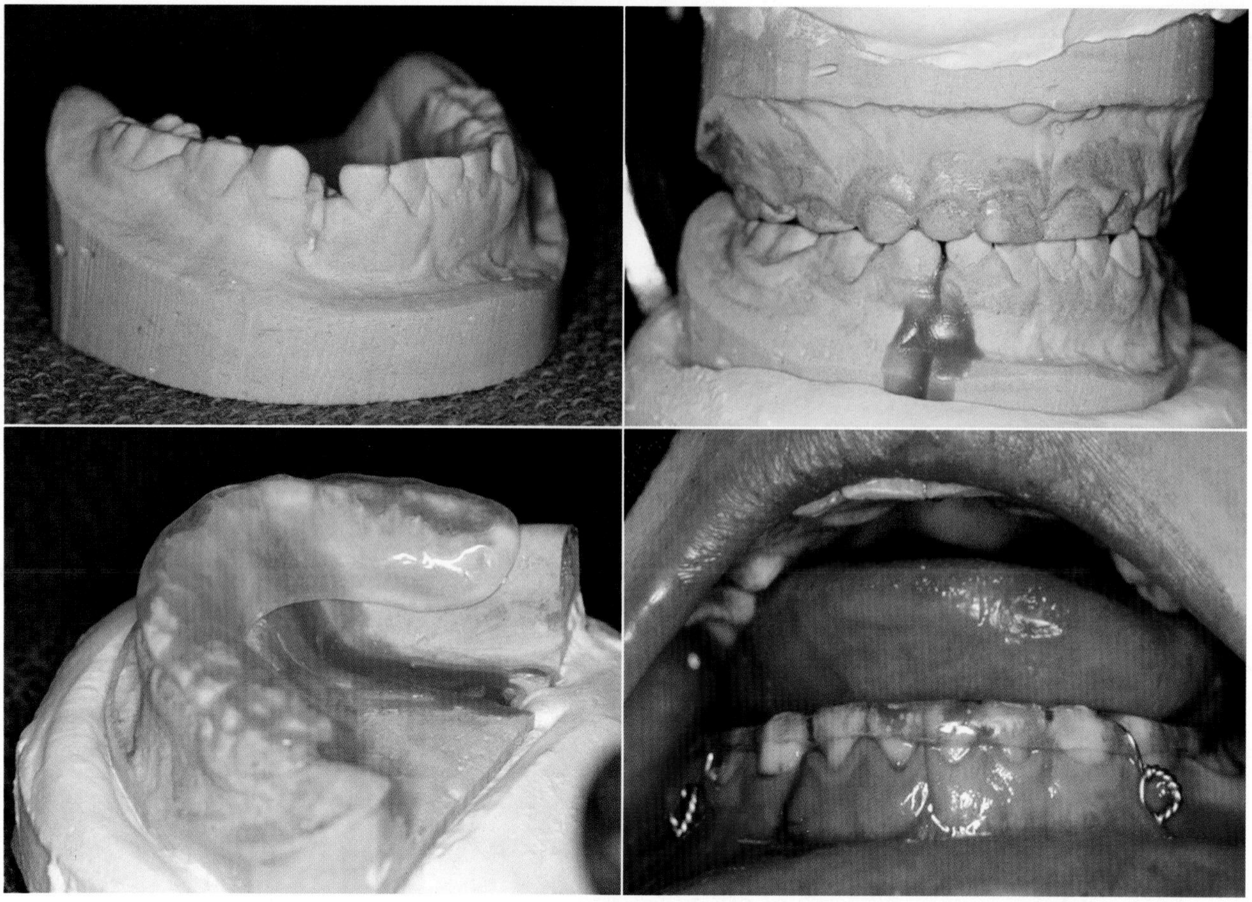

FIGURE 24-21 Five-year-old child with a right symphysis and bilateral intracapsular condyle fractures. **A**, Mandibular dental cast shows the degree of displacement of the right symphysis fracture. **B**, The lower cast is cut at the fracture site and reoriented into proper alignment by occluding with the maxillary cast. **C**, An occlusal/lingual acrylic splint is fabricated on the mandibular cast. **D**, Occlusal splint wired in place with circummandibular wires reducing and stabilizing the fractured mandible. Intermediate skeletal suspension wires were used to provide closed treatment (2 weeks) of the condylar fractures.

of the condylar fracture. In this fracture, minimal or moderate displacement of the condylar segment generally results in adequate postoperative function and occlusion (but only if a proper occlusal relationship was established during the period of healing of the fracture site). In these cases, IMF is used for a maximum of 2 to 3 weeks in adults and 10 to 14 days in children, after which there is a period of aggressive functional rehabilitation. Longer periods of IMF can lead to bony ankylosis or fibrosis and severe limited mouth opening. When there is significant anatomic displacement of the condylar segment, the outcome of treatment may be improved with open reduction and rigid fixation.[11]

When open reduction is performed, direct surgical access to the area of the fracture must be obtained. This access can be accomplished through several surgical approaches, depending on the area of the mandible fractured. Intraoral and extraoral approaches are possible. Generally, the symphysis and anterior mandible areas can be easily approached through an intraoral incision (Fig. 24-22), whereas posterior angle or ramus and condylar fractures are more easily visualized and treated through an extraoral approach (Fig. 24-23). In some cases, posterior body and angle fractures can be treated through a combination

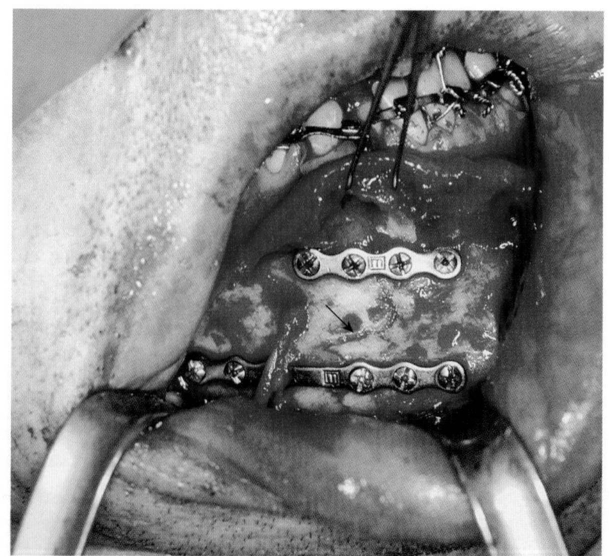

FIGURE 24-22 Intraoral exposure of reduced and fixated fracture in the right anterior body of the mandible (arrow shows fracture line). Preservation of mental nerve is demonstrated.

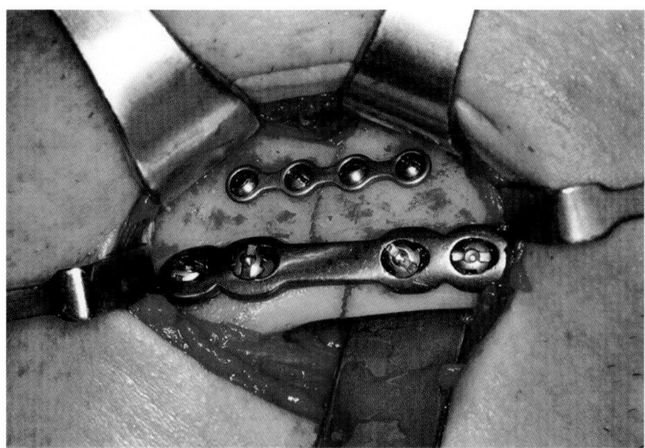

FIGURE 24-23 Extraoral exposure and plating of right posterior body fracture of the mandible.

approach using an intraoral incision combined with insertion of a small trocar and cannula through the skin to facilitate fracture reduction and fixation (Fig. 24-24). In either case a surgical approach should avoid vital structures such as nerves, ducts, and blood vessels and should result in as little scarring as possible.

The traditional and still acceptable method of bone fixation after open reductions has been the placement of direct intraosseous wiring combined with a period of MMF ranging from 3 to 8 weeks. This method of fixation can be accomplished through a variety of wiring techniques (e.g., wire osteosynthesis) and is often sufficient to maintain the bony segments in the proper position during the time of healing (Fig. 24-25). If wire osteosynthesis is used for fixation and stabilization of the fracture site, continued immobilization with IMF (generally 4 to 6 weeks) is required until adequate healing has occurred in the area of the fracture.

Currently, techniques for rigid internal fixation are widely used for treatment of fractures.[12] These methods use bone plates, bone screws, or both to fix the fracture more rigidly and stabilize the bony segments during healing (Figs. 24-26 and 24-27). Even with rigid fixation, a proper occlusal relationship must be established before reduction and fixation of the bony segments. Advantages of rigid fixation techniques for treatment of mandibular fractures include decreased discomfort and inconvenience to the patient because IMF is eliminated or reduced, improved postoperative nutrition, improved postoperative hygiene, greater safety for patients with seizures, and frequently, better postoperative management of patients with multiple injuries.

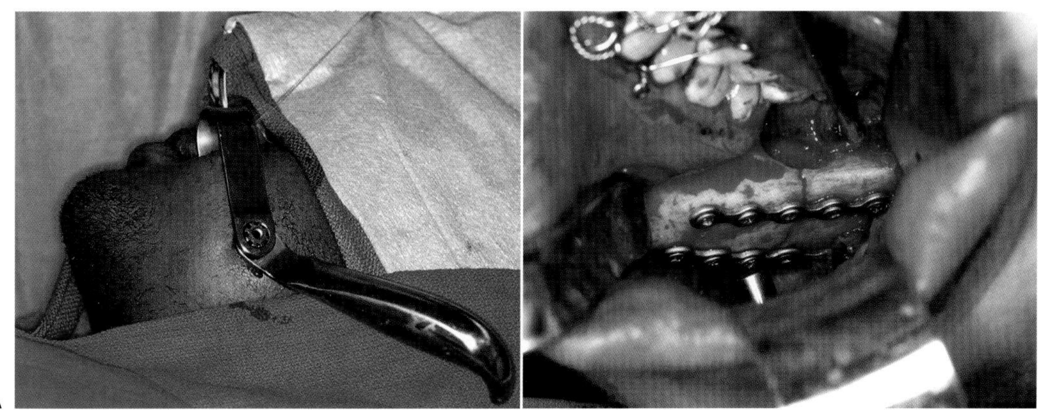

FIGURE 24-24 Use of intraoral incision combined with percutaneous cannula placement for access to mandibular angle region. A, View of left cheek with guarded cannula and handle in place. B, Intraoral view of the left angle fracture plates being percutaneously fixated with screws that are perpendicular to the lateral bone surface. Note that the impacted third molar that was in the line of fracture has been removed.

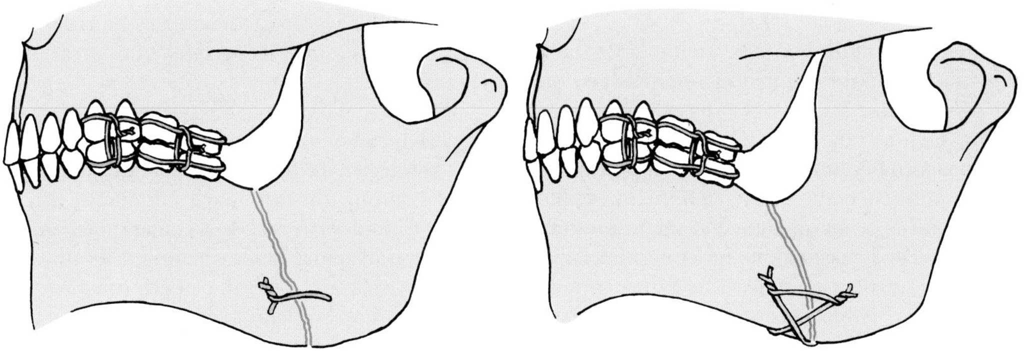

FIGURE 24-25 Surgical wiring of fracture sites for reduction and stabilization of mandible fractures (with wire osteosynthesis of fracture sites, patients must be maintained in intermaxillary fixation during the healing period).

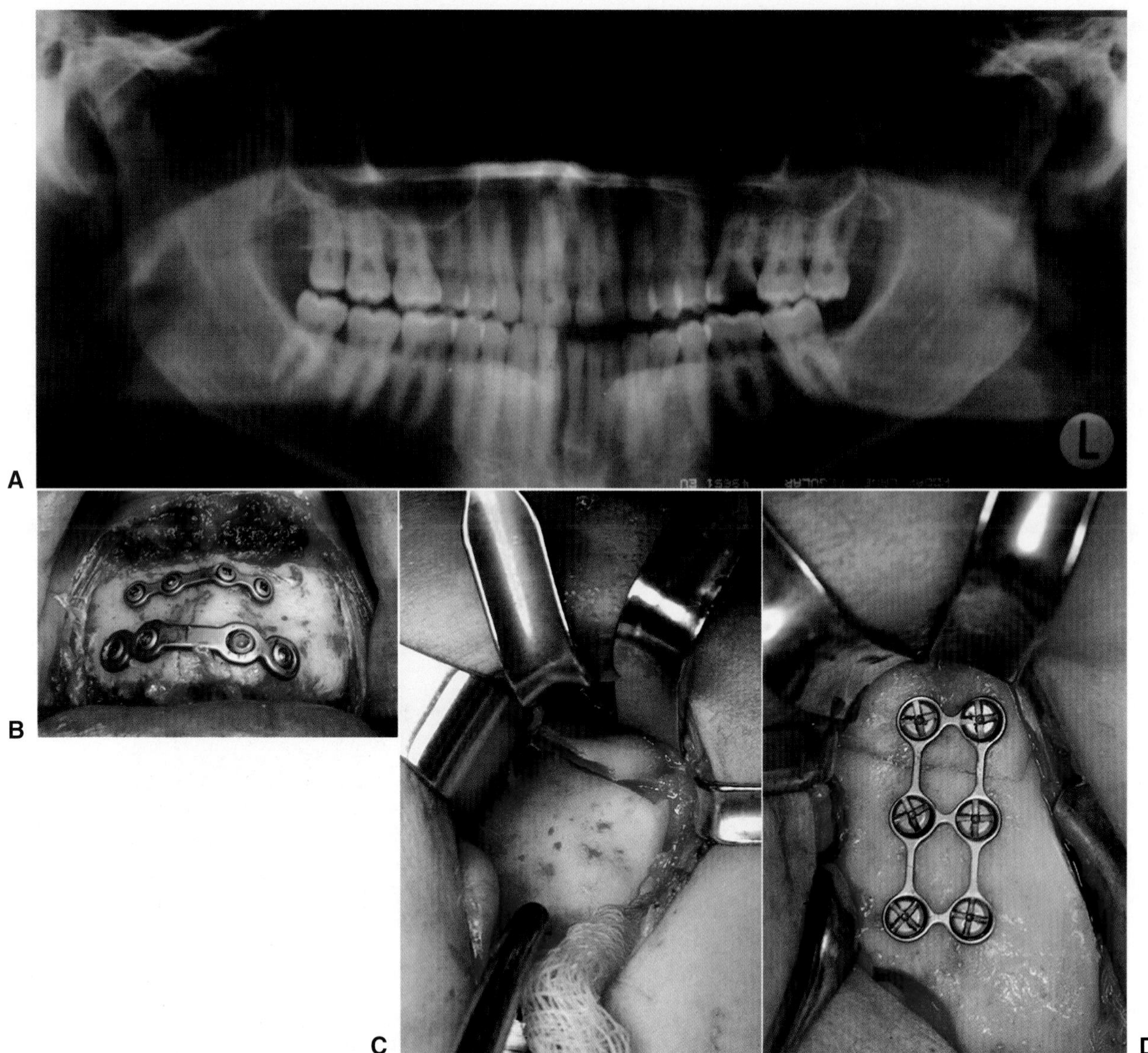

FIGURE 24-26 A, Preoperative panoramic radiograph with vertically displaced right symphysis and displaced and overlapped left condyle fractures. B, Clinical photograph of superior monocortical tension band plate and inferior bicortical plate fixating the right symphysis fracture. C, The left condyle fracture was approached extraorally and the displaced bony segments identified. D, The condylar fracture was reduced and fixated with a monocortical plate.

Midface Fractures

Treatment of fractures of the midface can be divided into those fractures that affect the occlusal relationship—such as Le Fort I, II, or III fractures—and those fractures that do not necessarily affect the occlusion, such as fractures of an isolated zygoma, zygomatic arch, or nasoorbital-ethmoid (NOE) complex.

In zygoma fractures, isolated zygomatic arch fractures, and NOE fractures, treatment is primarily aimed at the restoration of normal ocular, nasal, and masticatory function and facial esthetics. In an isolated zygoma fracture (the most common midfacial injury), an open reduction is generally performed through some combination of intraoral, lateral eyebrow or infraorbital approaches. An instrument is used to elevate and place the zygoma into the proper position. If adequate stabilization is not possible by simple manual reduction, bone plating of the zygomaticomaxillary buttress, zygomaticofrontal area, and the inferior orbital rim area may be necessary (Fig. 24-28).

In a zygomatic arch fracture, an extraoral or an intraoral approach can be used to elevate the zygomatic arch and return it to its proper configuration. In addition to restoring adequate facial contour, this approach eliminates the impingement on the coronoid process of the mandible and the subsequent limitation of mandibular opening. Elevation and reduction of the zygomatic arch should be performed within several days of the injury. Longer delays make maintaining the arch in a stable supported configuration difficult, and it tends to collapse or drift to its injured position.

The goal of treatment for NOE fractures is to reproduce normal nasolacrimal and ocular function while repositioning

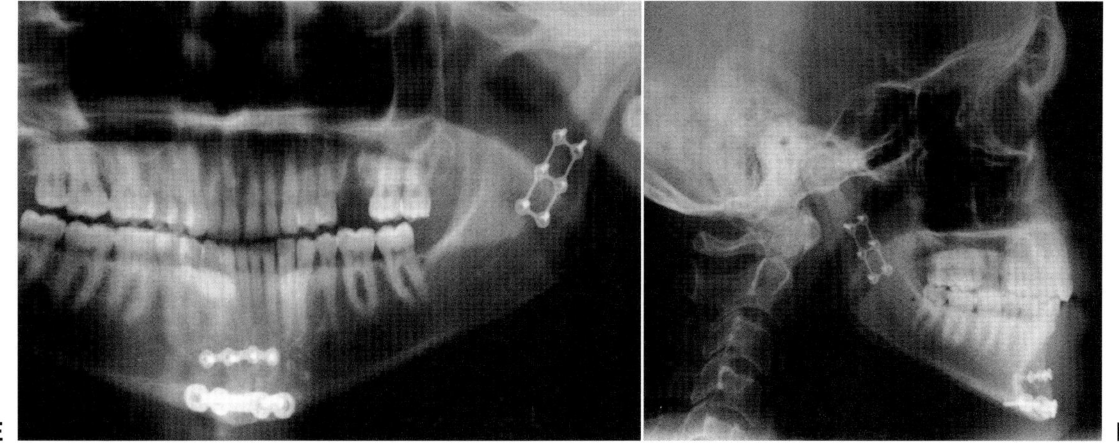

E F

FIGURE 24-26, cont'd E, Postoperative radiograph shows the fixated fractures and the removal of the nonsalvageable carious left maxillary first molar. F, Postoperative lateral cephalogram shows reestablishment of proper vertical dimensions and occlusion.

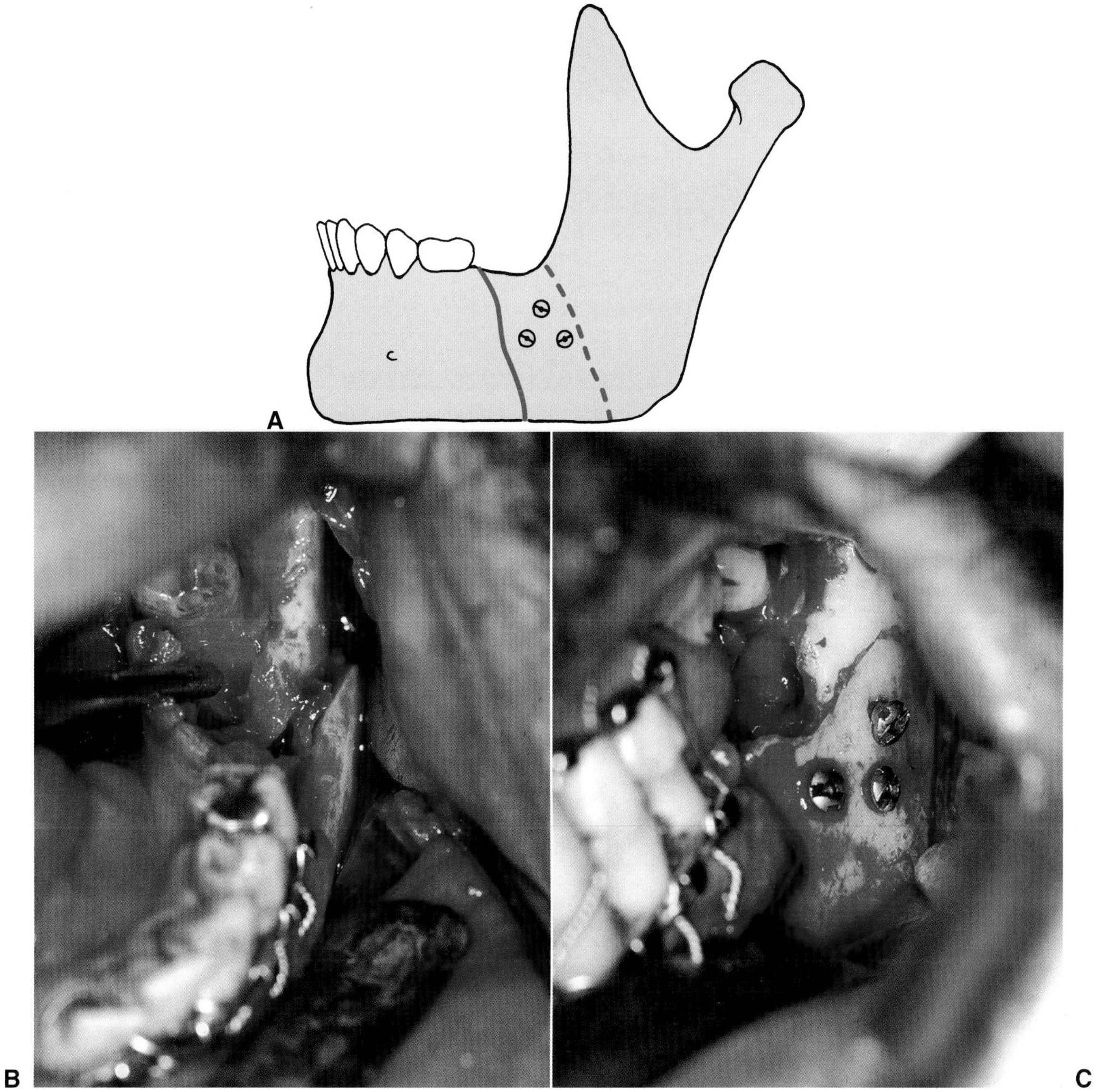

A

B C

FIGURE 24-27 A, Oblique fracture of mandible stabilized with three lag screws. B, Clinical photograph of oblique fracture. C, Clinical photograph of fixation.

Continued

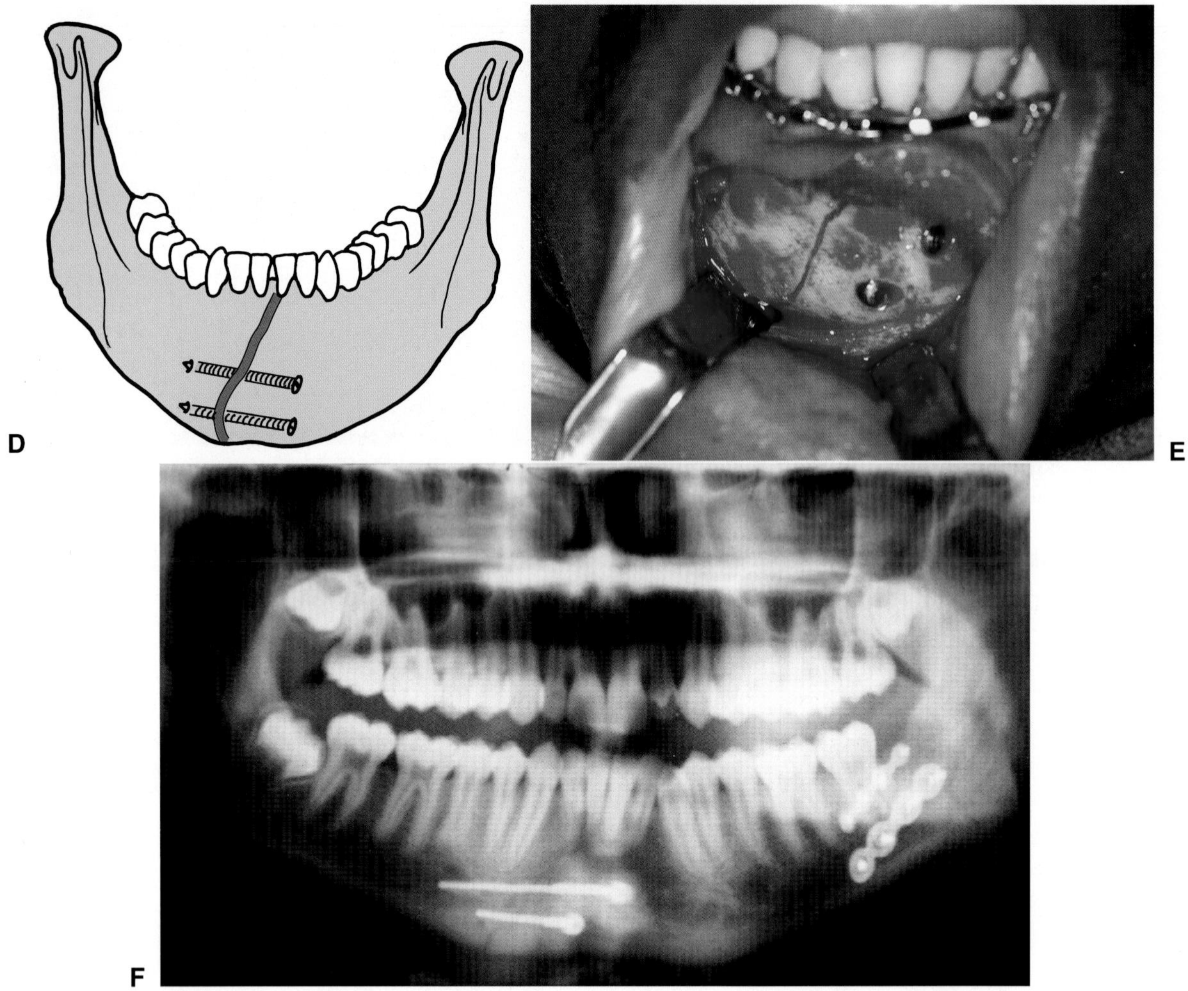

FIGURE 24-27, cont'd D, Two screws placed tangentially across symphysis, stabilizing anterior mandible by engaging facial cortex on both sides of fracture and applying compression across fracture site with lag screws. E, Clinical photograph of screw fixation. F, Radiograph.

the nasal bones and medial canthal ligaments into an appropriate position to ensure normal postoperative esthetics. In these situations, open reduction of the NOE area is usually necessary. Wide exposure to the supraorbital rim and nasal, medial canthal, and infraorbital rim areas can be achieved through a variety of surgical approaches. The most popular approach currently in use is the coronal flap, which allows exposure of the entire upper facial and nasoethmoidal complex through a single incision that can be easily hidden in the hairline (Fig. 24-29).[13] Small bone plates and direct transnasal wiring appear to be most effective in stabilizing and maintaining bony segments in these types of injuries.

In midfacial fractures involving a component of the occlusion, as in mandibular fractures, it is important *to reestablish a proper occlusal relationship* by placing the maxilla into the proper occlusion with the mandible. This step is accomplished by methods identical to the various types of IMF for mandibular fractures. However, as with mandibular fractures, reestablishing the occlusal relationship may not provide adequate reduction of the fractures in all areas. In addition to the need for anatomic reduction, additional stabilization of the fracture sites is often required.

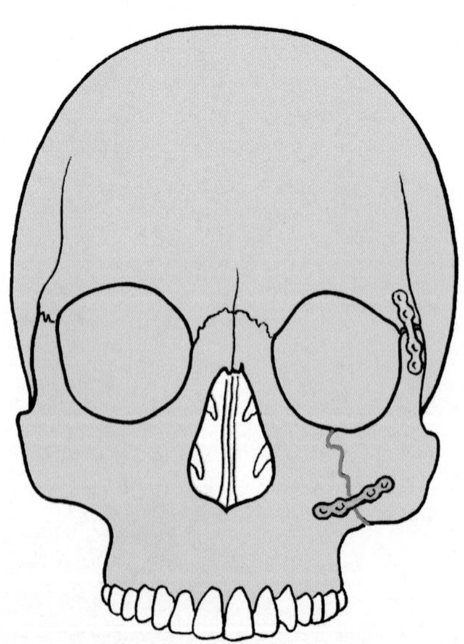

FIGURE 24-28 Plate stabilization of zygomatic complex fracture. Plates stabilize fractures at the zygomatic buttress and zygomaticofrontal suture area.

When adequate bony reduction occurs after IMF but the fracture remains unstable, direct wiring, suspension wiring techniques, or bone plates may be used to stabilize the fracture. An example of such a case is a Le Fort I, II, or III midfacial fracture with an intact mandible. By placing the patient in IMF, any movement of the mandible tends to dislodge the midfacial bones. Direct wiring techniques (i.e., wire osteosynthesis) or bone plates (i.e., rigid fixation) attempt to fixate the individual fractures directly.

Suspension wiring is sometimes used in addition to direct wiring or bone plating. The purpose of suspension wiring is to provide stabilization of fractured bones by suspending them to a more stable bone superiorly.[14] Suspension wiring techniques include those with wires attached to the piriform rim area, infraorbital rims, zygomatic arch, or frontal bone (Fig. 24-30). The suspension wires can be connected directly to the maxillary arch wire, or they can be connected with an intermediate wire to an interocclusal splint or to the mandible. These suspension

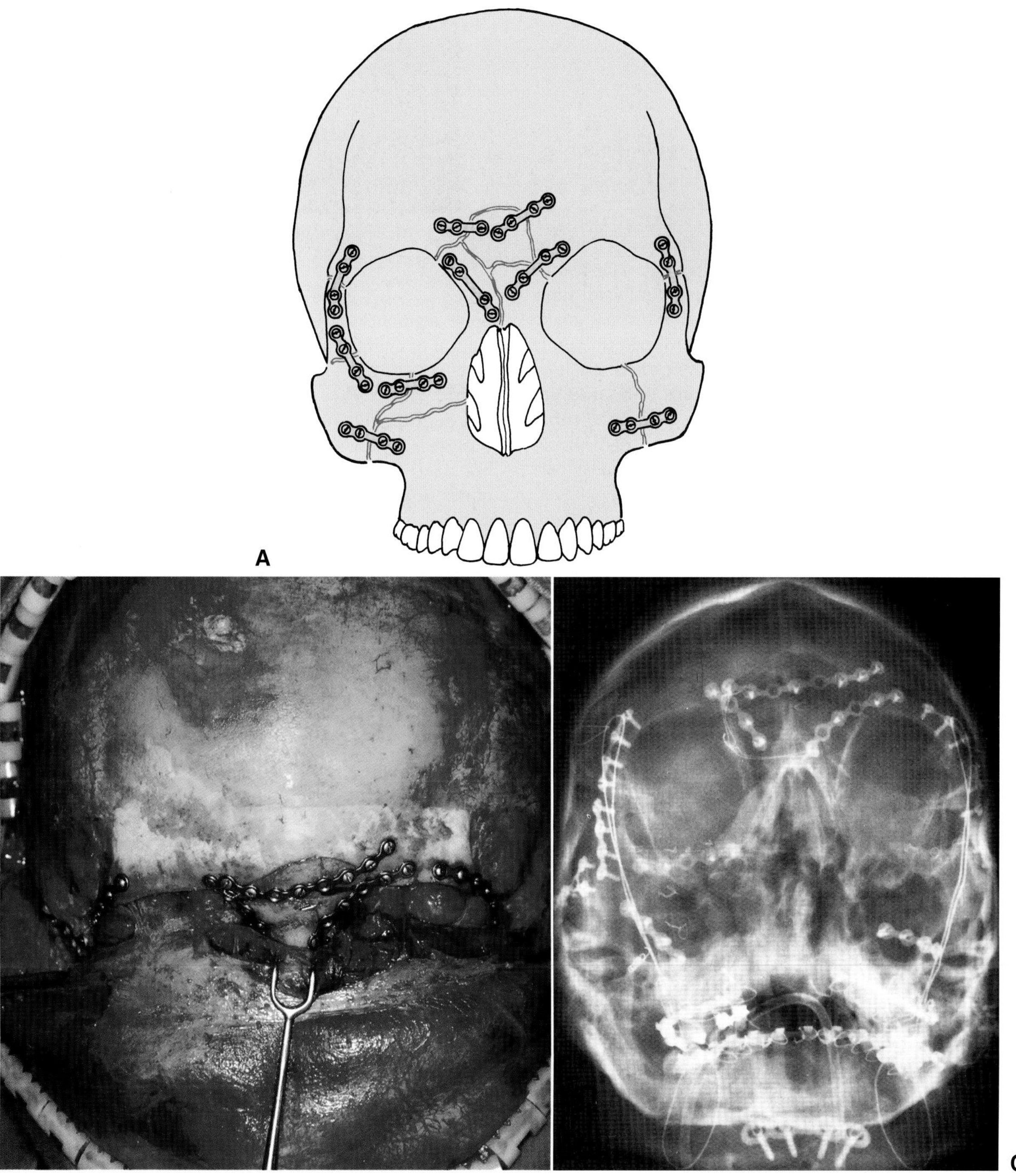

FIGURE 24-29 Plate stabilization of severe midface fracture. A, Diagrammatic representation. B, View of supraorbital area after stabilization of fragments with small bone plates. C, Postoperative Water's radiograph.

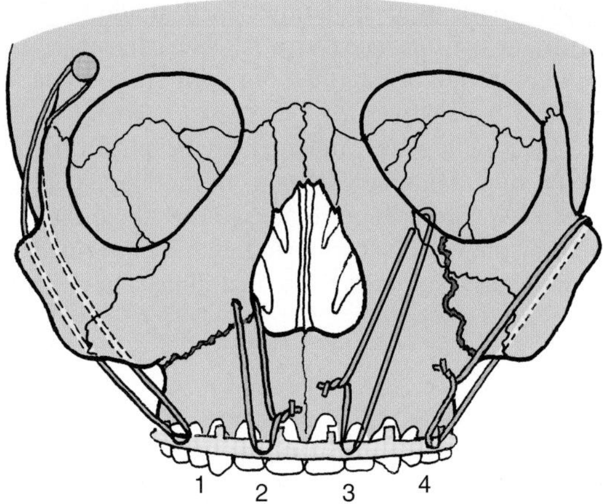

FIGURE 24-30 Suspension wiring techniques: *1*, Frontal bone suspension; *2*, piriform rim wiring; *3*, circumzygomatic suspension; *4*, circumzygomatic suspension.

wires prevent movement of the maxilla caused by the inferior pull of the mandible during attempted opening. The use of direct and suspension wire fixation does have significant limitations in many cases. The limited rigidity of wires may make it difficult to reconstruct and maintain the appropriate anatomic contours, particularly in concave and convex areas, such as orbital rims and the prominence of the zygoma. Wires may not provide adequate resistance to muscular forces during the entire healing period, eventually resulting in some fracture displacement. Rigid fixation using plating systems for the most part has eliminated the need for suspension wires.

The development and improvement in miniature and micro bone plate systems has greatly enhanced the treatment of midfacial fractures. These titanium alloy plates range in thickness from 0.6 to 1.5 mm and are secured by screws with 0.7- to 2.0-mm external thread diameters (Fig. 24-31). Each of the advantages listed for rigid fixation of mandibular fractures applies to midface fractures. In addition to these advantages, small bone plates have greatly improved the ability to obtain proper bony contours at the time of surgery. When limited to the use of direct-wiring or suspension-wiring techniques, reestablishing curve configurations of bony anatomy is nearly impossible, particularly in the areas of severely comminuted small bone fragments. Severely comminuted unstable midface fractures can now routinely be treated by wide exposure of all fractured segments combined with the use of bone plates to reestablish the facial pillars, develop adequate contours, and stabilize as many facial bone fragments as possible (Fig. 24-32). These titanium bone plates and screws are biocompatible and do not require removal at a second surgery unless they become palpable, infected, or interfere with secondary reconstructive surgery (e.g., bone grafting or implants).

Various polymers of polyglycolic acid and polylactic acid have been developed for resorbable plate and screw systems (Fig. 24-33).[15,16] Resorbable plating systems may be particularly desirable in pediatric and skull trauma, where growth and CT scan reimaging are considerations. However, because of the current designs, mechanical limitations, need for tapping, and cost, these systems are not routinely used. Use of bone plates and screws has also facilitated the use of immediate bone grafting to replace comminuted or missing bone segments at the time of surgery and to improve stabilization of comminuted segments.

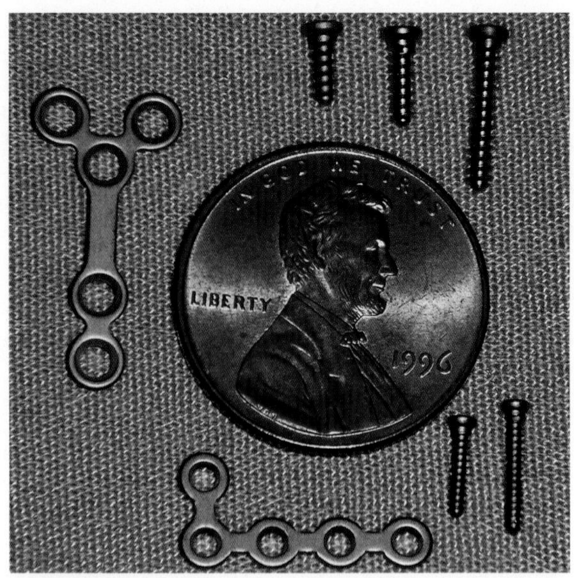

FIGURE 24-31 Microplates and microscrews adjacent to penny for size comparison.

Lacerations

The general guidelines for management of facial lacerations are outlined in Chapter 23. Frequently, fractures of the facial bones are associated with severe facial lacerations. The principles of laceration repair remain the same regardless of how small or large the injury.

Cleansing of the laceration and examination of the area for disruption of any vital structures is important. Possible injuries include lacerations of Stensen's duct, the facial nerve, or major vessels. In these cases, attempts mus0t be made to reanastomose the duct, identify and perform a primary repair of the severed nerve, or manage all associated bleeding (Fig. 24-34). Examination for these injuries before injection of local anesthesia or induction of general anesthesia is important because structural integrity and function (i.e., facial motion and salivary flow) may not be assessable after anesthesia.

The lacerations should be closed from the inside out, that is, from the oral mucosa to the muscle to the subcutaneous tissue and skin. All closures should be completed in layers to orient tissues properly and to eliminate any dead space within the wound to prevent hematoma formation. Easily identifiable landmarks, such as the vermilion border of the lip, ala of the nose, or areas of the laceration that can be easily identified and properly repositioned, should be sutured first (Fig. 24-35), after which the surgeon should close areas where wound margins are not so clearly reapproximated. All wounds should be cleansed periodically with hydrogen peroxide. Some surgeons advocate including the use of antibiotic ointment in wound care. However, use of dry occlusive dressings, such as Steri-Strip coverings can be equally effective. Sutures from facial wounds are generally removed in 5 to 7 days, depending on the location of the wound and the amount of tension necessary to provide adequate wound closure.

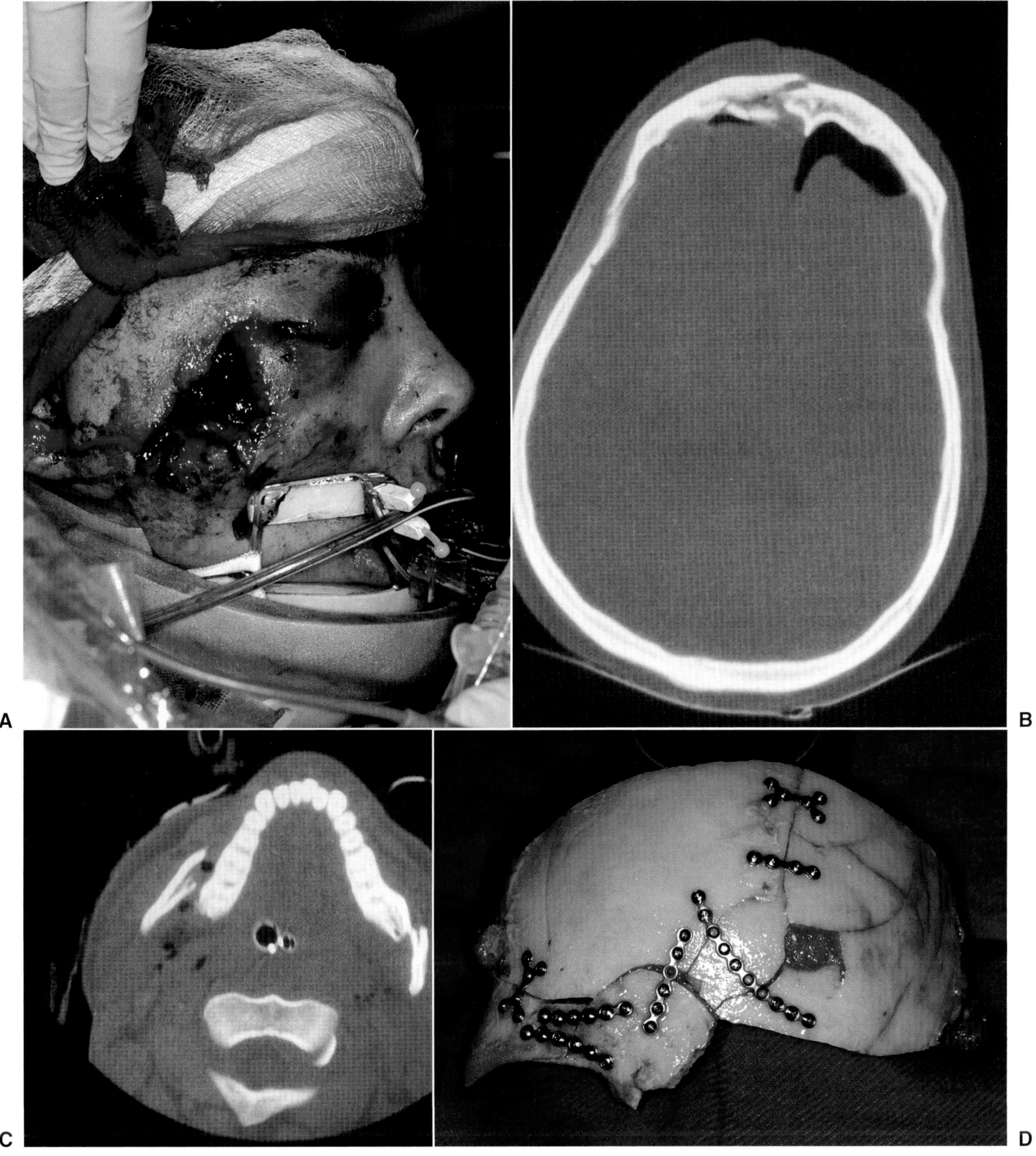

FIGURE 24-32 A, Patient (who sustained severe panfacial trauma from an industrial accident) in the operating department is shown in a cervical spine collar. B, Axial computed tomography scan reveals anterior skull fractures with intracranial air. C, Axial computed tomography scan with bilateral displaced mandible fractures. D, Operative view of skull vault plated while the neurosurgeon was repairing the dural tear.

Continued

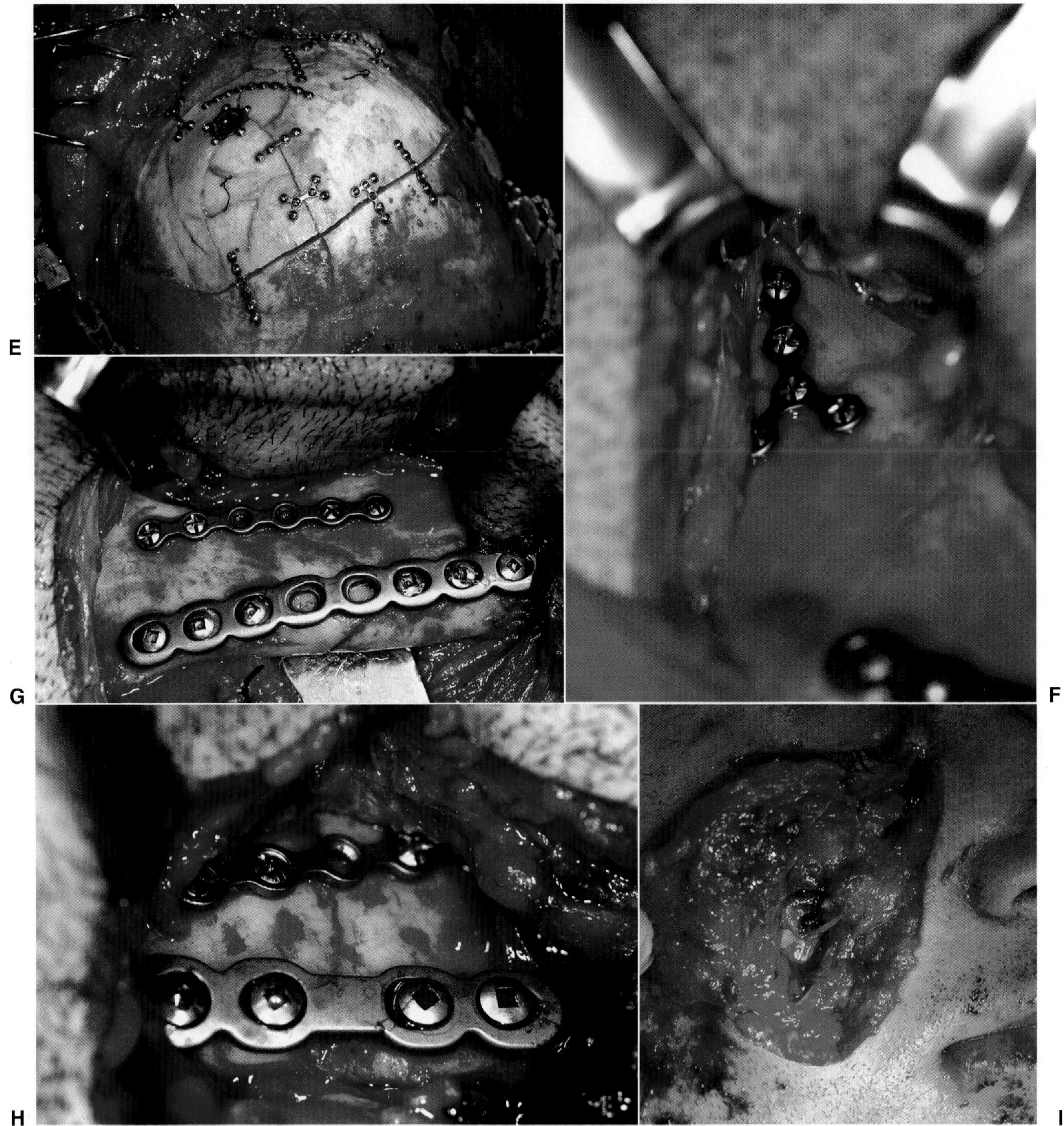

FIGURE 24-32, cont'd E, Cranial vault plated back in place. F, Right subcondylar fracture. G, Right body fractures plated through a large neck laceration. H, Left angle fracture. I, Revised wound of left cheek through which microplating of midfacial fractures was performed.

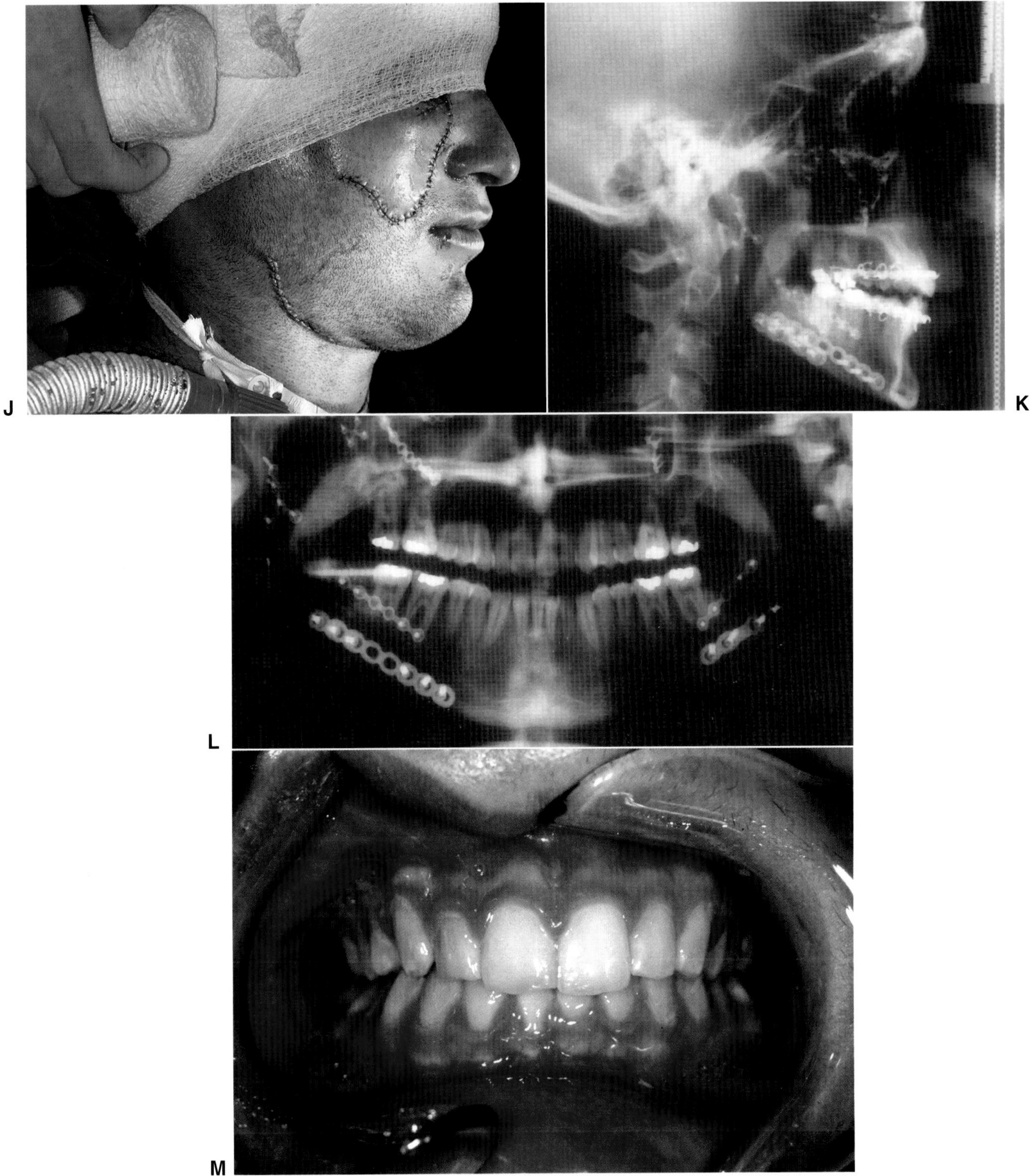

FIGURE 24-32, cont'd J, Repaired right cheek and neck lacerations and pressure head dressing being applied. K, Postoperative lateral cephalogram. L, Panoramic radiograph. M, Occlusion 6 weeks after surgery (see Fig. 26-30 for postoperative facial views and scar revision).

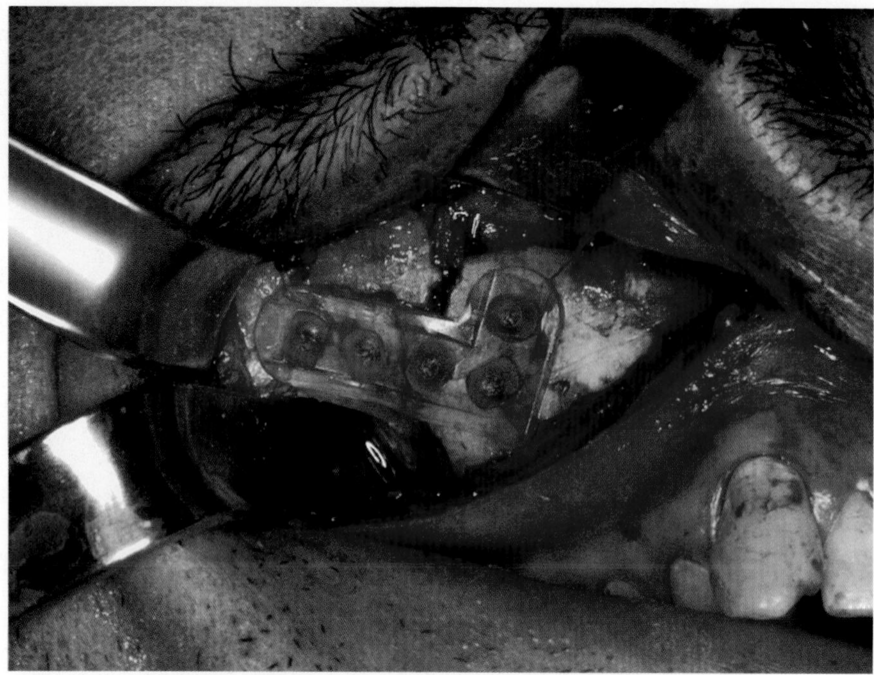

FIGURE 24-33 L-shaped resorbable (nonmetallic and almost translucent) plates and screws securing a right zygomaticomaxillary fracture.

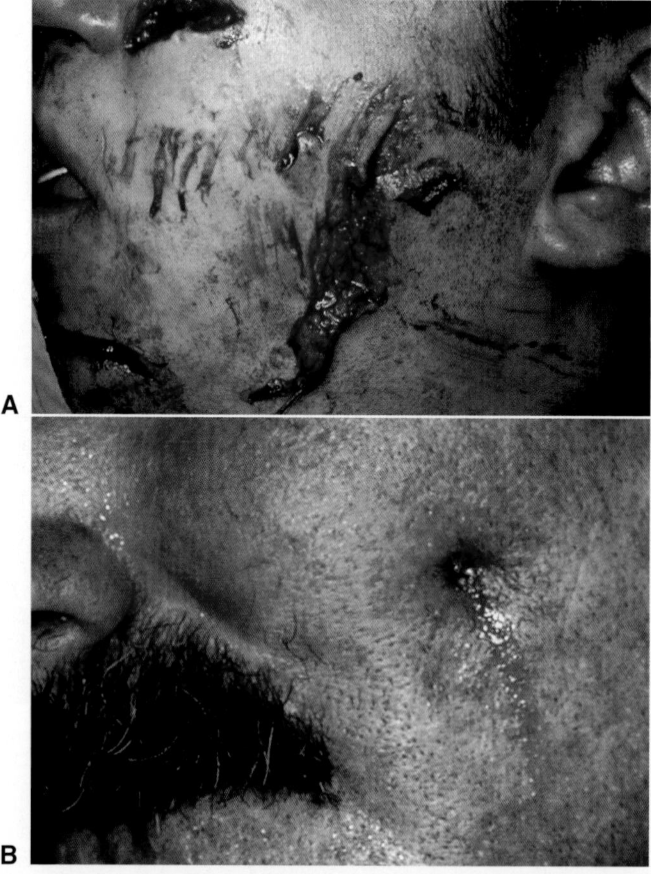

FIGURE 24-34 A, A deep penetrating laceration over the area of the facial nerve and parotid duct. Exploration may be necessary to locate and repair these structures. B, Postoperatively, the patient had breakdown of a wound margin with a persistent salivary fistula due to undetected injury of the parotid duct.

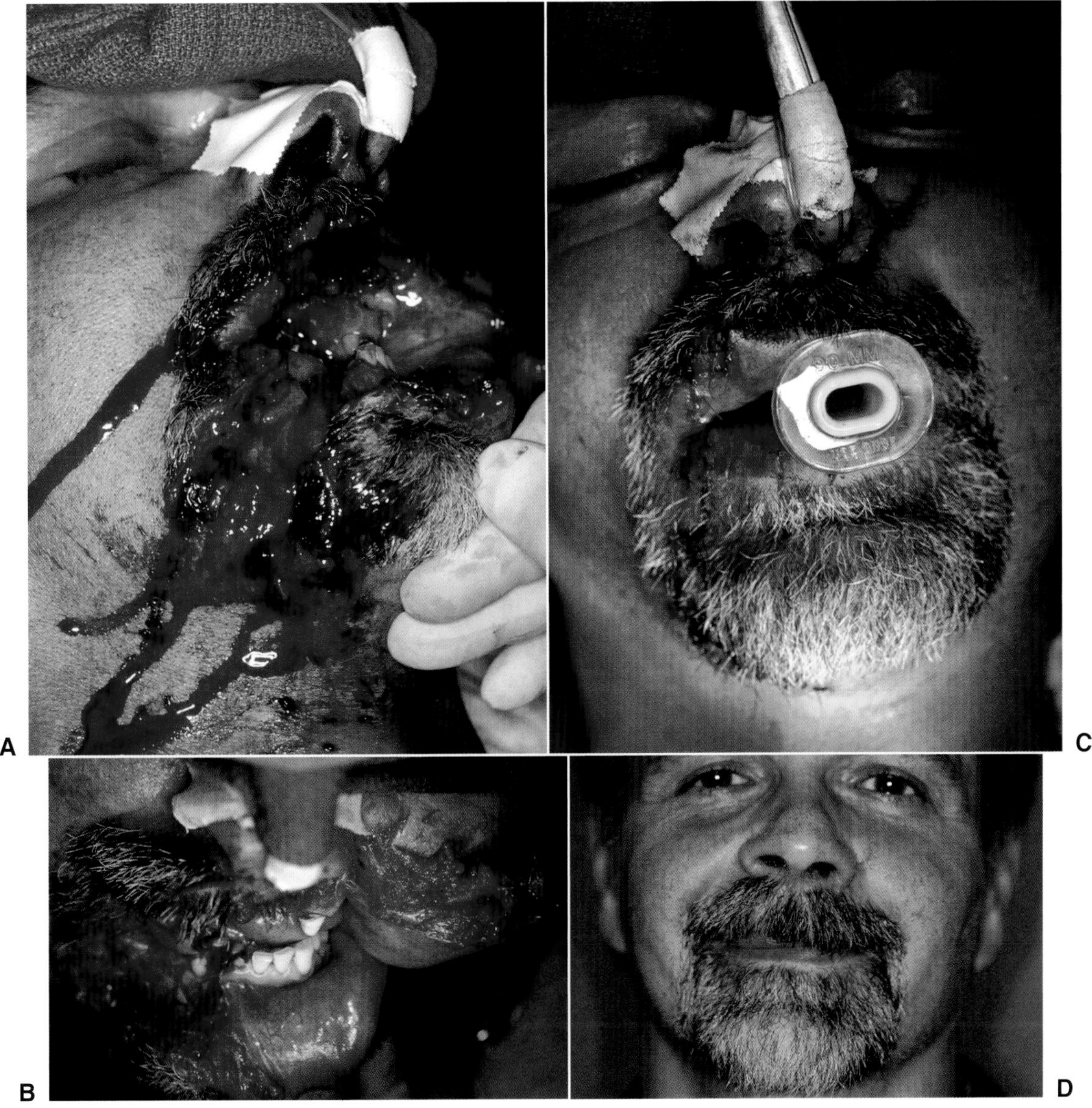

FIGURE 24-35 A, Chainsaw injury to the lips, jaws, and chin, resulting in loss of teeth and bone. B, View from above after hemostasis has been achieved and the wound has been débrided and trimmed. Note the nearly avulsed upper lip pedicled on the left side. C, View of repaired lacerations with patient nasally intubated and an oral airway in place. D, Three-month postoperative facial appearance.

REFERENCES

1. Batters Alvi A, Doherty T, Lewen G: Facial fractures and concomitant injuries in trauma patients, *Laryngoscope* 113:102, 2003.
2. Verschueren DS, Bell RB, Gagheri SC et al: Management of laryngo-tracheal injuries associated with craniomaxillofacial trauma, *J Oral Maxillofac Surg* 64:203, 2006.
3. Gerlock AJ, Sinn DP, McBride KL: *Clinical and radiographic interpretation of facial fractures,* Boston, 1981, Little, Brown.
4. Saigal K, Winokur RS, Finden S et al: Use of three-dimensional computerized tomography reconstruction in complex facial trauma, *Facial Plast Surg* 21:214, 2005.
5. Afzelius L, Rosen C: Facial fractures: a review of 368 cases, *Int J Oral Surg* 9:25, 1980.
6. Ellis E, El-Attar A, Moos K: An analysis of 2067 cases of zygomatical orbital fractures, *J Oral Maxillofac Surg* 43:417, 1985.
7. Olson RA, Fonseca RJ, Zeitler DL et al: Fractures of the mandible: a review of 580 cases, *J Oral Maxillofac Surg* 40:23, 1982.
8. Bagheri SC, Holmgren E, Kademani D et al: Comparison of the severity of bilateral LeFort injuries in isolated midface trauma, *J Oral Maxillofac Surg* 63:1123, 2005.
9. Manson PM, Hoopes JE, Su CT: Structural pillars of the facial skeleton: an approach to the management of Le Fort fractures, *Plast Reconstr Surg* 60:54, 1980.
10. Markowitz BL, Manson PM: Panfacial fracture: organization of treatment, *Clin Plast Surg* 16:105, 1989.
11. Villarreal PM, Monie R, Junquera LM et al: Mandibular condyle fractures: determinants of treatment and outcome, *J Oral Maxillofac Surg* 62:155, 2004.
12. Ochs MW, Tucker MR: Current concepts in management of facial trauma, *J Oral Maxillofac Surg* 51:42, 1993.
13. Van Sickels JE, White RP Jr: Rigid fixation for maxillofacial surgery. In Tucker MR, White RP Jr, Terry BC et al, editors: *Rigid fixation for maxillofacial surgery,* Philadelphia, 1991, JB Lippincott.
14. Bowerman JE: Fractures of the middle third of the facial skeleton. In Rowe NL, Williams JI, editors: *Maxillofacial injuries,* vol 1, New York, 1984, Churchill Livingstone.
15. Eppley BL, Prevel CD: Nonmetallic fixation in traumatic midfacial fractures, *J Craniofac Surg* 8:103, 1997.
16. Bell RB, Kindsfater CS: The use of biodegradable plates and screws to stabilize facial fractures, *J Oral Maxillofac Surg* 63:1576, 2005.

PART VII

Dentofacial Deformities

Patients with congenital or acquired abnormalities of facial bones and soft tissue generally require the assistance of many medical and dental specialists to achieve maximal rehabilitation. Patients with malocclusions and facial abnormalities resulting from an abnormal growth of facial bones usually require the services of general dentists, prosthodontists, periodontists, orthodontists, and oral and maxillofacial surgeons. The care of patients with cleft lips and palates involves most of the dental specialists, as well as pediatricians, plastic surgeons, otolaryngologists, speech and hearing therapists, and psychologists. Chapters 25 and 27 outline the treatments available for these patients, the sequence of treatment, and the need for participation of dental generalists and specialists.

Surgical procedures designed to enhance facial and total body esthetics are increasing in popularity. Patients of all ages are interested in procedures to improve abnormal or unesthetic facial features such as poorly proportioned noses, weak chins, and protruding ears. Aging patients are interested in procedures that restore a more youthful appearance to the face. Oral and maxillofacial surgeons perform facial cosmetic procedures and help coordinate other aspects of cosmetic dental treatment to provide the best possible esthetic improvement. Chapter 26 discusses these topics.

Facial trauma and pathologic anomalies often result in the loss of large portions of the jaws and associated structures. Reconstruction of missing portions of the jaws and associated facial bones and soft tissues usually necessitates comprehensive and often multiple surgical treatments to rehabilitate the patient adequately. Chapter 28 discusses the principles of maxillofacial reconstruction.

CHAPTER 25

Correction of Dentofacial Deformities

MYRON R. TUCKER, BRIAN B. FARRELL, AND BART C. FARRELL

CHAPTER OUTLINE

PREVALENCE OF DENTOFACIAL DEFORMITIES

Epidemiologic surveys demonstrate that a large percentage of the United States' population has a significant malocclusion.[1-3] Very little data describe the exact prevalence of significant skeletal facial deformity. This information can be extrapolated from studies that have evaluated the prevalence of severe malocclusion. The National Health and Nutrition Examination Survey (NHANES III) conducted from 1989 to 1994 obtained a sample of 14,000 individuals ages 8 through 50 that roughly approximates the general U.S. population. In this study, information was collected describing overjet/reverse overjet, vertical overlap (deep bite and open bite), and posterior crossbites.[1] It can be assumed that patients with extreme values in each of these categories have underlying facial deformities (Table 25-1). Because many patients have dental compensations for skeletal growth abnormalities (described later in this chapter), this study likely underestimates the severity of skeletal abnormalities. This type of data combined with other criteria that clearly define the most severe characteristics of a malocclusion, such as overjet versus crowding, can help to approximate more clearly the prevalence of skeletal abnormality that may require surgical correction as part of the treatment for malocclusion.[2]

It appears that about 2% of the U.S. population has mandibular deficiency and/or vertical maxillary excess that is severe enough to be considered handicapping.[3] Other abnormalities and their percentage of prevalence in the population include mandibular excess and/or maxillary deficiency, 0.3%; open bite, 0.3%; and asymmetry, 0.1%. Therefore, it appears that approximately 2.7% of the U.S. population may have a dentofacial deformity contributing to malocclusion that will require surgical treatment for correction.

Historically, treatment of malocclusions, even those associated with dentofacial deformities, has been aimed at correction of dental abnormalities, with little attention to the accompanying deformity of the facial skeleton. In the last 60 years, surgical techniques have been developed to allow positioning of the entire midface complex, mandible, or dentoalveolar segments to any desired position. The combining of surgical and orthodontic procedures for dentofacial deformities has become an integral part of the correction of malocclusions and facial abnormalities.

CAUSES OF DENTOFACIAL DEFORMITY

Malocclusion and associated abnormalities of the skeletal components of the face can occur as a result of a variety of factors, including inherited tendencies, prenatal problems, systemic conditions that occur during growth, trauma, and environmental influences. Although it is not within the scope of this book to present a detailed discussion of facial growth,

TABLE 25-1

Percentage of the U.S. Population with Severe/Extreme Malocclusion

	All Ages (Age Groups Combined)			All Racial/Ethnic Groups (Racial/Ethnic Groups Combined)		
Type of Malocclusion	**8-11**	**12-11**	**18-50**	**White**	**Black**	**Mexican-American**
CLASS II: OVERJET						
>10 mm (extreme)	0.2	0.2	0.4	0.3	0.4	0.4
7 to 10 mm (severe)	3.4	3.5	3.9	3.8	4.3	2.2
CLASS III: REVERSE OVERJET						
>-4 mm (extreme)	0.0	0.0	0.1	0.1	0.1	0.3
-3 to -4 mm (severe)	0.0	0.6	0.2	0.2	0.4	0.4
OPEN BITE						
>-4 mm (extreme)	0.3	0.2	0.1	0.1	0.7	0.0
-3 to -4 mm (severe)	0.6	0.5	0.5	0.4	1.3	0.0

Adapted from Proffit WR, White RP Jr: Dentofacial problems: prevalence and treatment need. In Proffit WR, White RP Jr, Sarver DM, editors: *Contemporary treatment of dentofacial deformity,* St Louis, 2003, Mosby.

an understanding of basic principles as they relate to the development of dentofacial deformities is essential. Enlow and Han's *Essentials of Facial Growth*[4] should be reviewed for a more complete discussion of the principles of facial growth.

General Principles of Facial Growth

The development of proper craniofacial form and function is a complex process affected by many factors. In the area of the craniofacial complex, areas exist that appear to have their own intrinsic growth potential, including the sphenooccipital and sphenoethmoidal synchondroses and the nasal septum. In addition, the majority of growth of the bones of the face occurs in response to adjacent soft tissue and the functional demands placed on the underlying bone. These soft tissue influences include the nasal, oral, and hypopharyngeal airway; facial muscles; and muscles of mastication.[5]

The general direction of normal growth of the face is downward and forward with lateral expansion. The maxilla and the mandible appear to grow by remodeling or differential apposition and resorption of bone, producing changes in three dimensions. Enlow and Hans[4] describe this phenomenon as *area relocation,* with the maxillary-mandibular complex enlarging in the downward and forward direction as an "expanding pyramid" (Fig. 25-1). The direction and amount of growth characterize an individual's growth pattern.[6] Alterations in the pattern of growth or in the rate at which this growth occurs may result in abnormal skeletal morphology of the face and an accompanying malocclusion.

Genetic and Environmental Influence

Genetic influence certainly plays a role in dentofacial deformities. Patterns of inheritance, such as a familial tendency toward a

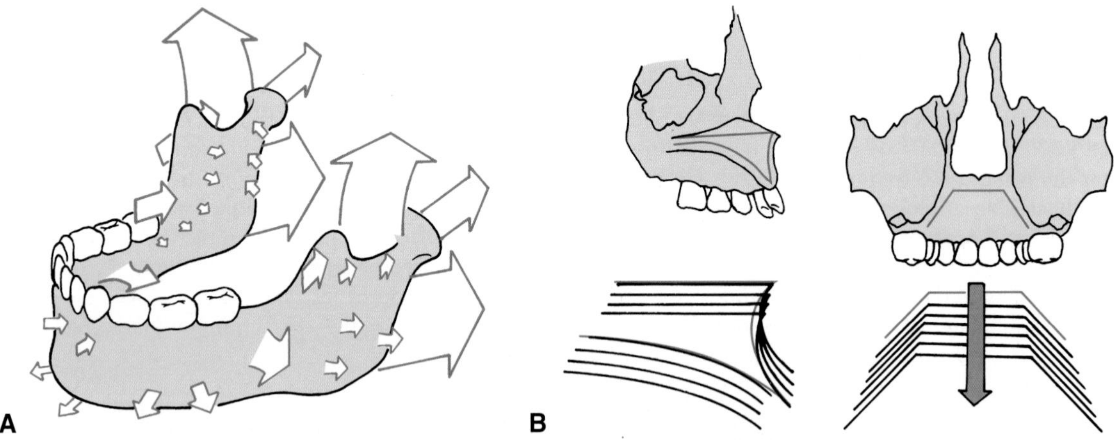

FIGURE 25-1 **A,** Mandibular growth resulting from apposition and resorption of bone. Primary areas of bony apposition include superior surface of alveolar process and posterior and superior surfaces of mandibular ramus. **B,** Forward and downward growth of nasal complex and maxilla in "expanding V." Resorption of bone at superior surface of palate occurs simultaneously with apposition at inferior surfaces of palate and alveolar processes. In addition, growth in posterior area of maxilla results in downward and forward expansion of maxilla. (From Enlow DH: *Handbook of facial growth,* Philadelphia, 1975, WB Saunders.)

prognathic or deficient mandible, are often seen in a patient with a dentofacial deformity. However, the multifactorial nature of facial development precludes the prediction of an inherited pattern of a particular facial abnormality.

Abnormal facial growth and associated malocclusions are sometimes associated with congenital abnormalities and syndromes. Some of these syndromes such as hemifacial microsomia and mandibulofacial dysostosis (Treacher Collins syndrome) are related to embryonic abnormalities of neural crest cells. Other congenital abnormalities affecting jaw growth include cleft lip and palate and craniosynostosis (premature fusions of craniofacial sutures). Facial growth abnormalities may be caused by maternal systemic influences such as fetal alcohol syndrome, which may result in hypoplasia of midface structures.

Environmental influences also play a role in the development of dentofacial deformities. As early as the prenatal stage, intrauterine molding of the developing fetal head may result in a severe mandibular deficiency. Abnormal function after birth also may result in altered facial growth because soft tissue and muscular function often influence the position of teeth and growth of the jaws. Abnormal tongue position or size can affect the position and growth of the maxilla and mandible (Fig. 25-2). Respiratory difficulty, mouth breathing, and abnormal tongue and lip postures can adversely influence facial growth.[7] Trauma to the bones of the face can result in severe abnormalities of the facial skeleton and the occlusion. In addition to the abnormality that occurs as an immediate result of trauma, further effects on the development of facial bones may occur. In the case of temporomandibular joint (TMJ) trauma in a growing child, significant restriction of jaw function may occur as a result of scarring or bony/fibrous ankylosis. Subsequent alteration of growth may result with deficient or asymmetric mandibular growth (Fig. 25-3).

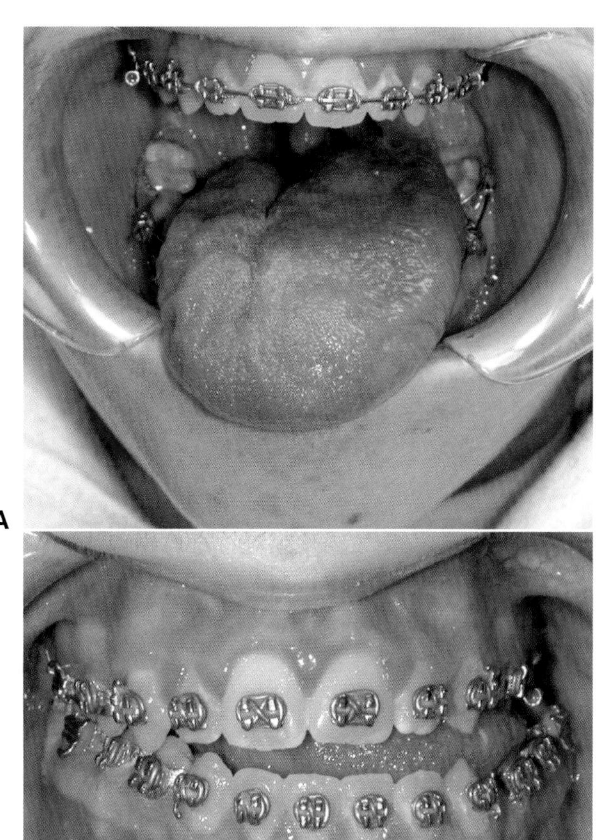

FIGURE 25-2 A, Tongue asymmetry with unilateral hypertrophy. B, Resulting unilateral open bite.

EVALUATION OF PATIENTS WITH DENTOFACIAL DEFORMITY

In the past, individual practitioners often treated patients with dentofacial deformities. Some patients have been treated with orthodontics alone, with a resultant acceptable occlusion but a compromise in facial esthetics. Other patients have had surgery without orthodontics in an attempt to correct a skeletal deformity, which resulted in improved facial esthetics but a less than ideal occlusion. In addition to orthodontic and surgical needs, these patients often have many other problems requiring periodontic, endodontic, complex restorative, and prosthetic considerations.

Many areas of dental practice, in addition to orthodontics and surgery, must be integrated to address the complex problems of patients with dental deformities. This integrated approach, used throughout the evaluation, presurgical, and postsurgical phases of patient care, provides the best possible results for these patients.[8]

The most important phase in patient care centers on evaluation of the existing problems and definition of treatment goals. At the initial appointment a thorough interview should be conducted with the patient to discuss the patient's perception of the problems and the goals of any possible treatment. The patient's current health status and any medical or psychological problems that may affect treatment are also discussed at this time.

The involved orthodontist and oral and maxillofacial surgeon should conduct a thorough examination of facial structure, with consideration of frontal and profile esthetics.

Evaluation of facial esthetics in the frontal view should assess the presence of asymmetries and evaluate overall facial balance. The evaluation should include assessment of the position of the forehead, eyes, infraorbital rims, and malar eminences; configuration of the nose, including the width of the alar base; paranasal areas; lip morphology; relationship of the lips to incisors; and overall proportional relationships of the face in the vertical and transverse dimensions. Figure 25-4 demonstrates normal facial proportions. The profile evaluation allows an assessment of the anteroposterior and vertical relationships of all components of the face. The soft tissue configuration of the throat should also be evaluated. Photographic documentation of the pretreatment condition of the patient should be a standard part of the evaluation. Video and digital computerized images have been introduced over the past decade as an additional aid in evaluating facial morphology.

A complete dental examination should include assessment of dental arch form, symmetry, tooth alignment, and occlusal

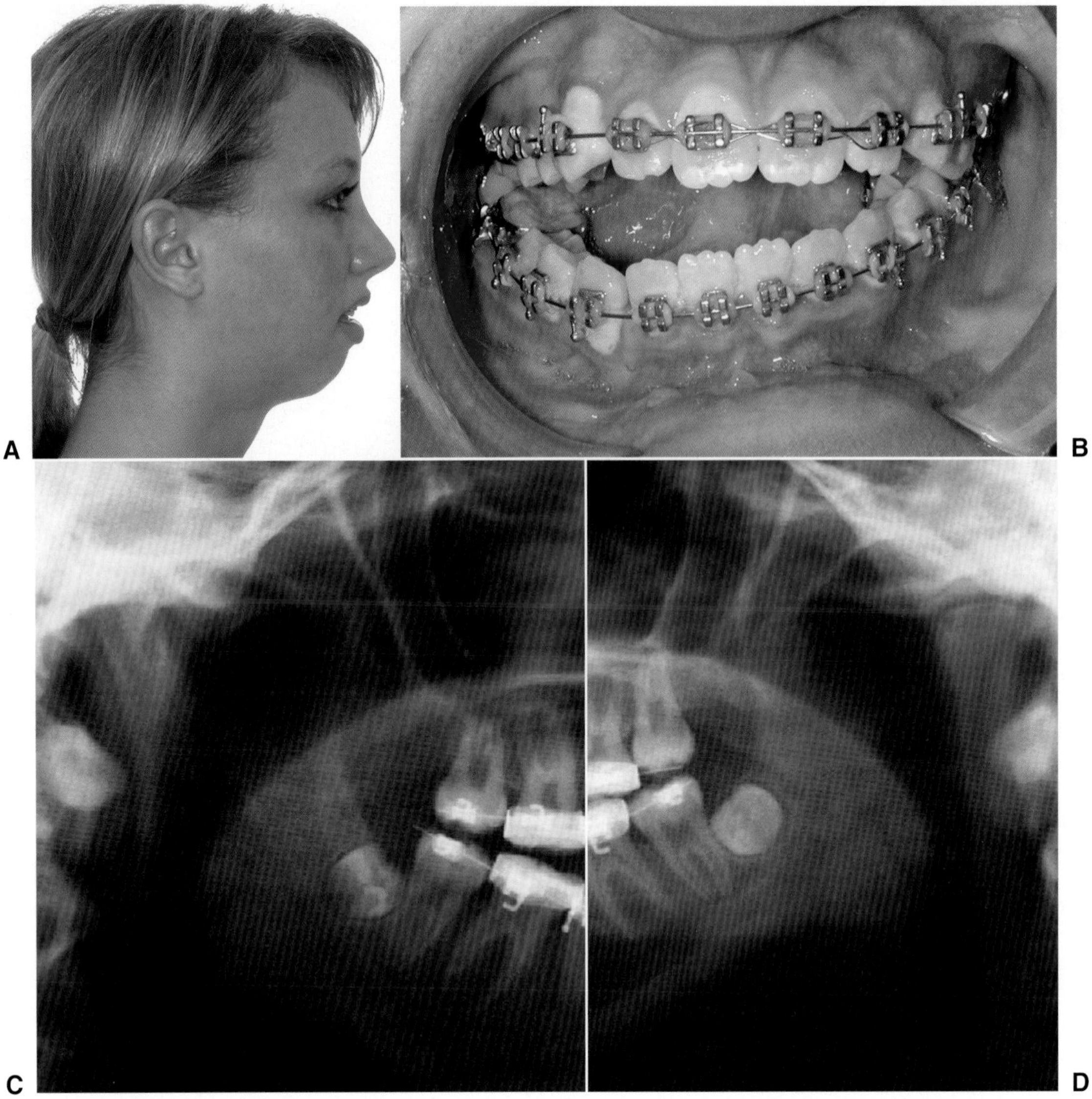

FIGURE 25-3 Condylar trauma at an early age resulting in restricted jaw function and subsequent deficient and asymmetric mandibular growth. A, Profile view. B, Occlusion with right side anterior open bite due to decreased growth in the left mandibular ramus area. C, Radiograph of right condyle and ramus (normal). D, Left side with decreased growth.

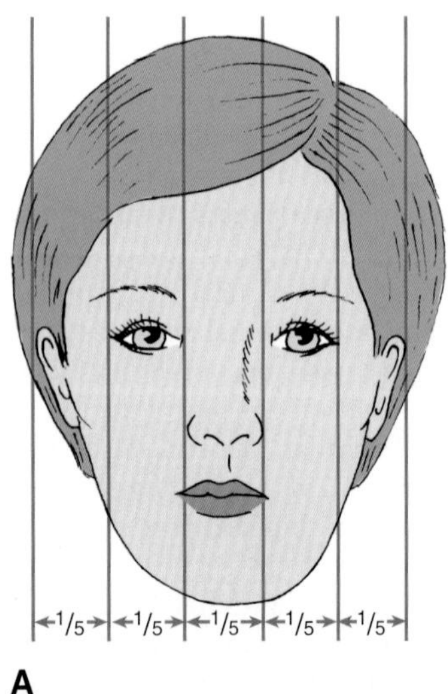

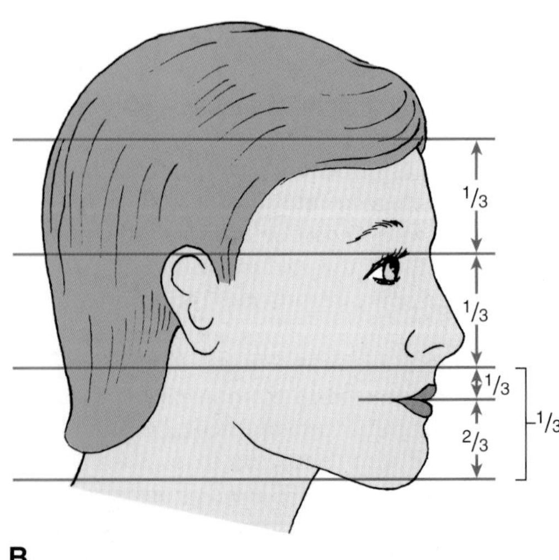

FIGURE 25-4 Normal facial proportions. A, Representation of proportional relationships of full-face view. Relationships of medial intercanthal distance, alar base width, and lip proportions to remainder of facial structures are demonstrated. B, Normal profile proportions demonstrates relationships of upper, middle, and lower thirds of face and proportional relationships of lip and chin morphology within lower third of face.

abnormalities in the transverse, anteroposterior, and vertical dimensions. The muscles of mastication and TMJ function should also be evaluated. A screening periodontal examination, including probing, should assess the patient's hygiene and current periodontal health status. Impressions and a bite registration for dental cast construction and evaluation should also be obtained at this time.

Lateral cephalometric and panoramic radiographs are routinely used in the patient evaluation and are an important part of the initial assessment. The cephalometric radiograph can be evaluated by several techniques to aid in the determination of the nature of the skeletal abnormality (Fig. 25-5; Table 25-2).[9,10] An important note, however, is that cephalometric radiographs are only a part of the evaluation process; they are used as adjunctive diagnostic tools in the clinical assessment of the patient's facial structure and occlusion. Other radiographic images may be helpful in evaluating patients for surgical correction. These may include posteroanterior facial films, TMJ images when indicated, and conventional and cone-beam computed tomography (Fig. 25-6). In difficult, complex cases, it may be helpful to obtain a stereolithic three-dimensional model constructed from computed tomography scan data. Computerized digital technology is currently available that helps to integrate the cephalometric data with digital images of the face to improve evaluation of the relationship of the underlying facial skeleton and overlying soft tissue. After careful clinical assessment and evaluation of the diagnostic records, a problem list and treatment plan should be developed that combines opinions from all practitioners participating in the patient's care, including the orthodontist, oral and maxillofacial surgeon, periodontist, and restorative dentist.

TABLE 25-2

Orthognathic Cephalometric Analysis

	Standard (Male)	Standard (Female)
HORIZONTAL (SKELETAL)		
N-A-Pg (angle)	3.9 degrees	2.6 degrees
N-A (II HP)	0.0 degrees	2.0 degrees
N-B (II HP)	-5.3 degrees	-6.9 degrees
N-Pg (II HP)	-4.3 degrees	-6.5 degrees
VERTICAL (SKELETAL, DENTAL)		
N-ANS (HP)	54.7 mm	50.0 mm
ANS-Gn (HP)	68.6 mm	61.3 mm
PNS-N (HP)	53.9 mm	50.6 mm
MP-HP (angle)	23.0 degrees	24.2 degrees
1-NF (NF)	30.5 mm	27.5 mm
1-MP (MP)	45.0 mm	40.8 mm
6-NF (NF)	26.2 mm	23.0 mm
6-MP (MP)	35.8 mm	32.1 mm
MAXILLA, MANDIBLE		
PNS-ANS (II HP)	57.7 mm	52.6 mm
Ar-GO (linear)	52.0 mm	46.8 mm
Go-Pg (linear)	83.7 mm	74.3 mm
Ar-Go-Gn (angle)	119.1 degrees	122.0 degrees
DENTAL		
OP upper-Hp (angle)	6.2 degrees	7.1 degrees
OP lower-Hp (angle)	—	—
A-B (II OP)	-1.1 mm	-0.4 mm
1-NF (angle)	111.0 degrees	112.5 degrees
1-MP (angle)	95.9 degrees	95.9 degrees

Modified from Burstone CJ, James RB, Legan H et al: Cephalometrics for orthognathic surgery, *J Oral Surg* 36:269, 1978.

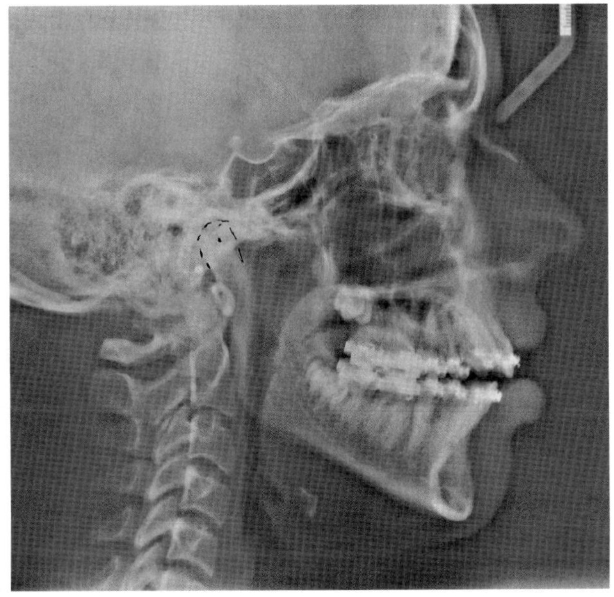

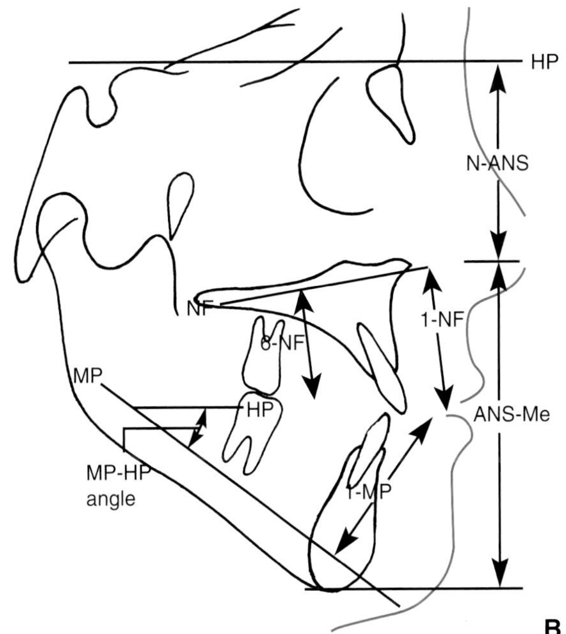

FIGURE 25-5 A, Lateral cephalometric radiograph. B, Tracing of lateral cephalometric head film, with landmarks identified for evaluating facial, skeletal, and dental abnormalities using system of cephalometrics for orthognathic surgery (Table 25-2). (B from Burstone CJ, James RB, Legan H et al: Cephalometrics for orthognathic surgery, *J Oral Surg* 36:269, 1978.)

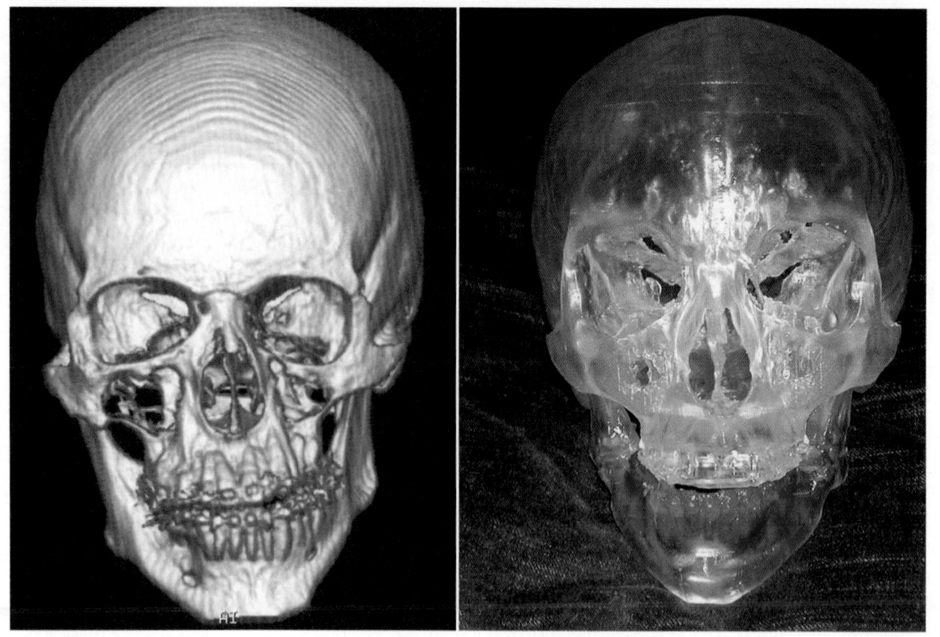

FIGURE 25-6 A, Three-dimensional reconstructed computed tomography scan. B, Stereolithic model.

PRESURGICAL TREATMENT PHASE

Periodontal Considerations

As the first step in treatment, gingival inflammation must be controlled and the patient's cooperation ensured. In patients who are unwilling or unable to clean their teeth properly before the placement of orthodontic appliances, oral hygiene procedures will be even less effective when complicated by orthodontic band placement.

Periodontal therapy includes oral hygiene instruction, scaling, and root planing; in certain instances, flap surgery to gain access for root planing may be necessary to provide proper tissue health. Whenever possible, it is desirable to delay comprehensive treatment until adequate patient compliance and control of inflammation are achieved.

As a result of the periodontal examination findings and proposed orthodontic and surgical plan, mucogingival surgery is often accomplished during this initial phase of therapy to provide a zone of attached keratinized tissue that is more resistant to potential orthodontic and surgical trauma. Soft tissue grafting is indicated in areas that have no keratinized gingiva or where only a thin band of keratinized tissue with little or no attachment is found when an increase in tissue trauma is likely (Fig. 25-7). Such trauma to these areas includes labial orthodontic movement of teeth or a surgical procedure such as an inferior border osteotomy or segmental osteotomies in interdental areas.

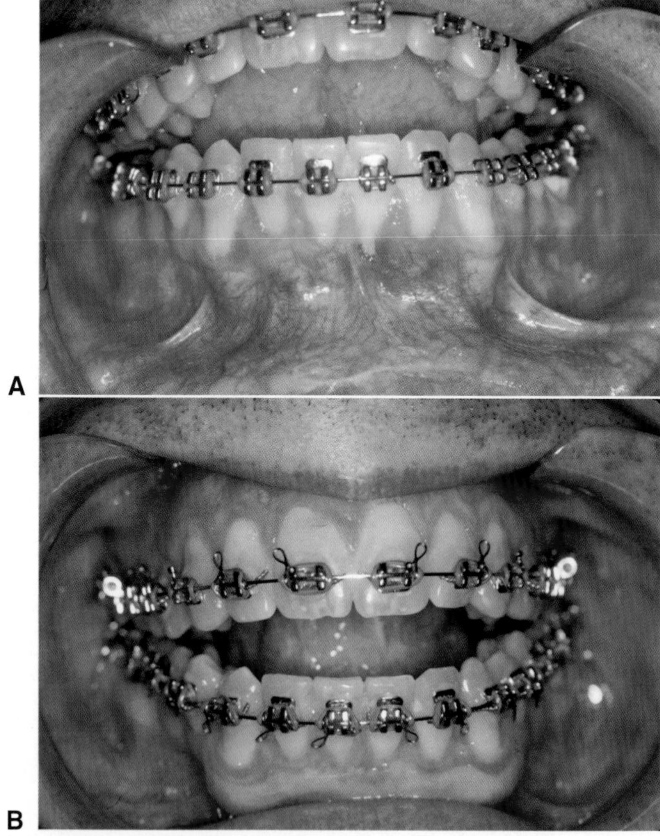

FIGURE 25-7 A, Presurgical appearance of gingival tissue labial to lower anterior teeth. Inadequate area of attachment and keratinization is visualized. B, Significant improvement in attachment and keratinization of labial gingival tissue after gingival grafting.

Restorative Considerations

During the presurgical restorative phase, the patient is evaluated for carious lesions and faulty restorations. Teeth should be evaluated endodontically and periodontally for restorability, and any nonrestorable teeth should be extracted before surgical intervention. All carious lesions must be restored early in the presurgical treatment phase. Existing restorations must function for 18 to 24 months during the orthodontic and surgical treatment phases, requiring that more durable restorative materials (i.e., amalgam and composite resin) be used, even though they may be replaced during the definitive postsurgical treatment phase. It is wise to delay final restorative treatment until the proper skeletal relationships are achieved and the finishing orthodontics is completed.

In the edentulous or partially edentulous patient, particular attention is paid to residual ridge shape and contour in denture-bearing areas. The distance between the maxillary tuberosity, posterior mandible, and ramus areas must be evaluated to ensure that adequate space is present for partial or complete dentures. Teeth that serve as removable partial denture abutments should be evaluated for potential retentive undercuts. If minor orthodontic movement can enhance undercuts, this information is conveyed to the orthodontist.

Presurgical Orthodontic Considerations

Obviously, not all malocclusions require correction with surgery. When the skeletal discrepancy is minimal and orthodontic compensation does not adversely affect dental or facial esthetics or posttreatment stability, orthodontic treatment alone may be the treatment of choice. However, in some cases an adequate occlusal relationship cannot be achieved because of the skeletal discrepancy; some patients may be treated with orthodontic compensation for a skeletal abnormality, resulting in an adequate occlusion but poor facial or dental esthetics or a poor long-term prognosis for posttreatment retention. These patients should be considered for surgery combined with orthodontic treatment.

Treatment Timing

Treatment of the stable adult deformity can be started without delay, but questions often arise about how best to manage the growing child who is identified as having a developing dentofacial deformity. If the facial pattern is favorable and significant growth potential remains, growth modification with techniques such as functional appliance therapy or headgear may be the preferred approach. For patients with unfavorable growth patterns or severe skeletal abnormalities or who are unwilling to undergo attempts at growth modification, surgery is usually the preferred treatment. As a general guideline, orthognathic surgery should be delayed until growth is complete in patients who have problems of excess growth, although surgery can be considered earlier for patients with growth deficiencies.

Orthodontic Treatment Objectives

Undesirable angulation of the anterior teeth occurs as a compensatory response to a developing dentofacial deformity. For example, a patient with maxillary deficiency and/or mandibular excess often has dental compensation for the skeletal abnormality with flared upper incisors and retracted or retroclined lower incisors (Fig. 25-8, *A* to *C*). Dental compensations for the skeletal deformity are corrected before surgery by orthodontically repositioning teeth properly over the underlying skeletal component, without considerations for the bite relationship to the opposing arch. This presurgical orthodontic movement accentuates the patient's deformity but is necessary if normal occlusal relationships are to be achieved when the skeletal components are properly positioned at surgery (Fig. 25-8, *D* to *F*). The surgical treatment then results in an ideal position of the skeletal and dental components (Fig. 25-8, *G* to *I*). The opposite dental compensation may occur in maxillary protrusion or mandibular deficiency (Fig. 25-9). Again, the decompensation is aimed at improving angulation of teeth over underlying bone, after which skeletal problems are corrected.

The essential steps in orthodontic preparation are to align the arches individually, achieve compatibility of the arches or arch segments, and establish the proper anteroposterior and vertical position of the incisors. The amount of presurgical orthodontics can vary, ranging from appliance placement with minimal tooth movement in some patients to approximately 12 to 18 months of appliance therapy in those with severe crowding and incisor malposition.

As the patient is approaching the end of orthodontic preparation for surgery, it is helpful to take impressions and evaluate progress models for occlusal compatibility. Minor interferences that exist can be corrected easily with arch wire adjustment and significantly enhance the postsurgical occlusal result. After any final orthodontic adjustments have been made, large stabilizing arch wires are inserted into the brackets, which provide the strength necessary to withstand the forces resulting from intermaxillary fixation (IMF) and surgical manipulation.

Final Treatment Planning

After the completion of the presurgical periodontics, restorative dentistry, and orthodontics, the patient returns to the oral and maxillofacial surgeon for final presurgical planning. The evaluation completed at the initial patient examination is repeated. The patient's facial structure and the malocclusion are re-examined. Presurgical digital photographs and radiographs are obtained. Presurgical models, a centric relation bite registration, and face-bow recording for model mounting are completed. Model surgery on a duplicated set of presurgical dental casts determines the exact surgical movements necessary to accomplish the desired postoperative occlusion (Fig. 25-10).

One of the most useful adjuncts to treatment planning for patients with dentofacial deformity is computerized imaging. This technology allows computerized digital images of the patient's face to be superimposed over bony landmarks obtained from the cephalometric radiograph. Cephalometric treatment planning can be completed with computer assistance. The computer can then produce a digital image that represents the facial esthetic result produced by the associated facial skeletal change (Fig. 25-11). The advantage of using this type of technology is the ability to predict more accurately the facial changes that may result from a particular surgical correction. The facial images are also more easily evaluated by patients, allowing them to assess the predicted results and provide input into the surgical treatment plan. The disadvantage of the technology is related to the inability of the computer to predict accurately every type of surgical change for every patient.[11] Different muscle tone and skin thickness and variable soft tissue response to bone change, for example, make it impossible for the computer to predict each individual variation precisely. However, with continued development, this technology will most likely become more common in the treatment planning and presurgical education for patients with dentofacial deformity. Although the current technology is primarily limited to isolated lateral or frontal views, three-dimensional predictive imaging capabilities will likely be available in the near future.

After completion of the model surgery, prediction tracings, and computer imaging evaluation, the orthodontist or general

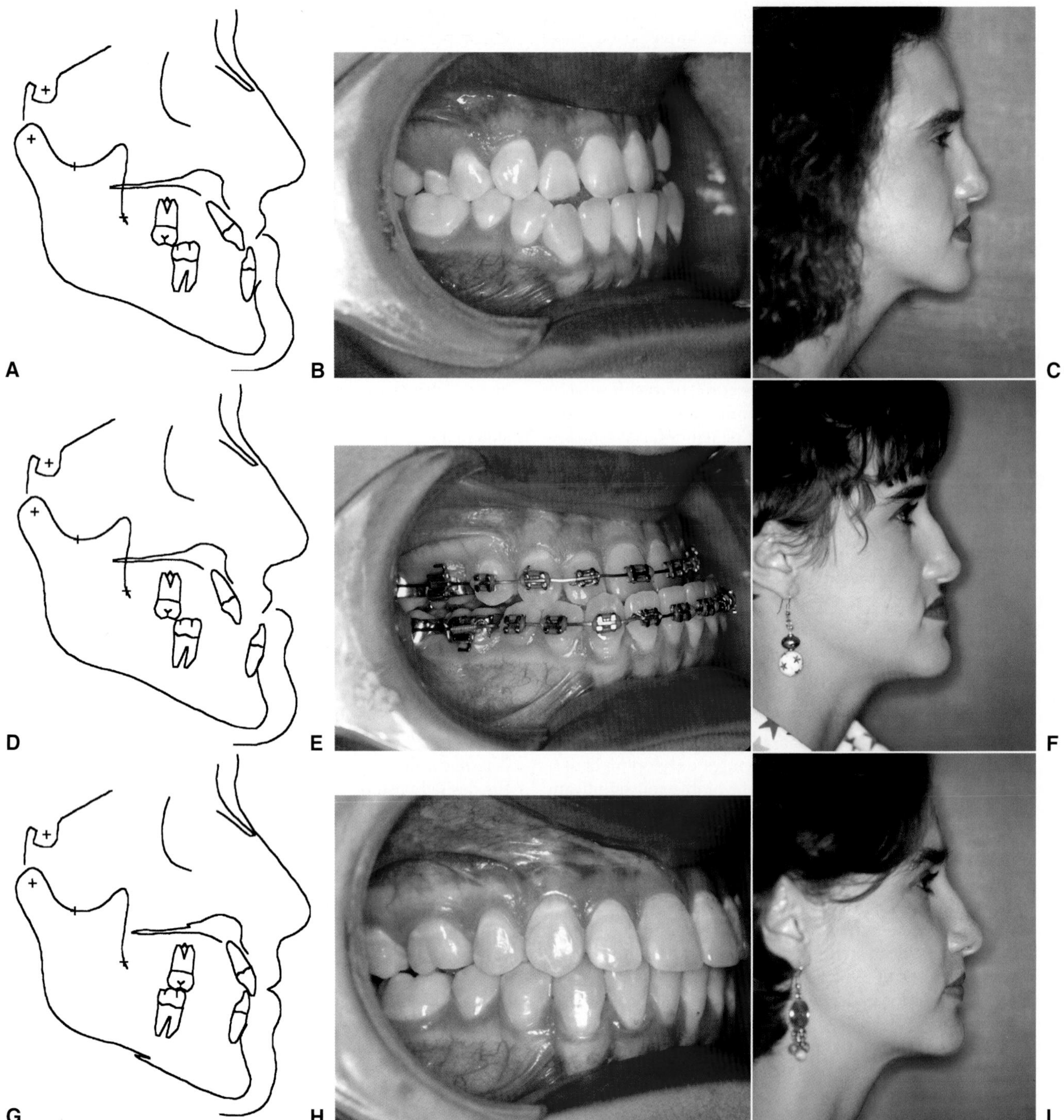

FIGURE 25-8 A, Class III skeletal malocclusion with maxillary deficiency and mandibular excess. B, Dental compensation includes retroclined lower incisors and proclined upper incisors. C, Facial profile. D, After initial orthodontic treatment before surgery. E, Dental compensation are removed with proclination of lower incisors and retroclination of upper incisors, which obviously increases the severity of malocclusion and facial discrepancy. F, Facial profile at this stage. G, Surgical correction with posterior positioning of mandible and advancement of maxilla. H, Ideal occlusion. I, Facial profile after treatment is complete.

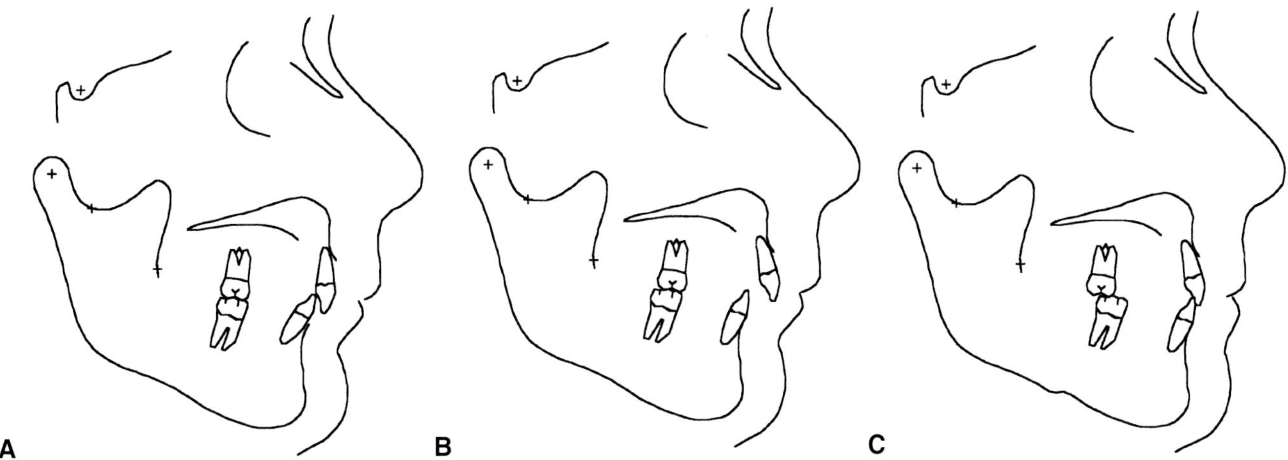

FIGURE 25-9 A, Class II occlusion with compensation demonstrating proclination of lower incisors and upright upper incisors. B, After orthodontic decompensation. C, After surgical correction with mandibular advancement.

dentist is often consulted to ensure that the predicted occlusal result is acceptable to all practitioners involved in the patient's treatment. Any orthodontic or restorative changes necessary to improve postsurgical position should be planned at this time.

SURGICAL TREATMENT PHASE

Dentofacial abnormalities frequently can be treated by isolated procedures in the mandible or maxilla and midface area. Because abnormalities can obviously occur in the maxilla and the mandible, surgical correction frequently requires a combination

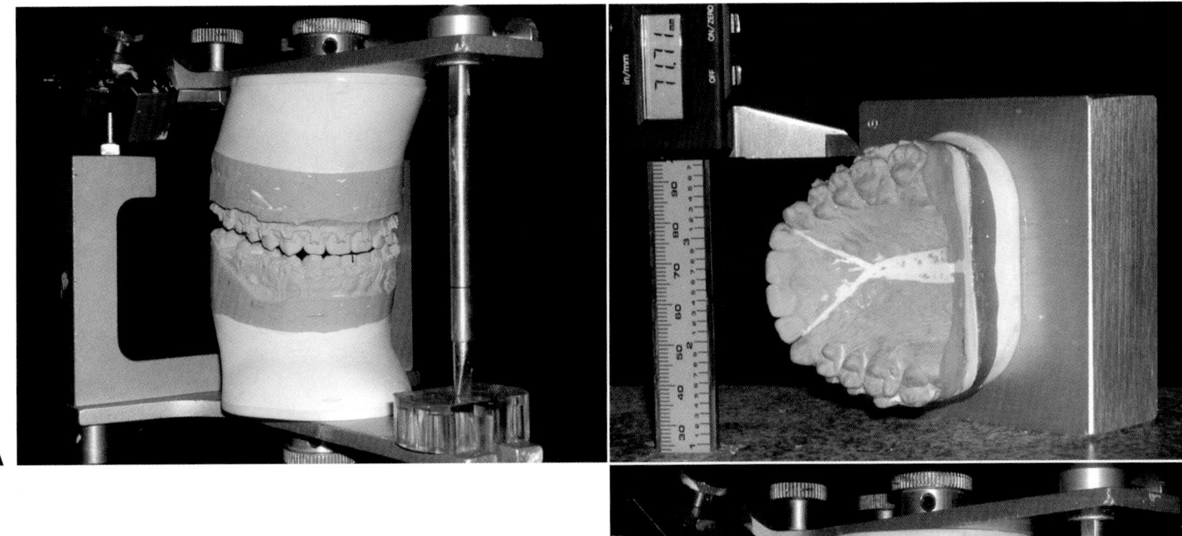

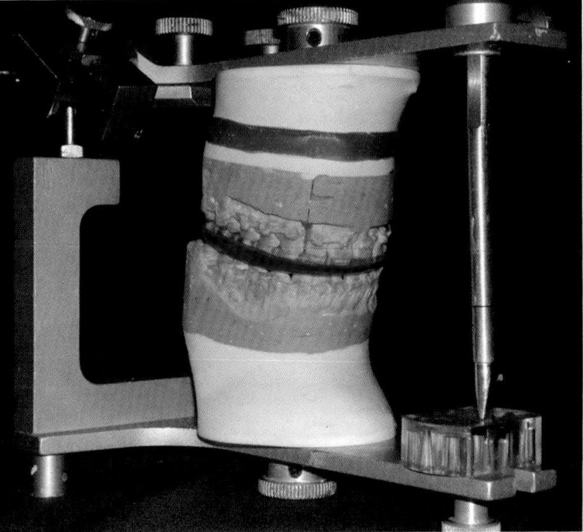

FIGURE 25-10 Model surgery used to determine direction and distance of surgical movement necessary to achieve desired postoperative occlusion and facial esthetics. A, Casts mounted on semiadjustable articulator. B, Repositioning of maxillary cast using precision measuring instrument. Distances of model surgical movements are coordinated between desired facial esthetics and movements necessary to create ideal postoperative occlusion. C, Maxillary cast remounted on semiadjustable articulator after precision movements have been completed and verified. Intraocclusal wafers are constructed on this final occlusal setup for use at time of surgery to align osteotomies and dental segments into desired postsurgical position.

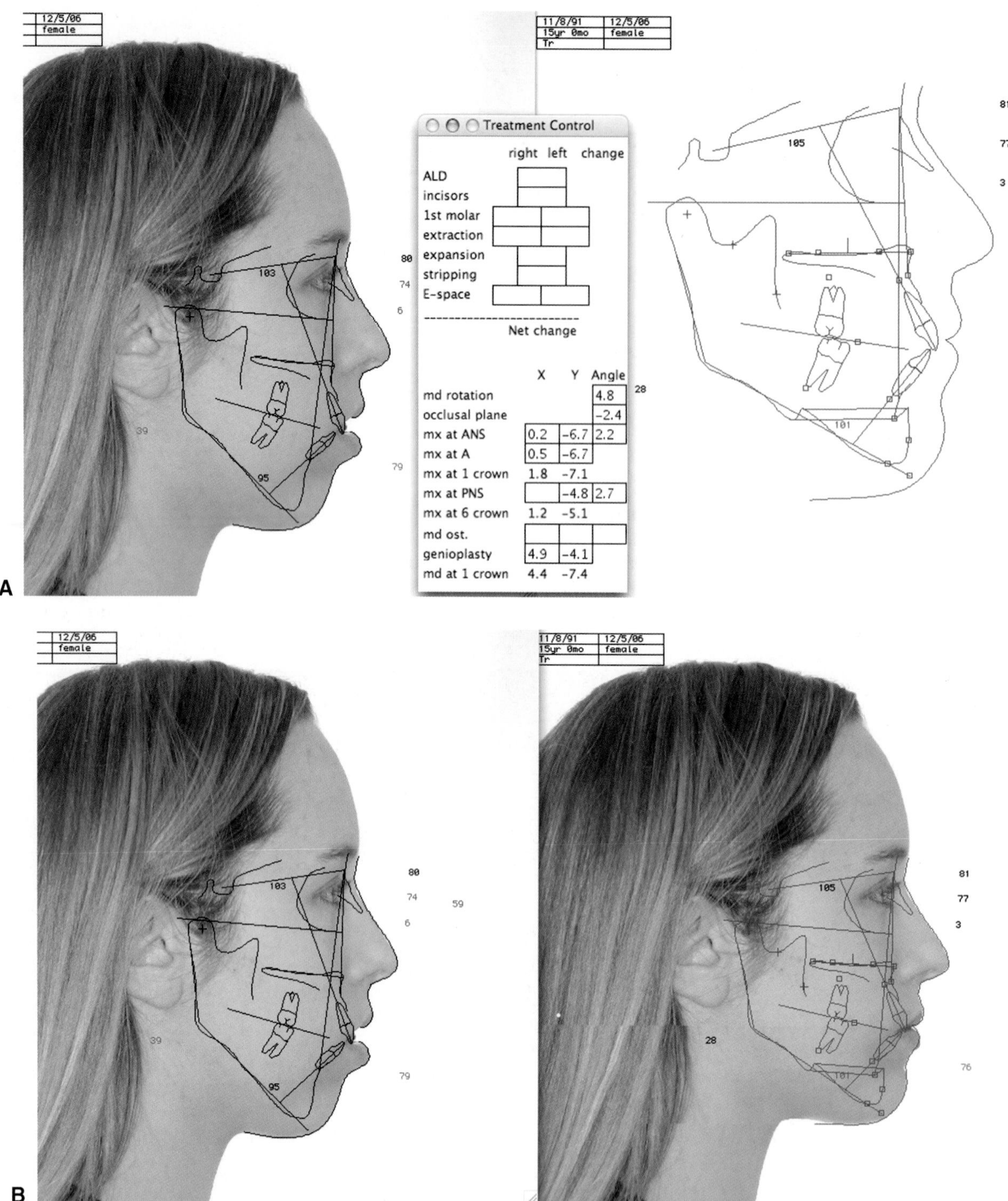

FIGURE 25-11 Computerized imaging for dentofacial surgical treatment planning. Digital image is obtained and placed in computer memory. Landmarks from cephalometric tracing are superimposed over digital image of face. **A**, Portions of cephalometric tracing can be moved to duplicate the anticipated surgical movements. The computer then manipulates the image to depict soft tissue changes. Digital images displayed on the computer monitor shows predicted facial changes (Quick Ceph Image System). **B**, View shows presurgical and estimated final images that would result from anticipated surgical procedure (in this case, maxillary superior repositioning and chin advancement).

of surgical procedures. The following sections describe a variety of surgical procedures completed as isolated osteotomies or as combination procedures.

Mandibular Excess

Excess growth of the mandible frequently results in an abnormal occlusion with Class III molar and cuspid relationships and a reverse overjet in the incisor area. An obvious facial deformity may also be evident. Facial features associated with mandibular excess include a prominence of the lower third of the face, particularly in the area of the lower lip and chin in the anteroposterior and vertical dimensions. In severe cases the large reverse overjet may preclude the patient's ability to obtain adequate lip closure without abnormal strain of the orbicularis oris muscles.

Mandibular excess was one of the first dentofacial deformities recognized as being best treated by a combination of orthodontics and surgery. Although surgical techniques for correction of mandibular excess were reported as early as the late 1800s, widespread use of currently acceptable techniques began in the middle of this century. Early techniques for treatment of mandibular prognathism dealt with the deformity by removing sections of bone in the body of the mandible, which allowed the anterior segment to be moved posteriorly (Fig. 25-12). When the reverse overjet relationship is isolated to the anterior dentoalveolar area of the mandible, a subapical osteotomy technique can be used for correction of mandibular dental prognathism.[12] In this technique, bone is removed in the area of an extraction site of a premolar or molar tooth, and the anterior dentoalveolar segment of the mandible is moved to a more posterior position (Fig. 25-13). Although these procedures are rarely used, they are occasionally performed in cases with unusual arch forms in combination with edentulous spaces.

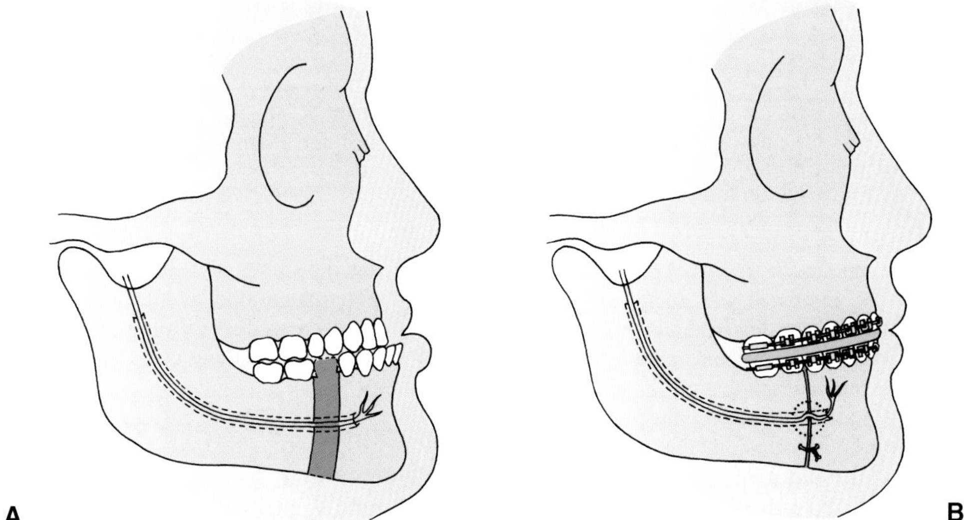

FIGURE 25-12 Body ostectomy with resection of portion of body of mandible followed by posterior repositioning of anterior segment. A, Preoperative view. B, Postoperative view.

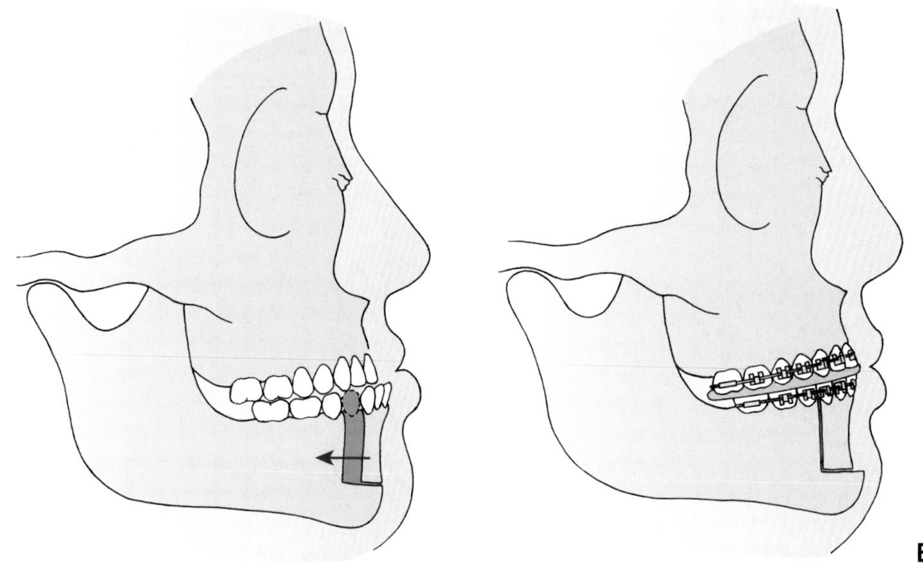

FIGURE 25-13 Anterior mandibular subapical osteotomy. A, Removal of premolar teeth and bone in area of extraction sites. B, After separation, anterior dentoalveolar segment is repositioned posteriorly, extraction sites are closed, and anterior reverse overjet relationship is corrected.

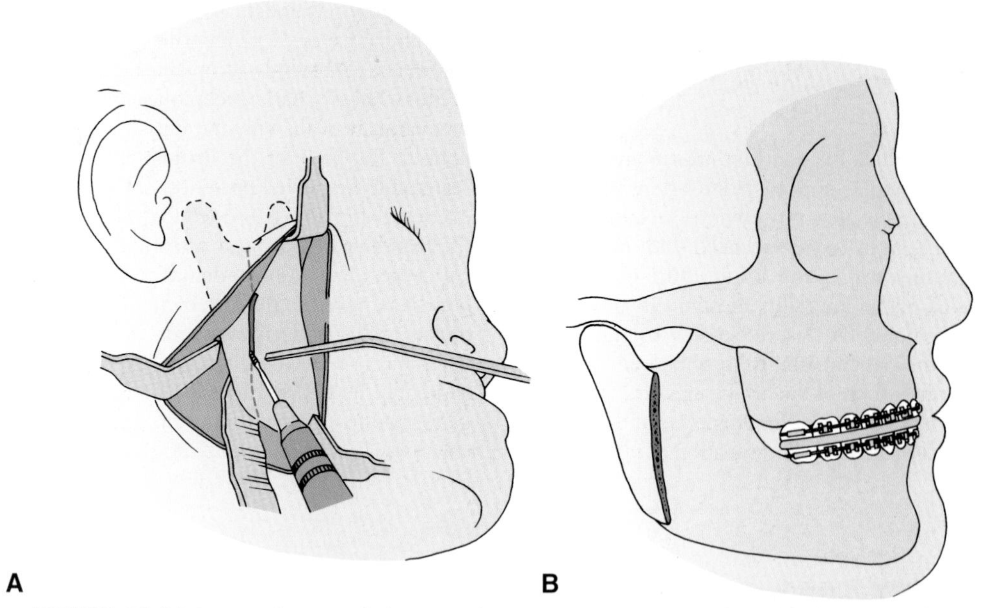

FIGURE 25-14 Extraoral approach for vertical ramus osteotomy. A, Submandibular approach to lateral aspect of ramus showing vertical osteotomy from sigmoid notch area to angle of mandible. B, Overlapping of segments after posterior repositioning of anterior portion of mandible. Proximal segment containing condyle is overlapped on lateral aspect of anterior portion of ramus.

In the early 1950s, Caldwell and Letterman[13] popularized an osteotomy performed in the ramus of the mandible for the correction of mandibular excess. In this technique the lateral aspect of the ramus is exposed through a submandibular incision, the ramus is sectioned in a vertical fashion, and the entire body and anterior ramus section of the mandible are moved posteriorly, which places the teeth in proper occlusion (Fig. 25-14).

The proximal segment of the ramus (i.e., the portion attached to the condyle) overlaps the anterior segment, and the jaw is stabilized during the healing phase with wiring of the bone segments combined with jaw immobilization using IMF. The extraoral approach is rarely used. A similar technique is performed with an intraoral incision and an angulated oscillating saw (Fig. 25-15).[14] The design of the osteotomy is identical to that performed through an extraoral incision. The bone segments can be stabilized using IMF, with or without direct wiring of the segments or using rigid fixation with bone plates or screws, eliminating the need for IMF. The advantages of the intraoral technique include elimination of the need for skin incision and decreased risk of damage to the mandibular branch of the facial nerve. Figure 25-16 demonstrates the clinical results of a patient treated with an intraoral vertical ramus osteotomy to correct mandibular excess.

Another popular technique for correction of mandibular prognathism is the bilateral sagittal split osteotomy (BSSO) first described by Trauner and Obwegeser[15] and later modified by Dalpont,[16] Hunsick,[17] and Epker.[18] The BSSO is accomplished through a transoral incision similar to that for the intraoral vertical ramus osteotomy. The osteotomy splits the ramus and posterior body of the mandible in a sagittal fashion, which allows setback or advancement of the mandible (Fig. 25-17). The telescoping effect in the area of the osteotomy produces large areas of bony overlap that have the flexibility necessary to move the mandible in several directions. The BSSO technique has become one of the most popular methods for treatment of mandibular deficiency and mandibular excess. Disadvantages include potential trauma of the inferior alveolar nerve, with subsequent decreased sensation in the area of the lower lip and chin during the immediate postoperative period. This may be permanent.

Mandibular Deficiency

The most obvious clinical feature of mandibular deficiency is the retruded position of the chin as viewed from the profile aspect. Other facial features often associated with mandibular

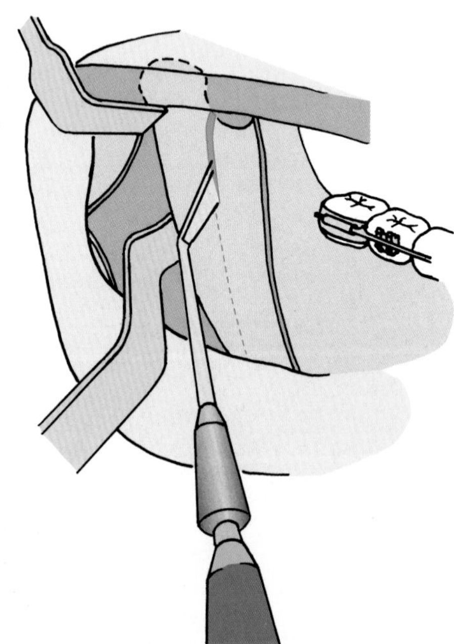

FIGURE 25-15 Intraoral technique for vertical ramus osteotomy through use of angulated oscillating saw.

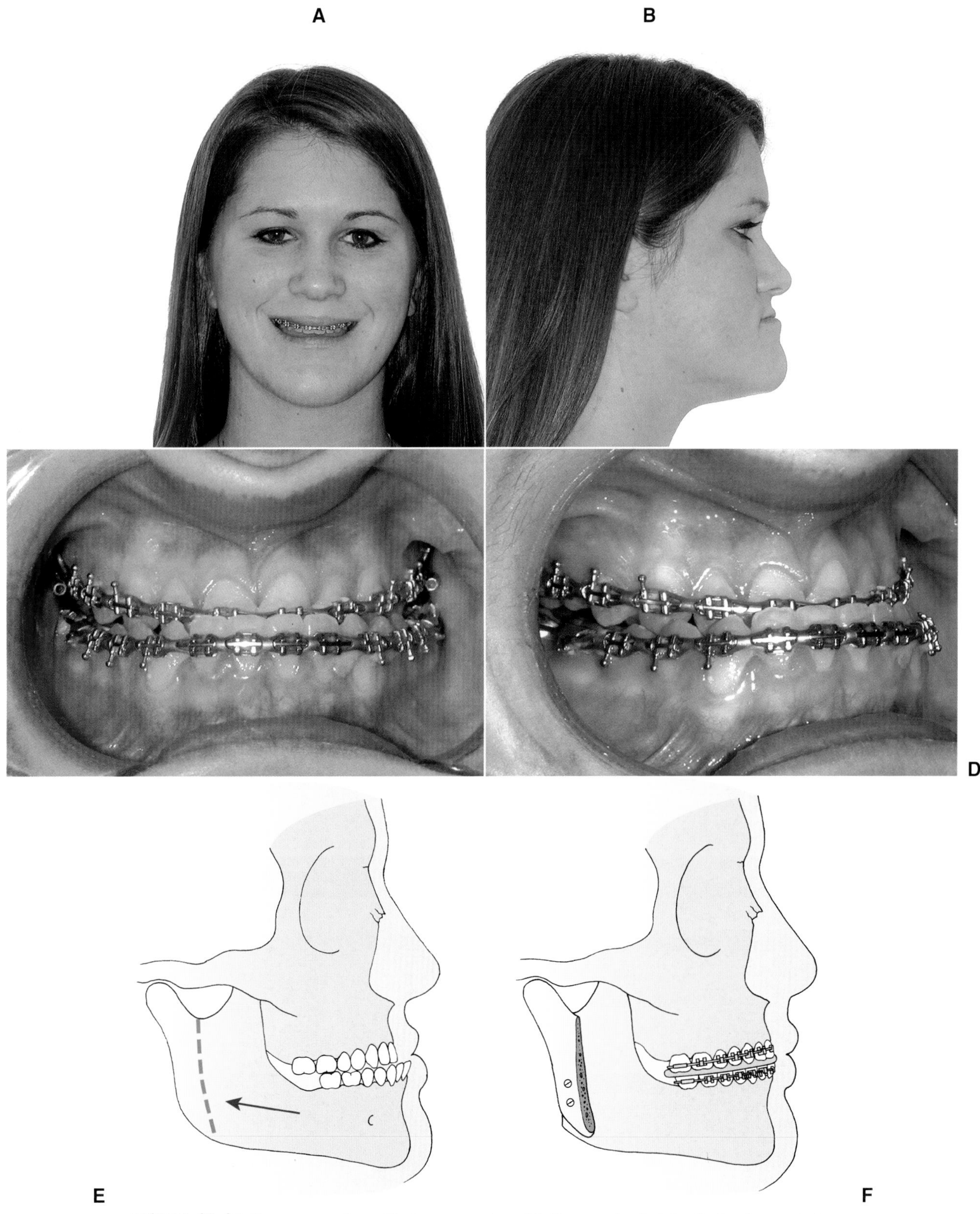

FIGURE 25-16 Case report of mandibular excess. A and B, Preoperative facial esthetics demonstrates typical features of Class III malocclusion resulting from mandibular excess. C and D, Presurgical occlusal photographs. E and F, Diagram of intraoral vertical ramus osteotomy with posterior positioning of mandible and rigid fixation.

Continued

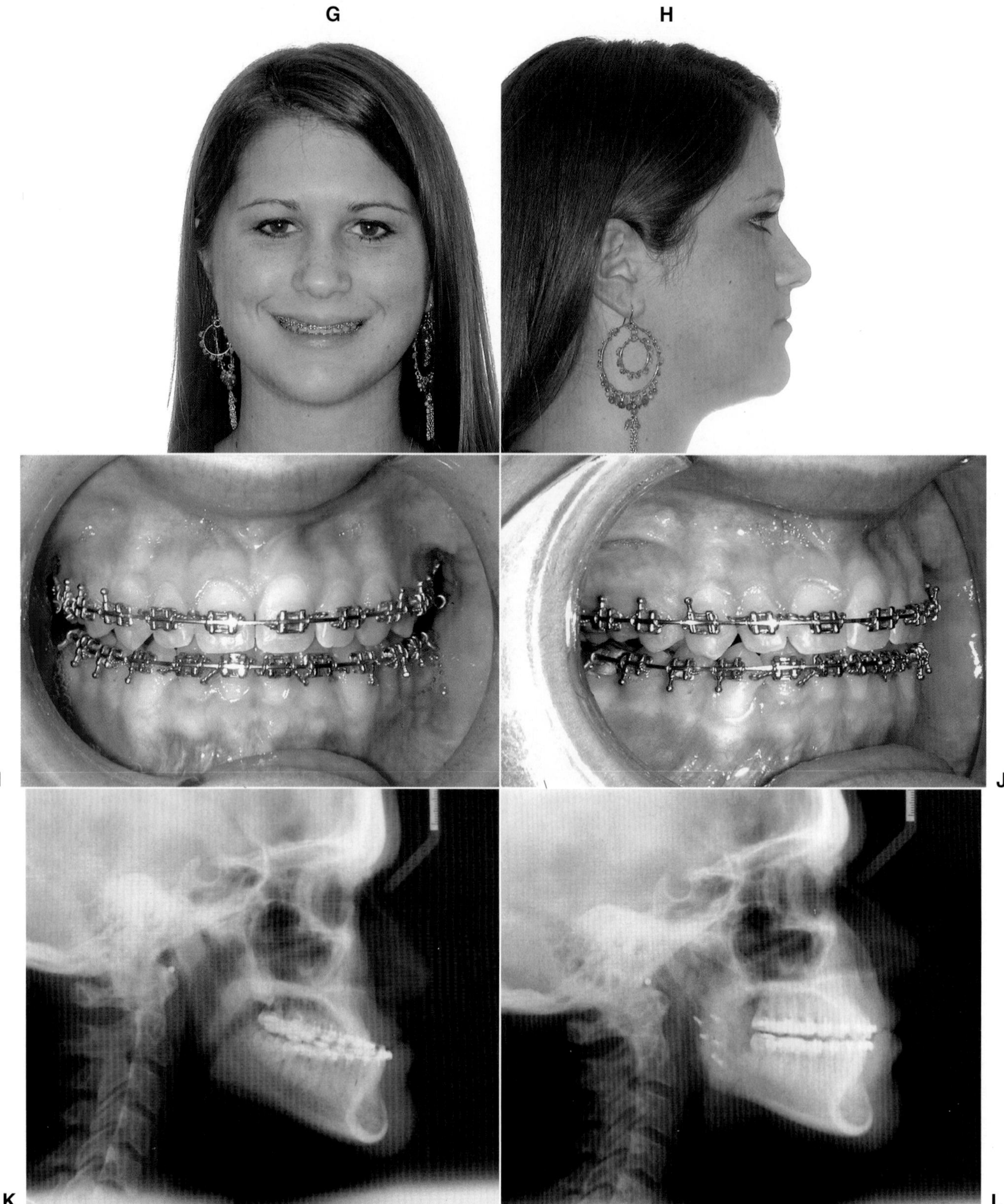

FIGURE 25-16, cont'd Postoperative frontal and profile view of patient seen in A and B. G and H, Postoperative occlusion seen in I and J. K and L show preoperative and postoperative radiographs.

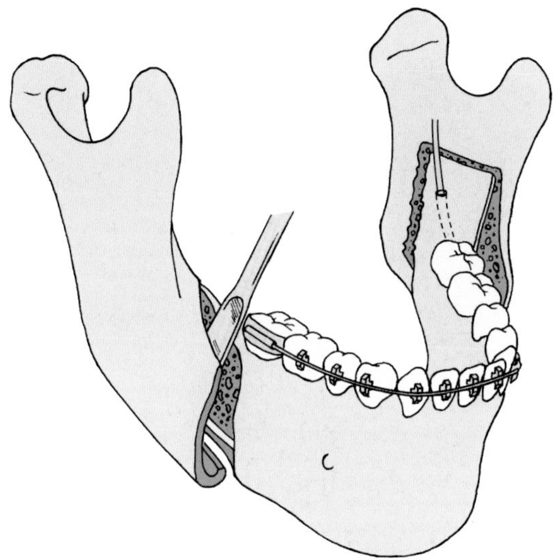

FIGURE 25-17 Sagittal split osteotomy. Ramus of mandible is divided by creation of horizontal osteotomy on medial aspect and vertical osteotomy on lateral aspect of mandible. These are connected by anterior ramus osteotomy. Lateral cortex of mandible is then separated from medial aspect, and mandible can be advanced or set back for correction of mandibular deficiency or excess, respectively.

deficiency may include an excess labiomental fold with a procumbent appearance of the lower lip, abnormal posture of the upper lip, and poor throat form. Intraorally, mandibular deficiency is associated with Class II molar and canine relationships and an increased overjet in the incisor area.

Surgical correction of mandibular deficiency was described as early as 1909. However, early results with surgical advancement of the mandible before the 1950s were extremely disappointing. In 1957, Robinson[19] described surgical correction of mandibular deficiency using an extraoral surgical approach, a vertical osteotomy, and iliac crest bone grafts in the area of the osteotomy defect. Several modifications of this technique were described over subsequent years. This type of extraoral approach may be useful in rare circumstances, including severely abnormal bony anatomy or for revision surgery (see Fig. 25-21). However, the extraoral incisions have the disadvantages of facial scarring and potential injury to branches of the facial nerve.

Currently, the BSSO, described previously in this chapter for mandibular setback, is the most popular technique for mandibular advancement (Fig. 25-18). This procedure is readily accomplished through an intraoral incision. The significant bony overlap produced with the BSSO allows for adequate bone healing and improved postoperative stability. The osteotomy is frequently stabilized with rigid fixation plates or screws, eliminating the need for IMF.

If the anteroposterior position of the chin is adequate but a Class II malocclusion exists, a total subapical osteotomy may be the technique of choice for mandibular advancement (Fig. 25-19). By combining the osteotomy with interpositioned bone grafts, this technique can be used to increase lower facial height.

When a proper occlusal relationship exists or when anterior positioning of the mandible would not be sufficient to produce adequate projection of the chin, an inferior border osteotomy (i.e., genioplasty) with advancement may also be performed. This technique is usually performed through an intraoral incision. The inferior portion of mandible is osteotomized, moved forward, and stabilized (Fig. 25-20, *A*, *C*, *D*, *E*, and *F*). In addition to anterior or posterior repositioning of the chin, vertical reduction or augmentation and correction of asymmetries can also be accomplished with inferior border osteotomies. Alloplastic materials can occasionally be used to augment chin projection; the material is onlayed in areas of bone deficiencies (Fig. 25-20, *B*).

Maxillary Excess

Excessive growth of the maxilla may occur in the anteroposterior, vertical, or transverse dimensions. Surgical correction of dentofacial deformities with total maxillary surgery (i.e., Le Fort I) has only become popular since the early 1970s. Before that time, maxillary surgery was performed on a limited basis, and most techniques repositioned only portions of the maxilla with segmental surgery. During the early years of maxillary surgery, many techniques were performed in two stages: facial or buccal cuts were performed during one operation; then sectioning of palatal bone was performed 3 to 4 weeks later. This staging was done under the assumption that this was necessary to maintain adequate vascular supply to the osteotomized segment. As experience and understanding of these techniques increased, several procedures for anterior and posterior segmental surgery evolved that used single-stage techniques.[20-22]

In the early 1970s, research by Bell et al.[23] demonstrated that total maxillary surgery could be performed without jeopardizing the vascular supply to the maxilla. This work showed that the normal blood flow in the bony segments from larger feeding vessels could be reversed under certain surgical conditions. If a soft tissue pedicle is maintained in the palate and gingival area of the maxilla, the transosseous and soft tissue collateral circulation and anastomosing vascular plexuses of the gingiva, palate, and sinus can provide adequate vascular supply, which allows mobilization of the total maxilla. Total maxillary osteotomies are currently the most common procedures performed for correction of anteroposterior, transverse, and vertical abnormalities of the maxilla.[24]

Vertical maxillary excess may result in associated facial characteristics, including elongation of the lower third of the face; a narrow nose, particularly in the area of the alar base; excessive incisive and gingival exposure; and lip incompetence (Fig. 25-21).

These patients may exhibit Class I, Class II, or Class III dental malocclusions. A transverse maxillary deficiency with a posterior cross-bite relationship, constricted palate, and narrow arch form is often seen with this deformity.

Vertical maxillary excess is frequently associated with an anterior open-bite relationship (i.e., apertognathia). This results from excessive downward growth of the maxilla, causing downward rotation of the mandible as a result of premature contact of posterior teeth. To correct this problem, the maxilla is repositioned superiorly (impacted), particularly in the posterior area. This allows the mandible to rotate upward and forward, establishing contact in all areas of the dentition. In some cases the occlusal plane of the maxilla is level after orthodontic preparation, and the open bite can be corrected by repositioning the maxilla in one piece (Fig. 25-22, *A* to *D*). In other cases, a step in the occlusal plane must be leveled to achieve the desired occlusion. This requires repositioning of the maxilla in segments (Fig. 25-22, *E* to *H*).

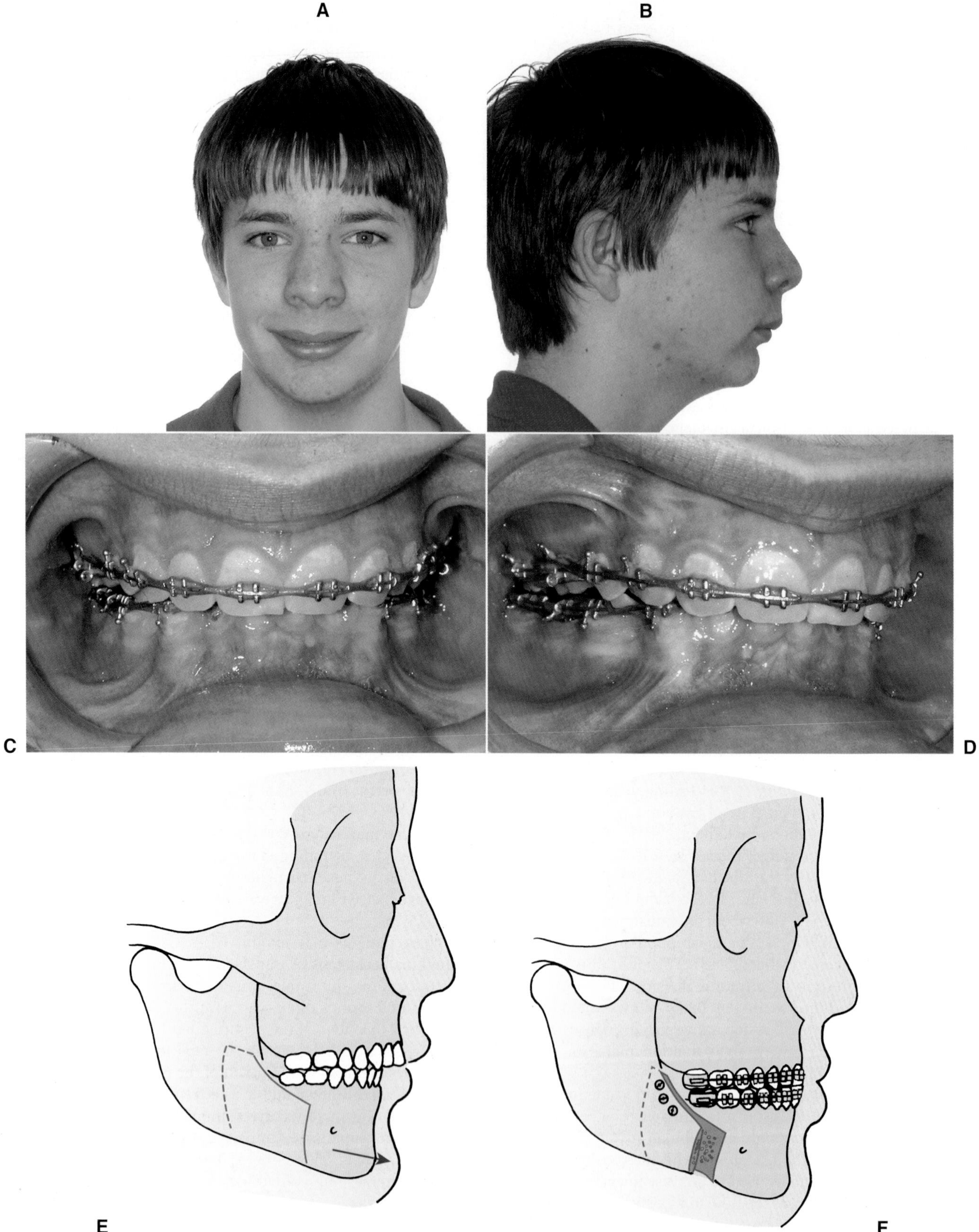

FIGURE 25-18 Case report of mandibular advancement. A and B, Preoperative facial esthetics demonstrating clinical features of mandibular deficiency. C and D, Preoperative occlusion demonstrating Class II relationship and overjet. E and F, Diagrammatic representation of bilateral sagittal split osteotomy with advancement of mandible.

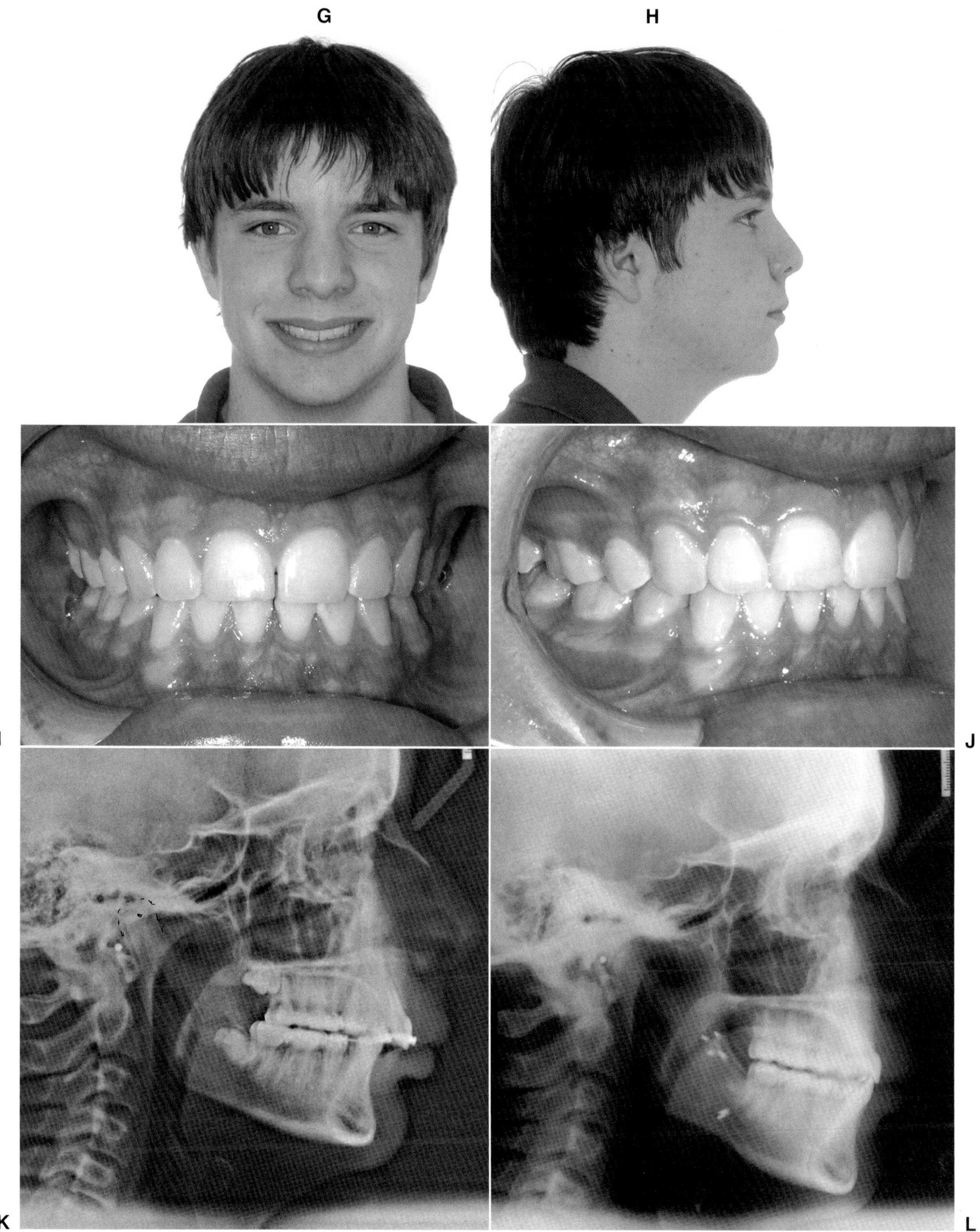

FIGURE 25-18, cont'd Case report of mandibular advancement. G and H, Postoperative facial appearance. I and J, Postoperative occlusion. K and L, Preoperative and postoperative radiographs.

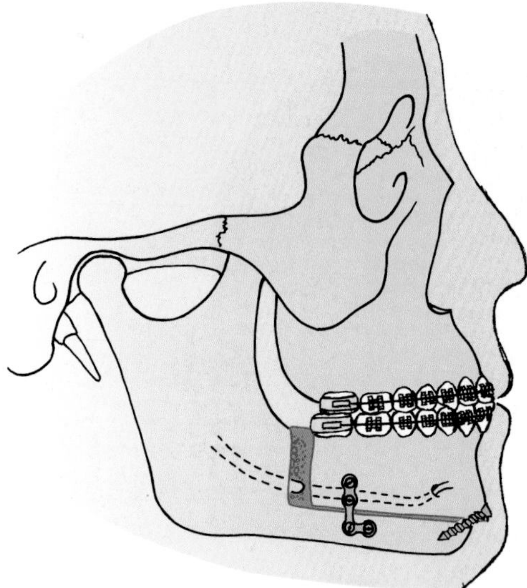

FIGURE 25-19 Total subapical osteotomy. Dentoalveolar segment of mandible is moved anteriorly, allowing correction of Class II malocclusion without increasing chin prominence.

Anteroposterior maxillary excess results in a convex facial profile usually associated with incisor protrusion and a Class II occlusal relationship. Total maxillary surgery can be completed to correct this problem.[25] In some cases the entire maxilla can be moved in one piece in a posterior direction. In addition to procedures in which the maxilla is moved in one piece, the bone can be sectioned into dentoalveolar segments to allow repositioning in the anteroposterior, superior, or inferior directions or to allow expanding in the transverse direction. Figure 25-23 demonstrates a three-piece maxillary osteotomy performed to correct anteroposterior maxillary excess combined with vertical deficiency.

Maxillary and Midface Deficiency

Patients with maxillary deficiency commonly appear to have a retruded upper lip, deficiency of the paranasal and infraorbital rim areas, inadequate tooth exposure during smile, and a prominent chin relative to the middle third of the face. Maxillary deficiency may occur in the anteroposterior, vertical, and transverse planes. The patient's clinical appearance depends on the location and severity of the deformity. In addition to the abnormal facial features, a Class III malocclusion with reverse anterior overjet is frequently seen.

The primary technique for correction of maxillary deficiency is the Le Fort I osteotomy. This technique can be used for advancement of the maxilla to correct a Class III malocclusion and associated facial abnormalities (Fig. 25-24). Depending on the magnitude of advancement, bone grafting may be required to improve bone healing and postoperative stability. In the case of vertical maxillary deficiency, elongation of the lower third of the face can be accomplished by bone grafting the maxilla in an inferior position with the Le Fort I osteotomy technique (Fig. 25-25). This technique improves overall facial proportion and normalizes exposure of the incisors during smiling. Also, in a large number of patients with Class III occlusions the jaw blamed by the patients and sometimes by dental providers is the mandible, when the problem is actually maxillary deficiency. Surgery in the wrong jaw in these cases can leave problematic facial esthetics, especially in male patients.

In severe midface deformities with infraorbital rim and malar eminence deficiency, a Le Fort III or modified Le Fort III type of osteotomy is necessary. These procedures advance the maxilla and the malar bones and, in some cases, the anterior portion of the nasal bones. This type of treatment is commonly required in patients with craniofacial deformities such as Apert's or Crouzon's syndrome (Fig. 25-26).

Combination Deformities and Asymmetries

In many cases the facial deformity involves a combination of abnormalities in the maxilla and the mandible.[26] In these cases, treatment may require a combination of maxillary and mandibular osteotomies to achieve the best possible occlusal, functional, and esthetic result (Figs. 25-27 and 25-28). In some cases, surgical treatment may involve a combination of standard surgical procedures described before in combination with more complicated osteotomies accomplished through extraoral approach using bone grafts harvested from the iliac crest (Fig. 25-29). Treatment of asymmetry in more than two planes of space frequently requires maxillary surgery, mandibular surgery, and inferior border osteotomies, as well as recontouring or augmentation of other areas of the maxilla and mandible (Fig. 25-30).

Orthognathic Surgery for Obstructive Sleep Apnea

Obstructive sleep apnea is the occurrence of apneic events (breathing stops) during sleep such that a patient has cessation of airflow for more than 10 seconds. This can be a serious condition with manifestations ranging from sleep disruption/deprivation and daytime somnolence to severe hypoxia during sleep and the potential of associated respiratory and cardiac abnormalities, and even death.[27]

The primary problem is a collapse of the airway during sleep. This can be a result of decreased muscle tone in the palate, tongue, or pharyngeal musculature. This condition can be associated with mandibular deficiency and the subsequent lack of forward suspension of the tongue and hypopharyngeal musculature (Fig. 25-31, *A*). This is usually accentuated in the supine position. Other factors such as obesity and alcohol or sedative drug use during sleep can aggravate the problem.

The complete workup for the patient with obstructive sleep apnea is beyond the scope of this chapter but usually includes a comprehensive physical evaluation, nasopharyngoscopy, a dentofacial evaluation, and polysomnography sleep study. Treatment may included nonsurgical measures such as weight loss, positional changes during sleep, jaw positioning devices, or continuous positive airway pressure using a facial or nasal mask during sleep.[28,29]

Surgical correction may include a limited uvulopalatoplasty or uvulopharyngealpalatoplasty in which varying portions of the soft palate, uvula, tonsils, and pharyngeal walls are resected to open the airway. Maxillary and mandibular advancement with orthognathic surgery has also been shown to be effective in improving the airway in many patients.[30] This improvement is a result of expanding the airway at the level of the soft palate, base of the tongue, and hypopharyngeal airway. This can be seen by comparing preoperative and postoperative radiographs (Fig. 25-31). The airway expansion resulting from surgery actually includes all dimensions, even lateral expansion.[31]

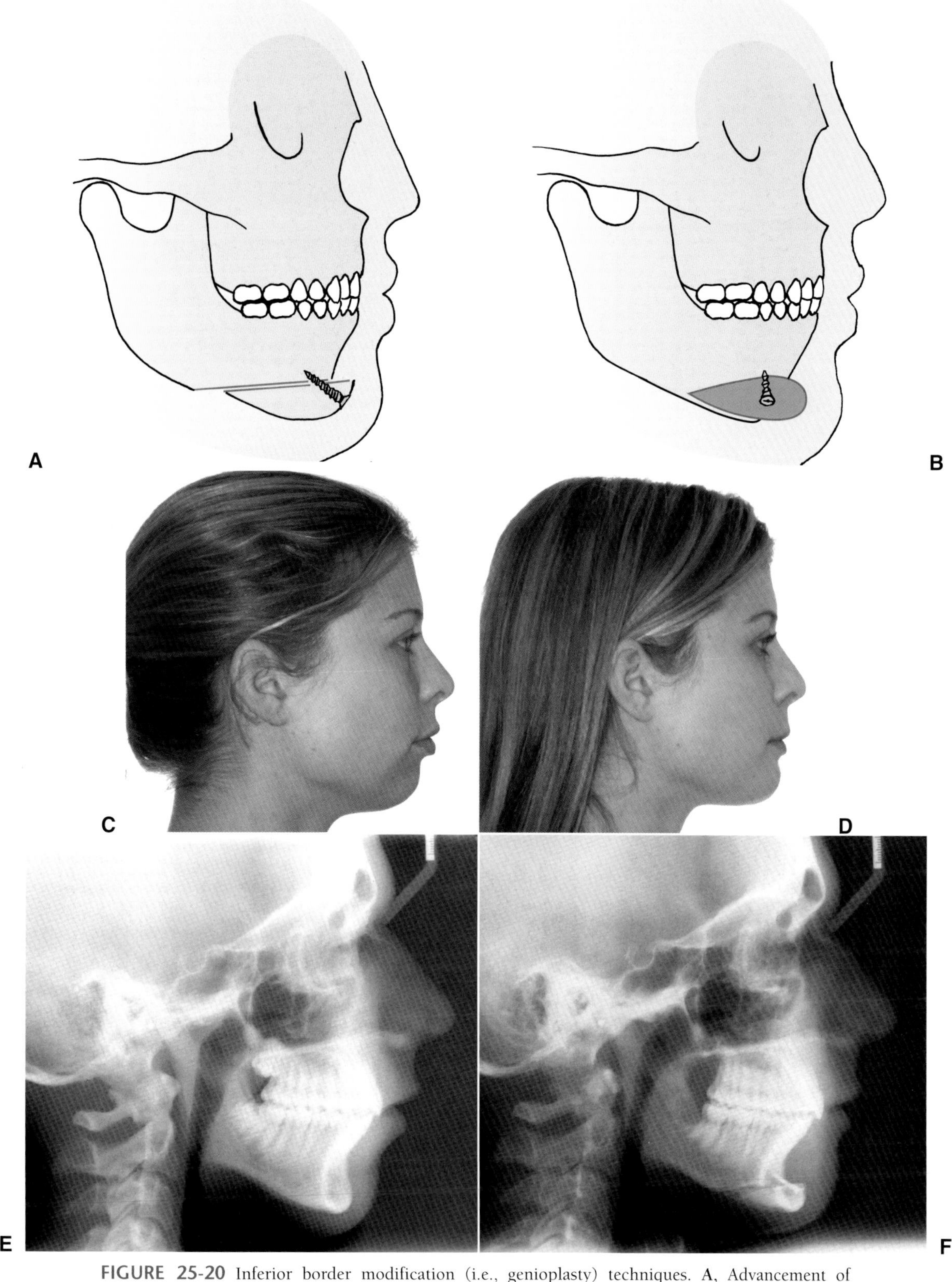

FIGURE 25-20 Inferior border modification (i.e., genioplasty) techniques. A, Advancement of inferior border of mandible to increase chin projection. B, Diagram of implant used to augment anterior portion of chin, eliminating need for osteotomy in this area. C, Clinical picture demonstrating chin deficiency. D, Postoperative photograph after advancement of inferior portion of anterior mandible. E, Preoperative radiograph. F, Postoperative radiograph.

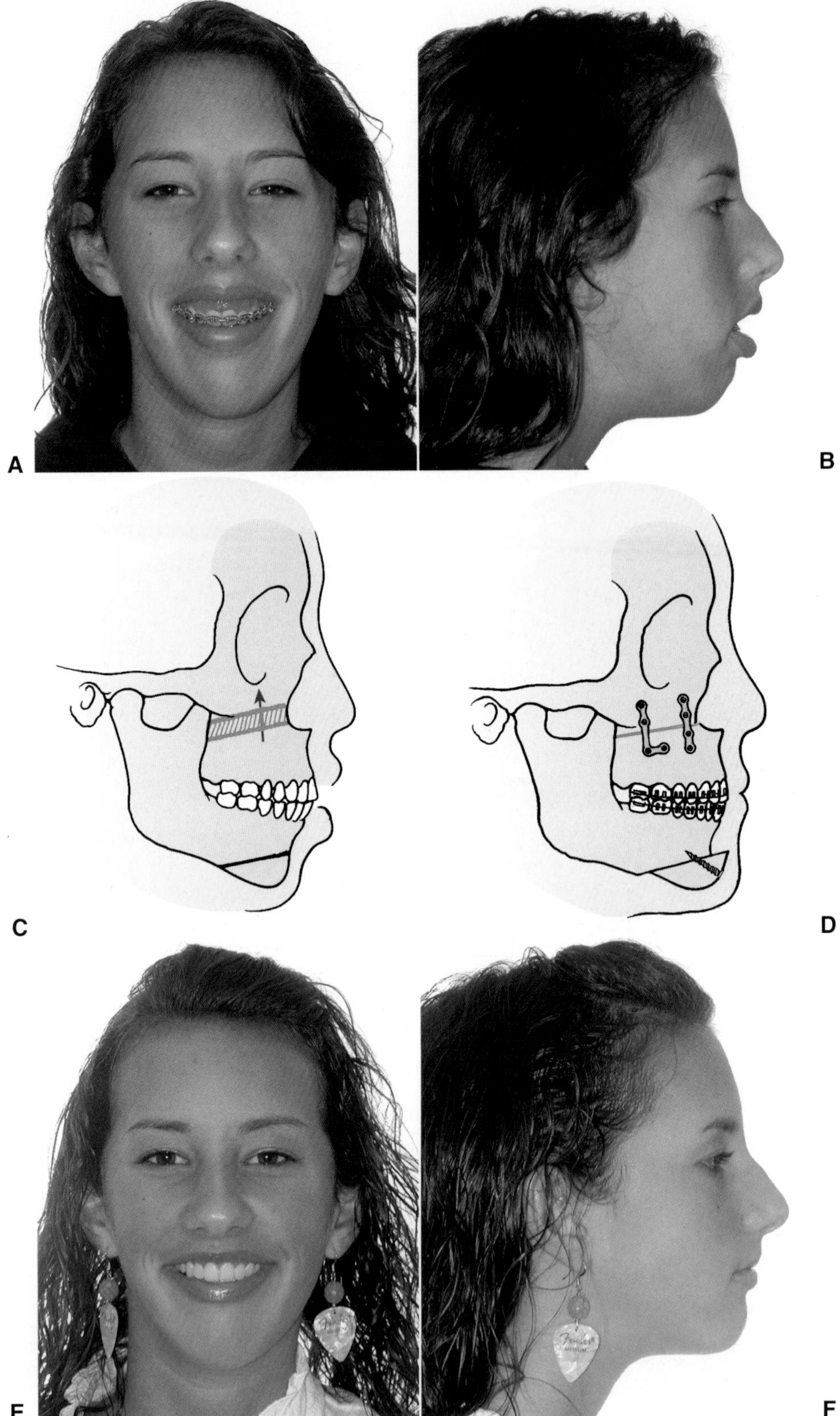

FIGURE 25-21 Typical clinical features of vertical maxillary excess. A and B, Full-face and profile views demonstrating elongation of lower third of face, lip incompetence, and excessive gingival exposure. C and D, Total maxillary osteotomy with superior repositioning combined with advancement genioplasty. E and F, Postoperative full-face and profile views after total maxillary osteotomy with superior repositioning and chin advancement.

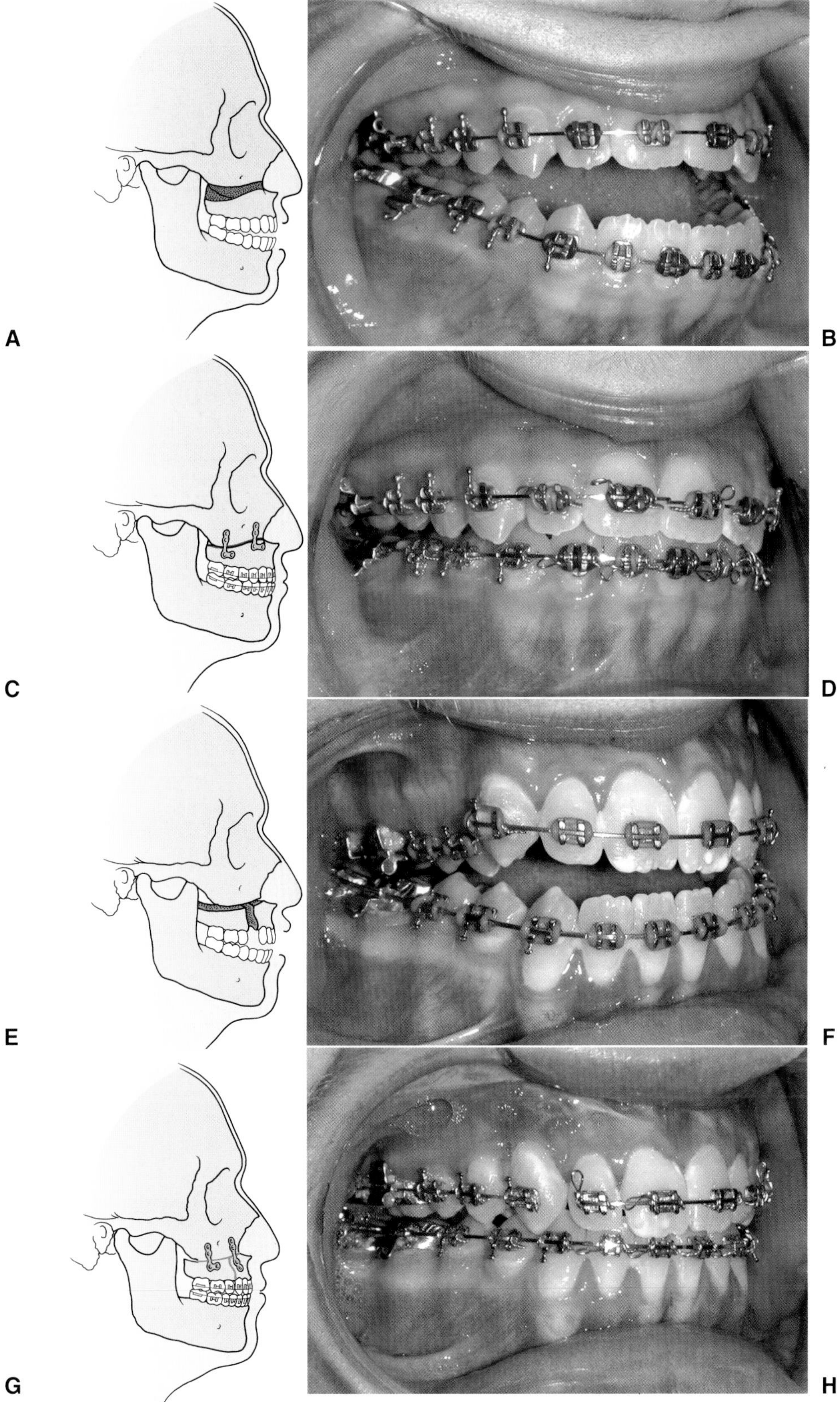

FIGURE 25-22 A, Anterior open bite as a result of vertical maxillary excess with entire maxillary occlusal plane on one level. B, Presurgical occlusion. C, Surgical correction with superior repositioning of maxilla in one piece. D, Postoperative occlusion. E, Open bite with maxillary occlusal plane on two levels. F, Presurgical occlusion. G, Segmental maxillary repositioning to close open bite and place segments on same plane of occlusion. H, Postoperative occlusion.

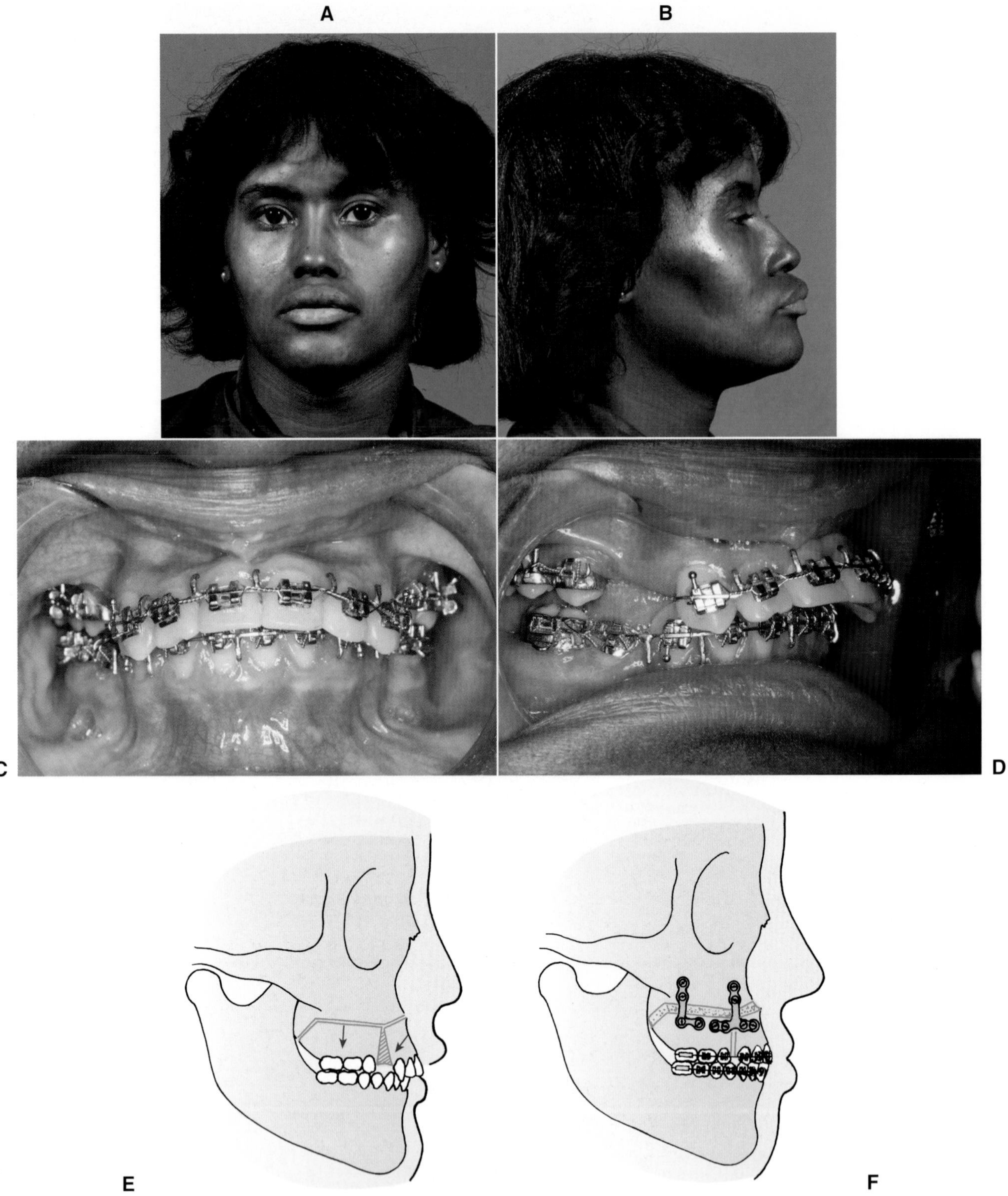

FIGURE 25-23 Case report of segmental maxillary osteotomy. A and B, Preoperative facial appearance demonstrates extreme protrusion of anterior maxillary segment and upper lip, decreased nasolabial angle, and decreased lower face height as a result of maxillary vertical deficiency. C and D, Preoperative occlusion demonstrates protrusive maxillary incisors and extraction space remaining after removal of maxillary premolar teeth bilaterally. E and F, Segmental maxillary osteotomy with closure of premolar extraction space, retraction of anterior segment of maxilla, and placement of bone graft in posterior maxillary area.

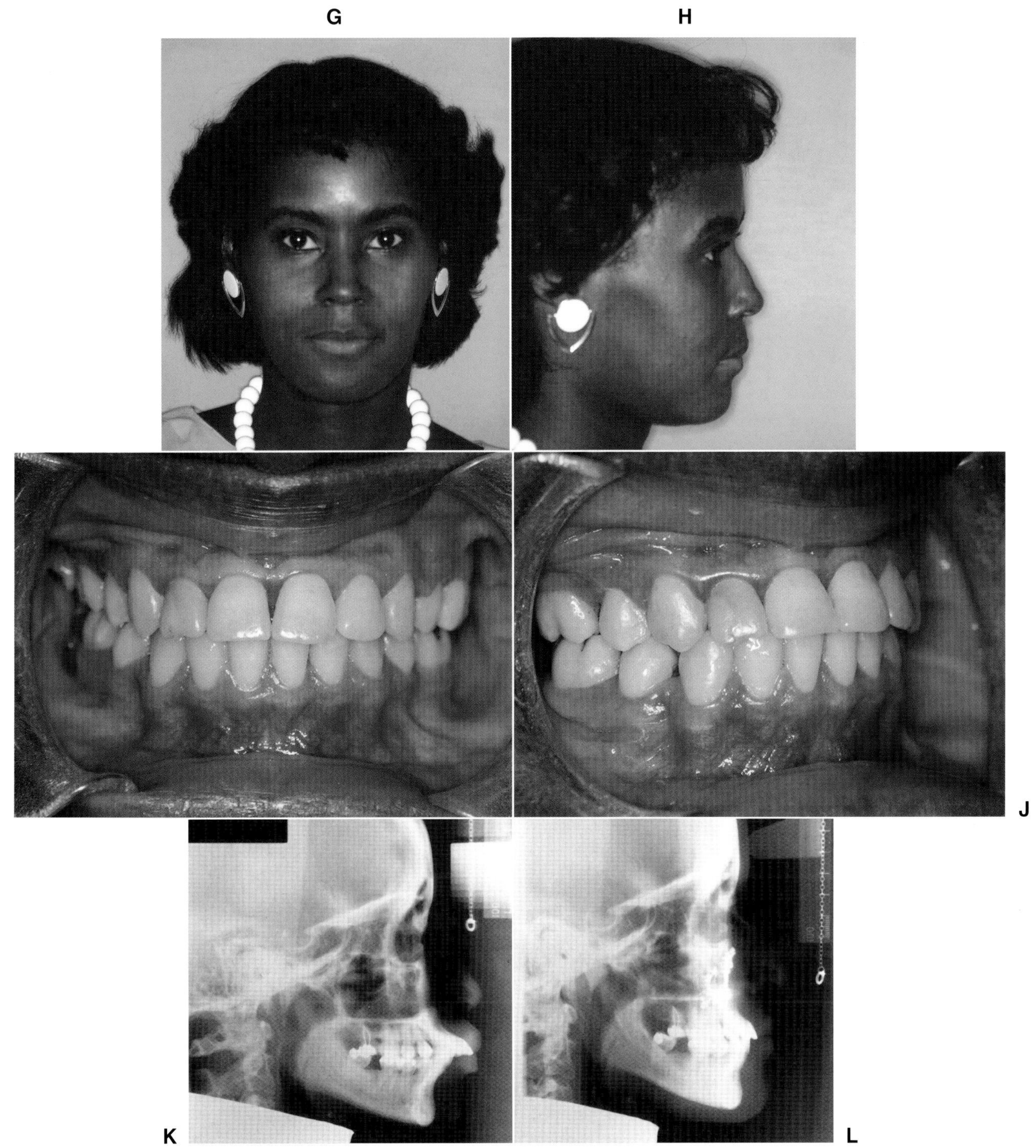

FIGURE 25-23, cont'd Case report of segmental maxillary osteotomy. G and H, Postoperative facial appearance. I and J, Postoperative occlusion. K and L, Preoperative and postoperative radiographs.

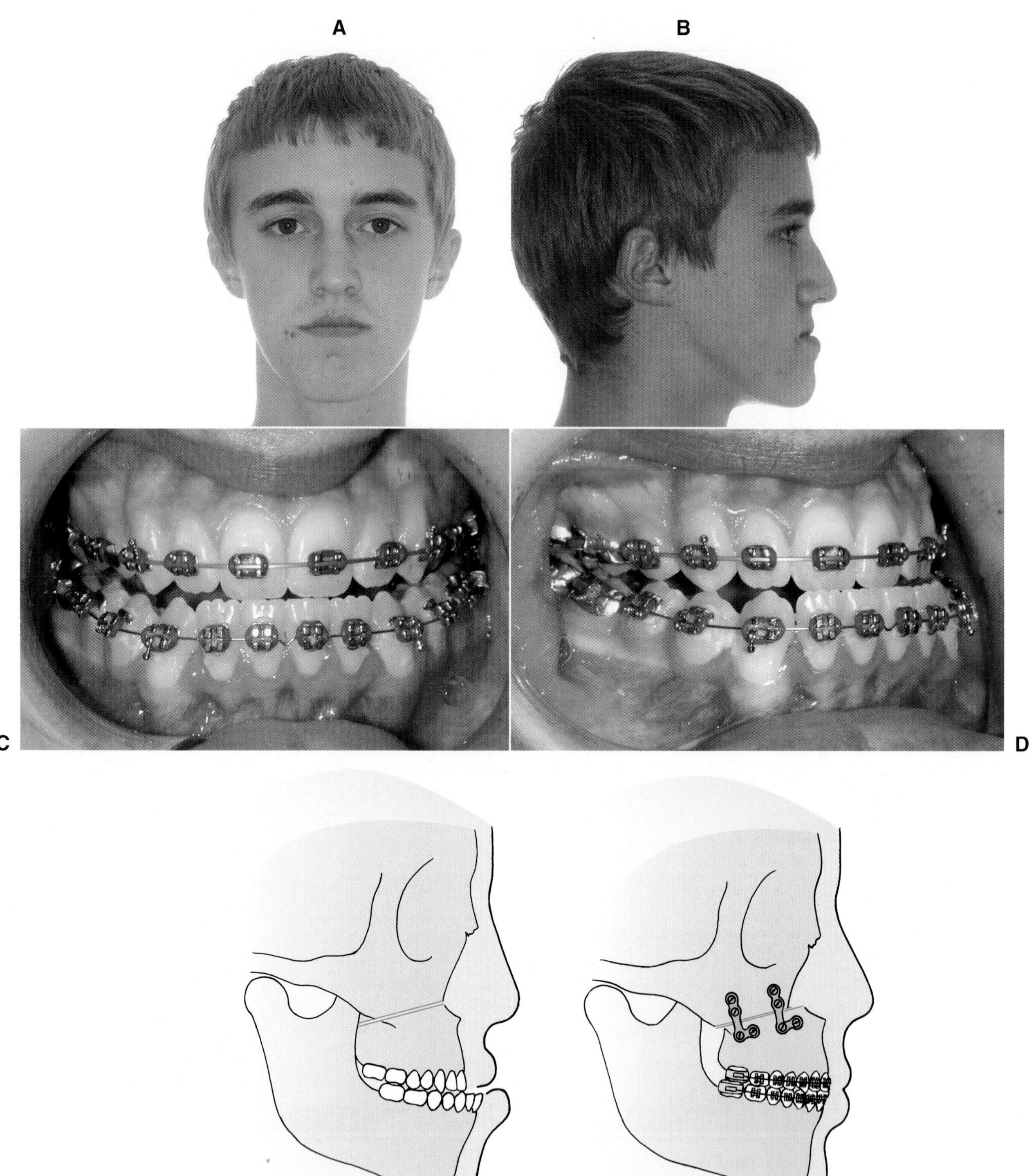

FIGURE 25-24 Case report of Le Fort I advancement. A and B, Preoperative facial esthetics demonstrating maxillary deficiency evident by facial concavity and paranasal deficiency. C and D, Preoperative occlusion demonstrating Class III relationship. E and F, Le Fort I osteotomy for maxillary advancement.

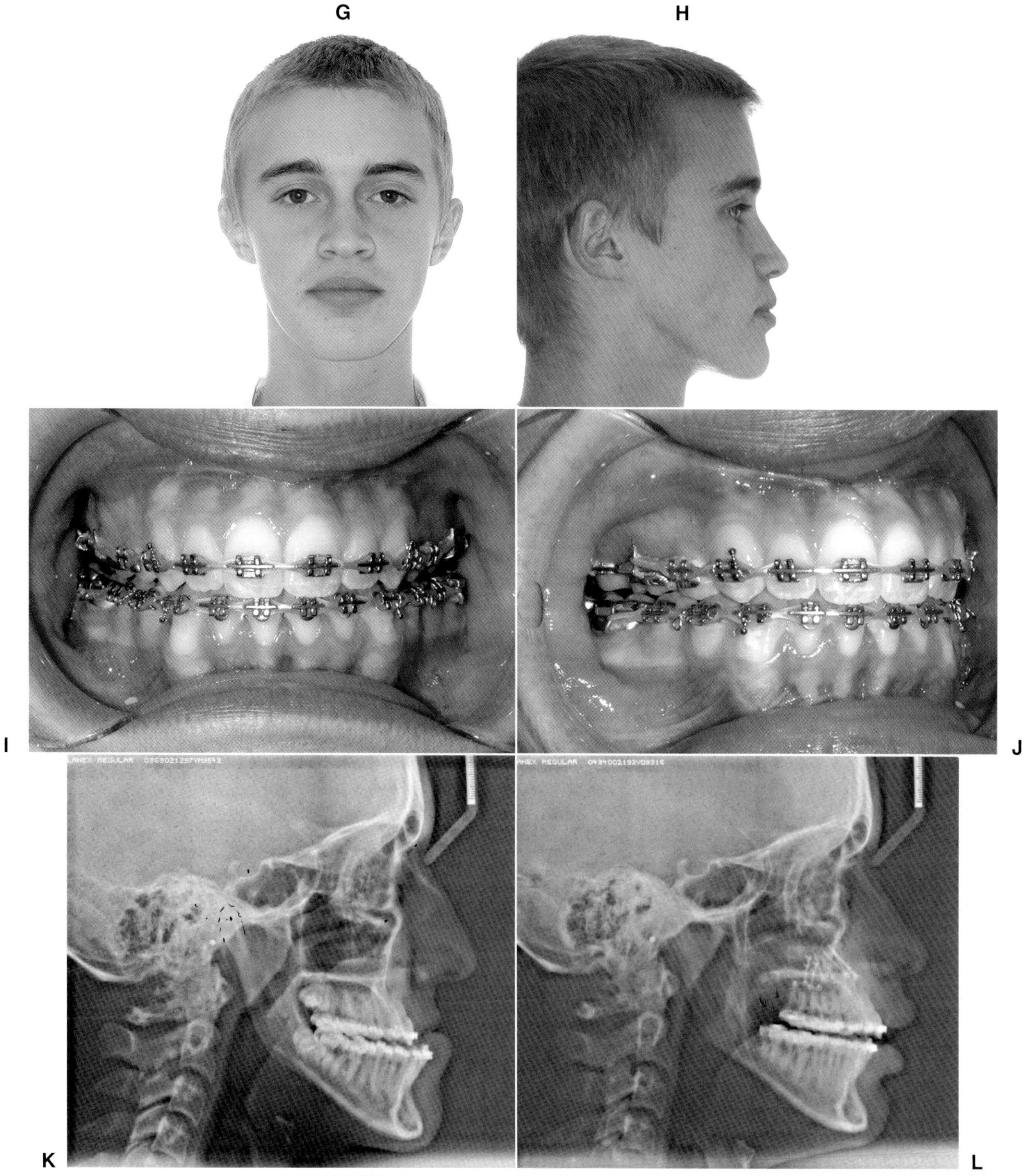

FIGURE 25-24, cont'd Case report of Le Fort I advancement. G and H, Postoperative facial appearance. (This patient also underwent a simultaneous rhinoplasty procedure.) I and J, Postoperative occlusion. K and L, Preoperative and postoperative radiographs.

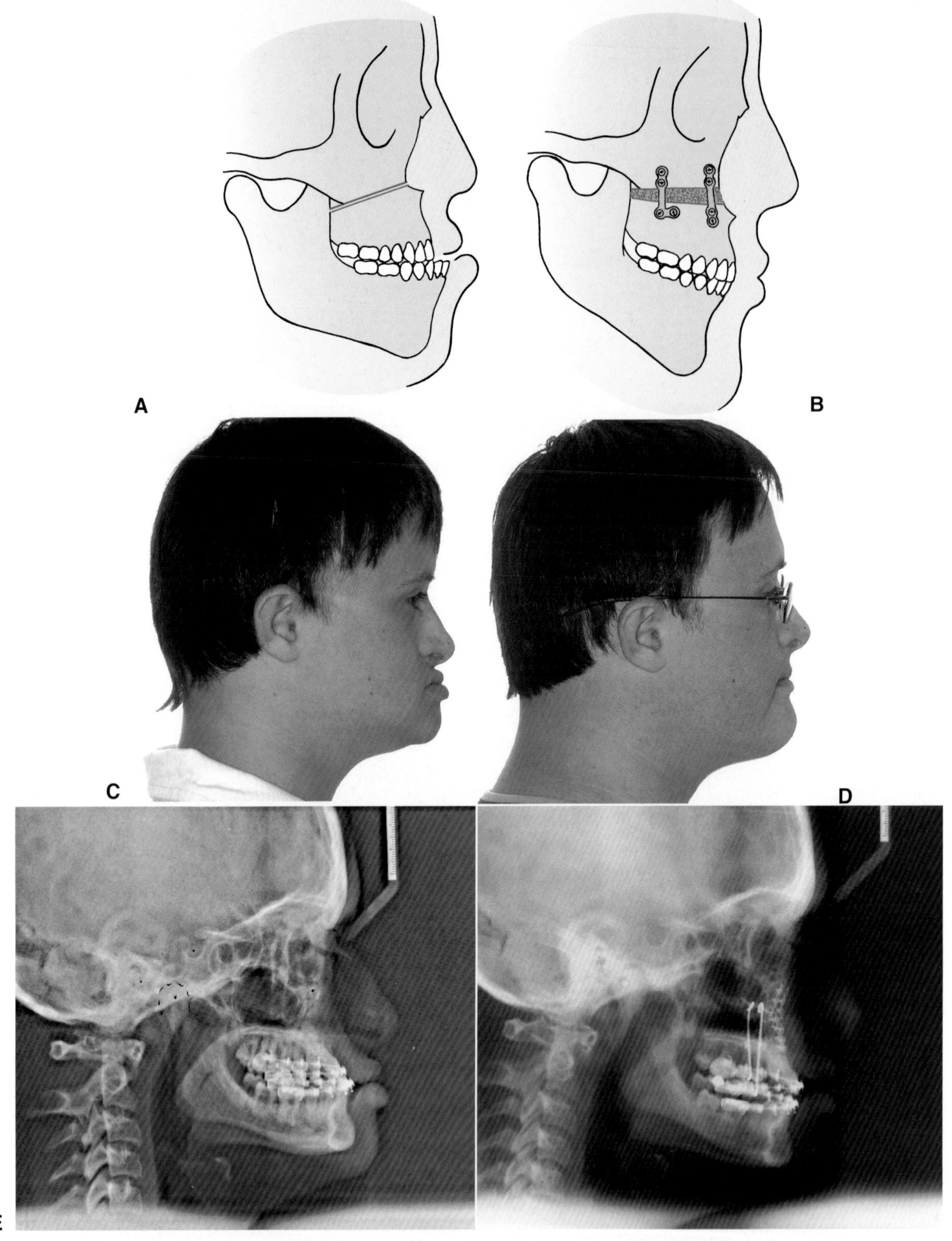

FIGURE 25-25 A and B, Inferior repositioning of maxilla and interpositional bone grafting. C, Preoperative profile view demonstrating vertical deficiency of lower third of face and resulting appearance of relative mandibular excess. D, Postoperative view after inferior repositioning of maxilla. Note normal facial vertical and anteroposterior relationships. E, Preoperative radiograph. F, Postoperative radiograph. Bone plates and auxiliary vertical struts are seen in this view.

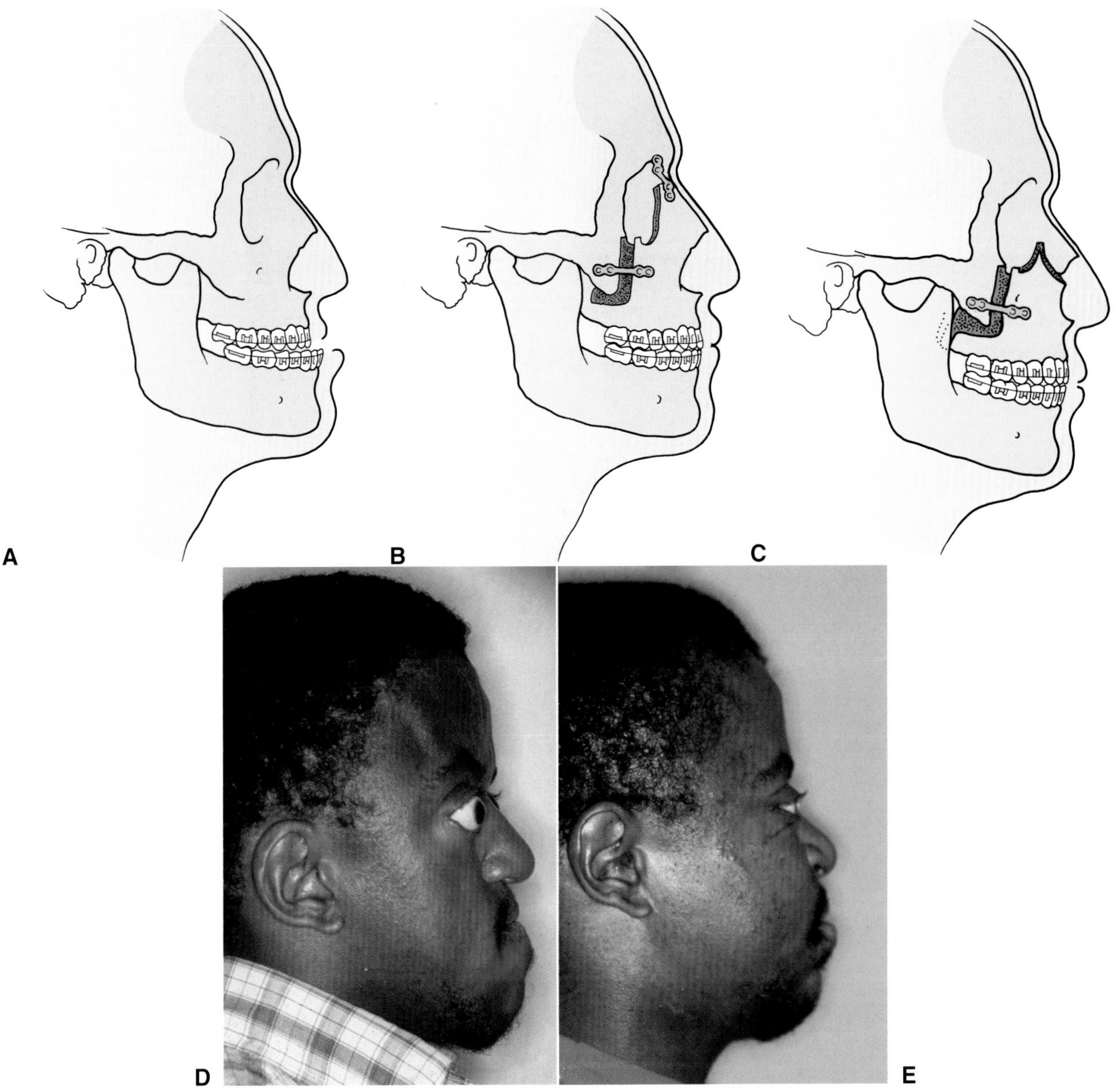

FIGURE 25-26 A, Severe midface deficiency. B, Le Fort III advancement. C, Modified Le Fort III advancement. D, Preoperative profile view of patient with Apert's syndrome. E, Postoperative profile view.

DISTRACTION OSTEOGENESIS

One new approach to correction of deficiencies in the mandible and the maxilla involves the use of distraction osteogenesis (DO). When correcting deformities associated with these deficiencies, the conventional osteotomy techniques have several potential limitations (described previously in this chapter). When large skeletal movements are required, the associated soft tissue often cannot adapt to the acute changes and stretching that result from the surgical repositioning of bony segments. This failure of tissue adaptation results in several problems, including surgical relapse, potential excessive loading of the TMJ structures, and increased severity of neurosensory loss as a result of stretching of nerves. In some cases the amount of movement is so large that the gaps created require bone grafts harvested from secondary surgical sites such as the iliac crest.

DO involves cutting an osteotomy to separate segments of bone and the application of an appliance that will facilitate the gradual and incremental separation of bone segments (Fig. 25-32). The gradual tension placed on the distracting bony interface produces continuous bone formation. Additionally, the surrounding tissue appears to adapt to this gradual tension, producing adaptive changes in all surrounding tissues, including muscles and tendons, nerves, cartilage, blood vessels, and skin. Because the adaptation involves a variety of tissue types in addition to bone, this concept should also include the term *distraction histogenesis*.

The concept of distraction is not new. Use of traction techniques to help bones heal to a correct length can be traced

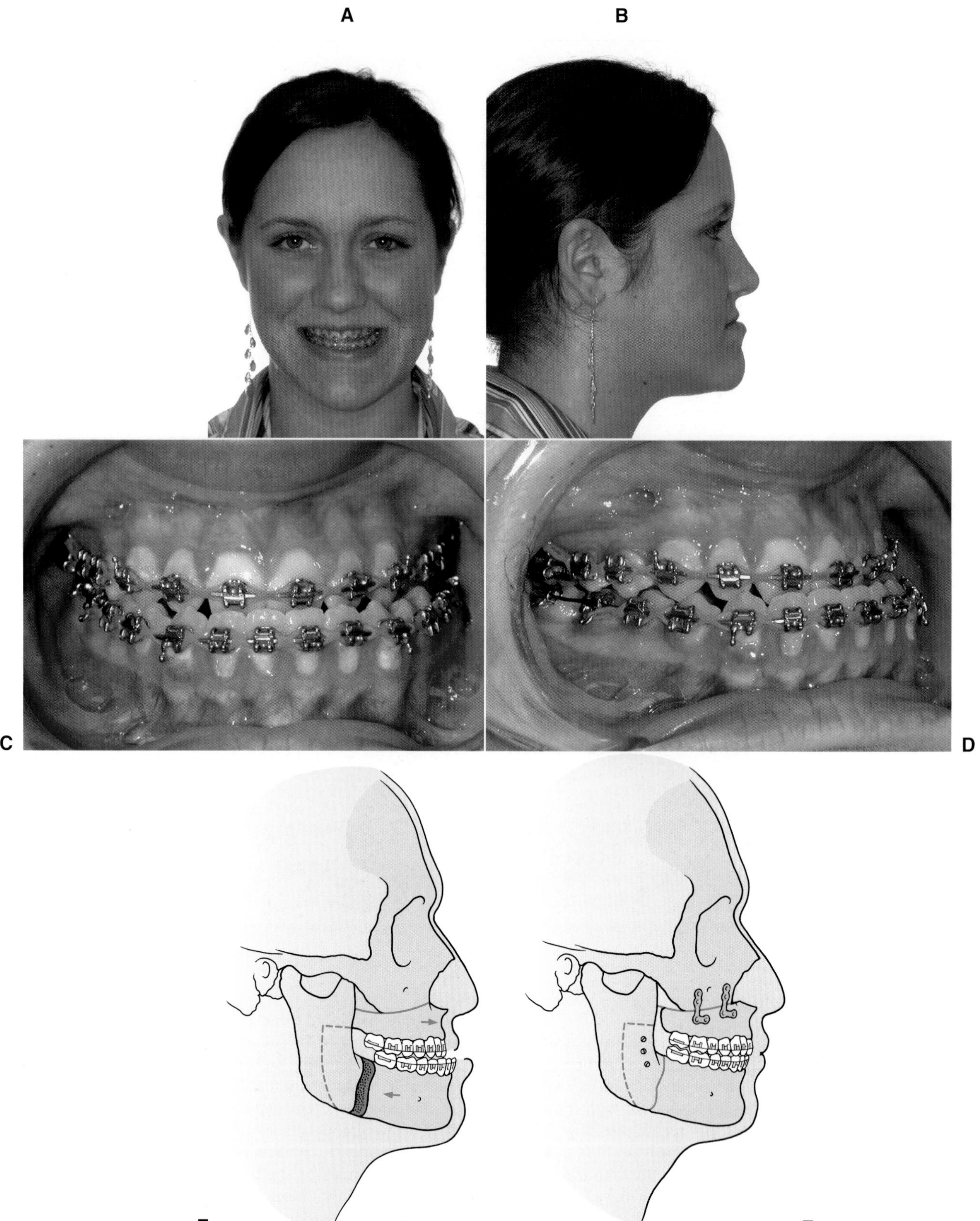

FIGURE 25-27 Case report of maxillary advancement and mandibular setback. A and B, Preoperative facial esthetics demonstrating severe maxillary deficiency combined with mandibular excess. C and D, Preoperative occlusion demonstrating Class III relationship. E and F, Le Fort I osteotomy for maxillary advancement and bilateral sagittal osteotomies for setback of the mandible.

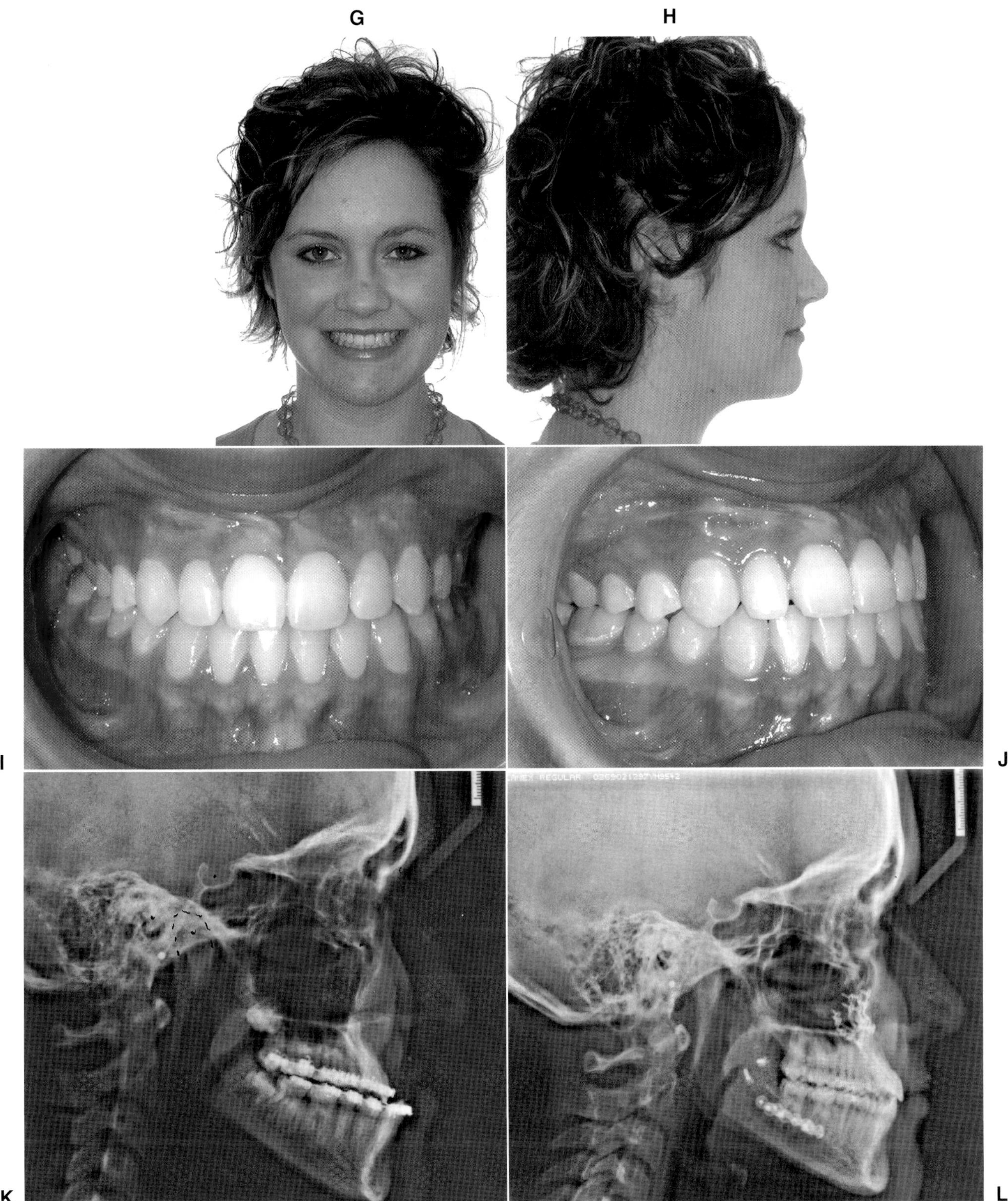

FIGURE 25-27, cont'd Case report of maxillary advancement and mandibular setback. G and H, Postoperative facial appearance. I and J, Postoperative occlusion. K and L, Preoperative and postoperative radiographs.

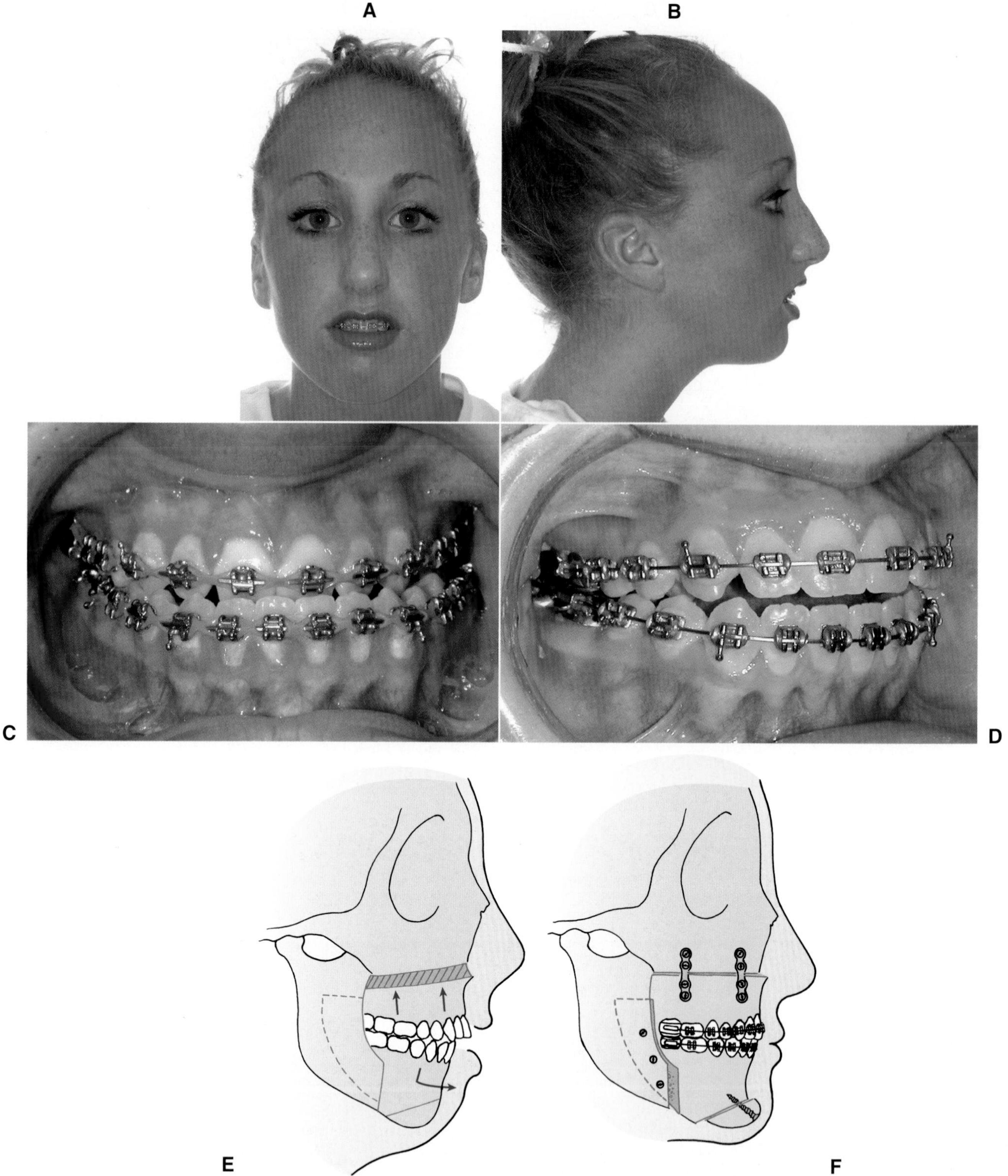

FIGURE 25-28 Case report of superior maxillary repositioning and advancement, mandibular advancement, and genioplasty. A and B, Preoperative facial esthetics demonstrating typical appearance of vertical maxillary excess and mandibular deficiency, including excess incisor exposure, lip incompetence, and lack of chin projection. C and D, Preoperative occlusion demonstrating Class II malocclusion. E and F, Diagram of Le Fort I osteotomy with superior repositioning of maxilla, sagittal osteotomies of mandible for advancement, and advancement genioplasty.

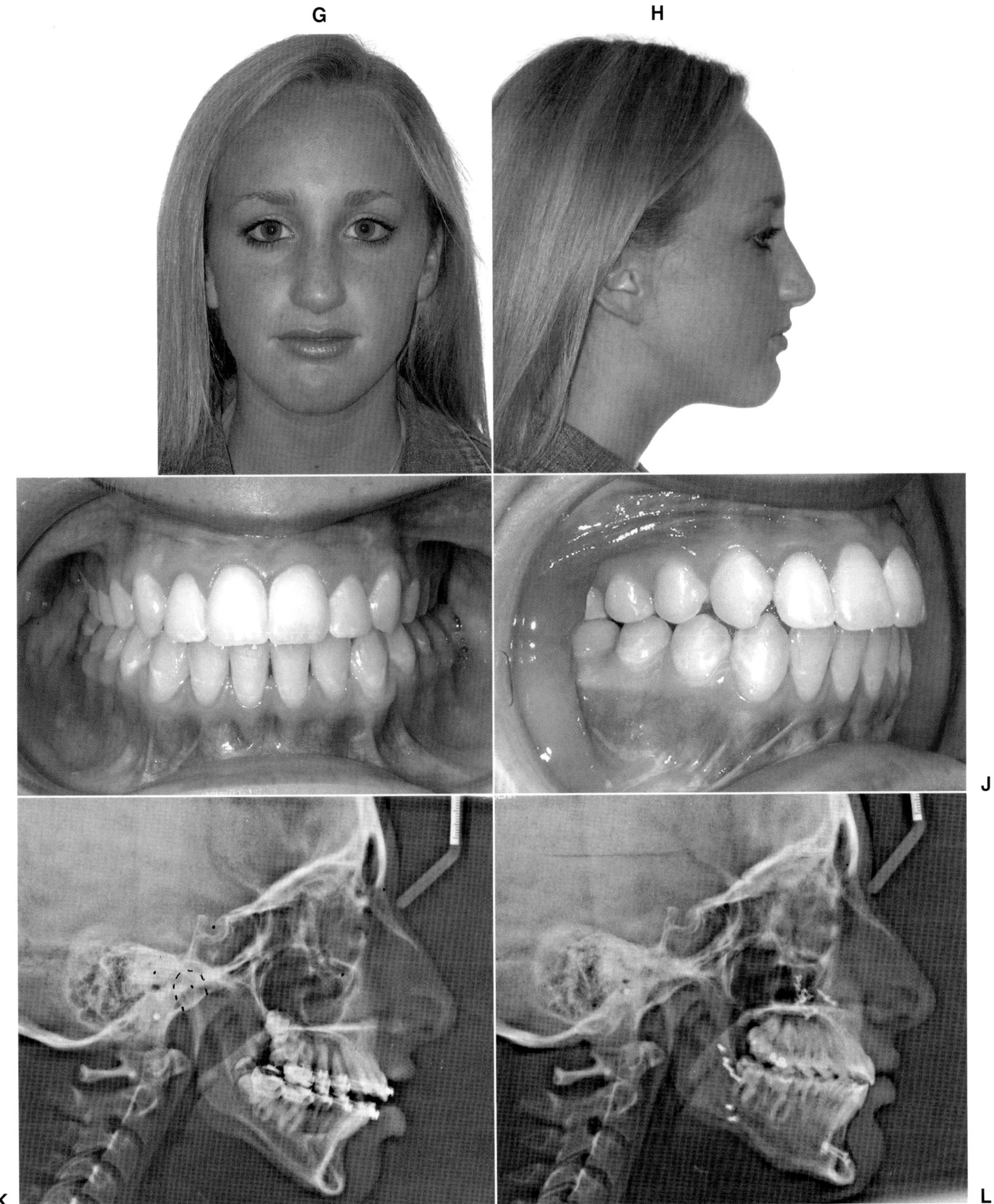

FIGURE 25-28, cont'd Case report of superior maxillary repositioning and advancement, mandibular advancement, and genioplasty. G and H, Postoperative facial appearance. I and J, Postoperative occlusion. K and L, Preoperative and postoperative radiographs.

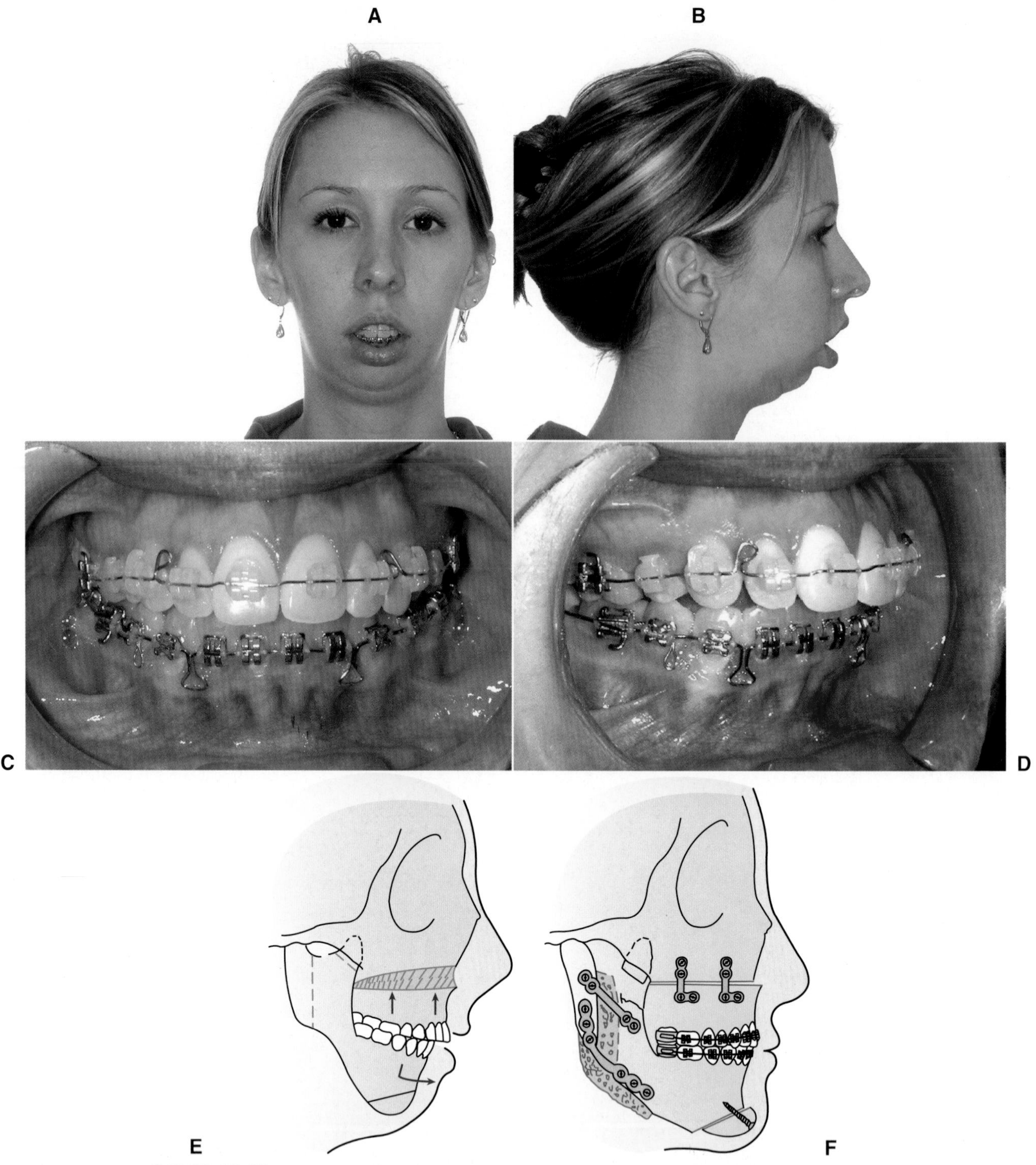

FIGURE 25-29 Case report of superior maxillary repositioning, extraoral approach for mandibular advancement, and genioplasty. A and B, Preoperative facial esthetics demonstrating typical appearance of vertical maxillary excess and mandibular deficiency, including excess incisor exposure, lip incompetence, and lack of chin projection. C and D, Preoperative occlusion demonstrating class II malocclusion. E and F, Diagram of Le Fort I osteotomy with superior repositioning of maxilla, extraoral osteotomies of mandible with bone grafts, and advancement genioplasty.

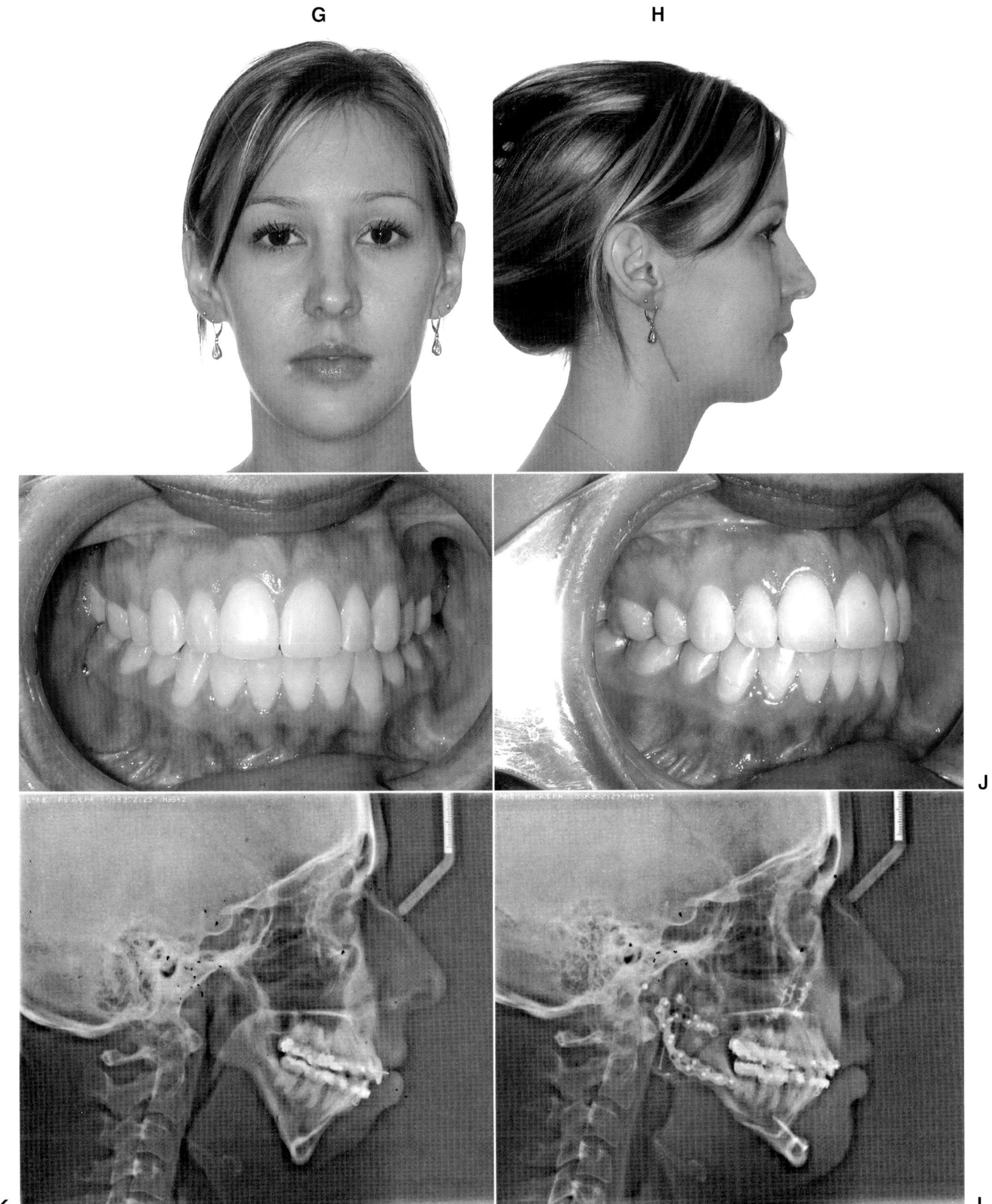

FIGURE 25-29, cont'd Case report of superior maxillary repositioning, extraoral approach for mandibular advancement, and genioplasty. G and H, Postoperative facial appearance. I and J, Postoperative occlusion. K and L, Preoperative and postoperative radiographs.

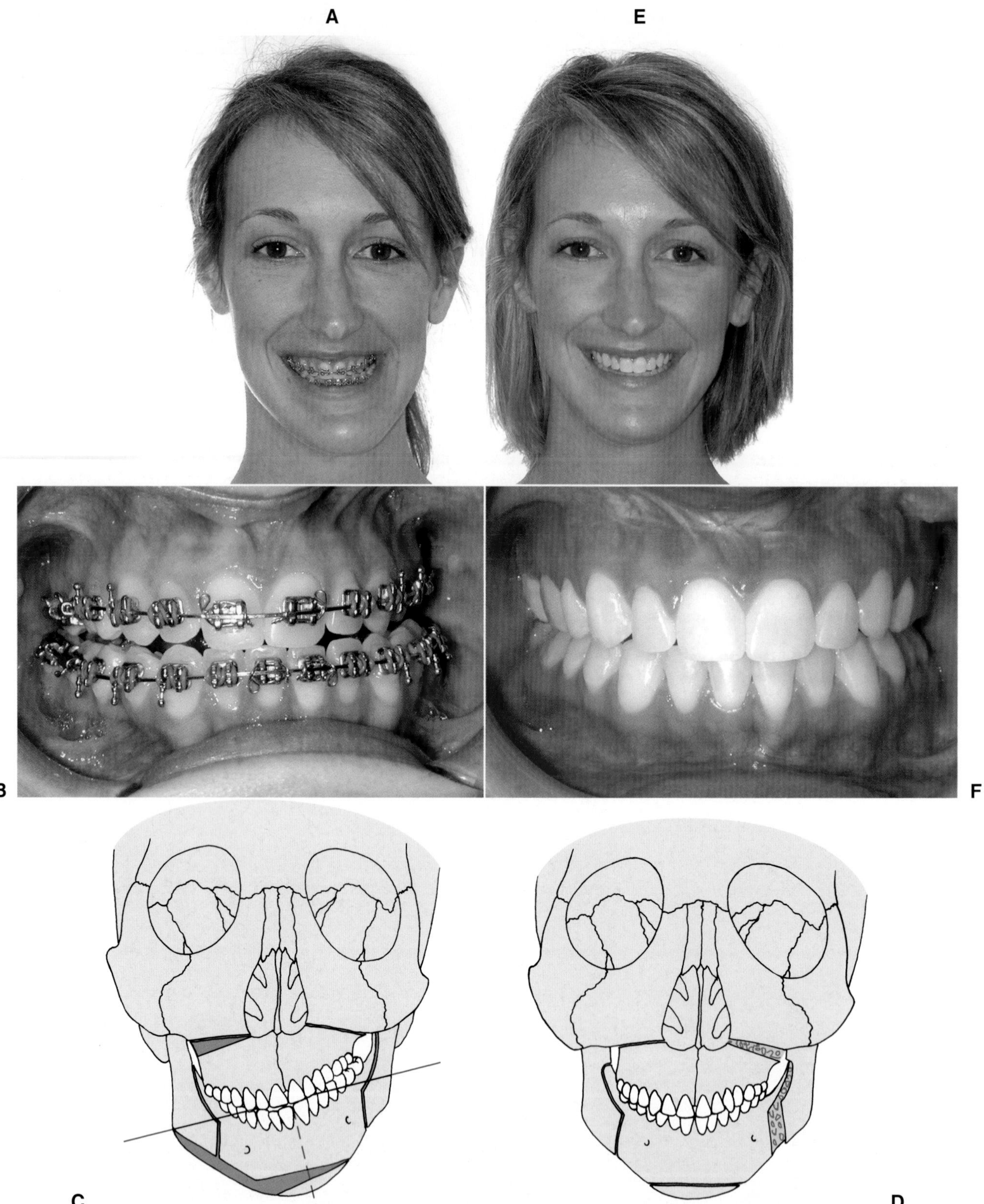

FIGURE 25-30 Facial asymmetry requiring maxillary and mandibular osteotomies, genioplasty, and inferior border recontouring for correction. A, Preoperative facial esthetics. B, Preoperative occlusion. C and D, Diagrams of Le Fort I osteotomy with inferior repositioning on left side and superior repositioning on right, sagittal osteotomies of mandible with advancement on left side and superior repositioning on right, asymmetric genioplasty, and right inferior border recontouring. E, Postoperative facial appearance. F, Postoperative occlusion.

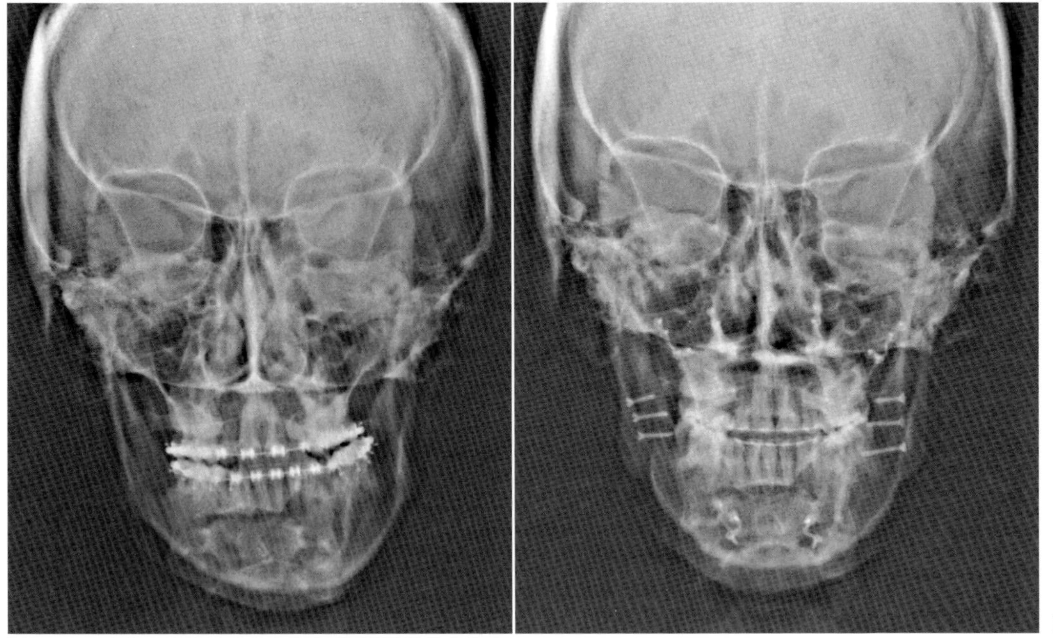

FIGURE 25-30, cont'd' Facial asymmetry requiring maxillary and mandibular osteotomies, genioplasty, and inferior border recontouring for correction. G, Preoperative radiograph. H, Postoperative radiograph.

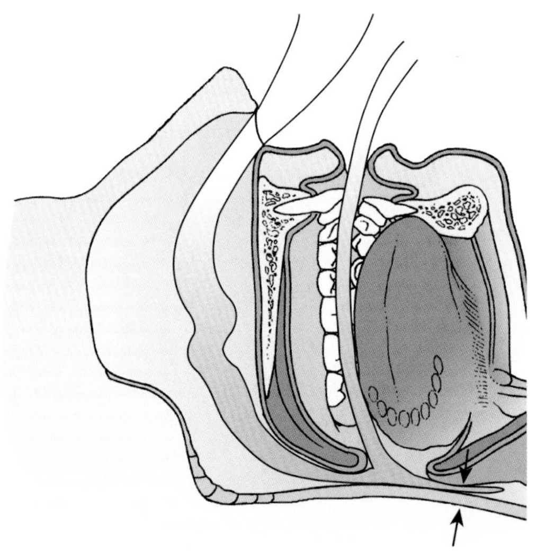

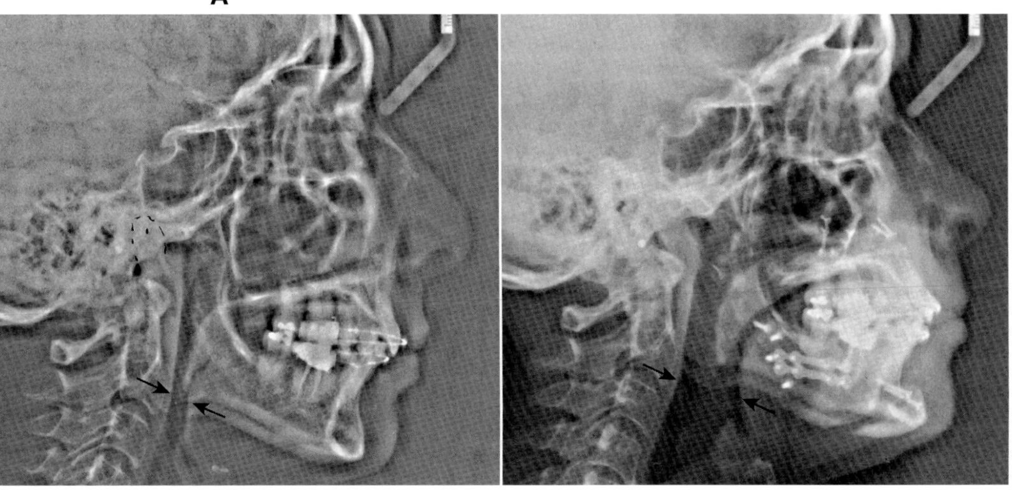

FIGURE 25-31 A, Narrow or collapsed airway as a result of mandibular deficiency. B, Preoperative cephalometric radiograph showing narrow hypopharyngeal airway. C, Postoperative cephalogram showing significant expansion of the airway.

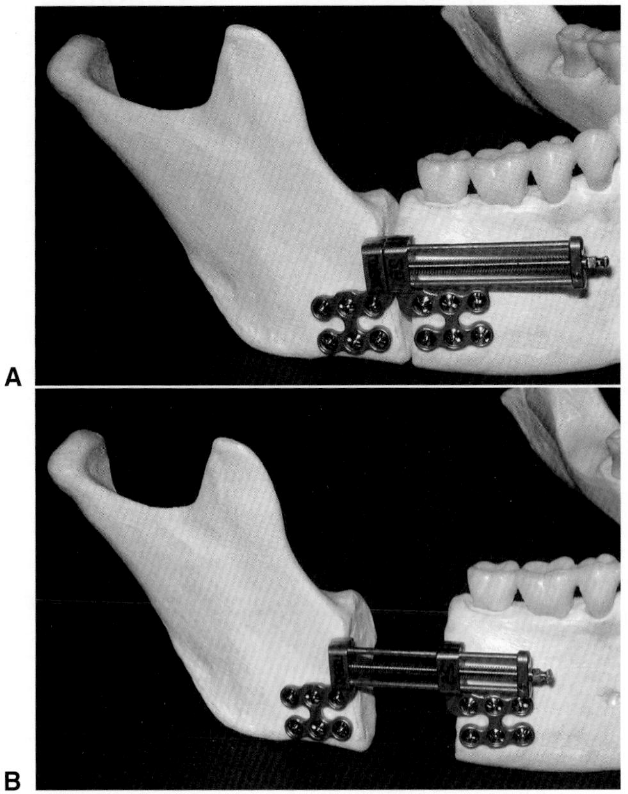

FIGURE 25-32 Distractor appliance used for mandibular advancement. A, Osteotomy of posterior mandibular body and ramus area with distractor in place. B, View showing distraction appliance fully expanded. Regenerate bone fills the intrabony gap during slow incremental activation of distractor that slowly separates the segments.

back to the time of Hippocrates when an external device was used to apply traction to a fractured and shortened leg.[32] A Russian surgeon, Gavril Ilizarov, developed the current concept of correcting bony deficiencies in the 1950s. The result of his work was not widely disseminated to the rest of the world until the late 1970s and early 1980s.[33,34] Since that time, the application of these principles has extended to all forms of orthopedic correction, including craniofacial surgery.[35,36]

DO involves several phases, including the osteotomy or surgical phase, latency period, distraction phase, consolidation phase, appliance removal, and remodeling. During the surgical phase an osteotomy is completed and the distraction appliance is secured. The latency phase is the period when very early stages of bone healing begin to take place at the osteotomy bony interface. The latency phase is generally 7 days during which time the appliance is not activated. After the latency period the distraction phase begins at a rate of 1 mm per day. This distraction rate is usually applied by opening or activating the appliance 0.5 mm twice each day. The amount of activation per day is termed the *rate of distraction;* the timing of appliance activation each day is termed the *rhythm.* During the distraction phase the new immature bone that forms is called the *regenerate.* Once the appropriate amount of distraction has been achieved, the appliance remains in place during the consolidation phase, allowing for mineralization of the regenerate bone. The appliance is then removed, and the period from the application of normal functional loads to the complete maturation of the bone is termed the *remodeling period.*

Because the use of these techniques in orthognathic surgery is relatively new, few long-term studies are available that document all of the potential benefits of DO. Possible advantages include the ability to produce larger skeletal movements, elimination of the need for bone grafts and the associated secondary surgical site, better long-term stability, less trauma to the TMJs, and decreased neurosensory loss. DO also has certain disadvantages: The placement and positioning of the appliance to produce the desired vector of bone movement is technique sensitive and sometimes results in less than ideal occlusal positioning, resulting in discrepancies such as small open bites or asymmetries. Other disadvantages include the need for two procedures: (1) placement and (2) removal of the distractors, as well as increased cost and longer treatment time, with more frequent appointments with the surgeon and the orthodontist.

One of the earliest uses of the DO concept in orthognathic surgery involved widening of the maxilla with a technique termed *surgical-assisted rapid palatal expansion.*[37] An adult maxilla with significant transverse deficiency is nearly impossible to correct with conventional orthodontic treatment. Even correction with segmental maxillary surgery to produce expansion has often shown disappointing results.[38] The use of surgical assisted palatal expansion, incorporating the concepts of DO, seems to produce better long-term results in these cases.[39] In these cases the expansion device is secured in place by the orthodontist. A surgical procedure is then completed by performing the bony cuts as described for a Le Fort I osteotomy, with the exception that the most posterior attachment of the lateral nasal wall and perpendicular plate of the palatine bone are not divided. A midline cut is also completed to create separation between the central incisors extending along the midpalatal suture. After a latency period the expansion device is activated 1 mm per day until the desired expansion takes place (Fig. 25-33). During this time a space develops between the central incisors, along the midpalatal suture, and at the area of the osteotomy along the lateral maxillary wall.

Bony regenerate gradually fills and matures in these areas. The appliance is then removed, and active orthodontic treatment is begun to close space between teeth, properly align the arch, and maintain the expansion.

In the case of mandibular deficiency, the initial surgical procedure involves performing an osteotomy and placement of the distraction appliance. After a latency period of 7 days, the distraction occurs with a rate and rhythm of 1 mm per day (completed by activating the appliance 0.5 mm twice each day). Once this distraction is complete, the appliance is left is place for the consolidation phase, which is usually 2 or 3 times the amount of time required for the distraction phase. The appliance is then removed, and active orthodontic treatment continues. Figure 25-34 demonstrates a case of DO of the mandible.

Distraction appliances are also available for maxillary and midface advancement. In some cases of traditional maxillary repositioning, autogenous bone may be required for grafting into the bony defect. The need for grafting obviously requires donor site surgery with the associated morbidities. DO eliminates the need for graft harvest in many of these patients. In patients with a cleft lip and palate there is often substantial scarring from multiple previous surgical procedures. This scarring combined with significant growth abnormalities creates soft tissue limitations that may prevent single-stage correction with conventional orthognathic surgical techniques.

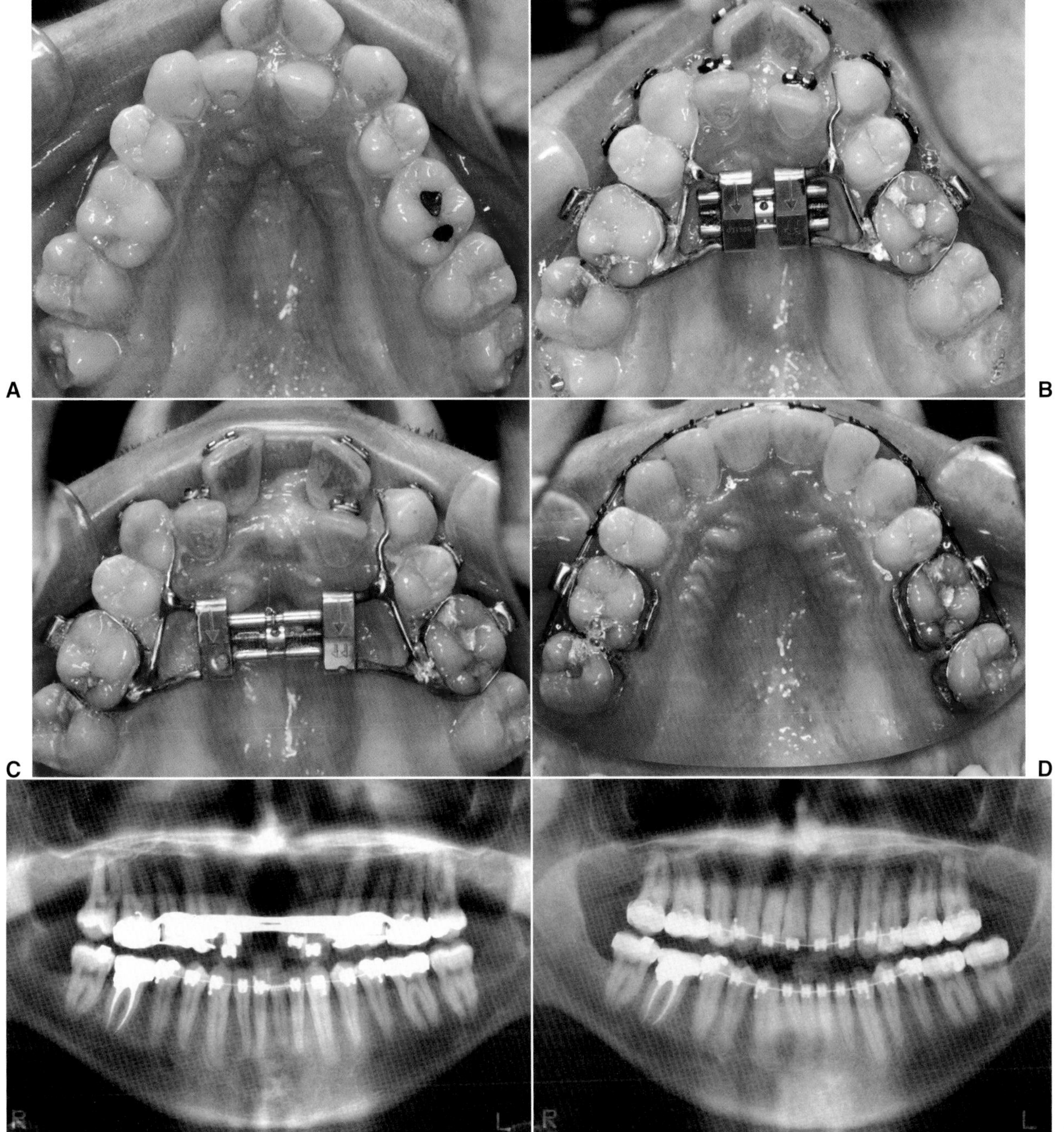

FIGURE 25-33 Distraction osteogenesis with surgically assisted palatal expansion for correction of transverse maxillary deficiency. A, Severe constriction of maxilla with inadequate arch length (note that severe crowding exists even though premolars have been extracted). B, Expansion device in place. C, Maxilla expanded (note space between central incisors). Osteogenesis, with bone formation, and histogenesis, with formation of gingival tissue, are occurring. D, Space closed with anterior teeth orthodontically aligned using newly formed regenerate bone. E, Radiograph showing expansion with immature regenerate bone in anterior space. F, Radiograph after orthodontic alignment.

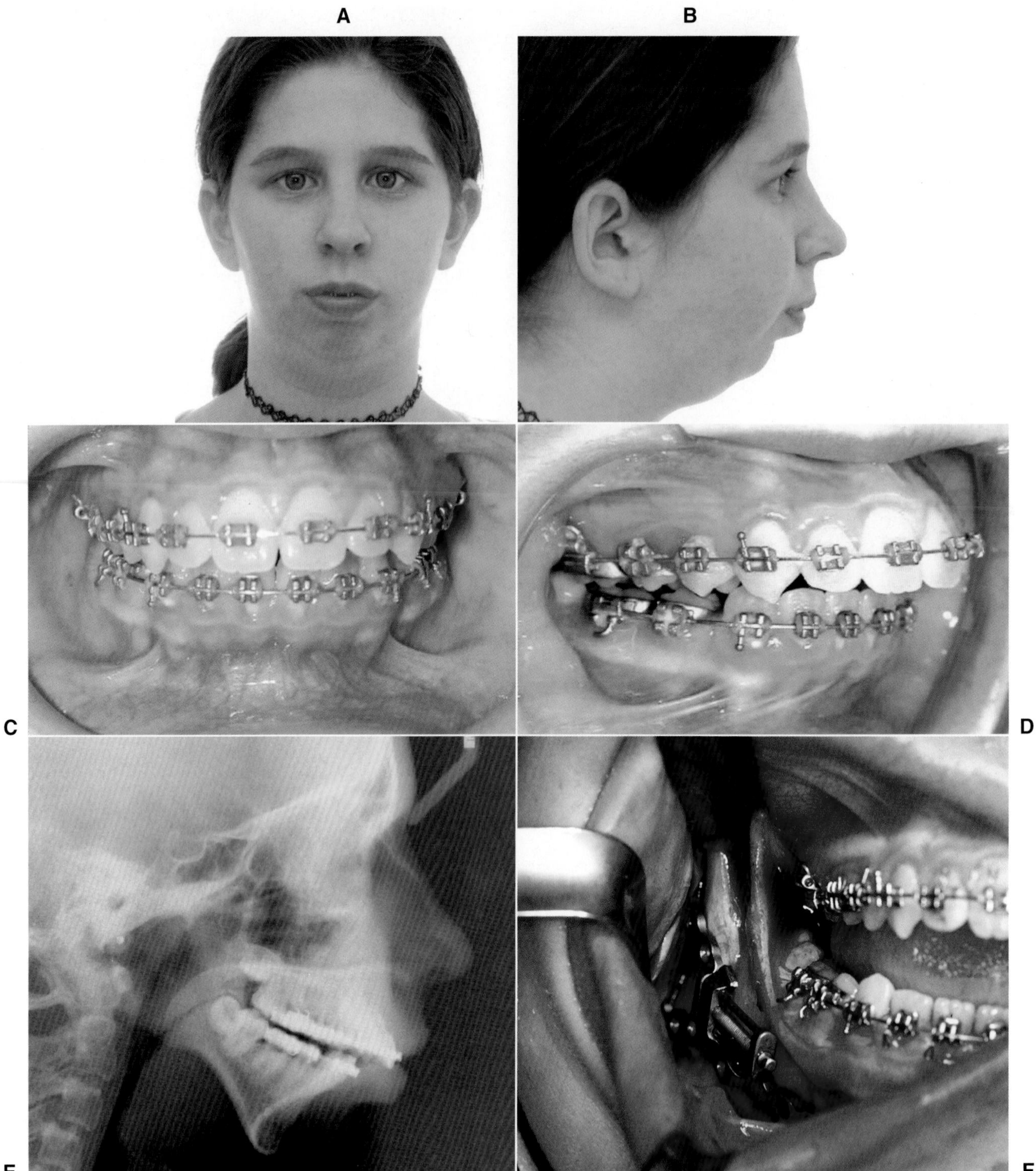

FIGURE 25-34 Case report of distraction osteogenesis to correct severe mandibular deficiency. A and B, Preoperative facial esthetics demonstrating severe mandibular deficiency. C and D, Preoperative occlusion demonstrating Class II relationship. E, Preoperative cephalometric radiograph. F, Surgical procedure to create osteotomy and place distraction appliance.

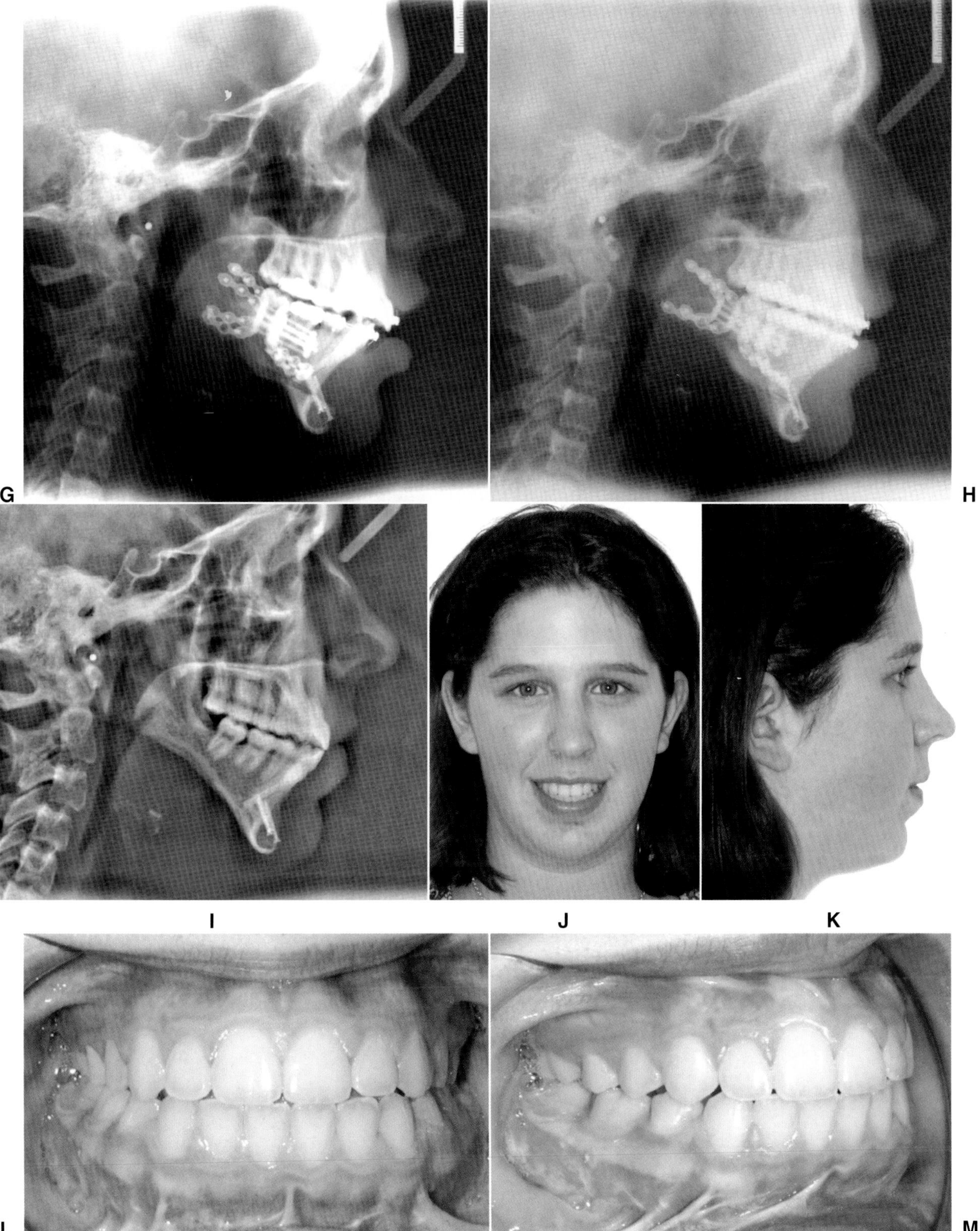

FIGURE 25-34, cont'd Case report of distraction osteogenesis to correct severe mandibular deficiency. G, Postoperative radiograph after latency phase complete and distraction started (chin advancement was completed at the same time distractors were applied). H, Radiograph after 16 days of distraction at 1 mm per day. I, Radiograph after distraction appliances removed, completion of orthodontic treatment, and debanding. J and K, Postoperative facial appearance. L and M, Postoperative occlusal views.

DO can be effective in treatment of these patients by gradually stretching the soft tissue envelope, generating new soft and hard tissue, eliminating the need for graft harvest, and providing good long-term stability.[40] Figure 25-35 demonstrates the effective use of DO for maxillary advancement in such a patient. Maxillary repositioning with DO may allow larger advancements with improved long-term stability.[41,42]

PERIOPERATIVE CARE OF THE ORTHOGNATHIC SURGICAL PATIENT

Patients undergoing orthognathic surgery are usually admitted to the hospital on the day of surgery. Before surgery the medical history, complete physical examination, preoperative laboratory tests, radiographic examinations, and consultation with the anesthesiologist are completed. Orthognathic surgery is accomplished in the operating room with the patient under general anesthesia. After surgery, the patient is taken to the postanesthesia care unit (i.e., recovery room) for an appropriate period, usually until alert, oriented, comfortable, and exhibiting stable vital signs; then the patient is returned to the hospital room. The nursing staff trained and experienced in the postoperative care of surgery patients continually monitor postoperative progress. The patient is discharged when feeling comfortable, urinating without assistance, taking food and fluid orally without difficulty, and ambulating well. The post-

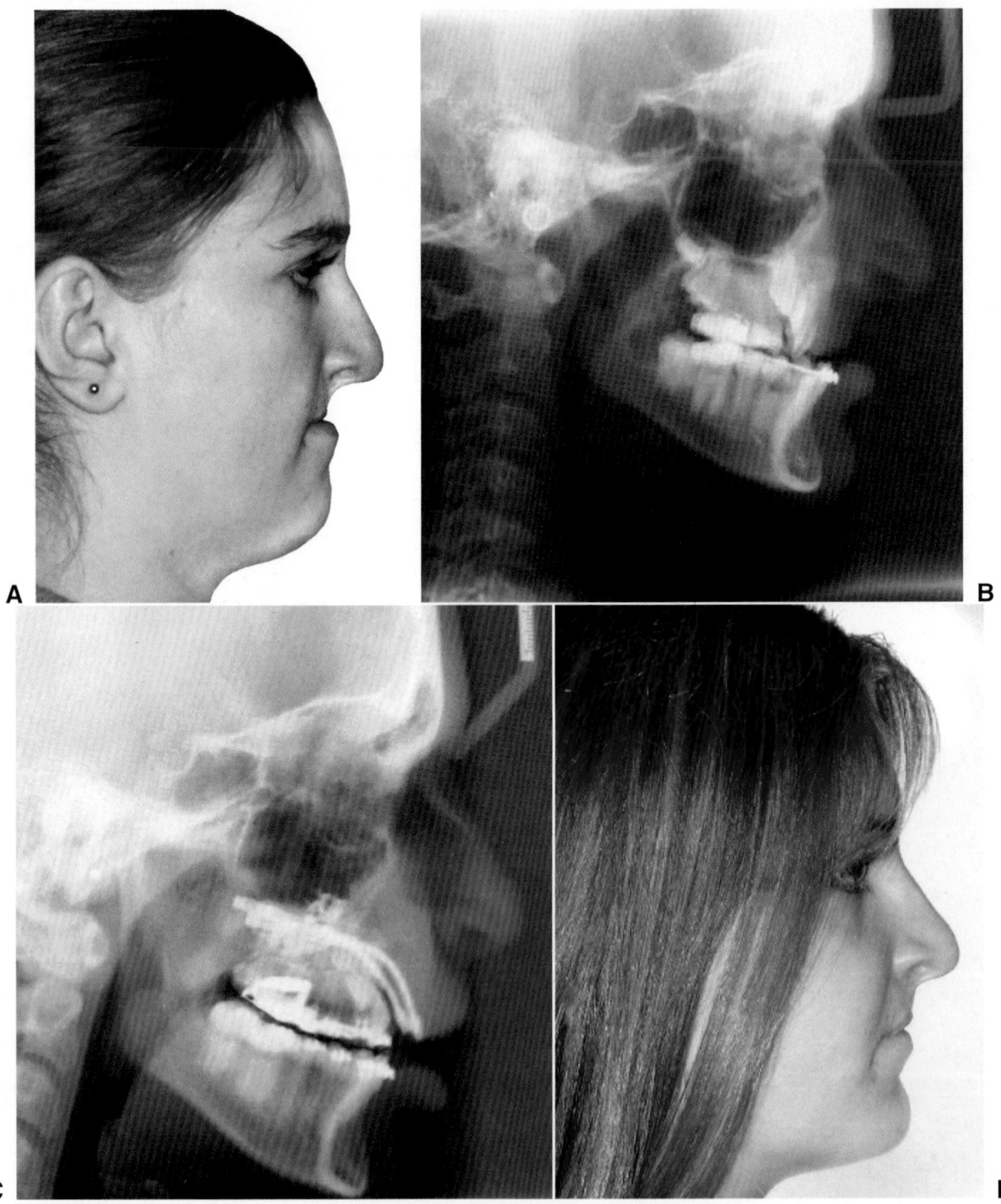

FIGURE 25-35 Distraction osteogenesis for correction of maxillary deficiency. **A**, Severe midface deficiency resulting from cleft lip and palate and multiple surgical interventions. **B**, Radiograph demonstrating maxillary hypoplasia and Class III malocclusion. **C**, Radiograph showing advancement of the maxilla using distractors. **D**, Final profile demonstrating improved facial balance and occlusion. (Photos courtesy Dr. Dan Spagnoli.)

surgical hospital stay usually ranges from 1 to 4 days. Patients generally require only mild to moderate pain medication during this time and often require no analgesics after discharge. As soon as is feasible, postoperative radiographs are obtained to ensure that the predicted bone changes have taken place and that stabilization devices are in the proper position.

The importance of postoperative nutrition should be discussed with patients and their families before the hospital admission for surgery. During the postoperative hospital stay, a member of the dietary staff may instruct the patient in methods of obtaining adequate nutrition during the period of IMF or limited jaw function. Special cookbooks designed for patients undergoing jaw surgery contain instructions for the preparation of diets in a blender.

In the past, one of the major considerations in the immediate postoperative period was the difficulty resulting from IMF. When the jaws are wired together, the patient has initial difficulties in obtaining adequate nutrition, performing necessary oral hygiene, and communicating verbally. The average IMF period ranges from 6 to 8 weeks.

During the past few years, several systems using small bone screws and bone plates have been developed to provide direct bony stabilization in the area of the osteotomies (Fig. 25-36).[43-46] The most recent development in rigid internal fixation is the use of screws and plates made of resorbable material. The materials are capable of maintaining adequate strength to stabilize bone during the healing period and are then resorbed by hydrolyzation. The use of these rigid fixation systems allows for early release from or total elimination of IMF, which results in improved patient comfort, convenience of speech and oral hygiene, and improved postsurgical jaw stability and function.

At the time of surgery, a small acrylic occlusal wafer is used to help position and stabilize the occlusion. When the IMF is released (usually in the operating room), the splint is wired to the upper or lower jaw. Light elastics are then placed on the surgical wires, and the combination of the splint and elastics

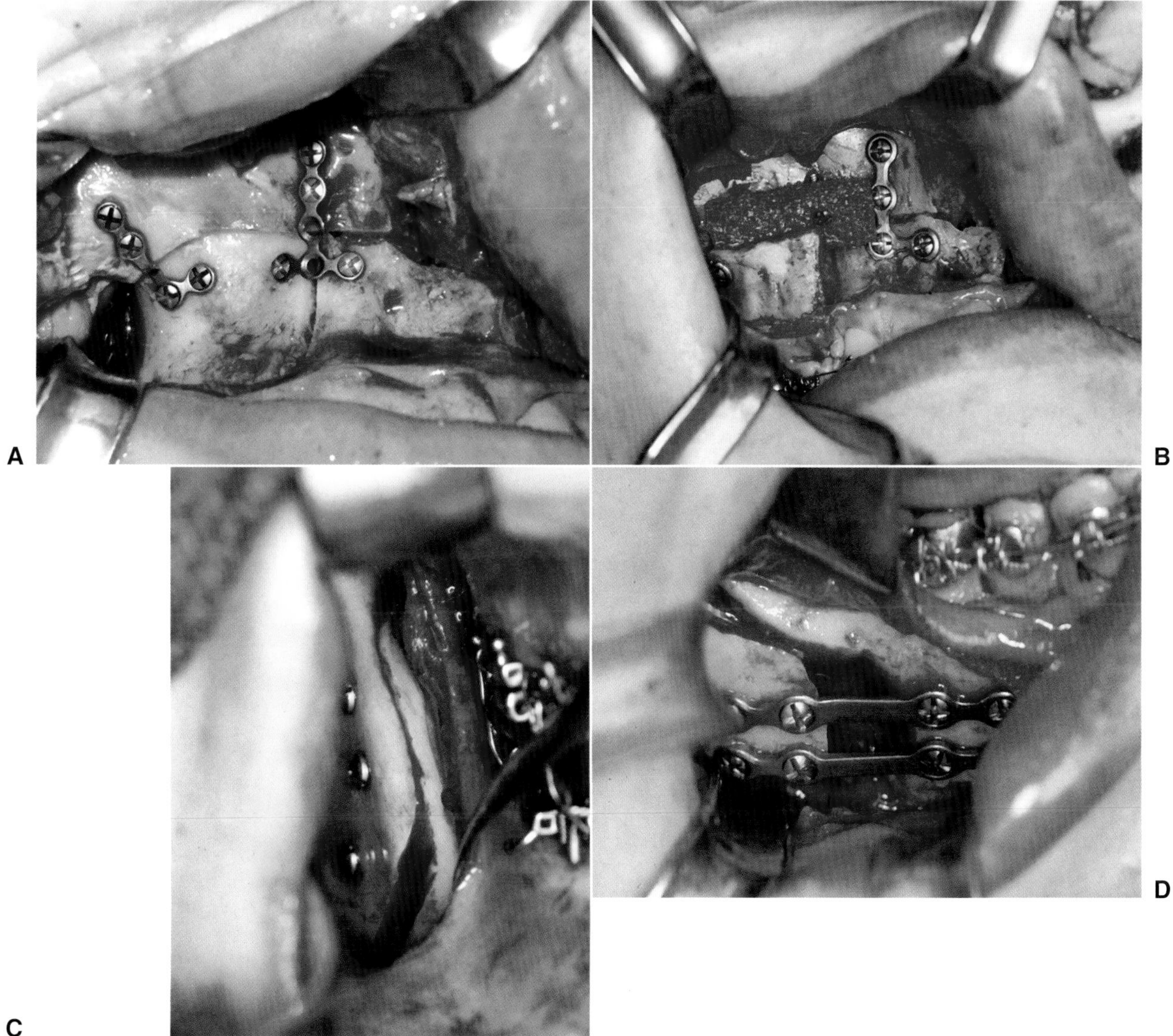

FIGURE 25-36 A, Use of small bone plates for stabilization of maxillary osteotomy. B, Maxillary advancement and downgraft with iliac crest bone graft stabilized with bone plates. C, Lag screws used to secure mandibular sagittal split osteotomy. D, Bone plates used to stabilize sagittal split osteotomy.

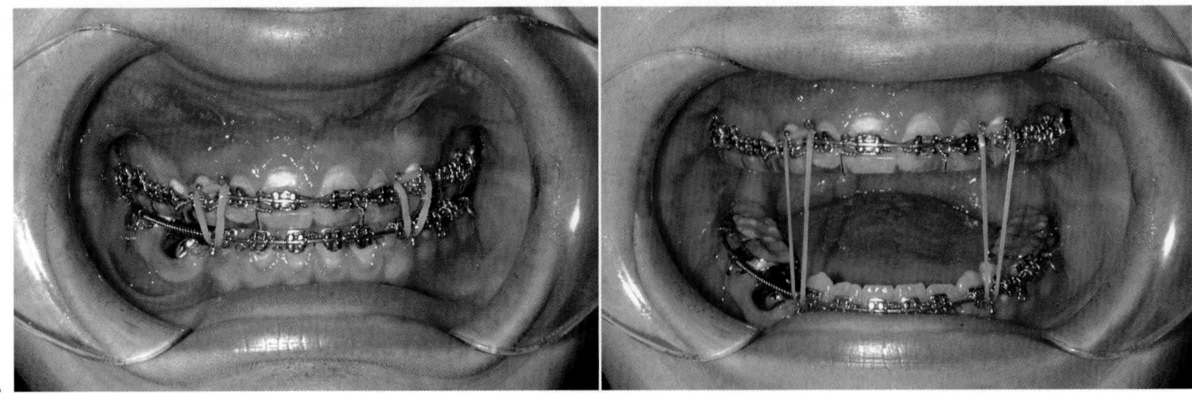

FIGURE 25-37 A, Interocclusal splint wired to maxilla. Light elastics are used to help guide patient into new postoperative occlusion. B, Patient 7 days after maxillary osteotomy.

serves to guide the jaw into the new postsurgical occlusion (Fig. 25-37). After an adequate accommodation period, the occlusal splint is removed and the patient is returned to the orthodontist's care.

POSTSURGICAL TREATMENT PHASE

Completion of Orthodontics

When a satisfactory range of jaw motion and stability of the osteotomy sites are achieved, the orthodontic treatment can be finished. The heavy surgical arch wires are removed and replaced with light orthodontic wire. Final alignment and positioning of the teeth is accomplished, as is closure of any residual extraction space. The light vertical elastics are left in place at this time to override proprioceptive impulses from the teeth, which otherwise would cause the patient to seek a new position of maximal intercuspation. The settling process proceeds rapidly and rarely takes longer than 6 to 10 months.

Retention after surgical orthodontics is no different from that for other adult patients, and definitive periodontal and prosthetic treatment can be initiated immediately after the final occlusal relationships have been established.

Postsurgical Restorative and Prosthetic Considerations

When patients require complex final restorative treatment, it is important to establish stable, full-arch contact as soon after orthodontic debanding as possible. Posterior vertical contacts are important in patients who have only anterior components of occlusion remaining. Well-fitting, temporary, removable partial dentures may suffice, and these appliances should be relined with tissue-conditioning materials as needed to maintain the posterior support during healing. When postsurgical orthodontics is complete, the remainder of restorative treatment can be accomplished in the same manner as for any nonsurgical patient.

Postsurgical Dental and Periodontal Considerations

The patient should be seen for a maintenance dental and periodontal evaluation approximately 10 to 14 weeks postoperatively. The mucogingival status is reevaluated, the mouth deplaqued, and areas of inflammation or pocketing lightly scaled. Frequent recall maintenance should continue during the remainder of orthodontic care when necessary. After the orthodontic appliances are removed, a thorough prophylaxis with a review of oral hygiene techniques is advisable. A thorough periodontal reevaluation 3 to 6 months after completion of the postsurgical orthodontics will determine future treatment needs. Periodontal surgery, including crown-lengthening or regenerative procedures, should be performed after the inflammation associated with orthodontic appliances has resolved. Areas of hyperplastic tissue should be observed for 3 to 6 months after orthodontic therapy, unless esthetic or restorative considerations necessitate earlier tissue removal. After completion of periodontal treatment, recall intervals should be adjusted to accommodate the individual patient's needs.

SUMMARY

The treatment of patients with dentofacial deformity involves the evaluation and treatment of many types of dental and skeletal problems. These problems require that all practitioners involved in patient care interact in a multidisciplinary team approach to treatment. This sequential, team approach yields the most satisfying results.

REFERENCES

1. Brunelle JA, Bhat M, Lipton JA: Prevalence and distributions of selected occlusal characteristics in the US population, 1988-1991, *J Dent Res* 75:706-713, 1996.
2. Proffit WR, Fields HW, Moray LJ: Prevalence of malocclusion and orthodontic treatment need in the United States: estimates from the N-HANES III survey, *Int J Adult Orthodon Orthognath Surg* 13:97-106, 1998.
3. Proffit WR, White RP Jr: Dentofacial problems: prevalence and treatment need. In Proffit WR, White RP Jr, Sarver DM, editors: *Contemporary treatment of dentofacial deformity,* St Louis, 2003, Mosby.
4. Enlow DH, Hans M: *Essentials of facial growth,* Philadelphia, 1996, WB Saunders.
5. Enlow DH: Wolff's law and factor of architectonic circumstance, *Am J Orthod* 54:803, 1968.
6. Enlow DH: Craniofacial growth and development. In Posnick JC, editor: *Craniofacial and maxillofacial surgery in children and young adults,* Philadelphia, 2000, WB Saunders.
7. Fields HW, Warren DW, Black K et al: Relationship between vertical dentofacial morphology and respiration in adolescents, *Am J Orthod Dentofacial Orthop* 99:147-154, 1991.

8. Tucker MR, Moriarty JM, Koth DL et al: Evaluation of treatment of patients with dentofacial deformities: a multidisciplinary approach, *North Carolina Dental Review* 3:13, 1985.
9. Burstone CJ, James RB, Legan H et al: Cephalometrics for orthognathic surgery, *J Oral Surg* 36:269, 1978.
10. Steiner CC: Cephalometrics in clinical practice angle, *Orthodontics* 28:8, 1959.
11. Smith JD, Thomas PM, Proffit R: A comparison of current prediction imaging programs, *Am J Orthod Dentofacial Orthop* 125:527, 2004.
12. Bell WH, Dann JJ: Correction of dentofacial deformities by surgery in the anterior part of the jaws, *Am J Orthod* 64:162, 1973.
13. Caldwell JB, Letterman GS: Vertical osteotomy in the mandibular rami for correction of prognathism, *J Oral Surg* 12:185, 1954.
14. Hall HD, Chase DC, Payor LG: Evaluation and realignment of the intraoral vertical subcondylar osteotomy, *J Oral Surg* 33:333, 1975.
15. Trauner R, Obwegeser H: The surgical correction of mandibular prognathism and retrognathia with consideration of genioplasty. I. Surgical procedures to correct mandibular prognathism and reshaping of the chin, *Oral Surg Oral Med Oral Pathol* 10:677, 1957.
16. Dalpont G: Retromolar osteotomy for the correction of prognathism, *J Oral Surg* 19:42, 1961.
17. Hunsuck EE: A modified intraoral sagittal splitting technique for mandibular prognathism, *J Oral Surg* 26:249, 1968.
18. Epker BN: Modifications in the sagittal osteotomy of the mandible, *J Oral Surg* 35:157, 1977.
19. Robinson M: Micrognathism corrected by vertical osteotomy of ascending ramus and iliac bone graft: new technique, *Oral Surg Oral Med Oral Pathol* 10:125, 1957.
20. Kufner J: Experience with a modified procedure for correction of open bite. In Walker RV, editor: *Transactions of the Third International Congress of Oral Surgery,* London, 1970, E&S Livingstone.
21. Schuchardt K: Experiences with the surgical treatment of deformities of the jaws: prognathia, micrognathia, and open bite. In Wallace AG, editor: *Second Congress of International Society of Plastic Surgeons,* London, 1959, E&S Livingstone.
22. Wunderer S: Erfahrungen mitder operativen Behandlung hochgradiger Prognathien, *Dtsch Zahn Mund Kieferheilkd* 39:451, 1963.
23. Bell WH, Fonseca RJ, Kenneky JW, Levy BM: Bone healing and revascularization after total maxillary osteotomy, *J Oral Surg* 33:253, 1975.
24. Tucker MR, White RP Jr: Maxillary orthognathic surgery. In Tucker MR, White RA Jr, Terry BC et al, editors: *Rigid fixation for maxillofacial surgery,* Philadelphia, 1991, JB Lippincott.
25. Jacobson R, Sarver DM: The predictability of maxillary repositioning in LeFort I orthognathic surgery, *Am J Orthod Dentofacial Orthop* 122:142, 2002.
26. Busby BR, Bailey LJ, Proffit WR et al: Long-term stability of surgical Class III treatment: a study of 5-year postsurgical results, *Int J Adult Orthodon Orthognath Surg* 17:159, 2002.
27. Guilleminault C: Obstructive sleep apnea: the clinical syndrome and historical perspective, *Med Clin North Am* 69:1187, 1985.
28. Veasey SC, Guilleminault C, Strohl KP et al: Medical therapy for obstructive sleep apnea: a review by the Medical Therapy for Obstructive Sleep Apnea Task Force of the Standards of Practice Committee of the American Academy of Sleep Medicine, *Sleep* 29:1036-1044, 2006.
29. Senn O, Bloch KE, Iseli A et al: Oral appliances for the treatment of snoring and obstructive sleep apnea, *Oto-Rhino-Laryngologia Nova* 11:168, 2001.
30. Waite PD, Vilos GA: Surgical changes of posterior airway space in obstructive sleep apnea, *Oral and Maxillofacial Surgery Clinics of North America* 14:385, 2002.
31. Fairburn SC, Waite PD, Vilos G et al: Three-dimensional changes in upper airways of patients with obstructive sleep apnea following maxillomandibular advancement, *J Oral Maxillofac Surg* 65:6, 2007.
32. Peltier LF: External skeletal fixation for the treatment of fractures. In *Fractures: a history and iconography of their treatment,* San Francisco, 1990, Norman Publishing.
33. Ilizarov GA: The principles of the Ilizarov method, *Bull Hosp Jt Dis* 56:49-53, 1997.
34. Ilizarov G, Devyatov A, Kameran V: Plastic reconstruction of longitudinal bone defects by means of compression and subsequent distraction, *Acta Chir Plast* 22:32, 1980.
35. Altuna G, Walker DA, Freeman E: Rapid orthopedic lengthening of the mandible in primates by sagittal split osteotomy and distraction osteogenesis: a pilot study, *Int J Adult Orthodon Orthognath Surg* 10:59, 1995.
36. Guerrero CA, Bell WH: Intraoral distraction. In *Distraction of the craniofacial skeletal,* New York, 1999, Springer-Verlag.
37. Lines PA: Adult rapid maxillary expansion with corticotomy, *Am J Orthod* 67:44, 1975.
38. Proffit WR, Turvey TA, Phillips C: Orthognathic surgery: a hierarchy of stability, *Int J Adult Orthodon Orthognath Surg* 11:191, 1996.
39. Betts NJ, Vanarsdall RL, Barber HD et al: Diagnosis and treatment of transverse maxillary deficiency, *Int J Adult Orthodon Orthognath Surg* 10:75, 1995.
40. Figueroa AA, Polley JW: Management of severe cleft maxillary deficiency with distraction osteogenesis: procedure and results, *Am J Orthod Dentofacial Orthop* 115:1-12, 1999.
41. Rachmiel A: Treatment of maxillary cleft palate: distraction osteogenesis verses orthognathic surgery. Part one: maxillary distraction, *J Oral Maxillofac Surg* 65:753-757, 2007.
42. Precious DS: Treatment of retruded maxilla in cleft lip and palate: orthognathic surgery verses distraction osteogenesis—the case for orthognathic surgery, *J Oral Maxillofacial Surg* 65:758-761, 2007.
43. Spiessl B: *New concepts of maxillofacial bone surgery,* Berlin, 1975, Springer-Verlag.
44. Borstlap WA, Stoelinga PJW, Hoppenreijs TJM, van't Hof MA: Stabilisation of sagittal split advancement osteotomies with miniplates: a prospective, multicentre study with two-year follow-up. I. Clinical parameters, *Int J Oral Maxillofac Surg* 33:433, 2004.
45. Sittitavornwong S, Waite PD, Dann JJ, Kohn MW: The stability of maxillary osteotomies fixated with biodegradable mesh in orthognathic surgery, *J Oral Maxillofac Surg* 64:1631, 2006.
46. Tucker MR, Frost DE, Terry BC: Mandibular surgery. In Tucker MR, White RA Jr, Terry BC et al, editors: *Rigid fixation for maxillofacial surgery,* Philadelphia, 1991, JB Lippincott.

CHAPTER 26

Facial Esthetic Surgery

MARK W. OCHS AND PETER N. DEMAS

CHAPTER OUTLINE

Patients are increasingly seeking procedures that enhance their appearance for personal and professional reasons. Esthetic oral and maxillofacial surgery is often included in a comprehensive treatment plan to complement restorative, prosthetic, and orthodontic treatment. Dental treatment plans, especially ones involving cosmetic therapy, are enhanced if dentists remain aware of the wide variety of esthetic surgical options available to patients. Orthodontists planning orthognathic surgery complete a careful evaluation of facial proportions that frequently includes the diagnosis of external nasal deformities and other hard and soft tissue abnormalities. Prosthetic rehabilitation often involves attempts to increase support to the perioral region and can be enhanced with facial rejuvenation procedures. Cosmetic restorative dentistry may provide the finishing touch to cosmetic surgical treatment. Pediatric dentistry patients with traumatic scars or congenital deformities can also be helped. Patients with oral and head and neck pathologic conditions such as skin cancers can be treated, reconstructed, and restored to adequate function and socially acceptable appearance.

Advances in medicine and nutrition, combined with increased public awareness of personal health care, enable patients to live longer, healthier, and more active lives. However, social pressure to maintain a youthful appearance as one ages encourages more individuals each year to undergo some form of esthetic enhancement. This trend is evident in members of the baby boomer generation, now in their 40s, 50s, and 60s, who have grown increasingly interested in these procedures.

Research from the American Academy of Cosmetic Surgery indicates that the number of patients undergoing esthetic procedures continues to increase yearly. Body liposuction is the most frequent surgical procedure, and it is surpassed by Botox (botulinum toxin) injections as the most popular nonsurgical cosmetic procedure. Facial procedures, such as eyelid rejuvenation, face-lifts, and facial skin rejuvenation, also continue to increase.

Women seeking esthetic surgery outnumber men approximately 9:1. However, men are increasingly seeking esthetic procedures, including eyelid and forehead rejuvenation and hair restoration. As expected, the popularity of specific procedures is age related. Patients under 35 years of age usually desire liposuction, rhinoplasty, chemical peels, and laser skin resurfacing. As patients age into their 40s, 50s and 60s, they seek liposuction, eyelid and forehead rejuvenation, face-lifts, and chemical or laser skin resurfacing.

Surgical technical advances also contribute to the growth of esthetic surgery. New techniques and technical advances in equipment reduce surgical risks, recovery time, and incision visibility. Technical innovations include endoscopic or minimally invasive procedures that use small incisions, liposuction with barely noticeable access sites, and lasers that enhance hemostasis and allow precise control over depth of skin removal.

Appearance matters more than many wish to admit, and interpersonal reactions are often influenced by appearance. Improved self-confidence occurs in many patients who have undergone successful esthetic surgical and cosmetic dental procedures. One commonly notices patients altering their wardrobe, makeup, and hairstyle after surgery; patients often are delighted in how others respond to their new image. However, it is important during the esthetic surgery consultation for the surgeon to attempt to determine whether the patient's desires for surgery are based on *personal* motivation, without undue outside influences or unrealistic expectations. Patients with external pressures and unrealistic expectations are more likely to be dissatisfied with the treatment outcome despite successful technical results.[1,2]

FACIAL AGING

Facial aging involves the changes to the skin itself and resultant effects on the appearance of the skin and on the underlying soft tissues. Natural aging combined with sun exposure produces a wide range of skin changes. Natural aging results in loss of skin elasticity and collagen, melanocyte pigmentations, and fat atrophy. Sun exposure adds photoaging caused by ultraviolet light. Ultraviolet light from sun tanning damages the skin and eventually causes a wrinkled, pigmented, and weathered appearance. Solar radiation also leads to an increased incidence of skin cancers. Gravitational changes on the skin and underlying tissues cause deep forehead lines, drooping brows, eyelid skin laxity and puffiness, loss of cheek roundness, and sagging neck and jaw lines (Fig. 26-1).

Although aging is an individual phenomenon, many factors can influence the appearance and rate of aging. These factors include general health, sedentary lifestyle, sun exposure, genetic influences, nutritional balance, alcohol consumption, and cigarette smoking. Cigarette use, with its vasoactive effects of nicotine, accelerates skin aging and reduces the ability of the body to repair wounds. The vasoactive effects can lead to poor healing in some esthetic surgical procedures.[3,4]

SURGICAL PROCEDURES

The procedures described in the following sections are presented as isolated surgical techniques. However, in practice, several of these are often combined and performed during a single surgical appointment.

Blepharoplasty

Blepharoplasty (i.e., eyelid rejuvenation) is one of the most common facial esthetic procedures performed on women and men. Aging eyelids exhibit a puffy, drooping, and baggy appearance. These effects are the result of eyelid skin laxity, orbicularis muscle hypertrophy, and orbital fat herniation out into the eyelids (Fig. 26-2). Redundant and folded skin of the upper eyelids is referred to as *dermatochalasis*. When extreme, the folded skin can extend beyond the eyelash margin and create a mechanical block to vision. Patients typically notice this later in the day when their "eyes are tired." This sagging, redundant, and folded upper eyelid skin over the lashes is termed *hooding*. The main cause of baggy lower eyelids is gradual thinning and laxity of the fine collagenous orbital septum. This structure normally separates the internal orbital contents from the eyelid. Over time this curtainlike structure bows outward like a sail, and then the intraorbital fat begins to herniate into the lower eyelids. The upper eyelid has two fat pads and the lower has three (Fig. 26-3). Besides the pouchlike filling of the lower eyelid, the outward shift of the orbital fat can create a subtle posterior settling of the globe (i.e., eyeball). This adds to the appearance of sunken in, tired, and baggy eyes.

During a blepharoplasty procedure, the surgeon removes excess skin and orbicularis oculi muscle and an appropriate amount of protruding orbital fat behind the bulging orbital septum (Fig. 26-4). The upper eyelid incision is hidden in the upper lid crease. The lower eyelid surgery can be performed in two ways: (1) with an incision just below the eyelashes (i.e., subciliary) or (2) from inside the lower lid (i.e., transconjunctival; Figs. 26-5 and 26-6). With the transconjunctival approach, the surgeon removes fat but does not excise any skin, and relies on a skin-tightening procedure, such as chemical peel or laser resurfacing, to treat any remaining skin laxity.

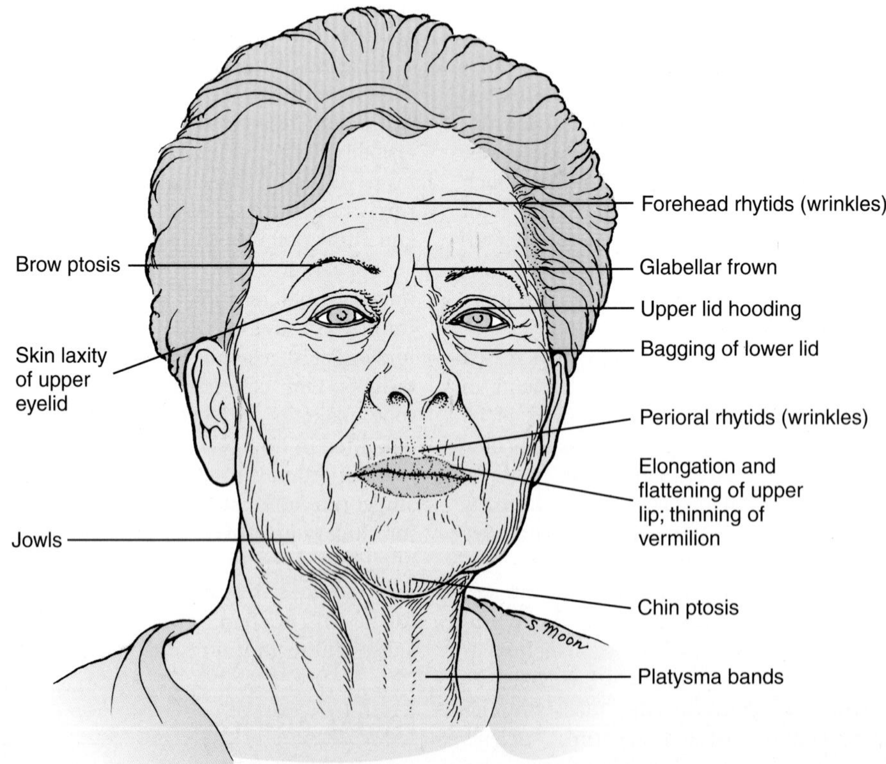

FIGURE 26-1 Facial changes associated with aging.

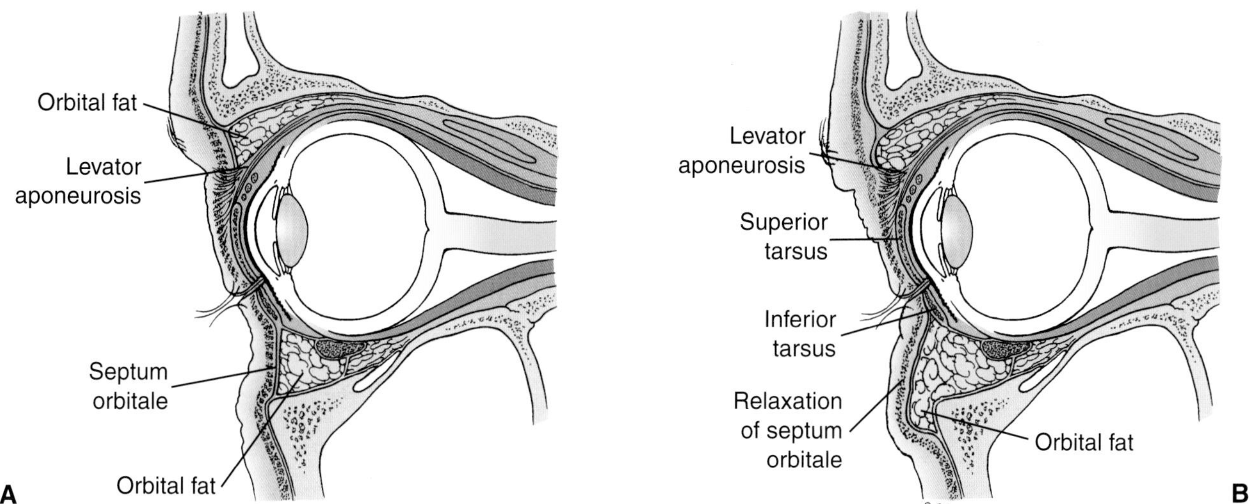

FIGURE 26-2 A, Normal sagittal view of the orbit and eyelids. B, With aging, orbital fat protrusion extends out into the upper and lower eyelids. This is due to a lax orbital septum. This gives a baggy appearance of the lids.

Recovery time from eyelid surgery is usually 7 to 10 days (Fig. 26-7).[5,6] Blepharoplasty can result in complications, which include excessive or inadequate skin removal, excessive or inadequate fat removal, dry-eye sensation, and intraorbital bleeding with rare but possible blindness.

Forehead and Brow Lift

A drooping forehead results in drooping eyebrows (i.e., brow ptosis), lateral upper eyelid fullness or hooding, and accentuated upper eyelid bagginess. Removing eyelid skin with blepharoplasty alone does not adequately address this problem if the brows are also ptotic. The normal or youthful eyebrow has the lower edge positioned at or slightly above the palpated bony supraorbital rim. The ideal esthetic female brow gently arches above the orbital rim lateral to the iris (Fig. 26-8). The peak of the arch of the brow should be aligned over the junction of the lateral edge of the iris and the sclera. Women often pluck their brows to reproduce this pattern. Male brows

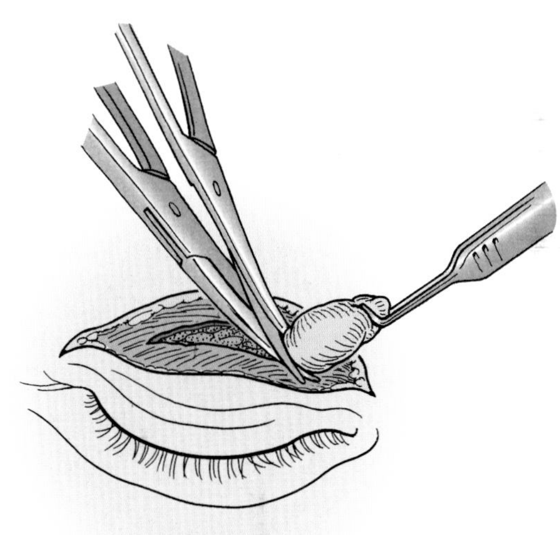

FIGURE 26-4 Clamping and excision of the right upper medial fat pad.

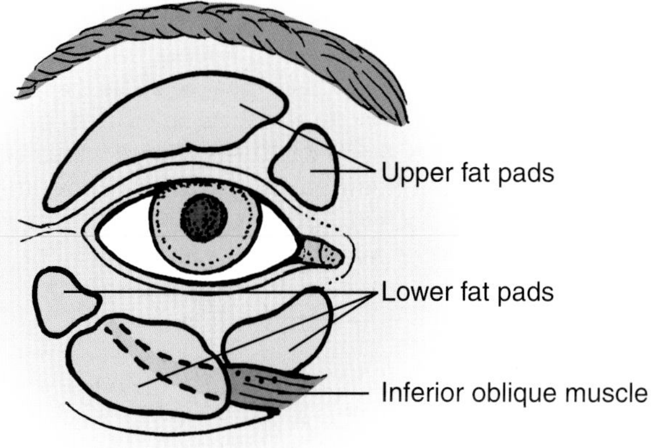

FIGURE 26-3 Orbital fat pads of the right eye. *Upper,* Medial and central. *Lower,* Medial, central, and lateral.

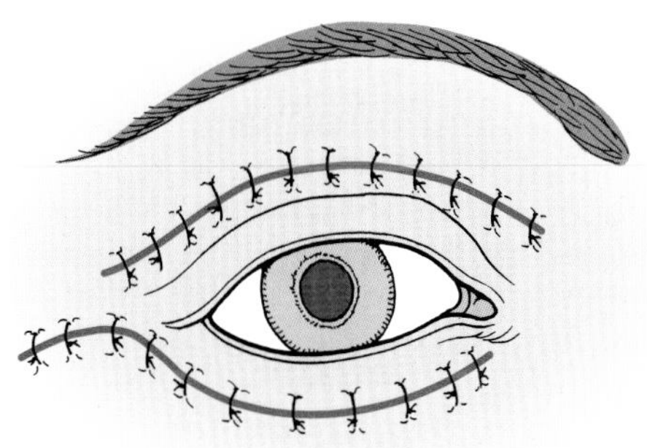

FIGURE 26-5 Sutured upper blepharoplasty and lower subciliary incisions.

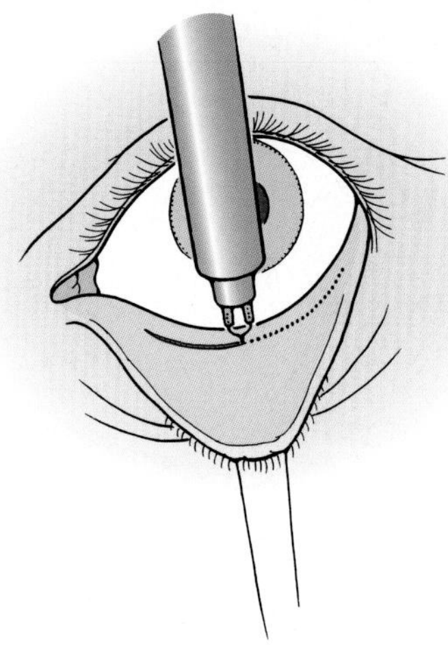

FIGURE 26-6 Left lower transconjunctival blepharoplasty incision with a handheld cautery.

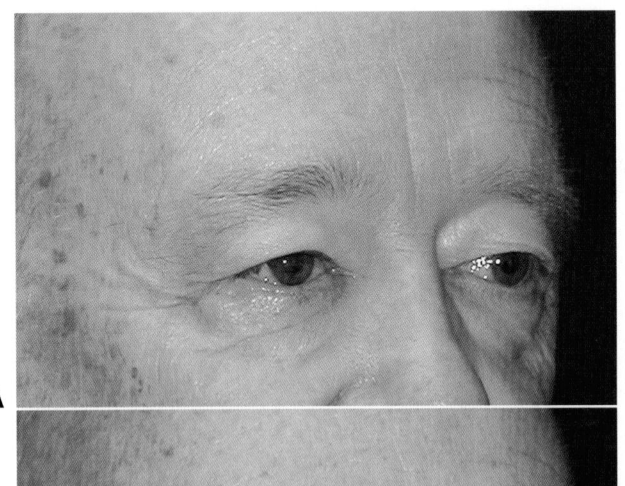

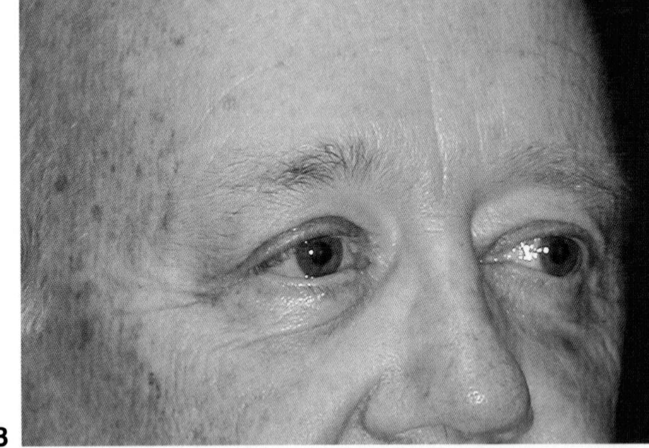

FIGURE 26-7 A, Preoperative view showing significant dermatochalasis of upper lids. B, After upper lid blepharoplasties, the patient shows improved definition to the upper lid crease and a more rested, youthful appearance. (Photos courtesy Dr. Todd Owsley.)

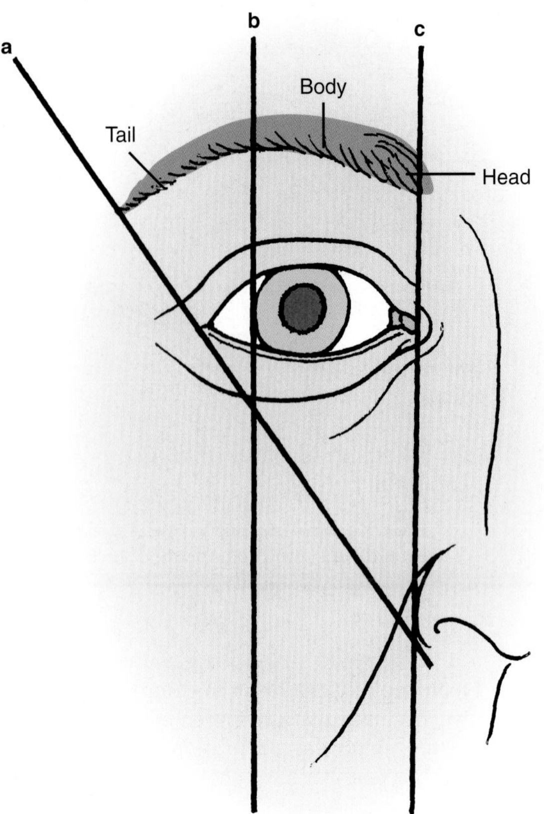

FIGURE 26-8 Right female eyebrow. The highest part of arch of brow occurs within the body (along *line b*), which transects the lateral limbus of the eye.

are generally flatter without an arch. Elevation of the brows to a rejuvenated position may eliminate or reduce the need to remove upper eyelid skin with blepharoplasty. Often a forehead and brow lift and upper lid blepharoplasty are combined during a single operation. Brow lifting reduces upper lid hooding by elevating the brow. Additionally, brow lifting reduces forehead and nasal bridge creases.

Most brow elevation surgeries are presently performed endoscopically with video camera assistance. This approach uses multiple small scalp incisions for access. After the scalp is undermined and mobilized, the forehead soft tissues are suspended and anchored in their new position (Fig. 26-9). A continuous full-thickness scalp incision within or at the hairline (i.e., pretrichial approach) is still used when required, such as with extreme brow ptosis or when one does not wish to elevate the hairline (Fig. 26-10). Care is taken to prevent injury to the sensory nerves (i.e., supraorbital and supratrochlear) and facial nerve branches of the scalp that supply motor innervation to the eyebrow region.

Postoperative recovery is 7 to 10 days (see Fig. 26-7).[7] Possible complications of brow lifting include asymmetric appearance, paresthesia, facial nerve deficits, and excessive lifting resulting in a "surprised" look.

Rhytidectomy

Rhytids are skinfolds, creases, or wrinkles. Rhytids can be referred to as coarse or fine depending on the depth and

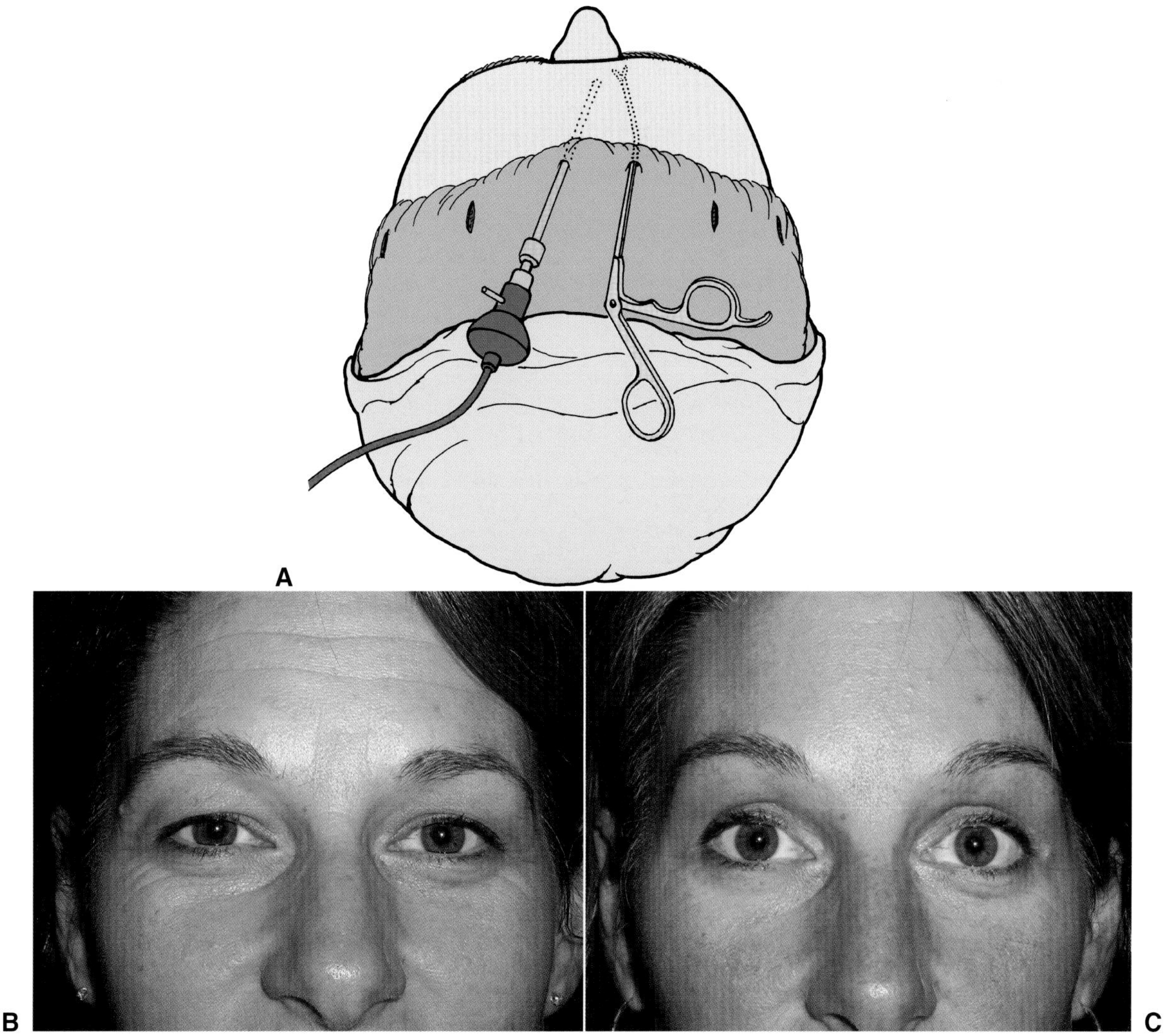

A

B C

FIGURE 26-9 A, Endoscopic forehead surgery with lighted endoscope *(left)* and scissors inserted on right. B, Preoperative view. C, Postoperative view after endoscopic forehead/brow lift. (Photos courtesy Dr. Todd Owsley.)

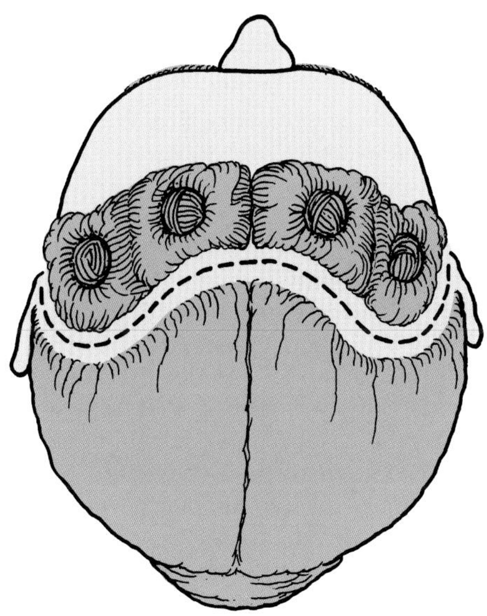

FIGURE 26-10 The coronal forehead lift incision is placed several centimeters behind the frontal hairline.

anatomic cause. Rhytidectomy, or "removal of skin wrinkles," is more commonly called *face-lift* surgery. This procedure rejuvenates sagging neck skin, jowls (i.e., sagging skin and fat posterior to the labiomental crease), nasolabial folds, and cheek laxity. Face-lift surgery can result in an elevated cheek contour and a refined mandibular neckline.

Numerous techniques are used for face-lift surgery. The most common technique uses a type of lazy S incision from the temple, around the ear, and into the posterior hairline (Fig. 26-11). The facial and neck skin is dissected and elevated in an upward and backward direction, and the underlying fascial layers are tightened (Fig. 26-12). The facial nerve must be protected during the dissection of the various layers (Fig. 26-13).

Frequently, the submuscular aponeurotic system layer is partially resected or is suspended superiorly (or both) and posteriorly to provide additional and longer-lasting effects. The excess skin is removed during wound closure (Fig. 26-14). To enhance neck contours, face-lift surgery often includes submental liposuction and platysma muscle tightening.

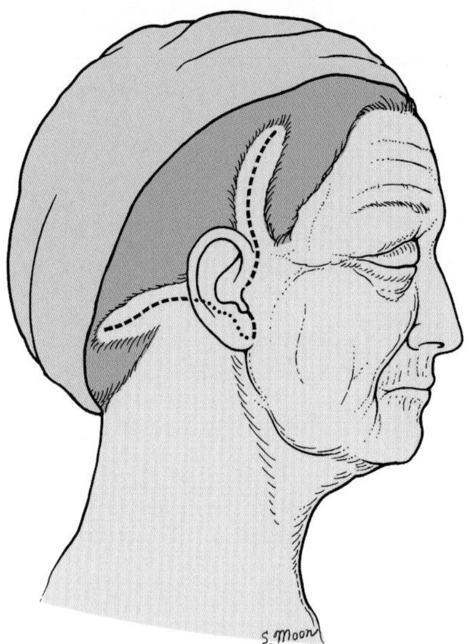

FIGURE 26-11 Incision line for face-lift.

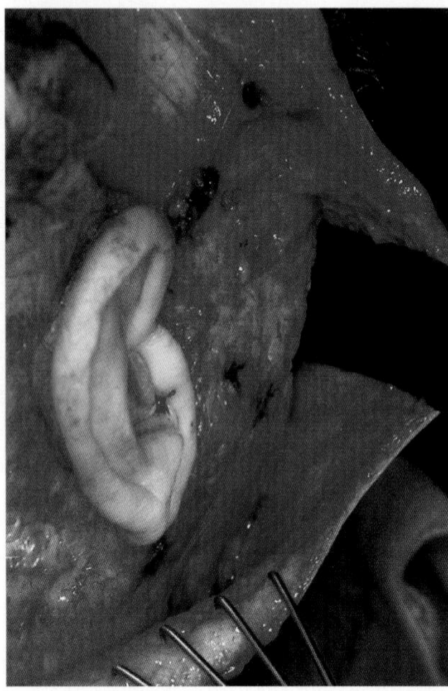

FIGURE 26-12 Face-lift dissection: Right posterior view of supine patient. A malleable retractor and tissue rake are seen adjacent to the ear.

Recovery from face-lift surgery takes about 14 days.[8,9] Potential complications include hematoma, facial nerve injury, and hypertrophic scar formation.

Septorhinoplasty

Nasal surgery, or rhinoplasty, can alter a patient's nasal appearance and correct nasal obstructive symptoms. When the nasal septum is also modified, the procedure is called a septorhinoplasty. Appearance changes may include modifying the nasal profile, the nasal bridge width, removing a dorsal hump, or improving nasal tip definition (Fig. 26-15). Patients of all ages may undergo nasal surgery. Younger patients usually seek to balance their nasal proportions with their existing facial features and eliminate nasal obstructive symptoms. Older patients

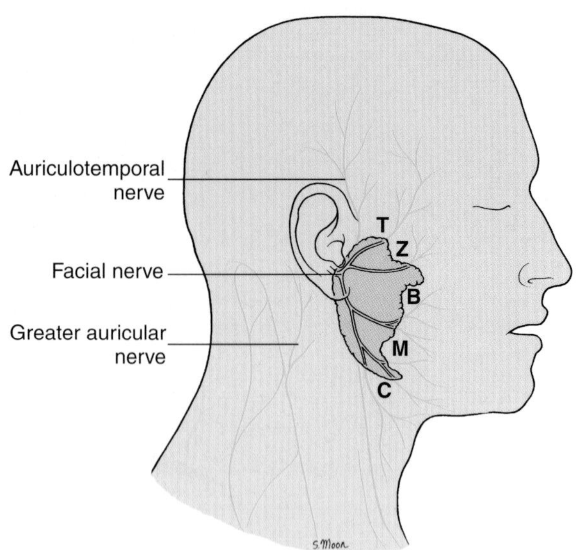

FIGURE 26-13 Nerves associated with face-lift surgery. Motor: facial nerve and branches—temporal (*T*), zygomatic (*Z*), buccal (*B*), marginal mandibular (*M*), and cervical (*C*). Sensory: auriculotemporal and greater auricular nerve.

often have rhinoplasty to rejuvenate a drooping nasal profile. With aging the upper lateral cartilages can separate and drift away from the nasal bones above them, causing an apparent nose lengthening and drooping nasal tip. This occurs more commonly in men.

Nasal surgery is performed most often with all internal nasal incisions (Fig. 26-16). More extensive nasal surgical procedures may require an open approach, which uses an additional columellar skin extension incision (Fig. 26-17). During nasal surgery, the nasal tip cartilages are refined and the dorsal profile is improved with hump reduction and thinning. This is accomplished with a combination of trimming the nasal cartilages and shaping of the nasal bones, with rasping and bony osteotomies (Fig. 26-18 and 26-19). Nasal dressings postoperatively include an external supportive splint and internal packing as required. These dressings are removed in 3 to 7 days depending on the surgery.

Initial recovery is 7 to 10 days, with final results more fully appreciated in about 3 months (Fig. 26-20).[10] Potential complications include bleeding, asymmetry, infection, septal hematoma, and overcorrection or undercorrection.

Skin Resurfacing

Skin resurfacing eliminates wrinkles and pigmentary discoloration and significantly tightens the skin, resulting in a more youthful appearance. Patients may begin to notice perioral rhytids during restorative or prosthetic treatment. They may complain to their dentist that anterior prosthetic restorations do not adequately fill out their lips. Women may remark that their lipstick "bleeds" or runs outward into the skin of the lips. This occurs in the fine channels of the vertical perioral rhytids. The dentist is limited by the supporting jaws and occlusal relationships as to how far the underlying frame (i.e., teeth) can stretch and support the overlying canvass (i.e., lips). Although excision methods such as blepharoplasty or face-lift eliminate skin excess and contours, skin resurfacing treats the fine rhytids or wrinkles. Skin resurfacing is often performed

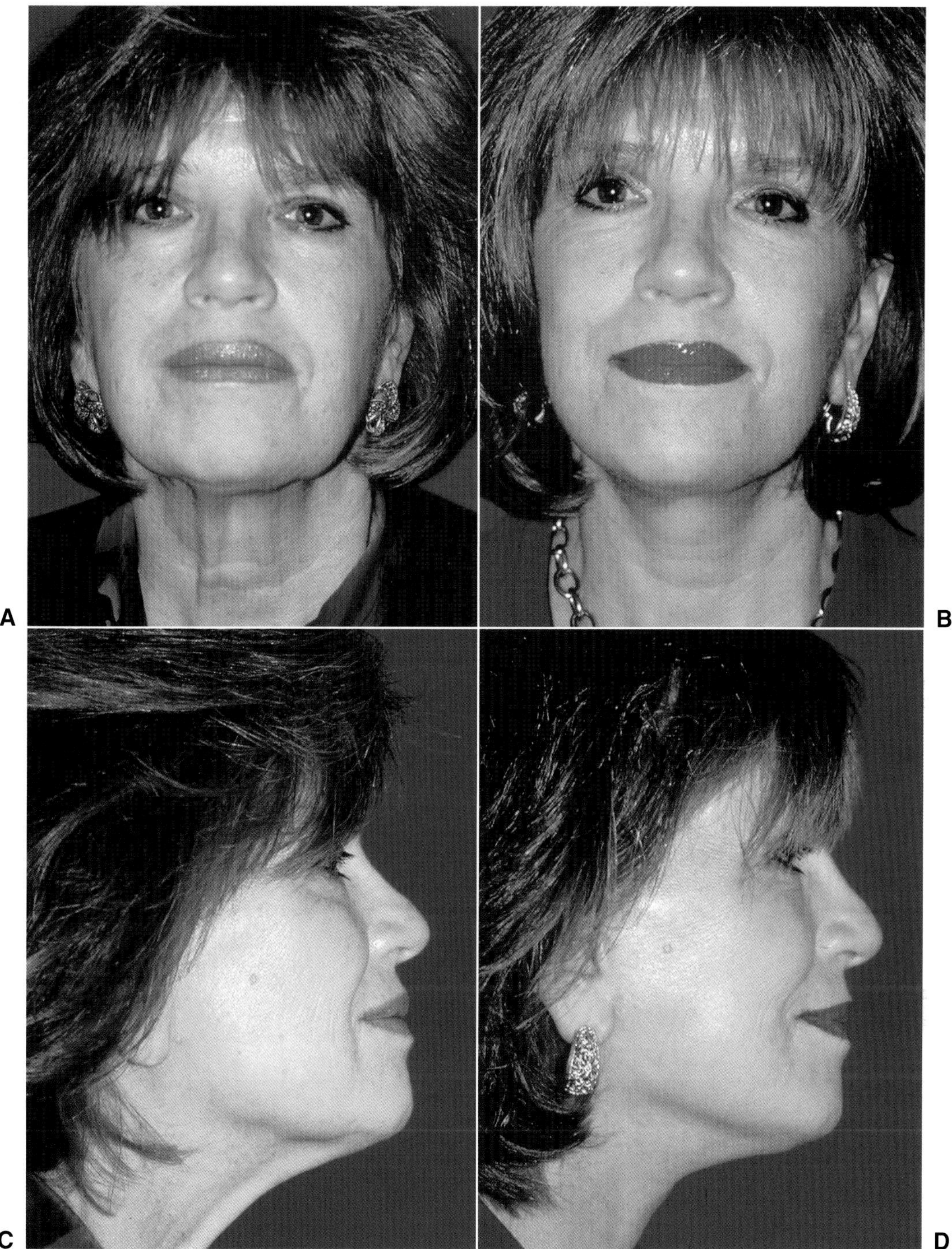

FIGURE 26-14 Face-lift surgery. A, Preoperative frontal view. B, Postoperative frontal view. C, Preoperative lateral view. D, Postoperative lateral view.

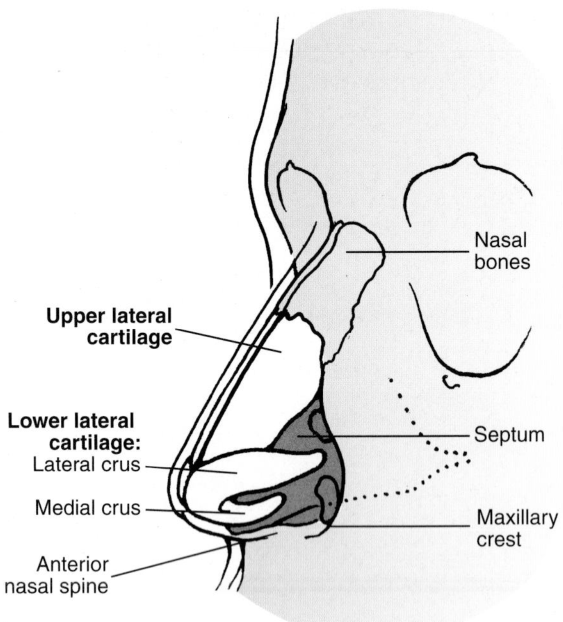

FIGURE 26-15 Nasal anatomy.

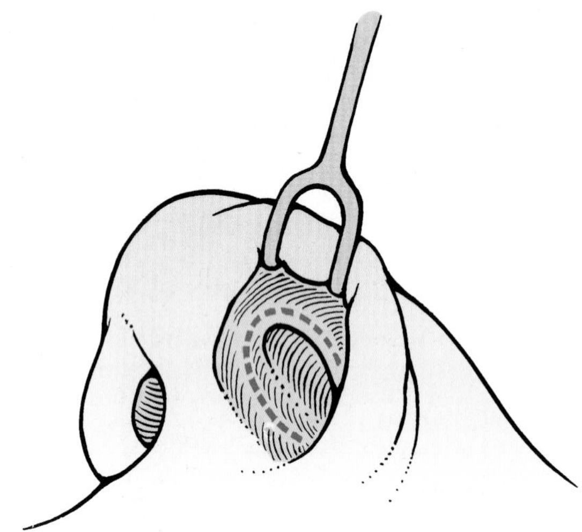

FIGURE 26-16 Intercartilaginous incision of the left side.

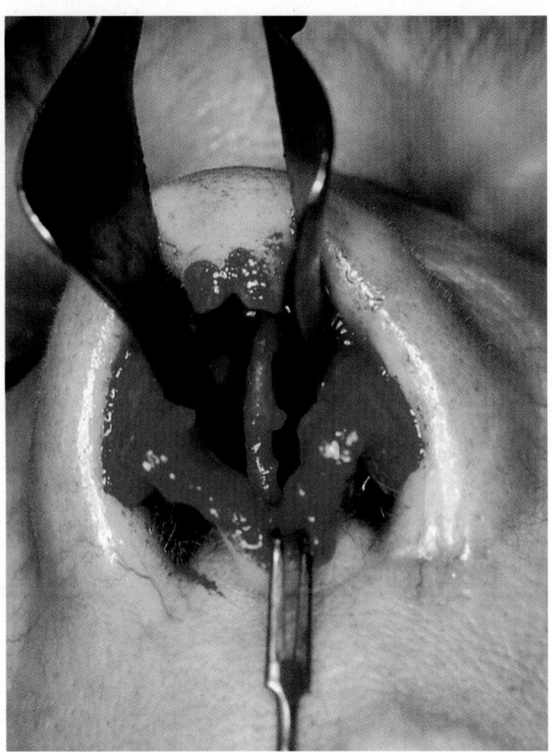

FIGURE 26-17 Open rhinoplasty with nasal speculum in place showing nasal septum and lower lateral cartilages.

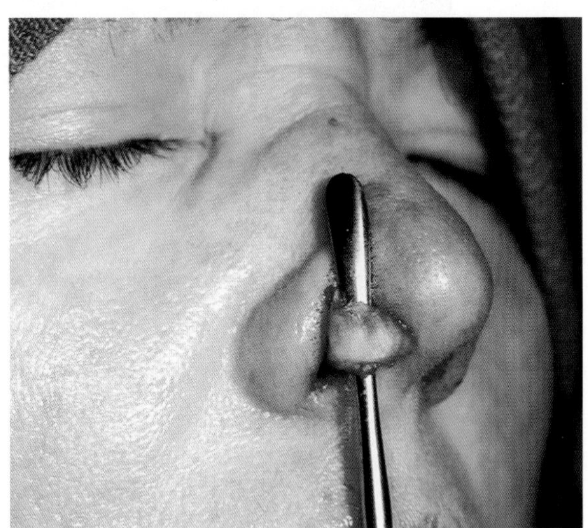

FIGURE 26-18 Delivery of right lower lateral cartilage for trimming in a "closed rhinoplasty."

after forehead lifts and face-lifts and blepharoplasties to achieve even more dramatic results.

Skin resurfacing collectively refers to chemical peels, dermabrasion, or laser skin resurfacing. Chemical peels use agents such as trichloroacetic acid, glycolic acid, or phenol. These chemicals cause the old superficial skin to peel off as if it were sunburned. This occurs after the new skin has reformed beneath the more superficial sloughing layers. Dermabrasion is a mechanical sanding performed with a diamond wheel or small wire wheel. Laser resurfacing vaporizes the skin and superficial layer of the dermis, usually with a carbon dioxide or erbium laser. Dermabrasion and laser have the advantage of recontouring irregular skin surfaces, such as traumatic or acne scars.

The chemical peel or laser or mechanical dermabrader typically penetrates from the papillary to midreticular layer of the skin (Fig. 26-21). The newly formed epithelium arises from the pores of the preserved deeper pilosebaceous units (i.e., hair, sebum, and sweat glands). The skin from these areas sprouts outward over the fresh, smooth, tightened surface. Surgeons frequently combine peeling with laser or dermabrasion on the same patient.

After the skin-resurfacing procedures are completed, various facial dressings are used to protect the skin during healing. The skin is healed or resurfaced in 5 to 14 days, depending on the

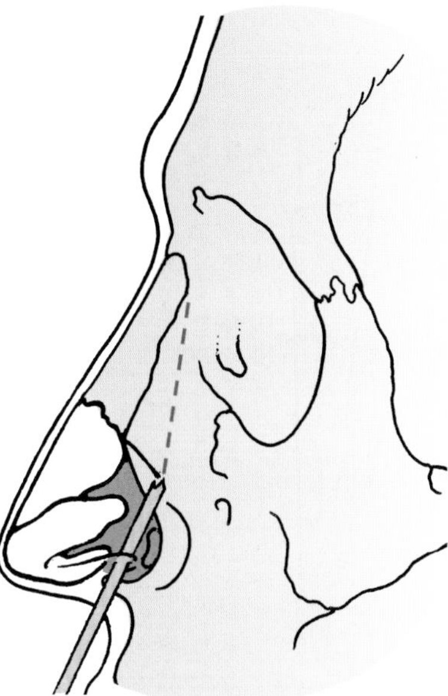

FIGURE 26-19 Lateral nasal osteotomy (*dotted line*) performed with an osteotome from the bony piriform rim to the proximal edge of the nasal bone. The nasal bones are then infractured, which narrows the nasal dorsum.

method used and the depth of the treatment. The new, more youthful skin is tighter, smoother, and less irregularly pigmented. The tightening is due to new collagen formation within the dermis. The color of the fresh skin progresses from red to pink and returns to normal as it fully matures in 2 to 3 months. Makeup can be used after initial healing to camouflage the fading erythema.

Possible complications of these procedures include hyperpigmentation with postoperative sun exposure, hypopigmentation, hypertrophic scarring, and infection (Fig. 26-22).[11,12]

Facial Liposuction

Facial liposuction is used to reduce submental and neck fullness. These excessive fat deposits are typically located superficial to the platysma. This can be detected by having patients "tense their neck" or attempt to move their chin inferiorly against finger resistance and then gently grasping the submental area or neck fold with the thumb and forefinger (i.e., pinch test). The purpose of liposuction is to remove the underlying coalesced fatty deposits, allowing the overlying skin to redrape over a newly formed neckline. This occurs partially because of the direct removal of fat. Further "shrinkage" of fat deposits occurs as a result of circumferential scarring of the fat as a result of instrumentation with the suction cannula during fat removal. Younger patients often have facial liposuction as a single procedure because they have good skin tone that redrapes and adapts well. Older patients with skin laxity can also benefit from facial liposuction but often also need additional face-lift and neck lift surgery to tighten the skin or a platysmal muscle plication (i.e., corsetlike tightening by suturing techniques) to repair or tighten a central platysmal dehiscence. Only small incisions are necessary under the chin or behind the ear lobes to reach the entire neck. The fat is removed using a tubular cannula under vacuum suction (Fig. 26-23).

After surgery a tight pressure dressing is applied to eliminate dead space and allow overlying skin to adapt closely to underlying soft tissue. Surgical recovery is 7 to 10 days, but 3 to 6 months are needed for the final results to be fully appreciated. This delay is due to the gradual process of remaining fat atrophy, remodeling, and skin tightening (Fig. 26-24).[13,14] Potential complications include uneven contours, infection, or marginal mandibular nerve injury (i.e., facial nerve motor branch).

Cheek Augmentation

Cheek augmentation provides for higher, more defined, prominent cheek bones and more youthful cheek fullness. Cheek augmentation is usually accomplished using a synthetic or

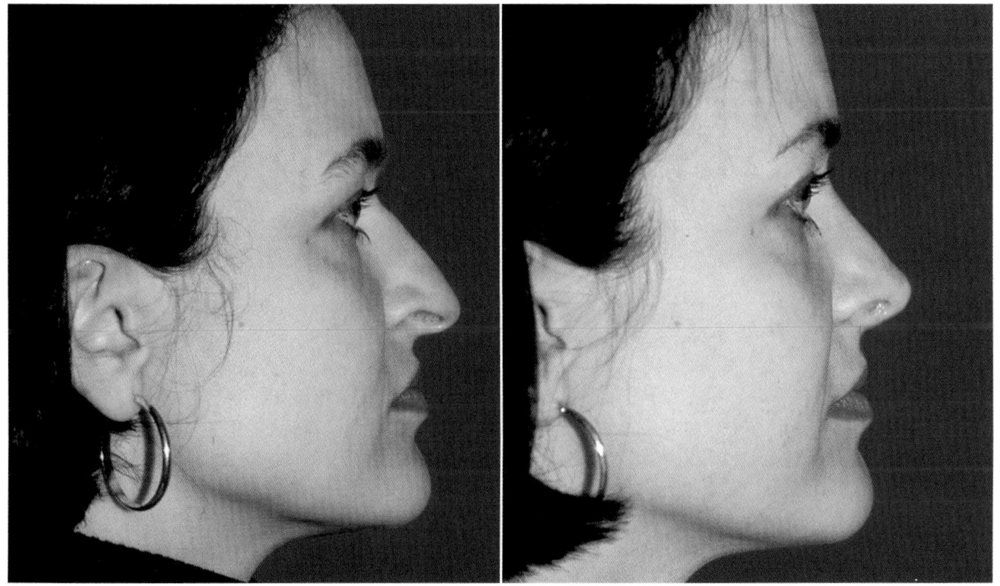

FIGURE 26-20 Rhinoplasty patient. A, Preoperative. B, Postoperative. View after dorsal hump reduction and tip elevation.

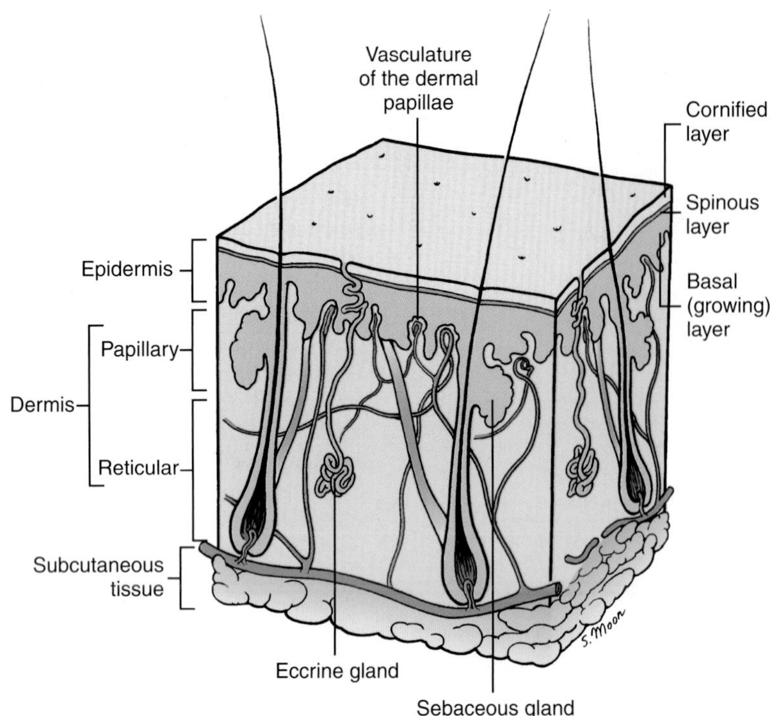

FIGURE 26-21 Cross-sectional anatomy of the skin layers.

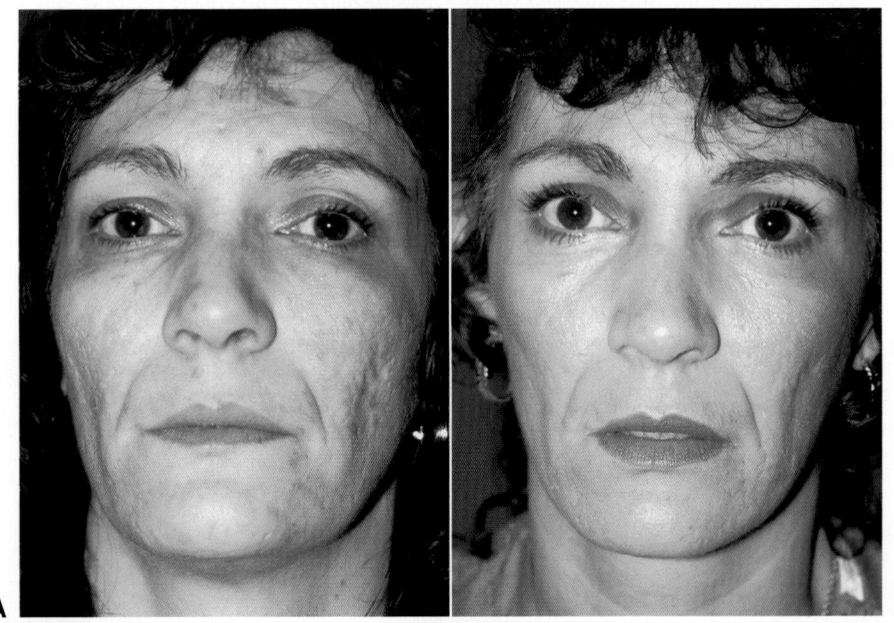

FIGURE 26-22 Laser skin resurfacing. The patient had acne scarring and rough skin texture. A, Preoperative. B, Postoperative.

alloplastic implant placed through a maxillary vestibular incision. The malar or cheek implants are supplied precontoured by the manufacturers and are available in varying sizes, thicknesses, and configurations (Fig. 26-25). These implants can also be custom made from three-dimensional models of the patient's facial bone structure made from reconstructed computed tomography scans. The surgeon selects the implants based on the patient's existing anatomy and desired result. Generally, the implants are partially malleable and can be custom contoured in situ and then stabilized with bone screws to the underling maxilla and zygoma or suture retained within the soft tissue pocket that has been created.

Surgical recovery is 1 to 2 weeks with final results fully appreciated in about 2 months.[15] Complications may include infection, overcontouring or undercontouring, or asymmetry. Transient infraorbital nerve paresthesia can be anticipated.

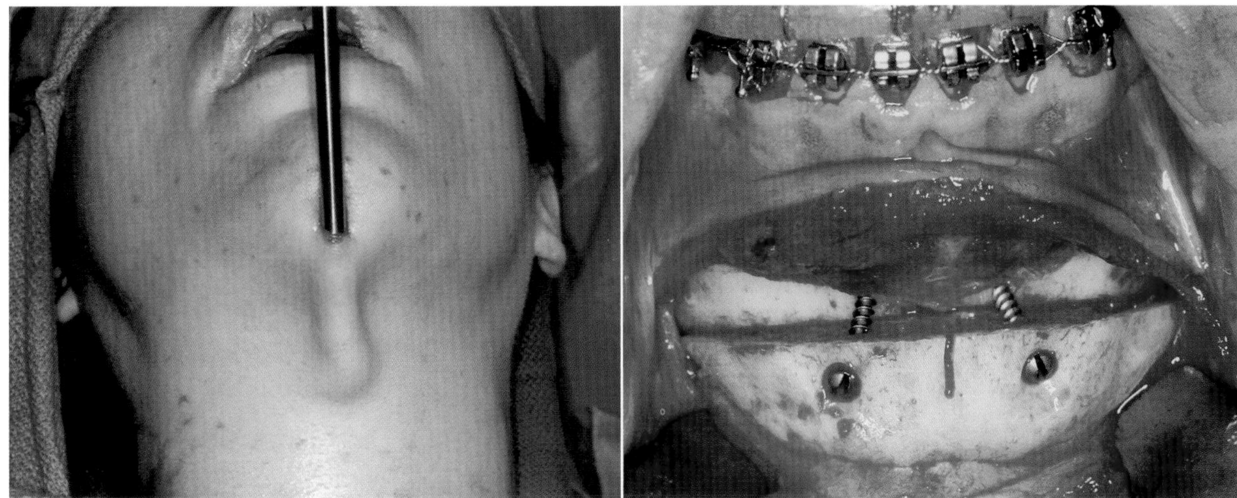

FIGURE 26-23 A, Submental liposuction with a cannula. B, Advancement genioplasty that can be done simultaneously with submental liposuction to enhance further the submental cervical form and definition.

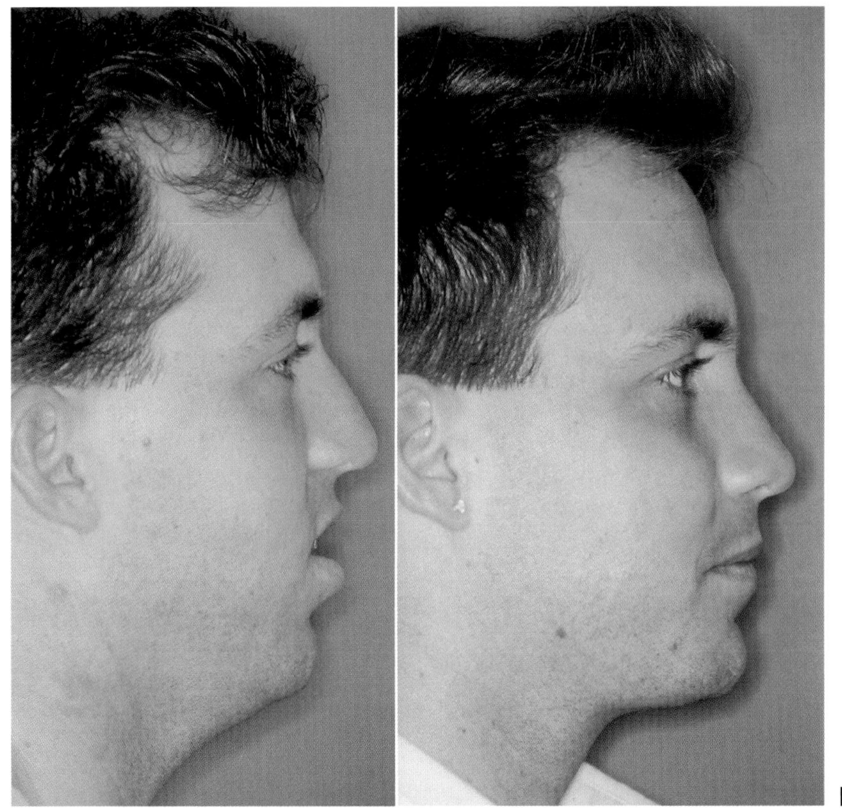

FIGURE 26-24 Submental liposuction and advancement genioplasty (8 mm). A, Preoperative profile view. B, Postoperative profile view.

Chin Augmentation or Reduction

Chin projection and contour influences neck definition and nasal size appearance. Noses look larger if the chin is recessive and necklines are more defined with a more prominent chin. Decisions to augment or reduce the chin are decided by evaluating the facial proportions, similar to the treatment planning that takes place with orthognathic surgery or a patient undergoing comprehensive prosthetic rehabilitation that alters the vertical dimension.

Augmentation of the chin can be performed using alloplastic implants or by advancement of the inferior border of the mandible (i.e., genioplasty) (see Fig. 26-23, *B*). Advancement genioplasty is discussed in Chapter 25. Alloplastic chin augmentation is not as popular with oral and maxillofacial surgeons because of lack of remodeling (i.e., edges may be felt), potential for underlying bone resorption, and increased risk of infection. Figure 26-26 demonstrates the use of an alloplastic implant for chin augmentation.

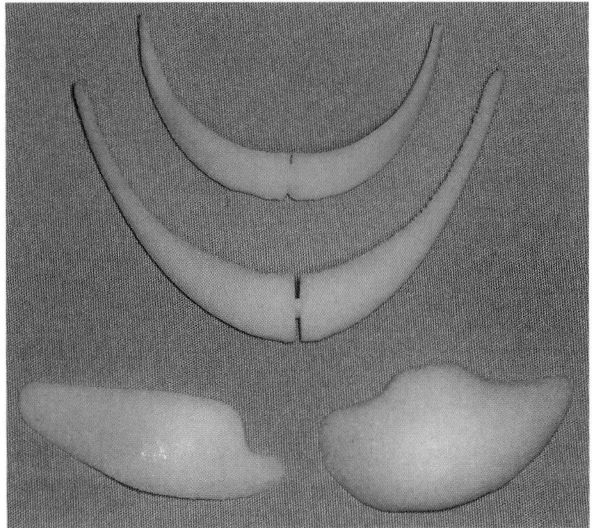

FIGURE 26-25 High-density porous polyethylene implants. Precontoured shapes for chin augmentation (*top, middle*) and cheek augmentation (*bottom, side by side*).

Simultaneous liposuction can enhance the esthetic results of chin advancements.

Potential genioplasty complications include infection and lip numbness. Recovery time is about 1 week, with the final result fully appreciated in about 6 weeks.[16,17]

Otoplasty

Otoplasty is altering the appearance of the ears. The most common ear deformity is overly prominent or protruding cupped ears. This deformity can be a source of awkwardness, especially in school-age children. Adults may also choose otoplasty for ear deformities not addressed while they were younger. Overly prominent ears are caused by hypertrophy of the conchal bowl cartilage (i.e., lower one half of the base) or lack of formation of the antihelical fold (Fig. 26-27, *A* and *B*).

Surgical correction involves exposing the ear cartilage through a postauricular incision. The cartilage is then partially excised or reshaped using cartilage scoring, sculpting techniques, and retention sutures (Fig. 26-27, *C* to *E*). A molded protective dressing is worn for 1 week, and the patient then uses a headband to protect the ears during sleeping for a number of months. Possible complications of otoplasty include infection, asymmetry, hematoma, and recurrence of the initial deformity.[18]

Lip Augmentation or Reduction

Lip augmentation can increase the thickness and vertical exposure of either the upper or lower lip. However, this procedure is most commonly performed on the upper lip to accent the perioral region. Generally, the lower lip is 30% larger in vertical dimension (i.e., vermilion to wet line) than the upper lip. Many methods for lip augmentation are available and include implantation of synthetic materials, bovine collagen, human cadaveric dermis, and autologous fat or dermis. Each material has its own advantages and disadvantages. The selected material is placed to plump the lip's central vermilion and to define the vermilion border (Fig. 26-28).

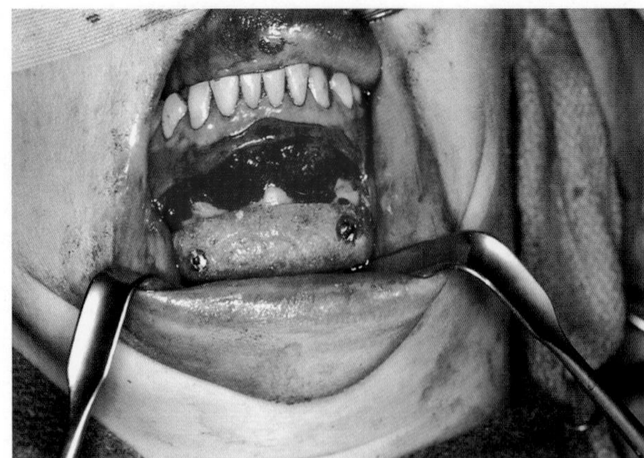

FIGURE 26-26 Placement and screw fixation of an alloplastic chin implant through a vestibular incision.

Although less commonly performed, lip reduction, or cheiloplasty, is also possible. Excess tissue is removed from the intraoral portion of the protuberant lip, and the lip mucosa is undermined and sutured in a more internally rotated position (Fig. 26-29). Recovery ranges from days to weeks, depending on the method used.[5]

Potential complications include infection, asymmetry, and overcorrection and undercorrection. Additionally, many of the natural materials placed in the lips resorb with time and may require further augmentation.

Botulinum Neurotoxin Therapy

Although first used for treatment of eye muscle spasms and eye muscle dysfunction, botulinum neurotoxin can also be used to reduce facial wrinkles of the forehead and the crow's-foot region (i.e., wrinkles emanating from the lateral canthus) around the eyes. Botulinum toxin is produced by the anaerobic microorganism *Clostridium botulinum* and is responsible for botulism food poisoning. The toxin blocks neurotransmitter release at the neuromuscular junction and thus temporarily paralyzes the muscle. The temporary paralysis creates long-term muscle weakness and atrophy. The most common region injected for facial rhytids is the forehead and glabellar region.

Very dilute doses can be safely injected with a 30-gauge needle selectively to paralyze specific facial muscles the animation of which has caused overlying skin wrinkles. The desired muscle paralysis occurs in 3 to 7 days and persists for 4 to 6 months (Fig. 26-30).

Retreatment with botulinum toxin injection may be necessary to further weaken or decrease muscle activity. Potential complications include diffusion into unintended muscles that can cause undesired eyebrow drooping or diplopia (i.e., double vision).[19,20]

Scar Revision

Facial scars can be caused by severe acne, facial trauma, or incisions needed for other surgery. Factors making scars noticeable include hypertrophy or keloids, uneven margins that cast shadows, color mismatch with surrounding skin, and tethering to underlying soft tissues that accentuates the scar during facial animation. Although a scar can never be totally eliminated, it can be altered and blended to significantly camouflage its appearance. Depending on the scar, it can be improved in

FIGURE 26-27 Teenage boy with prominent ears caused by conchal bowl hypertrophy. A, Preoperative frontal view. B, Postoperative frontal view. C, Lateral view of right ear before surgery. D, Postauricular dissection with excess cartilage removed. E, Sterile cotton roll sutured into place to bolster the shape and serve as part of the pressure dressing.

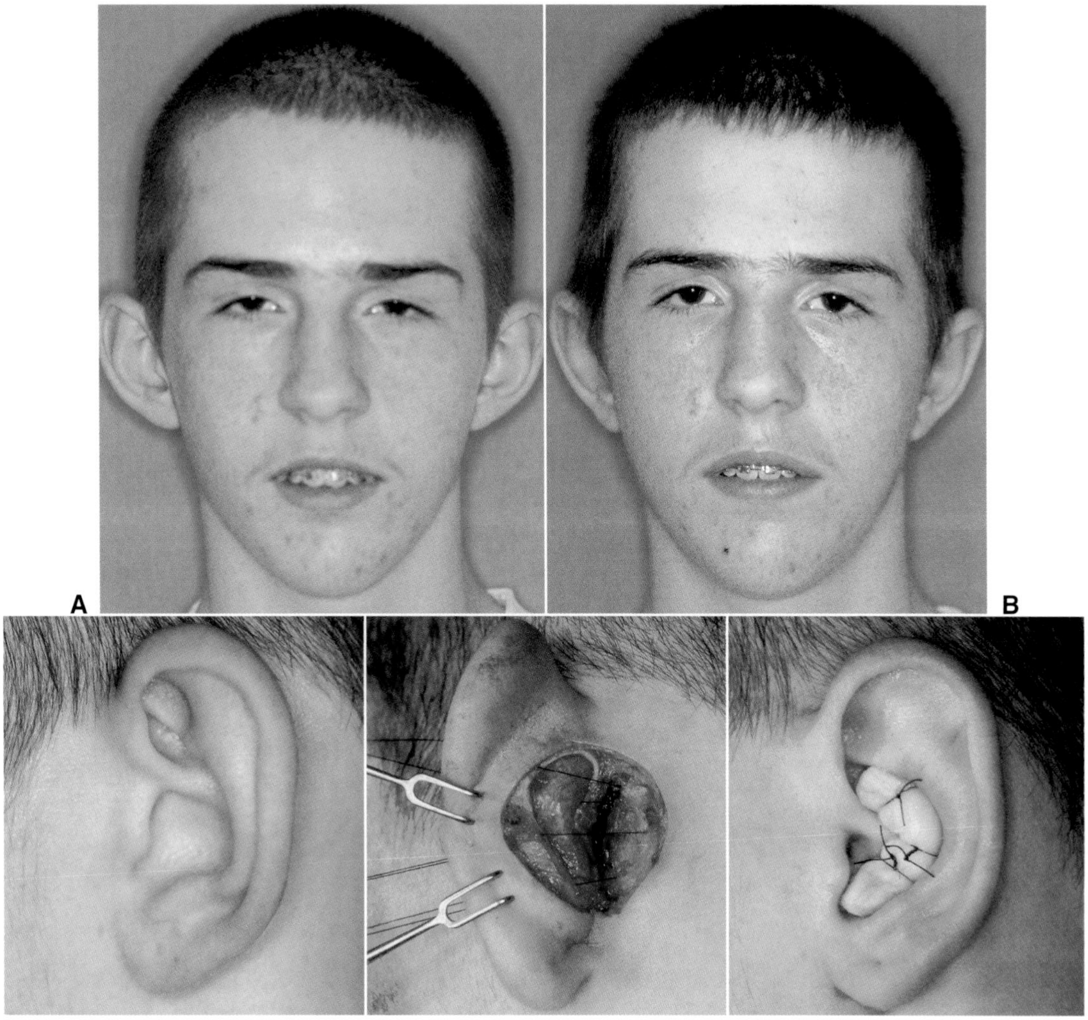

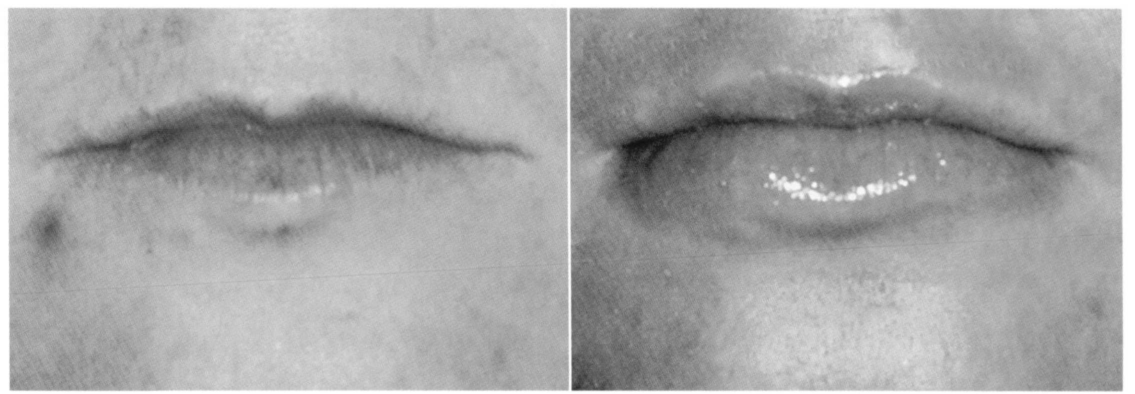

FIGURE 26-28 Lip augmentation. A, Preoperative view. B, Postoperative photo. Note the increased vertical dimension of the upper lip. (Photos courtesy Dr. Todd Owsley.)

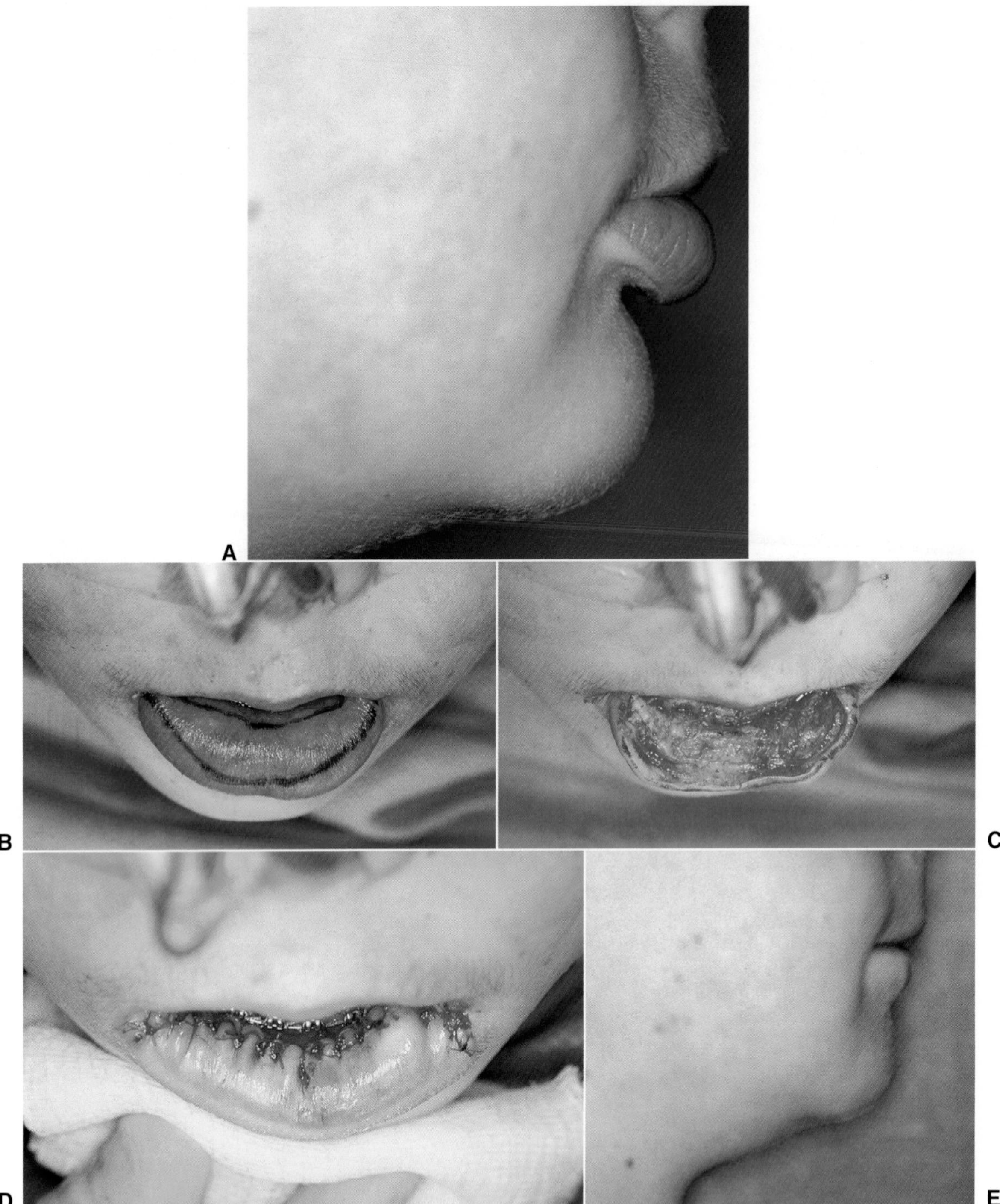

FIGURE 26-29 A, Profile view of severe protrusion/eversion of lower lip. B, Outline of mucosal tissue to be removed. C, Surgical site after excision of mucosa. D, Wound closure. E, Postoperative profile view showing improved lip position.

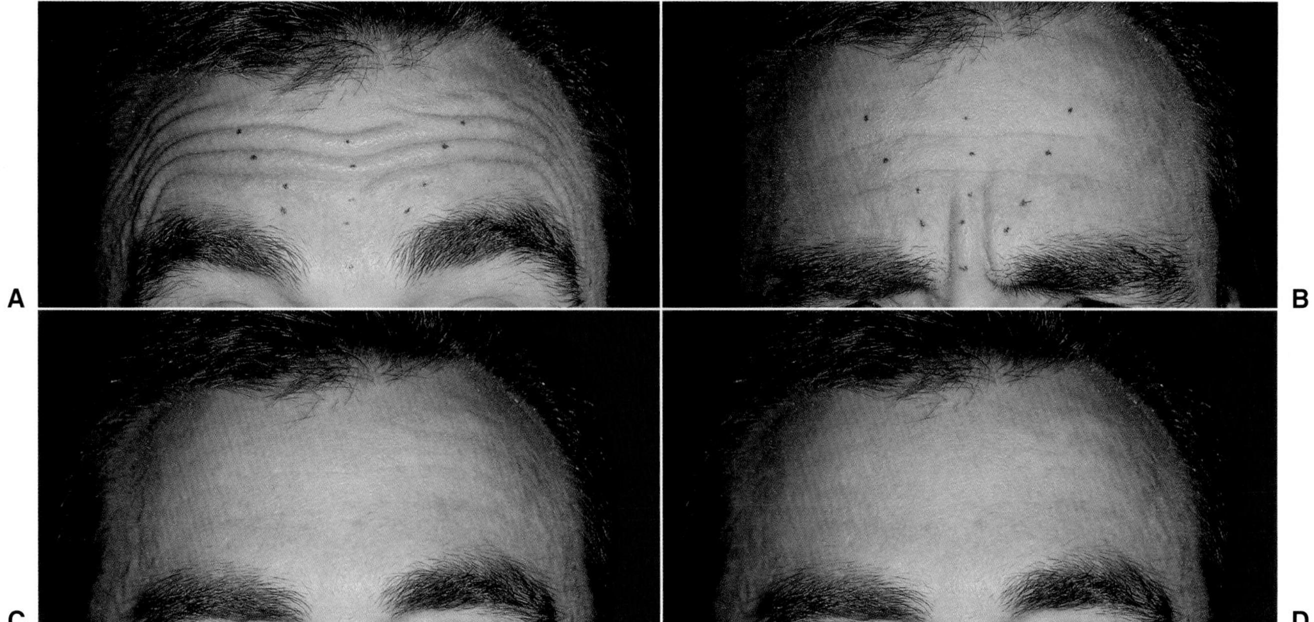

FIGURE 26-30 Botulinum toxin injection. **A**, Preoperative frontal view with eyebrows raised, accentuating heavy horizontal rhytids. Dots indicate planned injection sites. **B**, Forehead animated, causing vertical furrows in the glabellar region. **C**, Six weeks postinjection, showing residual upper forehead creases. **D**, Additional selective injection of the upper forehead yielded this 6-month postoperative result.

appearance by reexcision, altered by redirecting its alignment to better hide it in a natural facial crease, or blended with a skin-resurfacing procedure (Fig. 26-31). Recovery time varies with the extent of the scar and the method of treatment.[21,22] Possible complications include infection and hypertrophic scarring.

Hair Restoration

Although predominately associated with male pattern baldness, hair restoration can also be performed on women with alopecia. With improvement of surgical techniques that avoid a "plugged" appearance, hair restoration has increased in popularity.

Hair follicles are harvested from the posterior scalp below the vertex and are prepared into micrografts and minigrafts of one to four hairs per graft (Fig. 26-32). The grafts are then meticulously placed into the desired locations to restore the hairline. Preoperative planning is important to avoid an inappropriate looking hairline as the patient ages, and to ensure that the patient has adequate hair density to obtain a good result. Surgical treatment may need to be performed in stages to complete the treatment plan. The grafted hair units are typically more resistant to the balding hormonal effects of testosterone and androgens.

Postoperative healing is complete in about 2 weeks, but the transplanted hairs do not begin to grow until about 3 months, and a final mature result is not achieved until 9 to 12 months after surgery (Fig. 26-33, *A* and *B*).[23,24] Complications can include infection, loss of preexisting hair, poor graft growth, inappropriate hairline placement, and scarring.

SUMMARY

The current demand for facial esthetic surgery and cosmetic dentistry will continue to grow in popularity. The magnitude and appropriateness of any given comprehensive esthetic treatment plan should be carefully considered by the patient and dentist before initiation of any phase of the treatment. The oral and maxillofacial surgeon, trained in esthetic procedures and working with dental practitioners, can enhance the overall final esthetic result, leading to increased patient satisfaction.

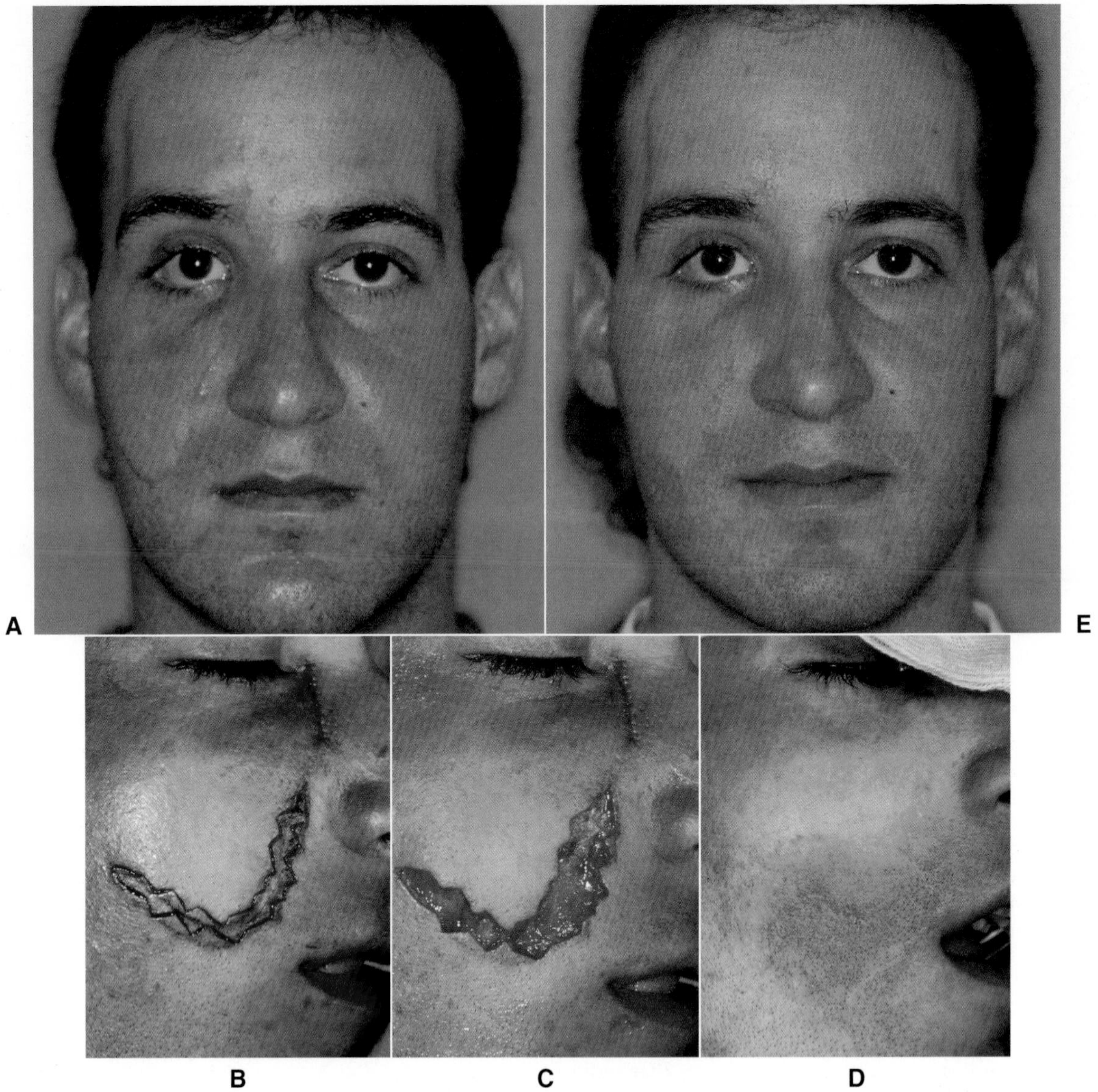

FIGURE 26-31 A, Patient who sustained multiple facial fractures and a full-thickness oblique laceration of the right cheek (has a tethered, thick, residual scar in this area). B, Intraoperative view of geometric outline. C, Excision of the scar that was undermined and sutured. D, Six weeks later the area was mechanically dermabraded. E, Postoperative appearance at 3 months.

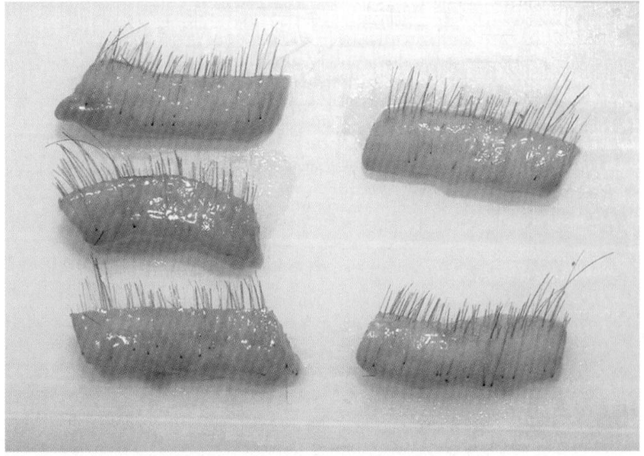

FIGURE 26-32 Harvested grafts from a strip of hair-bearing scalp.

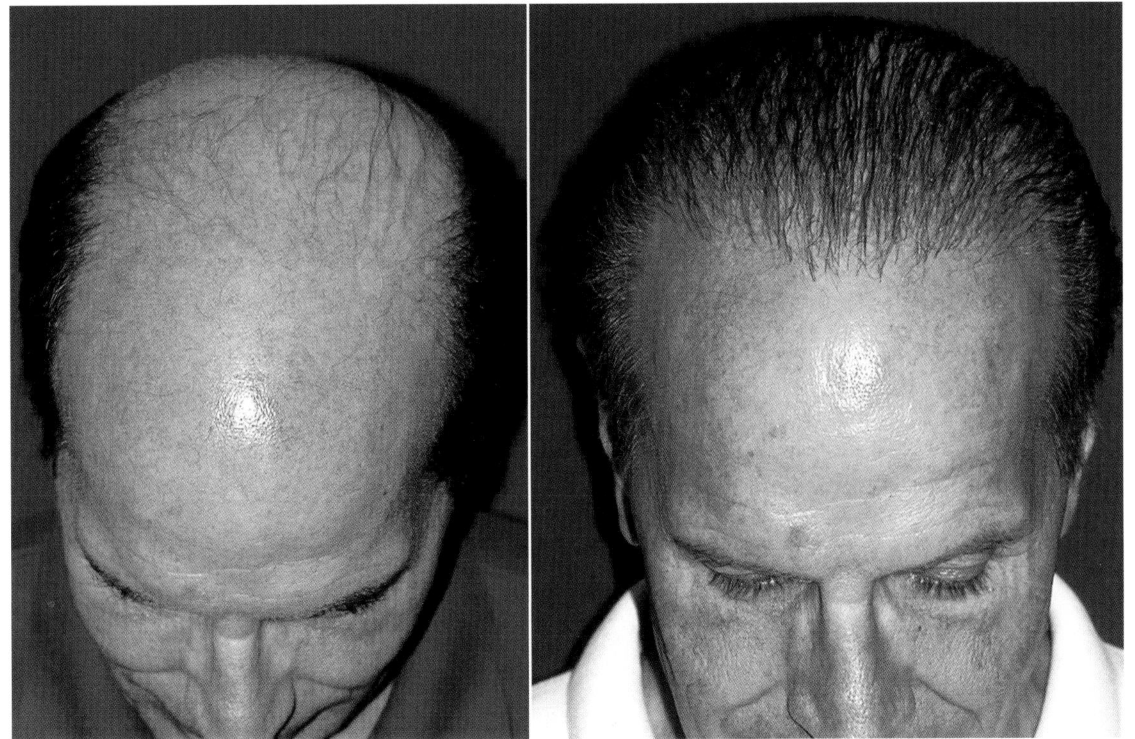

FIGURE 26-33 A, Preoperative view from above. B, Appearance after two surgical hair-grafting sessions and 6 months of graft maturation.

REFERENCES

1. von Soest T, Kvalem IL, Skolleborg KC et al: Psychosocial factors predicting the motivation to undergo cosmetic surgery, *Plast Reconstr Surg* 117:51, 2006.
2. Rankin M, Borah GL, Perry AW et al: Quality of life outcomes after cosmetic surgery, *Plast Reconstr Surg* 102:2139, 1998.
3. Rees TD, Liverett DM, Guy CL: The effect of cigarette smoking on skin flap survival in the facelift patient, *Plast Reconstr Surg* 73:911, 1984.
4. Rohrich RJ: Cosmetic surgery patients who smoke: should we operate? *Plast Reconstr Surg* 5:1137, 2000.
5. Niamtu J: Cosmetic oral and maxillofacial surgery options, *J Am Dent Assoc* 131:756, 2000.
6. Werther JR: Periorbital surgery as an adjunct to orthognathic surgery, *Atlas Oral Maxillofac Surg Clin North Am* 8:77, 1996.
7. Niamtu J: Endoscopic brow and forehead lift: a case for new technology, *J Oral Maxillofac Surg* 64:1129, 2006.
8. Alexander RW: Cosmetic alteration of the aging neck-rhytidectomy, *Atlas Oral Maxillofac Surg Clin North Am* 2:247, 1990.
9. Fulton JE, Saylan Z, Helton P et al: The S-lift facelift featuring the U-suture and the O-suture combined with skin resurfacing, *Dermatol Surg* 27:18, 2001.
10. Kuhn BS, Taylor CO: Rhinoplasty: contemporary management of the nasal tip, *J Oral Maxillofac Surg* 49:947, 1991.
11. Demas PN, Braun TW: Chemical skin resurfacing, *Atlas Oral Maxillofac Surg Clin North Am* 6:1, 1998.
12. Demas PN, Bridenstine JB, Braun TW: Pharmacology of agents used in the management of patients having skin resurfacing, *J Oral Maxillofac Surg* 55:1255, 1997.
13. Alexander RW: Liposculpture of the cervicofacial region, *Atlas Oral Maxillofac Surg Clin North Am* 6:73, 1998.
14. Ota BG: Cervicomental lipectomy as an adjunct to orthognathic surgery, *Atlas Oral Maxillofac Surg Clin North Am* 8:67, 1996.
15. Zide MF, Epker BN: Cosmetic augmentation of the cheeks: alloplasty, *Atlas Oral Maxillofac Surg Clin North Am* 2:359, 1990.
16. Strauss RA, Abubaker AO: Genioplasty: a case for advancement osteotomy, *J Oral Maxillofac Surg* 58:783, 2000.
17. Aziz SR, Ziccardi VB, Zweig BE: Biomaterials for post-traumatic maxillofacial reconstruction. In Fonseca RJ, Betts NJ, Barber HD, editors: *Oral and maxillofacial trauma,* ed. 3, Philadelphia, 2005, Elsevier Saunders, pp 1017-1033.
18. Donlon WC, Truta M: Simultaneous otoplasty and temporomandibular arthroplasty, *J Oral Maxillofac Surg* 50:951, 1992.
19. Niamtu J: Botulinum toxin A: a review of 1,085 oral and maxillofacial patient treatments, *J Oral Maxillofac Surg* 61:317, 2003.
20. Niamtu J: Aesthetic uses of botulinum toxin A, *J Oral Maxillofac Surg* 57:1228, 1999.
21. Horswell BB: Scar modification-techniques for revision and camouflage, *Atlas Oral Maxillofac Surg Clin North Am* 6:55, 1998.
22. Slavkin HC: The body's skin frontier and the challenges of wound healing: keloids, *J Am Dent Assoc* 131:362, 2000.
23. Hendler BH: Hair restoration surgery-hair transplantation and micrografting, *Atlas Oral Maxillofac Surg Clin North Am* 6:39, 1998.
24. Martin RJ, Mangubat EA: Hair transplantation: a review and case presentation, *J Oral Maxillofac Surg* 58:654, 2000.

CHAPTER 27

Management of Patients with Orofacial Clefts

EDWARD ELLIS III

CHAPTER OUTLINE

A cleft is a congenital abnormal space or gap in the upper lip, alveolus, or palate. The colloquial term for this condition is *harelip*. The use of this term should be discouraged because it carries demeaning connotations of inferiority. The more appropriate terms are *cleft lip, cleft palate,* or *cleft lip and palate.*

Clefts of the lip and palate are the most common serious congenital anomalies to affect the orofacial region. The initial appearance of clefts may be grotesque. Because clefts are deformities that can be seen, felt, and heard, they constitute a serious affliction to those who have them. Because of their location, clefts are deformities that involve the dental specialties throughout their protracted course of treatment. The general dentist will become involved in managing these patients' special dental needs because these patients may have partial anodontia and supernumerary teeth. Malocclusion is usually present, and orthodontic therapy with or without corrective jaw surgery is frequently indicated.

The occurrence of a cleft deformity is a source of considerable shock to the parents of an afflicted baby, and the most appropriate approach to the parents is one of informed explanation and reassurance. Parents should be told that the defects are correctable and need not adversely affect the child's future. However, parents should be prepared for a protracted course of therapy to correct the cleft deformities and to allow the individual to function with them.

The problems encountered in rehabilitation of patients with cleft deformities are unique. Treatment must address patient appearance, speech, hearing, mastication, and deglutition. A team manages most children currently affected with orofacial clefts.

Cleft teams are found in most cities of at least moderate size. These teams commonly comprise a general or pediatric dentist, an orthodontist, a prosthodontist, an oral and maxillofacial surgeon and a plastic surgeon, an audiologist, an otorhinolaryngologist, a pediatrician, a speech pathologist, a psychologist or psychiatrist, and a social worker. The number of specialists required reflects the number and complexity of the problems faced by individuals with orofacial clefts.

The occurrence of oral clefts in the United States has been estimated as 1 in 700 births.[1] Clefts exhibit interesting racial predilections, occurring less frequently in blacks but more so in Asians. Boys are affected by orofacial clefts more often than girls, by a ratio of 3:2. Cleft lip and palate (together) occurs about twice as often in boys as in girls, whereas isolated clefts of the palate (without cleft lip) occur slightly more often in girls.

Oral clefts commonly affect the lip, alveolar ridge, and hard and soft palates. Three fourths of clefts are unilateral deformities; one fourth are bilateral. The left side is involved more frequently than the right when the defect is unilateral. The cleft may be incomplete; that is, it may not extend the entire distance from lip to soft palate. Cleft lip may occur without clefting of the palate, and isolated cleft palate may occur without clefting of the lip (Fig. 27-1). A useful classification divides the anatomy into primary and secondary palates. The primary palate involves those structures anterior to the incisive foramen: the lip and alveolus; the secondary palate consists of those structures posterior to the incisive foramen: the hard and soft palates.[2] Thus an individual may have clefting of the primary palate, the secondary palate, or both (Fig. 27-2).

Clefts of the lip may range from a minute notch on the edge of the vermilion border to a wide cleft that extends into the nasal cavity and thus divides the nasal floor. Clefts of the soft palate may also show wide variations from a bifid uvula (Fig. 27-2, *D*) to a wide inoperable cleft. The bifid uvula is the most minor form of cleft palate, in which only the uvula is cleft. Submucosal clefts of the soft palate are occasionally seen. These clefts are also called *occult* clefts because they are not readily seen on cursory examination. The defect in such a cleft is a lack of continuity in the musculature of the soft palate. However, the nasal and oral mucosa is continuous and covers the muscular defect. To diagnose such a defect, the dentist inspects the soft palate while the patient says "ah." This action lifts the soft palate, and in individuals with submucosal palatal clefts, a furrow in the midline is seen where the muscular discontinuity is present. The dentist can also palpate the posterior aspect of the hard palate to detect the absence of the posterior nasal spine, which is characteristically absent in submucosal clefts. If a patient shows hypernasal speech without an obvious soft palatal cleft, the dentist should suspect a submucosal cleft of the soft palate.

EMBRYOLOGY

To understand the causes of oral clefts, a review of nose, lip, and palate embryology is necessary. The entire process takes place between the fifth and tenth weeks of fetal life.[3]

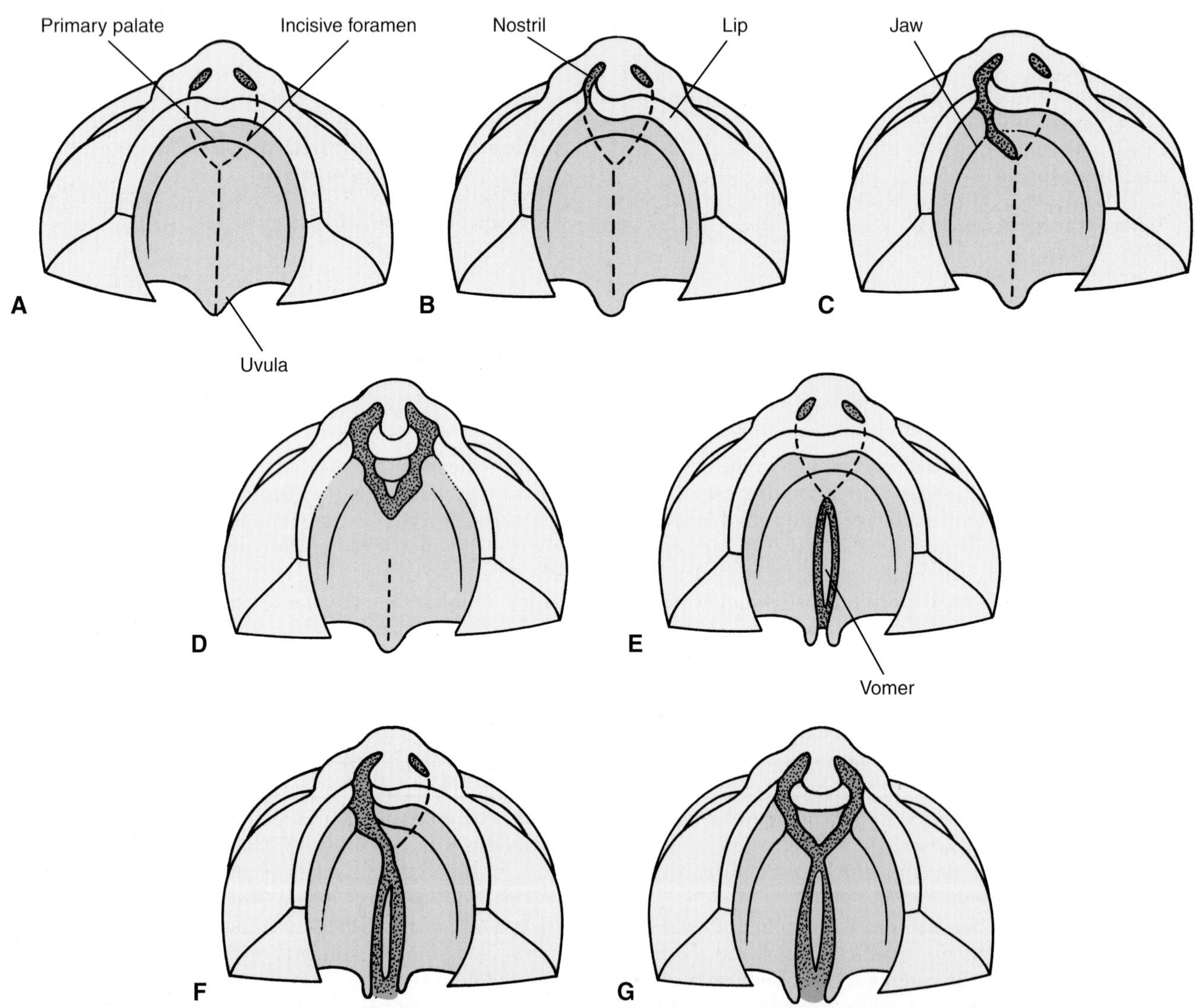

FIGURE 27-1 Ventral view of palate, lip, and nose showing variability of cleft lip and palate deformity. **A**, Normal. **B**, Unilateral cleft lip extending into nose. **C**, Unilateral cleft involving lip and alveolus, extending to incisive foramen. **D**, Bilateral cleft involving lip and alveolus. **E**, Isolated cleft palate. **F**, Cleft palate combined with unilateral cleft of alveolus and lip. **G**, Bilateral complete cleft of lip and palate. (From Langman J: *Medical embryology,* ed 3, Baltimore, 1975, Williams & Wilkins.)

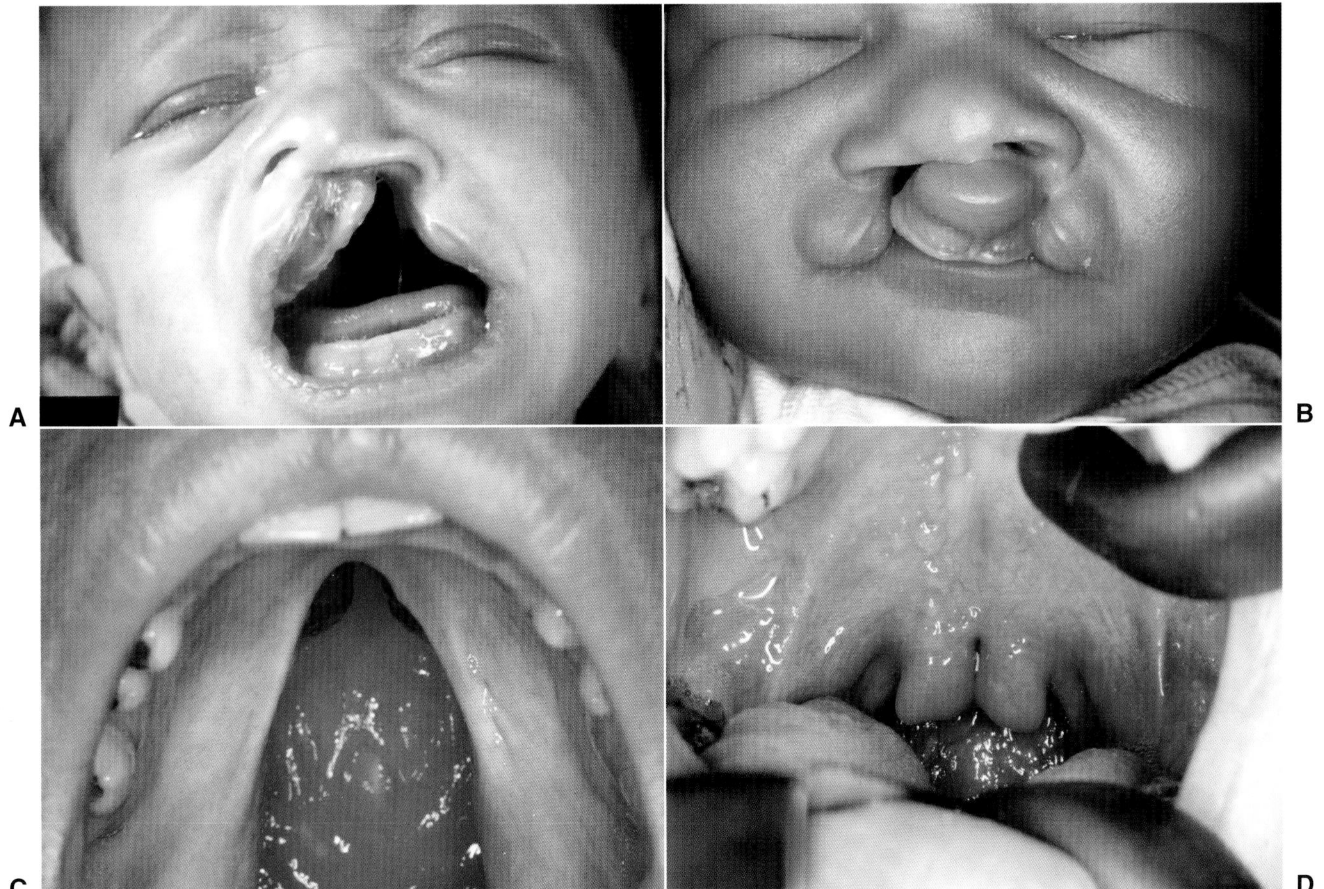

FIGURE 27-2 Photographs of various types of cleft deformities. Nasal deformities are also apparent. A, Unilateral complete cleft of lip and palate. B, Bilateral cleft lip and palate, complete on right, incomplete on left. C, Palatal view of isolated cleft palate. D, Bifid uvula.

During the fifth week, two fast-growing ridges, the *lateral* and *medial nasal swellings*, surround the nasal vestige (Fig. 27-3). The lateral swellings form the alae of the nose; the medial swellings give rise to four areas: (1) the middle portion of the nose, (2) the middle portion of the upper lip, (3) the middle portion of the maxilla, and (4) the entire *primary palate*. Simultaneously, the maxillary swellings approach the medial and lateral nasal swellings but remain separated from them by well-marked grooves.

During the next 2 weeks, the appearance of the face changes considerably. The maxillary swellings continue to grow in a medial direction and compress the medial nasal swellings toward the midline. Subsequently, these swellings simultaneously merge with each other and with the maxillary swellings laterally. Hence the upper lip is formed by the two medial nasal swellings and the two maxillary swellings.

The two medial swellings merge not only at the surface but also at the deeper level. The structures formed by the two merged swellings are known together as the *intermaxillary segment* (Fig. 27-4), which is composed of three components: (1) a labial component, which forms the philtrum of the upper lip; (2) an upper jaw component, which carries the four incisor teeth; and (3) a palatal component, which forms the triangular primary palate. Above, the intermaxillary segment is continuous with the nasal septum, which is formed by the frontal prominence.

Two shelflike outgrowths from the maxillary swellings form the secondary palate. These *palatine shelves* appear in the sixth week of development and are directed obliquely downward on either side of the tongue. In the seventh week, however, the palatine shelves ascend to attain a horizontal position above the tongue and fuse with each other, thereby forming the *secondary palate*. Anteriorly the shelves fuse with the triangular primary palate, and the incisive foramen is formed at this junction. At the same time, the nasal septum grows down and joins the superior surface of the newly formed palate. The palatine shelves fuse with each other and with the primary palate between the seventh and tenth weeks of development.

Clefts of the primary palate result from a failure of mesoderm to penetrate into the grooves between the medial nasal and maxillary processes, which prohibits their merging with one another. Clefts of the secondary palate are caused by a failure of the palatine shelves to fuse with one another. The causes for this are speculative and include failure of the tongue to descend into the oral cavity.

CAUSATIVE FACTORS

The causes of facial clefting have been extensively investigated. The exact cause of clefting is unknown in most cases. For most cleft conditions, no single factor can be identified as the cause.

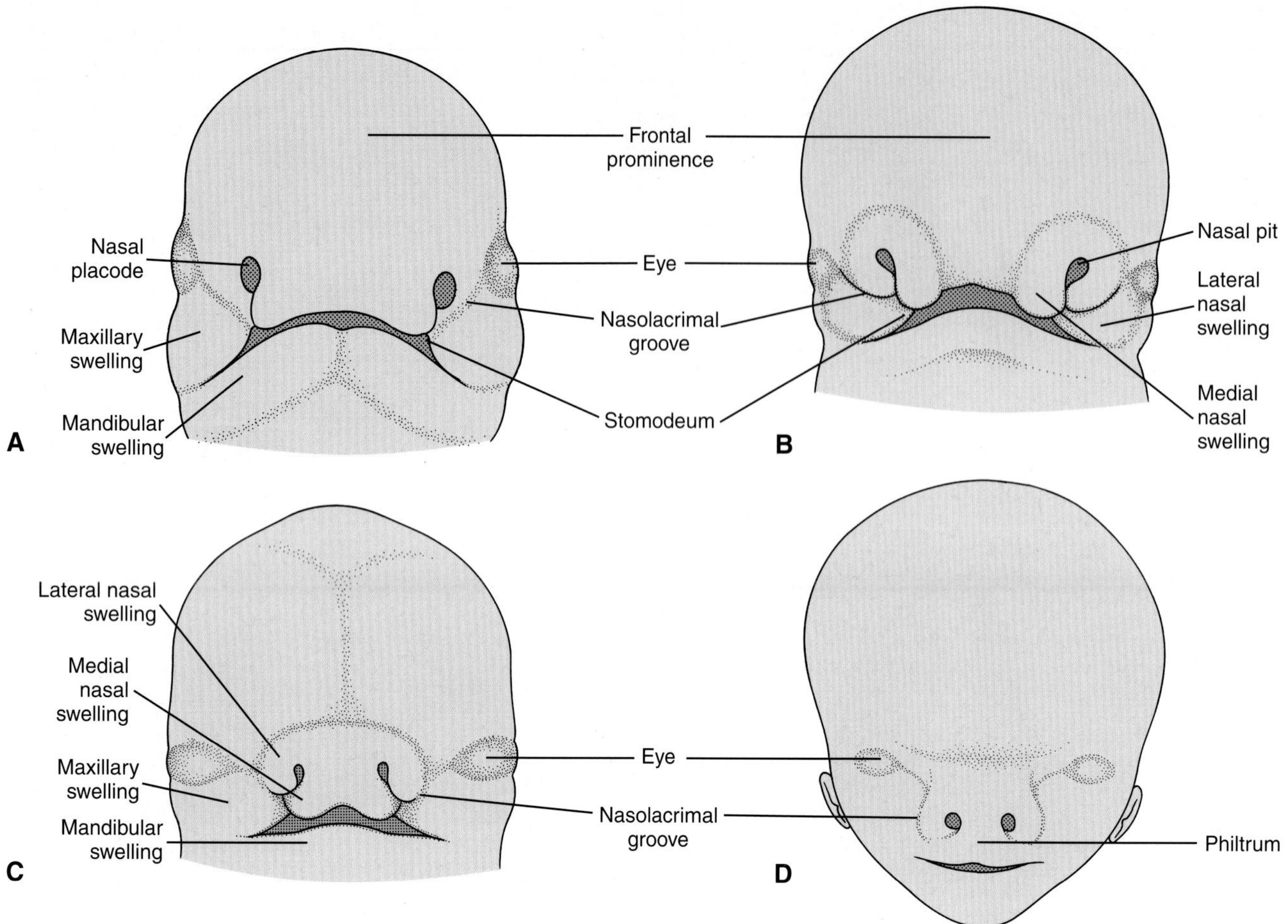

FIGURE 27-3 Frontal aspect of face. **A**, Five-week-old embryo. **B**, Six-week-old embryo. Nasal swellings are gradually separated from maxillary swelling by deep furrows. At no time during normal development does this tissue break down. **C**, Seven-week-old embryo. **D**, Ten-week-old embryo. Maxillary swellings gradually merge with nasal folds, and furrows are filled with mesenchyme. (From Langman J: *Medical embryology,* ed 3, Baltimore, 1975, Williams & Wilkins.)

However, it is important to distinguish between *isolated clefts* (in which the patient has no other related health problem) and *clefts associated with other birth disorders or syndromes.* A syndrome is a set of physical, developmental, and sometimes behavioral traits that occur together. Clefts have been identified as a feature in more than 300 syndromes, most of which are rare.[1] Syndromes account for approximately 15% of the total number of cases of cleft lip and cleft palate but nearly 50% of cases of isolated cleft palate. Medical geneticists are usually asked to consult with the family of children born with syndromes to identify the specific syndrome and to provide information to the parents about the likelihood of another child being affected.

For nonsyndromic clefts, it was initially thought that heredity played a significant role in the causation. However, studies have been able to implicate genetics in only 20% to 30% of patients with cleft lip or palate. Even in those individuals whose genetic backgrounds may verify familial tendencies for facial clefting, the mode of inheritance is not completely understood. The cause is not a simple case of mendelian dominant or recessive inheritance but is multigenetic. The majority of nonsyndromic clefts appear to be caused by an interaction between the individual's genes (i.e., genetic predisposition) and certain factors in the environment that may or may not be specifically identified.

Environmental factors seem to play a contributory role at the critical time of embryologic development when the lip and palatal halves are fusing. A host of environmental factors have been shown in experimental animals to result in clefting. Nutritional deficiencies, radiation, several drugs, hypoxia, viruses, and vitamin excesses or deficiencies can produce clefting in certain situations.

The risk for having another child with a cleft is based on a number of factors that are often unique in a particular family. These factors include the number of family members with clefts, how closely they are related, the race and sex of the affected individuals, and the type of cleft each person has. After a syndrome or complex disorder is excluded, recurrence risk counseling for a cleft can be offered to families. No genetic test can determine a person's individual chance of having a child with a cleft.

Every parent has approximately a 1 in 700 risk of having a child with a cleft. Once parents have a child with a cleft, the risk that the next child (and each succeeding child) will be affected is 2% to 5% (i.e., 2 to 5 chances in 100).[1] If more than

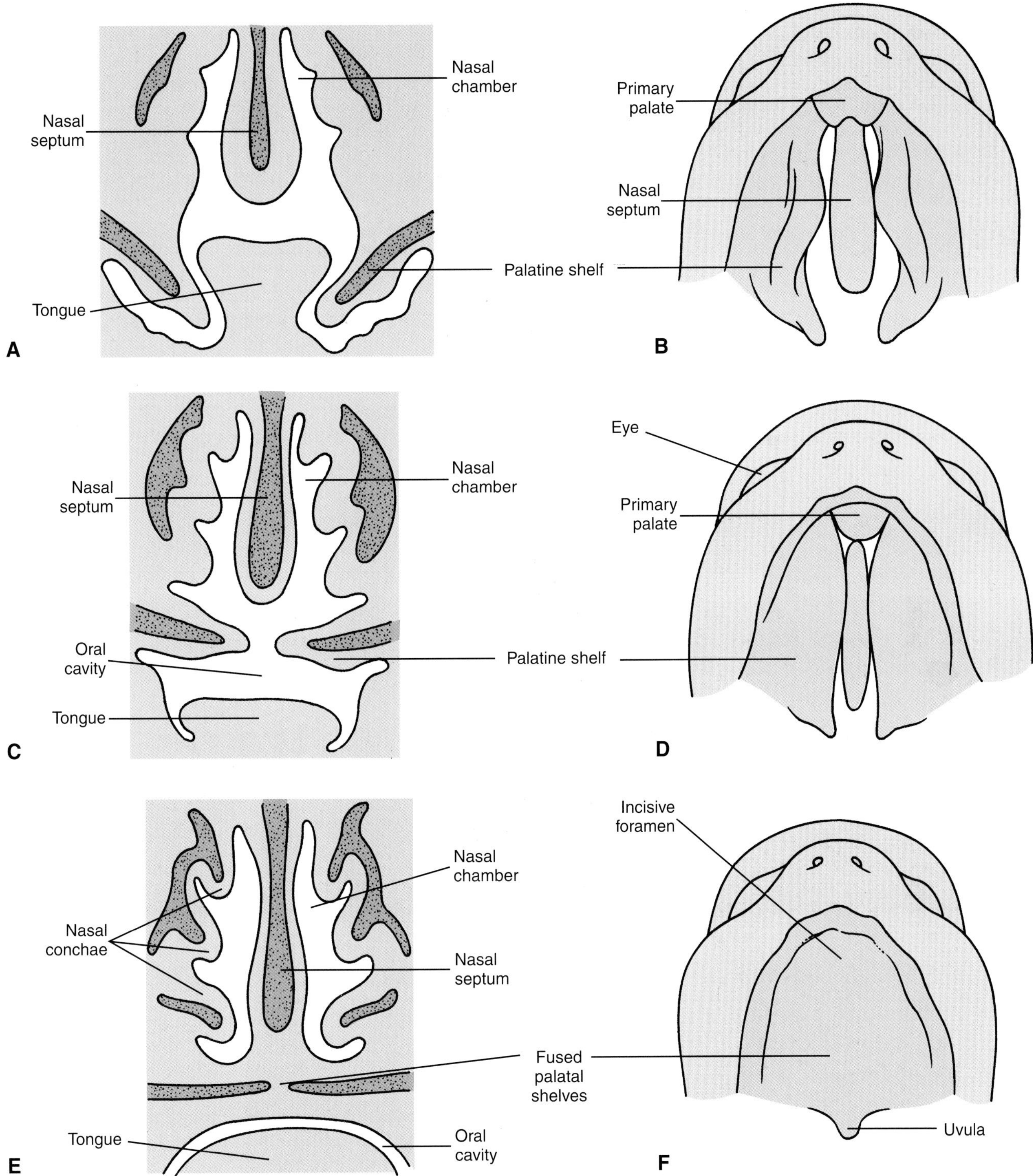

FIGURE 27-4 **A**, Frontal section through head of $6\frac{1}{2}$-week-old embryo. Palatine shelves are located in vertical position on each side of tongue. **B**, Ventral view of same. Note clefts between primary triangular palate and palatine shelves, which are still in vertical position. **C**, Frontal section through head of $7\frac{1}{2}$-week-old embryo. Tongue has moved downward, and palatine shelves have reached horizontal position. **D**, Ventral view of same. Shelves are in horizontal position. **E**, Frontal section through head of 10-week-old embryo. Two palatine shelves have fused with each other and with nasal septum. **F**, Ventral view of same. (From Langman J: *Medical embryology,* ed 3, Baltimore, 1975, Williams & Wilkins.)

one person in the immediate family has a cleft, the risk rises to 10% to 12% (i.e., roughly 1 chance in 10). A parent who has a cleft has a 2% to 5% chance that his or her child will have a cleft. If the parent with a cleft also has a close relative with a cleft, the risk increases to 10% to 12% for their child being born with a cleft. The unaffected siblings of a child with a cleft have an increased risk of having a child with a cleft (1% or 1 in 100, compared with 1 in 700 when no history of cleft exists). If a syndrome is involved, the risk for recurrence within a family can be as high as 50%.[1] Genetic counselors may be consulted for parents of children with clefts or for persons with clefts who would like to obtain more information on the relative risks for their offspring.

In summary, orofacial clefts are produced by incompletely understood mechanisms, genetic and environmental. With lack of complete knowledge of the causes, effective preventive measures, other than good prenatal practices (e.g., avoiding medications that are not absolutely necessary), are not available to prevent this deformity from developing.

PROBLEMS OF INDIVIDUALS WITH CLEFTS

Dental Problems

A cleft of the alveolus can often affect the development of the primary and permanent teeth and the jaw itself.[4] The most common problems may be related to congenital absence of teeth and, ironically, supernumerary teeth (Fig. 27-5). The cleft usually extends between the lateral incisor and canine area. These teeth, because of their proximity to the cleft, may be absent; when present, they may be severely displaced so that eruption into the cleft margin is common. These teeth may also be morphologically deformed or hypomineralized. Supernumerary teeth occur frequently, especially around the cleft margins. These teeth usually must be removed at some point during the child's development. However, these teeth may be retained if they can furnish any useful function in the patient's overall dental rehabilitation. Frequently, supernumerary teeth of the permanent dentition are left until 2 to 3 months before alveolar cleft bone grafting because these teeth, although non-

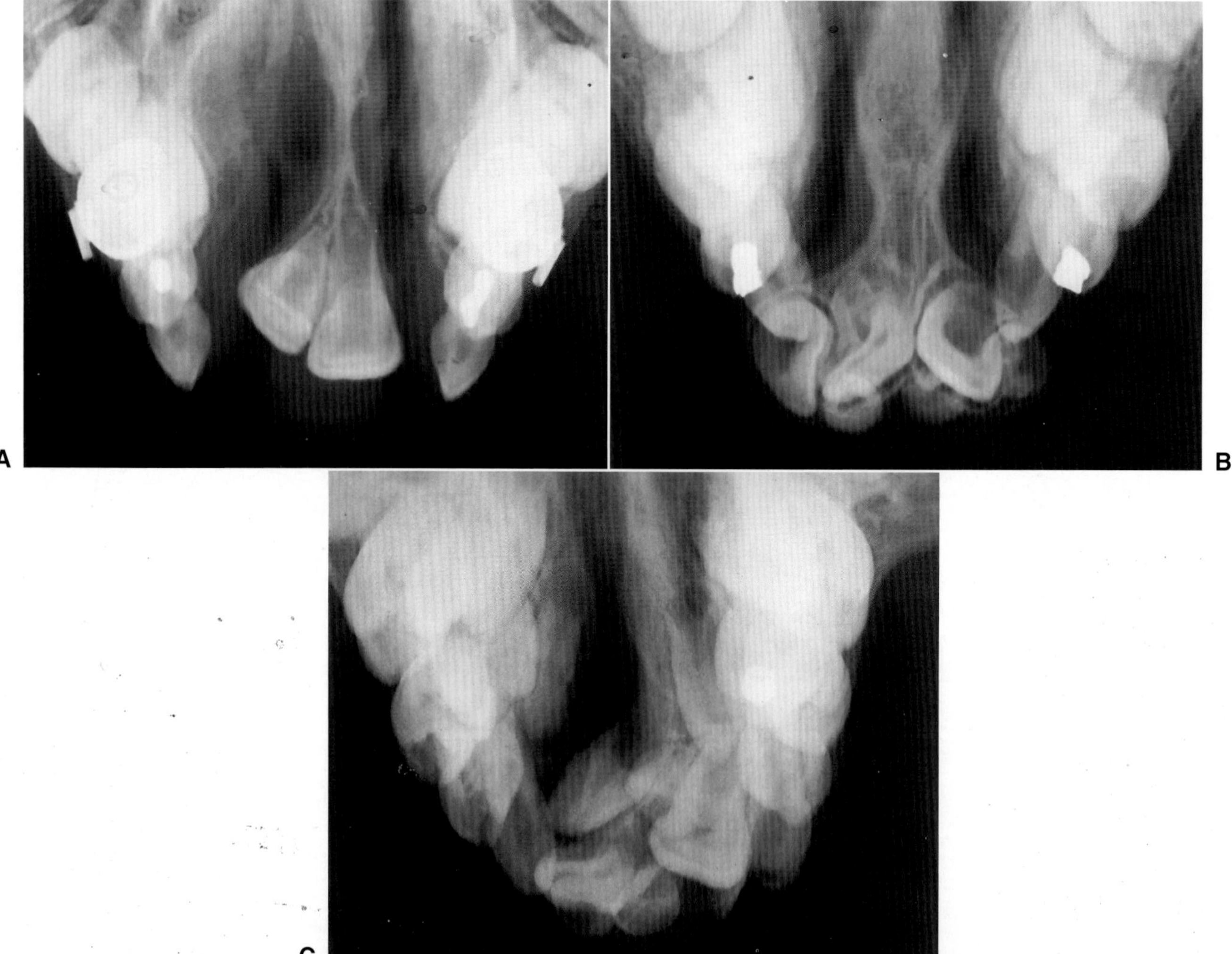

FIGURE 27-5 Occlusal radiographs from individuals with various types of cleft deformities. **A**, Bilateral complete cleft of alveolus and palate. Note absence of permanent lateral incisors. **B**, Bilateral complete cleft of alveolus and palate. Note absence of permanent lateral incisor on patient's left side. **C**, Unilateral complete cleft of alveolus and palate. Note supernumerary teeth within clefted area.

functional, maintain the surrounding alveolar bone. If extracted earlier, this bone may resorb, making the alveolar cleft larger.

Malocclusion

Individuals affected with cleft deformities, especially those of the palate, show skeletal discrepancies between the size, shape, and position of their jaws. Class III malocclusion, seen in most cases, is caused by many factors. A common finding is mandibular prognathism, which is frequently relative and is caused more by the retrusion of the maxilla than by protrusion of the mandible (i.e., pseudoprognathism; Fig. 27-6). Missing or extra teeth may partially contribute to the malocclusion. However, retardation of maxillary growth is the factor most responsible for the malocclusion. Generally, the operative trauma of the cleft closure and the resultant fibrosis (i.e., scar contracture) severely limit the amount of maxillary growth and development that can take place. The maxilla may be deficient in all three planes of space, with retrusion, constriction, and vertical underdevelopment common. Unilateral palatal clefts show collapse of the cleft side of the maxilla (i.e., the lesser segment) toward the center of the palate, which produces a narrow dental arch. Bilateral palatal clefts show collapse of all three segments or may have constriction of the posterior segments and protrusion of the anterior segment.

Orthodontic treatment may be necessary throughout the individual's childhood and adolescent years. Space maintenance and control is instituted during childhood. Appliances to maintain or increase the width of the dental arch are frequently used. This treatment is usually begun with the eruption of the first maxillary permanent molars.

Comprehensive orthodontic care is deferred until later, when most of the permanent teeth have erupted. Consideration for orthognathic surgical intervention for correction of skeletal discrepancies and occlusal disharmonies is frequently necessary at this time.

Nasal Deformity

Deformity of normal nasal architecture is commonly seen in individuals with cleft lips (see Fig. 27-2). If the cleft extends into the floor of the nose, the alar cartilage on that side is flared, and the columella of the nose is pulled toward the noncleft side. A lack of underlying bony support to the base of the nose compounds the problem.

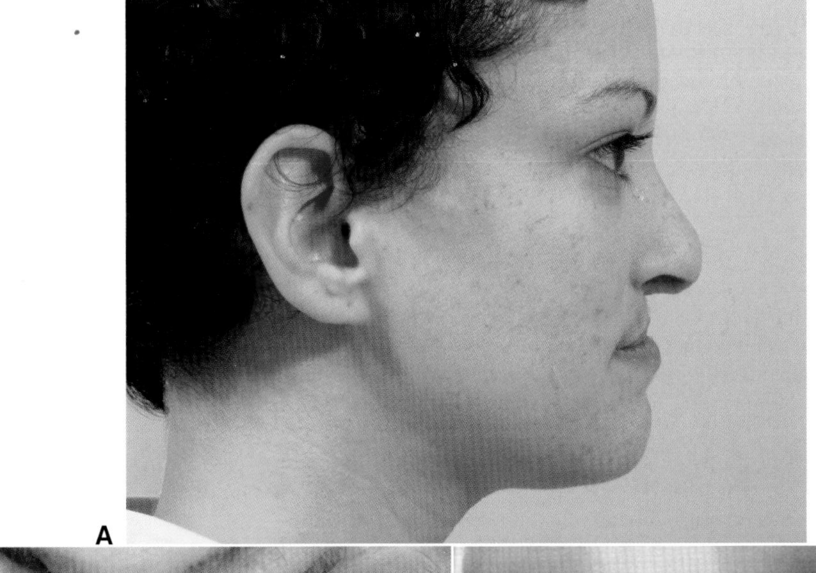

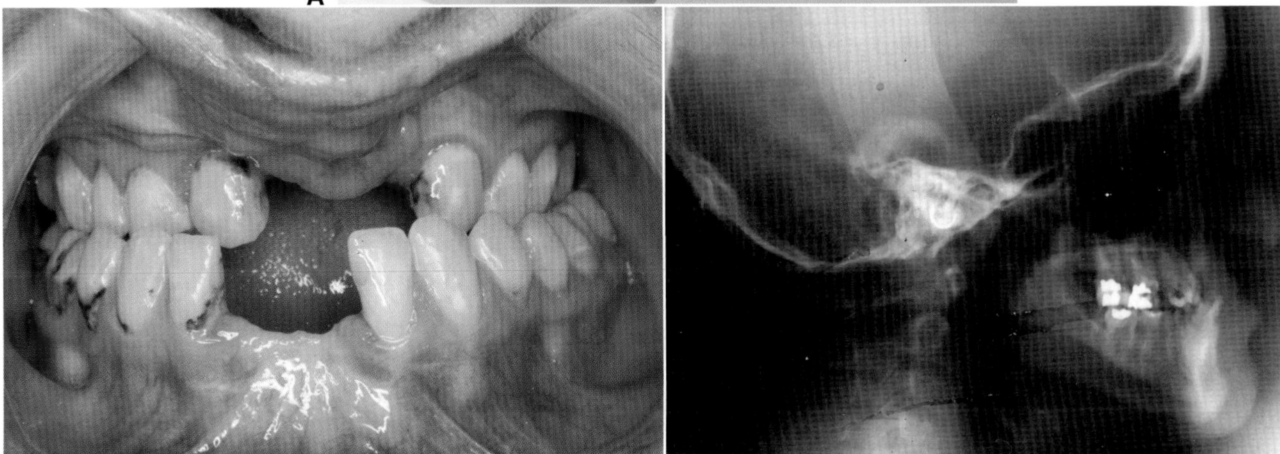

FIGURE 27-6 A, Facial profile of typical patient with a cleft. Note pseudoprognathic appearance of mandible. B, Occlusal relationship of patient showing Angle's Class III relationship with anterior crossbite. C, Lateral cephalogram showing maxillary skeletal sagittal deficiency contributing to Class III occlusal relationship.

Surgical correction of nasal deformities should usually be deferred until all clefts and associated problems have been corrected because correction of the alveolar cleft defect and the maxillary skeletal retrusion alters the osseous foundation of the nose. Improved changes in the nasal form therefore result from these osseous procedures. Thus nasal revision may be the last corrective surgical procedure the cleft-afflicted individual undergoes.

Feeding

Babies with cleft palates can swallow normally once the material being fed reaches the hypopharynx but have extreme difficulty producing the necessary negative pressure in their mouth to allow sucking breast or bottle milk. When a nipple is placed in the baby's mouth, he or she starts to suck just like any other newborn because the sucking and swallowing reflexes are normal. However, the musculature is undeveloped or not properly oriented to allow the sucking to be effective. This problem is easily overcome through the use of specially designed nipples that are elongated and extend further into the baby's mouth. The opening should be enlarged because the suck will not be as effective as in a normal baby. Other satisfactory methods are the use of eyedroppers or large syringes with rubber extension tubes connected to them. The tube is placed in the baby's mouth, and a small amount of solution is injected. These methods of feeding, while adequate for sustenance, require more time and care. Because the child will swallow a considerable amount of air when these feeding methods are used, the child is not usually fed while recumbent, and more frequent burping is necessary.

Ear Problems

Children with a cleft of the soft palate are predisposed to middle ear infections. The reason for this becomes clear on review of the anatomy of the soft palate musculature. The levator veli palatini and tensor veli palatini, which are normally inserted into the same muscles on the opposite side, are left unattached when the soft palate is cleft. These muscles have their origins directly on or near the auditory tube. These muscles allow opening of the ostium of this tube into the nasopharynx. This action is demonstrated when middle ear pressures are equalized by swallowing during changes in atmospheric pressure, as when ascending or descending in an airplane.

When this function is disrupted, the middle ear is essentially a closed space, without a drainage mechanism. Serous fluid may then accumulate and result in serous otitis media. Should bacteria find their way from the nasopharynx into the middle ear, an infection can develop (i.e., suppurative otitis media). To make matters worse, the auditory tube in infants is at an angle that does not promote dependent drainage. With age this angulation changes and allows more dependent drainage of the middle ear.

Children with cleft palate frequently need to have their middle ear "vented." The otorhinolaryngologist, who creates a hole through the inferior aspect of the tympanic membrane and inserts a small plastic tube, performs this procedure, which drains the ear to the outside instead of the nasopharynx (myringotomy).

Chronic serous otitis media is common among children with cleft palate, and multiple myringotomies are frequently necessary. Chronic serous otitis media presents a serious threat to hearing. Because of the chronic inflammation in the middle ear, hearing impairments are common in patients with cleft palate. The type of hearing loss experienced by the patient with cleft palate is conductive, meaning that the neural pathway to the brain continues to function normally. The defect in these instances is simply that sound cannot reach the auditory sensory organ as efficiently as it should because of the chronic inflammatory changes in the middle ear. However, if the problem is not corrected, permanent damage to the auditory sensory nerves (i.e., sensory neural loss) can also result. This type of damage is irreparable. The range of hearing impairment found in individuals with cleft palates is vast. The loss can be great enough so that normal-sounding speech is heard at less than one half of expected volume. In addition, certain sounds of speech (called *phonemes*), such as the *s*, *sh*, and *t* sounds, may be heard poorly. Audiograms are useful tools and are performed repeatedly on patients with cleft palates to monitor hearing ability and performance.

Speech Difficulties

Four speech problems are usually created by cleft lip and palate deformity. Retardation of consonant sounds (i.e., *p*, *b*, *t*, *d*, *k*, and *g*) is the most common finding. Because consonant sounds are necessary for the development of early vocabulary, much language activity is omitted. As a result, good sound discrimination is lacking by the time the palate is closed. Hypernasality is usual in the patient with a cleft of the soft palate and may remain after surgical correction. Dental malformation, malocclusion, and abnormal tongue placement may develop before the palate is closed and thus produce an articulation problem. Hearing problems contribute significantly to the many speech disorders common in patients with oral clefts.

In the normal individual, speech is created by the following scheme. Air is allowed to escape from the lungs, pass through the vocal cords, and enter the oral cavity. The position of the tongue, lips, lower jaw, and soft palate working together in a highly coordinated fashion results in the sounds of speech being produced. If the vocal cords are set into vibration while the airstream is passing between, then voice is superimposed on the speech sounds that result from the relationships of the oral structures. The soft palate is raised during speech production, preventing air from escaping through the nose.

For clear speech, it is necessary for the individual to have complete control of the passage of air from the oropharynx to the nasopharynx. The hard palate provides the partition between the nasal and oral cavities. The soft palate functions as an important valve to control the distribution of escaping air between the oropharynx and nasopharynx (Fig. 27-7). This is called the *velopharyngeal mechanism* (*velo* means *soft palate*). As the name implies, the two main components are (1) the soft palate and (2) the pharyngeal walls. When passive, the soft palate hangs downward toward the tongue, but during speech the muscles of the soft palate elevate it and draw it toward the posterior pharyngeal wall, which is what happens to the normal individual's soft palate when he or she is asked to say "ah." In normal speech, this action takes place rapidly and with an unbelievable complexity so that the valving mechanism can allow large amounts of air to escape into the nasopharynx or can limit the escape to none.

In individuals whose soft palate is cleft, the velopharyngeal mechanism cannot function because of the discontinuity of the

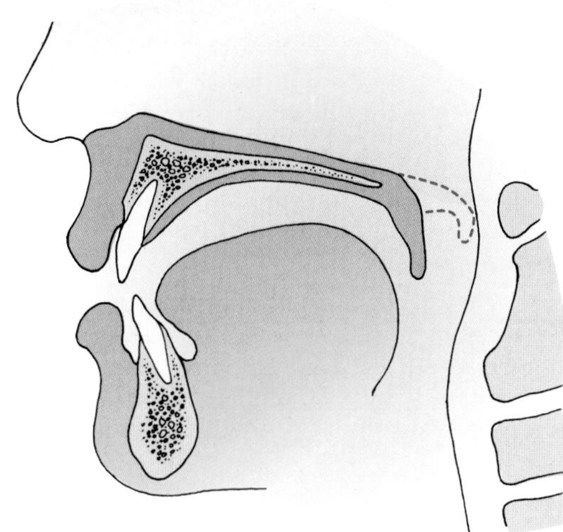

FIGURE 27-7 Upward and backward movement of soft palate during normal speech. Soft palate contact with posterior pharyngeal wall is shown.

musculature from one side to the other. The soft palate thus cannot elevate to make contact with the pharyngeal wall. The result of this constant escape of air into the nasal cavity is *hypernasal speech.*

Individuals with cleft palate have compensatory velopharyngeal, tongue, and nasal mechanisms in an attempt to produce intelligible speech. The posterior and lateral pharyngeal walls obtain great mobility and attempt to narrow the passageway between the oropharynx and nasopharynx during speech. A muscular bulge of the pharyngeal wall actually develops during attempts at closure of the passageway in some individuals with cleft palate and is known as *Passavant's ridge* or *bar.* Individuals with cleft palates develop compensatory tongue postures and positions during speech to help valve the air coming from the larynx into the pharyngeal areas. Similarly, the superficial muscles around the nose involved in facial expression are recruited to help limit the amount of air escaping from the nasal cavity. In this instance the valving is at the other end of the nasal cavity from the velopharyngeal mechanism. However, in an uncorrected cleft of the soft palate, it is literally impossible for compensatory mechanisms to produce a satisfactory velopharyngeal mechanism. Unfortunately, in surgically corrected soft palates, velopharyngeal competence is not always achieved with one operation, and secondary procedures are frequently necessary.

Speech pathologists are well versed in assisting children with cleft deformities to develop normal articulation skills. The earlier in life speech training is started in patients with cleft deformities, the better the eventual outcome. The patient may need to undergo speech counseling for several years to produce acceptable speech.

When hearing problems are also present, the speech problems are compounded. Hearing loss at an early age is especially detrimental to the development of normal speech skills. The child who is unable to hear is unable to imitate normal speech. Thus the parents must be cognizant of their child's development and ensure that regular visits to the pediatrician are undertaken.

Associated Anomalies

Although the child with an oral cleft is 20 times more likely to have another congenital anomaly than a normal child, no correlation is evident with specific anatomic zones of additional anomaly involvement.[2] Of those children who have associated anomalies, 38% have isolated cleft palate and 21% have cleft lip, with or without cleft palate. In the overall cleft-afflicted population, approximately 30% have other anomalies in addition to the facial cleft, ranging from clubfoot to neurologic disturbances. Of the overall cleft-afflicted population, 10% have congenital heart disease, and 10% have some degree of mental retardation. Thus the child with a facial cleft may require additional care beyond the scope of the cleft team.

TREATMENT OF CLEFT LIP AND PALATE

The aim of treatment of cleft lip and palate is to correct the cleft and associated problems surgically and thus hide the anomaly so that patients can lead normal lives. This correction involves surgically producing a face that does not attract attention, a vocal apparatus that permits intelligible speech, and a dentition that allows optimal function and esthetics. Operations begin early in life and may continue for several years. In view of the gross distortion of tissues surrounding the cleft, it is amazing that success is ever achieved. However, with modern anesthetic techniques, excellent pediatric care centers, and surgeons who have had a wealth of experience because of the frequency of the cleft deformity, acceptable results are commonplace.

Timing of Surgical Repair

The timing of the surgical repair has been and remains one of the most debated issues among surgeons, speech pathologists, audiologists, and orthodontists. To correct all of the defects as soon as the baby is able to withstand the surgical procedure is tempting. The parents of a child born with a facial cleft would certainly desire this mode of treatment, eliminating all of the baby's clefts as early in life as possible. Indeed, the cleft lip is usually corrected as early as possible. Most surgeons adhere to the proven "rule of 10" as determining when an otherwise healthy baby is fit for surgery (i.e., 10 weeks of age, 10 lb in body weight, and at least 10 g/dL hemoglobin in the blood). However, because surgical correction of the cleft is an elective procedure, if any other medical condition jeopardizes the health of the baby, the cleft surgery is postponed until medical risks are minimal.

Unfortunately, each possible advantage for closing a palatal cleft early in life has several possible disadvantages for the individual later in life. The six advantages for early closure of palatal defects are (1) better palatal and pharyngeal muscle development once repaired, (2) ease of feeding, (3) better development of phonation skills, (4) better auditory tube function, (5) better hygiene when the oral and nasal partition is competent, and (6) improved psychological state for parents and baby. The disadvantages of closing palatal clefts early in life are also several: The two most important are (1) surgical correction is more difficult in younger children with small structures, and (2) scar formation resulting from the surgery causes maxillary growth restriction.

Although different cleft teams time the surgical repair differently, a widely accepted principle is compromise. The lip is corrected as early as is medically possible. The soft palatal cleft is closed between 8 and 18 months of age, depending on a host of factors. Closure of the lip as early as possible is advantageous because it performs a favorable "molding" action on the distorted alveolus. Lip closure also assists the child in feeding and is of psychological benefit. The palatal cleft is closed next to produce a functional velopharyngeal mechanism when or before speech skills are developing. The hard palatal cleft occasionally is not repaired at the time of soft palate repair, especially if the cleft is wide. In such cases, the hard palate cleft is left open as long as possible so that maxillary growth proceeds as unimpeded as possible. Closure of the hard palatal cleft can be postponed at least until all of the deciduous dentition has erupted. This postponement facilitates the use of orthodontic appliances and allows more maxillary growth to occur before scarring from the surgery is induced. Because a significant portion of maxillary growth has already occurred by ages 4 to 5, closure of the hard palate at this time is usually performed before the child's enrollment in school. Removable palatal obturators can be fitted and worn in the meantime to partition the oral and nasal cavities.

The largest problem in evaluation of treatment regimens is the fact that the final results of surgical repair of clefts can only be judged conclusively when the individual's growth is complete. A surgical method used today cannot be put to careful scrutiny for 10 to 20 years, which, unfortunately, may allow many individuals with cleft deformities to be treated with procedures that may later be discarded, when follow-up examinations and studies show unsatisfactory or poor effects.

Cheilorrhaphy

Cheilorrhaphy is the surgical correction of the cleft lip deformity; this term is derived from *cheilo,* lip, and *rhaphy,* junction by a seam or suture. Cheilorrhaphy is usually the earliest operative procedure used to correct cleft deformities and is undertaken as soon as medically possible.

The cleft of the upper lip disrupts the important circumoral orbicularis oris musculature. The lack of continuity of this muscle allows the developing parts of the maxilla to grow in an uncoordinated manner so that the cleft in the alveolus is accentuated. At birth the alveolar process on the unaffected side may appear to protrude from the mouth. The lack of sphincteric muscle control from the orbicularis oris causes a bilateral cleft lip to exhibit a premaxilla that protrudes from the base of the nose and produces an unsightly appearance. Thus restoration of this muscular sphincter with lip repair has a favorable effect on the developing alveolar segments.

Objectives

The objectives of cheilorrhaphy are twofold: (1) functional and (2) esthetic. The cheilorrhaphy should restore the functional arrangement of the orbicularis oris musculature to reestablish the normal function of the upper lip. If muscle continuity is not restored across the area of the cleft, an esthetically unpleasing depression will result when the lip is brought into function. The second objective of cheilorrhaphy is to produce a lip that displays normal anatomic structures, such as a vermilion tubercle, Cupid's bow, and philtrum. The lip must be symmetric, well contoured, soft, and supple, and the scars must be inconspicuous. Another esthetic necessity is to correct (at least partially) the nasal deformity resulting from the cleft lip.

Despite the skill of the surgeon, these ideal objectives are rarely achieved. Hindrances are the poor quality of tissues in the cleft margins and the distortion of structures before surgical intervention. Several surgical techniques reproduce normal appearance immediately but do not maintain this appearance with growth. However, with careful selection of surgical technique, satisfactory results are obtainable.

Surgical Techniques

Because each cleft is unique, so must be the surgical procedure. Countless techniques can be used for cheilorrhaphy, each designed to elongate the cleft margins to facilitate closure (Figs. 27-8 and 27-9). In unilateral cases the unaffected side serves as a guide for lip length and symmetry. A key point in design is to break up lines of the scar so that with fibrosis and contracture, deformity of the lip is minimized. In lips closed in a linear fashion, scar contracture causes a characteristic notching of the upper lip. Attention to reorienting and reuniting the musculature of the lip is of paramount importance if normal function is to be established.

Cheilorrhaphy procedures serve to restore symmetry not only to the lip but also to the nasal tip. With the cleft extending through the floor of the nose, the continuity of the nasal apparatus is disrupted. Without the bony foundation for the alar cartilage, a collapse of the lateral aspect of the nose occurs. When the lip is closed, it is necessary to advance this laterally displaced tissue toward the midline. Thus cheilorrhaphy is the first and one of the most important steps in correcting the nasal deformity so common in patients with clefts.

Palatorrhaphy

Palatorrhaphy is usually performed in one operation, but occasionally it is performed in two. In two operations the soft palate closure (i.e., staphylorrhaphy) is usually performed first and the hard palate closure (i.e., uranorrhaphy) is performed second.

Objectives

The primary purpose of the cleft palate repair is to create a mechanism capable of speech and deglutition without significantly interfering with subsequent maxillary growth. Thus creation of a competent velopharyngeal mechanism and partitioning of the nasal and oral cavities are prerequisites to achieving these goals. The aim is to obtain a long and mobile soft palate capable of producing normal speech. Extensive stripping of soft tissues from bone creates more scar formation, which adversely affects maxillary growth. The precarious nature of the problem indicates the complexity of the surgical procedures designed and the ages at which they are instituted.

Surgical Techniques

Operative procedures for palatorrhaphy are as varied as techniques for cleft lip repair. Each cleft of the palate is unique. Repairs vary in width, completeness, amount of hard and soft tissue available, and palatal length. Thus the surgical techniques used to close cleft palate deformities are extremely varied, not just from one surgeon to another but from one patient to the next.

Hard Palate Closure

The hard palate is closed with soft tissues only. Usually no effort is made to create an osseous partition between the nasal

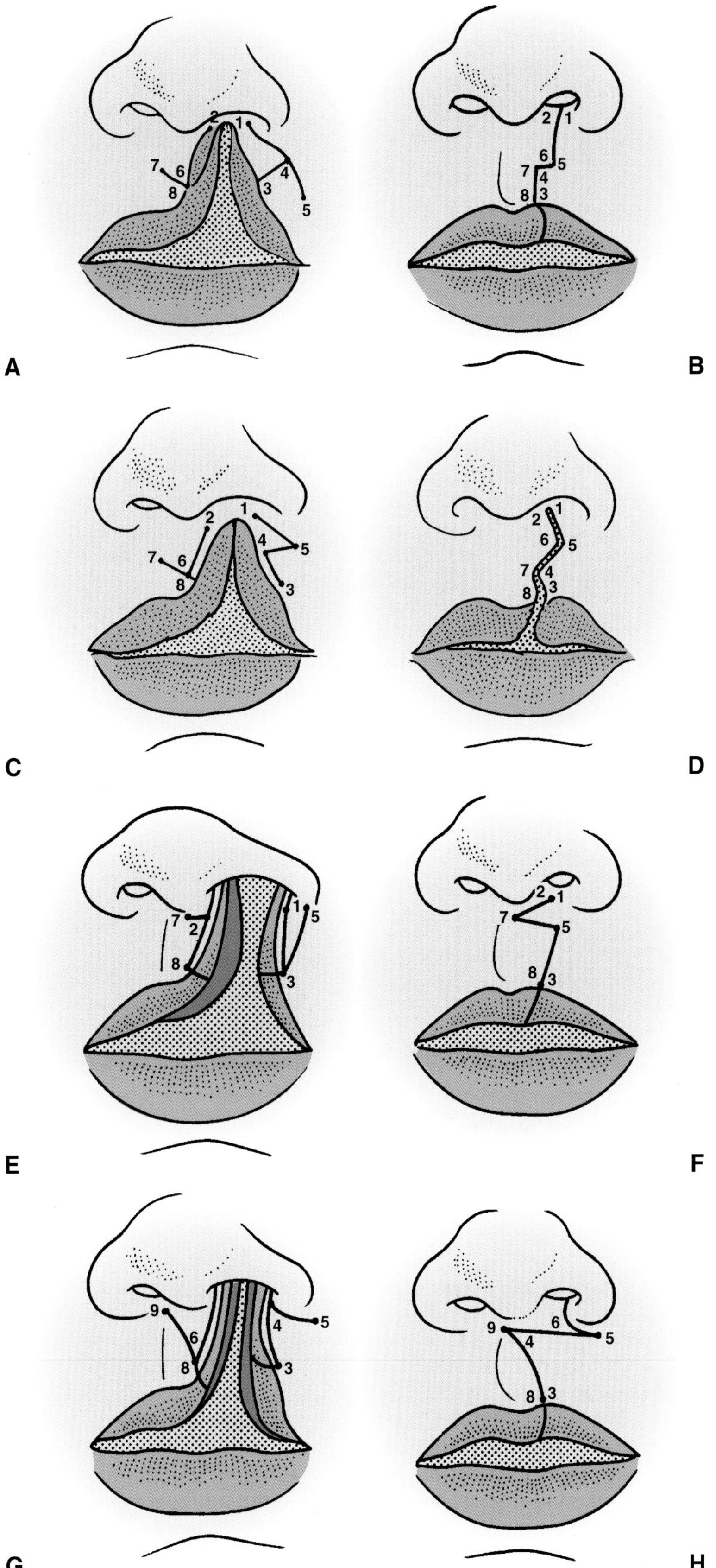

FIGURE 27-8 Several cheilorrhaphy techniques. A and B, Le Mesurier technique for incomplete unilateral cleft. C and D, Tennison operation. E and F, Wynn operation. G and H, Millard operation (i.e., rotation advancement technique).

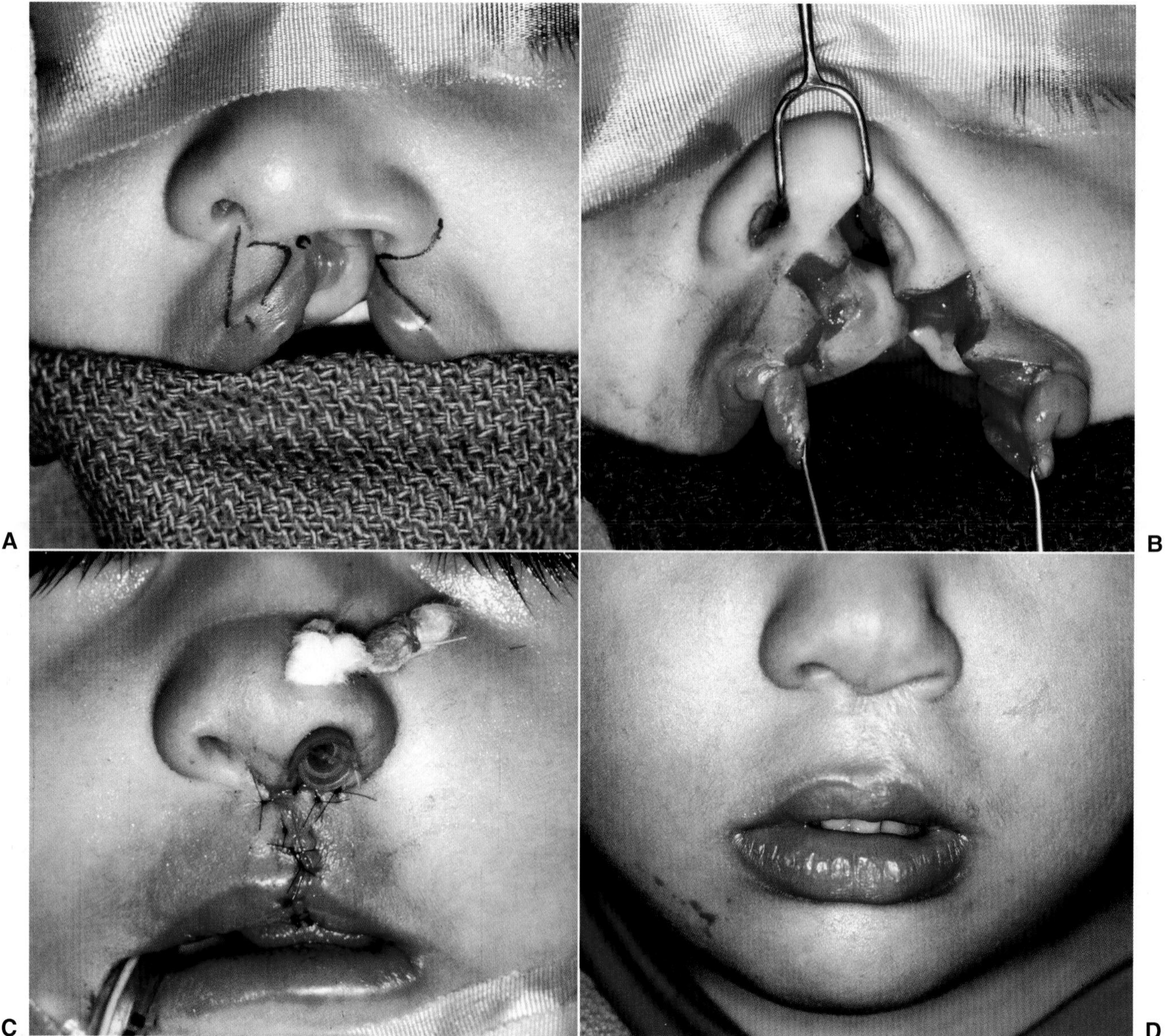

FIGURE 27-9 The Millard cheilorrhaphy technique. **A**, Incisions outlined. **B**, Flaps rotated. **C**, Closure. **D**, Result seen a few years later.

and oral cavities. The soft tissues extending around the cleft margin vary in quality. Some tissues are atrophic and not particularly useful. Other tissues appear healthy and readily lend themselves to dissection and suture integrity. In the most basic sense the soft tissues are incised along the cleft margin and are dissected from the palatal shelves until approximation over the cleft defect is possible. This procedure frequently necessitates the use of lateral relaxing incisions close to the dentition (Fig. 27-10). The soft tissues are then sutured in a watertight manner over the cleft defect and are allowed to heal. The areas of bone exposed by lateral relaxing incisions are allowed to heal by secondary intention. The superior aspect of the palatal flaps also reepithelializes with respiratory epithelium because this surface is now the lining of the nasal floor. When possible, it is advisable to obtain a two-layer closure of the hard palatal cleft (Fig. 27-11), which necessitates that the nasal mucosa from the floor, lateral wall, and septal areas of the nose be mobilized and sutured together before the oral closure.

When the vomer is long and attached to the palatal shelf opposite the cleft, a mucosal flap can be raised from it and sutured to the palatal tissues on the cleft side (Fig. 27-12). This procedure (i.e., vomer flap technique) requires little stripping of palatal mucoperiosteum and produces minimal scar contraction. The denuded areas of vomer and the opposite sides of the flap where no epithelium is present will reepithelialize. The vomer flap technique is useful in clefts that are not wide and where the vomer is readily available for use. The technique is a one-layer closure.

Soft Palate Closure

The closure of the soft palate is technically the most difficult of the operations yet discussed in the cleft-afflicted individual.

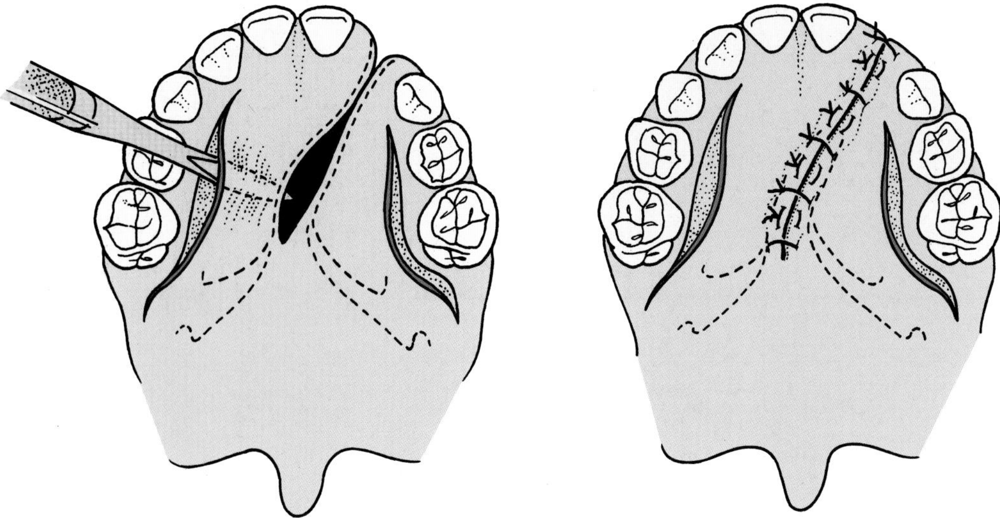

FIGURE 27-10 Von Langenbeck operation for closure of hard palate using lateral releasing incisions. This technique is one-layer closure. Nasal (i.e., superior) aspect of palatal flaps will epithelialize, as will denuded areas of palatal bone.

Access is the largest problem because the soft palate is toward the back of the oral cavity. The combination of difficulty with light, retraction, and the fact that the clinician can work only from the oral side yet must correct the oral and nasal sides of the soft palate leads to difficulties. In addition, the clinician may have to work with extremely thin, atrophic tissues yet produce a closure that will hold together under function while healing is progressing. To help accomplish this goal, the soft palate is always closed in three layers and in the same order: (1) nasal mucosa, (2) muscle, and (3) oral mucosa (Fig. 27-13). The margins of the cleft are incised from the posterior end of the hard palate to *at least* the distal end of the uvula (some surgeons carry the incision and closure down the palatopharyngeal fold to elongate the soft palate). The nasal mucosa is then dissected free from the underlying musculature and sutured to the nasal mucosa of the opposite side. The muscular layer requires special care. The musculature of the cleft soft palate is not inserted across to the opposite side but instead is inserted posteriorly and laterally along the margins of the hard palate. These muscular insertions must be released from their bony insertions and reapproximated to those of the other sides. Only then will the velopharyngeal mechanism have a chance to perform properly. If the quantity of muscular tissue is inadequate for approximation of the musculature in the midline, the pterygoid hamular processes can be infractured, thus releasing the tensor palatini muscles toward the midline. This maneuver is frequently necessary, especially in wide clefts.

Occasionally, the soft palate is found to be short, and articulation with the pharyngeal wall is impossible. This situation is especially prevalent in incomplete palatal clefts—those of the soft palate only. In these cases the palate can be closed in a manner that not only brings the two lateral halves together in the midline but also gains palatal length (Fig. 27-14). The so-called W-Y push-back procedure (Wardill) and U-shaped push-back procedure (Dorrance and Brown) are commonly used. The mucoperiosteum of the hard palate is incised and elevated in a manner that allows the entire soft tissue elements of the hard and soft palate to extend posteriorly, thus gaining palatal length.

Alveolar Cleft Grafts

The alveolar cleft defect is usually not corrected in the original surgical correction of the cleft lip or the cleft palate (Fig. 27-15). As a result, the cleft-afflicted individual may have residual oronasal fistulae in this area, and the maxillary alveolus will not be continuous because of the cleft. Because of this, five problems commonly occur: (1) oral fluids escape into the nasal cavity, (2) nasal secretions drain into the oral cavity, (3) teeth erupt into the alveolar cleft, (4) the alveolar segments collapse, and (5) if the cleft is large, speech is adversely affected.

Alveolar cleft bone grafts provide several advantages: First, they unite the alveolar segments and help prevent collapse and constriction of the dental arch, which is especially important if the maxilla has been orthodontically expanded. Second, alveolar cleft bone grafts provide bone support for teeth adjacent to the cleft and for those that will erupt into the area of the cleft. Frequently, the bone support on the distal aspect of the central incisor is thin, and the height of the bone support varies. These teeth may show slight mobility because of this lack of bone support. Increasing the amount of alveolar bone for this tooth helps to ensure its periodontal maintenance, especially if bone grafting occurs before the early stages of eruption of the tooth. The canine tends to erupt into the cleft site and, with healthy bone placed into the cleft, will maintain good periodontal support during eruption and thereafter. The third benefit of alveolar cleft grafts is closure of the oronasal fistula, which will partition the oral and nasal cavities and prevent escape of fluids between them. Augmentation of the alveolar ridge in the area of the cleft is a fourth advantage because it facilitates the use of dental prostheses by creating a more suitable supporting base. A fifth benefit is the creation of a solid foundation for the lip and alar base of the nose. It has become evident that the alveolar cleft-grafting procedure itself creates a favorable change in the nasal structure because the tissues at the base of the nose become supported after alveolar cleft grafting, whereas before the graft they had no solid osseous foundation. Therefore the alveolar graft should be performed before nasal revisions.

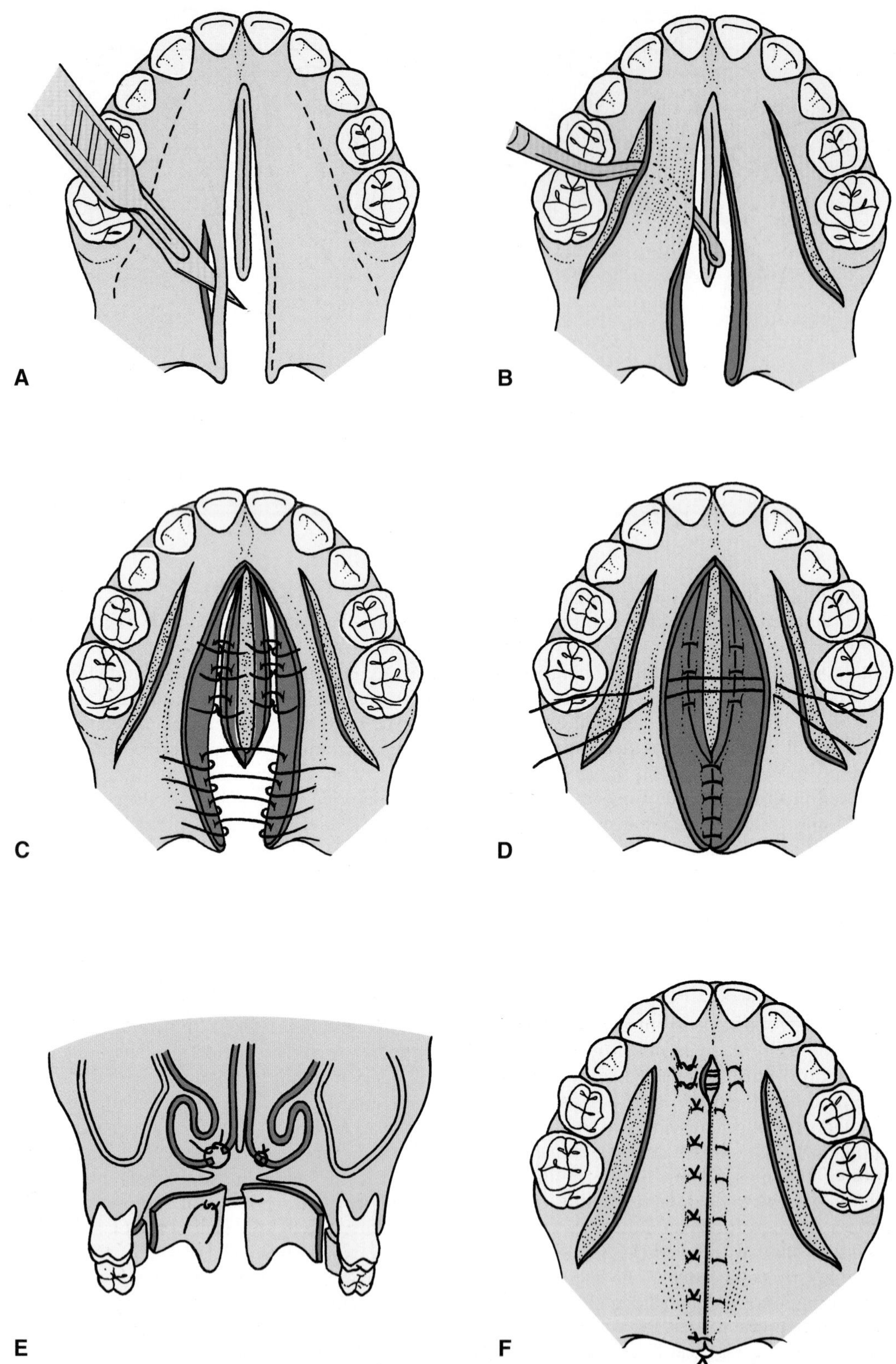

FIGURE 27-11 Variation of von Langenbeck operation for concomitant hard and soft palate closure. Operation uses three-layer closure for soft palate (i.e., nasal mucosa, muscle, oral mucosa) and two-layer closure for hard palate (i.e., flaps from vomer and nasal floor to produce nasal closure and palatal flaps for oral closure). **A**, Removing mucosa from margin of cleft. **B**, Mucoperiosteal flaps on hard palate are developed; note lateral releasing incisions. **C**, Sutures placed into nasal mucosa after development of nasal flaps from vomer and nasal floor. Sutures are placed so that knots will be on nasal side. **D**, Nasal mucosa has been closed. **E**, Frontal section showing repair of nasal mucosa. **F**, Closure of oral mucoperiosteum.

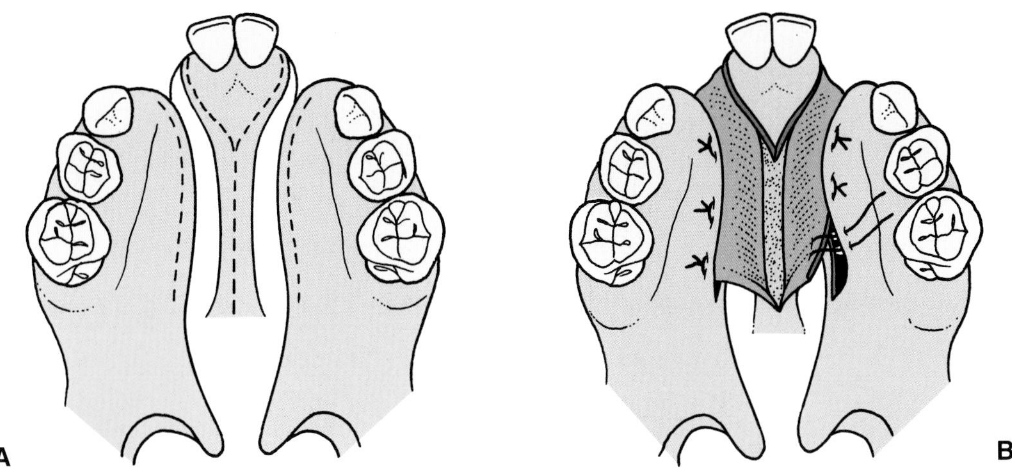

FIGURE 27-12 Vomer flap technique for closure of hard palate cleft (bilateral in this case). A, Incisions through nasal mucosa on underside of nasal septum (i.e., vomer) and mucosa of cleft margins. B, Mucosa of nasal septum is dissected off nasal septum and inserted under palatal mucosa at margins of cleft. This is a one-layer closure only. Connective tissue undersurface of nasal mucosa will epithelialize. This technique, because it does not require extensive elevation of palatal mucoperiosteum, produces less scarring with attendant growth restriction.

Timing of Graft Procedure

The alveolar cleft graft is usually performed when the patient is between ages 6 and 10. By this time a major portion of maxillary growth has occurred, and the alveolar cleft surgery should not adversely affect the future growth of the maxilla. It is important to have the graft in place before the eruption of the permanent canines into the cleft, thus ensuring their periodontal support. Ideally, the grafting procedure is performed when one half to two thirds of the unerupted canine root has formed. Some surgeons advocate that aleveolar grafting be performed nearer to the time when the maxillary central incisors are erupting.

Orthodontic expansion of the arch before or after the procedure is equally effective; however, some surgeons prefer to expand before bone grafting to facilitate access into the cleft area at surgery.

Surgical Procedure

Intact mucoperiosteal flaps on each side must cover bone grafts placed into the alveolar cleft. This means that flaps of nasal mucosa, palatal mucosa, and labial mucosa must be developed and sutured in a tension-free, watertight manner to prevent infection of the graft. The soft tissue incisions for alveolar cleft grafts vary, but in each procedure these conditions are met (Fig. 27-16).

The bone placed into the alveolar cleft is usually obtained from the patient's ilium or cranium; however, some surgeons are using allogeneic bone (i.e., homologous bone from another individual). The grafts are made into a particulate consistency and are packed into the defect once the nasal and palatal mucosa has been closed. The labial mucosa is then closed over the bone graft. In time these grafts are replaced by new bone that is indistinguishable from the surrounding alveolar process (see Fig. 27-15). Orthodontic movement of teeth into the graft sites is possible, and eruption of teeth into them usually proceeds unimpeded. Implants may also be placed.

Correction of Maxillomandibular Disharmonies

The individual with a cleft deformity usually exhibits maxillary retrusion and a transverse maxillary constriction resulting from the cicatricial contraction of previous surgeries. In many instances the associated malocclusion is beyond the scope of orthodontic treatment alone. In these cases, orthognathic surgery similar to the procedures outlined in Chapter 25 is indicated to correct the underlying skeletal malrelationships.

However, some differences exist in the technical aspects of maxillary surgery because of the other deformities and scarring that are present in the maxillas of individuals with clefts. In general, total maxillary osteotomies are necessary to advance and sometimes widen the maxilla. Closure of some of the space in the alveolar cleft area by bringing the alveolus of the cleft side anteriorly is also performed in several instances. These latter procedures necessitate the segmentation of the maxilla, which, because of the nature of the cleft, usually already has occurred. The differences between the cleft-afflicted patient and a non–cleft-afflicted patient, however, are the scar present across the palate and the decreased blood supply to the maxilla. Scarring from previous surgeries makes widening of the maxilla difficult, and frequently excision of some of this tissue is necessary. The clinician should try to be diligent and to maintain as much mucoperiosteum to the maxilla as possible because of the poor blood supply that the cleft maxilla receives. Care must also be taken not to create another oronasal fistula.

If the alveolar cleft had not been grafted previously, this can be done in the same operation. In bilateral clefts, however, the blood supply to the prolabial segment is very poor. It may be more prudent in these instances to perform the alveolar cleft grafts first and then perform a one-piece maxillary osteotomy after sufficient time has passed for revascularization of the prolabial segment.

One problem faced by the patient with a cleft palate when maxillary advancement procedures are planned is the effect this may have on the velopharyngeal mechanism. When the maxilla is brought forward, the soft palate is also drawn forward. A patient's preoperative marginal competence of the velopharyngeal mechanism may become incompetent in the postoperative period. Determination of which patients will have

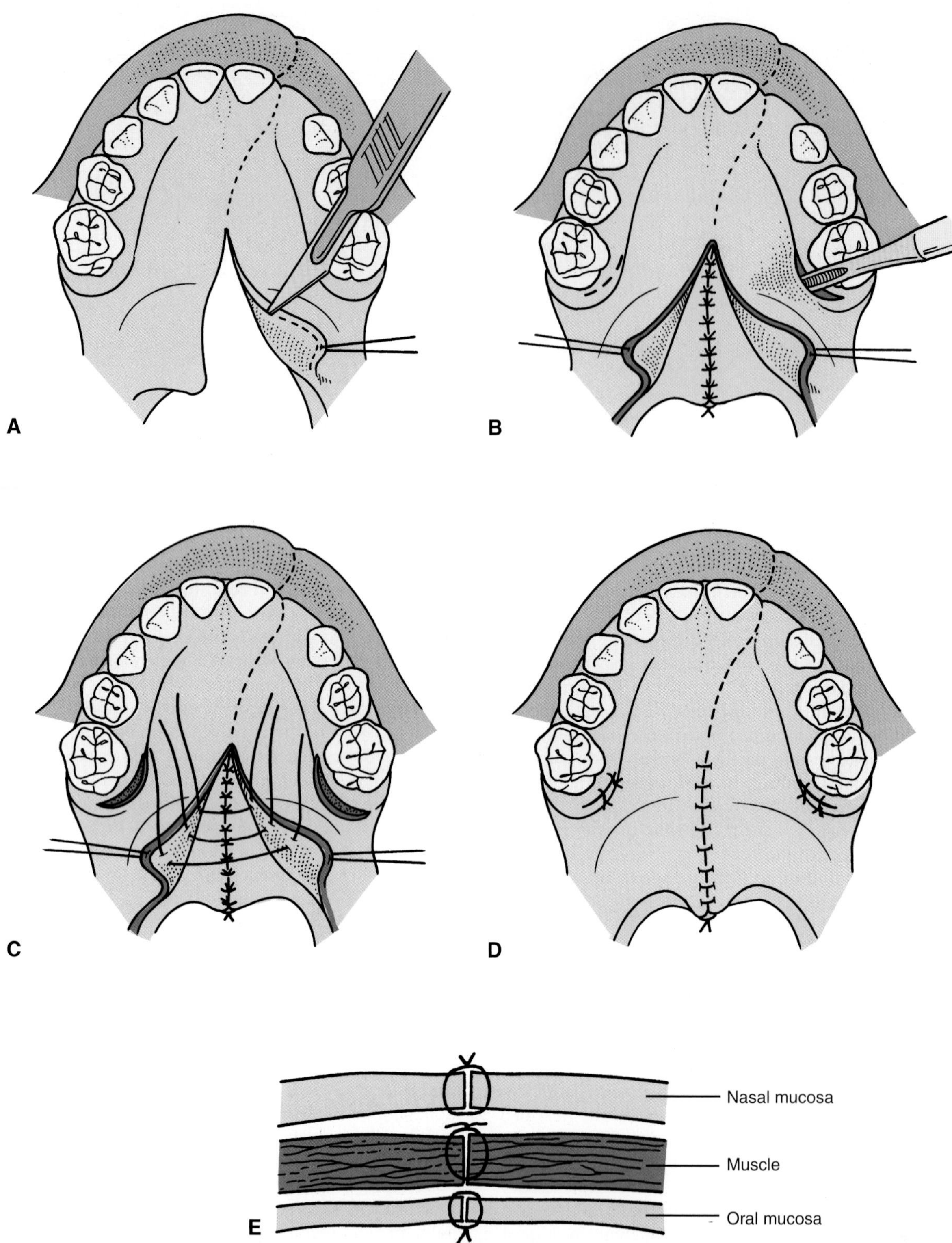

FIGURE 27-13 Triple-layered soft palate closure. **A**, Excision of mucosa at cleft margin. **B**, Dissection of nasal mucosa from soft palate to facilitate closure. Nasal mucosa is sutured together with knots tied on nasal (i.e., superior) surface. Note small incision made to insert instrument for hamular process fracture. This maneuver releases tensor veli palatini and facilitates approximation in midline. **C**, Muscle is dissected from insertion into hard palate, and sutures are placed to approximate muscle in midline. **D**, Closure of oral mucosa is accomplished last. **E**, Layered closure of soft palate. (From Hayward JR: *Oral surgery,* Springfield, IL, 1976, Charles C Thomas.)

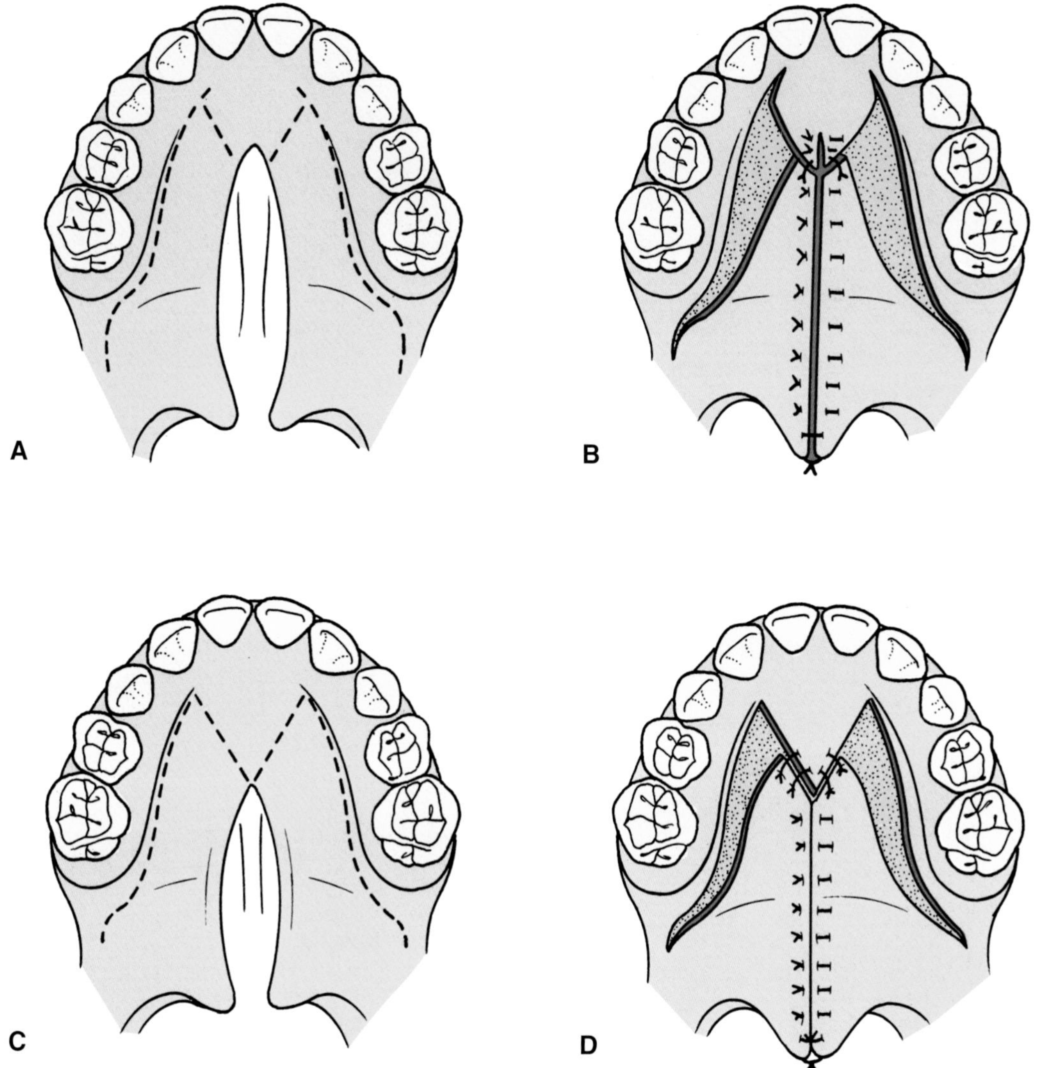

FIGURE 27-14 The Wardill operations for palatal lengthening on closure. **A** and **B**, Four-flap operation for extensive cleft. **C** and **D**, Three-flap operation for shorter cleft. Note amount of denuded palatal bone left after these operations.

this problem is difficult. Because of the possibility of this incompetence, however, secondary palatal or pharyngeal surgical procedures to increase velopharyngeal competence are discussed with the patient. These procedures can be performed later if necessary.

Secondary Surgical Procedures

Secondary surgical procedures are procedures performed after the initial repair of the cleft defects in an effort to improve speech or correct residual defects. The most commonly used technique to improve velopharyngeal competence secondarily is the pharyngeal flap procedure (Fig. 27-17). In this procedure a wide vertical strip of pharyngeal mucosa and musculature is raised from the posterior pharyngeal wall and inserted into the superior aspect of the soft palate. These flaps are most often based superiorly. The defect left in the posterior pharyngeal wall from elevation of the pharyngeal flap can be closed primarily or left to heal by secondary intention. Once inserted into the soft palate, the pharynx and the soft palate are joined, leaving two lateral ports as the opening between the oropharynx and nasopharynx, which reduces the airstream between the oropharynx and nasopharynx. The velopharyngeal mechanism then consists of raising the soft palate somewhat and medial constriction of the lateral pharyngeal walls.

Another technique that has recently had a resurgence of interest because of new biocompatible material is the placement of an implant behind the posterior pharyngeal wall to bring it anteriorly (Fig. 27-18). Thus the soft palate has less distance to traverse to close off the nasopharynx. The major problems with this technique in the past have been migration of the implant and infection, which usually results in the need for removal.

DENTAL NEEDS OF INDIVIDUALS WITH CLEFTS

Dentists will have patients with clefts in their practice because of the relatively large number of persons so affected. These patients should not pose any great problems because their dental needs do not differ dramatically from those of other individuals. However, because of the presence of the cleft,

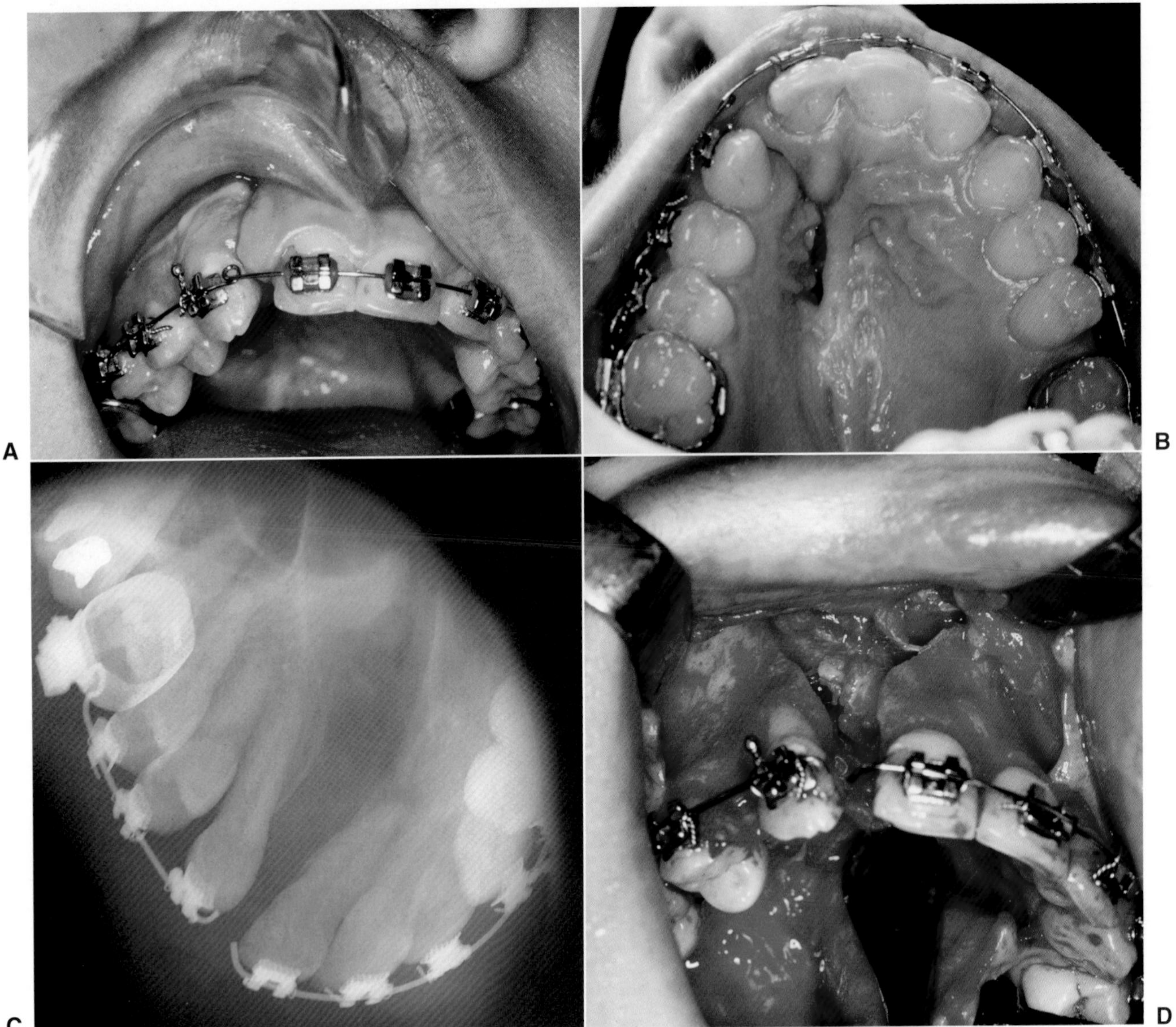

FIGURE 27-15 Labial (A), palatal, (B) and radiographic (C) views of a patent unilateral alveolar cleft that extends posteriorly along the hard palate. D, Photograph shows surgical closure of the nasal mucosa with inversion into the nasal cavity.

corrected or uncorrected, these individuals have a few special needs of which the dentist should be cognizant.

Because of the interdisciplinary approach that cleft-afflicted patients require, it behooves the dentist to be aware of the overall treatment plan formulated by the cleft team for the patient's treatment. Awareness of this plan precludes the performance of any irreversible or costly procedures on teeth that may be charted for extraction in the future. For instance, placing a bridge to replace a congenitally missing lateral incisor before alveolar bone grafting and orthodontic therapy is unwise. Similarly, extracting supernumerary teeth that may be temporarily retained to maintain alveolar bone support is also disadvantageous. All fixed bridgework should be delayed until after the orthodontic, orthognathic, and alveolar grafting procedures have been completed. Only then will the dentist be able to determine accurately the exact space and ridge form available for pontics. Furthermore, until the two halves of the maxillary arch have been united with bone grafts, the halves will move independently and bridgework spanning the cleft margin may become loose. Therefore the dentist must communicate freely with the other professionals who are managing the patient's other cleft problems, and coordination of services is of paramount importance.

Teeth adjacent to the cleft margins not only may be malformed or absent but also may have poor periodontal support because of lack of bone and their position in the cleft margin. This situation predisposes teeth to periodontitis and early loss if not kept in an optimal state of health. Because teeth are frequently malaligned and rotated, oral hygienic measures may be more difficult; these individuals may need more frequent prophylaxis and special oral hygienic instructions with careful reinforcement. Otherwise, rampant caries with premature loss

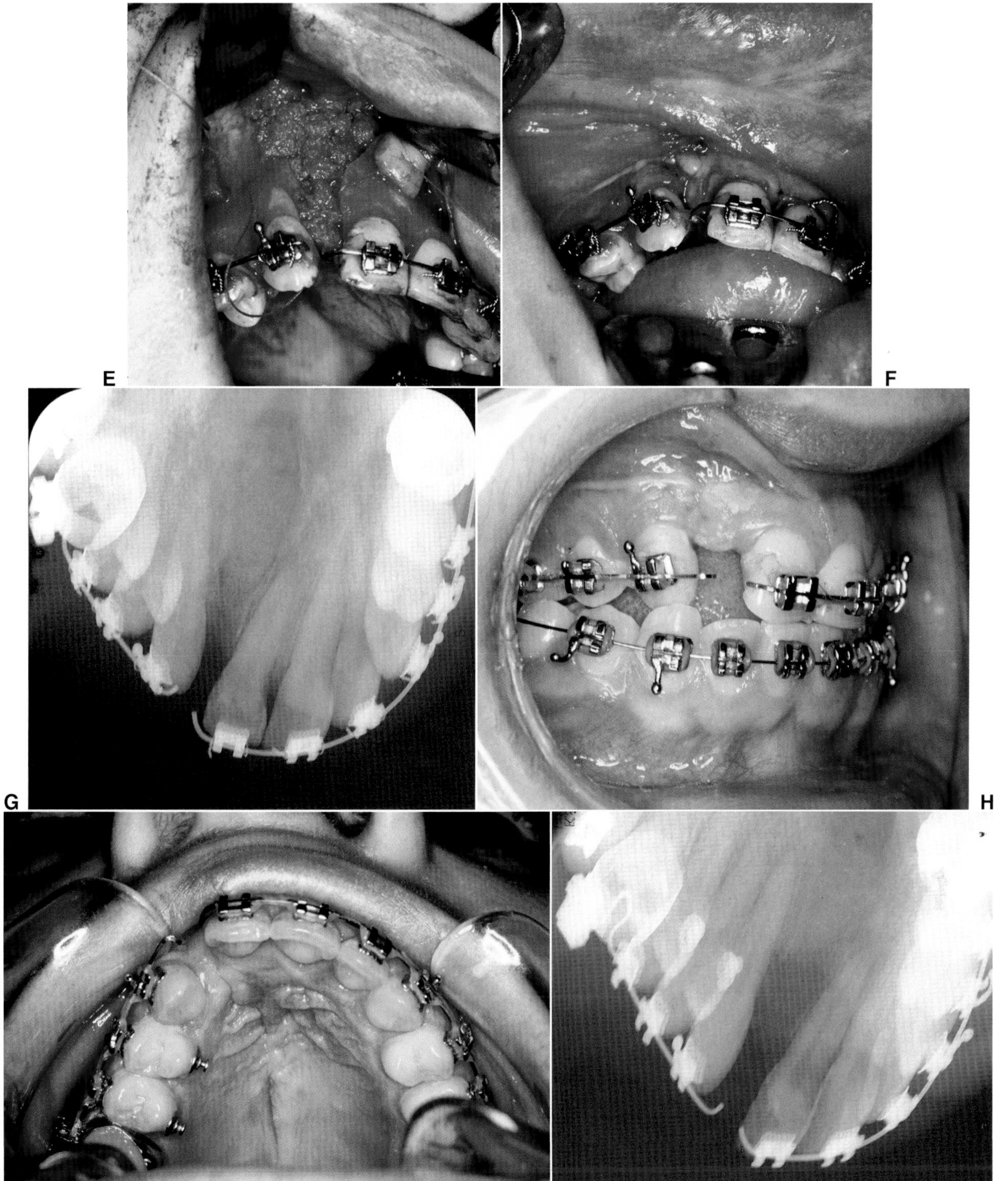

FIGURE 27-15, cont'd E, Particulate bone graft is placed into the defect. F, Closure of the palatal and labial mucosa over the bone graft. G, Radiographic result is demonstrated 3 days after surgery. H, Labial and (I) palatal views 3 months after surgery, showing healing of the soft tissues. J, Radiograph taken 3 months after surgery shows consolidation of the bone graft.

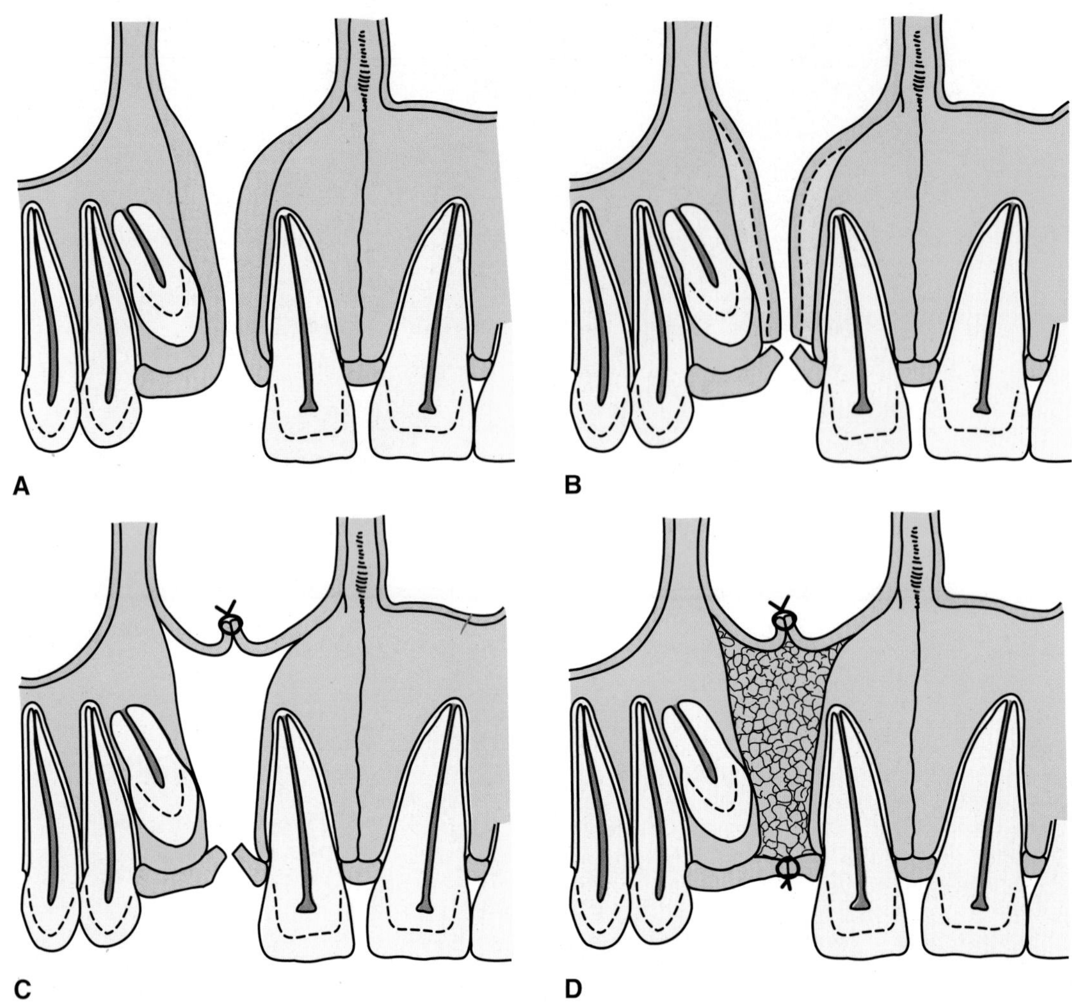

FIGURE 27-16 Technique for alveolar cleft bone grafting. A, Preoperative defect viewed from labial aspect. Fistula extends into nasal cavity. B, Incision divides mucosa fistula, which allows development of nasal and oral flaps. C, Mucosal flap developed from lining of fistula is turned inward, up into nasal cavity, and sutured in watertight manner. D, Bone graft material is packed into cleft, and oral mucosa is closed in watertight manner. Note partially developed canine and absence of lateral incisor.

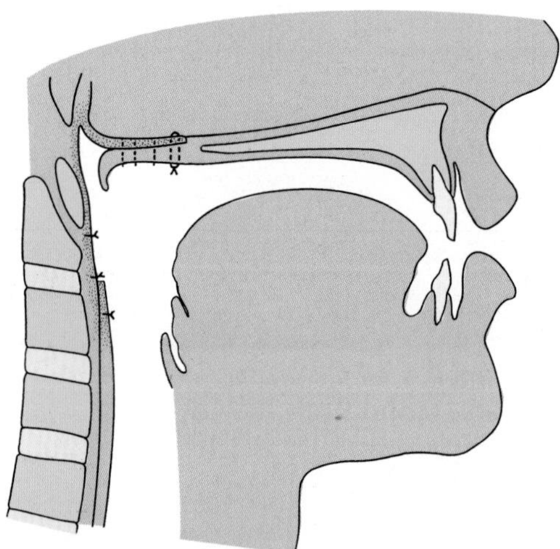

FIGURE 27-17 Superiorly based pharyngeal flap. Flap is sutured to superior aspect of soft palate, thus partially partitioning oral and nasal cavities from one another. Only nasal airway remaining after this operation is two lateral openings on each side of flap.

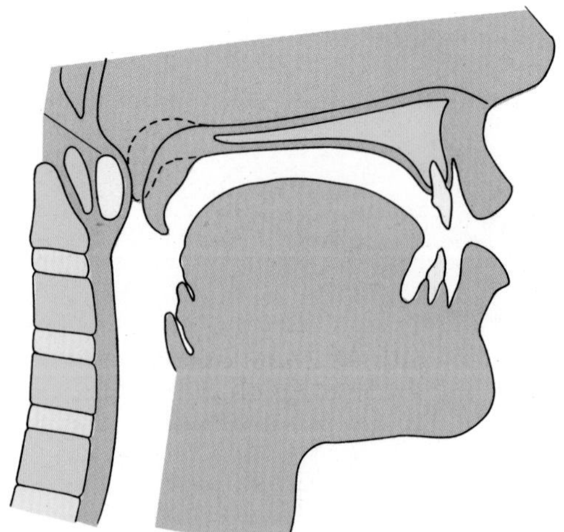

FIGURE 27-18 Posterior pharyngeal wall implant. This makes distance between soft palate and pharyngeal wall smaller so that velopharyngeal closure is facilitated.

may occur. This is a special tragedy in the cleft-afflicted individual because he or she may have fewer teeth to serve vital functions (e.g., retaining orthodontic, orthopedic, or speech appliances).

Prosthetic Speech Aid Appliances

Prosthetic care for the patient with a cleft may be necessary for two reasons: First, teeth that are so frequently missing in the cleft-afflicted patient should be replaced. Second, in patients who have failed to obtain velopharyngeal competence with surgical corrections, a speech aid appliance can be made by the dentist to decrease hypernasal speech. A speech aid appliance is an acrylic bulb attached to a tooth-borne appliance in the maxilla (Fig. 27-19). The bulb is fitted to project onto the undersurface of the soft palate and lifts the soft palate superiorly. If this bulb does not give adequate function, another projection of acrylic (i.e., bulb obturator) can be placed to extend to the posterior aspect of the palate. This narrows the pharyngeal isthmus, and the size can be adjusted for maximal effectiveness. The posterior pharyngeal wall then contacts this bulb in function. In many instances the size of the bulb can be reduced as the pharyngeal musculature becomes more active. This type of appliance is used in two instances: (1) before a pharyngeal flap procedure to develop muscle action or (2) if the secondary surgical procedures are not successful in producing velopharyngeal competence. The speech aid appliance is also useful concomitantly to hold prosthetic dental replacements, to cover hard palate defects, and to support deficient upper lips by a flange extending into the labial sulcus. Obviously, the maintenance of the residual dentition in an optimal state is prerequisite for successful speech aid appliance therapy.

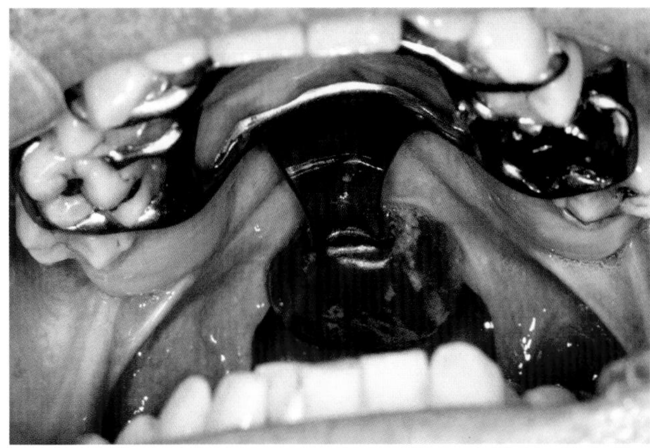

FIGURE 27-19 Prosthetic speech aid appliance. Appliance can be designed to lift soft palate and to obturate oral and nasal cavities if necessary.

REFERENCES

1. Jones C: *The genetics of cleft lip and palate: information for families,* Chapel Hill, NC, 2000, Cleft Palate Foundation.
2. Hayward JR: Cleft lip and palate. In Hayward JR, editor: *Oral surgery,* Springfield, IL, 1976, Charles C Thomas.
3. Langman J: *Medical embryology,* ed 3, Baltimore, 1975, Williams & Wilkins.
4. Ranta R: A review of tooth formation in children with cleft lip/palate, *Am J Orthod* 90:11, 1986.

CHAPTER 28

Surgical Reconstruction of Defects of the Jaws

EDWARD ELLIS III

CHAPTER OUTLINE

Defects of the facial bones, especially the jaws, have a variety of causes, such as eradication of pathologic conditions, trauma, infections, and congenital deformities. The size of the defects that are commonly reconstructed in the oral and maxillofacial region varies considerably from small alveolar clefts to mandibulectomy defects. Each defect poses a unique set of problems that reconstructive surgical intervention must address. In each of these instances, restoration of normal structure is usually possible, with resultant improvement in function and appearance.

When an osseous structure is defective in size, shape, position, or amount, reconstructive surgery can replace the defective structure. The tissue most commonly used to replace lost osseous tissue is bone. Bone grafting has been attempted for centuries with varying degrees of success. Recent advancements in the understanding of bone physiology, immunologic concepts, tissue-banking procedures, and surgical principles have made possible the successful reconstruction of most maxillofacial bony defects. As such, the biology and principles of transplantation of bone are presented in this chapter.

BIOLOGIC BASIS OF BONE RECONSTRUCTION

A tissue that is transplanted and expected to become a part of the host to which it is transplanted is known as a *graft*. Several types of grafts are available to the surgeon, which are discussed later. A basic understanding of how a bone heals when grafted from one place to another *in the same individual* (i.e., autotransplantation) is necessary to understand the benefits of the various types of bone grafts available.

The healing of bone and bone grafts is unique among connective tissues because new bone formation arises from tissue regeneration rather than from simple tissue repair with scar formation.[1] This healing therefore requires the element of cellular proliferation (i.e., osteoblasts) and the element of collagen synthesis. When bone is transplanted from one area of the body to another, several processes become active during the incorporation of the graft.

Two-Phase Theory of Osteogenesis

Two basic processes occur on transplanting bone from one area to another in the same individual[1-5]: The first process that leads to bone regeneration arises initially from transplanted cells in the graft that proliferate and form new osteoid. The amount of bone regeneration during this phase depends on the number of transplanted bone cells that survive the grafting procedure. Obviously, when the graft is first removed from the body, the blood supply has been severed. Thus the cells in the bone graft depend on diffusion of nutrients from the surrounding graft bed (i.e., the area where the graft is placed) for survival. A considerable amount of cell death occurs during the grafting procedure, and this first phase of bone regeneration may not lead to an impressive amount of bone regeneration when considered alone. Still, this phase is responsible for the formation of most of the new bone. The more viable cells that can be successfully transplanted with the graft, the more bone that will form.

The graft bed also undergoes changes that lead to a second phase of bone regeneration beginning in the second week. Intense angiogenesis and fibroblastic proliferation from the graft bed begin after grafting, and osteogenesis from host connective tissues soon begins. Fibroblasts and other mesenchymal cells differentiate into osteoblasts and begin to lay down new bone. Evidence shows that a protein (or proteins) found in the bone induces these reactions in the surrounding soft tissues of the graft bed.[6,7] This second phase is also responsible for the orderly incorporation of the graft into the host bed with continued resorption, replacement, and remodeling.

Immune Response

When a tissue is transplanted from one site to another in the same individual, immunologic complications usually do not occur. The immune system is not triggered because the tissue is recognized as "self." However, when a tissue is transplanted from one individual to another or from one species to another, the immune system may present a formidable obstacle to the success of the grafting procedure. If the graft is recognized as a foreign substance by the host, it will mount an intense response in an attempt to destroy the graft. The type of response the immune system mounts against "foreign" grafts is primarily a cell-mediated response by T lymphocytes. The response may not occur immediately, however, and in the early period the incorporation of a bone graft into the host may appear to be progressing normally. The length of this latent period depends on the similarity between the host and the recipient. The more similar they are (antigenically), the longer an immunologic reaction may take to appear. This type of immunologic reaction is the most common reason for rejection of hearts, kidneys, and other organs transplanted to another individual. Tissue-typing procedures, in which a donor and recipient are genetically compared for similarities before transplantation, are currently commonplace for organ transplantation but never for bone grafts.

Because of the immunologic rejection of transplants between individuals or between species, methods have been devised to improve the success of grafting procedures in these instances. Two basic approaches are used clinically: The first is the suppression of the host individual's immune response. Immunosuppression with various medications is most commonly used in organ transplant patients. This approach is not used routinely in oral and maxillofacial surgical bone grafting procedures because of the potential complications from immunosuppression.

Another approach that has been used extensively in oral and maxillofacial surgical procedures is the alteration of the antigenicity of the graft so that the host's immune response will not be stimulated. Several methods of treating grafts have been used, including boiling, deproteinization, use of thimerosal (Merthiolate), freezing, freeze-drying, irradiation, and dry heating. All of these methods, potentially helpful for use in bone grafts, are obviously not helpful in organ transplants.

TYPES OF GRAFTS

Several types of bone grafts are available for use in reconstructive surgery. A useful classification categorizes the bone grafts according to their origin and thus their potential to induce an immunologic response. Because of their origins and the preparations used to help avoid an intense immune response, the grafts have different qualities and indications for use.

Autogenous Grafts

Also known as *autografts* or *self-grafts*, autogenous grafts are composed of tissues from the same individual. Fresh autogenous bone is the most ideal bone graft material. The autogenous graft is unique among bone grafts in that it is the only type of bone graft to supply living, immunocompatible bone cells essential to phase I osteogenesis. The larger number of living cells that are transplanted, the more osseous tissue that will be produced.

Autogenous bone is the type used most frequently in oral and maxillofacial surgery. The bone can be obtained from a host of sites in the body and can be taken in several forms. Block grafts are solid pieces of cortical bone and underlying cancellous bone (Fig. 28-1). The iliac crest is often used as a source for this type of graft. The entire thickness of the ilium can be obtained, or the ilium can be split to obtain a thinner piece of block graft. Ribs also constitute a form of block graft. Particulate marrow and cancellous bone grafts are obtained by harvesting the medullary bone and the associated endosteum and hematopoietic marrow. Particulate marrow and cancellous bone grafts produce the greatest concentration of osteogenic cells, and because of the particulate nature, more cells survive transplantation because of the access they have to nutrients in the surrounding graft bed. The most common site for the procurement of this type of graft is the ilium. The iliac crest can be entered, and large volumes of particulate marrow and cancellous bone grafts can be obtained with large curettes. The diploic space of the cranial vault has recently been used as a site for obtaining this type of graft when small amounts of bone chips are needed (e.g., alveolar cleft grafts).

Autogenous bone may also be transplanted while maintaining the blood supply to the graft. Two methods can accomplish this: The first involves the transfer of a bone graft pedicled to a muscular (or muscular and skin) pedicle. The bone is not stripped of its soft tissue pedicle, preserving some blood supply to the bone graft. Thus the number of surviving osteogenic cells is potentially great. An example of this type of autogenous graft is a segment of the clavicle transferred to the mandible, pedicled to the sternocleidomastoid muscle. The second method by which autogenous bone can be transplanted without losing blood supply is by the use of microsurgical techniques. A block of ilium, tibia, rib, or other suitable bone is removed along with the overlying soft tissues after dissecting free an artery and a vein that supply the tissue (Fig. 28-2). An artery and a vein are also prepared in the recipient bed. Once the bone graft is secured in place, the artery and veins are reconnected using microvascular anastomoses. In this way the blood supply to the bone graft is restored.

Both of these types of autogenous grafts are known as *composite grafts* because they contain soft tissue and osseous elements. The first type described, in which the bone maintains a muscular origin, is a pedicled composite graft. The pedicle is the soft tissue remaining on it, which supplies the vasculature. The second type of composite graft is a free composite graft, meaning that it is totally removed from the body and immediately replaced, and its blood supply is restored by reconnection of blood vessels.

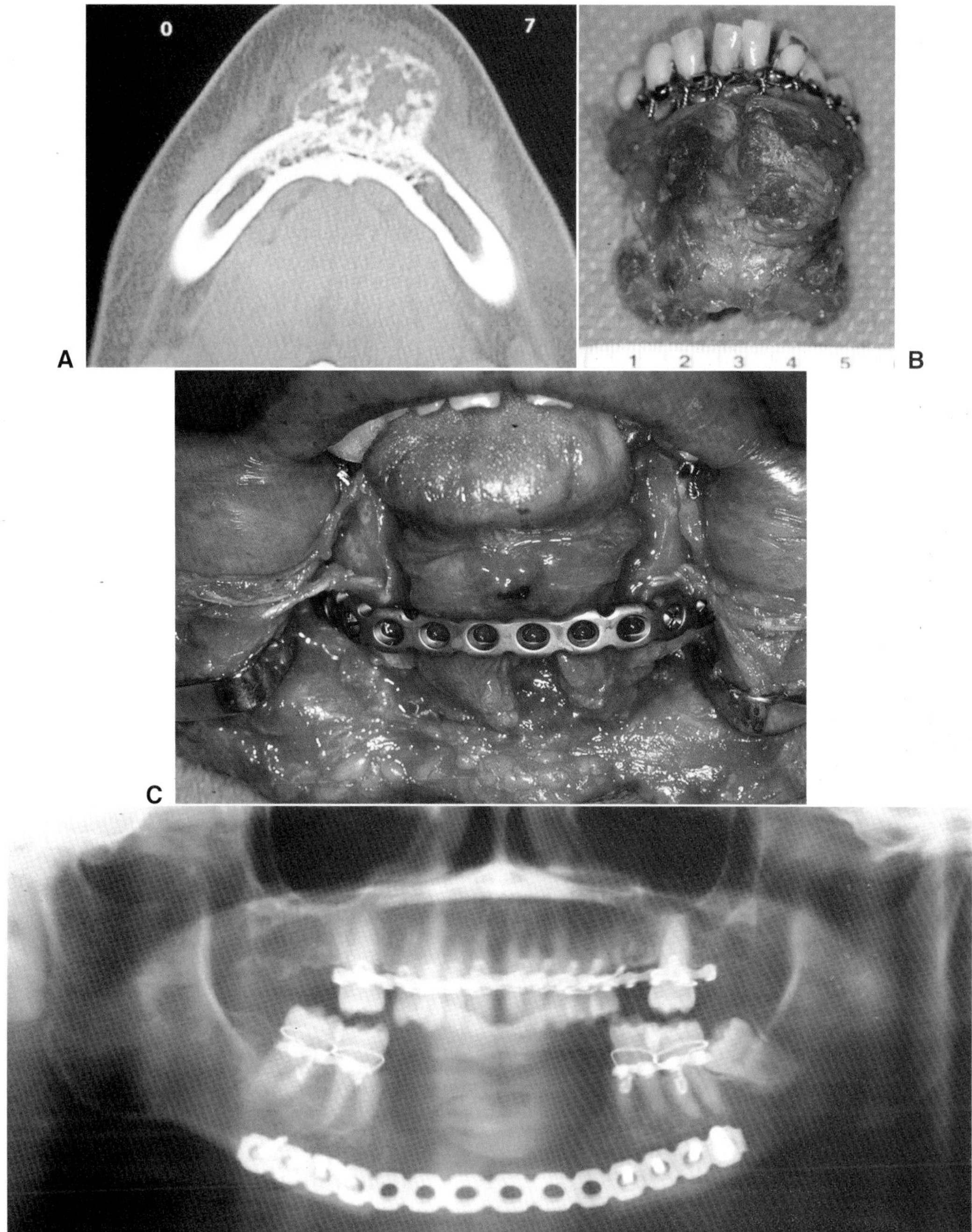

FIGURE 28-1 The use of autogenous corticocancellous block bone graft to replace defect in mandibular symphysis. This patient had an ameloblastoma of the anterior mandible. A, Computed tomography scan showing expansion and irregularity of bone. B, Specimen that was resected using an intraoral approach. C, Bone plate used to span the resection gap, controlling the position of the right and left mandibular halves, and allowing the patient to function postoperatively without the need for intermaxillary fixation. D, Panoramic radiograph taken immediately after resection. Three months later the oral soft tissues have healed, and the patient is prepared for bone graft reconstruction of the symphysis.

Continued

Although these types of grafts may seem ideal, they have some shortcomings when used to restore defects of the jaws. Because the soft tissues attached to the bone graft maintain the blood supply, there can be minimal stripping of the soft tissue from the graft during procurement and placement. Thus the size and shape of the graft cannot be altered to any significant degree. Frequently, inadequate bulk of bone is provided when these grafts are used to restore mandibular continuity defects. Another problem is the morbidity to the donor site. Instead of just removing osseous tissue, soft tissues are also removed with composite grafts, which causes greater functional and cosmetic defects.

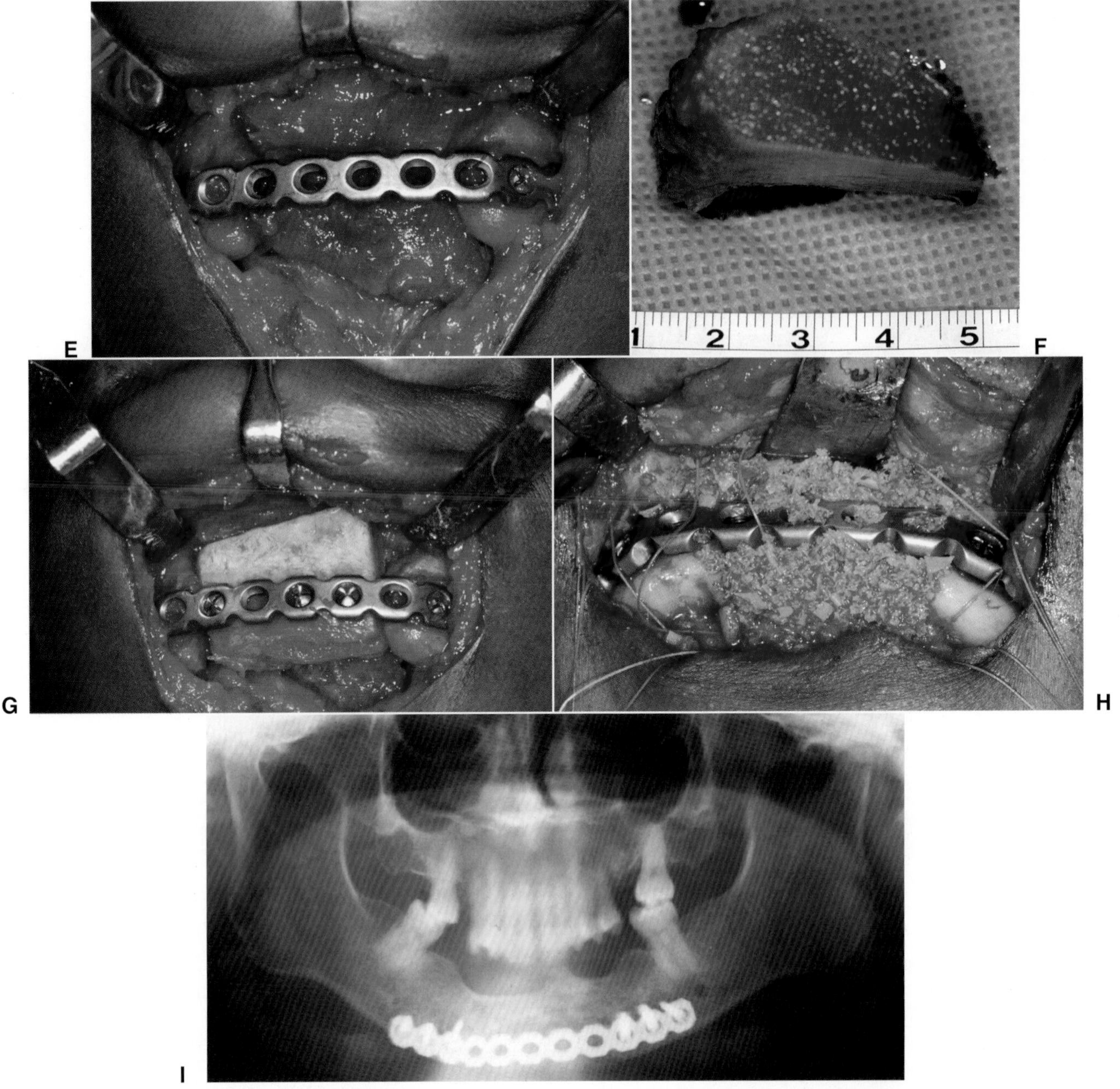

FIGURE 28-1, cont'd The use of autogenous block corticocancellous bone graft to replace defect in mandibular symphysis. **E**, Surgical exposure using an extraoral approach. **F**, Full-thickness bone graft harvested from the ilium along with particulate marrow and cancellous bone to use as "filler" and to provide osteocompetent cells. **G**, Bone graft attached to the bone plate. Particulate bone is then packed around the area to promote bone healing (**H**). **I**, Panoramic radiograph taken 2 years later showing bone fill and healing of graft to both mandibular halves.

Advantages

The advantages of autogenous bone are that it provides osteogenic cells for phase I bone formation, and no immunologic response occurs.

Disadvantages

A disadvantage is that this procedure necessitates another site of operation for procurement of the graft.

Allogeneic Grafts

Also known as *allografts* or *homografts,* allogeneic grafts are grafts taken from another individual of the same species. Because the individuals are usually genetically dissimilar, treating the graft to reduce the antigenicity is routinely accomplished. Today, the most commonly used allogeneic bone is freeze-dried. All of these treatments destroy any remaining osteogenic cells in the

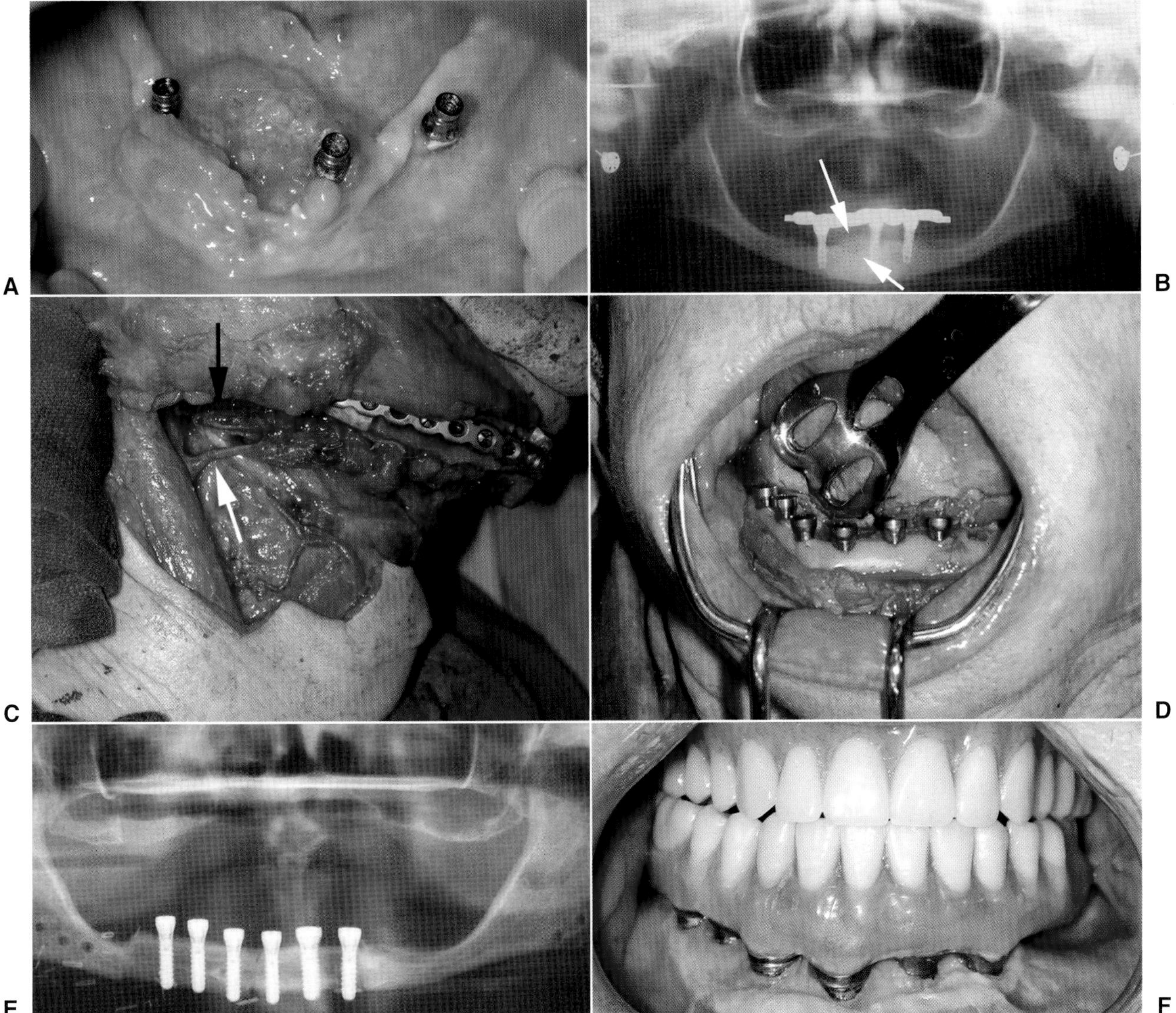

FIGURE 28-2 Example of a case reconstructed with a vascularized free flap. **A**, Squamous cell carcinoma located on the alveolar ridge and floor of mouth. **B**, Panoramic radiograph showing erosion of lesion into bone (*arrows*). **C**, Intraoperative photograph after mandible and surrounding soft tissues were resected, and a free fibular bone flap and reconstruction bone plate have been used to reconstruct the mandible. Note the venous anastomosis (*white arrow*). The arterial supply to the flap is also shown (*black arrow*), but the actual anastomosis is located more proximally, under the tissue, and is not visible. **D**, After the bone graft has healed, dental implants are inserted. **E**, Panoramic radiograph showing the reconstructed mandible after implants have been inserted. **F**, Intraoral view of prosthetic reconstruction of dental implants. The white tissue surrounding the implants is skin that was transferred with the bone flap. (Courtesy of Dr. Remy Blanchaert Jr.)

graft, and therefore allogeneic bone grafts cannot participate in phase I osteogenesis. The assistance of these grafts to osteogenesis is purely passive; they offer a hard tissue matrix for phase II induction.

Thus the host must produce all of the essential elements in the graft bed for the allogeneic bone graft to become resorbed and replaced. Obviously, the health of the graft bed is much more important in this set of circumstances than it is if autogenous bone were to be used.

Advantages

Advantages are that allogeneic grafts do not require another site of operation in the host and that a similar bone or a bone of similar shape to that being replaced can be obtained (e.g., an allogeneic mandible can be used for reconstruction of a mandibulectomy defect).

Disadvantages

The disadvantage is that an allogeneic graft does not provide viable cells for phase I osteogenesis.

Xenogeneic Grafts

Also known as *xenografts* or *heterografts*, xenogeneic grafts are taken from one species and grafted to another. The antigenic dissimilarity of these grafts is greater than with allogeneic bone. The organic matrix of xenogeneic bone is antigenically dissimilar to that of human bone, and therefore the graft must be treated more vigorously to prevent rapid rejection of the graft. Bone grafts of this variety are rarely used in major oral and maxillofacial surgical procedures.

Advantages

Advantages are that xenografts do not require another site of operation in the host, and a large quantity of bone can be obtained.

Disadvantages

Disadvantages are that xenografts do not provide viable cells for phase I osteogenesis and must be rigorously treated to reduce antigenicity.

Combinations of Grafts

The ideal graft would have the structural characteristics of a block graft with the osteogenic potential of particulate marrow and cancellous bone grafts. However, a large block graft necessitates removal of a large portion of the patient's anatomy and does not provide the high concentration of osteogenic cells that the particulate marrow and cancellous bone graft does. A commonly used technique to reconstruct defects of the mandible takes advantage of autogenous and allogeneic bone grafts (Fig. 28-3). An allogeneic block graft is obtained in the form of an ilium or mandible. This graft is used for its structural strength and protein, which induces phase II bone formation from the surrounding tissues. This graft is hollowed out until only the cortical plates remain.

Autogenous particulate marrow and cancellous bone is then obtained and packed into the shell to provide the osteogenic cells necessary for phase I bone formation. In this way the ingredients necessary for both phases of osteogenesis are provided without necessitating the removal of a large portion of the individual's anatomy. The allogeneic portion of the graft acts as a biodegradable tray, which in time is completely replaced by host bone.

Advantages

Advantages of this procedure are the same as those of autogenous and allogeneic grafts.

Disadvantages

The disadvantage is that this procedure necessitates a second site of operation in the host to obtain autogenous particulate marrow and cancellous bone graft.

ASSESSMENT OF PATIENT IN NEED OF RECONSTRUCTION

Patients who have defects of the jaws can usually be treated surgically to replace the lost portion. Each patient, however, must be thoroughly evaluated because no two patients have the exact same problems. Analysis of the patient's problem must take into consideration the hard tissue defect, any soft tissue defects, and any associated problems that will affect treatment.

Hard Tissue Defect

Several factors concerning the actual osseous defect must be thoroughly assessed to help formulate a viable treatment plan. Adequate radiographs are necessary to evaluate the full extent of the osseous defect. The site of the defect may be just as important as the size of the defect when dealing with mandibular osseous problems. For example, if the mandibular condyle is missing, treatment is relatively more difficult. A residual portion of the ramus with the condyle still attached makes osseous reconstruction easier because the temporomandibular articulation is difficult to restore.

The mandible has powerful muscles attached to it that usually direct functional movements. When the continuity of the mandible is broken, these muscles no longer work in harmony and may severely displace mandibular fragments into unnatural positions. Therefore the position of the residual mandibular fragments must be ascertained. For example, if a portion of the mandible in the area of the molars is missing, the muscles of mastication still attached to the mandibular ramus may rotate the ramus superiorly and medially, which may allow penetration into the oral cavity and compound the difficulty of planned treatment.

Soft Tissue Defect

Proper preparation of the soft tissue bed that is to receive the bone graft is just as important to the success of bone grafting as the bone graft material itself. The transplanted bone cells must survive initially by diffusion of nutrients from the surrounding soft tissues. Revascularization of the bone graft through the development of new blood vessels from the soft tissue bed must then occur. Thus an essential factor for the success of any bone-grafting procedure is the availability of an adequately vascularized soft tissue bed. Fortunately, this essential factor is usually obtainable in the lush vascular tissue of the head and neck region. However, occasionally the soft tissue bed is not as desirable as it could be, such as after radiotherapy or excessive scarring from trauma or infection. Therefore a thorough assessment of the quantity and quality of the

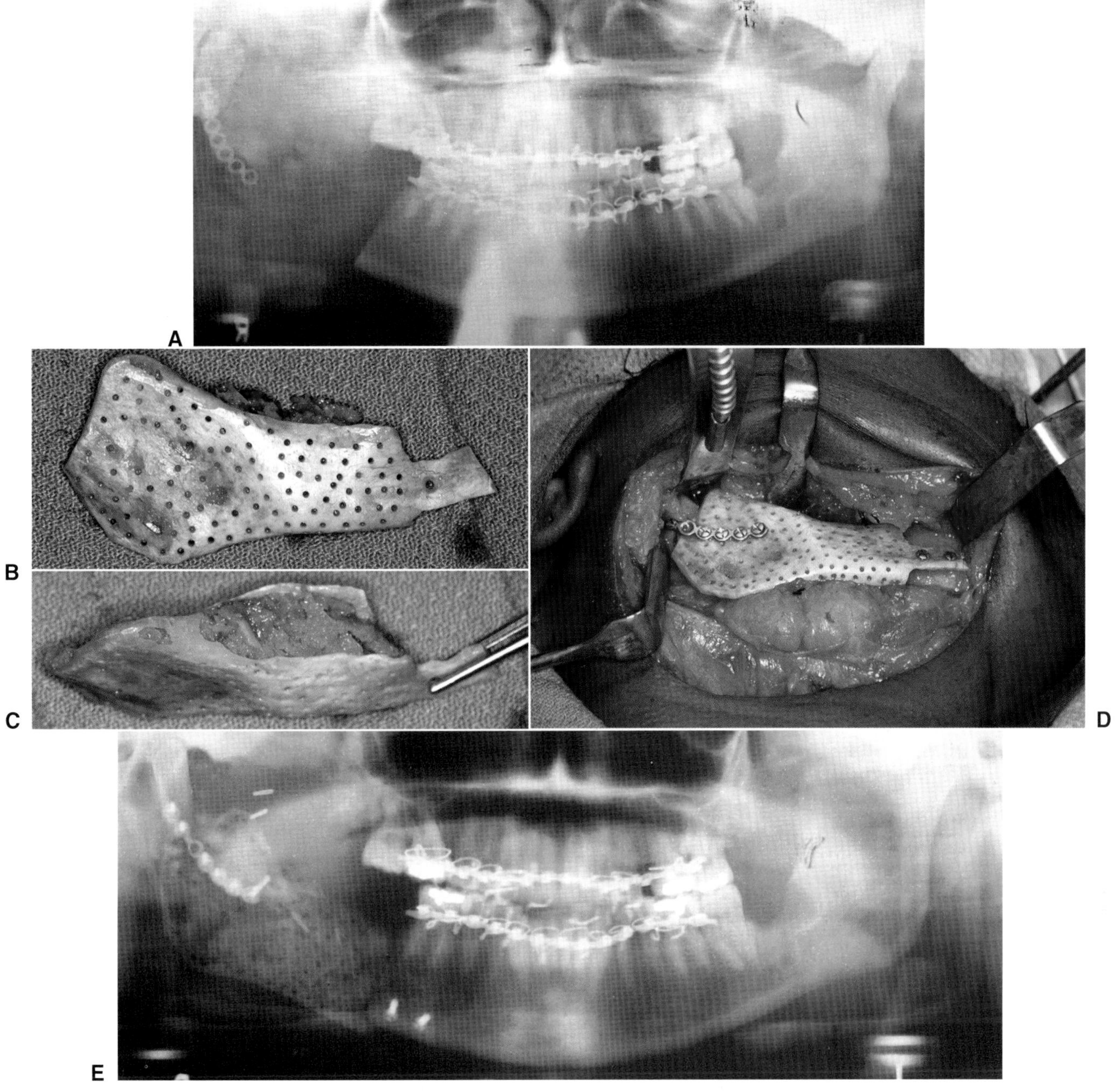

FIGURE 28-3 Use of a combination of allogeneic and autogenous bone grafts to reconstruct mandible after resection for ameloblastoma. A, Panoramic radiograph showing resected right mandibular ramus. A small bone plate was left attached to the condylar process to aid in later reconstruction. B and C, Allogeneic right mandible has been hollowed out and packed with autogenous particulate cancellous bone and marrow and fashioned to fit into defect. D, Graft has been secured to the mandibular condylar process and body. E, Postoperative panoramic radiograph showing graft in place.

surrounding soft tissues is necessary before undertaking bone graft procedures.

The reason for the osseous void often provides important information on the amount and quality of soft tissues remaining. For example, if the patient lost a large portion of the mandible from a composite resection for a malignancy, the chances are that the patient will have deficiencies in quantity and quality of soft tissues. During the initial surgery, many vital structures were probably removed, and denervation of the platysma muscle results in atrophy of the muscular fibers. An intraoral examination helps the clinician determine how much oral mucosa was removed with the mandibular fragment.

Frequently, the tongue or floor of the mouth appears to be sutured to the buccal mucosa, with no intervening alveolar ridge or buccal sulcus, because the gingiva is sacrificed with the osseous specimen.

If the patient received cancericidal doses of radiation to the area of the osseous defect, the clinician can assume that the patient's soft tissues have undergone extreme atrophy and scarring and will be nonpliable and fragile. The soft tissues in this instance will provide a poor bed for a bone graft because the environment is hypovascular, hypoxic, and hypocellular.[1] Similarly, if the patient's defect was caused by a severe infection, it is likely that an excess of scar tissue formation occurred, which will result in nonpliable, poorly vascularized tissue.

After a thorough evaluation, a decision must be made about the adequacy of the soft tissues. If the *quantity* of tissue is deficient, soft tissue flaps from the neck containing muscle and skin can be used to enhance the amount of tissue available to close over the bone graft. If the soft tissues are deficient in *quality,* one of two basic methods can be used to reconstruct a patient's defects: The first is to supply an autogenous bone graft with its own blood supply in the form of a free or pedicled composite graft.

The second method is to improve the quality of the soft tissues already present by the use of hyperbaric oxygen (HBO). The HBO method improves tissue oxygenation by the administration of oxygen to the patient under higher-than-normal atmospheric pressures. Tissue oxygenation has been shown to improve to acceptable levels after 20 HBO treatments.[8]

After HBO treatment, bone-grafting procedures can be performed with good success. Another course of HBO treatment is then recommended after the bone-grafting procedure.[8]

Associated Problems

The clinician must always remember that the cure should be less offensive to the patient than the disease process. In other words, if a reconstructive procedure will significantly risk the individual's life or is associated with a very high incidence of complications that may make life worse for the patient, it would probably be in the patient's best interest to forgo the procedure. As with any type of therapy, significant factors must be assessed, such as the patient's age, health, psychological state, and most important perhaps, the patient's desires. Thorough understanding by the patient of the risks and benefits of any treatment recommendation is imperative so that the patient can make an informed decision.

GOALS AND PRINCIPLES OF MANDIBULAR RECONSTRUCTION

Marx and Sanders[1] have identified several major goals for mandibular reconstruction that one should strive for and achieve before considering any grafting procedure a success.

Restoration of Continuity

Because the mandible is a bone with two articulating ends acted on by muscles with opposing forces, restoration of continuity is the highest priority when reconstructing mandibular defects. Achieving this goal provides the patient with better functional movements and improved facial esthetics by realigning any deviated mandibular segments.

Restoration of Alveolar Bone Height

The functional rehabilitation of the patient rests on the ability to masticate efficiently and comfortably. Prosthetic dental appliances are frequently necessary in patients who have lost a portion of their mandible. To facilitate prosthetic appliance usage, an adequate alveolar process must be provided during the reconstructive surgery. The ideal ridge form outlined in Chapter 13 for the edentulous patient applies equally to patients undergoing mandibular reconstructive surgery.

Restoration of Osseous Bulk

Any bone-grafting procedure must provide enough osseous tissue to withstand normal function. If too thin an osseous strut is provided, fracture of the grafted area may occur.

SURGICAL PRINCIPLES OF MAXILLOFACIAL BONE-GRAFTING PROCEDURES

Several important principles should be followed during any grafting procedure. They must be strictly adhered to if a successful outcome is desired. The following are a few that pertain to reconstructing mandibular defects:

1. *Control of residual mandibular segments.* When a continuity defect is present, the muscles of mastication attached to the residual mandibular fragments will distract the fragments in different directions unless efforts are made to stabilize the remaining mandible in its normal position at the time of partial resection. Maintaining relationships of the remaining mandible fragments after resection of portions of the mandible is a key principle of mandibular reconstruction. This is important for occlusal and temporomandibular joint positioning. When the residual fragments are left to drift, significant facial distortions can occur from deviation of the residual mandibular fragments (Fig. 28-4). Metal bone plates inserted at the time of resection are useful for controlling the position of the mandibular fragments (Figs. 28-1 and 28-5). These plates are of sufficient strength to obviate the need for intermaxillary fixation, permitting active use of the mandible in the immediate postoperative period. In older individuals or those with significant medical compromise, this may be the final form of reconstruction. Use of bone plates provides soft tissue support to maintain facial symmetry. When the mandibular symphysis has been removed, the tongue can be sutured to the plate, maintaining its forward position to prevent airway obstruction (Fig. 28-1, *E*). The bone plate can be left in place when the mandible is secondarily reconstructed with bone grafts, permitting mobility of the mandible during the healing phase of the bone graft (Figs. 28-1 and 28-5).

When the position of the residual mandibular fragments have not been maintained during the resection, realignment is more difficult during the reconstructive surgery. Over time the muscles of mastication become atrophic, fibrotic, and nonpliable, which makes realignment of the fragments extremely difficult. During the reconstructive surgery, it may be necessary to strip several muscles off the mandibular fragments to release the bone from their adverse pull. A coronoidectomy is usually performed to remove the superior pull of the temporalis muscle. Before inserting a bone graft, the clinician must be sure to reach the desired position of the remaining mandibular fragments because what is achieved at surgery is what the patient must live with in the future.

If the mandibular condyle has been resected or is unusable, reconstruction of the condyle with a costochondral junction of a rib or alloplastic condyle is necessary to maintain the forward position of the reconstructed mandible (Fig. 28-5).

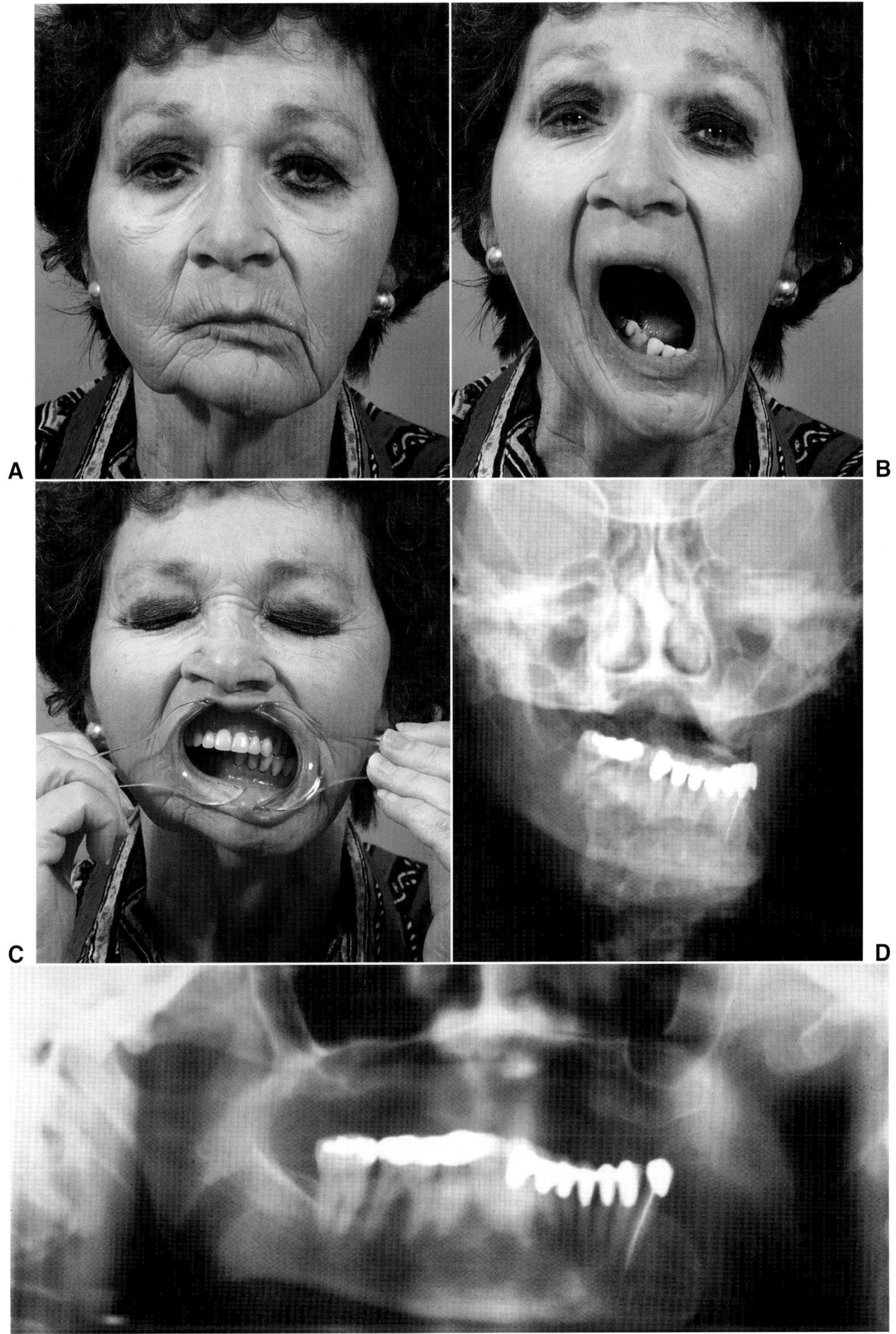

FIGURE 28-4 Patient whose left mandibular ramus and posterior body were removed 10 years previously because of malignant disease (**A**). The deviation of the chin to the left side is visualized. **B**, She deviated to the left side when opening her mouth. **C**, The mandibular deviation also causes a severe malocclusion. **D**, Posteroanterior cephalogram showing deviation of the mandible to the left. **E**, Panoramic radiograph showing residual mandible.

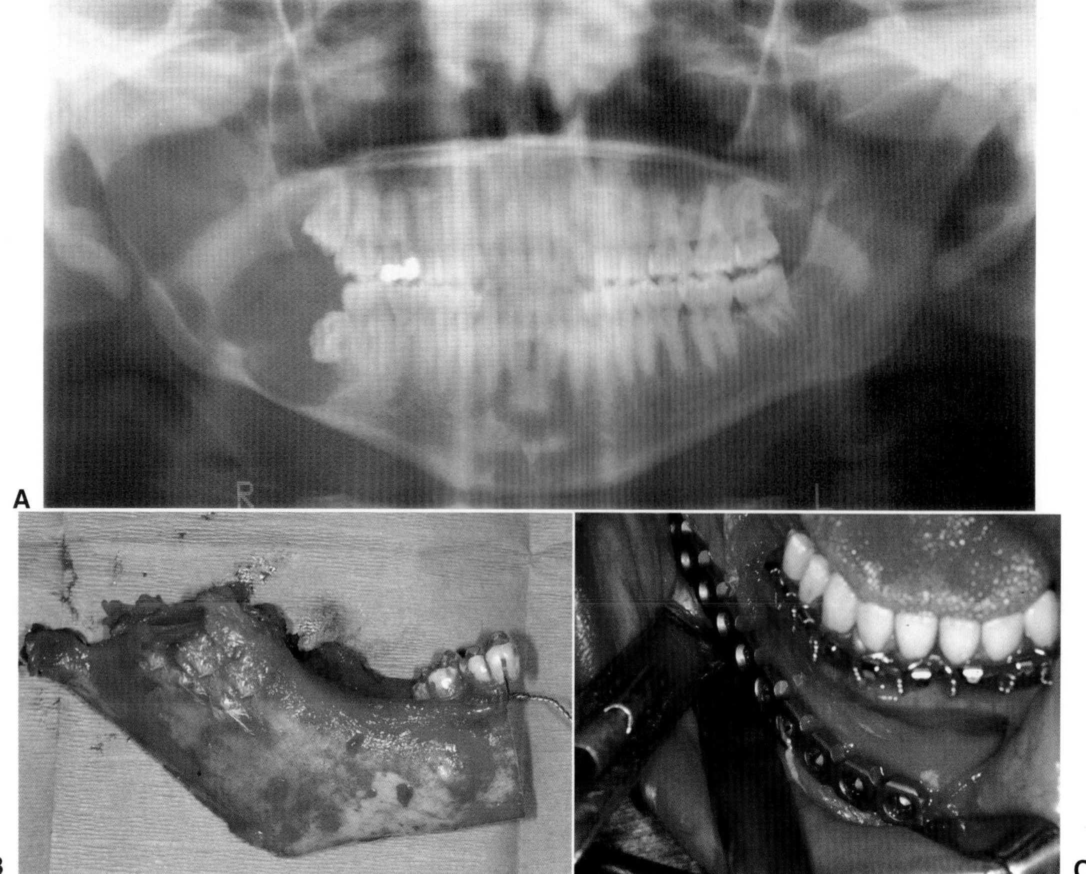

FIGURE 28-5 Example showing the use of a reconstruction bone plate temporarily to maintain the position of the mandible before bony reconstruction. A, Panoramic radiograph showing radiolucent lesion of the mandible that proved to be an ameloblastoma. B, Resection specimen. C, Because the condylar process had to be excised, a reconstruction bone plate with a condylar prosthesis attached to the end has been secured to the mandibular body and symphysis.

2. *A good soft tissue bed for the bone graft.* All bone grafts must be covered on all sides by soft tissues to avoid contamination of the bone graft and to provide the vascularity necessary for revascularization of the graft. Areas of dense scar should be excised until healthy tissue is encountered. Incisions should be designed so that when the wound is closed, the incision will not be over the graft, which means that the initial incision may be very low in the neck. A multilayered soft tissue closure is performed to reduce any space that might allow collection of blood or serum and to provide a watertight closure.
3. *Immobilization of the graft.* Immobilization of bone is necessary for osseous healing to progress, which is why orthopedic surgeons apply a cast to a fractured extremity. In dealing with mandibular defects, the graft must be secured to remaining mandibular fragments, and these fragments must be rigidly immobilized to ensure that no movement exists between them. This immobilization is most often provided by the use of intermaxillary fixation, in which the mandible is secured to the maxilla. However, several other methods are possible, such as using a bone plate between the residual bone fragments. Immobilization for 8 to 12 weeks is usually necessary for adequate healing between the graft and the residual mandibular fragments.
4. *Aseptic environment.* Even when transplanting autogenous osseous tissue, the bone graft is basically avascular, which means that the graft has no way of fighting any amount of infection. Therefore a certain percentage of bone grafts become infected and must be removed. Several measures can be taken to improve the success of bone-grafting procedures. The first is to use an extraoral incision where possible. The skin is much easier to cleanse and disinfect than is the oral cavity. Bone grafts inserted through the mouth are exposed to the oral flora during the grafting procedure.

Furthermore, the intraoral incision may dehisce and again expose the bone graft to the oral flora. Bone grafts placed through a skin incision are more successful than those inserted transorally. However, it is important that during the extraoral dissection the oral cavity is not inadvertently entered. Ideally, dissection to the level of the oral mucosa without perforation is preferred.
5. *Systemic antibiosis.* The prophylactic use of antibiotics may be indicated when transplanting osseous tissue. Prophylaxis may be beneficial in helping reduce the incidence of infection (see Chapter 15).

Because of the many muscles attaching to and providing mobility to the mandible, it is the facial bone that is the most difficult to reconstruct. Other facial bones are reconstructed on similar principles.

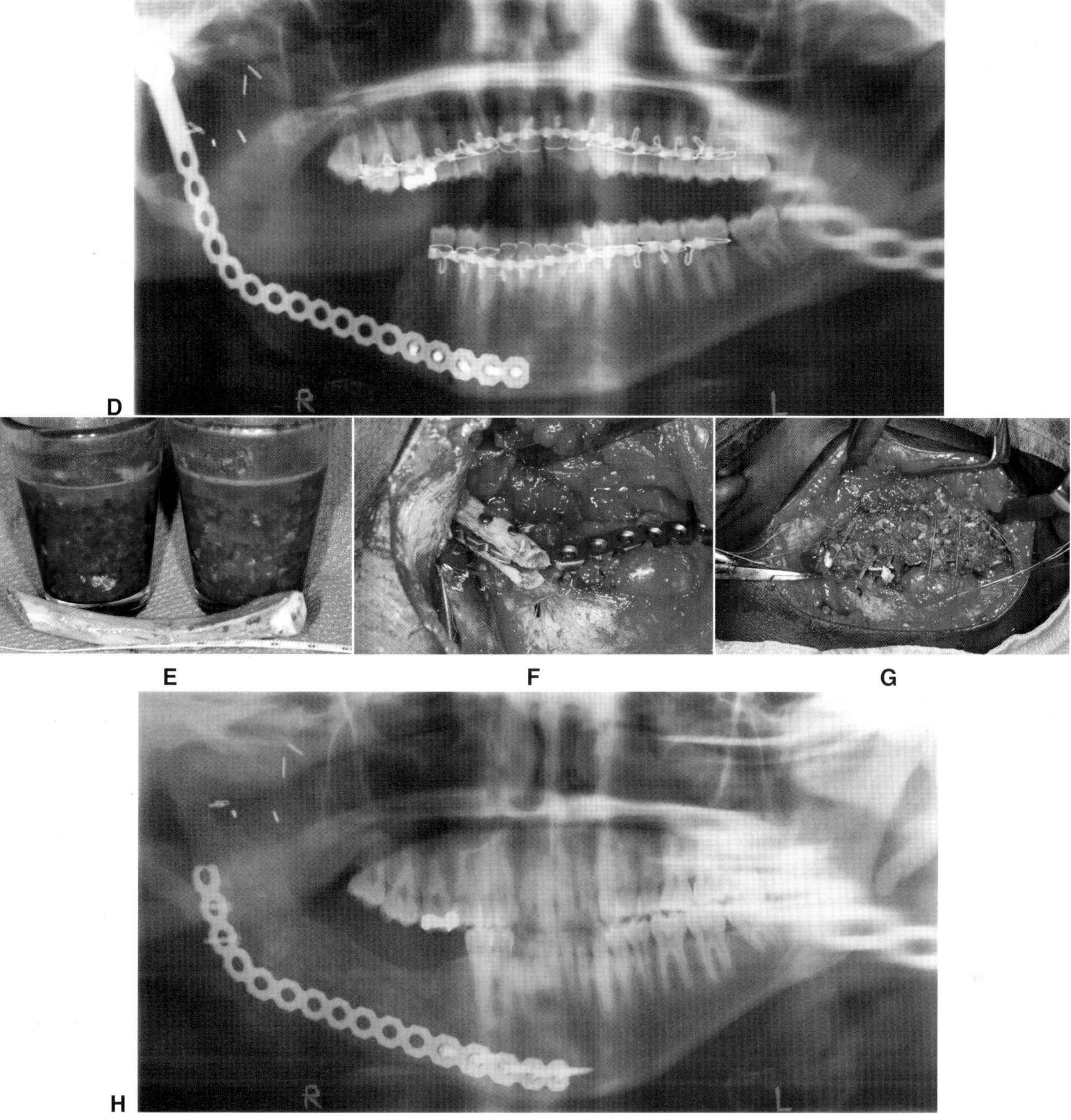

FIGURE 28-5, cont'd Example showing the use of a reconstruction bone plate temporarily to maintain the position of the mandible before bony reconstruction. D, Postoperative panoramic radiograph showing bone plate in place. After 6 to 8 weeks for healing of the oral soft tissues, mandibular reconstruction was undertaken. A rib with some of the costal cartilage attached to one end and particulate bone from the ilium were obtained (E). The condylar prosthesis was removed from the end of the bone plate, and the body of the rib was grooved and placed into the glenoid fossa, surrounding the bone plate (F). The mandibular ramus and posterior body were reconstructed by packing particulate bone into the defect (G). H, Panoramic radiograph taken 6 months later shows good consolidation of the graft.

REFERENCES

1. Marx RE, Saunders TR: Reconstruction and rehabilitation of cancer patients. In Fonseca RJ, Davis WH, editors: *Reconstructive preprosthetic oral and maxillofacial surgery,* Philadelphia, 1986, WB Saunders.
2. Axhausen W: The osteogenetic phases of regeneration of bone: a historical and experimental study, *J Bone Joint Surg Am* 38:593, 1956.
3. Burwell RG: Studies in the transplantation of bone: the fresh composite homograft-autograft of cancellous bone, *J Bone Joint Surg Br* 46:110, 1964.
4. Elves MW: Newer knowledge of immunology of bone and cartilage, *Clin Orthop Relat Res* 120:232, 1976.
5. Gray JC, Elves M: Early osteogenesis in compact bone, *Calcif Tissue Int* 29:225, 1979.
6. Urist MR: Osteoinduction in undermineralized bone implants modified by chemical inhibitors of endogenous matrix enzymes, *Clin Orthop Relat Res* 78:132, 1972.
7. Urist MR: The substratum for bone morphogenesis, *Dev Biol* 4(suppl):125, 1970.
8. Marx RE, Ames JR: The use of hyperbaric oxygen therapy in bony reconstruction of the irradiated and tissue-deficient patient, *J Oral Maxillofac Surg* 40:412, 1982.

PART VIII

Temporomandibular Disorders and Facial Pain

The dentist is commonly perceived as the health care provider with the most expertise in facial neuropathic conditions, whether facial pain or altered nerve function, as well as disorders of the temporomandibular joints. Dentists receive extensive professional education in facial and temporomandibular joint anatomy, physiology, and pathologic conditions. Painful disorders of the maxillofacial region, whether neurologic or musculoskeletal, are common reasons for obtaining a dental opinion. Therefore, it is important for dentists to become knowledgeable about facial neuropathologic conditions and temporomandibular joint disorders.

Chapter 29 presents an overview of facial neuropathologic conditions. The neurophysiology of pain, differential diagnosis of facial pain disorders, and methods of managing various neurogenic facial pain problems are discussed. Then the evaluation and management of altered sensory nerve function are considered.

Temporomandibular joint physiology and pathology is a broad topic, and entire, comprehensive books exist on this topic. Chapter 30 is a concise, up-to-date discussion of the ever-changing field of temporomandibular joint disorders from the viewpoint of oral and maxillofacial surgeons. The chapter is designed to provide the reader with knowledge of the evaluation and management of patients with functional disorders of the temporomandibular joint, including internal derangements, ankylosis, and arthritides.

CHAPTER 29

Facial Neuropathology

JAMES R. HUPP

CHAPTER OUTLINE

The dentist is frequently called on to diagnose pain in the oral and maxillofacial region. Although pain in the mouth is most frequently of odontogenic origin, many facial pains arise from other sources. The diversity of structures in the head and neck region (e.g., eyes, ears, salivary glands, muscle, joints, sinus membranes, intracranial blood vessels) can make arriving at an accurate diagnosis challenging. Even typical toothache symptoms may occur in a healthy tooth because of referred pain or a damaged pain transmission system.

BASICS OF PAIN NEUROPHYSIOLOGY

Pain is a complex human psychophysiologic experience. The sensory-discriminative aspect enables dentists to localize and quantify the pain, but it should be appreciated that this unpleasant experience is influenced by factors such as past experience, cultural behaviors, and emotional and medical states. As the term implies, the pain experience has psychological and physiologic aspects. The physiologic aspects involve several processes: transduction, transmission, and modulation. The sum of these processes, when integrated with higher thought and emotional centers, yields the human experience of pain. Transduction refers to activation of specialized nerves, namely A-delta and C fibers, which transmit information to the spinal cord, or in the case of the trigeminal nerve, to the trigeminal nucleus.

Table 29-1 lists peripheral nerve fibers and their individual characteristics. Chemical, thermal, and mechanical stimuli can activate the free nerve endings of nociceptors, the peripheral nerves indicated previously that transmit pain information. Once in the central nervous system (CNS), information regarding pain is transmitted to the thalamus and hence to cortical centers that process the sensory-discriminative and the emotional-affective aspects of the experience. Modulation systems are activated with pain transmission to varying degrees. The pain modulation system limits the rostral flow of pain information from the spinal cord and trigeminal nucleus to higher cortical centers. A schematic representation of these pain pathways is shown in Fig. 29-1. The chemical and receptor milieu in which transmission and modulation activity occurs is complex. The primary neurochemicals for transmission pathways involve glutamate and substance P, although dozens of neurochemicals have been implicated in pain transmission. The brainstem and spinal cord are the predominant structures involved in modulation. The related primary chemicals include the endogenous opioids, along with serotonin and norepinephrine. Alterations in receptor function are now thought to be critical to the generation of many chronic painful states.

Although the system appears hardwired as described previously, the psychological influences on pain perception should not be underestimated. For the dentist, this influence is a daily part of clinical practice. All dentists are well aware of the extensive variability of the pain response that different patients display to similar procedures. For instance, for some patients, the sound of the dental drill evokes true pain perception, despite the fact that the bur has not yet touched the tooth. Psychological influences are particularly important in determining perceived pain intensity and patient response to pain. When pain becomes chronic, generally defined as greater than 4 to 6 months in duration, attention to psychological influences can become particularly important when treating the pain experience.

CLASSIFICATION OF OROFACIAL PAINS

Numerous classification systems exist for orofacial pain conditions. At the most basic level, it is appropriate to classify orofacial pains as primarily somatic, neuropathic, or psychological.

TABLE 29-1

Relationship Between Sensory Nerve Fiber Size (Diameter) and Conduction Velocity

Fiber Type	Diameter (μm)	Velocity (m/s)
Aα	13-22	70-120
Aβ	8-13	40-70
Aγ	4-8	15-40
Aδ	1-4	5-15
B	1-3	3-14
C	0.5-1.0	0.5-2.0

Somatic pain arises from musculoskeletal or visceral structures interpreted through an *intact* pain transmission and modulation system. Common orofacial examples of musculoskeletal pains are temporomandibular disorders or periodontal pain. Examples of visceral orofacial pains include salivary gland pain and pain caused by dental pulpitis, the tooth pulp behaving like a visceral structure. *Neuropathic pain* arises from damage or alteration to the pain pathways, most commonly a peripheral nerve injury from surgery or trauma. Other causes may involve CNS injury as in thalamic stroke.

Orofacial pains of true *psychological origin* are so rare as not to be included in the differential diagnosis of orofacial pain for the general practitioner. Although psychological influences frequently modify the patient's perception of pain intensity and the patient's response to pain, an actual pain symptom generated by intrapsychic disturbance (e.g., conversion disorder or psychotic delusion) is exceedingly rare. *Malingering,* a term used to identify behavior in which a patient consciously feigns illness or the extent of illness for personal gain, can and does occur, although the literature suggests that the incidence is low. However, a dental patient complaining of chronic pain should be presumed to have a real pain problem unless definitively proved otherwise.

The term *atypical facial pain* is still seen in the literature and is used as a diagnosis primarily by physicians and some dentists; therefore a medical diagnosis code (i.e., *International Classification of Diseases,* ninth revision, code) is associated with it. When reviewing the literature regarding atypical facial pain, a psychological cause is frequently implied. Because true psychogenic pain is rare, this term should be abandoned. For those undiagnosed facial pains, the appropriate term should be *facial pain of unknown cause* until a definitive diagnosis has been established. As a practical matter, these patients unfortunately continue to be labeled with the diagnosis of atypical facial pain for coding purposes, but the dentist should be aware that this is a "diagnosis" awaiting further clarification.

This chapter covers neuropathic facial pains and common headache disorders. Temporomandibular disorders are discussed in Chapter 30. A glossary of pain terminology is listed in Box 29-1.

NEUROPATHIC FACIAL PAINS

Neuropathic pains arise from an injured pain transmission or modulation system. Surgical intervention or trauma is frequently the cause. For example, trauma to the infraorbital region may lead to numbness or pain in the distribution of the infraorbital nerve. In oral and maxillofacial surgery, extraction of mandibular third molars carries a slight but measurable risk of

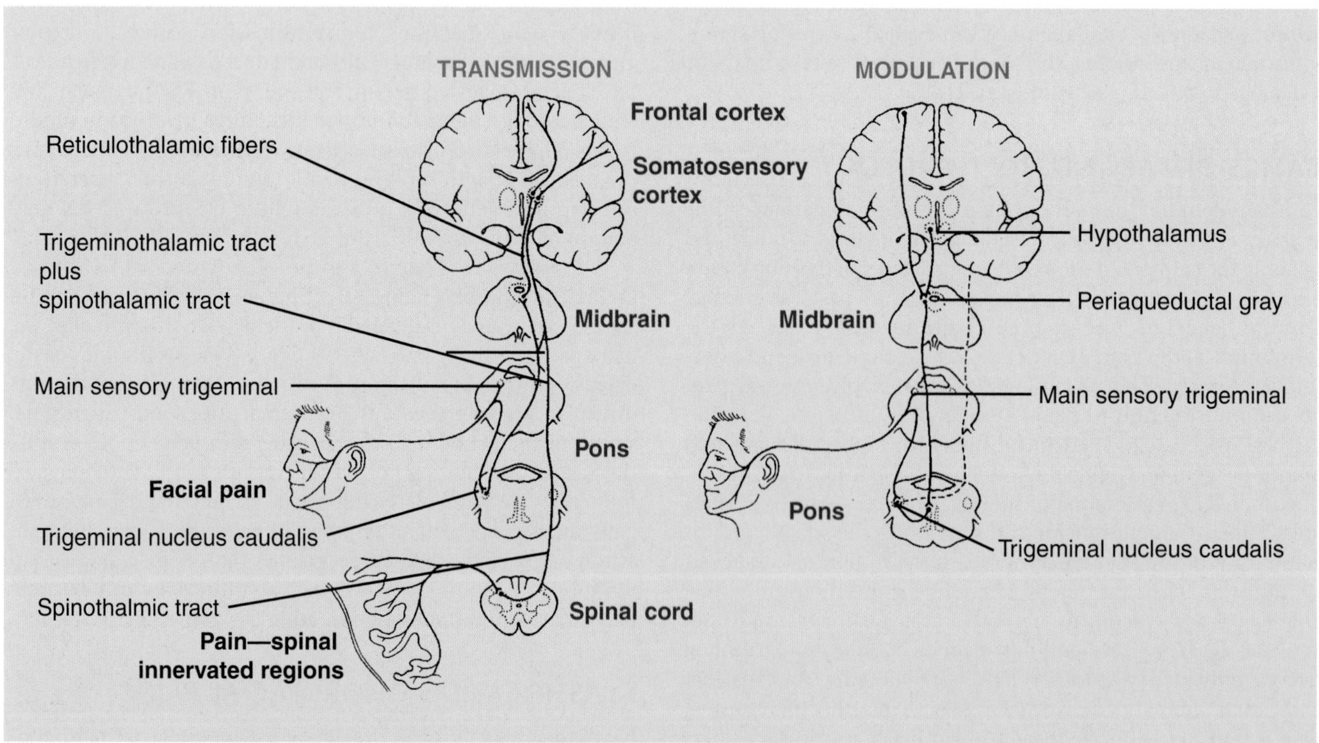

FIGURE 29-1 Trigeminal and spinal pain transmission pathways *(left)*. Trigeminal pain modulation system *(right)*. Dotted line indicates decreased pain transmission.

BOX 29-1

Glossary of Pain Terms

Allodynia	Pain caused by a stimulus that does not normally provoke pain
Analgesia	Absence of pain in response to stimulation that would normally be painful
Anesthesia	Absence of all sensation
Deafferentation pain	Pain caused by loss of sensory input into the central nervous system
Dysesthesia	Unpleasant abnormal sensation, whether spontaneous or evoked (Note: Dysesthesia includes paresthesia but not vice versa.)
Hyperalgesia	Increased sensitivity to noxious stimulation
Hyperesthesia	Increased sensitivity to all stimulation, excluding special senses (Note: When the sensation is painful, the terms *allodynia* and *hyperalgesia* may be appropriate.)
Hypoalgesia	Diminished sensitivity to noxious stimulation
Hypoesthesia	Diminished sensitivity to all stimulation, excluding the special senses (Note: When the sensation is pain, the terms *hypoalgesia* and *analgesia* may be appropriate.)
Neuralgia	Pain in the distribution of a nerve or nerves
Neuropathy	Disturbance of function or pathologic change in a nerve
Paresthesia	Abnormal sensation, whether spontaneous or evoked

nerve damage to the mandibular or lingual nerves. In the majority of these cases, damage leads to paresthesia, an abnormal sensation in the dermatome of the affected nerve. Typically, this sensation is one of mild numbness or tingling. Loss of all sensation may occur when the nerve is transected. In a subset of cases, dysesthesia—an abnormal, unpleasant sensation—can result; it is often described as a burning or sharp electric shocklike sensation. When a patient complains of burning or sharp shocklike pain in the face or mouth, pain of neuropathic origin should be included in the differential diagnosis. One should appreciate that the oral cavity is the most common site of amputation, if one recognizes amputations to include the teeth and the dental pulp (i.e., endodontics). As in phantom limb pain after extremity amputation, "phantom" sensations can also arise, albeit rarely, after dental and pulpal trauma or extraction. Neuropathic pains may also give rise to the sensation of tooth pain, which often is a diagnostic dilemma for the dentist. Referral of patients for management of these disorders to dentists focusing on orofacial pain diagnosis and management or to the patient's personal physician or a neurologist is customary.

Neuropathic Facial Pains Presenting as Toothache

Trigeminal Neuralgia

The prototypic neuropathic facial pain is trigeminal neuralgia (TN; Box 29-2), literally nerve pain arising from the trigeminal nerve. Although this could refer to any neuropathic pain of trigeminal nerve origin, TN or tic douloureux (i.e., painful tic) has specific inclusion criteria. Occurring most frequently in patients over 50 years of age (incidence 8:100,000; female-to-

BOX 29-2

Trigeminal Neuralgia: Clinical Characteristics

- Severe paroxysmal pain
- Unilateral location (96%); *r* > *l*
- Mild superficial stimulation provokes pain
- V2 and V3 dermatomes most affected
- Frequently pain free between attacks
- No neurologic deficits
- No dentoalveolar cause found
- Local anesthesia of trigger zone temporarily arrests pain

male ratio 1.6:1.0), TN usually occurs with sharp, electric shocklike pain in the face or mouth. The pain is intense, lasting for brief periods of seconds to 1 minute, after which there is a refractory period during which the pain cannot be reinitiated. At times, a background aching or burning pain is present. Usually a trigger zone is present where mechanical stimuli such as soft touch may provoke an attack. Firm pressure to the region is generally not as provocative. Common cutaneous trigger zones include the corner of the lips, cheek, ala of the nose, or lateral brow. Any intraoral site may also be a trigger zone for TN, including the teeth, gingivae, or tongue. Trigger zones in the V2 and V3 distributions are most common, after which they occur alone (and in decreasing order of incidence) in the V3, V2, and V1 distributions. The pain of TN illustrates an important distinction of many neuropathic pains as opposed to somatic pains—the lack of a typical graded response to increasing stimulation. If light stimulation produces a pain response out of proportion to the stimulus, a neuropathic process should be considered. This also holds true for pain that has a burning or electric shocklike quality. Sometimes a background aching pain accompanies TN, making it difficult to distinguish from the pain of acute pulpitis or possibly periapical periodontitis. Importantly, local anesthetic block of the trigger zone arrests the pain of TN for the duration of anesthesia and sometimes longer, which can lead the dentist to ascribe a "dental" cause to the pain complaint.

The cause of TN is not entirely clear, but the consensus is that pressure on the root entry zone of the trigeminal nerve by a vascular loop leads to focal demyelination. This demyelination in turn precipitates ectopic or hyperactive discharge of the nerve. The site of demyelination determines the trigeminal division involved and hence the clinical presentation. Other diseases such as multiple sclerosis, tumors, and Lyme disease can produce pain similar to that produced by TN. The treatment of TN is medical or surgical. Medical treatment is generally undertaken with anticonvulsants.

The classical medication for the condition is carbamazepine, but newer anticonvulsants (e.g., gabapentin and oxcarbazepine) and the antispastic baclofen, are commonly used as well. Table 29-2 lists commonly used TN and neuropathic facial pain medications. Many of these medications have significant, even life-threatening, side effects; therefore, only dentists focusing on orofacial pain diagnosis and management use them in dental practice. Surgical treatment includes microvascular decompression of the offending vascular loop (so-called Janetta procedure), GammaKnife radiosurgery, percutaneous needle thermal rhizotomy, or balloon compression of the root

TABLE 29-2

Common Medications for Trigeminal Neuralgia and Neuropathic Facial Pains

Medications	Dosage (mg/d)
ANTICONVULSANTS	
Carbamazepine (Tegretol)	400-1200
Gabapentin (Neurontin)	600-3200
Clonazepam (Klonopin)	2-8
Divalproex (Depakote)	500-2000
Oxcarbazepine (Trileptal)	300-2400
Lamotrigine (Lamictal)	50-500
Topiramate (Topamax)	50-400
Phenytoin (Dilantin)	300-600
TRICYCLIC ANTIDEPRESSANTS	
Amitriptyline	10-300
Doxepin	10-300
Nortriptyline	10-150
Imipramine	10-300
ANTISPASTIC	
Baclofen (Lioresal)	15-80

entry zone. For the dentist, the critical issue is recognizing TN so that unneeded dental treatment or extraction is avoided. Unfortunately, when the trigger zone is located in an intraoral, dental, or periodontal site, unnecessary dental treatment is common.

Pretrigeminal Neuralgia

Although a rare condition, pretrigeminal neuralgia (pre-TN) has been recognized for some time. The presenting condition is typically an aching dental pain in a region where physical and radiographic examination reveals no abnormality. Local anesthetic block of the tooth (or extraction site, if applicable) arrests pain for the duration of anesthetic action. A number of patients with this condition have been demonstrated to go on to have typical TN symptoms (i.e., sharp electric shock pains the area). Pre-TN responds to similar treatments as TN, beginning with anticonvulsant therapy. To avoid unnecessary dental treatment, the dentist must have a high index of suspicion for secondary diagnoses for those pains that are inconsistent with physical examination or do not respond in a predictable way after treatment. Clinical features of pre-TN are listed in Box 29-3.

Odontalgia Resulting from Deafferentation (Atypical Odontalgia)

Pain resulting from deafferentation refers to pain that occurs when there has been damage to the afferent pain transmission system. Usually this condition is caused by trauma or surgery, including extraction and endodontic treatment. By definition, extraction and endodontics are deafferentating because they involve amputation of tissue that contains the nerve supply of a human structure, the tooth. Limb amputation is another example of a deafferentation procedure. As with phantom limb pain, a similar picture of oral deafferentation pain may occur, but only in a small subset of patients are the symptoms severe enough to warrant treatment. These pains may be maintained by various mechanisms, some readily appreciated and others complex and not yet completely understood. Peripheral hyperactivity at the site of nerve damage is easily understandable. At the site of dental alveolar nerve damage, neuronal hyperactivity leading to persistent pain occurs. In this form, the pain is frequently arrested with local anesthetic block. CNS hyperactivity, however, also can be responsible for persistent pain experienced in the tooth site. In this model, peripheral neural damage leads to changes in the second-order nerve in the trigeminal nucleus that synapsed with the primary peripheral nociceptor. Changes occur centrally in which ongoing pain transmission to higher cortical centers can occur despite minimal or even no peripheral input. Local anesthetic block does not arrest pain in this circumstance.

Additionally, patients may exhibit both forms of compromise simultaneously (i.e., only a portion of pain may be arrested by local anesthetic block). Sympathetic nervous system activity has also been shown to augment some of these complex neuropathic processes. Clinical features of deafferentation pains are listed in Box 29-4. Interestingly, for many deafferentation pains, further peripheral surgical procedures frequently intensify symptoms and lead to a broader area of perceived pain. If pain resulting from deafferentation is suspected, further surgical procedures should be undertaken cautiously.

The key to recognizing all of these conditions, and avoiding unnecessary and potentially harmful dental treatment, frequently lies in obtaining an excellent description of the chief complaint, including quality of pain, duration, alleviating factors, and aggravating factors. The history of the complaint and how the symptoms have changed over time can also be valuable. A more complete discussion follows in the section Evaluation of Patient with Orofacial Pain.

Other Neuropathic Facial Pains

Although the following pains share common mechanisms with those discussed previously, it is appropriate to list

BOX 29-3

Pretrigeminal Neuralgia: Clinical Characteristics

- Aching or burning pain
- Continuous or intermittent
- Unilateral location
- Local anesthesia of painful region temporarily arrests pain
- Neurologic examination normal
- No dentoalveolar cause found
- Frequently responsive to anticonvulsant therapy

BOX 29-4

Odontalgia Resulting from Deafferentation

Burning or aching pain is continuous or almost continuous
Sharp paroxysms may occur
Allodynia, hyperesthesia, or hypoesthesia may be present
No dentoalveolar cause is found
History of surgical or other trauma exists
History of symptoms greater than 4 to 6 months exists
Local anesthetic block equivocal

them separately because they possess some unique characteristics.

Postherpetic Neuralgia

Postherpetic neuralgia (PHN) is a potential sequela of herpes zoster infection. Shingles, or herpes zoster, may occur at any stage in a person's life. Herpes zoster is the clinical manifestation of the reactivation of a lifelong latent infection with varicella zoster virus, usually contracted after an episode of chicken pox in early life. Herpes zoster occurs more commonly in later life and in immunocompromised patients. Each year in the United States, shingles strikes at least 850,000 persons. Most are over 60 years of age. By age 85, 50% of persons will have had a bout. Of those who do, 60% to 70% will have PHN. Varicella zoster virus tends to be reactivated only once in a lifetime, with the incidence of second attacks being less than 5%. PHN occurs after reactivation of the virus, which can lay dormant in the ganglia of a peripheral nerve. Most commonly, this is a thoracic nerve, but approximately 10% to 15% of the time the trigeminal nerve is involved, with the V1 dermatome affected in approximately 80% of cases. When reactivated, the virus travels along the nerve and is expressed in the cutaneous dermatome of that nerve. For a thoracic nerve, for example, the patient has a unilateral patch of vesicular eruption closely outlining the classical dermatome for that nerve. In the ophthalmic division of the trigeminal nerve, the V1 dermatome is outlined by rash. In the V2 or V3 distribution, intraoral and cutaneous expression is commonly seen. The acute phase is painful but subsides within 2 to 5 weeks. However, a subset of patients develops a deafferentation pain that, as discussed previously, can have peripheral, central, or mixed features. The pain is typically burning, aching, or shocklike (consistent with a pain caused by a neuropathic condition). Treatment is undertaken with anticonvulsants or the tricyclic or other antidepressants. Tramadol, a mild opioid with mild antidepressant effects, can be a useful adjunct. Local injection of painful sites, sympathetic block, or both is sometimes of value. Most importantly, preventive treatment of PHN with antivirals, analgesics, and frequently corticosteroids very early after rash presentation can significantly reduce the expression of PHN.

A related condition, Ramsay Hunt syndrome, is a herpes zoster infection of the sensory and motor branches of the facial nerve (VII) and in some cases the auditory nerve (VIII). Symptoms include facial paralysis, vertigo, deafness, and herpetic eruption in the external auditory meatus.

Neuroma

After peripheral nerve transection, the proximal portion of the nerve generally forms sprouts in an effort to regain communication with the severed distal component. When sprouting occurs without distal segment communication, a stump of neuronal tissue, Schwann cells, and other neural elements can form. This stump, or neuroma, can become exquisitely sensitive to mechanical and chemical stimuli.

The pain is commonly burning or shocklike. Frequently, a positive Tinel's sign is present. In this test, tapping over the suspected neuroma produces sharp, shooting electric shocklike pain. Damage to the mandibular or lingual nerve after third molar surgery is another source for neuroma formation. Some oral and maxillofacial surgeons provide microneurosurgical treatment, which can be beneficial for some patients.

Although it is difficult to predict which patients will benefit from nerve repair, clearly neurosurgical intervention should be accomplished within 3 to 6 months to improve the likelihood of success. Again, the commonality of symptom presentation in multiple nerve injury models suggests the importance of eliciting the patient's description of pain when facing a diagnostic dilemma.

Burning Mouth Syndrome

In this condition the patient perceives a burning or aching sensation in all or part of the oral cavity. The tongue is the most frequently involved site. Perceived dry mouth and altered taste are common. The cause is unknown, but a defect in pain modulation may be the most promising theory. Most patients are postmenopausal women, although hormone replacement therapy does not consistently affect symptoms. Approximately 50% of patients improve without treatment over a 2-year period, indicating the importance of placebo-controlled trials when scientifically testing any treatment modality. The predominant treatment approach is with anticonvulsants or antidepressants, although neither avenue, even in combination, shows consistent results.

Other Cranial Neuralgias

As with TN, any of the cranial nerves with a sensory component appears capable of a neuralgic presentation. The most common of the other cranial nerves to present this way is the glossopharyngeal nerve (IX). The presenting symptom is typically sharp, electric shocklike pain on swallowing with a trigger zone in the oropharynx or the base of the tongue. Pain is usually experienced in the throat or tongue but may be referred to the lower jaw. The facial nerve (VII) has a small somatic component on the anterior wall of the external auditory meatus in which shocklike pains are experienced (sometimes associated with symptoms of tinnitus, dysgeusia, and dysequilibrium). The vagus nerve (X) also has the potential for neuralgic activity manifesting as pain in the laryngeal region shooting deep to the mandibular ramus or even to the region of the temporomandibular joint. Most often, treatment of cranial neuralgias, like TN, involves the use of anticonvulsants; however, in some cases intracranial surgery is necessary.

CHRONIC HEADACHE

Headache has many causes and is one of the most common complaints made to the primary care physician. When headaches recur regularly, the majority are diagnosed as one of the primary (no other cause) headaches: migraine, tension-type headache, or cluster headache. Although most headaches are centered in the orbits and temples, many may present in the lower half of the face, teeth, or jaws.

Migraine

Migraine is a common headache afflicting approximately 18% of woman and 8% of men. The first migraine headache typically occurs in the teenage years or in young adulthood but may begin in very young children as well. Before puberty, migraine occurs equally in both sexes. After puberty the ratio changes so that women are at least twice as likely as men to have migraines. Migraine headaches are unilateral in approximately 40% of cases. An "aura" may develop several minutes to 1 hour before headache onset in approximately 40% of patients. The aura is a neurologic disturbance, frequently expressed as flashing or shimmering lights or a partial loss of vision.

Complicated auras may produce transient hemiparesis, aphasia, or blindness. Upward of 80% of migraineurs have nausea and photophobia (intolerance to light) during attacks. Migraines typically last 4 to 72 hours. The International Headache Society criteria for migraine are listed in Boxes 29-5 and 29-6. Headache triggers include menstruation, stress, certain vasoactive foods or drugs and certain musculoskeletal disorders that produce pain in the trigeminal system (e.g., temporomandibular disorders). The mechanism for migraine headache, although not completely understood, appears to involve neurogenic inflammation of intracranial blood vessels resulting from neurotransmitter imbalance in certain brainstem centers. Migraine is a referred pain process, and the intracranial vessel involved determines the site of perceived pain (e.g., the orbit, temple, jaw, or vertex of the head). Preventive treatment is directed at normalizing neurotransmitter imbalance with antidepressants, anticonvulsants, β-blockers, and other drugs. Biofeedback and other therapies are also helpful. Treatment of acute attacks is with the "triptans" (e.g., sumatriptan [Imitrex], zolmitriptan [Zomig], rizatriptan [Maxalt], naratriptan [Amerge], and almotriptan [Axert]), ergots, nonsteroidal antiinflammatory drugs, opioid analgesics, antiemetics, and other agents.

For the dentist, knowledge of migraine is important because temporomandibular disorders may precipitate a migraine attack in a migraine-prone patient. Likewise, cervical spine and cervical muscular disorders may precipitate migraine. Also important is for the dentist to recognize that cervical and masticatory muscle hyperactivity often occurs during a migraine headache. Migraine may therefore be a perpetuating factor in some temporomandibular disorders or a reason for misdiagnosis. Although toothache and jaw pains are not a common expression of migraine, a number of cases have been reported in the literature and are seen with some frequency by pain specialists. When migraine is a cause of jaw or face pain, the key to the diagnosis is recognizing that nausea, sonophobia, and photophobia are not accompaniments of masticatory musculoskeletal disorders or jaw and tooth pain of dental origin.

BOX 29-5

International Headache Society Criteria for Migraine Headache Without Aura

A. Two of the following:
  - Unilateral headache pain location
  - Headache pain has pulsating quality
  - Moderate to severe intensity
  - Aggravation by routine physical activity

B. At least one of the following:
  - Nausea
  - Photophobia and phonophobia

C. Headache, untreated, lasting 4 to 72 hours

D. Both of the following:
  - Similar pain in the past
  - No evidence of organic disease

BOX 29-6

International Headache Society Criteria for Migraine Headache with Aura

Headache pain is preceded by fully reversible neurologic symptoms, occurring over 5 to 60 minutes, such as the following:

◆ Visual
  - Scintillating scotoma
  - Fortification spectra
  - Photopsia

◆ Sensory
  - Paresthesia
  - Numbness
  - Unilateral weakness
  - Speech disturbance

Common migraine characteristics:

◆ Duration: usually 12 to 72 hours
◆ Sex: female/male ratio >2:1
◆ Neurologic aura: ~40%

Tension-Type Headache

The majority of patients who report to the physician with a chief complaint of headache are diagnosed with tension-type headache. The name can be misleading because "muscle tension" or "tension from stress" is not always present, alone or in combination. Tension-type headache is common in the general population, and most individuals experience at least one tension-type headache at some point.

Chronic tension-type headache is more common in women than in men. The headache is generally bilateral. Pain is frequently bitemporal or frontal-temporal in distribution. Patients commonly describe their pain as though their head is "in a vice" or a "squeezing hatband" is around their head. Headache can occur with or without "pericranial muscle tenderness" (i.e., tenderness to palpation of the masticatory and occipital muscles). To be defined as chronic tension-type headache, symptoms must be present longer than 15 days per month. The International Headache Society criteria for tension-type headache are listed in Box 29-7. Treatment of tension-type headache is commonly with tricyclic or other antidepressants.

BOX 2F9-7

International Headache Society Criteria for Episodic Tension-Type Headache

A. Headache pain accompanied by two of the following symptoms:
  - Pressing/tightening (nonpulsating) quality
  - Mild to moderate intensity
  - Bilateral location
  - Not aggravated by routine physical activity

B. Headache pain accompanied by both of the following symptoms:
  - No nausea or vomiting
  - Photophobia and phonophobia not present or only one present

C. Fewer than 15 days per month with headache (Note: *If more than 15 days/month, headache is termed a* chronic tension-type headache.)

D. No evidence of organic disease

When tension-type headache occurs in migraineurs, migraine treatments are usually beneficial.

Psychosocial factors are often a contributing factor influencing tension-type headache. In this situation, cognitive-behavioral and other psychological therapies are frequently beneficial.

For the dentist, it is important to distinguish tension-type headache from masticatory myofascial pain. This can be confusing because both conditions have similar symptoms. It is significant that in myofascial pain, pressure to various head or neck muscles refers to the site of head pain, whereas in tension-type headache, pressure identifies the site of pain. Importantly for either condition, identifying the site of pain does not always imply the source of pain. Additionally, in tension-type headache, pain does not proportionally increase with increasing pressure to the headache site nor refer pain to other areas.

Cluster Headache

Cluster headache is an overwhelmingly unilateral head pain typically centered around the eye and temporal regions. The pain is intense, frequently described as a stabbing sensation (i.e., as if an ice pick was being driven into the eye). Some component of parasympathetic overactivity is present (commonly lacrimation, conjunctival injection, ptosis, or rhinorrhea). Headaches last 15 to 180 minutes and may occur once or multiple times per day, commonly with precise regularity (e.g., awakening the patient at the same time night after night). The headaches occur in clusters such that they may be present for some months and then remit for several months or even years. Alcohol ingestion consistently triggers headache, but only during cluster episodes. As opposed to most other chronic headaches, men are much more likely to have cluster headaches than are women (Box 29-8). International Headache Society criteria are listed in Box 29-9. Treatment, as in migraine, is preventive or symptomatic. Preventive treatment is accomplished with verapamil, lithium salts, anticonvulsants, corticosteroids, and certain ergot compounds. Symptomatic treatment is with "triptans," ergots, and analgesics. Oxygen inhalation at 7 to 10 L/min may be an effective abortive treatment.

Dentists must be aware that cluster headache frequently produces pain in the posterior maxilla, mimicking severe dentoalveolar pain in the posterior maxillary teeth. The pain is frequently stabbing and intense, although background aching may occur. Unnecessary dental therapy is, unfortunately, common. Common features can distinguish a toothache resulting from cluster headache from a toothache produced by a dental problem:

- Rapid emergence and discontinuation of symptoms unlike typical toothache
- Toothache precipitated by alcohol ingestion
- Toothache accompanied by unilateral rhinorrhea or other parasympathetic symptoms
- Toothache that occurs with periodicity

BOX 29-8

Common Cluster Headache Features

Sex: Mainly male
Frequency: Up to 8 per day
Quality: Throbbing/stabbing
Intensity: Severe

BOX 29-9

International Headache Society Criteria for Cluster Headache

A. Severe unilateral orbital, supraorbital, or temporal pain (or a combination) lasting 15 to 180 minutes (Note: Frequently in posterior maxillary dentoalveolar region as well)
B. At least one of the following on the headache side:
   - Conjunctival injection
   - Facial sweating
   - Lacrimation
   - Miosis
   - Nasal congestion
   - Ptosis
   - Rhinorrhea
   - Eyelid edema
C. No evidence of organic disease

OTHER CHRONIC HEAD PAINS OF DENTAL INTEREST

Temporal Arteritis (Giant Cell Arteritis)

Temporal arteritis, more properly termed *giant cell arteritis*, is literally an inflammation (i.e., vasculitis) of the cranial arterial tree that can affect any or all vessels of the aortic arch and its branches. The condition is most prevalent in those over 50 years of age. The inflammation results from a giant cell granulomatous reaction. Polymyalgia rheumatica, the most common nonarticular rheumatologic condition causing diffuse muscle inflammation, is frequently a comorbid condition. Dull aching or throbbing temporal or head pain is a common complaint affecting 70% of patients and is the presenting symptom in one third of patients. Jaw claudication (i.e., increasing weakness and pain in the jaw or tongue with ongoing mastication) may lead the patient to visit the dentist for diagnosis. Any older patient reporting jaw or face pain not obviously of odontogenic origin and whose symptoms suggest temporal arteritis should be referred for an erythrocyte sedimentation rate test—a standard laboratory blood test. Although a negative test does not rule out temporal arteritis, a significantly elevated erythrocyte sedimentation rate may help confirm the diagnosis. A temporal artery biopsy may also be obtained, but again a negative test does not conclusively rule out the condition. Treatment is with high-dose corticosteroids, frequently for many months, and early treatment is necessary to avoid blindness caused by extension of the disease process to the ophthalmic artery.

Indomethacin-Responsive Headaches

A number of head pains respond primarily or exclusively to the nonsteroidal antiinflammatory drug indomethacin. One of these headaches, chronic paroxysmal hemicrania, is similar in presentation to cluster headache, although the attacks are short lived (lasting several minutes) and occur many times per day. Unlike cluster headaches, women are more often affected than men. Again toothache may be the initial presentation. Exertional headaches, as in weight lifting or during intercourse, may also produce intense, rapid-onset headache responsive to indomethacin. Hypnic headache, waking the patient from sleep generally within 2 to 4 hours of sleep onset and lasting 15 minutes to 3 hours, is frequently indomethacin responsive, but hypnic headache is not accompanied by symptoms of parasympathetic overactivity.

EVALUATION OF PATIENT WITH OROFACIAL PAIN

Evaluation of the dental patient who has jaw or face pain of nonodontogenic origin is an important skill for the dentist to master. Obtaining an accurate history is the most important component of information gathering. For chronic headache disorders and many neuropathic disorders, such as TN, pre-TN, and other cranial neuralgias, as well as burning mouth syndrome, generally no abnormality is found on physical examination; therefore the clinician must rely on the verbal history to arrive at an accurate diagnosis. Chronic headache disorders based on symptom description are presented in Table 29-3.

The pain history should include the chief complaint, including the current description of pain quality (e.g., aching, throbbing, burning, shocklike, paroxysmal, or some combination), intensity, when it occurs, how long it lasts, if it changes in character over time, precipitating factors, and alleviating factors. The history of the present illness should include date of onset, circumstances surrounding onset, how the pain evolved over time, diagnostic tests undertaken, diagnoses rendered, what treatments were instituted in the past, and the response to those treatments. Finally, a comprehensive medical and dental history should be taken. Most commonly a short differential diagnostic list can be made at this time. The physical examination attempts to narrow this list to obtain a working diagnosis.

The physical evaluation should include all aspects of the normal dental evaluation, including vital signs determination, intraoral examination with oral cancer screening, and head and neck examination with an evaluation of the temporal and carotid arteries, lymph nodes, skin, head, and neck, as well as myofascial and temporomandibular joint examination. In addition, a cranial nerve screening examination should be performed. It is understood that most dentists would not include all aspects of the formal neurologic examination, such as fundoscopic examination and testing of ability to smell, in this screening. See Table 29-4 for cranial screening evaluation. This latter examination is frequently an attempt to detect areas of hyperesthesia or hyperalgesia, allodynia, a trigger zone for TN, or an area of decreased sensation. In addition, it is important to define whether the pain follows normal neuroanatomic boundaries and, if so, to define these areas. Diagnostic anesthetic testing, usually with a vasoconstrictor-free solution, is appropriate to help define whether a suspected neuropathic pain condition has a significant peripheral component perpetuating pain.

When a peripheral component occurs, local anesthesia may arrest the pain for the duration of anesthesia. Most commonly, local anesthesia is applied to increasingly larger neuroanatomic regions. For instance, with a pain in the region of the mandibular canine, topical anesthesia in the anterior mandibular gingiva is applied. If pain is not arrested, the response to infiltration anesthesia is assessed. If no response is seen, a mental block (sparing the lingual nerve) is attempted, and finally, inferior alveolar and lingual nerve block anesthesia is undertaken if pain has not yet been alleviated. At each test, any alteration in pain response is noted.

Imaging is appropriate for many disorders to rule out an odontogenic, sinus, or bony pathologic conditions. The orthopantograph is helpful when supported by selected dental periapical radiographs as needed. For most neuropathic and headache disorders, intracranial imaging is important to rule out a CNS demyelinating process (e.g., multiple sclerosis in which TN may be the presenting symptom), vascular malformation, tumor, or other abnormality. Except for specially trained dentists, it is appropriate for the primary care physician or neurologist to order these studies. Other specialized studies (e.g., magnetic resonance arteriography, bone scan, and scintigraphy) may be indicated. With the information obtained from these studies, the dentist may elect to treat the patient or refer the patient to an oral and maxillofacial surgeon, general dentist focusing on orofacial pain diagnosis and management, or an appropriate physician. The role of the primary care dentist is mainly to establish a proper diagnosis and avoid unnecessary treatment, which may jeopardize the patient's health.

TABLE 29-3

Differential Diagnoses of Common Headaches

	Temporal Arteritis	Migraine	Cluster	Tension
Onset	Acute or chronic	Acute	Acute	Chronic
Location	Localized	Unilateral (40%)	Unilateral	Global, unilateral
Associated symptoms	Weight loss, polymyalgia rheumatica, fever, decreased vision, jaw claudication	Nausea, vomiting, photophobia, phonophobia	Rhinorrhea, lacrimation of ipsilateral side	Multisomatic complaints
Pain character	Severe throbbing over area affected	Throbbing	Sharp stabbing	Aching
Duration	Prolonged	Prolonged	30 minutes-2 hours	Daily
Prior history	(–)	(+)	(+)	(+)
Diagnostic test	Erythrocyte sedimentation rate (+)	None—history	None—history	None—history
Physical examination	Tender temporal arteries, myalgias, fever	Nausea, vomiting, photophobia, phonophobia	Unilateral, rhinorrhea, lacrimation, partial Horner syndrome	(–)

TABLE 29-4

Rapid Cranial Nerve Examination for the General Dentist

The examination begins with patient seated in the dental chair. The clinician asks if patient has any severe problems with seeing, hearing, or dizziness and observes patient for signs of visual or auditory problems, including whether the eyes move consensually. The clinician also checks for eyelid ptosis and mouth symmetry when patient smiles.

Next, the patient tries to hold eyelids tightly closed while the clinician tries to open them with the fingers. While the patient's eyes are closed, the clinician holds coffee or cloves to the patient's nose and asks patient to identify the odor. The patient then opens the eyes widely while raising the eyebrows. The clinician shines a bright light into each eye individually and observes the reaction of each pupil. The patient looks directly left and right and then tries to look at each shoulder without moving the head.

The clinician then asks the patient to show the teeth, then pucker, and then evert the lower lip. Next the patient clenches the jaw closed while the clinician palpates each masseter muscle. The patient then opens the mouth and sticks the tongue straight out. While the tongue is out, the clinician uses a cotton-tipped applicator to stroke each side of the uvula briefly. With the clinician's hands on the lateral aspects of the patient's chin, the patient then tries to push laterally against the hands. The clinician then rubs the fingers in front of each of the patient's ears and asks what the patient hears.

Finally, areas of hypoesthesia or hyperesthesia should be identified and recorded. Areas of the pain complaint should receive special attention if nerve injury is suspected. Trigger areas for trigeminal neuralgia should also be investigated if symptoms warrant.

Cranial Nerve (CN)	Abnormal Test Results
I—Olfactory	Failure to identify odor may indicate nasal obstruction or CN I problem.
II—Optic	Failure of pupil to constrict or presence of nonconsensual gaze may indicate CN II problem.
III—Oculomotor	Failure of pupil to constrict or presence of ptosis may indicate CN III problem.
IV—Trochlear	Inability of eye to look to ipsilateral shoulder may indicate CN IV problem.
V—Trigeminal	Inability to feel light touch may indicate sensory CN V problem. Weakness of masseter may indicate motor CN V problem. Areas of hypoesthesia or hyperesthesia should be identified and recorded. Areas of pain complaint should receive special attention if nerve injury is suspected. Trigger areas for trigeminal neuralgia should also be investigated if symptoms warrant.
VI—Abducent	Inability of eye to look to ipsilateral side may indicate CN VI problem.
VII—Facial	Inability to raise eyebrows, hold eyelids closed, symmetrically smile, pucker, or evert lower lip may indicate CN VII problem.
VIII—Acoustic	Poor hearing or symptoms of vertigo may indicate CN VIII problem.
IX—Glossopharyngeal	Failure of uvula to elevate on stroked side may indicate CN IX problem.
X—Vagus	Failure of uvula to elevate on stroked side may indicate CN X problem.
XI—Accessory	Weakness in turning head against resistance may indicate CN XI problem.
XII—Hypoglossal	Deviation of tongue to one side may indicate CN XII problem on that side.

Bibliography

Bates RE, Stewart CM: Atypical odontalgia: phantom tooth pain, *Oral Surg Oral Med Oral Pathol* 72:479, 1991.

Campbell RL, Parks KW, Dodds RN: Chronic facial pain associated with endodontic neuropathy, *Oral Surg Oral Med Oral Pathol Oral Radiol Endod* 69:287, 1990.

Dalessio DJ, Silberstein SD: *Wolff's headache and other head pain,* ed 6, New York, 1996, Oxford University.

Delcanho RE, Graff-Radford SB: Chronic paroxysmal hemicrania presenting as toothache, *J Orofac Pain* 7(3):300, 1993.

Diamond ML: Emergency department treatment of the headache patient, *Headache Quarterly* 3(suppl):28, 1992.

Fromm GH, Graff-Radford SB, Terrence CF et al: Pre-trigeminal neuralgia, *Neurology* 40:1493, 1990.

Fromm GH, Sessle BJ: *Trigeminal neuralgia,* Boston, 1991, Butterworth-Heinemann.

Graff-Radford SB, Solberg WK: Atypical odontalgia, *J Craniomandib Disord* 6:260, 1992.

Headache Classification Committee of the IHS: Classification and diagnostic criteria for headache disorders, cranial neuralgias and facial pain, *Cephalalgia* 8:1, 1988.

Loeser JD, Butler SH, Chapman CR et al: *Bonica's management of pain,* ed 3, Philadelphia 2000, Lippincott Williams & Wilkins.

Maciewicz R: Neurologic aspects of chronic facial pain, *Anesth Prog* 37:129, 1990.

Mitchell RG: Pretrigeminal neuralgia, *Br Dent J* 149:167, 1980.

Moncada E, Graff-Radford SB: Benign indomethacin-responsive headaches presenting in the orofacial region: eight case reports, *J Orofac Pain* 9:276, 1995.

Moncada E, Graff-Radford SB: Cough headache presenting as a toothache: a case report, *Headache* 33:240, 1993.

Okeson JP: *Bell's orofacial pains,* ed 5, Carol Stream, IL, 1995, Quintessence.

Okeson JP: *Orofacial pain: guidelines for assessment, classification and management,* Carol Stream, IL, 1996, Quintessence.

Raskin NH: *Headache,* ed 2, New York, 1988, Churchill Livingstone.

CHAPTER 30

Management of Temporomandibular Disorders

MYRON R. TUCKER, BRIAN B. FARRELL, AND BART C. FARRELL

CHAPTER OUTLINE

Patients frequently consult a dentist because of pain or dysfunction in the temporomandibular region. The most common causes of temporomandibular disorders (TMDs) are muscular disorders, which are commonly referred to as *myofascial pain and dysfunction*. These muscular disorders are generally managed with a variety of reversible nonsurgical treatment methods.

Other causes of temporomandibular pain or dysfunction originate primarily within the temporomandibular joint (TMJ). These causes include internal derangement, osteoarthritis, rheumatoid arthritis, chronic recurrent dislocation, ankylosis, neoplasia, and infection. Although most of these disorders respond to nonsurgical therapy, some patients may eventually require surgical treatment. If a successful result is to be achieved, management of these patients requires a coordinated plan between the general dentist, oral and maxillofacial surgeon, and other health care providers.

EVALUATION

The evaluation of the patient with temporomandibular pain, dysfunction, or both is like that in any other diagnostic workup. This evaluation should include a thorough history, a physical examination of the masticatory system, and problem-focused TMJ radiography.

Interview

The patient's history may be the most important part of the evaluation because it furnishes clues for the diagnosis. The history begins with the chief complaint, which is a statement of the patient's reasons for seeking consultation or treatment. The history of the present illness should be comprehensive, including an accurate description of the patient's symptoms, chronology of the symptoms, description of how the problem affects the patient and information about any previous treatments (including the patient's response to those treatments). To have patients complete a general questionnaire is often useful to help provide information about the history of their problem. The use of a visual analog pain scale may also help obtain an understanding of the patient's perception of the severity of their pain.

Examination

The physical examination consists of an evaluation of the entire masticatory system. The head and neck should be inspected for soft tissue asymmetry or evidence of muscular hypertrophy. The patient should be observed for signs of jaw clenching or other habits. The masticatory muscles should be examined systematically. The muscles should be palpated for the presence of tenderness, fasciculations, spasm, or trigger points (Fig. 30-1).

The TMJs are examined for tenderness and noise (Fig. 30-2). The location of the joint tenderness (e.g., lateral or posterior) should be noted. If the joint is more painful during different areas of the opening cycle or with different types of functions, this should be recorded. The most common forms of joint noise are clicking (a distinct sound) and crepitus (i.e., scraping or grating sounds). Many joint sounds can be easily heard without special instrumentation or can be felt during palpation of the joint; however, in some cases auscultation with a stethoscope may allow less obvious joint sounds, such as mild crepitus, to be appreciated.

The mandibular range of motion should be determined. Normal range of movement of an adult's mandible is about 45 mm vertically (i.e., interincisally) and 10 mm protrusively and laterally (Fig. 30-3). The normal movement is straight and symmetric. In some cases, tenderness in the joint or muscle areas may prevent opening. The clinician should attempt to ascertain not only the painless voluntary opening but also the maximum opening that can be achieved with gentle digital pressure. In some cases the patient may appear to have a mechanical obstruction in the joint causing limited opening but with gentle pressure may actually be able to achieve near normal opening. This may suggest muscular rather than intracapsular problems.

The dental evaluation is also important. Odontogenic sources of pain should be eliminated. The teeth should be examined for wear facets, soreness, and mobility, which may be evidence of bruxism. Although the significance of occlusal abnormalities is controversial, the occlusal relationship should be evaluated and documented. Missing teeth should be noted, and dental and skeletal classification should be determined. The clinician should note any centric relation and centric occlusion discrepancy or significant posturing by the patient. The examination findings can be summarized on a TMD evaluation form and included in the patient's chart. In many cases a more detailed chart note may be necessary to document adequately all of the history and examination findings described previously.

Radiographic Evaluation

Radiographs of the TMJ are helpful in the diagnosis of intra-articular, osseous, and soft tissue pathologic conditions. The use of radiographs in the evaluation of the patient with TMD should be based on the patient's signs and symptoms instead of routinely ordering a standard set of radiographs. In many cases the panoramic radiograph provides adequate information as a screening radiograph in evaluation of TMD. A variety of other radiographic techniques are available that may provide useful information in certain cases.

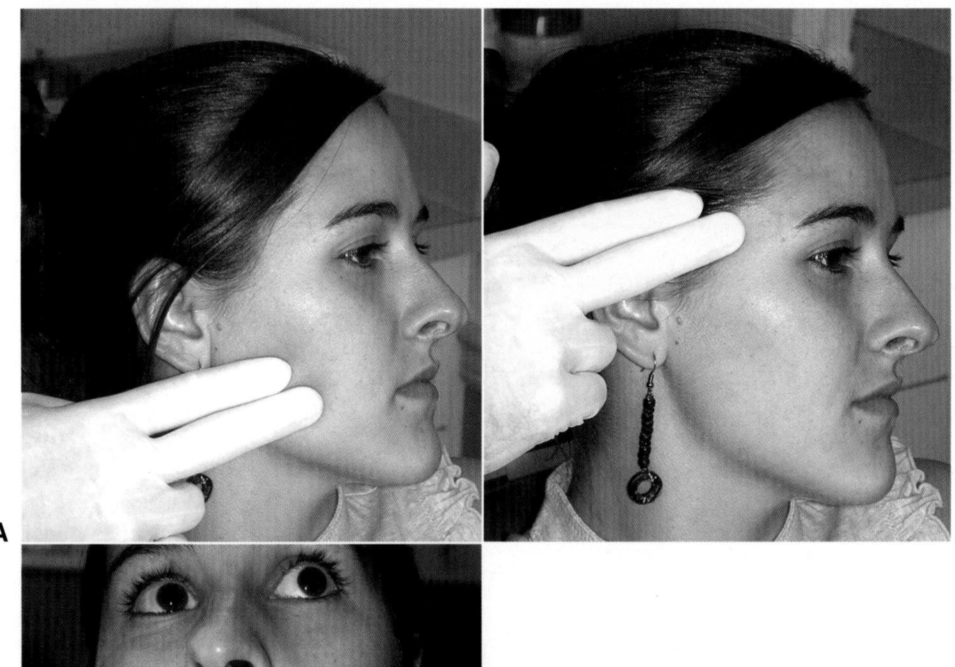

FIGURE 30-1 Systematic evaluation of muscles of mastication. A, Palpation of masseter muscle. B, Palpation of temporalis muscle. C, Palpation of temporalis tendon attachment on coronoid process and ascending ramus.

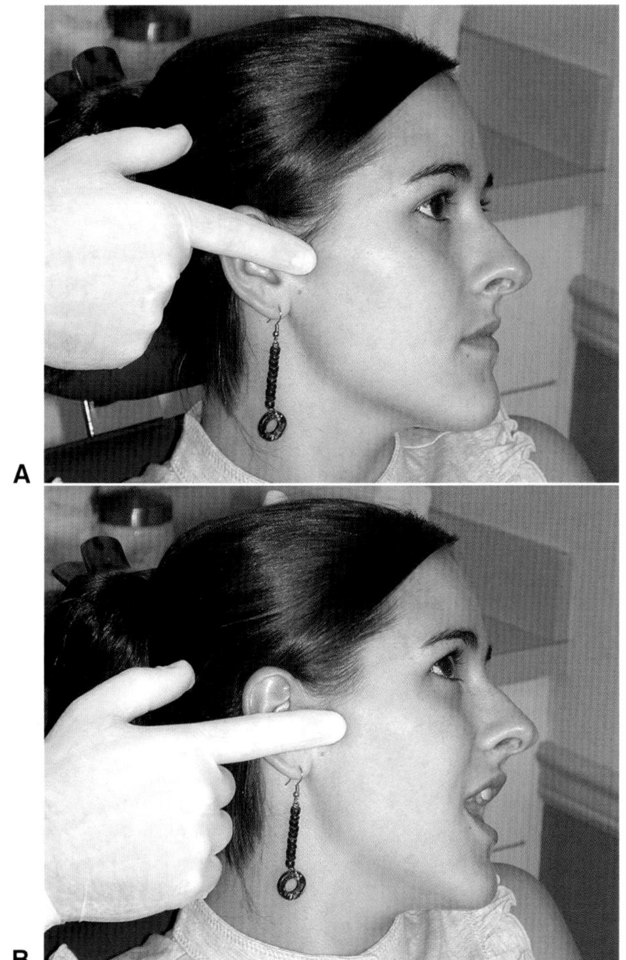

FIGURE 30-2 Evaluation of temporomandibular joint for tenderness and noise. Joint is palpated laterally in closed position (**A**) and open position (**B**).

Panoramic Radiography

One of the best overall radiographs for screening evaluation of the TMJs is the panoramic radiograph. This technique allows visualization of both TMJs on the same film. Because a panoramic technique provides a tomographic-type view of the TMJ, this can frequently provide a good assessment of the bony anatomy of the articulating surfaces of the mandibular condyle and glenoid fossa (Fig. 30-4); and other areas, such as the coronoid process, can also be visualized.[1] Many machines are equipped to provide special views of the mandible, focusing primarily on the area of the TMJs. These radiographs can often be completed in the open and closed position.

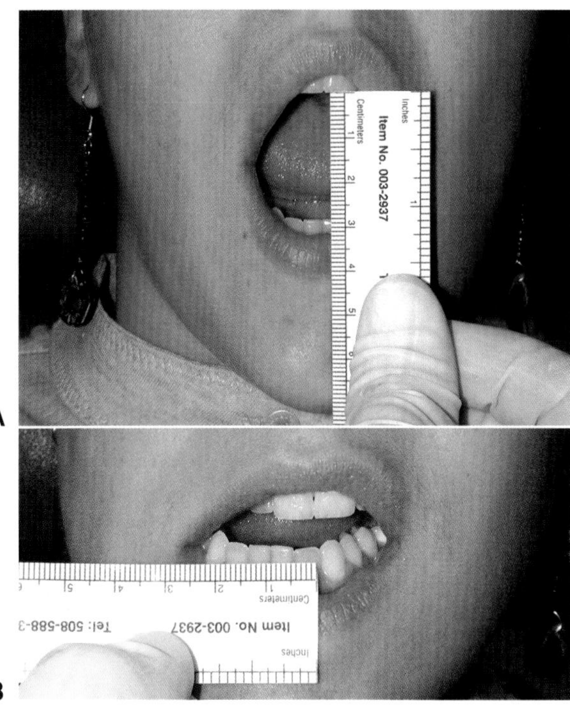

FIGURE 30-3 Measurement of range of jaw motion. **A**, Maximum voluntary vertical opening. **B**, Evaluation of lateral excursive movement (should be approximately 10 mm). Protrusive movements should be similar to excursion.

Tomograms

The tomographic technique allows a more detailed view of the TMJ.[2] This technique allows radiographic sectioning of the

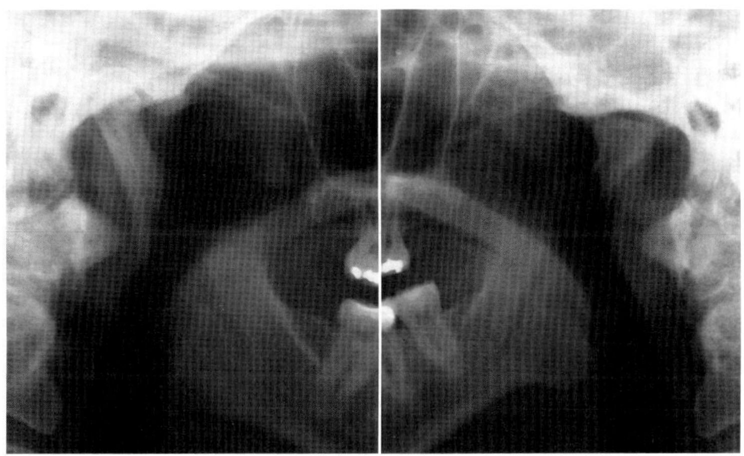

FIGURE 30-4 Panoramic imaging. **A**, Normal anatomy of right condyle. **B**, Imaging illustrates degenerative changes of left condyle via remodeling.

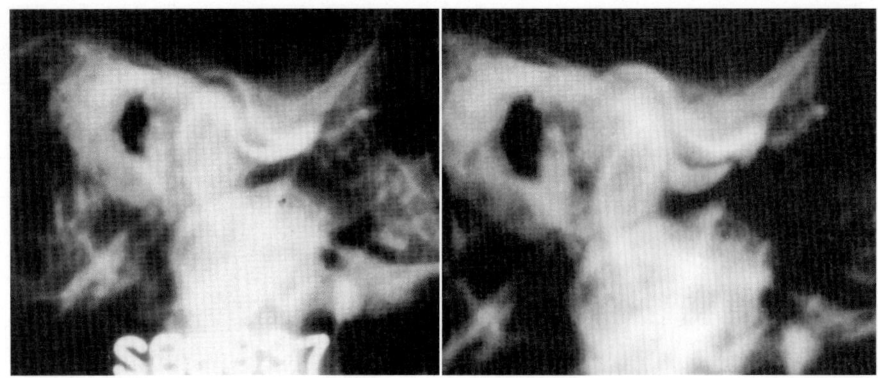

FIGURE 30-5 Arthrogram shows dye in inferior and superior joint spaces. Anatomy and location of disk is indirectly interpreted from dye pattern observed after injection of joint spaces above and below disk. This arthrogram demonstrates anterior disk displacement without reduction. A, Closed position. B, Open position.

joint at different levels of the condyle and fossa complex, which provides individual views visualizing the joint in "slices" from the medial to the lateral pole. These views eliminate bony superimposition and overlap and provide a relatively clear picture of the bony anatomy of the joint.

Temporomandibular Joint Arthrography

This imaging method was the first technique available that allowed visualization (indirect) of the intraarticular disk. Arthrography involves the injection of contrast material into the inferior or superior spaces of a joint, after which the joint is radiographed.[3] Evaluation of the configuration of the dye in the joint spaces allows evaluation of the position and morphology of the articular disk (Fig. 30-5). This technique also demonstrates the presence of perforations and adhesions of the disk or its attachments. With the availability of more advanced, less invasive techniques, arthrography is rarely used.

Computed Tomography

Computed tomography (CT) provides a combination of tomographic views of the joint, combined with computer enhancement of hard and soft tissue images.[4] This technique allows evaluation of a variety of hard and soft tissue pathologic conditions in the joint. CT images provide the most accurate radiographic assessment of the bony components of the joint (Fig. 30-6). CT scan reconstruction capabilities allow images obtained in one plane of space to be reconstructed so that the images can be evaluated from a different view. Thus evaluation of the joint from a variety of perspectives can be made from a single radiation exposure.

Magnetic Resonance Imaging

The most effective diagnostic imaging technique to evaluate TMJ soft tissues is magnetic resonance imaging (MRI; Fig. 30-7).[5] This technique allows excellent images of intraarticular soft tissue, making MRI a valuable technique for evaluating disk morphology and position. MRI images can be obtained showing dynamic joint function in a cinematic fashion, providing valuable information about the anatomic components of the joint during function. The fact that this technique does not use ionizing radiation is a significant advantage.

Nuclear Imaging

Nuclear medicine studies involve intravenous injection of technetium-99, a γ-emitting isotope that is concentrated in areas of active bone metabolism. Approximately 3 hours after injection of the isotope, images are obtained using a gamma camera. Single-photon emission computerized tomography images can then be used to determine active areas of bone metabolism (Fig. 30-8).[6] Although this technique is extremely sensitive, the information obtained may be difficult to interpret. Because bone changes, such as degeneration, may appear identical to repair or regeneration, this technique must be evaluated cautiously and in combination with clinical findings.

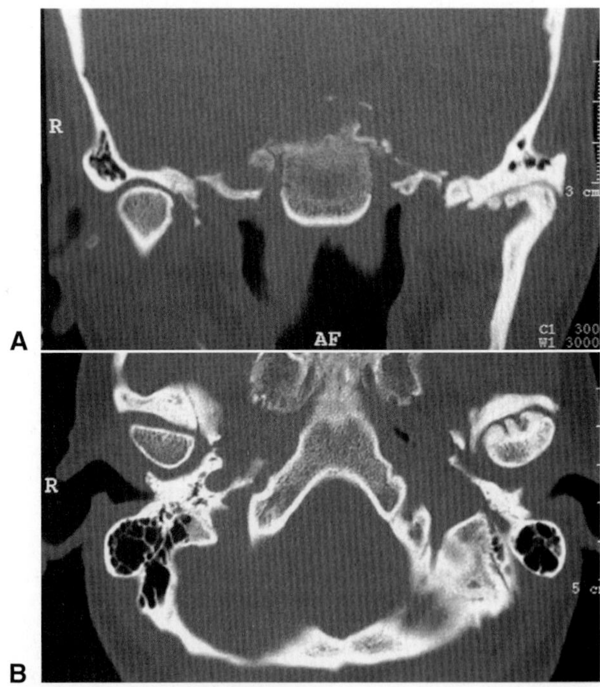

FIGURE 30-6 Computerized tomography. A, Coronal images illustrate normal architecture of the right (*R*) condyle with alteration of the left condyle resulting from a history of trauma. B, Axial views depict the altered condylar anatomy referenced against the contralateral joint.

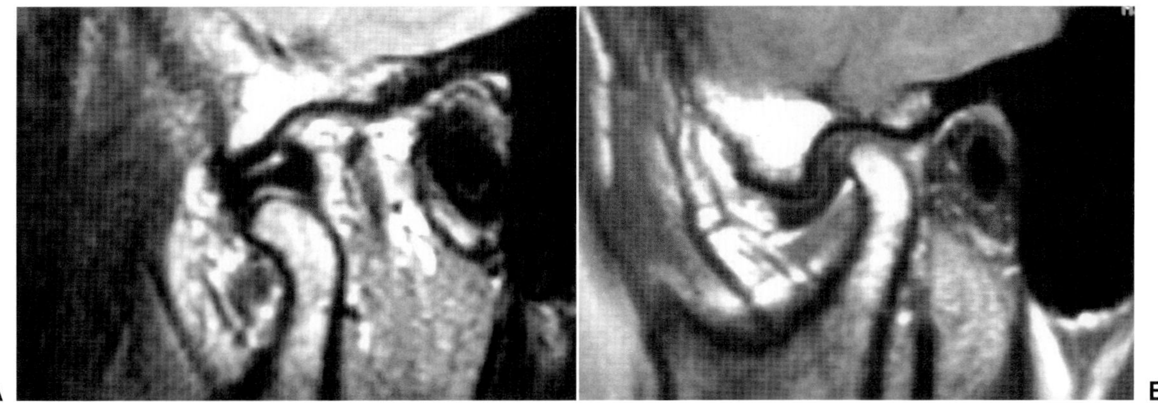

FIGURE 30-7 Magnetic resonance image. **A**, Normal positioning of the articular disk between the articular eminence and condyle during translation. **B**, Image demonstrates anterior disk displacement without reduction, limiting range of motion.

Psychological Evaluation

Many patients with temporomandibular pain and dysfunction of long-standing duration develop manifestations of chronic pain syndrome behavior. This complex may include gross exaggeration of symptoms and clinical depression.[7,8] The comorbidity of psychiatric illness and temporomandibular dysfunction can be as high as 10% to 20% of patients seeking treatment.[9] A third of these patients is suffering from depression at the time on initial presentation, whereas more than two thirds have had a severe depressive episode in their history.[10] Psychiatric disorders may elicit somatic components through parafunctional habits resulting in dystonia and myalgia, and individuals with chronic pain commonly have a higher incidence of concomitant anxiety disorders.[11-13] Behavioral changes associated with pain and dysfunction can be elicited in the history through questions regarding functional limitation that results from the patient's symptoms.[14] If the functional limitation appears to be excessive compared with the patient's clinical signs or the patient appears to be clinically depressed, further psychological evaluation may be warranted.[15]

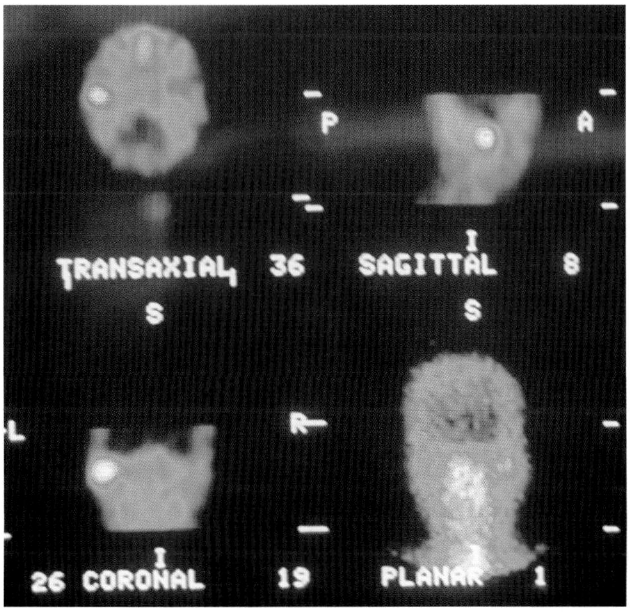

FIGURE 30-8 Single-photon emission computed tomography (bone scan). Area of increased activity is apparent in both temporomandibular joints.

CLASSIFICATION OF TEMPOROMANDIBULAR DISORDERS

Myofascial Pain

Myofascial pain and dysfunction (MPD) is the most common cause of masticatory pain and limited function for which patients seek dental consultation and treatment. The source of the pain and dysfunction is muscular, with masticatory muscles developing tenderness and pain as a result of abnormal muscular function or hyperactivity. The muscular pain is frequently, but not always, associated with daytime clenching or nocturnal bruxism. The cause of MPD is multifactorial. One of the most commonly accepted causes of MPD is bruxism resulting from stress and anxiety, with occlusion being a modifying or aggravating factor. MPD may also occur because of internal joint problems, such as disk displacement disorders or degenerative joint disease (DJD).

Patients with MPD generally complain of diffuse, poorly localized, preauricular pain that may also involve other muscles of mastication, such as the temporalis and medial pterygoid muscles. In patients with nocturnal bruxism, the pain is frequently more severe in the morning. Patients generally describe decreased jaw opening with pain during functions such as chewing. Headaches, usually bitemporal in location, may also be associated with these symptoms. Because of the role of stress, the pain is often more severe during periods of tension and anxiety.

Examination of the patient reveals diffuse tenderness of the masticatory muscles. The TMJs are frequently nontender to palpation. In isolated MPD, joint noises are usually not present. However, as mentioned previously, MPD may be associated with a variety of other joint problems that may produce other TMJ signs and symptoms. The range of mandibular movement in patients with MPD may be decreased and is associated with deviation of the mandible toward the affected side. The teeth frequently have wear facets. However, the absence of such facets does not eliminate bruxism as a cause of the problem.

Radiographs of the TMJs are usually normal. Some patients have evidence of degenerative changes, such as altered surface contours, erosion, or osteophytes. These changes, however, may result from or be unassociated with the MPD problem.

Disk Displacement Disorders

In a normally functioning TMJ the condyle functions in a hinge and a sliding fashion. During full opening the condyle not only rotates on a hinge axis but also translates forward to a position near the most inferior portion of the articular eminence (Fig. 30-9). During function the biconcave disk remains interpositioned between the condyle and fossa, with the condyle remaining against the thin intermediate zone during all phases of opening and closing.

Anterior Disk Displacement with Reduction

In anterior disk displacement the disk is positioned anterior and medial to the condyle in the closed position. During opening the condyle moves over the posterior band of the disk and eventually returns to the normal condyle and disk relationship, resting on the thin intermediate zone. During closing the condyle then slips posteriorly and rests on the retrodiskal tissue, with the disk returning to the anterior, medially displaced position (Fig. 30-10).

Examination of the patient usually reveals joint tenderness, and muscle tenderness may also exist. Joint noise (i.e., clicking) is commonly heard with opening, when the condyle moves from the area posterior to the disk into the thin concave area in the middle of the disk. In some cases, clicking can be heard or palpated during the closing cycle. Maximal opening can be normal or slightly limited, with the click occurring during the opening movement. Anatomically, the opening click corresponds to the disk reducing to a more normal position. The closing click (i.e., reciprocal click) corresponds to the disk failing to maintain its normal position between the condylar head and the articular eminence and slipping forward to the anteriorly displaced position. Crepitus may be present and is usually a result of articular movement across irregular surfaces.

The images obtained from plain TMJ radiography in patients with anterior disk displacement may be normal or may demonstrate slight bone abnormalities. MRI images usually demonstrate anterior displacement of the disk.

Anterior Disk Displacement Without Reduction

In this type of internal derangement the disk displacement cannot be reduced, and thus the condyle is unable to translate to its full anterior extent, which prevents maximal opening and causes deviation of the mandible to the affected side (Fig. 30-11).

In these patients no clicking occurs because they are unable to translate the condyle over the posterior aspect of the disk. This lack of translation may result in restricted opening, deviation to the affected side, and decreased lateral excursions to the contralateral side. Some evidence suggests that the limitation of motion may not be directly related to the actual dis-

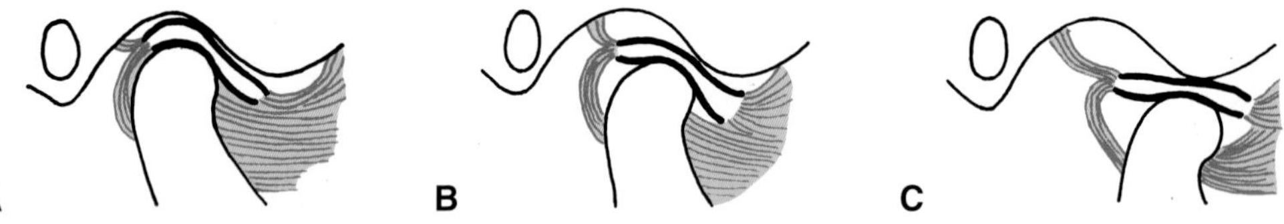

FIGURE 30-9 Normal disk and condyle relationship. **A**, Biconcave disk is interpositioned between fossa and condyle in closed position. **B**, When condyle translates forward, thin intermediate zone stays in consistent relationship with condyle. **C**, Maximum open position.

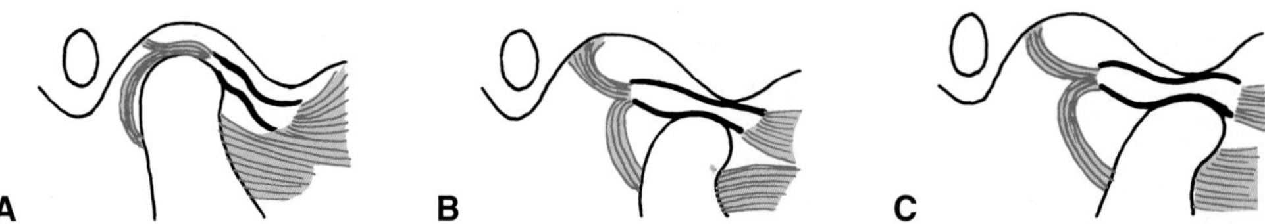

FIGURE 30-10 Anterior disk displacement with reduction. **A**, Biconcave disk is situated anterior to articulating surface of condyle. When condyle translates forward, it eventually passes over thickened posterior band of disk, creating clicking noise. **B**, After click occurs, disk remains in appropriate relationship with condyle through remainder of opening cycle. **C**, Maximum opening position. When mandible closes, condyle and disk relationship return to position as shown in **A**.

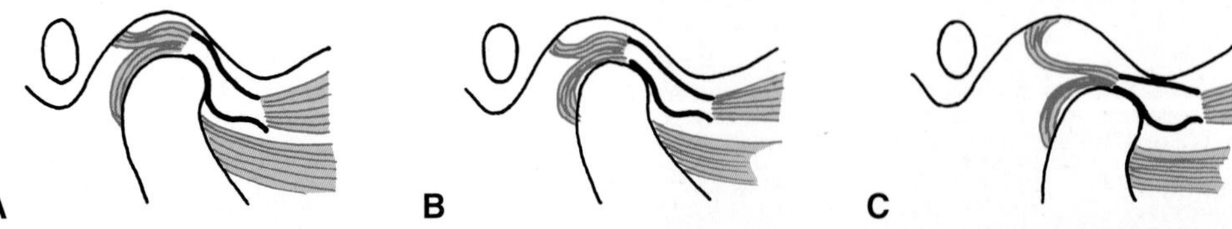

FIGURE 30-11 Anterior disk displacement without reduction. **A**, Disk that has been chronically anteriorly displaced now has amorphous shape rather than distinct biconcave structure. **B**, When condyle begins to translate forward, disk remains anterior to condyle. **C**, In maximum open position, disk tissue continues to remain anterior to condyle, with posterior attachment tissue interposed between condyle and fossa.

placement of the disk but rather to the adherence of the disk to the fossa, causing a restriction of the sliding function of the joint.[16]

Radiographic evaluation of disk displacement without reduction is similar to findings in anterior disk displacement with reduction. Plain TMJ radiography may appear normal, whereas CT scans and MRIs generally demonstrate anteromedial disk displacement. However, in this disorder, images taken in the maximal open position continue to show anterior disk displacement within the open position.

Degenerative Joint Disease (Arthrosis, Osteoarthritis)

DJD includes a variety of anatomic findings, including irregular, perforated, or severely damaged disks in association with articular surface abnormalities, such as articular surface flattening, erosions, or osteophyte formation (Fig. 30-12). The mechanisms of TMJ degenerative diseases are not clearly understood but are thought to be multifactorial. Current concepts of DJD incorporate three possible mechanisms of injury: (1) direct mechanical trauma, (2) hypoxia reperfusion injury, and (3) neurogenic inflammation.[17]

Mechanical trauma may result from significant and obvious trauma to the joint or much less obvious microtrauma, such as excessive mechanical loading. The excessive stress produced in the joint can lead to molecular disruption and the generation of free radicals, with resulting oxidative stress and intracellular damage. Excess loading can also affect local cell populations and reduce the reparative capacity of the joint.

The hypoxia-reperfusion theory suggests that excessive intracapsular hydrostatic pressure within the TMJ may exceed the blood vessel perfusion pressure, resulting in hypoxia.

This type of increased intracapsular pressure has been clearly demonstrated in patients during clenching and bruxing.[18] When the pressure in the joint is decreased and perfusion is reestablished, free radicals are formed. These free radicals may interact with other substances in the joint (e.g., hemoglobin) to produce even more damage.

Neurogenic inflammation results when a variety of substances are released from peripheral neurons. It is hypothesized that in cases of disk displacement, the compression or stretching of the nerve-rich retrodiskal tissue may result in release of proinflammatory neuropeptides.[17,19] The release of cytokines results in the release and activation of a variety of substances including prostaglandins, leukotrienes, and matrix-degrading enzymes. These compounds not only have a role in the disease process but also may serve as biologic markers that may help to diagnose and eventually treat pathologic conditions of the joint.[20,21] It must be emphasized that it is impossible to predict the progression of pathologic conditions of the joint.

Patients with DJD frequently experience pain associated with clicking or crepitus located directly over the TMJ. Usually, an obvious limitation of opening is present, and symptoms usually increase with function. Radiographic findings are variable but generally exhibit decreased joint space, surface erosions, osteophytes, and flattening of the condylar head. Irregularities in the fossa and articular eminence may also be present.

Systemic Arthritic Conditions

A variety of systemic arthritic conditions are known to affect the TMJ. The most common of these is rheumatoid arthritis. Other processes, such as systemic lupus, can also affect the TMJ. In these cases, symptoms are rarely isolated to the TMJs, and several other signs and symptoms of arthritis are usually present in other areas of the body.

In the case of rheumatoid arthritis, an inflammatory process results in abnormal proliferation of synovial tissue in a so-called pannus formation (Fig. 30-13).

TMJ symptoms that result from rheumatoid arthritis may occur at an earlier age than those associated with DJD. As opposed to DJD, which is usually unilateral, rheumatoid arthritis (and other systemic conditions) usually affects the TMJs bilaterally.

Radiographic findings of the TMJ initially show erosive changes in the anterior and posterior aspects of the condylar heads. These changes may progress to large eroded areas that leave the appearance of a small, pointed condyle in a large fossa. Eventually, the entire condyle and condylar neck may be destroyed. Laboratory tests, such as rheumatoid factor and erythrocyte sedimentation rate, may be helpful in confirming the diagnosis of rheumatoid arthritis.

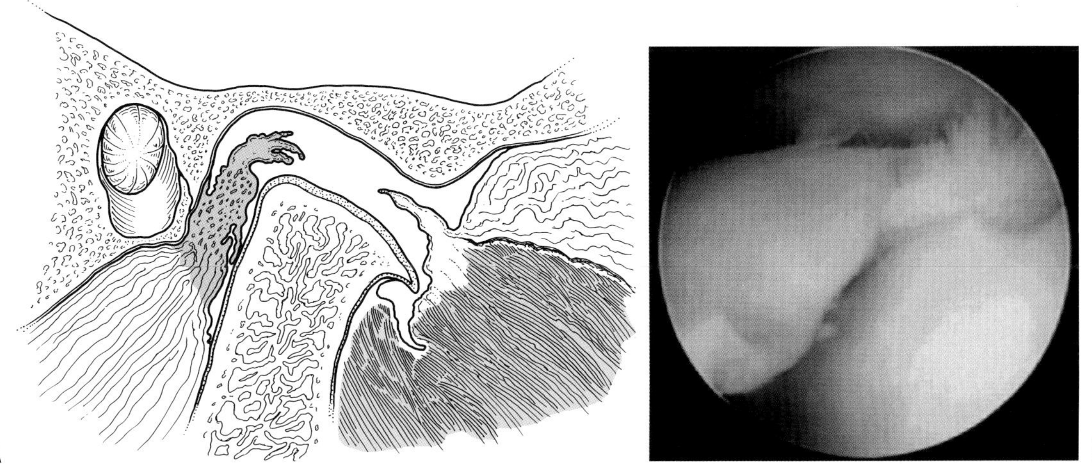

FIGURE 30-12 A, Degenerative joint disease demonstrates large perforation of disk tissue and erosion and flattening of articulating surfaces of condyle and fossa. B, Arthroscopic visualization of disk perforation with exposure of condyle in superior joint space.

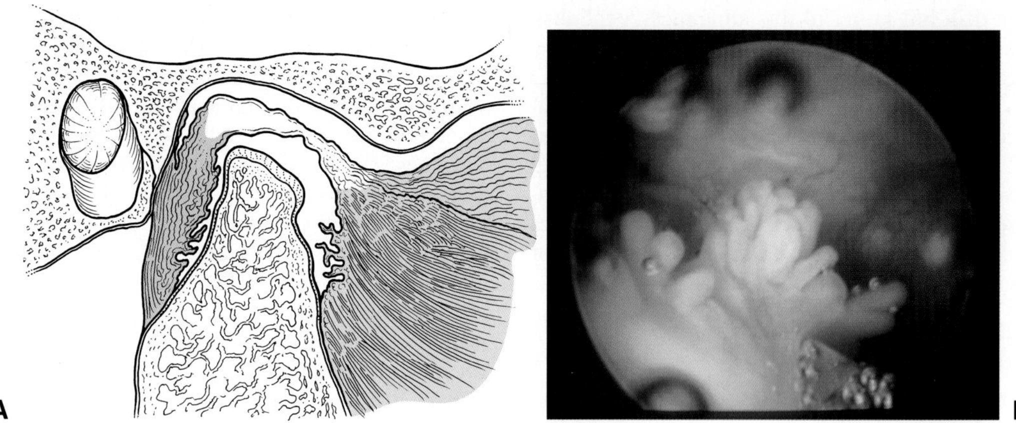

FIGURE 30-13 A, Changes seen in rheumatoid arthritis of temporomandibular joint. These changes include proliferation of synovial tissue, creating resorption in anterior and posterior areas of condyle. Irregularities of disk tissue and articulating surface of condyle eventually occur. B, Arthroscopic view of synovial hyperplasia.

Chronic Recurrent Dislocation

Dislocation of the TMJ occurs frequently and is caused by mandibular hypermobility. Subluxation is a displacement of the condyle, which is self-reducing and generally requires no medical management. A more serious condition occurs when the mandibular condyle translates anteriorly in front of the articular eminence and becomes locked in that position (Fig. 30-14). Dislocation may be unilateral or bilateral and may occur spontaneously after opening the mouth widely, such as when yawning, eating, or during a dental procedure. Dislocation of the mandibular condyle that persists for more than a few seconds generally becomes painful and is often associated with severe muscular spasms.

Dislocations should be reduced as soon as possible. This reduction is accomplished by applying downward pressure on the posterior teeth and upward pressure on the chin, accompanied by posterior displacement of the mandible. Usually reduction is not difficult. However, muscular spasms may prevent simple reduction, particularly when the dislocation cannot be reduced immediately. In these cases, anesthesia of the auricular temporal nerve and the muscles of mastication may be necessary. Sedation to reduce patient anxiety and provide muscular relaxation may also be required. After reduction the patient should be instructed to restrict mandibular opening for 2 to 4 weeks. Moist heat and nonsteroidal antiinflammatory drugs (NSAIDs) are also helpful in controlling pain and inflammation.

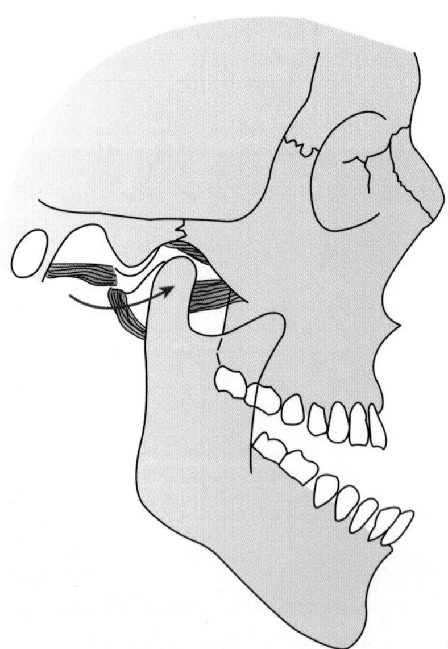

FIGURE 30-14 Diagram demonstrating hypermobility of joint allowing dislocation of condyle anterior to articular eminence.

Ankylosis

Intracapsular Ankylosis

Intracapsular ankylosis, or fusion of the joint, leads to reduced mandibular opening that ranges from partial reduction in function to complete immobility of the jaw. Intracapsular ankylosis results from a fusion of the condyle, disk, and fossa complex as a result of the formation of fibrous tissue, bone fusion, or a combination of the two (Fig. 30-15). The most common cause of ankylosis involves macrotrauma, most frequently associated with condylar fractures. Other causes of ankylosis include previous surgical treatment that resulted in scarring and, in rare cases, infections.

Evaluation of the patient reveals severe restriction of maximal opening, deviation to the affected side, and decreased lateral excursions to the contralateral side. If the ankylosis is the result primarily of fibrous tissue, jaw mobility will be greater than if the ankylosis is a result of bone fusion.

Radiographic evaluation reveals irregular articular surfaces of the condyle and fossa, with varying degrees of calcified connection between these articulating surfaces.

Extracapsular Ankylosis

Extracapsular ankylosis usually involves the coronoid process and temporalis muscle. Frequent causes of extracapsular ankylosis are coronoid process enlargement, or hyperplasia, and trauma to the zygomatic arch area. Infection around the temporalis muscle may also produce extracapsular ankylosis (Fig. 30-16).

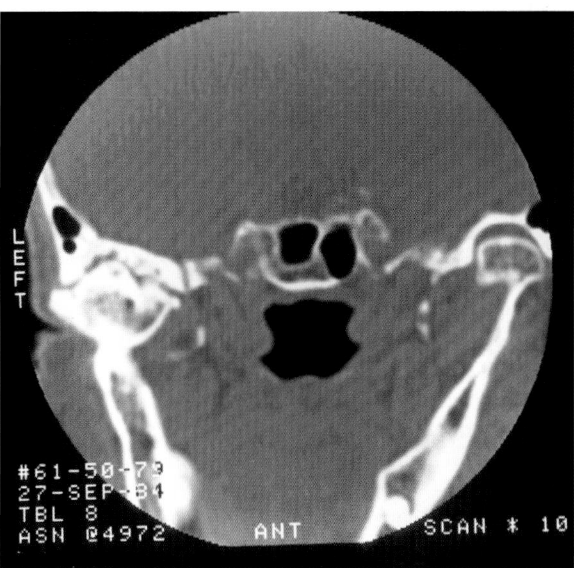

FIGURE 30-15 Bony ankylosis. Computed tomography scan imaging illustrating partial bony fusion of condyle and glenoid fossa.

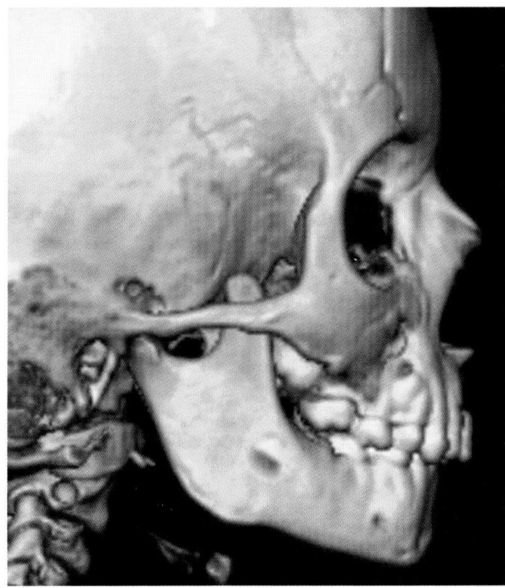

FIGURE 30-16 Extracapsular ankylosis resulting from coronoid hypertrophy. Elongation of coronoid process results in impingement against the posterior aspect of the maxilla during opening, limiting mandibular range of motion.

Patients initially have limitation of opening and deviation to the affected side. In these cases, complete restriction of opening is rare, and limited lateral and protrusive movements can usually be performed, indicating no intracapsular ankylosis. Panoramic radiography generally demonstrates the elongation of a coronoid process. A submental vertex radiograph may be useful in demonstrating impingement caused by a fractured zygomatic arch or zygomaticomaxillary complex.

Neoplasia

Neoplasms in the TMJ are rare. Neoplasms can occasionally result in restriction of opening and joint pain. Tumors within the TMJ may result in an abnormal condyle and fossa relationship or an intracapsular ankylosis. A complete discussion of the neoplastic processes known to occur in the TMJ area is beyond the scope of this chapter.

Infections

Infections in the TMJ area are rare, even in the case of trauma or surgical intervention in this area. In third world countries where antibiotic therapy of middle ear infections is not available, extension of infectious processes may occasionally involve the TMJ and result in intracapsular ankylosis.

REVERSIBLE TREATMENT

Although the cause of temporomandibular pain and dysfunction can arise from several different sources, initial treatment is frequently aimed at nonsurgical methods of reducing pain and discomfort, decreasing inflammation in muscles and joints, and improving jaw function. In some cases, such as ankylosis or severe joint degeneration, surgical treatment may be the preferred initial course of therapy. However, in most cases—including MPD, disk displacement disorders, and degenerative and systemic arthritic disorders—a nonsurgical, reversible treatment phase may provide significant reduction in pain and improvement in function. Most patients with MPD and internal derangements do well without any type of long-term or invasive treatment. In the case of anterior disk displacement without reduction (i.e., closed lock), most patients experience a gradual progression of increased opening and decreased discomfort without extensive treatment. This is apparently the result of physiologic and anatomic adaptation of tissue within the joint. It appears that in many patients the posterior attachment tissue undergoes fibrous adaptation and adequately serves as interpositioning tissue between the condyle and fossa.[22] This is often termed *pseudodisk adaptation* (Fig. 30-17). This pseudodisk formation, combined with other normal healing capabilities of joints, is most likely responsible for clinical improvement in many patients.

Patient Education

The first step in involving patients in their own treatment is to make them aware of the pathologic condition producing their pain and dysfunction and to describe the prognosis or possible progression of their pain and dysfunction. Many problems of masticatory pain and dysfunction stabilize or improve with conservative therapy, despite patients' concerns that they may be on a continually deteriorating course. In the case of a patient with MPD, a precise, confident explanation should attempt to assure the patient that muscular pain usually improves with minimal treatment. The clinician should also explain that although symptoms may recur on occasion, they generally can be controlled with the treatment (described later in this chapter).

In some cases, such as DJD, the patient should be made aware of the long-term spectrum of outcomes of this problem. Warning signs of further deterioration, including increased pain, limitation of motion, and increased joint noise, should be emphasized to the patient.

Patients who have an awareness of the factors associated with their pain and dysfunction can actively participate in their own improvement. Myofascial pain often results from para-

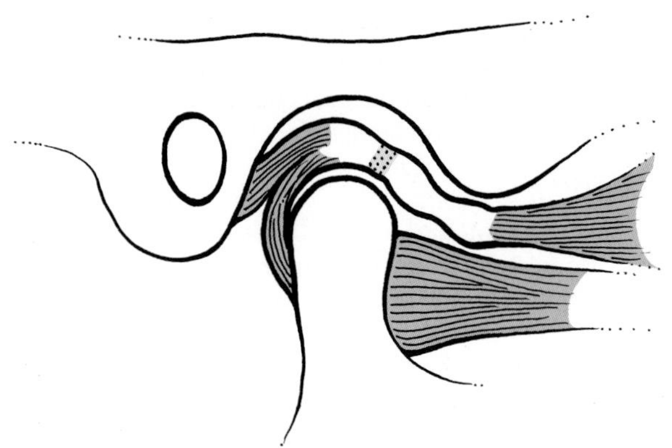

FIGURE 30-17 Anteriorly displaced disk results in stress on retrodiskal tissue. Subsequent fibrosis provides adaptation, producing a functional, although anatomically different, interpositional disk.

functional habits or muscular hyperactivity resulting from stress and anxiety. Patients who are aware of these factors are often able to control their activity and thereby reduce discomfort and improve function. Biofeedback devices provide information to patients to help them control their muscular activity. For example, the output from surface electrodes over the masseter or temporalis muscle can be used to indicate clenching or grinding during daytime activity.[23] Electromyographic recordings can also be useful in evaluating nocturnal bruxism and associated pain and can be used to monitor the effectiveness of splint therapy and medication to control muscular hyperactivity. Other forms of stress control, such as physical exercise, reducing exposure to stressful situations, and psychological counseling, can also be explored. When the patient becomes aware of the relationship between personal actions and the symptoms of pain and dysfunction, behavior modification can follow.

Modification of diet combined with home exercise routines are also an important part of the patient's educational process. Patients who experience temporomandibular pain or dysfunction frequently find that it is most apparent when chewing hard food. Temporary alteration of the diet to a softer consistency may result in a significant reduction in symptoms. A gradual progression to a more normal diet over a period of 6 weeks may be sufficient to reduce joint or muscle symptoms. Aggravating factors including chewing of gum, fingernails, or ice should be reviewed, and cessation or limitation of these activities should be encouraged.

Medication

Pharmacologic therapy is an important aspect of nonsurgical management of TMD. Medications typically used in the treatment of TMDs include NSAIDs; (2) occasionally, stronger analgesics; (3) muscle relaxants; and (4) antidepressants.

NSAIDs not only reduce inflammation but also serve as an excellent analgesic. Categories of nonsteroidal antiinflammatory medications include propionic acid derivatives (ibuprofen, naproxen), salicylates (aspirin, diflunisal), and acetic acid compounds (indomethacin, sulindac). These medications can be effective in reducing inflammation in muscles and joints and in most cases provide satisfactory pain relief. These drugs are not associated with severe addiction problems, and their use as an analgesic is strongly preferred over narcotic medications. Dosing of antiinflammatory medications is most effective when they are administered on a time-regulated schedule rather than on a pain-dependent schedule. Patients should be instructed to take the medicine regularly, obtaining an adequate blood level that should then be maintained for a minimum of 7 to 14 days. Discontinuation or tapering of the medicine can then be attempted.

The cyclooxygenase-2 (COX-2) inhibitors such as celecoxib (Celebrex) have gained popularity in the treatment of inflammation and pain. Prostaglandins produced by COX-1 activity appear to be required for normal physiologic function, whereas those produced by COX-2 activation mediate pain and inflammation. The COX-2 inhibitors are intended to reduce pain and inflammation without affecting prostaglandin-dependent functions. Some COX-2 inhibitors have recently been associated with the potential for significant side effects including cardiac complications, and they should be used with the appropriate caution and monitoring of the patient. Consultation with the patient's physician may be warranted.

Analgesic medicines for patients with TMJ disorders may range from acetaminophen to potent narcotics. One important principle of treatment for all pain and dysfunction in patients is to remember that the problem may be chronic and that medication could produce long-term addiction. Because of the sedative and depressive effects of narcotics and their potential for addiction, these medications should be restricted to short-term use for episodes of severe, acute pain or in a postoperative setting. In such instances, medications such as acetaminophen with codeine should be sufficient. This medication should not be used for longer than 10 days to 2 weeks if possible.

Muscle relaxants may provide significant improvement in jaw function and relief of masticatory pain through control of dystonia. However, muscle relaxants have a significant potential for depression and sedation and can produce long-term addiction. In many patients with acute pain or exacerbation of muscular hyperactivity, muscle relaxants can be considered for short periods, such as 10 days to 2 weeks. The lowest effective dose should be used. Diazepam (Valium), carisoprodol (Soma), cyclobenzaprine (Flexeril), and tizanidine (Zanaflex) are examples of commonly used muscle relaxants. Pharmacologic therapy often provides adequate relief of muscular symptoms in patients with TMD.

Antidepressants, most commonly tricyclic antidepressants used in low doses, appear to be useful in the management of patients with chronic pain.[24,25] Tricyclic antidepressants prevent the reuptake of amine neurotransmitters, such as serotonin and norepinephrine, causing an inhibition of pain transmission. Recently, anecdotal evidence has suggested that these antidepressants may be effective in decreasing nocturnal bruxism. It appears that nighttime bruxing may be in part a result of disruption of normal sleep patterns.[26,27] Amitriptyline (Elavil) used in small doses (10 to 25 mg at bedtime) may improve sleep patterns, decrease bruxism, and result in decreased joint and muscle pain.

Medications that must be administered by injection may occasionally be helpful in managing muscular and joint pain and inflammation. Recently, the use of botulinum toxin A has shown promise in decreasing masticatory muscle hyperactivity.[28,29] Botulinum toxin (Botox) is a neurotoxin produced by the bacterium *Clostridium botulinum*. This neurotoxin produces a paralytic effect on muscles by inhibiting the release of

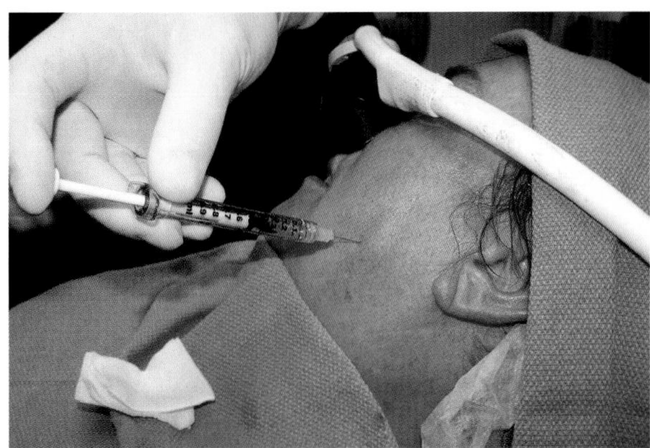

FIGURE 30-18 Botulinum toxin infiltration into muscles of mastication.

acetylcholine at the neuromuscular junction. In very low doses, Botulinum toxin can be safely administered by injection directly into the affected muscle area, decreasing muscle contraction activity and the associated pain (Fig. 30-18). The effect of Botulinum toxin is temporary, lasting from a few weeks to several months. In many cases, injection of Botulinum toxin must be repeated to obtain long-term pain relief.

Injection of local anesthetic combined with steroids into the temporalis tendon and the joint has been shown to be an effective way to decrease pain and inflammation. Tendinitis in areas such as the insertion of the temporalis tendon along the ascending ramus and coronoid process often responds favorably to trigger point injection. Local anesthetic provides temporary relief of pain, and steriods exert their effect through the inhibition of proinflammatory cytokines.[30] There continues to be some debate about the long-term effect of steroids in the joint and the possibility that further degeneration may be associated with steroid injection.[31] Further research is required in this area.

Physical Therapy

Physical therapy can be useful in the management of patients with temporomandibular pain and dysfunction. A variety of techniques have been used successfully as adjunctive therapy for treatment of temporomandibular dysfunction. The most common modalities used include range of motion exercises, relaxation training, ultrasound, spray and stretch, and pressure massage.[32,33]

Although the patient is generally encouraged to reduce the functional load placed on the joint and muscles, it is important to remember that maximizing range of motion is also an important aspect of treatment of all TMDs.[34] Limited mandibular range of motion may lead to problems in the TMJ and muscles of mastication. The lack of mobility may limit the lubrication of the joint via changes in the synovial membrane and contribute to degenerative changes of the articular surfaces. Limited muscular movement can result in fibrosis, further restriction of motion and an increase in pain. Physical therapy is initially implemented through a home regimen. These exercises include gentle stretching exercises done within pain tolerance through passive opening or active exercise routines. Establishing a baseline is a valuable resource to gauge progress and can be measured via the number of fingers positioned between the incisal edges or dispensing a plastic ruler. Simple methods for passive therapy include stretching by exerting a scissor effect with the thumb and forefinger or interval increases in tongue blades placed between the upper and lower teeth (Fig. 30-19). The force is exerted until resistance or pain is encountered and is maintained for several seconds. Appliances are also available that provide easy and efficient methods for improving jaw mobility through passive exercise. Consultation with a physical therapist may be required to provide a regimen to assist in overcoming persistent immobilization.[35,36]

Relaxation training, although perhaps not physical therapy in the strictest sense, can be effective in reducing symptoms caused by muscular pain and hyperactivity. During the educational phase, patients are made aware of the contribution of stress and muscular hyperactivity to pain. Relaxation techniques can be used to reduce the effects of stress on muscle and joint pain. Electromyographic monitoring of the patient's muscular activity can be used as an effective teaching tool by providing instant feedback demonstrating relaxation therapy, reduction of muscular hyperactivity, and the resultant improvement in symptoms of pain.

Ultrasound is an effective way to produce tissue heating with ultrasonic waves, which alter blood flow and metabolic activity at a deeper level than that provided by simple surface moist-heat applications.[37] The effect of ultrasonic tissue heating is theoretically related to increase in tissue temperature, increase

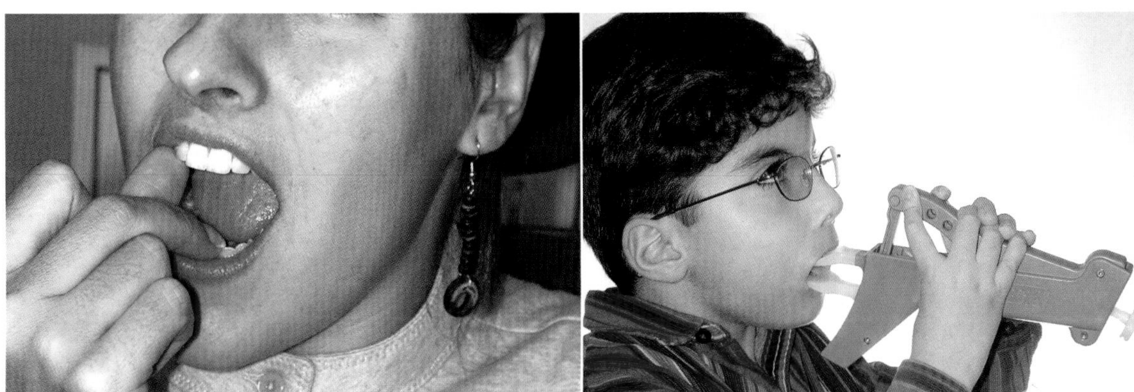

FIGURE 30-19 Jaw exercising. A, Passive stretch applied through scissoring of thumb and forefinger. B, Physical therapy through Therabite appliance to increase range of jaw motion.

in circulation, increase in uptake of painful metabolic by-products, and disruption of collagen cross-linking, which may affect adhesion formation. All of these effects may result in a more comfortable manipulation of muscles and a wider range of motion. In addition, intraarticular inflammation may also be reduced with ultrasonic applications. Ultrasonic treatments are usually provided by a physical therapist in combination with other treatment modalities.

Spray and stretch is an effective method for improving range of motion. The theory behind spray and stretch is the concept that significant superficial skin stimulation can produce an overriding or distracting effect on pain input that originates in the muscles and joints.[38] By spraying a vapocoolant material, such as fluoromethane, over the lateral surface of the face, the muscles of mastication can be passively or actively stretched with a reduced level of pain.

Friction massage involves the use of firm cutaneous pressure sufficient to produce a temporary degree of ischemia. This ischemia and the resultant hyperemia have been described as a method for inactivation of trigger points, which are areas responsible for pain referred to muscles in the head and neck area.[38] More frequently, this technique may be useful in disrupting small fibrous connective tissue adhesions that may develop within the muscles during healing after surgery and injury or as a result of prolonged muscular shortening from restricted motion.

Physical therapists and other practitioners sometimes use transcutaneous electrical nerve stimulation (TENS) to provide pain relief for chronic pain patients when other techniques have been unable to eliminate or reduce pain symptoms. The exact mechanism of action of TENS is not completely understood. The technique was initially based on the concept that stimulation of superficial nerve fiber with TENS may be responsible for overriding pain input from structures such as masticatory muscles and the TMJs. Interestingly, many patients who use TENS units experience pain relief that is longer in duration than the time during which the unit is actually applied. This may be a result of the release of endogenous endorphin compounds that can provide extended periods of decreased pain.

Each of the physical therapy modalities may be useful in the reduction of TMJ pain and increasing range of motion. The low cost of physical therapy compared with other medical treatment, the likelihood that some benefit will occur, and the minimal risk associated with these techniques are strong arguments for frequent use of physical therapy in the management of patients with TMD.

Splint Therapy

Occlusal splints are generally considered a part of the reversible or conservative treatment phase in the management of patients with TMD. Splint designs vary; however, most splints can be classified into two distinct groups: (1) autorepositioning splints and (2) anterior repositioning splints.

Autorepositioning Splints

The autorepositioning splint, also called *anterior guidance splints, superior repositioning splints,* or *muscle splints.* The splints are most frequently used to treat muscle problems or eliminate TMJ pain when no specific internal derangement or other obvious pathologic condition can be identified. However, these splints may be used in some cases, such as anterior disk displacement or DJD, in an attempt to unload or reduce the force placed directly on the TMJ area. These splints are designed to provide a flat surface with even contact in all areas of the occlusion. The splint provides full-arch contact without working or balancing interferences and without ramps or deep interdigitation that would force the mandible to function in one specific occlusal position (Fig. 30-20). This splint allows the patient to seek a comfortable muscle and joint position without excessive influence of the occlusion. Nitzan[18] has shown that properly designed splints can be effective in reducing intraarticular pressure. An example of this type of splint would be in a patient with a Class II malocclusion and significant overjet who continually postures forward to obtain incisor contact during mastication. Many of these patients complain of muscular symptoms and describe a feeling that they do not have a consistent, repeatable bite relationship. Wearing an autorepositioning splint allows full-arch dental contact with the condyles in a more posterior retruded position, which frequently results in reduction of muscle and joint symptoms.

Anterior Repositioning Splints

Anterior repositioning splints are constructed so that an anterior ramping effect forces the mandible to function in a protruded position (Fig. 30-21). This type of splint is most useful in providing temporary relief and, in rare cases, a long-term cure for anterior disk displacement with reduction. In these cases the anterior position is determined by protrusion of the mandible necessary to produce the proper disk and condyle relationships (after the protruding or opening click has occurred).

The splint is usually worn 24 hours a day for several months. Theoretically, after the disk is repositioned for a long period, the posterior ligaments may shorten and maintain the disk in proper relationship to the condyle. Despite theoretical expectations, these splints are generally ineffective in producing permanent reduction of disk displacement. However, even when the splints are not curative, they often provide significant relief of discomfort in the acute stages of TMJ dysfunction.

PERMANENT OCCLUSION MODIFICATION

After completion of a course of reversible treatment, many patients may be candidates for permanent modification of the occlusion. This permanent modification appears to be most appropriate when patients have had significant improvement in masticatory function and reduction in pain as a result of temporary alteration of occlusal position with splint therapy. Permanent occlusion modification may include occlusal equilibration, prosthetic restoration, orthodontics, and orthognathic surgery. Although the relationship between occlusion abnormalities and TMD is unclear, it does appear that permanent modification of the occlusion in indicated patients may provide long-term improvement in symptoms of pain and dysfunction.

TEMPOROMANDIBULAR JOINT SURGERY

Despite the fact that many patients with internal pathologic conditions of the joint improve with reversible nonsurgical treatment, some patients eventually require surgical intervention to improve masticatory function and decrease pain.

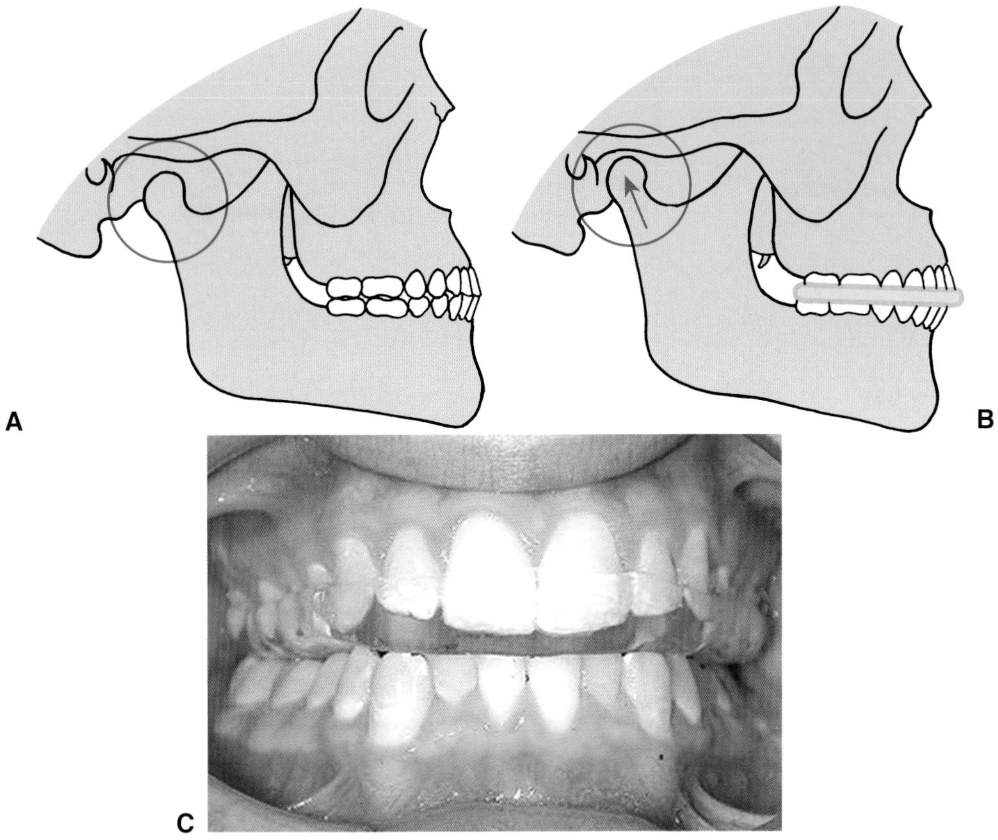

FIGURE 30-20 Autorepositioning splint. A, Diagram representing maximum interdigitation obtained with condyle slightly down and forward. B, Repositioning of mandible by eliminating forced interdigitation of teeth results in posterior and superior repositioning of condyle. C, Clinical photograph of occlusal splint.

Several techniques are currently available for correction of a variety of TMJ derangements.

Arthrocentesis

Arthrocentesis is a minimally invasive technique that involves placing ports (needles or small cannulas) into the TMJ to lavage the joint and to break up fine adhesions. Most patients undergoing arthrocentesis do so with intravenous sedation and an auriculotemporal nerve block. Several techniques have been described for TMJ arthrocentesis.[16,39] The most common method involves initially placing one needle into the superior joint space (Fig. 30-22). A small amount of lactated Ringer's solution is injected to distend the joint space and release fine adhesions that may be limiting disk mobility. With the joint insufflated, a second needle is placed into the superior joint space, allowing thorough lavage with large amounts of fluid (approximately 200 ml).

During the arthrocentesis the jaw can be gently manipulated. At the conclusion of the procedure, steroids, local anesthesia, or a combination of both can be injected into the joint space before the needles are withdrawn. Discomfort after the procedure is managed with mild analgesics or NSAIDs. Some type of exercise regimen or physical therapy is accomplished during the recovery period.

Many types of internal pathologic conditions of the joint appear to respond well to arthrocentesis. The most common use appears to be in patients with anterior disk displacement without reduction. Treatment appears to be effective, with results similar to or better than other types of arthroscopic and open surgical procedures. Nitzan[39] demonstrated that arthrocentesis produced significant improvement in incisal opening and reduction of pain in patients with persistent and severe closed lock.

The success seen with arthrocentesis has several potential explanations. When disk displacement occurs, negative pressure may develop within the joint, causing a "suction cup" effect between the disk and fossa. Distending the joint obviously eliminates the negative pressure. In some cases of more chronic disk displacement, some adhesion may develop between the disk and fossa. With arthrocentesis the distention under pressure can release these adhesions. Capsular constriction may occur as a result of joint hypomobility and can be stretched with pressure distention. Finally, there may be an accumulation of some of the chemical mediators described previously. The simple flushing action in the joint may eliminate or decrease biochemical factors contributing to inflammation and pain.

Arthroscopy

Arthroscopic surgery has become one of the most popular and effective methods of diagnosing and treating TMJ disorders.[40] The technique involves placement of a small cannula into the superior joint space, followed by insertion of an arthroscope to

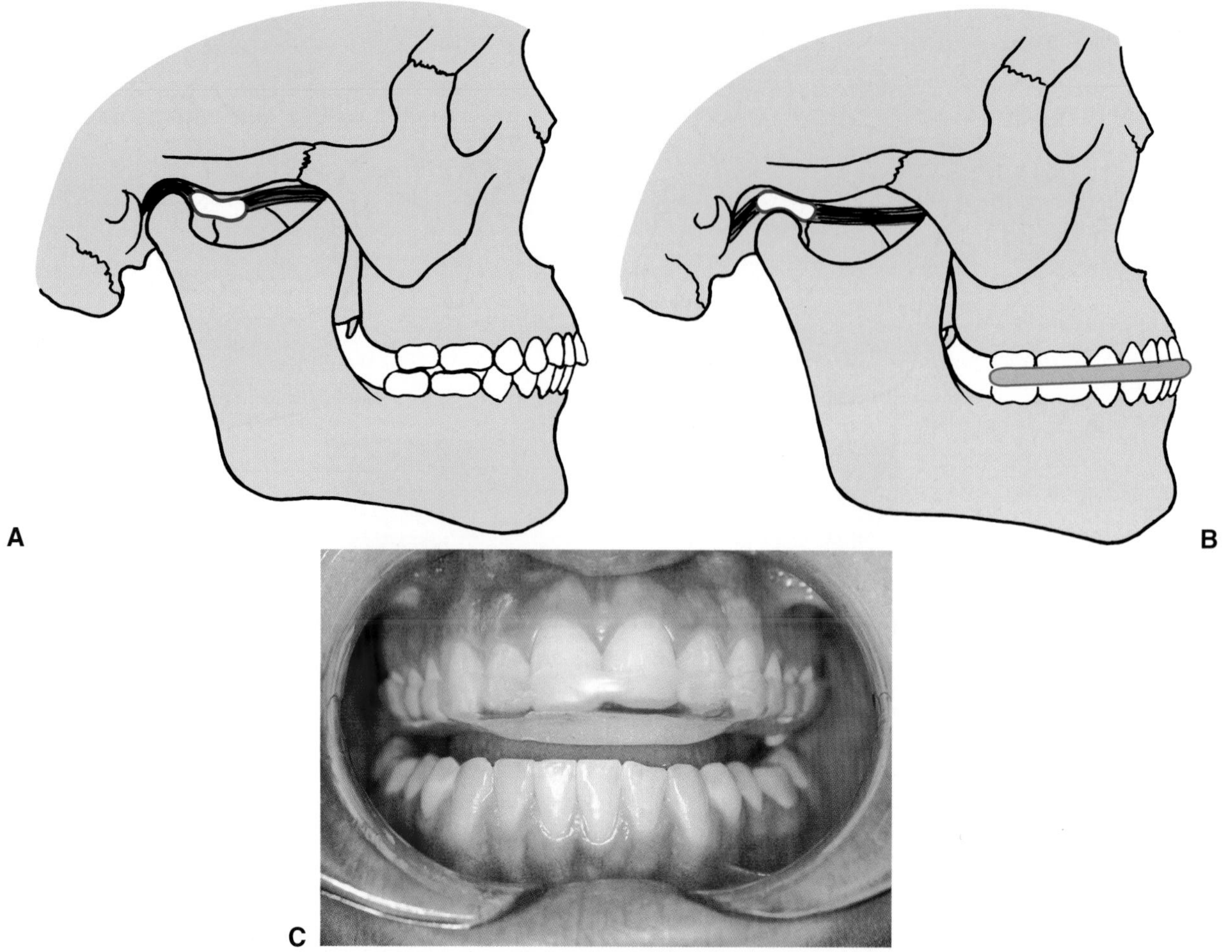

FIGURE 30-21 Anterior repositioning splint. A, Diagram of anteriorly displaced disk. B, Disk interposition between condyle and articular eminence, with anterior repositioning splint in place. Anterior position of mandible allows function with condyle in appropriate condyle and disk relationship. C, Clinical photograph of anterior repositioning splint.

allow direct visualization of all aspects of the glenoid fossa, superior joint space, and superior aspect of the disk. Arthroscopic evaluation enables the surgeon to visualize the joint and therefore contributes to the diagnosis of the internal pathologic condition of the joint. Lysis of adhesions and lavage of the joint are also completed.

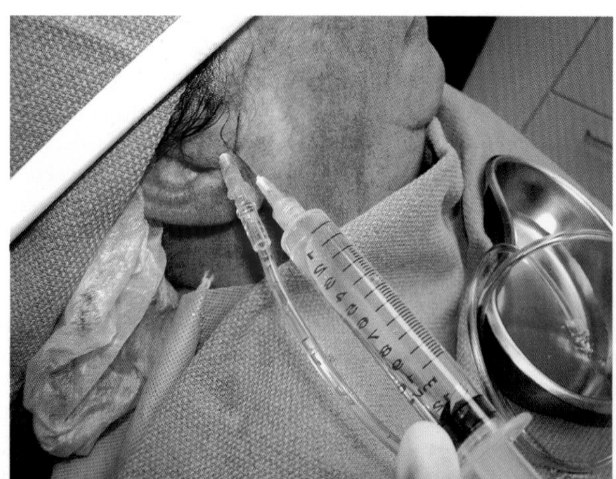

FIGURE 30-22 Arthrocentesis. Port placement into superior joint space paralleling the external auditory meatus to allow lavage and lysis of fine adhesions.

More sophisticated arthroscopic operative techniques have been developed, increasing the ability of the surgeon to correct a variety of intracapsular disorders. Current surgical techniques usually involve the placement of at least two cannulas into the superior joint space. One cannula is used for visualization of the procedure with the arthroscope, whereas instruments are placed through the other cannula to allow instrumentation in the joint (Fig. 30-23). Instrumentation used through the working cannula includes forceps, scissors, sutures, medication needles, cautery probes, and motorized instrumentation such as burs and shavers. Laser fibers can also be used to eliminate adhesions and inflamed tissue and incise tissue within the joint. Disk manipulation, disk attachment release, posterior band cautery, and suture techniques have been developed in an attempt to reposition or stabilize displaced disks.[41] Although it appears that attempts to reposition displaced disks do not result in anatomic restoration of normal disk position, patients undergoing this type of treatment appear to have significant clinical improvement after arthroscopic surgery.[42]

Arthroscopic surgery has been advocated for treatment of a variety of TMJ disorders, including internal derangements,

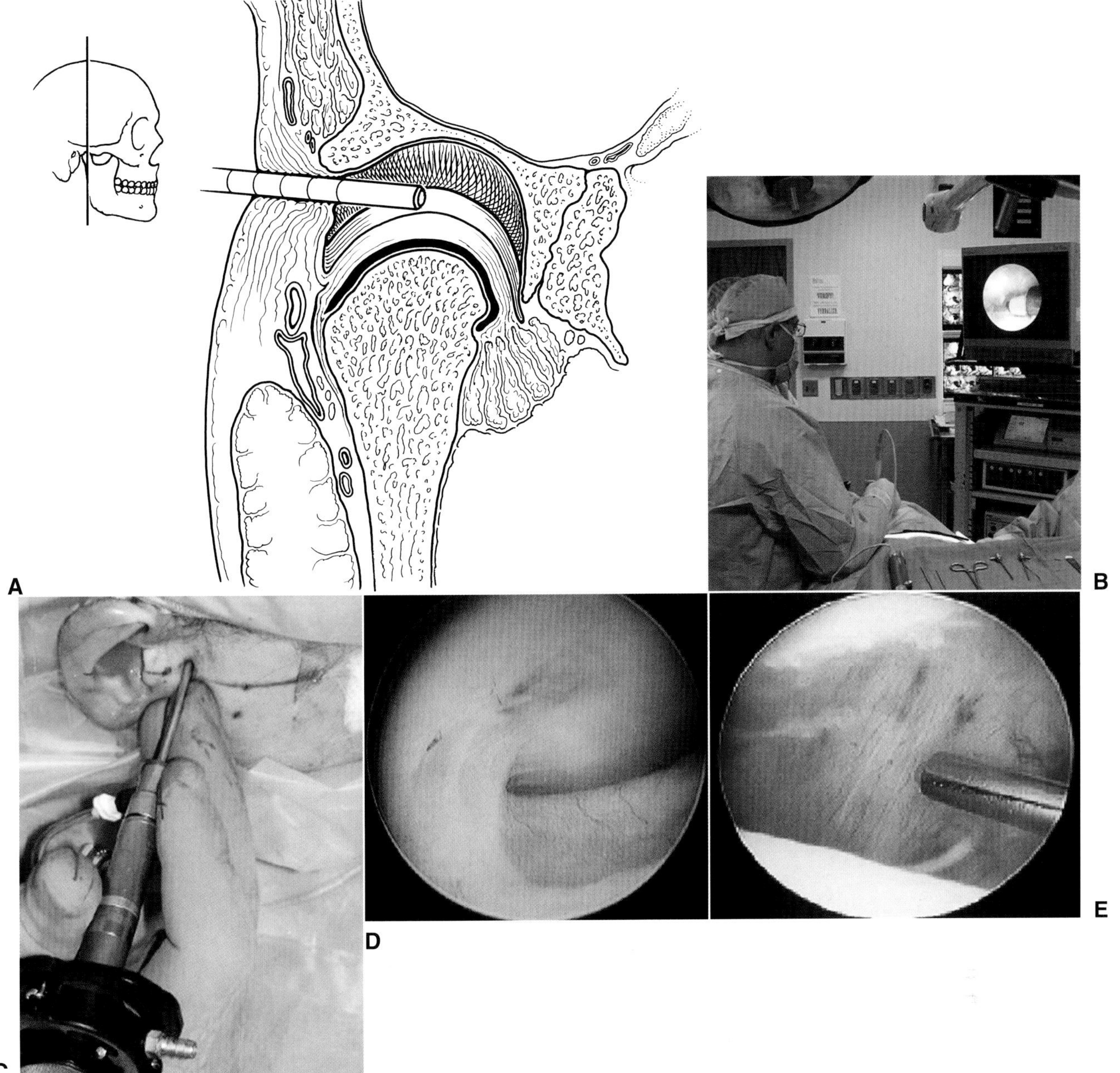

FIGURE 30-23 Temporomandibular joint arthroscopy. A, Diagram depicting arthroscope placement in superior joint space. B, Operating room orientation for arthroscopy. C, Arthroscope orientation for visualization of the temporomandibular joint. D, View of superior joint space with disk inferiorly and fibrous adhesions limiting disk mobility. E, Instrumentation through a second port (radio frequency, laser, motorized shaver) allows surgical manipulation within the joint space.

hypomobility as a result of fibrosis or adhesions, DJD, and hypermobility. The removal of disks with gross perforations can be accomplished with the arthroscope while preserving the surrounding synovial tissue for lubrication.[43] The efficacy of arthroscopic treatment appears to be similar to that of open joint procedures, with the advantage of less surgical morbidity and fewer and less severe complications.[41-44]

As with most TMJ surgical procedures, patients are placed on some type of physical therapy regimen and often continue splint therapy to help decrease loading on the joint during healing.[45]

Disk-Repositioning Surgery

Open joint procedures are generally reserved for individuals who have not responded favorably to other measures. Open surgical exploration of the TMJ traditionally proceeds after conservative techniques have been maximized. Disk plication and repositioning through an variety of open approaches has been a common surgical procedure performed to correct anterior disk displacement that has not responded to nonsurgical treatment and that most frequently results in persistent painful clicking joints or closed locking. Although these disorders are often managed surgically with arthrocentesis or arthroscopy, many surgeons still prefer this type of surgical correction. In this operation, the displaced disk is identified and repositioned into a more normal position by removing a wedge of tissue from the posterior attachment of the disk and suturing the disk back to the correct anatomic position (Fig. 30-24). In some cases this procedure is combined with recontouring of the disk, articular eminence, and mandibular condyle. After surgery, patients generally begin a nonchew diet for several weeks, progressing to a relatively normal diet in 3 to 6 months. A progressive regimen of jaw exercises is also instituted in an attempt to obtain normal jaw motion within 6 to 8 weeks after surgery.

In general, the results of open arthroplasty have been favorable, with a majority of patients experiencing less pain and improved jaw function.[46] Unfortunately, this surgery does not produce improvement in all patients, with 10% to 15% of patients describing no improvement or a worsening of the condition.

Disk Repair or Removal

In some cases the disk is so severely damaged that the remnants of disk tissue must be removed. Diskectomy without replacement was one of the earliest surgical procedures described for treatment of severe TMJ internal derangements.[47] With current technology, the diskectomy procedure can be performed through arthroscopic techniques to minimize scar tissue formation and preserve lubrication provided by the synovium. Although this technique has been widely used, there seems to be a wide variation in clinical results, with some joints showing minimal anatomic changes and significant clinical improvement and some joints demonstrating severe degenerative changes with continued symptoms of pain and dysfunction.

In advanced internal pathologic conditions of the joint, the disk may be severely damaged and perforated but may have adequate remaining tissue so that a repair or patch procedure can be accomplished. Autogenous grafting techniques include the use of dermis, auricular cartilage, or temporalis fascia.[48,49] Dermis harvested from the abdomen or upper lateral thigh placed into the joint functions as an interpositional disk (Fig. 30-25). The dermal graft with associated adipose tissue provides lubrication and coverage of the articular surfaces.

Another alternative to the use of a free graft involves rotation of a temporalis muscle flap into the joint to provide interpositional tissue between the condyle and fossa.[50] The posterior fibers of the temporalis are mobilized from the temporal bone with an anterior pedicle originating from the coronoid process (Fig. 30-26). The maintenance of the anterior aspect of the temporalis muscle provides a blood supply to the flap, enhancing

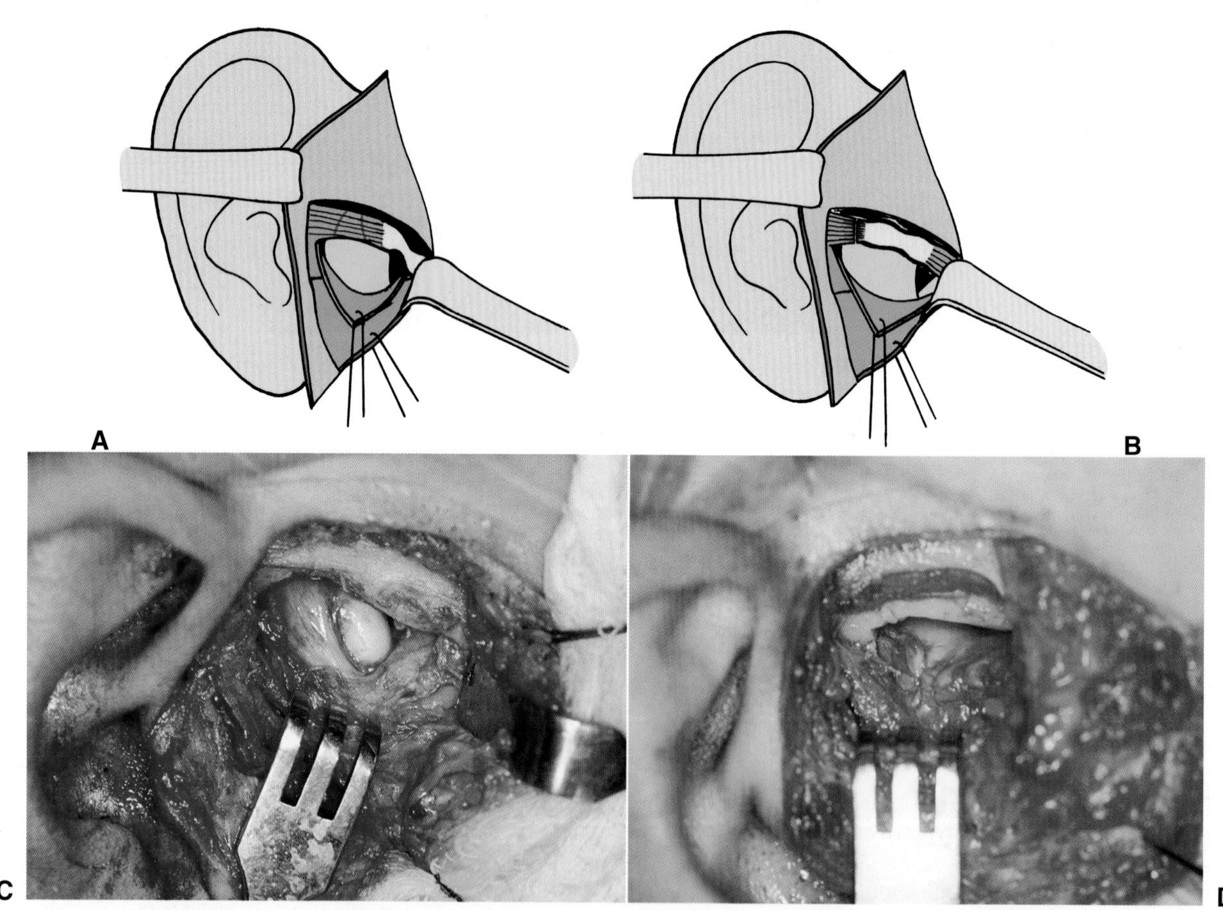

FIGURE 30-24 Open temporomandibular joint surgery. **A**, Preauricular incision through skin subcutaneous tissue and temporomandibular joint capsule, exposing anteriorly displaced disk. **B**, Wedge of tissue is removed from posterior attachment area, and disk is repositioned and sutured into its correct position. **C**, Displaced disk anterior to mandibular condyle. **D**, Disk repositioning and plication via open arthrotomy.

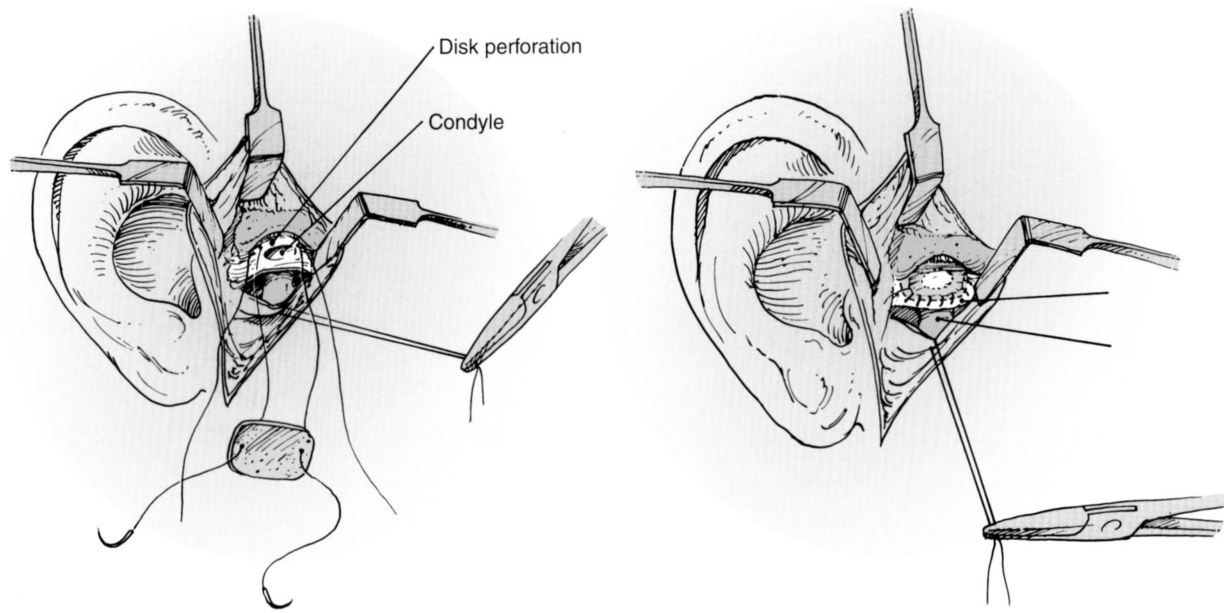

FIGURE 30-25 Dermal graft used to patch small perforation of disk.

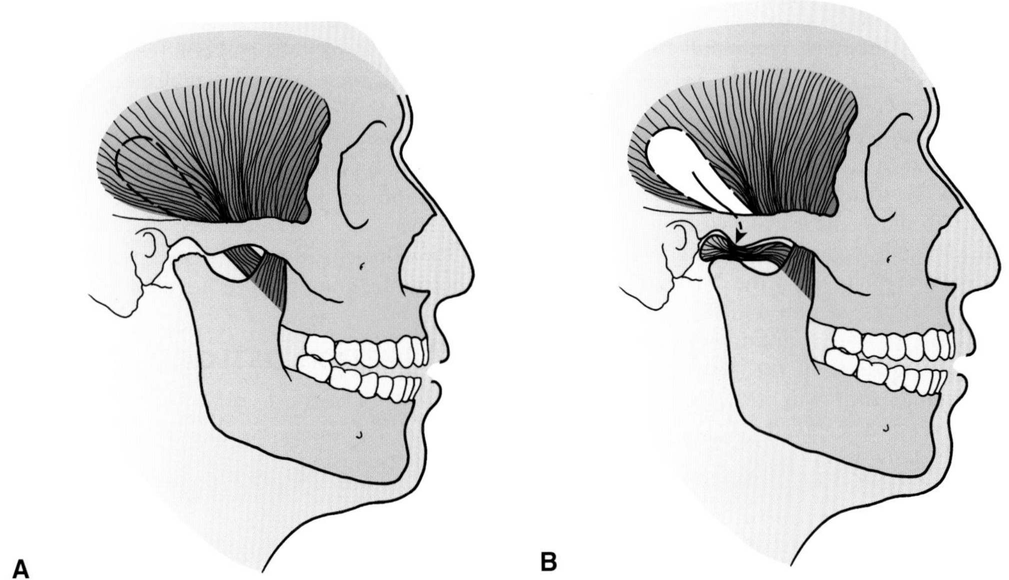

FIGURE 30-26 **A**, Temporalis muscle flap. **B**, Rotation of temporalis muscle flap recreating articular surface for condyle. The preservation of the overlying fascia allows lubrication of joint space.

viability. The fascia, muscle, and periosteum are ligated to prevent separation and are rotated under the zygomatic arch. The flap is positioned over the condyle and sutured to the residual retrodiskal tissue. The preservation of the overlying fascia may aid in continued lubrication of the obliterated joint.

Condylotomy for Treatment of Temporomandibular Joint Disorders

The condylotomy is an osteotomy completed in a manner identical to the vertical ramus osteotomy described in Chapter 25 (Fig. 30-27). When used for treatment of TMJ problems, the osteotomy is completed, but no wire or screw fixation is placed, and the patient is placed into intermaxillary fixation for a period ranging from 2 to 6 weeks. The theory behind this operation is that muscles attached to the proximal segment (i.e., segment attached to the condyle) will passively reposition the condyle, resulting in a more favorable relationship between the condyle, disk, and fossa.[51,52]

This technique has been advocated primarily for treatment of disk displacement with or without reduction. DJD and subluxation or dislocation have also been suggested as possible indications for use of this technique. Although this method of surgical treatment has been controversial, it appears to provide significant clinical improvement in a variety of TMJ disorders.

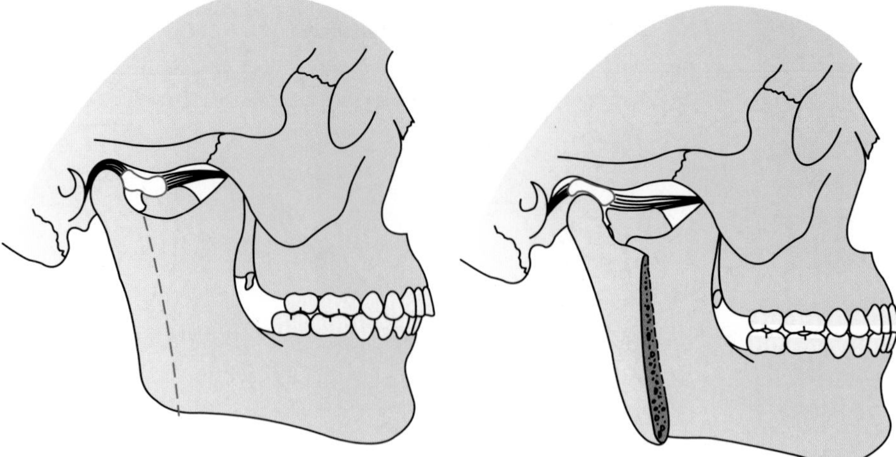

FIGURE 30-27 Condylotomy allowing condylar sag to correct internal derangement.

Total Joint Replacement

In some cases, a pathologic condition of the joint results in destruction of joint structures and in loss of vertical dimension of the condyle and posterior ramus, malocclusion, limited opening, and severe pain. In these cases, reconstruction or replacement of condylar and fossa components of the TMJ may be necessary. Surgical techniques may involve replacement of the condyle or fossa but most commonly include both elements.

One method of joint reconstruction involves grafting autogenous tissue using a costochondral bone graft.[53] These grafts are most frequently used in growing individuals but also can be used effectively in the treatment of a variety of adult disorders. Figure 30-28, *B*, shows the use of a costochondral graft for replacement of a severely degenerated mandibular condyle. In this situation the graft replaces only the condylar portion of the joint and does not address significant abnormalities of the fossa. Problems with costochondral grafting include recurrent ankylosis, degenerative changes of the graft, and (in some cases) excess and asymmetric growth of the graft.

In the past, several types of prosthetic joint replacement have been available.[54] Long-term results of prosthetic joint replacements have been disappointing because of a variety of engineering and biologic problems. However, for many patients with significant destruction of TMJ structures who have had poor results from other surgical treatment, no other viable surgical options exist. In these cases the joint destruction results in severe pain, limited motion or complete ankylosis, and severe malocclusions.

Total joint replacement in severe TMJ disease, such as a severely degenerative or multiply operated joint with excessive scarring, aims to restore function through improved range of motion and reduction in pain. Older joint prostheses met with limited success because of the excessive scar tissue associated with multiple previous open joint surgeries, mechanical failure, and foreign body reaction from wear debris. Newer-generation joint prostheses have improved engineering, better biocompatibility, and materials with greater wear resistance. Total joint replacement can be completed with standard preformed fossa and condyle parts or with custom fabrication of joint components. Custom joints are generated from a stereolithic model based on three-dimensional CT scan imaging of the articular fossa and mandibular anatomy (Fig. 30-28, *C*).

Access to the joint and ramus are achieved through a preauricular and retromandibular incision, respectively. A nerve simulator is used during the dissection to ensure preservation of the facial nerve to the muscles of facial expression. Soft tissue dissection is completed to expose the TMJ capsule, condyle, coronoid, and ramus. Removal of the diseased condyle is completed, followed by débridement of the articular fossa. The joint fossa and condylar prosthesis are placed after the occlusion has been established with maxillomandibular fixation and secured with bone screws. The established occlusion is verified while maintaining sterility of the surgical field. Manipulation of the mandible intraoperatively allows for evaluation of joint function in the absence of muscular influences.

These recent advantages have provided significant improvement in the outcome after total joint replacement.[55,56]

DISTRACTION OSTEOGENESIS

The loss of vertical ramus height is a consequence of a condylar pathologic condition and may result in asymmetry and malocclusion, as well as dysfunction and pain. Severe alteration of condylar anatomy may result from a variety of conditions such as hemifacial microsomia, growth disturbances, trauma, or a pathologic condition. Until recently, skeletally immature patients were treated primarily with costochondral grafts.[57] The need for donor site surgery and unpredictable results including asymmetric growth and ankylosis yielded less than ideal results in many patients. More recently, distraction osteogenesis has been used successfully to reconstruct the mandibular condyle.[58]

Distraction osteogenesis of the mandibular condyle involves exposing the mandibular ramus, usually through an extraoral approach. The distractor is temporary stabilized on the lateral surface of the mandible, an osteotomy of the posterior ramus is completed, and the distraction appliance is attached to the osteotomized (condyle) segment and to the stable portion of the ramus (Fig. 30-29). Following an initial latency period of 5 to 7 days, the distraction appliance is activated, producing approximately 1 mm of bone movement per day. This process creates regenerate bone formation in response to distraction of the condylar segment. Range of motion is maintained during distraction, and control of the occlusion and molding of the

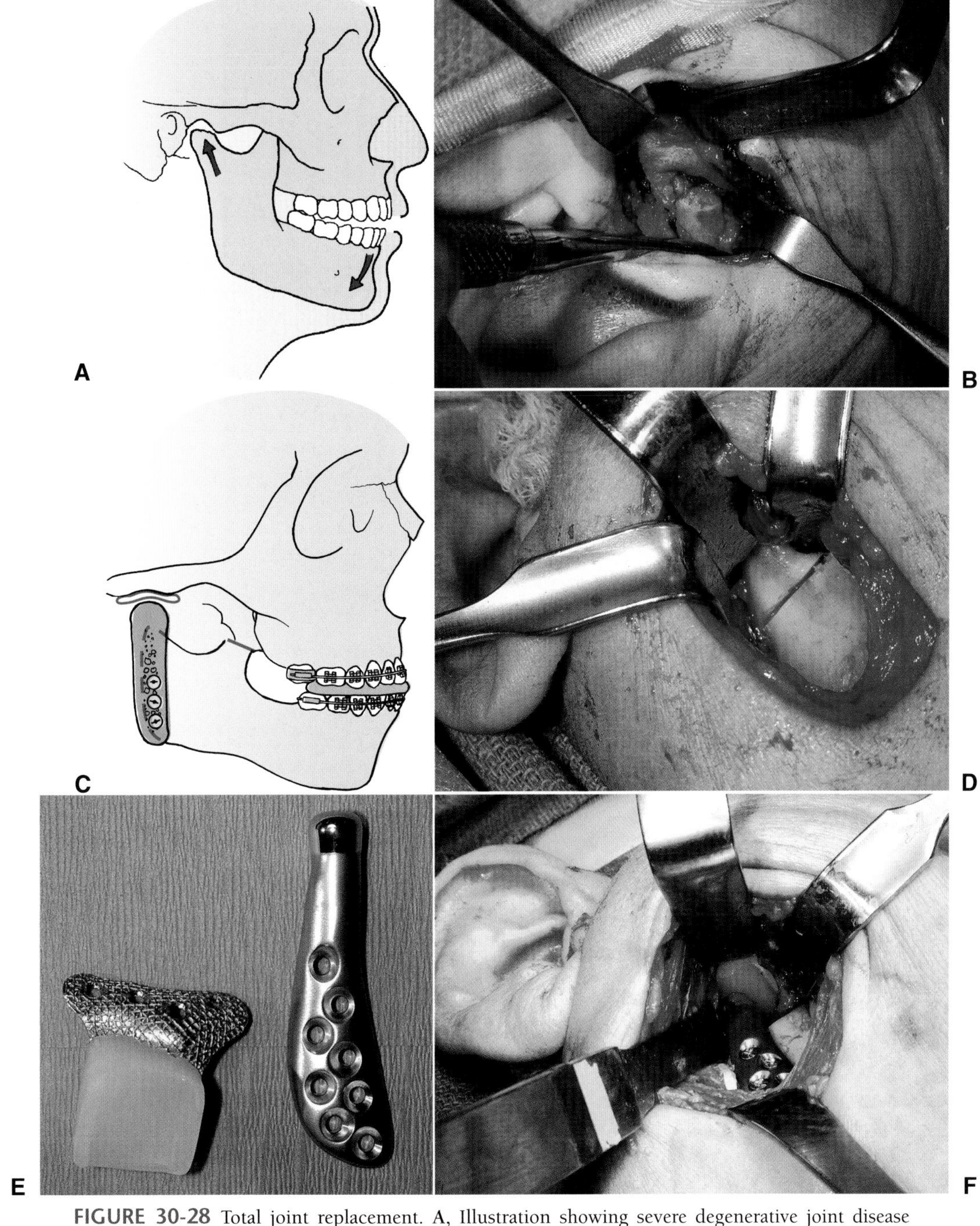

FIGURE 30-28 Total joint replacement. **A**, Illustration showing severe degenerative joint disease resulting in open bite malocclusion caused by resorption of condyle. **B**, Exposure via a preauricular approach confirms severe degeneration of the condyle. **C**, Illustration of costochondral bone graft placed along posterior aspect of mandible to reconstruct severely damaged condyle. This technique is usually reserved for growing patients. **D**, Bone cut for condylectomy completed with sagittal saw while protecting important adjacent neurovascular structures. **E**, Custom condylar and fossa prosthesis fabricated from a stereolithic model. **F**, Positioning of condyle and fossa in total joint reconstruction.

regenerate can be completed with elastic traction guidance. The consolidation period is typically calculated as 3 times the period of distraction. During this time the structural integrity over the regenerate is maintained with the distraction appliance. A second intervention is required to remove the distractor, and a stabilizing bone plate can be placed over the regenerate gap. Surgical access to remove the distractor is through the existing incision. The reestablishment of vertical ramus height and increased mandibular continuity allows for reestablishment of symmetry and occlusion. Finalizing the occlusion often requires orthodontic detailing or equilibration to aid in providing a stable, balanced interdigitation.

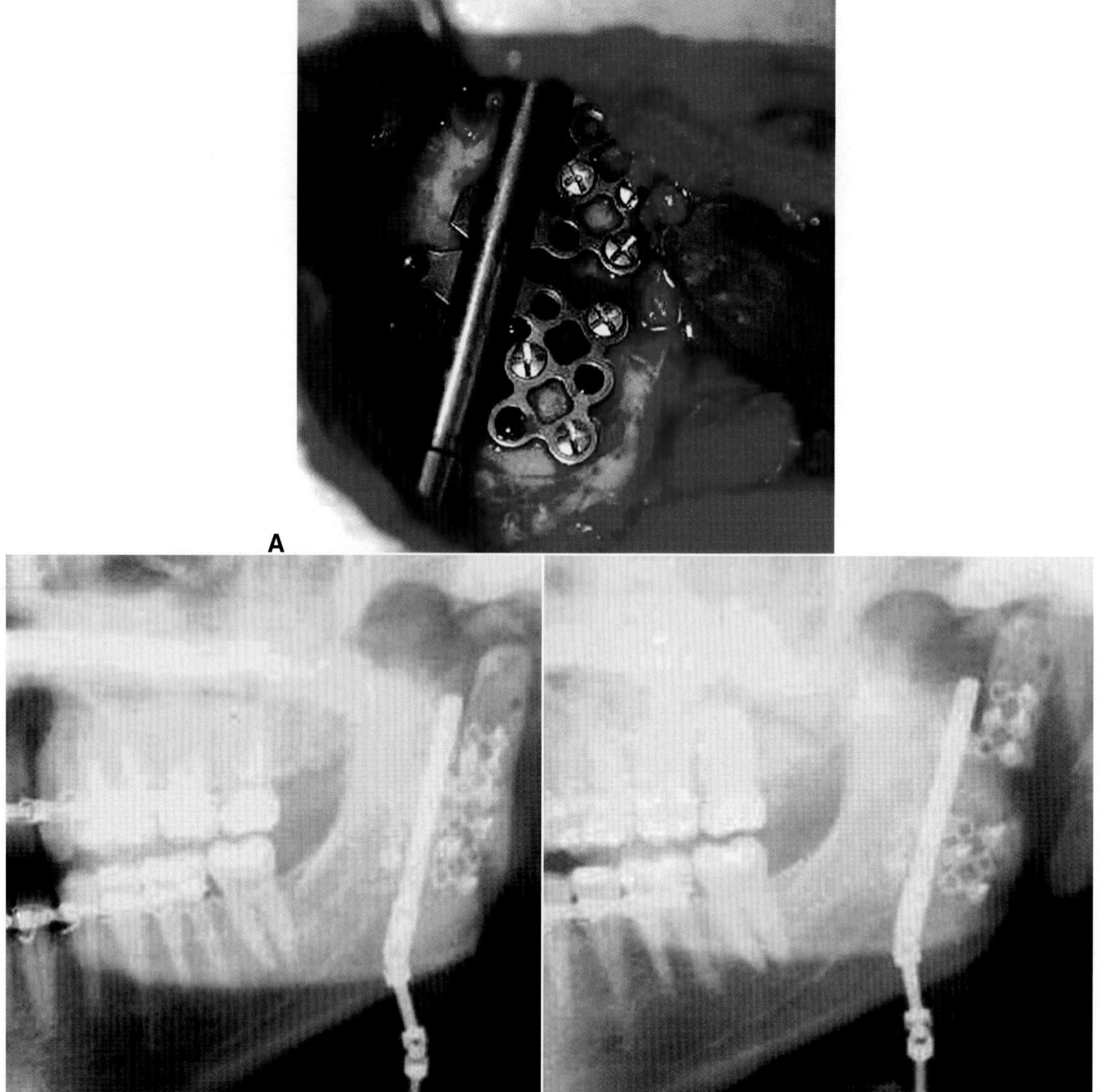

FIGURE 30-29 Distraction osteogenesis. **A**, Distractor placement on mandibular ramus with orientation and vector toward glenoid fossa. **B**, Panoramic radiograph before distraction of ramus to recreate the mandibular condyle. **C**, Pseudocondyle formation following distraction.

REFERENCES

1. Blaschke DD, White SC: Radiology. In Sarnat BG, Laskin DM, editors: *The temporomandibular joint: biological diagnosis and treatment,* ed 3, Springfield, IL, 1980, Charles C Thomas.
2. Blair GS, Chalmers IM, Leggat TG et al: Circular tomography of the temporomandibular joint, *Oral Surg Oral Med Oral Pathol* 35:416, 1973.
3. Dolwick MF, Katzberg RW, Helms CA et al: Arthrotomographic evaluation of the temporomandibular joint, *J Oral Surg* 37:793, 1979.
4. Helms CA, Morrish RB Jr, Kircos LT et al: Computed tomography of the meniscus of the temporomandibular joint: preliminary observations, *Radiology* 145:719, 1982.
5. Manzione JV, Katzberg RW, Tallents RH et al: Magnetic resonance imaging of the temporomandibular joint, *J Am Dent Assoc* 113:398, 1986.
6. Oesterreich FU, Jend-Rossmann I, Jend HH et al: Semi-quantitative SPECT imaging for assessment of bone reaction to internal derangements of the temporomandibular joint, *J Oral Maxillofac Surg* 45:1022, 1987.
7. Sternback RA: Varieties of pain games. In Bonica JJ, editor: *Advances in neurology: international symposium on pain,* vol 4, New York, 1973, Raven.
8. Yap AU, Chua EK, Tan KB et al: Relationship between depression/somatization and self-reports of pain and disability, *J Orofac Pain* 18:220-225, 2004.
9. Green CS: Orthodontics and temporomandibular disorders, *Dent Clin North Am* 32:529-538, 1988.
10. Kinney RK, Gatchel RJ, Ellis E et al: Major psychological disorders in chronic TMD patients: implications for successful management, *J Am Dent Assoc* 123:49-54, 1992.

11. Rugh JD: Psychological components of pain, *Dent Clin North Am* 31:579-594, 1987.
12. Moss RA, Adams HE: The assessment of personality, anxiety and depression in mandibular pain dysfunction subjects, *J Oral Rehabil* 11:233-237, 1984.
13. Katon W, Egan K, Miller D: Chronic pain: lifetime psychiatric diagnosis and family history, *Am J Psychiatry* 142:1156-1160, 1985.
14. Turner JA, Whitney C, Dworkin SF et al: Do changes in patients beliefs and coping strategies predict temporomandibular disorder treatment outcomes? *Clin J Pain* 11:177-188, 1995.
15. Rugh JD, Solberg WK: Psychological implications in temporomandibular pain and dysfunction, *Oral Sci Rev* 7:3, 1976.
16. Nitzan DW, Samson B, Better H: Long-term outcome of arthrocentesis for sudden onset, persistent severe closed lock of the temporomandibular joint, *J Oral Maxillofac Surg* 55:151, 1997.
17. Milam SB, Schmitz JP: Molecular biology of temporomandibular joint disorders: proposed mechanisms of disease, *J Oral Maxillofac Surg* 53:1445, 1995.
18. Nitzan DW: Intraarticular pressure in the functioning human temporomandibular joint and its alteration by uniform elevation of the occlusal plane, *J Oral Maxillofac Surg* 52:671, 1994.
19. Holmlund A, Ekblom A, Hansson P et al: Concentrations of neuropeptide substance P, neurokinin A, calcitonin gene-related peptide, neuropeptide Y, and vasoactive intestinal polypeptide in synovial fluid of human temporomandibular joint: a correlation with symptoms, signs, and arthroscopic findings, *Int J Oral Maxillofac Surg* 20:228, 1991.
20. Israel HA, Saed-Nejad R, Ratliffe A: Early diagnosis of osteoarthrosis of the temporomandibular joint: correlation between arthroscopic diagnosis and keratan sulfate levels in the synovial fluid, *J Oral Maxillofac Surg* 49:708, 1991.
21. Quinn JH, Bazan NG: Identification of prostaglandin E_2 and leukotriene BA_4 in the synovial fluid of painful dysfunctional temporomandibular joints, *J Oral Maxillofac Surg* 48:968, 1990.
22. Blaustein D, Scappino RP: Remodeling of the temporomandibular joint disk and posterior attachment in disk displacement specimens in relation to glycosaminoglycan content, *Plast Reconstr Surg* 78:756, 1986.
23. Riggs RR, Rugh JD, Borghi W: Muscle activity of MPD and TMJ patients and nonpatients, *J Dent Res* 61:277, 1982 (abstract).
24. Plesh O, Curtis D, Levine J et al: Amitriptyline treatment of chronic pain in patients with temporomandibular disorders, *J Oral Rehabil* 27:834-841, 2000.
25. Kreisberg MK: Tricyclic antidepressants: analgesic effect and indications in orofacial pain, *J Craniomandib Disord* 2:171-177, 1988.
26. Raigrodski AJ, Mohamed SE, Gardiner DM: The effect of amitriptyline on pain intensity and perception of stress in bruxers, *J Prosthodont* 10:73-77, 2001.
27. Cohen SP, Mullins R, Abdi S: The pharmacologic treatment of muscle pain, *Anesthesiology* 101:495-526, 2004.
28. Erg-King T, Jankovic J: Treating severe bruxism with botulinum toxin, *J Am Dent Assoc* 131:211, 2001.
29. Von Lindern JJ: Type A botulinum toxin in the treatment of chronic facial pain associated with temporomandibular dysfunction, *Acta Neurol Belg* 101:39, 2001.
30. Kopp S, Carlsson GE, Haraldson T et al: Long-term effect of intra-articular injections of sodium hyaluronate and corticosteroid on temporomandibular joint arthritis, *J Oral Maxillofac Surg* 45:929, 1987.
31. Poswillo D: The effects of intraarticular deposition of betamethasone in the goat temporomandibular joint: discussion, *J Oral Maxillofac Surg* 52:1440, 1995.
32. Medlicott MS, Harris SR: A systematic review of the effectiveness of exercise, manual therapy, electrotherapy, relaxation training, and biofeedback in the management of temporomandibular disorder, *Phys Ther* 86:955-973, 2006.
33. Sturdivant J, Fricton JR: Physical therapy for temporomandibular disorders and orofacial pain, *Curr Opin Dent* 1:485-496, 1991.
34. Maloney G: Effect of a passive jaw motion device on pain and range of motion in TMD patients not responding to flat plane intraoral appliances, *J Craniomandibular Pract* 20:55-56, 2002.
35. Hertling D, Kessler R: *Management of common musculoskeletal disorders: physical therapy principles and methods*, ed 2, Philadelphia, 1990, JB Lippincott.
36. Richardson JK, Iglarsh AI: *Clinical orthopaedic physical therapy*, Philadelphia, 1994, WB Saunders.
37. Griffin JE, Karselis GD, Terrence C: *Ultrasonic energy in physical agents for physical therapists*, Springfield, IL, 1979, Charles C Thomas.
38. Travell JG, Simons DJ: *Myofacial muscles in myofascial pain and dysfunction: the trigger point manual*, Baltimore, 1983, Williams & Wilkins.
39. Nitzan DW: Arthrocentesis for management of severe closed lock of the temporomandibular joint: current controversies in surgery for internal derangement of the temporomandibular joint, *Atlas Oral Maxillofac Surg Clin North Am* 6:245, 1994.
40. Sanders B, Buoncristiani R: Diagnostic and surgical arthroscopy of the temporomandibular joint: clinical experience with 137 procedures over a two year period, *J Craniomandib Disord* 1:202, 1987.
41. McCain J, Podrasky A, Zabiegalskin NA: Arthroscopic disc repositioning and suturing: a preliminary report, *J Oral Maxillofac Surg* 50:568, 1992.
42. Moses J, Sartoris D, Glass R et al: The effect of arthroscopic surgical lysis and lavage of the superior joint space on TMJ disk position and mobility, *J Oral Maxillofac Surg* 47:674, 1989.
43. Mazzonetto R, Spagnoli DB: Long-term evaluation of arthroscopic diskectomy of the temporomandibular joint using holmium YAG laser, *J Oral Maxillofac Surg* 59:1018-1023, 2001.
44. Zeitler D, Porter B: A retrospective study comparing arthroscopic surgery with arthrotomy and disc repositioning. In Clark G, Sanders B, Bertolami C, editors: *Advances in diagnostic and surgical arthroscopy of the temporomandibular joint*, Philadelphia, 1993, WB Saunders.
45. Bertolucci LE: Postoperative physical therapy in temporomandibular joint arthroplasty, *Cranio* 10:211-220, 1992.
46. Dolwick MF: Disc preservation surgery for the treatment of internal derangements of the temporomandibular joint, *J Oral Maxillofac Surg* 59:1047, 2001.
47. McKenna SJ: Discectomy for the treatment of internal derangements of the temporomandibular joint, *J Oral Maxillofac Surg* 59:1051, 2001.
48. Tucker MR, Jacoway JR, White RP Jr: Use of autogenous dermal graft for repair of TMJ meniscus perforations, *J Oral Maxillofac Surg* 44:781, 1986.
49. Tucker MR, Kennady MC, Jacoway JR: Autogenous auricular cartilage implantation following discectomy in the primate temporomandibular joint, *J Oral Maxillofac Surg* 48:38, 1990.
50. Sanders B, Buoncristiani RO: Temporomandibular joint arthrotomy: management of failed cases, *Oral Maxillofac Surg Clin North Am* 1:944, 1989.
51. Bell WH, Yamaguchi Y, Poor MR: Treatment of temporomandibular joint dysfunction by intraoral vertical ramus osteotomy, *Int J Adult Orthodon Orthognath Surg* 5:9, 1990.
52. Hall HD, Navarro EZ, Gibbs SJ: One- and three-year prospective outcome study of modified condylotomy for treatment of reducing disk displacement, *J Oral Maxillofac Surg* 58:7-17, 2000.
53. Lindqvist C, Jokinen J, Paukku P et al: Adaptation of autogenous costochondral grafts used for temporomandibular joint reconstruction, *J Oral Maxillofac Surg* 46:465, 1988.
54. Kent JN, Misiek DJ, Akin RK et al: Temporomandibular joint condylar prosthesis: a ten-year report, *J Oral Maxillofac Surg* 41:245, 1983.
55. Mercuri LG: The use of alloplastic prostheses for temporomandibular joint reconstruction, *J Oral Maxillofac Surg* 58:70, 2000.
56. Mercuri LG: Considering total temporomandibular joint replacement, *Cranio* 17:44, 1999.
57. Ko EW, Huang C, Chen Y: Temporomandibular joint reconstruction in children using costochondral grafts, *J Oral Maxillofac Surg* 57:789-800, 1999.
58. Stucki-McCormick SU: Reconstruction of the mandibular condyle using transport distraction osteogenesis, *J Craniofacial Surg* 8:48-53, 1997.

PART IX

Management of the Hospitalized Patient

The willingness and ability of the dental practitioner to manage hospitalized patients can be a fulfilling experience for the dentist and a tremendous service to the dentist's patients and community. Patients with serious medical problems requiring dental care sometimes need the facilities and staff support available only in a hospital or surgical center. Institutionalized patients frequently find hospitals the only setting in which dental care can be provided. In addition, patients hospitalized for nondental reasons occasionally develop dental problems for which definitive care cannot be deferred until they are discharged. Finally, patients with dental emergencies or facial trauma commonly go to hospital emergency departments and immediately require someone with dental expertise to provide proper evaluation and therapy.

Effective dental practice in a hospital requires more than common sense. Although each hospital is unique, there are common administrative concepts that must be learned to practice in a hospital effectively. Chapter 31 is designed to inform the reader of the common protocols used in hospitals to facilitate communication among care providers and between health care providers and agencies outside of the hospital. This chapter also describes some of the basic problems hospitalized patients may experience, whether they are there for dental care or for other problems.

CHAPTER 31

Management of the Hospitalized Patient

JAMES R. HUPP

CHAPTER OUTLINE

Most dentists find that they can practice without hospital facilities, but the ability to care for patients in a hospital setting adds a stimulating dimension to a dentist's professional life.

As a vital member of a community health care team, the hospital-affiliated dentist is consulted about the dental needs of patients in the emergency room and of those admitted to the hospital by other doctors or the dentist. Dentists who join a hospital medical staff are permitted to perform dental consultations for hospitalized patients and to bring patients to the hospital to perform procedures best done there. In addition, for dentists seeking to provide care with their patients under general anesthesia, community surgery centers are often the ideal answer.

HOSPITAL GOVERNANCE

Administrative Organization

Hospital organization varies from institution to institution, but most are based on standards of The Joint Commission. The mission of this national organization is to set standards for hospitals and ambulatory care centers, to monitor these facilities to ensure that those standards are being met, and then to accredit hospitals and ambulatory centers meeting the standards.

Most general, acute care community hospitals have a board of trustees that include community leaders who make up the highest governing body of the institution. These trustees are advised in health matters by a joint conference committee, which is a liaison group that includes members from hospital management, the medical staff, and the board of trustees. The hospital chief executive officer is in charge of the daily operation of the hospital and typically reports to the board of trustees. Hospital governance from this point is divided into two major organizational bodies: medical staff and hospital administration.

The medical staff includes all the health care professionals who work at the hospital. The chief of staff is the most senior governing member of the medical staff and reports to the hospital president and joint conference committee and chairs the medical board. The medical board or executive committee commonly includes the chiefs of all the medical departments of the hospital and often includes representatives from nursing and hospital administration. Dentists who join the medical staff typically become members of the dental department or division. Although at some large hospitals, dentistry is on equal footing with other major departments, such as psychiatry or pediatrics, it is more often made a division, or section, of the department of surgery, similar to other surgical disciplines, such as urology and neurosurgery. As a member of the medical staff, a dentist is usually asked to serve on committees in which dental expertise is needed, such as on infection control and oversight of the pharmacy and therapeutics.

Hospital administration is managed by the hospital chief executive officer, who has several vice presidents or assistant directors to direct various areas of hospital operations, such as nursing, support services, and finance (Fig. 31-1).

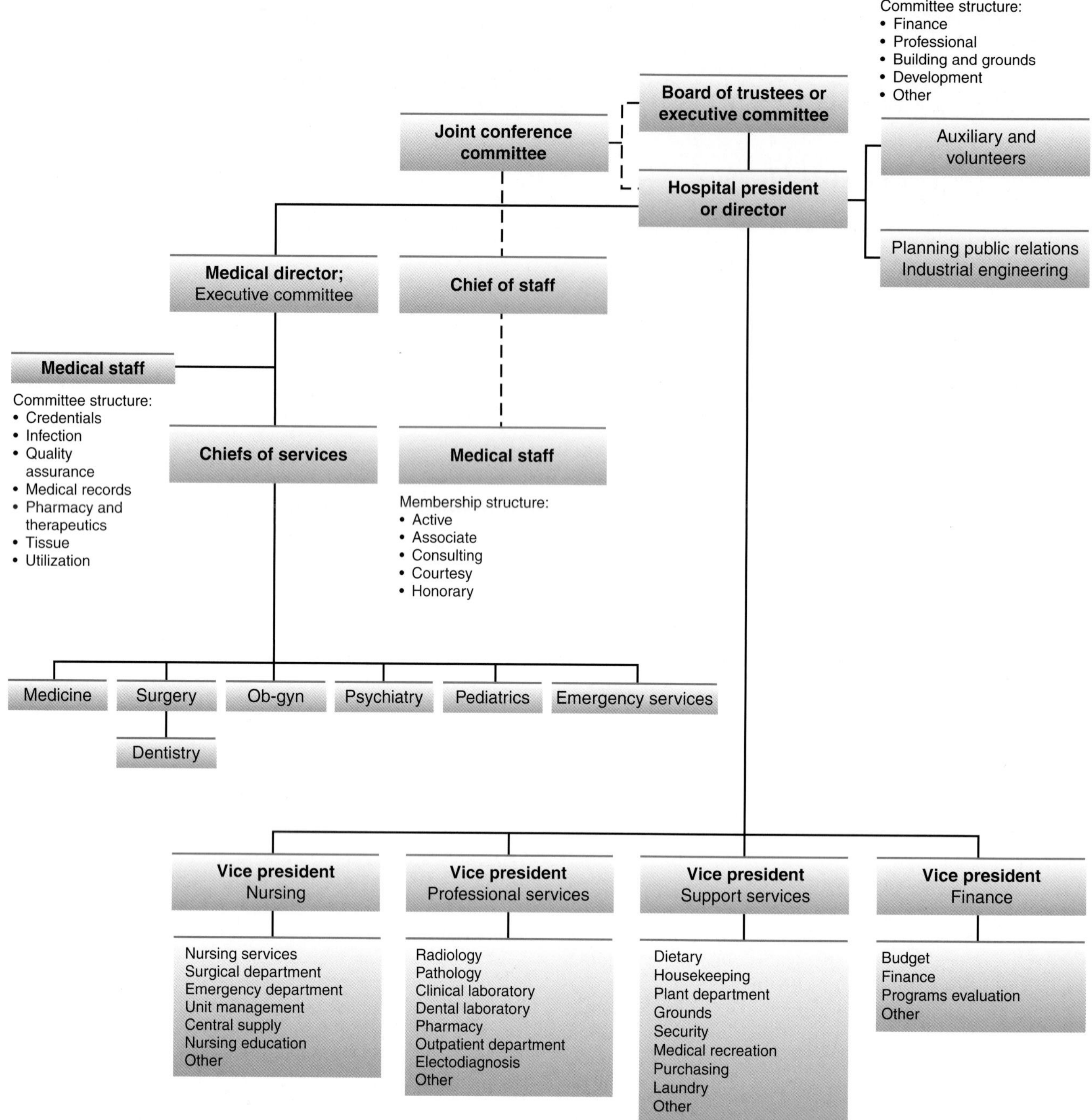

FIGURE 31-1 Typical hospital organization flow diagram. Although dentistry is commonly part of the surgery department, it may be a separate department in some hospitals.

Medical Staff Membership

Membership on a hospital medical staff is not usually gained by simple request. The hospital credentials committee, consisting of physicians and dentists on the medical staff and their administrative support staff, carefully review the qualifications of doctors applying for staff membership to ensure that individuals granted privileges are competent to practice in the hospital environment and have no evidence of criminal, ethical, or other problems in their past.

Various levels of medical staff membership exist (e.g., active, associate, and courtesy), each carrying certain privileges and restrictions. Staff membership, however, never automatically gives the dentist the privilege to admit patients to the hospital or to use the operating room facilities. These privileges are granted based on a review of the applying dentist's education and experience. Dentists who have completed a general practice residency or dental specialty training that provided hospital experience usually have little difficulty gaining medical staff membership and some admitting privileges.

However, because of hospital regulations, most dental patients admitted to a hospital by dentists other than oral and maxillofacial surgeons require a physician's participation in the admission process.

HOSPITAL DENTISTRY

Consultations

The request for consultation carries different connotations among health care professionals. To some, the consultant is only expected to render an opinion and not to begin implementing any advice until given permission by the patient's attending physician or, in the case of the emergency room, by the patient's designated emergency department physician. However, many physicians allow consultants to perform any test or procedure necessary to act on their opinion. Therefore the dental consultant must clarify with the requesting doctor whether only an opinion is being sought or whether the dentist can proceed to order tests and render treatment before conducting the consultation. In some cases, the consultation request form provides a section in which the requesting doctor can indicate the type of consultation desired.

Emergency Room Consultations

Emergency room consultations are usually requested verbally because of the urgency of the situation. The dentist should make use of any history and physical examination, laboratory, and radiographic results already available to avoid excessive duplication. However, the dentist still needs to do a careful, comprehensive history and physical examination of the oral and maxillofacial region and order special imaging as necessary to allow a complete, well-organized assessment of the patient's dentofacial problems. All of this information is recorded in the medical record on a consultation form, in the progress notes, or in the emergency room record. A recommendation should be offered that considers other medical problems, acute or long-standing, and the urgency of the treatment. Guidelines for answering consultations are shown in Box 31-1, and a sample of a written emergency suite dental consultation is shown in Figure 31-2.

The way emergency suites are equipped for dental therapy varies. If the dentist cannot offer high-quality care in the emergency setting, the problem should be temporized and an appointment made for definitive care in the dental office. Dentists who are frequently called to hospital emergency rooms sometimes find it useful to carry in their car a set of instruments and supplies necessary for initially handling common oral emergencies.

If more than one dentist serves as a dental consultant to an emergency room, a call schedule is usually established to designate, on a daily, weekly, or monthly basis, which dentist is expected to be available in case of an emergency. When on call, the dentist should keep the hospital aware of how to be contacted quickly.

BOX 31-1

Guidelines for Answering Consultations

- State reason for consultation in opening sentence.
- State that chart has been reviewed and patient examined.
- Be brief but thorough, particularly with dentofacial portion of the examination.
- Be specific with recommendations.
- Provide contingency plans.
- Follow up written consultation with verbal contact with requesting doctor.
- Follow patient's progress until dental problem is resolved.

Inpatient Consultations

Dental consultation for a hospitalized patient is similar to consultations for emergency room patients: the dentist is expected to evaluate the oral and maxillofacial region, offer an assessment, and formulate a dental treatment plan that considers the overall clinical situation. Dental consultation requests should be written on standard hospital consultation forms or in the appropriate portion of the electronic medical record on which the requesting physician states the question or questions to be answered by the dental consultant. The requesting doctor should also provide a brief statement of other active problems the patient may have. If a dentist receives an unwritten or unclearly written consultation request, the dentist should make an effort to clarify what is desired. The dentist should make every attempt to answer all consultation requests within 12 to 24 hours.

The recorded results of consultations should be sufficiently complete to document all significant findings (positive and negative). The assessment should read as a concise dental problem list, and the treatment plan should be clearly recorded, with an indication of the priority and urgency of any necessary care. The terms used should be those physicians and nurses can understand, rather than technical dental terms. Excessive verbiage should be avoided. If the dentist finds it impossible to finish the evaluation without additional tests, arrangements should be made to obtain necessary tests in the near future, and a preliminary consultation note should be made to inform the requesting physician of the findings and preliminary recommendations. After seeing the patient, it is good practice to call the physician who requested the consultation to inform the physician of the findings and recommendations. However, it is still necessary to record a formal answer directly on the consultation form or on a progress note or in the electronic medical record, with an indication in the response of where the answer has been written. In addition, if the consultation request asks for care to be provided, the dentist should carefully document that care. In addition, as in any care provided in the hospital setting, the dentist should collect enough data about the patients to allow the office staff to bill properly for services rendered. Codes for such care and consultations are available in standard medical coding manuals. An example of a dental consultation form is presented in Figure 31-3.

Requesting a Consultation

When a patient has a problem the dentist does not feel qualified to evaluate or manage alone, a formal consultation request can be made. When requesting a medical consultation, the dentist should indicate whether the consultant is free to order necessary tests and to proceed with any necessary treatment. Preferably, the requesting dentist should personally call to ask the consultant for an opinion. Alternatively, an order can be written directing a hospital clerk to call the consultant's office.

CONSULTATION REPORT

NORTHSIDE GENERAL HOSPITAL

Patient Identification

Diaz Walter D.
YOO 109876 DOB 5/5/95
Admit 12/8/07 Scott

TO: (Consultant and/or Service)	FROM: (Physician and/or Service)	Date Requested
Dr. Brown - Dental	Dr. Scott - ER	12/8/07

Summary and Reason for Request:

9 year old boy hit in face with ball today. Please evaluate and treat dental injuries. Thank You.

James Scott M.D.

CONSULTANT: Findings and Recommendations:

Consultation Date 12/8/07

Thank you for asking me to provide a dental consultation for this unfortunate 9 year old male baseball pitcher who was struck in the nasal area by a line-drive about two hours ago. His parents state that he fell to the ground striking the back of his head and had a 4-5 second long loss of consciousness but the patient claims he remembers being hit by the ball. Epistaxis occurred initially, but spontaneously ceased in about 10 minutes. Since the accident, the patient has been alert and seemed to his parents to be fully oriented. The patient now complains of pain in the nose and upper lip as well as a mild generalized headache.

The patient has no pertinent medical, family or social history. Patient received last tetanus booster 5 yrs. ago. He last saw his dentist 2 months ago.

The patient denies any occlusal change or oral bleeding but thinks both of his maxillary central incisors are loose. He denies any visual disturbance, problems breathing through either nasal passage, or neck pain.

My H & N exam reveals a 2x2 cm abrasion in the occipital region of his scalp. There are no palpable steps or areas of ecchymosis in the facial bones but he is tender to palpation of the nasal tip and upper lip. Inspection of the nasal septum reveals no hematoma but a fresh blood clot is present on the anterior septum of the right nares.

Use one side only: For additional space, use 2nd sheet

CONSULTATION REPORT (continued next page) M.D.

FIGURE 31-2 Example of dental consultation form written for a patient who suffered sports injury to the face. The dentist was asked to examine the patient in the hospital emergency department.

CONSULTATION REPORT

NORTHSIDE GENERAL HOSPITAL

Patient Identification

Diaz Walter D.
YOO 109876 DOB 5/5/95
Admit 12/8/07 Scott

TO: (Consultant and/or Service)	FROM: (Physician and/or Service)	Date Requested

Summary and Reason for Request:

______________ M.D.

CONSULTANT: Findings and Recommendations: (continued)	Consultation Date

Intraorally the occlusion is class I and all teeth are stable except #8 & 9 which are in good alignment but can be moved slightly in an A-P direction but cannot be intruded or rotated with gentle pressure. The inside of the upper lip has a 1cm long superficial laceration of the mucosa and the upper lip is mildly edematous. The crowns of all teeth and restorations appear intact. Neck was normal to exam.

I obtained an oblique occlusal film of the maxillary anterior teeth that shows mild enlargement of the periodontal ligament space around teeth #8 & 9 but no root fractures are visible.

Impression: ① Subluxation teeth #8 & 9
② Small laceration mucosal upper lip
③ Contusion upper lip and nose
④ Abrasion scalp
⑤ ? Concussion

Recommendations: ① Avoid biting anything with front teeth
② Intraoral laceration this size doesn't require repair, but pt. should rinse c̄ NS p̄ meals and hs vigorously
③ Shave hair in area of scalp abrasion. Clean c̄ betadine scrub. Keep scalp clean
④ Tetanus booster
⑤ See family dentist within 5 days
⑥ Advise parents & pt. that injured teeth may eventually require endodontic care.

Use one side only: For additional space, use 2nd sheet

CONSULTATION REPORT John Brown D. M.D.

Note: I have gone ahead and carried out these recommendations and will let you make the discharge decision.

FIGURE 31-2, cont'd Example of dental consultation form written for a patient who suffered sports injury to the face. The dentist was asked to examine the patient in the hospital emergency department.

CONSULTATION REPORT

Patient Identification

Frost David E.
A000 65432 DOB 2/6/88
Admit 6/30/07

NORTHSIDE GENERAL HOSPITAL

TO: (Consultant and/or Service)	FROM: (Physician and/or Service)	Date Requested
Dr. Cole - Dental	Dr. Smith - Heme - Oncology	7/3/07

Summary and Reason for Request:

Right-sided oral pain for past 3 days. Patient presently receiving chemotherapy for leukemia. Please evaluate and recommend treatment.

Drew Smith M.D.

CONSULTANT: Findings and Recommendations: Consultation Date 7/3/07

Thank you for asking me to see this seriously ill 19 year old leukemic who has a three day history of pain in the area of his lower right posterior teeth. The patient denies any previous problems in this area until a dull pain began 3 nights ago. The pain has gradually worsened and now requires narcotic analgesics for relief. The pain is well localized in the molar region, worsened by chewing, and radiates to his ear. Robert has had a metallic taste in his mouth for 2 days and reports that his gums bleed during brushing. On examination I found the dentition to be well restored but the lower right 3rd molar is only partly erupted. The tissue over-lying that tooth appears inflamed but I was unable to express pus from it on palpation. The opposing tooth tends to impinge on the inflamed tissue when Robert bites. The patient has moderate trismus and I note that although his WBC is only 500, that he is afebrile.

Impression: I believe Mr. Miller has a severe pericoronitis (inflammation of soft tissue over an impacted tooth) which is exacerbated by his immunodeficient state and trauma from the opposing tooth.

Recommendations:

① Panorex radiograph to examine entire tooth and local anatomy
② Coagulation screen including platelet count and bleeding time
③ Oral hygiene with 50:50 mix of NS and H_2O_2
④ Hold antibiotics unless patient becomes febrile
⑤ If coagulation studies OK, extract tooth #1 under local anesthesia
⑥ Defer removal of involved lower 3rd molar until inflammation resolves

Use one side only: For additional space, use 2nd sheet

CONSULTATION REPORT Neal Cole D.M.D.

and pts. general condition improves. Thank you for letting me see this poor young gentlemen. Please let me know if you want me to carry out my recommendations.

FIGURE 31-3 Example of dental consultation form for hospital inpatient in hematology and oncology department, whom dentist was asked to see for problem with pericoronitis.

A consultant's recommendations should be viewed as an educated opinion. A dentist is under no obligation to follow a consultant's advice in its entirety or at all. The patient's attending doctor must make the final decision of which diagnostic tests to perform and what care the patient will receive, including when the attending doctor is a dentist.

Hospitalizing Patients for Dental Care

Deciding on Hospitalization

The vast majority of patients needing routine dental care, including oral and maxillofacial surgery, can be safely managed in the dental office. However, occasionally some patients require that dental care be provided in a hospital or surgery center.

A patient may be better treated in a hospital for several reasons. One of the most common reasons is behavioral management. Patients unable to cooperate (e.g., because of mental retardation), unwilling to cooperate (e.g., uncontrollable children), or who refuse dental care while awake can be deeply sedated or placed under general anesthesia; this allows routine dental care to be delivered to these individuals quickly and safely. An operating room setting for dental treatment may also be necessary for the physically handicapped patient who is unable to gain access to a dental office or is unable to remain relatively motionless during procedures.

An operating room is also often needed to provide dental care for patients with high-risk medical conditions, such as patients requiring care that cannot be delayed until the medical condition is alleviated or improved, or patients requiring emergency dental care shortly after a serious myocardial infarction. In some cases a patient's physician may be able to provide guidance as to the safety of office-based dental care. A final reason for planning a procedure in an operating room is for patients in whom acceptable local anesthesia cannot be attained, such as those requiring care on teeth in an area of severe infection. Usually these patients are best referred to an oral and maxillofacial surgeon, but hospitalization may be an alternative if the dentist feels capable of managing the surgical problem.

Day Surgery Facilities

In the past, operating room facilities were available only in hospitals, and patients had to be admitted the day before dental surgery and remain in the hospital until the dentist believed discharge was indicated (commonly 1 to 2 days postoperatively). However, changes have occurred in methods of delivering operating room care. Free-standing or hospital-based surgical centers now exist that offer staffed operating and recovery rooms and anesthesiologists for patients not needing preoperative or postoperative hospitalization. Many hospitals also offer the use of their operating room and staff without requiring hospital admission. A dentist may find that many patients unable to be cared for in the dental office can be effectively treated in day surgery facilities without hospitalization.

Preoperative Patient Evaluation

Once the decision to use an operating room facility has been made, several steps must be taken before the operation. The operating room staff must be contacted, and the operating time scheduled. Most facilities need some biographic information about the patient, the reason for the procedure, the procedure planned, who will perform the procedure, how long the operating room will be in use, the type of anesthesia required (i.e., sedation only or general anesthesia), and whether special equipment will be required. A hospital-based operating room must also know whether the patient will be admitted; patients to be admitted must have a room reservation made and an estimated length of stay.

All operating room facilities require that a medical history and physical examination be performed before the operation. See Chapter 1 for guidelines for recording the history and physical examination results in the medical record. This recording can be performed by the patient's physician before the day of the operation or, in some facilities, by the anesthesiologist during the preanesthetic consultation. Most facilities also require that any medically indicated laboratory tests, radiographs, or electrocardiograms be done at a time proximate to the surgery. Requirements vary from place to place, but the usual minimal testing necessary is a hematocrit.

"Doctor's orders" communicate patient care instructions to nurses and other hospital staff members. The dentist's orders should be accurate, clearly written if not using an electronic medical record, and comprehensive.

Preoperative orders are necessary for patients being admitted to a hospital or scheduled to be treated in an operating room without hospital admission. Orders are best written by the dentist but may be given to nurses over the telephone (dentists must eventually sign telephone orders). An example of admission and preoperative orders is given in Figure 31-4.

Before surgery the operating dentist should place a note in the patient's record that briefly describes the nature of the patient's medical and dental problems and the expected operating room and hospital course. The hospital staff can then use this note to familiarize themselves with the patient's general condition and reason for admission (Fig. 31-5).

Care of Hospitalized Patient

Operating Room Protocols

The patient's operating dentist bears the ultimate responsibility for any mishaps that occur in the operating room other than those relating to duties relegated to anesthesiology. Therefore the dentist must be meticulous in monitoring all that is done to the patient and should take charge if anything is being done that may harm the patient.

The operating team usually consists of the operating surgeon and an assistant. The assistant should have sufficient familiarity with the planned procedure to help the dentist by suctioning, retracting, and cutting sutures. Many hospitals allow the dentist to bring an office assistant to assist in the operating suite. Anesthesia may be provided by an anesthesiologist (a medical physician) or by an anesthetist (a nurse with special training in anesthesiology who usually must work under an anesthesiologist's supervision). A scrub nurse, who is sterilely gowned and gloved, passes instruments to the surgeon during the procedure and, among other duties, keeps track of the sponges and needles used. The circulating nurse remains ungowned and assists in setting up equipment, retrieving supplies, and completing nursing records of the operation.

The dentist should try to see the patient in the preoperative area before anesthetic premedication to help clarify any final questions the patient may have, learn whom the patient wants notified at the completion of the operation, and give emotional support to the patient.

During final preanesthetic patient preparation, the dentist should review the operative plans with the anesthesiologist.

ORDER SHEET

NORTHSIDE GENERAL HOSPITAL

Patient Identification

Frost David E.
A000 65432 DOB 2/6/88
Admit 6/30/07

USE BALLPOINT PEN. BEAR DOWN.
You are making up to four copies.

Unless an order is specifically noted, authorization is hereby given for the dispensing of drugs by non-proprietary nomenclature as set forth by The Pharmacy and Therapeutics Committee.

AUTOMATIC STOP ORDERS Narcotics and anticoagulants must be rewritten within 48 hours of original order; all other drugs within 7 days.

DATE AND TIME	ORDERS	SIGNATURE	TRANSCRIBED BY
10/1/07	Admission / Preoperative Orders		
	① Admit to 6th floor, - Dental Service		
	Dr. Brown : attending		
	office # 555-8427		
	② Cond - Good		
	③ Dx - Impacted third molars		
	Cerebral palsy		
	Penicillin allergy please label chart		
	④ NPO		
	⑤ Med: Lorazepam 2mg PO @ 6:30 c̄		
	small sip of H_2O		
	⑥ Void on call to OR		
	⑦ Ambulate c̄ asst only p̄ pre med given		
	⑧ Solumedrol 125 mg on chart to OR with		
	patient		
	Thank You		
	Dr. John Brown		

ORIGINAL — CHART COPY ORDER SHEET

FIGURE 31-4 Example of admission preoperative doctor's orders written for patient with cerebral palsy admitted to hospital on day of third molar surgery. Because patient is coming to hospital on day of surgery, admission orders and preoperative orders can be combined.

CLINICAL RECORD—IN-PATIENT

NORTHSIDE GENERAL HOSPITAL

Patient Identification

Schultz, Carl A.
X00012345 DOB 6/6/82
Admit 10/7/07 Brown

DATE / TIME	DOCTOR'S NOTES	ALL OTHER NOTES BEGIN — ALL ENTRIES MUST BE SIGNED AND POSITION NOTED
10/7/07	◄ BEGIN HERE	◄ HERE Admission note
0730	This is the third admission to this hospital for this 25 yr. old cerebral palsy victim for elective surgical removal of four impacted 3rd. molars in the operating room this morning. Performance in OR found necessary due to patients inability to stay relatively immobile for the surgery without general anesthesia. Patient has penicillin allergy but no other medical problems. Patient and parents advised in lay terms of reasons for potential problems including infection, nerve damage, bleeding, mandibular fracture, damage to other teeth, and dry socket and they consent to my plans	
	Dr. John Brown	

CLINICAL RECORD IN-PATIENT

FIGURE 31-5 Example of hospital admission note that attending surgeon uses to document (in record) reason for hospitalization and projected hospital course.

These plans include surgical site, length of procedure, oral hazards (e.g., loose teeth or restricted opening), route of intubation desired, and whether the patient will be admitted to the hospital. The dentist should remain near the patient's head during intubation to assist if necessary.

Once the patient is under general anesthesia, the dentist should ensure that steps are taken to prevent accidental injuries. Dental patients are usually operated on in a supine position, with the head end of the operating table raised about 15 degrees. The extremities must be placed in physiologic positions (i.e., positions patients would find comfortable for long periods if they were not anesthetized). Proper positioning helps prevent nerve injuries and excess loading of any part of the anatomy. In addition, padding should be placed in any area of pressure concentration, such as under heels and around elbows, particularly if the dental procedure is likely to last longer than 1 hour. Most hospitals currently place all patients on foam or gel-filled cushions or air mattresses during surgery to help prevent pressure sores. The head should be placed on a contoured cushion to help prevent excessive movement of the head during surgery.

Patient protection during anesthesia is also provided by several other means. If the procedure is expected to last more than 4 hours, a urinary (Foley) catheter should be placed to prevent overdistention of the bladder. The anesthesiologist may want this done even for shorter operations to monitor urinary output. If an electrocautery unit will be used, a grounding pad must be placed. To protect the patient's eyes, a lubricating ointment should be applied and the eyelids should be taped closed. Patients who are intubated nasally require close attention to proper tube stabilization; tubes that place excess pressure on the nasal alar cartilage can easily cause pressure sores that result in an unsightly deformity (Fig. 31-6).

The final step before surgery is preparation of the patient's operative site. If necessary, any facial hair can be shaved. Then the skin in the maxillofacial and anterior neck regions should be prepared by scrubbing with a soap-containing solution and painting with a disinfecting solution, such as iodophor. The patient is then draped with two layers of linen material or one layer of waterproof paper material to cover all portions of the body except the operative site. The oral cavity is prepared for the procedure by first gently suctioning the pharynx, placing a moist throat pack, and using large volumes of irrigation solution to help decrease the bacterial count by dilution. The use of a sterile toothbrush and chlorhexidine improves the effectiveness of oral cavity preparation. The anesthesiologist and circulating nurse should be asked to make a note that the throat has been packed so they can help remind the surgeon to remove the pack after the surgery is complete. Local anesthesia is typically administered even when patients will be under general anesthesia to help lessen the amount of general anesthetic drugs required and delay the onset of postoperative discomfort.

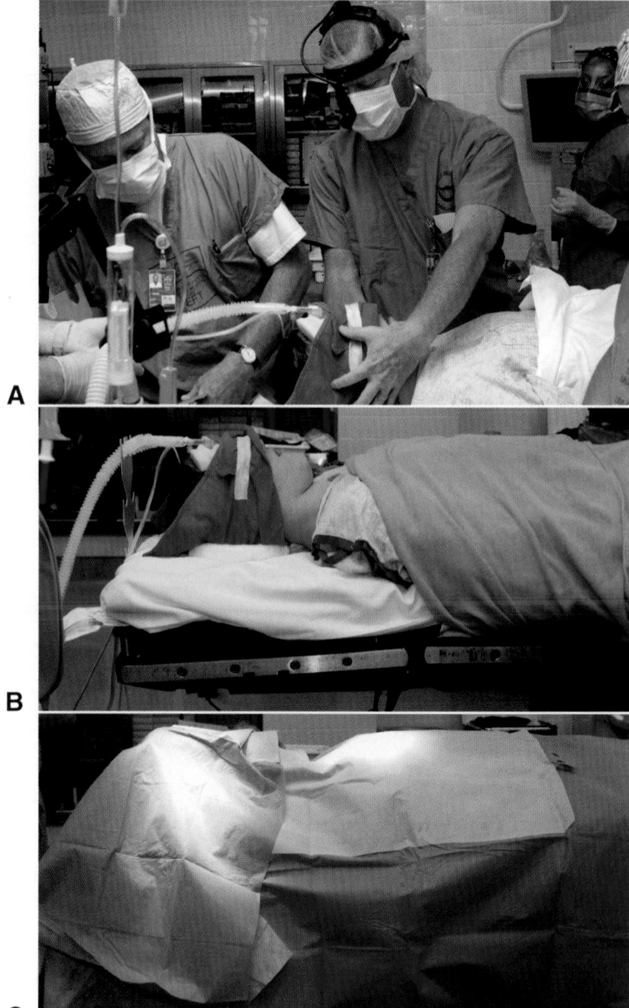

FIGURE 31-6 Preparing (prepping) patient for operating room oral and maxillofacial surgery. **A**, Surgeon helps anesthesiologists by guiding placement of tubes and tapes used to secure tubes. Surgeon also helps hold the patient's head to help stabilize while the device is placed behind the patient's head. **B**, Patient before draping, with padding of pressure points. Nasoendotracheal tube is supported to prevent alar damage, eyes are lubricated, pads are placed to protect eyes, and then eyes are covered with a towel. An antiseptic solution is applied on face to reduce number of bacteria not indigenous to patient's facial region. **C**, Same patient after draping is complete. Only the operative site is exposed.

Dental Surgeon and Assistant Preparation

The dental surgeon prepares for surgery by first checking that all instruments and patient records required to perform the surgery successfully are available. This preparation should be done before the day of surgery if the dentist does not regularly use a particular facility (in case any essential equipment or records must be brought from the surgeon's office on the day of surgery).

Before entering the operating room suite, the surgical team changes from street clothes into surgical scrub uniforms in a locker room. Shoes worn outside of the operating suite are covered with shoe covers. Scalp hair is covered with a cap. Members of the surgical team with long beards should wear head covers that extend across the chin and anterior neck. All jewelry, including watches, rings, necklaces, and earrings, should be removed before scrubbing. A mask that covers the nose and mouth should be tied in place before the surgeon enters the operating room. Before the surgical scrub, the surgeon should check the patient's records, place radiographs on the view box, adjust overhead lights, check the patient's position, apply defogging solution to eyeglasses, and adjust the headlight.

The surgical hand and arm scrub is then performed to lessen the chance of contaminating a patient's wound. Although sterile gloves are worn, gloves are frequently torn during oral and maxillofacial surgical procedures, thereby exposing the patient to the surgeon's skin. By proper scrubbing with antiseptic solutions, the hand and arm bacterial counts are reduced.

Several acceptable methods may be used to perform a surgical hand and arm scrub. Most hospitals have a surgical scrub protocol that should be followed when doing surgery. Standard in most techniques is the use of an antiseptic soap solution, a moderately stiff brush, and a fingernail cleaner. The hands and forearms are wetted in a scrub sink, keeping the hands above the level of the elbows until the hands and arms are dried. A copious amount of antiseptic soap from a wall dispenser or from an antiseptic-impregnated scrub brush is applied to the hands and arms up to the elbows. The antiseptic soap is allowed to remain on the arms, while all visible debris is removed from underneath each fingernail tip with the sharp-tipped fingernail cleaner. Then more antiseptic soap is applied and scrubbing is begun using repeated firm strokes of the scrub brush on every surface of the hands and arms, stopping about 5 cm below the elbow (Fig. 31-7). Scrub techniques based on the number of

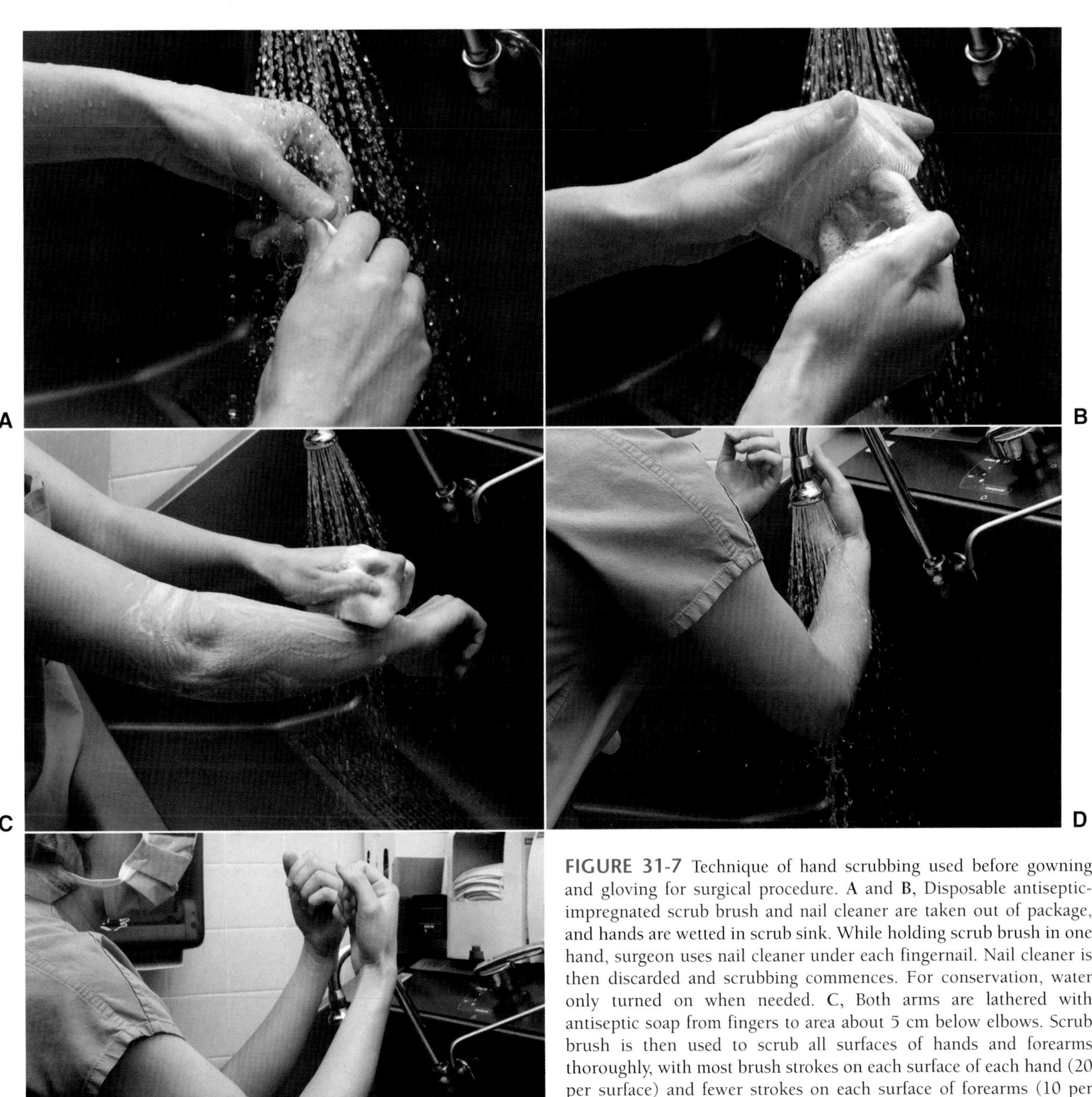

FIGURE 31-7 Technique of hand scrubbing used before gowning and gloving for surgical procedure. **A** and **B**, Disposable antiseptic-impregnated scrub brush and nail cleaner are taken out of package, and hands are wetted in scrub sink. While holding scrub brush in one hand, surgeon uses nail cleaner under each fingernail. Nail cleaner is then discarded and scrubbing commences. For conservation, water only turned on when needed. **C**, Both arms are lathered with antiseptic soap from fingers to area about 5 cm below elbows. Scrub brush is then used to scrub all surfaces of hands and forearms thoroughly, with most brush strokes on each surface of each hand (20 per surface) and fewer strokes on each surface of forearms (10 per surface). **D**, After scrubbing is completed, brush is discarded and arms are rinsed completely. During rinsing, arm is put through the water, starting at fingertips, then pushing through to elbow. **E**, Arms are then allowed to drain for several seconds over scrub sink. During scrubbing and rinsing, hands and forearms are kept raised above level of elbows until scrub gown is in place.

strokes to each surface rather than a set time for scrubbing are more reliable. An individual's scrub technique should follow a set routine designed to ensure that all forearm and hand surfaces are properly prepared. However, scrubbing too long and too firmly can be as detrimental as inadequate scrubbing because skin that is excessively traumatized by scrubbing develops a much higher resident bacterial flora. Once scrubbing is completed, the hands and forearms should be rinsed free of soap solution under running water, moving the arm through the stream from fingertips to elbow. The hands must be kept higher than the elbows during the entire scrub and rinse to allow all excess fluid to drip off the arm at the elbow.

Once scrubbing is completed, the surgeon should enter the operating room, taking care to avoid contaminating scrubbed hands and arms. Drying commences with a sterile towel handed to the surgeon by the scrub nurse. The towel is held in one hand to dry the other hand, advancing up the forearm and stopping short of the elbow. The towel is then transferred to the dry hand, and the process is repeated on the wet hand with an unused portion of the towel. Next, the scrub nurse fully opens the sterile surgical gown, and the surgeon introduces the hands into the openings for the arms of the gown.

While the scrub nurse helps push the gown up the surgeon's arm, the circulating nurse pulls the gown on from the rear of the surgeon and ties it securely (Fig. 31-8). The scrub nurse then holds the surgical gloves open while the surgeon places one hand into each glove. The gloves should completely cover the hands and wrists and completely overlap the cuff of the surgical gown (Fig. 31-9). The surgeon must not allow the hands to fall beneath waist level from this point until ungowning (Fig. 31-10).

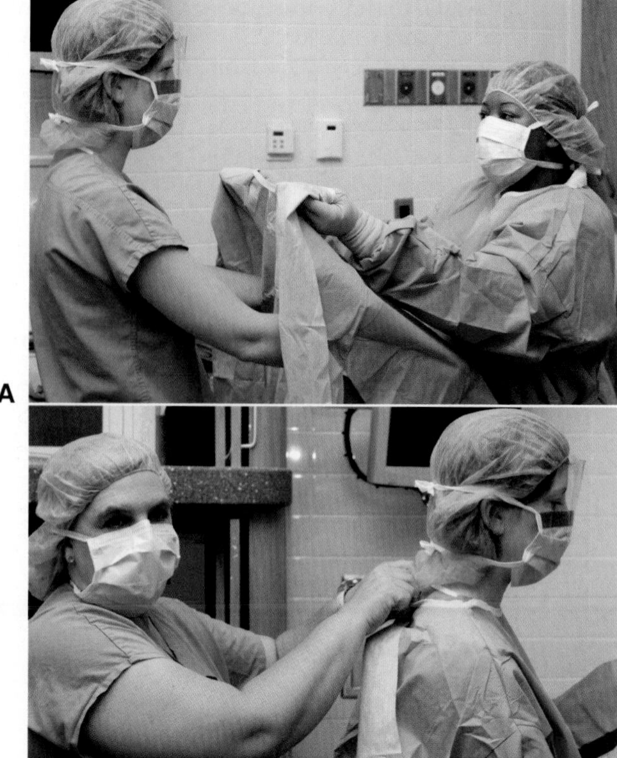

FIGURE 31-8 Gowning for operating room surgery. **A**, Scrub nurse holds sterile gown open for surgeon to place arms into sleeves. The scrub nurse has hands on front side of gown to prevent possibility of accidentally touching ungowned surgeon. Surgeon pushes arms into sleeves of gown, taking care not to thrust through cuff of gown, potentially contaminating scrub nurse. While surgeon is placing arms into sleeves, scrub nurse is pushing gown onto surgeon. **B**, Unsterile circulating nurse then ties back of surgeon's gown, taking care to touch only inside surfaces of gown.

Postoperative Responsibilities

Once the operative procedure is completed, the oral cavity is again irrigated and cleared by suction of the accumulated fluids. Before throat pack removal, the scrub nurse should be asked whether all sponges and needles used during the surgery are accounted for; if they are not, a search must be made to find them. If necessary, intraoral gauze packs should be placed for hemostasis, and the packs should have long ends that trail out of the mouth for easy retrieval.

Nurses (under the supervision of anesthesiologists) make many of the immediate postoperative decisions in the post-anesthesia care unit. However, the dentist should write postoperative orders immediately after the completion of surgery to ensure that any special instructions can be initiated in the postanesthesia care unit.

Postoperative orders should include statements of the diagnosis, procedure performed, patient allergies, and general condition of the patient after surgery. Nursing actions, such as vital sign monitoring, wound care, and medication administration schedule, should be clearly spelled out. The patient's diet, activity level, bed positioning, and allowable personal hygiene should be delineated. Finally, parameters should be outlined that, if breached, make immediate notification of the dentist or physician mandatory. An outline for postoperative orders is listed in Box 31-2; a sample of postoperative orders is shown in Figure 31-11.

BOX 31-2

Principal Components of Postoperative Orders

- Diagnosis (or diagnoses) and surgical procedure
- Condition
- Allergies
- Instructions for monitoring vital signs
- Activity and positioning
- Diet
- Medications
- Intravenous fluids
- Wound care
- Parameters for notification of physician or dentist
- Special instructions (e.g., ice packs, lip protection, and hygiene)

Shortly after the surgical procedure is completed, a brief operative note should be placed in the patient's record. This note is usually in a relatively standard format that includes listing the preoperative and postoperative diagnoses, the names of the procedures performed during surgery, the name or names of the surgeon or surgeons, the type of anesthesia, the placement of any drains, the estimated blood loss, and whether any specimens were sent for pathologic examination.

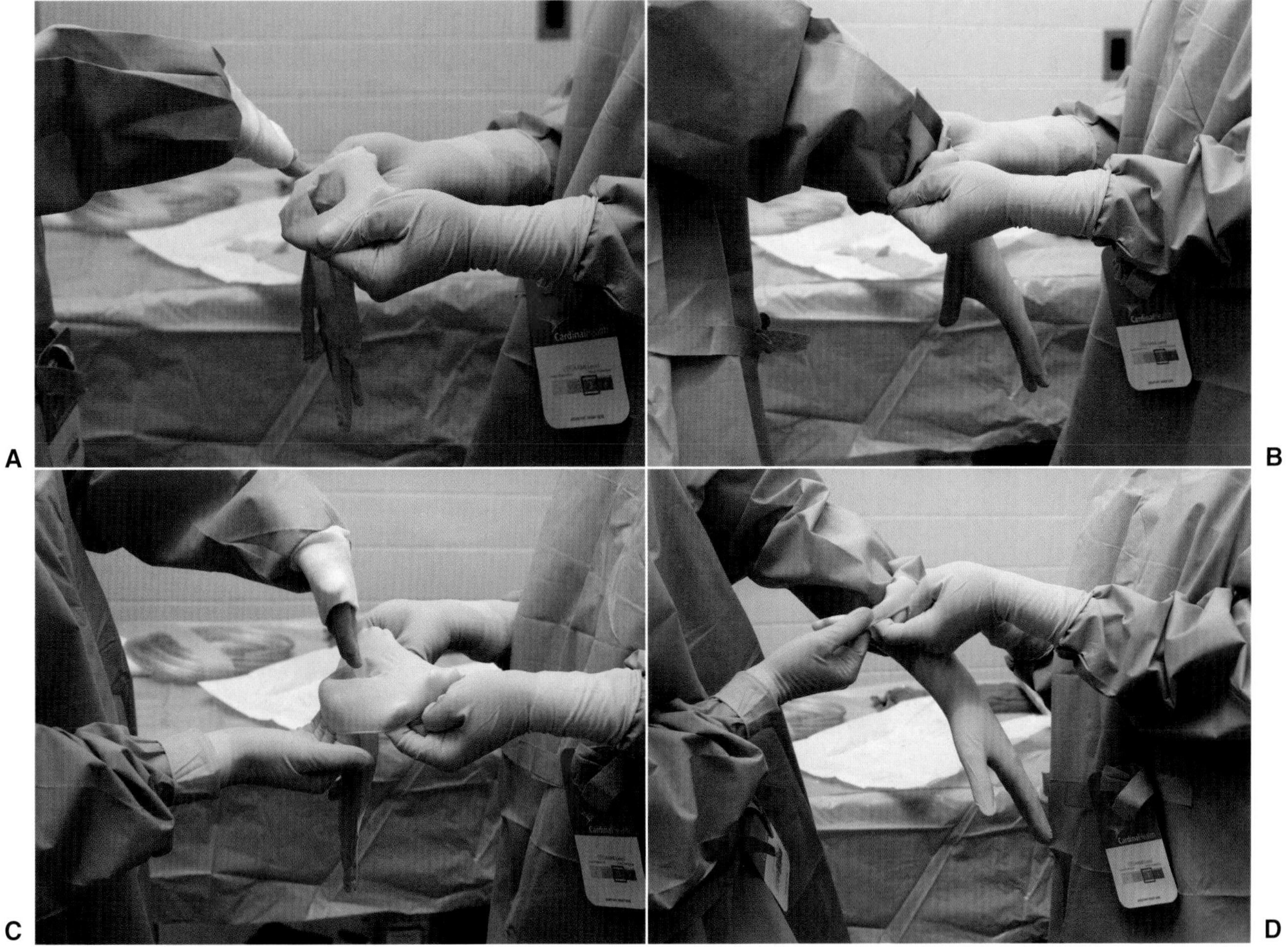

FIGURE 31-9 Gloving for operating room surgery. **A**, Scrub nurse holds open first glove to allow surgeon to insert hand into glove while surgeon's wrist is in flexion. Surgeon pushes hand into glove with fingers adducted, while nurse pulls glove onto surgeon's hand. **B**, Once surgeon's hand is into palm region of glove, fingers are partially abducted and slipped into appropriate finger holes. Nurse continues to pull glove on until cuff of glove is above cuff of surgeon's gown. Nurse then releases glove. No further adjustments of first glove are made at this time. **C**, Scrub nurse then holds second glove open in same manner that first glove was presented to surgeon. Surgeon can now help hold cuff of glove open while inserting other hand. **D**, Hand being gloved is pushed into glove while other hand assists nurse in pulling glove into place. Once both gloves are in place, they can be used to adjust each other, pulling all slack out of area of fingertips.

The hospital staff uses this note to learn quickly the general information about the operative procedure.

In addition, before leaving the operating suite, a full report of the operation should be dictated using the designated format of the facility at which the surgery was performed. The general outlines and examples of a brief operative note and transcribed operative report are shown in Boxes 31-3 and 31-4 and in Figure 31-12.

Patients generally remain in the postanesthesia care unit until they are sufficiently alert and unlikely to injure themselves and their vital signs are stable within acceptable limits. An anesthesiologist usually makes the decision about discharge to a hospital room or home, unless it is specified that the dentist will make that decision. The discharged patient should be placed directly under the care of a competent adult and not be allowed to go home unescorted.

BOX 31-3

Common Format for Recording Brief Operative Note

- Preoperative diagnosis
- Postoperative diagnosis
- Procedure
- Surgeon or surgeons
- Type of anesthesia
- Unusual, unexpected, or significant findings at surgery
- Fluid status, including estimated fluid loss and amount of fluid administered to patient
- Description of anything left in operative site, such as drains or packing
- Specimens (Was specimen sent to pathology or microbiology laboratory?)

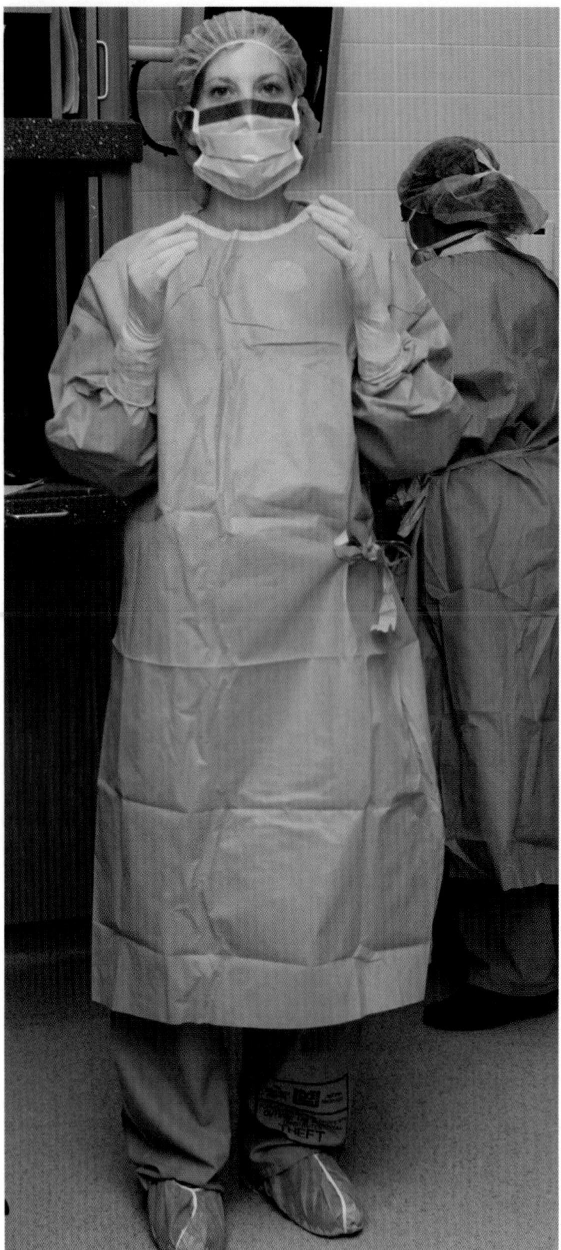

FIGURE 31-10 Surgeon ready for operating room surgery. Hands should not be allowed to fall below waist level from this point until the surgery is completed and all surgical wounds are closed and dressed.

Hospital rounds (i.e., patient visits) give the surgeon the opportunity to check the patient's postoperative recovery personally and to revise orders as necessary. Unstable hospitalized patients require frequent visits; stable patients are usually seen twice a day during the first week after surgery and once daily thereafter. Each patient visit by the surgeon warrants a brief notation (i.e., progress note) in the record that documents the patient's progress and any new plans for further care. Notes are usually written using a record format that includes a brief description of how the patient is progressing *subjectively* and *objectively,* an *assessment* of the patient's condition, and a *plan* for further care (SOAP). Figure 31-13 shows a typical postoperative progress notation in the SOAP format.

BOX 31-4

Common Format for Dictating Operative Note

- Identify dictator.
- State that operative note is being dictated.
- State patient's name, spelling out last name.
- State patient's medical record (hospital) number.
- State date of operation.
- State preoperative diagnosis.
- State postoperative diagnosis.
- Give name of procedure performed.
- Give name of surgeon and any surgical assistants.
- Completely describe surgical procedure, including how the patient was prepared for surgery in the operating room.
- Reidentify dictator.
- State to whom copies of the dictation should be sent.

Discharge planning should begin as soon as the surgical procedure is completed and includes making arrangements for any necessary patient education, such as oral hygiene, wound care, and dietary instructions. In addition, the patient should be told of acceptable activity levels and plans for follow-up office visits. Necessary prescriptions for medications should be provided, as well as instructions on how to contact the appropriate physician or dentist should problems arise. A written discharge note should be included in the progress note section of the medical record (Fig. 31-14 and Box 31-5).

A dictated discharge summary is necessary for hospitalized patients, whereas surgical centers generally accept a written discharge summary on a special form. The dictated summary should include a brief narrative, including the reason for hospital admission and the pertinent history that led to admission. The significant positive and negative findings of the history and physical examination should be described, including any laboratory results. The hospital course, including the name of the operative procedure, should be in the summary. Finally, discharge instructions, prescriptions, and follow-up appointments should be detailed in the report. Arrangements should be made to send copies of the discharge summary to other doctors who may find the information useful, including the patient's family physician (Fig. 31-15 and Box 31-6).

BOX 31-5

General Information to Include in Written Discharge Note

- Complete a standard SOAP progress note and include the following under *P* (plans) section:
  - Deposition (to where and with whom patient will be discharged)
  - List of medications that the patient is prescribed or instructed to take, dosing regimen, and instructions for use
  - Dietary instructions
  - Activity instructions
  - Hygiene instructions
  - Follow-up appointment

ORDER SHEET

NORTHSIDE GENERAL HOSPITAL

Patient Identification

Schultz, Carl A.
X00012345 DOB 6/6/82
Admit 10/7/07 Brown

USE BALLPOINT PEN. BEAR DOWN.
You are making up to four copies.

Unless an order is specifically noted, authorization is hereby given for the dispensing of drugs by non-proprietary nomenclature as set forth by The Pharmacy and Therapeutics Committee.

AUTOMATIC STOP ORDERS Narcotics and anticoagulants must be rewritten within 48 hours of original order; all other drugs within 7 days.

DATE AND TIME	ORDERS	SIGNATURE	TRANSCRIBED BY
10/7/07	Post op orders		
9:20	(1) S/P Surgical extraction 4 third molars		
	(2) Condition: Good		
	(3) Allergy: Penicillin, please label chart		
	(4) Vital signs: q 15 min until stable		
	then q 1° x 2, then q 4°		
	Oral Temps q 4° w/a		
	(5) HOB at least 30°, OOB c̄ assistance only		
	(6) Ice packs to face if patient desires, please inquire		
	(7) Diet: clear cool liquids, advance to full		
	cool liquids as tolerated		
	(8) I & O q shift		
	(9) Meds:		
	(a) M.S. 4 mg. & Phenergan 50 mg IM q 4° prn mod-		
	severe pain or		
	(b) Tylox ī po q 4° prn mod-severe pain		
	(c) Acetaminophen 500 mg po q 3° prn mild pain		
	(d) Decadron 0.75 mg PO BID		
	(e) Compazine 5 mg IM prn N or V. May repeat in		
	30 min. x1. Call surgeon if nausea persists		
	thereafter.		
	(f) Mediinhaler ii puffs q 4° prn wheezing		
	(10) IV: D5 1/4 NS @ 100 cc/hr		
	Change to Hep lock when PO > 400 cc/8 hr		
	(11) Bite on moistened 4x4 gauze placed over op		
	sites continuously for 45 min prn bleeding		
	(12) Keep lips thinly coated with Vaseline		
	(13) Call surgeon – office 674-1212, home - 525-6666		
	if BP > 180/10 < 90/60, P > 120 < 55, T > 101°,		
	uncontrollable bleeding, wheezing or if pt. fails		
	to void by 1700.		
	Thank You Dr. John Brown		

ORIGINAL — CHART COPY ORDER SHEET

FIGURE 31-11 Example of postoperative orders written after removal of third molars in operating room.

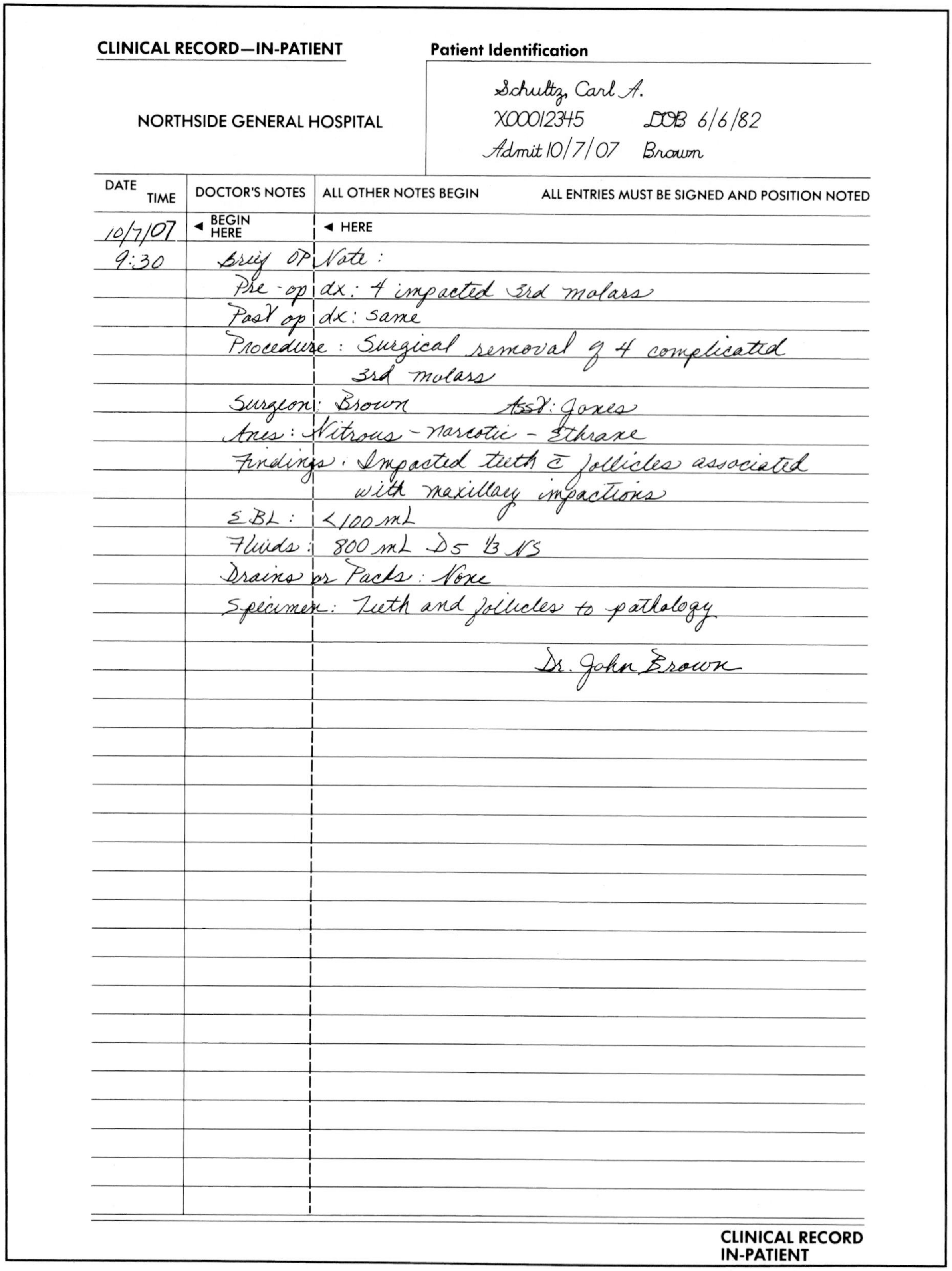

CLINICAL RECORD—IN-PATIENT

NORTHSIDE GENERAL HOSPITAL

Patient Identification

Schultz, Carl A.
X00012345 DOB 6/6/82
Admit 10/7/07 Brown

DATE TIME	DOCTOR'S NOTES	ALL OTHER NOTES BEGIN	ALL ENTRIES MUST BE SIGNED AND POSITION NOTED
10/7/07	◄ BEGIN HERE	◄ HERE	
9:30	Brief OP Note:		
	Pre-op dx: 4 impacted 3rd molars		
	Post op dx: same		
	Procedure: Surgical removal of 4 complicated 3rd molars		
	Surgeon: Brown Asst: Jones		
	Anes: Nitrous - narcotic - Ethrane		
	Findings: Impacted teeth c̄ follicles associated with maxillary impactions		
	EBL: <100 mL		
	Fluids: 800 mL D5 1/3 NS		
	Drains or Packs: None		
	Specimen: Teeth and follicles to pathology		
	Dr. John Brown		

CLINICAL RECORD IN-PATIENT

FIGURE 31-12 A, Example of brief operative note for quick documentation in hospital record of what was performed, whether in operating room or elsewhere in hospital.

NORTHSIDE GENERAL HOSPITAL

OPERATIVE REPORT

NAME: SCHULTZ, Carl
UNIT NUMBER: X00012345
OPERATIVE DATE: 10-07-07
DOB: 06-06-82

PREOPERATIVE DIAGNOSIS: Full bony impacted teeth Nos. 1, 16
Partial bony impacted teeth Nos. 17, 32
POSTOPERATIVE DIAGNOSIS: Same
SURGEON: John Brown, D.M.D.
ASSISTANT SURGEON: William Jones, D.D.S.
OPERATIONS: Surgical extraction of impacted third molars Nos. 1, 16, 17, and 32

PROCEDURE: The patient was brought to the operating room without premedication and placed onto the operating table in the supine position. After attaching monitoring equipment and checking the vital signs the patient was placed under general anesthesia induced by a combination of inhalational and intravenous agents. A right nasal endotracheal intubation was performed and the tube secured into position after good breath sounds were heard bilaterally on auscultation. The operating table was placed into a 15-degree head-up position, and then the patient was prepped and draped in the usual fashion for intraoral oral surgery.

The oral cavity was inspected and suctioned free of gross secretions, and a moist throat pack was placed. 0.5% Marcaine with 1:200,000 epinephrine was infiltrated in the maxillary posterior buccal vestibules, the greater palatine nerve regions, and the inferior alveolar, lingual, and buccal nerves were blocked bilaterally with a total of 45 mg of Marcaine and 0.045 mg of epinephrine. The oral cavity was then irrigated with copious amounts of normal saline irrigation and suctioned free of gross liquid. A medium sized rubber bite block was carefully placed between the arches on the left side. Attention was first directed to the right retromolar region of the mandible, where a No. 15 blade was used to make an incision beginning in the lower fourth of the external oblique ridge of the mandible, bringing the incision forward to the distal line angle of tooth No. 31. The incision was then continued in the buccal gingival sulcus to the distal aspect of tooth No. 30. A No. 9 dental periosteal elevator was then used to create a full-thickness mucoperiosteal envelope type of flap, exposing the buccal aspect of the retromandibular region of the mandible. A right angle retractor was placed into the depth of the envelope flap to protect it, and the assistant used a tongue retractor to protect the tongue. The mesio-angularly impacted tooth No. 32 was identified, and a straight tissue burr in an air-driven handpiece under continuous saline irrigation was used to remove sufficient bone on the buccal and distal aspects of tooth No. 32 to expose the height of contour. The burr was then used to section the tooth along its long axis through the furcation. A large, straight

FIGURE 31-12, cont'd B, Example of dictated operative note to describe in detail exact procedure performed in operating room.

dental elevator was used to complete the tooth sectioning. The Crane pick was then used to remove the distal aspect of the tooth, and a small straight dental elevator was used to remove the mesial aspect. The roots of both tooth segments appeared intact. A dental curette was used to gently remove the small remnant of dental follicle remaining in the socket. A bone rasp was used to smooth the bone in regions where elevators had been used, and the sockets and areas under the flaps were irrigated with copious amounts of saline irrigation. Little bleeding was present at that time, so half a capsule of tetracycline was poured into the socket, and the flap was reapproximated with two 4-0 black silk sutures.

Attention was next directed to the right maxillary tuberosity region, where a new No. 15 blade was used to create a crestal incision beginning on the disto-superior aspect of the tuberosity, continuing the incision anteriorly to the posterior aspect of tooth No. 2. The incision was then continued in the buccal gingival sulcus anteriorly to the distal line angle of tooth No. 3. A No. 9 dental periosteal elevator was then used to create a full-thickness mucoperiosteal flap on the buccal aspect of the tuberosity. The Minnesota retractor was used to remove a small amount of thin bone overlying the full bony impacted tooth No. 1. A Potts elevator was used to elevate tooth No. 1 out of the socket along with the attached dental follicle. The root of the tooth appeared to be intact. The socket was inspected and then irrigated with normal saline. The flap was then reapproximated with two 4-0 black silk sutures. A large gauze was then placed over the fresh extraction sites, and attention was directed to the left side of the mouth, where teeth Nos. 16 and 17 were extracted in an identical fashion to teeth Nos. 1 and 32.

The oral cavity was then suctioned free of all gross fluids, and the throatpack was removed. The hypopharynx was then suctioned with a tonsil suction. The patient was extubated in the operating room and taken to the postanesthesia care unit in good condition for recovery.

ESTIMATED BLOOD LOSS:	50 mL
FLUIDS RECEIVED:	1,200 mL Dextrose 5%/Lactated Ringers
DRAINS:	None
DRESSINGS:	Bilateral oral packs that trailed out of the mouth
COMPLICATIONS:	None

John Brown D.M.D.

John Brown, D.M.D.
Attending Surgeon

c: Dr. William Jones

FIGURE 31-12, cont'd B, Example of dictated operative note to describe in detail exact procedure performed in operating room.

Management of Postoperative Problems

Airway Problems

Routine dentoalveolar surgery is unlikely to cause airway compromise unless a condition such as Ludwig's angina is present. However, patients in whom an endotracheal tube has been placed during general anesthesia are at risk for postextubation (i.e., after removal of the endotracheal tube) airway narrowing or obstruction, which is caused by trauma to the mucosal lining of the upper respiratory tract that produces edema. The narrowest portion of the upper respiratory tract is the region of the vocal cords through which the endotracheal tube must be passed and on which the tube rests during anesthesia. The amount of respiratory tract mucosal injury depends on the patient's anatomy, the size of tube used, the type of tube, and care used during placement. Injuries caused by tube type have been lessened by the use of tubes with high-volume, low-pressure cuff designs. Patients generally do well after extubation, except for mild to moderate throat discomfort during

CLINICAL RECORD—IN-PATIENT

NORTHSIDE GENERAL HOSPITAL

Patient Identification

Schultz, Carl A.
X00012345 DOB 6/6/82
Admit 10/7/07 Brown

DATE TIME	DOCTOR'S NOTES	ALL OTHER NOTES BEGIN — ALL ENTRIES MUST BE SIGNED AND POSITION NOTED
10/7/07	◄ BEGIN HERE	◄ HERE
20:00		Post-op check
	S-	Pt. feels drowsy. Moderate pain well
		controlled with oral narcotic
		Denies nausea
	O-	Vital signs WNL & stable
		Mild facial edema
		Operative sites show slight ooze
		Chest clear to auscultation
		IV site benign
		Intake last 8 hrs. - 1450 mL (250 mL PO)
		Ambulated to BR with assistance
		Voided 600 mL
	A-	Doing well, needs to increase PO intake
	P-	Encourage PO intake
		Slow IV rate to 75 mL/hr.
		Bite on moistened gauze if bleeding
		increases during the night
		John Brown DMD

CLINICAL RECORD IN-PATIENT

FIGURE 31-13 Example of hospital progress note made to document patient's course in hospital and to inform others of future plans for patient. Note SOAP format used: *S* is any comments made by patient (subjective), *O* is objective findings by dentist, *A* is assessment by dentist of how patient is doing, and *P* is plans for future care.

CLINICAL RECORD—IN-PATIENT

NORTHSIDE GENERAL HOSPITAL

Patient Identification

Schultz, Carl A.
X00012345 DOB 6/6/82
Admit 10/7/07 Brown

DATE TIME	DOCTOR'S NOTES ◄ BEGIN HERE	ALL OTHER NOTES BEGIN ◄ HERE — ALL ENTRIES MUST BE SIGNED AND POSITION NOTED
10/8/07 7[45]	P.O.D. – Discharge Note	
	S- Pt. complains of moderate pain – well controlled with oral narcotic. Denies nausea and able to swallow liquids without difficulty	
	O- Vital signs WNL and stable Mild facial edema and moderate trismus Operative sites without ooze Chest clear to auscultation Able to ambulate without assistance P.O. intake for past 8 hours – 400cc	
	A- Doing well, Ready for D/C	
	P- D/C to home escorted by father Rx Decadron 0.75 mg PO bid x 2 days Tylox ∓ PO q 4° prn pain x 25 Liquids advanced to soft diet as tolerated Limit activities for 2 days then increase as tolerated Saline rinses p̄ meals and h.s. RTC 10/14/07 at 11 am and prn	
	John Brown DMD	

CLINICAL RECORD IN-PATIENT

FIGURE 31-14 Example of written discharge note in SOAP format to document patient's progress. Discharge instructions are documented under P.

```
NORTHSIDE GENERAL HOSPITAL          Schultz, Carl
                                    X00012345   DOB: 6/6/82

Discharge Summary

Admitted: 10/7/07        Discharged: 10/8/07

     This was the third admission at Northside General for this
25 year old male with cerebral palsy.  Elective admission was
necessary for surgical removal of four impacted third molars
which had recently become symptomatic necessitating extraction
under general anesthesia.
   PMH: Hospitalizations: 1986-restorative dentistry under GA
                          1990-appendectomy without problems
                          1994-restorative dentistry under GA
        Illnesses: Cerebral palsy due to birth anoxia
                   Asthma, never needed hospitalization
        Medications: Medi-inhaler as needed.
        Allergies: Penicillin
        Social: Lives at home with parents
   Past medical, family and social history otherwise
unremarkable.

   ROS: Pertinent findings-Intermittent pain and swelling around
partially erupted lower third molars.  Denies other oral
discomfort.  Patient claims inability to maintain upright posture
without the use of body brace.  Weakness in leg asnd back muscles
bilaterally.  ROS otherwise unremarkable.
   PE: Pertinent findings-
      HEENT- nasal airways patent, Class I occlusion with well-
restored dentition, no mucosal lesions. No adenopathy. All teeth
except #1 and 16 visible. Teeth #17 and 32 partially erupted with
operculums present.
      Chest- Clear to percussion and auscultation without
wheezes or rales.  Heart had regular rate and rhythm without
murmurs or extra sounds present.

Hospital course:  On morning of admission patient was placed
under general anesthesia in the operating room and had surgical
removal of 4 third molars.  Surgery and anesthesia tolerated well
and patient was discharged to home on the first postoperative
day in good condition.

Discharge instructions:
     Rx-Decadron 0.75mg PO bid for 2 days
     Rx-Tylox 1 PO q4hr prn pain X 25
     Cool liquid advanced to soft diet as tolerated
     Warm saline rinses after meals and hs
     Restrict normal activities for 2 days
     Return to office on 10/14/07 at 11am.

                                            John Brown D.M.D.
                                            John Brown, D.M.D.
                                            Attending Surgeon
```

FIGURE 31-15 Example of dictated hospital discharge summary.

swallowing for 1 to 2 days. However, occasionally, laryngeal edema of sufficient severity to compromise the patient's ability to breathe is produced. The first symptom is usually a crowing sound during attempts to inspire and expire. The patient may also need to use accessory muscles of respiration to force air through the cords.

Prevention of airway trauma is the best form of care. If trauma is known to have occurred during intubation or extubation (or in patients having prolonged intubation), postoperative orders should include the delivery of cooled, humidified air or oxygen, administration of racemic epinephrine through an aerosol, and placement of tracheotomy equipment near the patient's bed. These patients should be closely monitored, preferably under close supervision by an anesthesiologist, until the dentist is comfortable that airway problems are under control.

Nausea and Vomiting

Nausea and vomiting occur commonly after general anesthesia, which is part of the rationale for fasting patients pre-

BOX 31-6

Common Format for Dictating the Hospital Discharge Summary

- Identify dictator.
- State that discharge summary is being dictated.
- State patient's name, spelling out last name.
- Give patient's medical record (hospital) number.
- State date(s) of hospital admission and discharge.
- State final diagnosis(ses).
- Give patient's chief complaint on admission.
- Describe history of illness or problem requiring surgery.
- List any significant findings on history and on physical, radiographic, and laboratory examinations.
- Briefly describe hospital course, including the following:
  - Description of all therapy rendered
  - Any complications that occurred
  - Outcome of any therapy provided
- Describe discharge instructions given to the patient, including the following:
  - Disposition (to where and with whom the patient is being discharged)
  - Medications
  - Activity
  - Diet
  - Hygiene
  - Follow-up plans
- Describe patient's condition on discharge.
- Reidentify dictator.
- State to whom copies of the summary should be sent.

operatively. The symptoms are primarily related to anesthetic drugs and occasionally to excessive air that might have been forced into the stomach during induction of anesthesia. Nausea and vomiting usually resolve with time but can be a serious problem if the patient is not fully in control of laryngeal reflexes, is in intermaxillary fixation, or is unable to begin taking needed medications and sustenance orally. Swallowed blood can also stimulate nausea and vomiting.

Vomiting in a patient with depressed reflexes is best handled by placing the patient in a horizontal position on the right side until reflexes are recovered. Patients in intermaxillary fixation but with normal airway reflexes should be able to eliminate any vomitus through the nose and mouth because postoperative stomach contents should be of liquid consistency. Even so, constant retching can disrupt a properly set facial fracture or a delicate wound repair, so awake patients in or out of fixation may need to receive antiemetic medications to relieve nausea. However, before giving antiemetic agents, the possibility of depressed gastrointestinal motility or brain injury should be ruled out. If a patient develops airway problems while in intermaxillary fixation, an instrument capable of releasing fixation should be readily available. Many dentists have a pair of wire cutters taped to the head of a patient's bed.

Fever

Fever is generally defined as an oral temperature of greater than 99° F (37.2° C) or rectal temperature higher than 99.8° F (38° C). A postoperative fever may be produced by a variety of factors. However, based partially on when in the postoperative period fever occurs, it may be attributed to one of a few common causes. For example, fever the night after surgery is usually attributed to bacteremias resulting from organisms in surgical wounds. Fevers occurring in the first or second postoperative day after general anesthesia or major surgery are generally attributed to insufficient depth of breathing, which produces atelectasis (collapse of terminal lung alveoli), or, less commonly, to dehydration. Fever 2 days after surgery can be an early sign of a wound infection or, if the patient had the bladder catheterized or has prolonged atelectasis, it may be caused by a bladder infection or pneumonia.

No matter when a fever arises, an investigation should be undertaken to discover the cause. The patient should be questioned about wound pain, swelling, foul taste, productive cough, and dysuria. On examination, particular reference should be made to the surgical wound, sites of intravenous (IV) catheters, and lungs. Studies such as a white blood cell count, urinalysis, and chest radiographs may be useful in determining an explanation for a postoperative fever, if clinically indicated. A medical consultation may be necessary if a cause for a persistent fever remains obscure. Once it is documented that a fever exists, the patient's symptoms and increased metabolic expenditure from the fever can be lessened by administration of acetaminophen.

Atelectasis

Atelectasis is a common problem in patients who have undergone abdominal surgery and fail to fill their lungs to normal capacity because of the incisional pain provoked by deep breathing. In patients who have had dentoalveolar surgery under general anesthesia, atelectasis can result from (1) inactivity that allows the patient to breathe without filling the lungs to normal capacity; (2) postoperative narcotic analgesics that depress the sigh reflex, which normally functions to prevent atelectasis; or (3) an endotracheal tube misplacement so that only one lung was aerated during surgery.

Prolonged atelectasis can lead to pneumonia; thus prevention of atelectasis is important. Instructing patients to take deep sustained inspirations periodically during the postoperative period and to begin ambulation as soon as possible after surgery lessens the possibility of developing atelectasis. Limiting the use of unnecessarily large doses of narcotic analgesics can also prevent atelectasis.

Fluids and Electrolytes

Hypovolemia can be found in patients after surgery because of insufficient fluid intake to match fluid loss. Fluids are lost through the obvious routes of urination, vomiting, and nasogastric suctioning, as well as by insensible routes, such as expired air and perspiration. The primary source of replacement fluids is normally oral ingestion. However, postoperative patients who are unable or unwilling to maintain necessary fluid intake orally require IV supplementation until oral fluid intake resumes. The usual volume of fluid intake necessary (combination of oral and IV) for a nonfebrile adult in the postoperative period is between 2500 and 3000 mL daily, with a higher volume for patients with higher-than-normal fluid loss and a lower volume for patients susceptible to fluid overloading, such as those with renal or myocardial insufficiency.

The choice of IV fluid type is based on the knowledge that human serum must have certain electrolytes kept within a narrow range to maintain vital physiologic functions. Sodium, potassium, and chloride are the three electrolytes considered when choosing an IV solution. Three standard IV crystalloid solutions are available for use individually or in combination. Dextrose 5% in water is a 5% glucose solution that provides free water, a source of calories in a fluid that is isotonic with plasma, and no electrolytes. Normal saline, or 0.9% sodium chloride solution, provides 154 mEq each of sodium and chloride per liter of water, which makes the solution roughly isotonic but actually functions to draw interstitial fluid into the intravascular compartment.* Lactated Ringer's solution contains generally physiologic electrolyte concentrations (Na^+, 130 mEq; Cl^-, 109 mEq; K^+, 3 mEq) and lactate, which buffers serum acidity by providing a substrate that can be metabolized into bicarbonate.

In general, the otherwise healthy patient requires a relatively physiologic IV solution with some calories during and after surgery, which can be provided by combination crystalloid solutions, such as 5% dextrose in a 0.45% sodium chloride solution to which 20 mEq of potassium chloride per liter has been added. Patients with special medical problems likely to cause electrolyte abnormalities, such as those receiving potassium-wasting diuretics or prolonged IV fluid infusions, will need their serum electrolytes monitored to guide IV fluid choice.

Blood Component Transfusion

Blood transfusions are rarely required after dentoalveolar surgery, which is fortunate because of the potential for spread of infectious diseases in the course of transfusions and the risk of incompatibility reactions. The primary reason why transfusions are unnecessary is the nature of oral surgery, which if properly performed, is unlikely to allow significant blood loss. In addition, placement of patients in reverse Trendelenburg's position* and the use of hypotensive anesthetic techniques have further lessened blood loss.

Occasionally, circumstances arise in which blood components are necessary, such as for trauma patients who have lost blood from serious injuries or patients with thrombocytopenia. In the past, patients requiring transfusions were given whole blood; however, modern blood banks currently separate donated blood into its various components (i.e., plasma, red blood cells, platelets, and white blood cells). Patients with a low hematocrit and therefore lowered oxygen-carrying capacity of the blood can be given only the portion of blood that they require—packed red blood cells. Similarly, patients who are thrombocytopenic from chemotherapy but require emergency oral surgery can be given platelet concentrates.

Another means of transfusion therapy—autogenous blood transfusion—is available in most centers. This technique is used when it is suspected that an intraoperative blood transfusion may be required. Patients can donate a unit of their own blood before surgery. The blood is then stored and made available for their personal use during surgery.

Various criteria exist to help determine when red cell or platelet transfusions are necessary. In general, a healthy patient with normal red cell mass can tolerate an acute fall in hematocrit to 25% to 30% without suffering significant ill effects. A chronically anemic patient can easily tolerate an even lower concentration of red blood cells. Dentists managing patients with thrombocytopenia should seek the advice of a hematologist when deciding whether platelet transfusion is warranted.

*Saline is commonly available in several dilutions (0.9% [normal], 0.45%, 0.33%, and 0.25%).

*Patient is supine on operating table, with the head end of the table raised.

APPENDIX I

Instrument List and Typical Retail Prices (2007)

Basic Tray

Local anesthesia syringe	$48.00
Woodson elevator	$47.50
Periapical curette	$44.29
Small straight elevator	$59.99
Large straight elevator	$59.99
College pliers	$26.50
Curved hemostat	$42.50
Towel clip	$39.95
Austin retractor	$77.75
Suction	$36.00
TOTAL	**$482.47**

Forceps

No. 150 upper universal	$131.95
No. 151 lower universal	$131.95
No. 53L upper molar	$129.95
No. 53R upper molar	$129.95
No. 23 lower cowhorn	$129.95
No. 17 lower molar	$129.95
No. 286 root	$118.95
TOTAL	**$902.65**

Surgical Tray

Needle holder	$60.00
Suture	$8.99/dozen
Suture scissor	$57.00
Periosteal elevator	$31.25
No. 3 blade handle	$5.49
No. 15 blade	$0.26
Adson tissue forceps	$13.29
Bone file	$55.99
Tongue retractor	$55.00
Root tip pick	$43.99
Russian tissue forceps	$49.50
Cryer elevator R	$55.49
Cryer elevator L	$55.49
Rongeur	$211.00
TOTAL	**$647.25**

Biopsy Tray

No. 3 blade handle	$5.49
No. 15 blade	$0.26
Needle holder	$60.00
Suture	$8.99/dozen
Suture scissors	$57.00
Metzenbaum scissors	$50.00
Allis tissue forceps	$54.44
Adson tissue forceps	$13.29
Curved hemostat	$42.50
TOTAL	**$291.97**

Postoperative Tray

Suture scissors	$57.00
College pliers	$26.50
Suction	$36.00
TOTAL	**$119.50**

Miscellaneous

Molt mouth prop	$154.50
Silicone bite block	$32.00
Minnesota retractor	$32.60
TOTAL	**$219.10**

GRAND TOTAL **$2662.94**

Note: The foregoing prices are average prices from 2007 catalogs from the following companies: Sullivan-Schien, Melville, N.Y.; Patterson Dental, St. Paul, Minn. Actual prices may vary.

APPENDIX II

Operative Note (Office Record) Component Parts

1. Date
2. Patient identification
3. Diagnosis
4. Review of medical history, medications, and vital signs
5. Oral examination
6. Anesthesia (dose and block technique used)
7. Procedure, including statement of progress of procedure and complications
8. Discharge instructions
9. Medications prescribed (drug and amount or copy of prescription)
10. Return appointment (scheduling)
11. Signature (legible or printed underneath)

DATE: July 1, 2008

ID and DX: This 52 y.o.m requires extraction of mandibular left second premolar and first molar. Both teeth are nonrestorable because of extensive caries.

MEDICAL HISTORY: Patient has chronic hypertension for which a thiazide diuretic has been prescibed. Reminder of history is unremarkable. Pulse 84; BP 130/85.

ORAL EXAMINATION: Soft tissue of cheeks, lips, tongue, floor of mouth, and palate are WNL. No palpable nodes or masses. Carious, nonrestorable teeth #19 and 20.

ANESTHESIA: Lidocaine 36 mg with 0.018 mg epinephrine via mandibular and long buccal blocks.

PROCEDURE: Routine forceps extraction of teeth #19 and 20. Distal root of first molar fractured—retrieved with Cryer elevator. No flap required. Patient tolerated procedure without difficulty.

DISCHARGE: Copy of routine postoperative instructions given and reviewed.

MEDICATIONS: Tylenol #3—24 caps. 1 or 2 caps q4h prn pain.

RETURN: Patient asked to return in 1 week for postoperative checkup.

John Jay Jones

FIGURE A-1 Example of an oral surgery note.

APPENDIX III

Drug Enforcement Administration Schedule of Drugs and Examples

A. Schedule I Drugs

These drugs are not available for clinical use in the United States.

Examples: Heroin, marijuana, LSD (lysergic acid diethylamide)

B. Schedule II Drugs

These drugs have high abuse liability. They require written prescription and DEA number. Prescription cannot be refilled without a new prescription. Prescription cannot be telephoned to pharmacy.

Examples: Morphine, meperidine, plain codeine, oxycodone compounds, pentobarbital

C. Schedule III Drugs

These drugs have lower abuse potential. Prescriptions may be telephoned in to pharmacy but require DEA number. The prescription can be refilled up to 5 times in 6 months.

Examples: Codeine compounds, hydrocodone compounds, dihydrocodeine compounds, pentazocine

D. Schedule IV Drugs

Nonnarcotic drugs with lower abuse potential. DEA number required.

Examples: Chloral hydrate, diazepam

E. Schedule V Drugs

Note: Nonsteroidal antiinflammatory drugs are not scheduled drugs.

APPENDIX IV

Examples of Useful Prescriptions

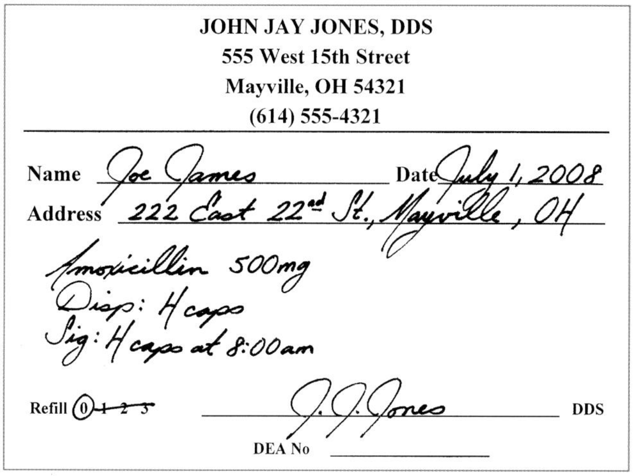

JOHN JAY JONES, DDS
555 West 15th Street
Mayville, OH 54321
(614) 555-4321

Name Joe James Date July 1, 2008
Address 222 East 22nd St., Mayville, OH

Amoxicillin 500mg
Disp: 4 caps
Sig: 4 caps at 8:00am

Refill (0) 1 2 3 J.J. Jones DDS
DEA No

FIGURE A-2 Prescription for oral bacterial endocarditis prophylaxis with amoxicillin.

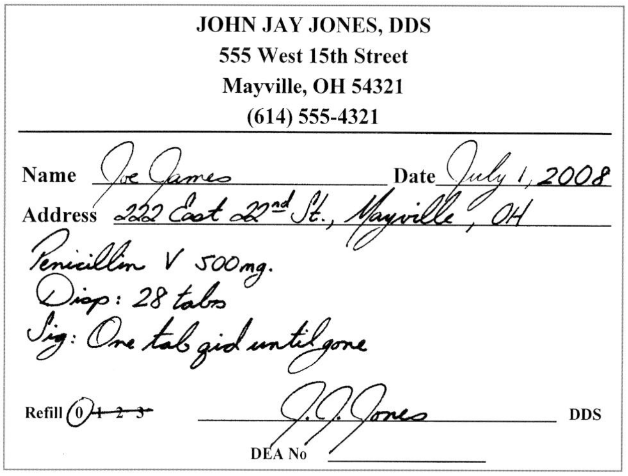

JOHN JAY JONES, DDS
555 West 15th Street
Mayville, OH 54321
(614) 555-4321

Name Joe James Date July 1, 2008
Address 222 East 22nd St., Mayville, OH

Penicillin V 500mg.
Disp: 28 tabs
Sig: One tab qid until gone

Refill (0) 1 2 3 J.J. Jones DDS
DEA No

FIGURE A-3 Prescription for oral penicillin therapy of odontogenic infection.

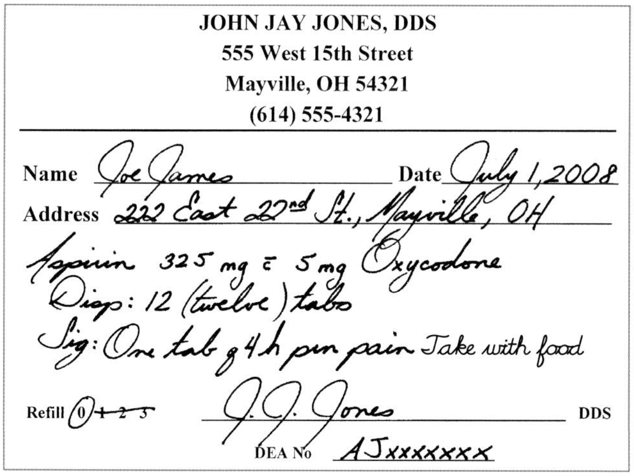

JOHN JAY JONES, DDS
555 West 15th Street
Mayville, OH 54321
(614) 555-4321

Name Joe James Date July 1, 2008
Address 222 East 22nd St., Mayville, OH

Aspirin 325 mg c̄ 5 mg Oxycodone
Disp: 12 (twelve) tabs
Sig: One tab q 4 h prn pain Take with food

Refill (0) 1 2 3 J.J. Jones DDS
DEA No AJXXXXXXX

FIGURE A-4 Prescription for aspirin with oxycodone. This prescription must have a Drug Enforcement Administration number and cannot be telephoned in to the pharmacy.

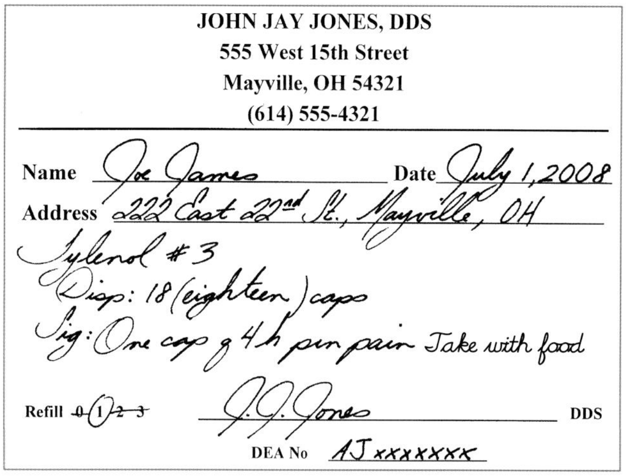

JOHN JAY JONES, DDS
555 West 15th Street
Mayville, OH 54321
(614) 555-4321

Name Joe James Date July 1, 2008
Address 222 East 22nd St., Mayville, OH

Tylenol #3
Disp: 18 (eighteen) caps
Sig: One cap q 4 h prn pain Take with food

Refill 0 (1) 2 3 J.J. Jones DDS
DEA No AJXXXXXXX

FIGURE A-5 Typical brand name prescription. This compound has 300 mg of acetaminophen and 30 mg of codeine.

APPENDIX V

Consent for Extractions and Anesthesia

1. I, ____________________, give my permission for Dr. ________________ and any assistants deemed necessary, to perform the procedure(s) discussed below in #2.

2. The reason(s) for the surgery and anesthesia have been explained to me and I understand the procedure(s) to consist of:

   Lay terminology ____

   Medical terminology ____

   Sensible alternative procedures including not doing surgery at all have been discussed with me.

3. I have been advised of potential complications of this procedure that are able to be reasonably anticipated which are:

   ____

   ____

4. I understand that anesthesia will be necessary for my surgery and give permission for the use of medications the doctors feels are necessary except those to which I am allergic that are listed below:

   ____

5. I understand that no guarantees can be given of the results of surgery on the human body, but that the doctor and office staff will do their best to achieve excellent results.

6. All my questions concerning this procedure have been answed to my satisfaction.

Patients signature indicating agreement with statements 1 through 6:

____ Date ____________

Witness of the consent signature:

____ Date ____________

FIGURE A-6 Example of a patient consent form.

APPENDIX VI

Antibiotic Overview

I. Cephalosporins

The cephalosporins are a group of β-lactam antibiotics that are effective against gram-positive cocci and many gram-negative rods. A large number of cephalosporins are available and are roughly divided into three generations, based on their activity against gram-negative organisms. The first-generation antibiotics have a similar activity, including activity against gram-positive cocci, *Escherichia coli, Klebsiella* organisms, and *Proteus mirabilis*.

The second-generation cephalosporins have broader activity against gram-negative bacteria and increased activity against the anaerobic bacteria. The second generation has less activity against the gram-positive cocci than the first generation.

The third-generation cephalosporins are much more active against enteric gram-negative rods but are decidedly less active than first- and second-generation cephalosporins against gram-positive cocci.

Two useful oral cephalosporins are effective in odontogenic infections: (1) cephalexin (Keflex) and (2) cefadroxil (Duricef). Although neither of these is the drug of first choice for odontogenic infections, the drugs may be useful in certain situations in which a bactericidal antibiotic is necessary.

The toxicity of the cephalosporin group is primarily related to allergy. Patients who are allergic to penicillin drugs should be given the cephalosporin antibiotics *with caution*. Patients who have had anaphylactic reactions to penicillin should not be given the cephalosporins.

II. Clindamycin

The antibacterial spectrum of clindamycin includes the gram-positive cocci and almost all anaerobic bacteria. Clindamycin is effective for streptococci, staphylococci, and anaerobic infections. The drug is more expensive than penicillin and erythromycin and may have increased gastrointestinal toxicity in susceptible patients.

III. Metronidazole

Metronidazole is an antibiotic that is effective *only* for anaerobic bacteria. Metronidazole has no effect on aerobic bacteria such as streptococci. The drug is primarily used in periodontal disease therapy but may also be useful in the management of anaerobic odontogenic infections alone or in combination with antiaerobic antibiotics such as penicillin.

IV. Penicillin

Penicillin is the drug of choice for odontogenic infections because its antibacterial spectrum includes the gram-positive cocci (except staphylococci) and oral anaerobes. Penicillin G is the form given parenterally, and penicillin V is preferred for oral administration. Penicillin has little toxicity except for allergic reactions, which occur in about 3% of the population.

Penicillinase-resistant penicillins are a group of drugs that are useful for penicillinase-producing staphylococci. Dicloxacillin is the preferred penicillinase-resistant penicillin for oral use. These drugs should be used only for culture-documented infection caused by staphylococci.

Several extended-spectrum penicillins exist. The ampicillin-amoxicillin group is effective against more gram-negative rods than penicillin. Amoxicillin is absorbed better from the GI tract than ampicillin and is thus preferred when the drug is given orally. Amoxicillin is the drug of choice for prevention of bacterial endocarditis because of its excellent GI absorption and slow renal elimination.

V. Tetracyclines

The tetracyclines are available for oral and parenteral administration and are generally considered to be broad-spectrum antibiotics. However, common bacterial resistance to these drugs exists. At this time, tetracyclines are useful only against anaerobic bacteria, which forms the basis for their use in odontogenic infections.

The toxicities of tetracyclines are generally low but include staining of developing teeth if given to children or to pregnant or lactating women. Minocycline and doxycycline are preferred because they need to be taken only once or twice daily.

The tetracyclines have an anticollagenase effect. This activity may make them useful for treatment of periodontal and periimplant disease. Doxycycline 100 mg qd may be especially useful.

VI. Fluoroquinolones

This family of antibiotics includes ciprofloxacin (Cipro) and ofloxacin (Floxin). The fluoroquinolones are broad-spectrum, bactericidal, orally taken antibiotics. Unfortunately, these drugs are only marginally effective against streptococci and have little or no effect against anaerobic bacteria. Therefore, the usefulness of fluoroquinolones in odontogenic infections is low. The drugs should rarely, if ever, be used empirically for a patient with an odontogenic infection.

The third generation of fluoroquinolones has high antistreptococcal and antianaerobic activity. These drugs may be especially useful when a bactericidal antibiotic is necessary for a patient with severe penicillin allergy. Drugs such as moxifloxacin and levofloxacin are examples of this drug group.

VII. Antifungal Drugs

Mucosal candidosis, or oral thrush, should be treated with the topical application of antifungal agents. The two drugs of choice are (1) nystatin and (2) clotrimazole. Both drugs are available as lozenges that are held in the mouth until they dissolve. The patient should use one lozenge 4 to 5 times daily for 10 days for effective control and to prevent relapse of the candidosis.

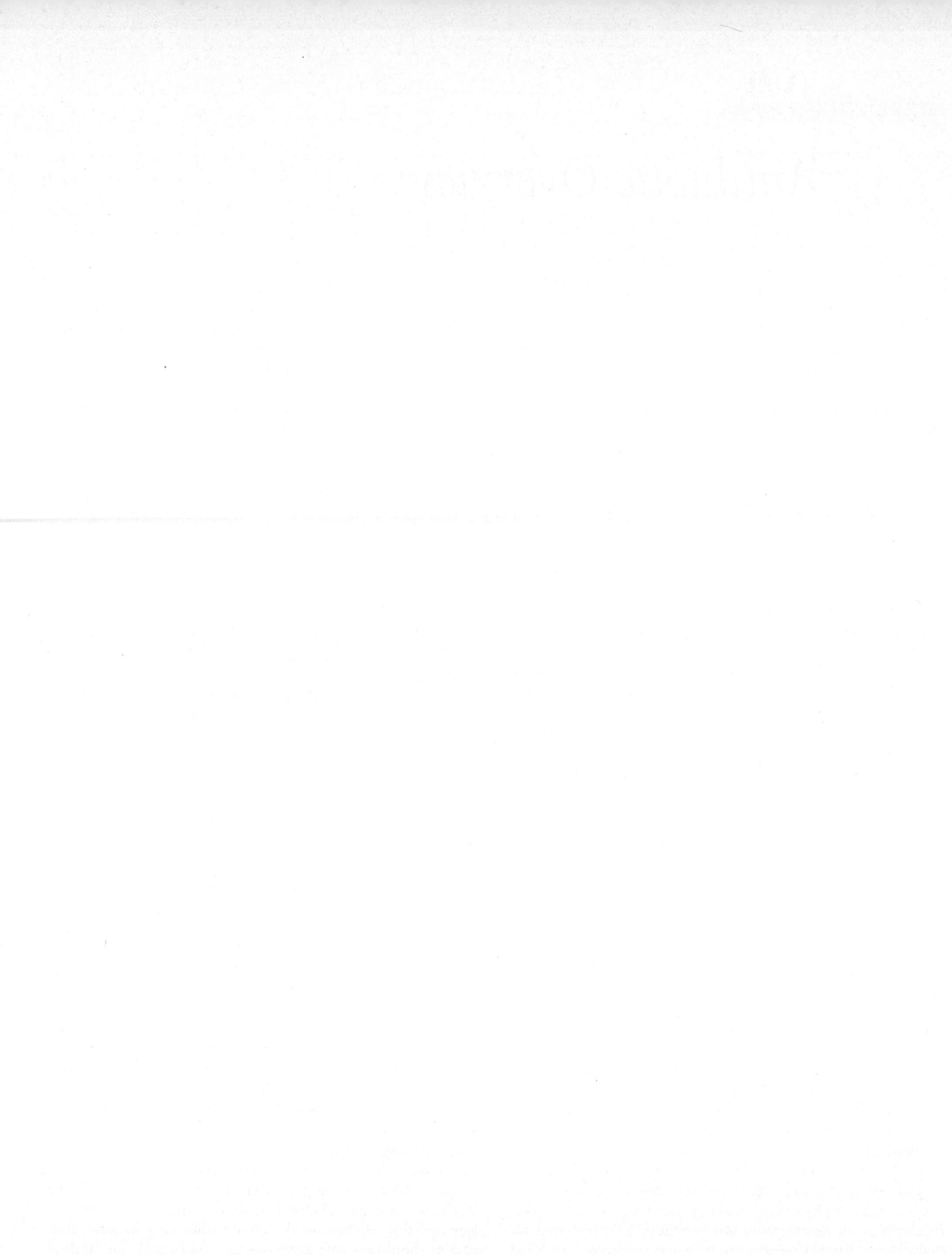

Index

Page numbers followed by b indicate boxes; f, figures; t, tables.

B

C

D

E

F

G

H

I

M

N

P

R

S

T

U

V

W

X

Y

Z